Tumor Ecosystem

Erwei Song

Editor

Tumor Ecosystem

An Ecological View of Cancer Growth
and Survival

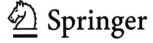

Editor
Erwei Song
Guangdong Provincial Key Laboratory of
Malignant Tumor Epigenetics and Gene
Regulation, Guangdong-Hong Kong Joint
Laboratory for RNA Medicine, Medical
Research Center
Sun Yat-sen Memorial Hospital, Sun Yat-sen University
Guangzhou, China

Nanhai Translational Innovation Center of Precision Immunology
Sun Yat-sen Memorial Hospital, Sun Yat-sen University
Foshan, China

Breast Tumor Center
Sun Yat-sen Memorial Hospital, Sun Yat-sen University
Guangzhou, China

ISBN 978-981-99-1182-0   ISBN 978-981-99-1183-7   (eBook)
https://doi.org/10.1007/978-981-99-1183-7

"Dedicated to Dr. Hinkar Au, who is a monument of surgeon and scientist. Also, to my daddy..."—Erwei Song

Foreword

I would like to express my heartiest congratulations to Erwei on the successful completion of this book *Tumor Ecosystem: An Ecological View of Cancer Growth and Survival*. I first knew Erwei on the Expert Panel of Future Generations Therapy Conference San Francisco more than a decade ago. I still vividly remember glancing across the room, my mind remembering the names of the "big shots," and my eyes rested on a young post-doc among the experts. Although at that time this name is unfamiliar to me, I was duly impressed by his lecture that day. Erwei proved himself to be a passionate, brilliant, and vigorous young surgeon and a visionary pioneer in breast cancer research. Parallel to my belief, Erwei firmly supports the notion that personalized cancer immunotherapy is the future of cancer therapy. Fast forward, we now get a clear picture of how cancer immunotherapy is shaping the diagnosis and therapy of malignant cancers.

Greek physician Hippocrates (460–370 BC), who is considered the "Father of Medicine," was the first to define cancer. Hippocrates used the terms carcinos and carcinoma to describe non-ulcer forming and ulcer-forming tumors. Through the years, our definition of cancer has been refined with revolutionary eras that "re-define" our conceptual understandings of cancer. The first revolution in cancer is that "cancer is a regional disease." In 1894 Halsted described his procedure for treating breast cancer by removing the breast tissue, chest muscles, and lymph nodes in the armpit, a procedure he named radical mastectomy, and that became the standard of care for treating breast cancer until 1970.

In 1971, Dr. Fisher led the NSABP in a landmark clinical trial in women with primary breast cancer comparing radical mastectomy with less extensive total mastectomy. In 1976, he initiated a study comparing total mastectomy with less disfiguring lumpectomy, with or without breast irradiation. For over 10 years, Dr. Fisher and his research team carried out "a multitude of investigations regarding the biology of tumor metastasis." These studies showed that the addition of systemic, adjuvant chemotherapy or hormonal therapy provided a survival advantage over surgery alone and led to the first trial of tamoxifen as a breast cancer prevention agent in 1992. That trial showed that tamoxifen decreased the incidence of breast cancer by half in women with increased risk for the disease. What he found was that there was no survival advantage in removing more tissue. Less invasive surgeries resulted in similar survival rates as the more extensive surgeries. Therefore, Fisher proposes the first primary systemic treatment, or now famously known as Neoadjuvant Chemotherapy (NAC). NAC is given to patients prior to surgery to reduce the tumor size, and to halt tumor progression and metastasis. These studies provided a scientific basis for considering cancer from a systemic point of view, where drugs given to the host is effective against a solid tumor. This finding leads to the second revolution: "cancer is a systemic disease."

The third revolution is the realization that "cancer is a heterogenous disease." Traditionally, breast cancer is associated with four major subtypes, which in most cases are determined by testing for the estrogen receptor (ER) and HER2. For example, trastuzumab (a HER-2 targeting antibody) has been introduced as an active antibody-targeting HER2 overexpressed breast cancer. However, disparities existed in the clinical outcomes of patients within each of these four subtypes, suggesting molecular heterogeneity. In 2000, Dr. Perou and his team employ a sequencing technology that analyzes genetic information from individual cells (single cell sequencing). Dr. Perou is known for developing assays which identify breast cancer subtypes, and that information is converted into a "risk score" that guides a patient's clinical care.

The twenty-first century presented the dawn of personalized precision therapy for cancer. Cancer therapy should consider a comprehensive approach: cancer origin, subtypes, immunoscore, patient's sex, age, comorbidity, inherent diseases, among others, to precisely define and diagnose cancer patients. The core idea of this book, as proposed by Erwei, is that "cancer is an ecological disease." The concept of cancer ecology or cancer ecosystem is a most comprehensive consideration of the interaction of cancer cells with its local environment, interaction of disseminated metastatic cancer seed with their metastatic niche, while considering the impact of host towards cancer cell growth and survival as a unique ecosystem. This concept provides insights beyond the conventional tumor-stromal interactions in its microenvironment.

In each chapter, they detailed the in-depth crosstalks between the interactions and inter-relationship of various cells in local *onco-spheres*, interactions between different organs in distal *onco-spheres*, and interactions between host and guests (*i.e.,* microbes, virus, tumor cells) in systemic *onco-spheres*. Having understood the cancer ecology concept, they utilize ecology principles to further delineate the features of the dynamics of the tumor ecosystem through calculation of Eco and Evo index, which ultimately reveals that cancer growth and survival is indeed parallel to the living ecosystem. Considering all the factors above, they summarize the technological advances that enable successful visualization, modeling, and subtyping of cancer ecosystem. Finally, they depicted how therapeutic strategies could be successfully designed, guided by the understanding of the concept of cancer ecosystem and its dynamics.

I personally believe that this book would pave the way for the fourth revolution in cancer. We must now consider cancer from a holistic point of view, taking into consideration the intrinsic and extrinsic factors that could encourage tumor growth: the solid tumor microenvironment, their interactions with their local microenvironment (local *onco-sphere*), the process of pre-metastatic niche formation, the interactions of these metastatic seeds with their new "soil" in other organs (distal *onco-sphere*), and how the host (immune, metabolic, neuron, digestive system etc.; *systemic oncosphere*) could modulate cancer.

This revolutionary concept lays a foundation for the development of tumor ecology, a new discipline, and provides basic theories and methods for precise cancer prevention and treatment. Predicting the arrival of a new era of cancer treatment that targets the fragility of the tumor ecosystem is of great significance for accelerating the development of tumor ecological therapies. I strongly recommend this book for all clinicians, researchers, and medical students to clearly understand the concept of tumor as an ecosystem, looking at cancer with an ecological view. This could revolutionize the way we diagnose and treat solid tumors, realizing personalized precision treatment in the near future.

Laboratory of Molecular and Tumor   Bernard A. Fox
Immunology, Robert W. Franz Cancer
Center, Earle A. Chiles Research
Institute, Providence Cancer Institute,
Portland, OR, USA

Preface

Cancer cells can be conceived as "living organisms," interacting with cellular or noncellular components in the host internal environment, not only with the local tumor microenvironment (TME) but also constantly communicating with a distant organ niche as well interacting with the host's nervous, endocrine, and immune systems, to construct a self-sustainable "biosphere," as we termed the *tumor ecosystem*. This ecological concept extends and deepens our understanding of cancer pathobiology beyond its local interaction with stromal cells within the TME. With increasing features of the systemic tumor-host interplay being disclosed, we propose that a new era of cancer therapy targeting the ecosystemic vulnerability of human malignancies has come.

Herein we propose a new concept of *onco-spheres* in cancer ecosystem. *Onco-spheres* are defined as where cancer cells (living organisms) dynamically interact with nontumor cellular (other living organisms) and noncellular components (nonliving environmental factors) in the "host" internal environment (habitat) to construct a self-sustainable cancer ecosystem, which can be scoped at three different levels: primary/regional, distal, and systemic *onco-spheres*.

By looking at the interaction of cancer and host as a unique ecosystem, we will use ecology principles to further delineate the features of the dynamics of the tumor ecosystem. In this book, we will delve deeper into the interactions and inter-relationship of various cells in primary *onco-spheres*, interactions between different organs in distal *onco-spheres*, and interactions between host and guests (*i.e.,* microbes, virus, tumor cells) in systemic *onco-spheres*. Recent advances in technologies that enable successful visualization, modeling, and subtyping of tumor ecosystem would be discussed. Finally, we will address how the understanding of the tumor ecosystem components and its dynamics could guide successful design of therapeutic strategies.

As the pioneer in proposing this concept, we feel that this full-scale overview of the tumor ecosystem is able to inform readers about this concept, and to pave the way for designing novel therapeutic strategies on actionable targets within the tumor ecosystem.

Guangzhou, China   Erwei Song
Foshan, China

Acknowledgments

To all authors who we were unable to cite in this book, and to all colleagues who helped with wonderful suggestions and criticism during the process of writing this book. This work was supported by grants from the Natural Science Foundation of China (81621004, 92159303, 81720108029, 81930081, 91940305), Guangdong Science and Technology Department (2020B1212060018, 2020B1212030004), Department of Natural Resources of Guangdong Province (GDNRC[2021]51), Clinical Innovation Research Program of Bioland Laboratory (2018GZR0201004), Bureau of Science and Technology of Guangzhou (20212200003), the Program for Guangdong Introducing Innovative and Entrepreneurial Teams (2019BT02Y198).

Contents

Part III   Systemic *Onco-Sphere*

Contributors[1]

Phei Er Saw Guangdong Provincial Key Laboratory of Malignant Tumor Epigenetics and Gene Regulation, Guangdong-Hong Kong Joint Laboratory for RNA Medicine, Medical Research Center, Sun Yat-sen Memorial Hospital, Sun Yat-sen University, Guangzhou, China
Nanhai Translational Innovation Center of Precision Immunology, Sun Yat-sen Memorial Hospital, Sun Yat-sen University, Foshan, China

Erwei Song Guangdong Provincial Key Laboratory of Malignant Tumor Epigenetics and Gene Regulation, Guangdong-Hong Kong Joint Laboratory for RNA Medicine, Medical Research Center, Sun Yat-sen Memorial Hospital, Sun Yat-sen University, Guangzhou, China
Nanhai Translational Innovation Center of Precision Immunology, Sun Yat-sen Memorial Hospital, Sun Yat-sen University, Foshan, China
Breast Tumor Center, Sun Yat-sen Memorial Hospital, Sun Yat-sen University, Guangzhou, China

---

[1] This book is wholly written by Phei Er Saw and Erwei Song, with Erwei Song being the sole editor of this book.

Part I
Local *Onco-Sphere*

Chapter 1
Introduction to Tumor Ecosystem

Phei Er Saw and Erwei Song

"Host internal environment is for cancer cells what the ecosystem is for living organisms, as an interplay between tumor cells and cellular as well as noncellular factors in the local TME and distal premetastatic niche impacts upon cancer progression and therapeutic responses."
Erwei Song, Nature Cancer, 2021 [1]

Abstract Cancer is a systemic disease. Cancer growth and survival depends on not only the communication between tumor cells and its surrounding, they are also constantly communicating with host inflammatory, immune, endocrine, and neuronal system. These communications create networks and crosstalks that enables a pro-tumoral environment, ultimately leading to cancer growth. Understanding the comprehensive view of tumor ecosystem will enable us to obtain precious information on how to reverse cancer growth by targeting various components in these communications.

P. E. Saw
Guangdong Provincial Key Laboratory of Malignant Tumor Epigenetics and Gene Regulation, Guangdong-Hong Kong Joint Laboratory for RNA Medicine, Medical Research Center, Sun Yat-sen Memorial Hospital, Sun Yat-sen University, Guangzhou, China

Nanhai Translational Innovation Center of Precision Immunology, Sun Yat-sen Memorial Hospital, Sun Yat-sen University, Foshan, China

E. Song (✉)
Guangdong Provincial Key Laboratory of Malignant Tumor Epigenetics and Gene Regulation, Guangdong-Hong Kong Joint Laboratory for RNA Medicine, Medical Research Center, Sun Yat-sen Memorial Hospital, Sun Yat-sen University, Guangzhou, China

Nanhai Translational Innovation Center of Precision Immunology, Sun Yat-sen Memorial Hospital, Sun Yat-sen University, Foshan, China

Breast Tumor Center, Sun Yat-sen Memorial Hospital, Sun Yat-sen University, Guangzhou, China
e-mail: songew@mail.sysu.edu.cn

Ecological Principles in Cancer

According to the American Cancer Society, the global incidence of cancer is projected to reach 29.4 million cases by 2040—an increase of more than 60% from 18.1 million cases in 2018. The eight hallmarks of cancer, defined by Hanahan and Weinberg in their pivotal articles from 2000 and 2022, are an organizational framework to understand the intricacy of carcinogenesis [2–4]. The hallmarks of carcinogenesis constitute self-sustainability in growth signals, unresponsiveness to growth inhibition, apoptosis evasion, endless cell replication, angiogenesis, tissue invasion and metastasis, immune escape, and metabolic deregulation. Genetic instability and proinflammatory cytokines, in part, also contribute to attaining the hallmarks, by inducing tumor heterogeneity and sustaining cellular injury [5–9].

Ecological principles can be applied in vivo to conceptualize the interactions between cancer cells and the environment within human body. The place where a group of organisms live and interact among themselves and with the physical environment is termed "ecosystem." The complex in vivo interaction between cancer cells and bodily host cells mirrors that of an ecosystem, consisting of biotic factors such as fibroblast, endothelial cells, and white blood cells and environmental factors including the extracellular matrix [10–12]. Adopting an ecological approach in cancer therapeutics and combining the use of sequencing technology may help to identify therapeutic targets and drive precision medicine in oncology [13, 14].

An ecosystem—as described by pioneering ecologist Eugene Odum—is a unit consisting of the living community (organisms) and nonliving constituents (environment) in a given area where energy is transferred and cycled through biotic interactions and the nonliving environment [15]. Under the ecological hierarchy, the ecosystem is the smallest unit that fulfills all the basic needs of survival. Even so, ecosystems are not isolated; instead, they are interconnected with other ecosystems in a complex network, which forms the biosphere [16] Drawing parallels between the ecosystem and the human body, tumor cells developing in an organ can be thought of as a novel species living alongside other host cells in the complicated habitat, which, together, forms an ecosystem. Moving up the ecological hierarchy, the patient can be considered as the biosphere, a place where the cancer ecosystem alongside other ecosystems exists within. The study of ecology in the context of tumor biology is likely to uncover new understanding of cancer development, especially in the field of metastasis research [10, 17].

Tumor heterogeneity is a widely recognized concept among scientists today, that a tumor is made up of heterogeneous cancer cell populations rather than a group of genetically identical cancer cells [18, 19]. If genetic heterogeneity in tumor could encode for phenotypic traits that impact survival and are passed onto the next generation, then the cancer cell population would evolve, resulting in competition for resources and selection for a more adaptable species under natural selection. This may explain why acquired therapeutic resistance occurs. Resistant cancer cells, the more well-adapted species across the heterogeneous cell population, are selected for during natural selection. Furthermore, studies have linked tumor heterogeneity in pre-malignancy to poorer patient prognosis [20]. Younger cancer patients, on the other hand, have a better prognosis, partly because younger tumors are less genetically diverse and hence less prone to acquire therapeutic resistance. In addition, tumor heterogeneity potentially results in a phenomenon known as evolutionary suicide [21]: cancer cells disregard the physiological regulations obeyed by normal tissue to pursue greater tumor proliferation through metastasis, which ultimately leads to the death of their host and to its self-destruction. Every cancer patient unknowingly provides the battle ground for this phenomenon to occur, sacrificing their lives at times as evolutionary suicide takes place within [22].

Researchers have long considered cancer as an evolutionary disease due to its diverse genetic makeup and limitless clonal expansion. Genetic drift can occur in parts of a single tumor, which may confer selective advantage to the intratumor cells, allowing for swift adaption to host cell defense and invasion into novel tissue; in other words, the fittest cells survive [19]. In general, cancer cells in its environment mimic the functioning pattern of an ecosystem, where a cancer cell's fitness is determined by how it interacts with the local niche and the systemic environment in the host body. We can think of the cancer ecosystem as an inter-crossing biosphere, a place where cancer growth is jointly supported by several players: living organisms (cancer cells and non-cancerous cells), nonliving habitats (local or distant tissue), and growth stimuli (neuroendocrine signals and nutrients). Here, we can adopt an ecological viewpoint to understand the expansion and proliferation of cancer cells within a tissue. Cancer cells, as the emerging species, employ different metabolic and reproductive tactics to compete with somatic cells, the existing population, in occupying a novel habitat, which we now termed the local *onco-sphere*. A primary solid tumor will develop if cancer cells thrive in the tissue [22].

By integrating ecological concepts with cancer pathophysiology, cancer cells can be viewed as the novel species armed with highly evolved metabolic and reproductive tactics. These intruders take over the host cells' habitat and resources, resist predation by host immunity, populate and expand into the system, and then plant themselves into the newly conquered habitat. Once cancer cells evolve and grow in the local niche, they spread out to metastasize distant tissues. Cancer cells are all-rounders in contrast to the highly specialized host cells, allowing it to outsmart the local immune responses and successfully establish new *onco-sphere*s. Energy— derived from glucose, proteins, lipids, and chemical elements—is necessary for cell growth and survival. Cancer cells could invade and disrupt the microenvironment, which is the region occupied by cells, including the extracellular matrix. Cell-to-cell interaction may influence the cells' ecological functions in the microenvironment, such that immune cells would assume the role of predators to hunt down cancer cells, or the other way around. In addition, factors that may alter a niche within the body include pH, metabolism, oxygen saturation, hemodynamics, chemical intoxication, or infection. As cancer and somatic cells compete in the same niche, any substantial changes might potentially introduce a new niche that is conducive to cancerous growth. The ecological roles of cancer cells in the *onco-sphere* are essentially determined by cellular interactions that either promote or inhibit cancer progression. Using the ecological analogy, tumor-promoting cellular interactions include mutualism and commensalism; tumor-inhibiting relationships include predation, parasitism, and competition. Throughout this book, we will delve deeper into the detailed interactions in each level of cancer ecology.

Box 1.1 *Onco-Sphere*: A New Concept in Cancer Ecosystem

Cancer ecosystem is the self-sustaining biosphere occupied by cancer cells, with its creation depending on how cancer cells, as the living component, interact with its surroundings, which include other cells occupying the same microenvironment, structural components of the microenvironment, even distal tissues and organ systems such as the neuroendocrine and immune systems. This concept provides insights beyond the conventional tumor stromal interactions in cancer biology. Extending the cancer ecosystem's concept beyond the tumor microenvironment (TME), we herein introduce a new term called *onco-sphere*, a biosphere that is self-sustainable for cells to multiply and proliferate. Primary *onco-sphere* refers to niches where tumor initiates, regional *onco-sphere* refers to lymph nodes migration of cancer cells, while distal *onco-sphere* is where the tumor expands and spreads in their pre/post-metastatic niche. Systemic *onco-sphere* considers the relationship among the above relationships with the host as a whole. In this book, we will fully uncover the mechanisms of cancer growth and metastasis in the light of the concept of cancer ecosystem.

In each chapter, we will highlight the cross talk and multidirectional communications between cancer cells, their stromal cells, infiltrated immune cells, including physiological changes, biochemical changes, and biophysical changes in the local *onco-sphere*; and how these changes dictate changes in the regional and distal *onco-sphere*. Furthermore, in Part III of this book, we will look at how the host behaves as a systemic *onco-sphere* to influence cancer growth and vice versa (Fig. 1.1).

Interactions in Local *Onco-Sphere*

At different phases of tumor growth, different types of cells reside and aggregate within the TME. Early stage of tumor growth is characterized by infiltration of inflammatory cells, hematopoietic and endothelial progenitor cells from the bone marrow, and tumor-associated fibroblasts [23]. To subdue tumor growth, it is critical to recruit immune cells to the site of malignancy as early as possible, which include antigen-presenting cells such as dendritic cells, lymphocytes such as natural killer cells, and macrophages [24]. However, immunosuppressive cells, such as myeloid-derived suppressors cells (MDSC), regulatory T cells (Tregs), and type 2-polarized macrophages (M2), which are inherently connected with the growing TME, block the anti-tumor immune response [25]. Cancer cells can interact with the cellular or structural components of TME with or without contact: contact-dependent that

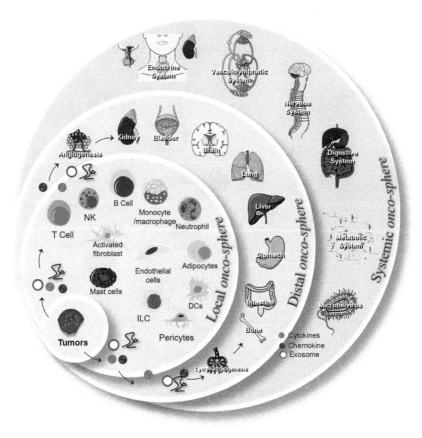

Fig. 1.1 New *onco-sphere* concept in tumor ecology. The local *onco-sphere* is established from the interaction of tumor with its microenvironment, which include cytokines, chemokines, and other factors in driving cancer development in the niche. Cells adapt and shed from the primary tumor to invade the secondary organs in organotrophic metastasis, to create a new distal *onco-sphere*. At the same time, the local, distal (regional), and systemic *onco-spheres* (the host) constantly communicate within each other, contributing to the sustainability of the cancer

requires physical interaction of binding sites, and contact-independent interaction via signaling molecules such as cytokines, lipids, and growth factors. Bone-marrow-derived stromal cells populate the TME and contribute to its development; these stromal cells are endothelial cells, mesenchymal cells, fibroblasts, and inflammatory cells of myeloid and lymphoid origin [26, 27]. During chronic inflammation, the stromal cells residing in the TME are capable of transforming into another cell type to support cancerous growth [28, 29]. All these interactions will be detailed in Chaps. 2, 3, 4, 5, 6, 7, 8, and 9 (Fig. 1.2).

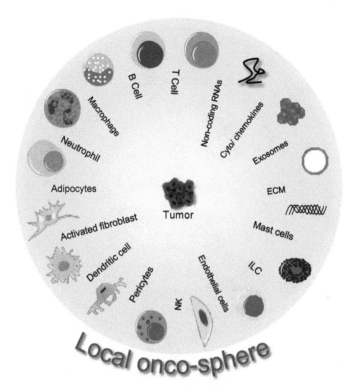

Fig. 1.2 The interaction within the local *onco-sphere*, dictating the close relationship of tumor cells with every component in the local *onco-sphere*, including immune cells, stromal cells, extracellular matrix, exosomes, non-coding RNAs, and cytokines and chemokines. This inter-connecting network reveals the complexity of a solid tumor

Interaction in Distal *Onco-Sphere*

Among a number of mechanisms suggested by various studies, habitat modification is the most widely agreed mechanism that elucidates the susceptibility of a tissue to cancer invasion [30, 31]. Cancer cells usually behave like generalists as compared to resident cells, which are more specialized. This characteristic of cancer cells allows it to outsmart the resident cells by hijacking more resources within the niche at one time, which ultimately favors its invasion of the new habitat [32, 33]. David Tilman and his research team studied ecosystem stability and how it affects the biodiversity. They proposed that a more diversified ecosystem utilizes the resources more extensively and thus are more resistant to invasion [34–36]. If the resources in the ecosystem are inadequately consumed by its existing population, a new niche may be established and invaded by a new species. A process known as niche construction may arise if the new niche is left unexploited for some time by the existing population, intruders could then hijack the resources of the new niche and "coevolve with it," while altering the niche according to its metabolic needs [22]. Such alterations may be unsuitable or even hostile to the host. Moreover, instead of cohabitating in harmony with other species, the intruders can transform the niche to accommodate to its demands only and facilitate its migration and exploitation. Perhaps this ecological understanding may explain the development of metastases.

Healthy cells in tissue are conventionally thought to be in a stable state and hence should not be vulnerable to "evolutionary unstable" cancer cells that utilize different metabolic or reproductive strategy in its invasion. In other words, these healthy cells have attained the greatest extent of evolutionary adaptation [37]. So, it is theorized that certain mechanism must have taken place to destabilize the evolutionary state of these healthy cells for tissue invasion and metastasis to occur. Aging is one of the proposed mechanisms [38, 39] by which healthy cells eventually drift away from the peak of their evolutionary adaptation, enabling cancer cells to invade and colonize distal *onco-sphere*. Aging is usually associated with the gradual loss of cellular function and gradual accumulation of molecular damage due to a plethora of internal of external factors, such as mutations or carcinogen exposure, which impairs the fitness of cells and usurps it from its adaptive peak.

Another effect of aging is the decline of mitochondrial function, presumably as a result of cumulative damage from reactive oxygen species exposure over the course of a person's life [40–43]. This decline in mitochondrial function would reduce fitness in normal cells because mitochondrion is the powerhouse of aerobic respiration that sustains cellular metabolism. Cancer is a multistep process that requires time and various factors to attain all the hallmarks of cancer. Aging provides more time for precancerous cells to grow toward becoming full-fledge tumors. At the same time, the study of cancer genetics strives to investigate the various factors (cancer clones and pathways) that drive cancer development [22]. Herein, we summarize important interactions in distal *onco-spheres*; which will also be discussed in detail in respective chapters in this book.

Malignant Transformation of Aberrant Stroma: Field Cancerization

Field cancerization is a malignant transformation process of the stroma that are in close proximity to the parental tumor. This phenomenon is especially observable in epithelial cancers such as skin cancer, breast cancer, ovarian cancer, and others. Past researchers had also observed that if a tumor is resected, a secondary tumor that possess similar genetical component can develop in nearby epithelium, given that these epithelia had been altered beforehand to welcome these precancerous lesions. This observation also proved that mutagen or carcinogen can indeed lead to carcinogenesis, as repeated or prolonged exposure of these leads to an irreversible change in the stroma, which can encourage cancer growth. This concept will be discussed in Chap. 10.

Pre-metastatic Niche

Primary tumors provide a favorable milieu in distal organs and tissues for eventual metastases, known as pre-metastatic niche, which is conditioned and formed through a complicated web of interactions between tumor secretory factors, bone-marrow-derived cells, and local stromal cells. A pre-metastatic niche is defined by six fundamental traits that allow tumor cells to colonize and drive metastasis: suppress immune responses, induce inflammation, promote angiogenesis, instigate lymphangiogenesis, initiate organotropism, and drive reprogramming of stromal cells [44]. We will discuss this further in Chap. 11. In light of the cancer ecosystem concept, the first route to metastasis is angiogenesis and lymphangiogenesis to the closest lymph node, which we termed as regional *onco-sphere*. We will discuss specific mechanisms of lymph node metastasis in Chap. 12. We will also discuss the overview of metastasis and their molecular mechanism (Chaps. 13 and 14).

Cluster Metastasis

During metastasis, cancer cells frequently takeover stem cell functions to obtain sternness—a characteristic that initiates cancer development. While many genetic and epigenetic studies had explored cancer cells' stemness from solid tumors found in situ and distantly, little is known about the functions and roles of circulating tumor cells (CTCs) in cancer development [45]. Interestingly, when connections between cells are disrupted, transcriptional regulation is modified by reconditioning DNA methylation and inhibiting transcriptional factor binding to stem cells. This provokes us to contemplate what is the minimal condition for cells to exhibit stemness from an epigenetic perspective. CTC clusters are usually heterogeneous in nature, varying in size and type, including tumor-associated macrophages, fibroblasts, and white blood cells. An issue worth investigating is how these CTC clusters with considerable heterogeneity impact epigenetic state. Another question is when did these CTC clusters acquire their epigenetic states: while separating from the primary tumor or while circulating in the system? It would be meaningful to find out if these CTC clusters were responsible for activating the epigenetics state during metastasis. It is yet unknown how cell clustering regulates the development and maintenance of low DNA methylation state in cluster-specific areas from a molecular standpoint. Some embryonic stem cell transcription factors (for example, OCT4 [46]) are known to operate as pioneer factors in reprogramming by altering chromatin accessibility. As a result, researchers still do not know if these stem cell transcription factors contribute to maintaining a low DNA methylation state at the target sites. Identifying the intricate mechanisms underpinning this dynamic regulation in epigenetics might help to design cluster-specific targeted therapies. Single-cell analysis is a set of novel technologies that has been employed for analyzing molecular characteristics of cells [47]. We will further explore the emerging concepts and mechanism of cluster metastasis in Chap. 15.

Organotrophic Metastasis

Most cancers in advance stages metastasize to a particular organ or organs, in a process termed as "organotropism," which is the greatest contributing factor to cancer deaths. To improve prognosis of patients, it is crucial to study the mechanisms of metastasis in hope of identifying therapeutic targets and developing treatment modalities [48]. Metastatic organotropism, a process where cancer cells spread and colonize distant tissues, does not occur by chance. It is a process orchestrated by multiple players: immune responses of host TME, cell-to-cell interactions, epigenetics, and molecular subtypes of cancer [49]. Cancer cells modify the distal tissue site into a pre-metastatic niche (PMN) that is conducive for cancer development by secreting growth factors, recruiting host cells from other tissues, and altering host cells functional machinery to suit its metabolic needs [44]. To aid metastasis, cancer cells can interact with components of the extracellular matrix of the TME. A "seed and soil" theory was first proposed in 1889 by Steven Paget, to explain how tumors metastasize [50]. To understand metastasis, we may consider the analogy of cancer cells to seeds and host microenvironment to soil. Cross-talk interactions between the cancer cells with the host microenvironment are crucial to tumor growth. The presence of physiological barriers in host body—such as the blood–air barrier and blood–brain barrier (BBB)—is another key player in organotrophic metastasis. The cellular and molecular mechanisms in which the cancer cells penetrate these physiological barriers to extravasate in secondary organs may help us understand organotrophic metastasis. The blood–air barrier, the site of gas exchange in the lungs, is made up of the capillary endothelium, capillary basement membrane, and alveolar epithelium. The blood–brain barrier (BBB), lined with endothelial tight junctions and astrocytic foot processes, protects the brain from circulating pathogens and is harder to penetrate [51]. In contrast to the BBB, the fenestrated sinusoidal endothelia in the liver and bone marrow are less selective and easily allow passage of larger molecules into the organ niches [52]. In Chap. 16, we will be exploring the molecular and cell biological processes underlying organotrophic metastasis [53]. In an emerging concept of local metastasis, the term "field cancerization" has been introduced. In Chap. 17, we will discuss the inter-communication between local and distal oncosphere via potent communicators such as cancer stem cells (CSCs).

Systemic *Onco-Spheres*: The Host Factor

Interactions in Systemic Onco-Spheres

Inflammation and Immune System

Inflammation is one of the greatest contributors to carcinogenesis and is actively involved in the entire process of tumor growth. Inflammation is a notable characteristic of the TME, which is generated from the interactions between cancer cells, stromal cells, and inflammatory cells within the microenvironment. These cells exhibit high plasticity and are capable of regularly altering their phenotypes and functions. We will discuss how inflammation is initiated in cancer and study the underlying mechanisms of inflammation-related carcinogenesis and development. Pathological pro-tumor inflammation is highly similar to physiologic inflammation usually involved in tissue repair. The differences between this "good" and "bad" inflammation will be discussed in detail, especially on the account of spatiotemporal factors. The discovery of cancer therapeutics relies on understanding the mechanistic interactions between cells and molecules involved in the pro-tumor process [54].

Pro-tumor inflammation destabilizes genome, modifies epigenetics, induces cancer cells multiplication, enhances pathways that resist apoptosis, stimulates angiogenesis, and leads to metastasis [3]. Previous studies had proven that inflammatory immune cells are indispensable in pro-tumor inflammation. Further experiments had been conducted to study immune cell behavior and its effect on varying stages of tumor growth, during early malignant changes, formation of primary tumors, metastasis, and after treatment [55]. (Please see Chaps. 18, 19, 20, and 21 for detailed description).

Endocrine System

Abnormal neuroendocrine signaling facilitates cancer growth and progression in the body. A mass of tumor, akin to a fully developed organ, can be sympathetically innervated by nerve fibers, which synthesize and disperse neurotransmitters (for example, norepinephrine) to support tumor growth [56]. At the same time, the sympathetic nervous system regulates tumor biology by secreting epinephrine from the adrenal glands [57, 58]. The neuroendocrine molecules bind to its cognate receptors in the TME, which triggers the signaling cascades involved in mediating stress responses, leading to far-reaching and substantial effects on the local and systemic *onco-spheres* [59]. Psychiatric disorders and emotional disturbances can cause neuroendocrine dysfunction and dysregulation by altering the hypothalamic-pituitary-adrenal axis and sympathetic nervous system activity, and as a result, stress hormones—such as cortisol and norepinephrine—are produced and released excessively into the body macroenvironment [60, 61]. Several studies had shown that chronic stress is a result of excessive stimulation sustained in the SNS and HPA axis, which causes extensive DNA damage and genomic instability, encourages cancer growth, induces angiogenesis, hampers host immunity, and eventually escalates cancer [57, 62, 63]. The sympathetic (adrenergic) nerves were proven to have a pro-tumor involvement in prostate cancer [58]. On the other hand, as demonstrated in pancreas cancer, the parasympathetic (cholinergic) nerves of the peripheral autonomic nervous system were involved in the suppression of cancer initiation and development [64]. Neuroendocrine molecules produced by cancer may worsen emotional distress in patients, which may set off "vicious cycle" in the TME and in the host systemically by reducing immunity, driving metabolic reprogramming, and generating a conducive milieu at distant sides. Currently, the scientific community is in great need of a comprehensive understanding of how tumor and the neuroendocrine system communicate within the systemic *onco-sphere* and the detailed mechanism of how the chemical signals are relayed between tumor, neural, endocrine, and immune system. This would be highly conducive to developing novel treatment strategies to manage cancer. We will further discuss how the host neuroendocrine system drives cancer progression and the other way around in Chap. 22.

Neuronal System

Throughout our body, nerves travel alongside lymph and blood vessels to different anatomical regions. Although much has been learned about angiogenesis and lymphangiogenesis in cancer, less is known about the biological implications of "neo-neurogenesis," the formation of new innervation induced by tumor growth. The factors secreted by nerve fibers can be hijacked by cancer cells to create a favorable milieu for its survival and growth. Cancer cells can release factors that promote neurite and axonal growth, eventually leading to neurogenesis. The impact of neuronal growth on tumorigenesis was first studied several decades ago, and later more studies had emerged and implied that cancer cells and the neuronal system have reciprocal connections. The interaction between cancer cells and the neuronal system was proven as a survival strategy employed by the cancer cells. However, much more research is needed to fully understand the function of neurotransmitters, neuropeptides, and their related receptor-initiated signaling pathways in tumorigenesis, as well as treatment response. The functional mapping of neurotransmitters and neuropeptides in the TME would be valuable to understand how the neuronal system influences cancer development [65].

The local tumor environment (*local onco-sphere*), which plays an important role in the formation, development, and metastasis of cancer, is made up of cellular components (such as fibroblasts, immune cells, inflammatory cells, and adipocytes), structural components (extracellular matrix), and lymph and blood vessels [66]. Oncogenes and tumor suppressor genes have long been known to have roles in carcinogenesis. But the focus of cancer biology has switched from the study of cancer genetics to the study of dynamic interactome between cancer cells and TME. Angiogenesis, in this aspect, has been extensively studied in previous research [67]. Extrapolating the findings of angiogenesis, more research had been conducted on the interactions between neuronal cells and TME, with findings in cancers of the pancreas, prostate, breast, head, neck, and bile duct [68–72]. These studies demonstrated that neuronal cells, as part of the TME, control abnormal tissue behavior and modulate cancer growth, which is often associated with poor patient prognosis. Key concerns in neuronal system and cancer development, including how neuroactive chemokines affect cancer, how nerves stimulate cancer growth, and how neurons communicate with cancer cells, were explored by many research groups previously. Furthermore, researchers are able to study the molecular pathways of cancer–nerve cross talk at greater clarity owing to improvement in technologies, such as increased precision in imaging techniques and neural manipulation [73]. The interaction between host nervous system and cancer progression will be detailed in Chap. 23.

Metabolic System

Before the study of cancer biology shifted its focus to cancer genetics on oncogenes and tumor suppressor genes, scientists had been investigating the cancer metabolic system since earlier days. Cancer metabolism is founded on the notion that cancer cells' metabolic processes differ from those of normal cells, and these differences aid in tumorigenesis and sustain malignancy. The modification of metabolism, termed "reprogrammed metabolism," is recognized as a hallmark of cancer as many cancer types exhibit such property [74]. However, the exact mechanism of metabolism reprogramming remains unknown, as well as the effect of such programming on allowing cancer progression or sustaining malignancy. Another key concern is if scientists can leverage these metabolic modifications for therapeutic advantage.

Reprogramming of cancer metabolism is often thought to increase fitness, which gives rise to selective advantage during cancer formation. Many classic examples from past experiments demonstrated that cancer reprogramming "strengthens" cells by conditioning them to survive under stress or to thrive and multiply at abnormally high rates. Changes in bioenergetics, increased biosynthesis, and redox balance are explored in depth below. If some of the metabolic modifications benefit the cancer cells, then it stands to reason that some of these metabolic processes might be good therapeutic targets. Many experiments illustrated that inhibiting increased metabolic activity in tumors impedes cancer growth [75, 76]. This finding has been applied into successful therapeutics in human cancer in some circumstances, as demonstrated in the indispensable use of enzyme asparaginase in the treatment of acute lymphoblastic leukemia (ALL). Asparaginase catalyzes the conversion of asparagine into aspartic acid and ammonia [77]. A steady supply of asparagine is required to sustain the elevated rates of protein synthesis in ALL since the cancer cells are inefficient in generating asparagine de novo. Hence, administering enzyme asparaginase systemically effectively removes this supply of asparagine. To maximize the effectiveness of metabolic interventions in cancer treatment, it is necessary to determine which metabolic pathways are responsible for conferring survival advantage at different stages of tumor growth. Because some modifications in metabolic pathways are critical in early stages of carcinogenesis to counter nutrient limitations [78] while other modifications are only essential in later stages of cancer progression, such as during metastasis [79, 80]. It is important to test the new treatment targets in models that reflect cancer pathophysiology more accurately as the targets were proposed from simplified models such as in vitro cell culture [81]. We will detail this in Chap. 24.

Microbes (Bacterial/Virus)-Induced Cancer

About one-fifth of all deadly human cancers were caused by microbes [82], implying that managing microbe-related processes might help prevent cancer. The source of these cancer-causing microbes may be endogenous or exogenous. While many types of microorganisms induce cancer [83–87], but several notable microorganisms are responsible for the majority of human cancers linked to microbes, namely, human papilloma viruses (HPV), which cause cancer of the anogenital region, Helicobacter pylori, which causes gastric cancers, and hepatitis B and C viruses, which cause hepatic carcinomas [88, 89]. Dealing with HPVs and hepatitis viruses, cancer prevention has seen remarkable results with the introduction of vaccines. For instance, the Food and Drug Administration (FDA) of the United States had approved the use of a quadrivalent HPV vaccine (against four HPV subtypes, i.e., type 6, 11, 16, 18) in preventing cervical cancer [90]. Our knowledge of these cancer-causing microbes in human just begun in the last few decades and is still growing, even though microorganisms, particularly viruses, have long been recognized to cause cancer in animals [91, 92].

Consider this phenomenon wherein a population of heavy smokers, whom all have major risk factor to develop lung cancer, but some of them never in fact got the disease. Many research studies point to genetic differences among these heavy smokers to account for who actually develops lung cancer and who has greater risk for it. The human microbiota, the native microorganisms that we carry within ourselves, may also contribute to cancer risk as they affect our metabolism and constitute our body. These microbes, largely bacteria found in human tissues such as the gastrointestinal tract, can share a mutualistic or pathogenic relationship with our body and temporarily or permanently inhabit our body [93–96]. How susceptible we are to certain diseases may be influenced by the genetic differences between the microorganisms each individual carry, which encodes for varying traits [97] that interact with our body, subtly or explicitly, by altering endocrinal homeostasis and cancer risk [98, 99]. Similarly, differences in exposure to or contact with microorganism predispose to differential risk of lung cancer among individuals with identical smoking habits. Hence, the microbiota genotype in the host may hold equal significance as the human genotype of host itself in modulating disease risk [93, 97, 100]. To support this notion, recent discovery pointed to Merkel cell polyomavirus as a pathologic microbe that has been linked to causing an aggressive form of skin cancer known as Merkel cell carcinoma [101]. Microbes play a role in both cancer initiation and progression, and understanding such roles—although its distinction unclearly defined yet—may help scientists formulate treatment and prevention strategies against microbe-related cancers [100]. We will delve deeper into the discussion of how microbes and virus interact systemically with cancer in Chaps. 25 and 26, respectively.

Finally, we will give a detailed account on the state-of-the-art technology used in visualizing and subtyping cancer ecosystem (detailed in Chap. 27). We also summarized the timeline of the utilization of bio-engineering methods to mimic cancer ecosystem (i.e., patient-derived xenograft models, organoids, 3D bioprinting) in Chap. 28. This is followed by a detailed summary of how we see the evolution of cancer ecosystem in Chap. 29 and wrap up the book with an outlook of cancer ecosystem-based therapeutic modality in Chap. 30.

Ecological Concepts in Cancer *Onco-Spheres*

Through this book, readers will be introduced to cancer ecosystem, an analogical concept to the natural ecosystem. For example, in a natural environment, host immune system always preys on tumor cells, being a good predator and keeping the host in a healthy homeostatic condition. However, in cancerous environment, cancer could make use of their surroundings to create an environment that could lead to a symbiotic relationship, for example, to change fibroblasts into CAFs that could secrete pro-tumoral factors to support tumor growth, while the tumor can also secrete pro-survival factor that can sustain CAFs phenotype. In other method, cancer cell induces a "commensal" relationship with the immune system, by overexpression checkpoint inhibitors, which reduces the ability of the immune cells to recognize them as foe. These are just a few of the examples that we will introduce over the book, also summarized below in Fig. 1.3.

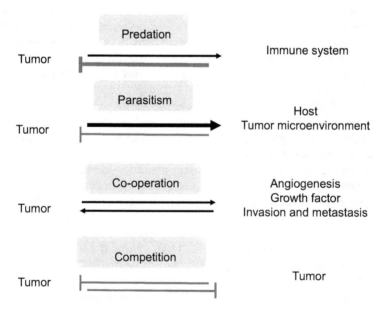

Fig. 1.3 Ecological parallelism in cancer ecology

Predation

We could draw parallels between the tumor–immune system relationship and the predator–prey model. In the latter, the predators grow and thrive by feeding on and denting the prey population. The immune system may be portrayed as the predators while cancer cells play the role of the prey population, as it constantly develops a wide range of counter-adaptations to flee from predation. One such adaptation is by downregulating the major histocompatibility complex [102]. An evolving escape mechanism in cancer cells may be problematic to the effectiveness of immune therapy. Tumors with low genetic heterogeneity are more likely to benefit from immune therapy than those with high genetic heterogeneity. Although the death of tumor cells does not directly favor or promote the development of immune cells, but in the presence of a tumor, antigen-presenting cells activate clonal expansion and T-cells differentiation, causing cytotoxic T lymphocytes to proliferate. This obser-vation fits with the predator–prey model. However, we noted that the predator–prey model is not a perfect fit to what occurs within the body. In nature, if the prey population is wiped out, or perhaps goes into extinction, predators would run out of food source and follow suit. In contrast, if tumor cells (prey) are fully purged, the immune system (predator) is still intact and functioning. We can apply the knowl-edge of the predator–prey model or a population bottleneck to make sense of conditions such as minimal residual disease (where a small amount of cancer cells remains even after treatment and leads to relapse). Therefore, it can be confirmed that the immune system is on constant vigilance to curb the residual cancer cells [103].

How Cancer Escapes Predation?

The presence of tumors is usually accompanied by elevated level of inflammation in the body system [104–107]. It is speculated that pre-cancerous cells synthesize growth factors—just like immune cells—during an infection, together producing a microenvironment saturated with growth factors [108, 109]. A small population of cancer cells can multiply quickly if growth factors become available for an extended period. Growth factors may well be the catalyst for tumor growth. Some tumors are even capable of synthesizing their own growth factors (e.g., hormone-secreting tumors) or acquire the ability to obtain growth factors from other cells. Therefore, once inflammation had begun, attempts to reduce the inflammatory response may be insufficient to halt cancer development.

Expression of Self-Antigen T-cell tolerance may develop as tumors often express self-antigens such as p53 or MDM2 [110]. A transcriptionally mutant form of p53 is discovered in about 50% of human cancers while in the rest of the cases, normal p53 function is disrupted by other mechanisms such as MDM2 amplification [111]. Mutant p53 demonstrates enhanced stability and is overexpressed in cancerous tissue in comparison to the wild-type p53 present in normal tissues. Therefore, it is suggested that mutant p53 antigens can be utilized in targeted immunotherapy [112].

Downregulation of MHC Class I in Tumor Major histocompatibility complex (MHC) molecules play an integral role in both T-cell priming and effector phase of adaptive immunity. It has been shown that tumors are capable of modifying the antigen processing mechanisms in MHC class I and II. In cancer, one or multiple genes encoded in the MHC class I antigen presentation pathway are mutated and/or dysregulated. This interferes with the antigen presentation pathway, leading to complete loss or downregulation of surface MHC proteins [113, 114]. The downregulation of MHC class I in tumor induces two consequences: cancer evasion from the classical T-cell-dependent immunity and activation of NK cell-mediated surveillance. A cooperative, interrelated process is shown to exist between the innate and adaptive immune system against tumors. When antigens are detected, the innate immunity rapidly reacts by activating non-specific MHC class I immunosurveillance (NK/$\gamma\delta$ T cells). NK cells secrete IFN-γ that upregulates MHC class I expression on tumor cell surface. As a result, the adaptive immunity is mobilized to fight the tumor cells specifically and efficiently [115]. MHC specific to human is called human leukocyte antigen (HLA) complex, located on chromosome 6p21.3. Studies have shown that downregulating or disrupting HLA class I expression on tumor cells can lead to immune evasion by cancer cells [116]. The most common mechanism for missing HLA haplotype in cancer is the loss of heterozygosity (LOH), especially at the HLA locus (LOH-6p21) [117]. However, the absence of some HLA alleles (such as HLA-Cw6, HLA Cw7) may sensitize cancer cells to cytotoxic T lymphocytes (CTLs) due to their function as inhibitory ligands that bind to CTL receptors [118].

Expression of NK Cells Inhibitory Receptors NK cells can distinguish cancer cells from normal cells through expressing various HLA class I receptors [119]. TIGIT and CD96 receptors expressed on NK cells have regulatory functions in the adhesion of NK cells to their target cells (tumors) and in migration/homing [120]. Since tumor cells expressed ligands such as PVR (CD155) and Nectin-2 (CD112), we can learn the migration of NK cells with the corresponding receptors by studying the tissue distribution of these ligands [121]. NK and T cells that are competent in infiltrating and occupying healthy tissues or tumors could be determined by the presence of other tissue retention receptors such as CD69 and CD103 [122]. Cytolytic function of NK cells is suppressed by the expression of NK cell inhibitory receptors. Two major classes of NK inhibitory receptors have been discovered: the type I transmembrane proteins of the IG superfamily (e.g., p58.2 13 or Ig-like transcript 2) [123] and the type II transmembrane proteins with C-type lectin domain (e.g., CD94/NK2 heterodimer) [124]. Suppression of the cytolytic function of NK cells is induced when NK inhibitory receptors bind to MHC class I molecules of the target cells. Majority of NK receptors are found on NK cells while some are expressed on CD8$^+$ T cells, although any given NK receptors only exist in less than 10% of the human CD8$^+$ T cells population [125].

Resistance to Apoptosis Apoptosis—a physiological process of programmed cell death common to many species—is crucial in maintaining tissue growth and homeostasis throughout life [126]. Cancer cells often exhibit the ability to resist apoptosis and proceed with uncontrolled proliferation. Studies have demonstrated that cancer cells often overexpress proteins that inhibit the apoptotic process [127]. One such mechanism employed by cancer cells to resist apoptosis is by synthesizing increased levels of anti-apoptotic proteins. The Korsmeyer rheostat model of apoptosis was derived from early studies of the BH3 protein pathway [128]. According to this model, the death or survival of a cell is regulated by antagonistic activities of killer and survival proteins in the BH3 pathway. Apoptosis occurs when activities of killer proteins exceed survival proteins (anti-apoptotic molecules). Conversely, if survival proteins become overexpressed and surpass killer proteins, the signals for programmed cell death will be disregarded, resulting in cancerous growth. With the understanding of this rheostat model, targeted anti-cancer strategies using small-molecule inhibitors (SMI) are designed to selectively inhibit anti-apoptotic proteins including B-cell lymphoma 2 (Bcl-2), B-cell lymphoma extra-large (Bcl-xL), myeloid cell leukemia 1 (Mcl-1), Bcl-2-like-protein-2 (BCL2L2/Bcl-2), and Bcl-2 related protein A1 (A1/Bfl1) [129].

Tumor Microenvironment Not Permissive to T-Cell Infiltration Immunosuppressive cytokines such as IL-10 and TGF β are released by cancer cells against T-cell infiltration [130–132]. Cancer-associated IL-10 undermines T-cell-mediated immune response by inhibiting the functions of dendritic cells and downregulating MHC class I expression via transporter associated with antigen processing (TAP) protein complex. IL-10 also inhibits transcription of antigen-processing machinery (APM) gene in T cells, leading to defective APM components [133]. Moreover, cancer cells express Fas ligands on its surface membrane, which bind to T cells, triggering T-cell apoptosis and rendering T-cell infiltration unsuccessful [134].

Cooperation: Mutualism and Commensalism

Currently, scientists are still groping the concept of cooperative relationships (*e.g.,* mutualism and commensalism) within cancer cells. A study noted that commensal behavior exists between neoplastic clones. It was observed that neoplastic clones help other clones by inducing increased fitness and conferring the ability to migrate and colonize distant tissues [135–137]. Another case of cooperative relationship was demonstrated in a study done by Axelrod and his team, which suggested that cancer cells work together by sharing diffusible factors. This allowed individual cell to bypass the need to collect all the hallmarks of cancer one by one [138]. So far, in human cancers, mutualism has only been found between cancer epithelium and activated fibroblasts. The mutualistic relationship granted fitness advantage [139–141] to both types of cells and appeared to be co-evolving [142–144]. It is widely suggested that tumors interact with their macroenvironment (host) via endocrine signaling, as demonstrated in paraneoplastic syndromes [145].

Conventionally, scientists deem it necessary that every single cell has to gather all the mutations required in order for cancer to develop in human. This process of accumulating all the "hallmarks of cancer" is equivalent to ticking all the boxes of carcinogenesis. However, it is suggested that cancer may occur without obtaining all the mutations required. Instead of working independently to tick off all the boxes of cancer, cells establish a cooperative relationship with other pre-malignant cells to share the hallmarks they each acquired, and together, they create a microenvironment equipped with the necessary phenotypes for malignancy to take place [138]. Cooperative relationships between cells may explain the prevalence of cancer. With cooperation, cells could ultimately gather all the hallmarks in accordance with the conventional view of cancer development. Therefore, the first cancer cell that manages to possess all hallmarks will likely multiply much faster than other cells that did not. We hypothesized that a cooperative relationship between cells accelerates the process of carcinogenesis. Conventionally, cells that have yet to tick all the boxes are thought to be incapable of malignant growth. On the contrary, such cells can in fact display rapid tumor development by sharing resources, implying that pre-malignant cells—cells that are few steps away from ticking all the boxes—can also proliferate quickly, potentially contributing to cancer formation.

Angiogenesis Cancer cells can release vascular endothelial growth factor (VEGF), a key mediator of blood vessel formation, into the tumor site, which stimulates neo-angiogenesis and provides extra blood supplies for tumor growth [146, 147]. This observation illustrated commensalism between tumor cells and other cells in the vicinity, as neo-angiogenesis brings increased nourishment (an abundant supply of blood, oxygen, diffusible factors for growth) to both types of cells. An example of commensalism can be seen in the interactions between cancer cells and stromal cells; cancer cells express *ras* oncogene, which downregulates thrombospondin-1, an angiogenesis-inhibitor secreted by stromal fibroblasts. This promotes angiogenesis and consequently benefits all neighboring cells; the cancer cells achieve increased tumor growth while fibroblasts thrive as evidenced by the occurrence of desmoplasia [146].

Self-Sufficiency of Certain Growth Signals Cancer cells are often self-sufficient as they are capable of synthesizing growth factors such as VEGF, platelet-derived growth factor (PDGF), and transforming growth factor β (TGF-β). These growth factors play a role in tissue damage repair and are regulated by stromal cells [139, 148]. Commensal behavior is displayed when these cancer-associated growth factors interact with stromal cells via paracrine signaling, which activate stromal cells, leading to angiogenesis, inflammation, and production of more growth factors and proteases [149–151]. These cancer-associated growth factors also help with tumor proliferation and growth via autocrine signaling. Also, cancer cells may express growth factor receptors that correspond to the growth factors produced by adjacent cancer cells within a tumor; although not yet confirmed, this can be seen as a form of mutualism [152]. Examples of paracrine signaling between cancer cells and their adjacent cells were illustrated in TGF-β-EGF receptor, PDGFA-PDGFαR, and VEGF-Flt-1 in breast cancer using immunohistochemical/immunofluorescence double-staining techniques of GFs/GF receptors [153]. This suggested that pre-malignant cells cooperate by distributing the resources each has acquired (the tumor growth factors), forming a heterogeneous community working toward the same goal.

Tissue Invasion and Metastasis The cooperative relationship between cancer cells and stromal cells builds a well-conditioned tumor microenvironment that aids in tissue invasion and metastasis. Under usual circumstances, when cancer cells invade tissues of anchorage-dependent cells such as epithelial cells, the loss of contact with the basement membrane would trigger anoikis, a type of programmed cell death at the site of invasion. A general explanation for how tumors can successfully invade tissue and achieve anchorage-independent growth was the development of a specific mutation that confers the ability to survive without anchorage. In contrast to the general view, it was found that tumors are capable of tissue invasion without developing a specific mutation against anoikis. Instead, peritumor fibroblasts cooperate with cancer cells by secreting stromelysin-3, a factor that allows tumors to survive through the invasion into adjacent tissues [154]. Also, it was proven that cancer cells and their accomplices such as fibroblasts, inflammatory cells, and endothelial cells all participate in the pathways of cancer development. Stromal cells present proteases that aid in breaking down extracellular matrix around the tumor site, thus resulting in tissue invasion and further migration [141].

Competition

Competition occurs within heterogeneous population of cancer cells as they compete for resources such as oxygen and fight for growth factors [155]. Previous studies that inoculated neoplastic clones into both flanks of mice [136] and rats [156] demonstrated that the relationships between tumors may be competitive (when tumor growth in both flanks was inhibited) and sometimes, amensal (when only one side was affected). Neoplastic clones displayed unmistakable competition when they trigger an immune reaction that eliminates the other tumor clones. By applying the Lotka–Volterra competition equations in the understanding of cancer development, we can postulate several ways that may wipe out cancer cells: alleviate stressful effects of cancer cells on normal tissues, intensify normal tissues' ability to compete with tumors, and decrease tissue support for cancer cells (e.g., prevent angiogenesis) [157].

Competition in Neoplastic Clones

Subpopulations of tumor cells were injected into both flanks of mice to compare the growth rate at each injection site. It was found that growth rate of the subpopulations is associated to the relationship shared between tumors on opposite sides. Consider

Table 1.1 Different ecological relationship between each "*onco-sphere*" revealing a unique and intriguing relationship in an inter-"*onco-spherical*" manner

Cell injection site		Growth rate		
Flank 1	Flank 2	Flank 1	Flank 2	Relationship
Subline 66	Subline 66	Increase	Increase	Symbiosis
Subline 67	Subline 67	Increase	Increase	Symbiosis
Subline 66	Subline 67	Decrease	Decrease	Competition
Subline 168	Subline 168	Increase	Increase	Symbiosis
Subline 168	–	Increase	–	–
Subline 168	Subline 68H	Decrease	Increase	Competition
Subline 68H	–	Slow growing		–
Subline 68H	Subline 68H	Slow growing	Slow growing	Competition
Subline 68H	Subline 168	Increase	Decrease	Commensalism
Subline 168	Subline 410	Decrease	No effect	Amensalism
Subline 410	–	Increase	–	–
Subline 410	Subline 410	Increase	Increase	Symbiosis
Subline 410 + 2000 rads	Subline 168	–	Abrogate effect on subline 168	Commensalism

the following experiment. In this experiment, the researcher used the same cell line to both flanks, same parental origin but clonally different cell line (denoted by H), or two different cell lines. Note that in this experiment, the negative control is to inject the cells on only one side (at Flank 1). Also, the injection was done at a constant number of cells into the right and left flank of the same mouse. The findings are summarized in Table 1.1 below.

Surprisingly, the aggressive neoplastic clones are more likely to be selected for over the healthy population during an immune response, possibly due to genetic heterogeneity in tumors. Although not yet proven, the immune response is therefore speculated to be cooperating with cancer cells rather than being a predator in such cases. Observing that subpopulations of neoplastic clones can affect each other's growth in varied ways, we can conclude that solely examining the genetic composition of a tumor is insufficient to predict its progression [136].

Parasitism

Parasitism very much resembles predation in the sense that one (perpetrator species) gains benefit while the other (victim species) is harmed, but parasitism is characterized by its ability to propagate without causing the immediate death of their host (victim). Parasitic relationships among cancer cells of a tumor are rarely found. But it is common to find cancer cells hijacking their neighboring tissues for metabolic benefits, such as exploiting growth factors produced by fibroblasts, commanding neo-angiogenesis for increased tumor growth, and breaking down extracellular matrix [158, 159].

Cachexia Cachexia, often seen in cancer, is considered as a paraneoplastic syndrome (simply put, it refers to the abnormal state of health in response to cancer). Cachexia leads to poorer prognosis and lower quality of life in cancer patients. It is a complex wasting disorder characterized by the gradual loss of muscles and fat tissues found in almost half of the cancer patient population. Cachectic patients are often anorexic, suffering from this eating disorder characterized by the involuntary loss of appetite. Although both conditions contribute to weight loss, but anorexia is not the culprit for loss of lean body mass. In cancer patients, tumor cells stimulate increased gene expression and protein production within the body, raising the biochemical work load of the Cori cycle. This leads to an increase in thermogenesis and the basal metabolic rate. Lipolysis often occurs to provide the energy needed by both tumor cells and host cells, thereby accounting for the loss of adipose tissue. Meanwhile, the loss of lean body mass is mainly due to an imbalance in protein metabolism: increased protein breakdown and decreased protein synthesis. Ubiquitin-proteasome pathways and lysosomes are excessively activated in cachexia, leading to increased protein breakdown. Protein synthesis is downregulated via the following mechanisms: First, the concentration of eIF4F complexes is lowered, hindering translation initiation. Second, elongation phase of translation is blocked. Third, dsRNA-dependent protein kinase is activated, causing increased downstream eIF2-induced phosphorylation, and hence reduces methionyl-tRNA binding to the smaller ribosomal subunit. Furthermore, tumor cells produce proteolysis-inducing factors, and the body simultaneously produces tumor necrosis factor-α and glucocorticoids, leading to severe muscle wasting in cancer patients [160].

Cancer Cells Stimulating CAFs to Secrete Growth Factor [161] A significant level of chemokine is believed to be secreted by cancer-associated fibroblasts (CAFs); these chemokines include C-C motif chemokine ligand (CCL) and C-X-C motif chemokine ligand (CXCL). CCL and CXCL play important roles in the development and metastasis of melanoma, by associating with their respective chemokine receptors and modifying gene expression in CAFs and melanoma cells [162]. Co-culture studies of CAFs with tumor cells demonstrated elevated level of CCL2, CXCL1, CXCL2, CXCL8 (IL-8) in cancers of the breast, pancreas, mouth, and skin [163]. A study revealed that CXCL14 stimulates prostate cancer progression and metastasis both in vitro and in vivo by paracrine signaling [164]. Co-culture studies of CAFs with melanoma cells exhibited increased expression of CXCL8, IL-1, and CCL2, thereby contributing to angiogenesis and cancer migration [163]. CAFs also secrete growth factors such as HGF and TGF- β that stimulate cancer cell growth. In advance melanoma, TGF-β stimulates cancer progression and migration via paracrine signaling [165, 166]. HGF promotes the proliferation and metastasis of melanoma cells via several mechanisms: regulating tyrosylphosphorylation of MET and other proteins such as MAPK and ERK2 [167], inducing expression of fibronectin that leads to increased matrix assembly [168], and mediating E-cadherin to N-cadherin switch through changing the expression of transcriptional factors SNAI1, SNAI2, and TWIST1 in a stage-specific manner [169, 170]. Furthermore, growth factors from CAFs such as VEGFs interact with stromal cells in many ways and facilitate further tumor development [171]. Studies have demonstrated that CAFs in melanoma produce increased level of cytokines and GFs such as VEGF, CXCL 12, and IL-6 in response to oxidative stress caused by hypoxia and to the presence of chemical factors released by melanoma cells, resulting in melanoma chemotaxis and metastasis [172, 173].

Breakdown of the Extracellular Matrix and the Release of Growth Factors for Cancer Metastasis MMPs play essential role in angiogenesis by breaking down the ECM to facilitate endothelial cell invasion into nearby tissue. Recent studies have revealed that MMPs' involvement in angiogenesis is evidently more than just breaking down components of the ECM for endothelial cell invasion. MMPs also contribute to the release of growth factors for cancer, by generating proangiogenic factors, structurally modifying growth factors and receptors such as integrins and adhesion receptors, and releasing antiangiogenic factors [174–176]. Furthermore, MMPs degrade or cleave inactive precursors into active forms of growth signals. For example, insulin-like growth factor (IGF)-binding proteins are degraded by MMP to generate active IGFs, proteoglycan perlecan in vascular basement membranes is degraded to yield FGFs, and latent TGFβ-binding proteins (e.g. decorin) are degraded to release latent TGFβ. Specifically MMP-2 and MMP-9 are known to proteolytically degrade latent TGF β1 and TGF β2 into their respective active forms [177]. Heparin-binding EGF (HB-EGF) is activated by MMP-3 and MMP-7 via cleavage of its precursor from the cell membrane; TNFα is also activated in a similar manner by MMP-1, -3, and -7 [175]. MMP-9 promotes angiogenesis by activating IL-8, an inflammation- and angiogenesis-promoting cytokine via cleavage, and by inactivating platelet factor-4, an angiogenesis inhibitor via degradation [178].

Conclusion

All the above examples are excellent proofs that human body acts as a natural reservoir for cancer to grow, invade, and metastasize. By utilizing principles found in the natural ecological world, cancer cells manipulate their microenvironment (local *onco-sphere*) to conquer more niches for them to grow (distal *onco-sphere*) and manipulate the host system (systemic *onco-sphere*). In the coming chapters, we will discuss in detail how and why cancer should be seen from an ecosystem point of view in order for cancer patients to be given precise and personalized cancer therapeutics. This book will provide a comprehensive ecological view of a cancer ecosystem. In the beginning of each chapter, we will detail the underlying molecular mechanism of each discussed subject and then reveal the close intra-, inter-, *oncospheric* relationship with cancer. To date, many researchers are looking at cancer similar to the blind men encountering different parts of an elephant. Specialized researchers have seen only one aspect of tumor aggressiveness and determined its mechanisms accordingly, which is indeed important; nevertheless, insufficient to properly address the core problems in cancer growth and progression. We aim to achieve a holistic and comprehensive view of cancer, taking local, distal, and systemic *onco-spheric* interactions into account.

References

1. Liu J, Lao L, Chen J, Li J, Zeng W, Zhu X et al (2021) The IRENA lncRNA converts chemotherapy-polarized tumor-suppressing macrophages to tumor-promoting phenotypes in breast cancer. Nat Cancer 2(4):457–473
2. Hanahan D, Weinberg RA (2000) The hallmarks of cancer. Cell 100(1):57–70
3. Hanahan D, Weinberg RA (2011) Hallmarks of cancer: the next generation. Cell 144(5): 646–674
4. Hanahan D (2022) Hallmarks of cancer: new dimensions. Cancer Discov 12(1):31–46
5. Smithers DW (1962) An attack on cytologism. Lancet 1(7228):493–499
6. Cavallo F, De Giovanni C, Nanni P, Forni G, Lollini PL (2011) 2011: the immune hallmarks of cancer. Cancer Immunol Immunother 60(3):319–326
7. Colotta F, Allavena P, Sica A, Garlanda C, Mantovani A (2009) Cancer-related inflammation, the seventh hallmark of cancer: links to genetic instability. Carcinogenesis 30(7):1073–1081
8. Pietras K, Ostman A (2010) Hallmarks of cancer: interactions with the tumor stroma. Exp Cell Res 316(8):1324–1331
9. Camacho DF, Pienta KJ (2012) Disrupting the networks of cancer. Clin Cancer Res 18(10): 2801–2808
10. Pienta KJ, McGregor N, Axelrod R, Axelrod DE (2008) Ecological therapy for cancer: defining tumors using an ecosystem paradigm suggests new opportunities for novel cancer treatments. Transl Oncol 1(4):158–164
11. Beltrao P, Cagney G, Krogan NJ (2010) Quantitative genetic interactions reveal biological modularity. Cell 141(5):739–745
12. Mareel M, Constantino S (2011) Ecosystems of invasion and metastasis in mammary morphogenesis and cancer. Int J Dev Biol 55(7–9):671–684
13. Ziogas DE, Katsios C, Roukos DH (2011) From traditional molecular biology to network oncology. Future Oncol 7(2):155–159
14. Roychowdhury S, Iyer MK, Robinson DR, Lonigro RJ, Wu Y-M, Cao X et al (2011) Personalized oncology through integrative high-throughput sequencing: a pilot study. Sci Transl Med 3(111):111ra21-ra21
15. Chen KW, Pienta KJ (2011) Modeling invasion of metastasizing cancer cells to bone marrow utilizing ecological principles. Theor Biol Med Model 8:36
16. Barrett GW, Brewer R, Odum E (2004) Fundamentals of ecology, 5th edn. Brooks/Cole
17. Pienta KJ, Loberg R (2005) The "emigration, migration, and immigration" of prostate cancer. Clin Prostate Cancer 4(1):24–30
18. Stratton MR, Campbell PJ, Futreal PA (2009) The cancer genome. Nature 458(7239):719–724
19. International Cancer Genome Consortium, Hudson TJ, Anderson W, Artez A, Barker AD, Bell C et al (2010) International network of cancer genome projects. Nature 464(7291):993–998
20. Merlo LMF, Pepper JW, Reid BJ, Maley CC (2006) Cancer as an evolutionary and ecological process. Nat Rev Cancer 6(12):924–935

21. Rankin DJ, López-Sepulcre A (2005) Can adaptation lead to extinction? Oikos 111(3): 616–619
22. Kareva I (2011) What can ecology teach us about cancer? Transl Oncol 4(5):266–270
23. Albini A, Sporn MB (2007) The tumour microenvironment as a target for chemoprevention. Nat Rev Cancer 7(2):139–147
24. Gajewski TF, Schreiber H, Fu YX (2013) Innate and adaptive immune cells in the tumor microenvironment. Nat Immunol 14(10):1014–1022
25. Marvel D, Gabrilovich DI (2015) Myeloid-derived suppressor cells in the tumor microenvironment: expect the unexpected. J Clin Invest 125(9):3356–3364
26. Hanahan D, Coussens LM (2012) Accessories to the crime: functions of cells recruited to the tumor microenvironment. Cancer Cell 21(3):309–322
27. Bergfeld SA, DeClerck YA (2010) Bone marrow-derived mesenchymal stem cells and the tumor microenvironment. Cancer Metastasis Rev 29(2):249–261
28. Coussens LM, Zitvogel L, Palucka AK (2013) Neutralizing tumor-promoting chronic inflammation: a magic bullet? Science 339(6117):286–291
29. Pitt JM, Marabelle A, Eggermont A, Soria JC, Kroemer G, Zitvogel L (2016) Targeting the tumor microenvironment: removing obstruction to anticancer immune responses and immunotherapy. Ann Oncol 27(8):1482–1492
30. Didham RK, Tylianakis JM, Gemmell NJ, Rand TA, Ewers RM (2007) Interactive effects of habitat modification and species invasion on native species decline. Trends Ecol Evol 22(9): 489–496
31. Sax DF, Stachowicz JJ, Brown JH, Bruno JF, Dawson MN, Gaines SD et al (2007) Ecological and evolutionary insights from species invasions. Trends Ecol Evol 22(9):465–471
32. Parker JD, Burkepile DE, Hay ME (2006) Opposing effects of native and exotic herbivores on plant invasions. Science 311(5766):1459–1461
33. Callaway RM, Thelen GC, Rodriguez A, Holben WE (2004) Soil biota and exotic plant invasion. Nature 427(6976):731–733
34. Tilman D, Wedin D, Knops J (1996) Productivity and sustainability influenced by biodiversity in grassland ecosystems. Nature 379(6567):718–720
35. Tilman D (2004) Niche tradeoffs, neutrality, and community structure: a stochastic theory of resource competition, invasion, and community assembly. Proc Natl Acad Sci U S A 101(30): 10854–10861
36. Tilman D, Lehman CL, Thomson KT (1997) Plant diversity and ecosystem productivity: theoretical considerations. Proc Natl Acad Sci U S A 94(5):1857–1861
37. Marusyk A, DeGregori J (2008) Declining cellular fitness with age promotes cancer initiation by selecting for adaptive oncogenic mutations. Biochim Biophys Acta 1785(1):1–11
38. DeGregori J (2011) Evolved tumor suppression: why are we so good at not getting cancer? Cancer Res 71(11):3739–3744
39. Henry CJ, Marusyk A, Zaberezhnyy V, Adane B, DeGregori J (2010) Declining lymphoid progenitor fitness promotes aging-associated leukemogenesis. Proc Natl Acad Sci U S A 107(50):21713–21718
40. Benz CC, Yau C (2008) Ageing, oxidative stress and cancer: paradigms in parallax. Nat Rev Cancer 8(11):875–879
41. Druzhyna NM, Wilson GL, LeDoux SP (2008) Mitochondrial DNA repair in aging and disease. Mech Ageing Dev 129(7–8):383–390
42. Lin MT, Beal MF (2006) Mitochondrial dysfunction and oxidative stress in neurodegenerative diseases. Nature 443(7113):787–795
43. Balaban RS, Nemoto S, Finkel T (2005) Mitochondria, oxidants, and aging. Cell 120(4): 483–495
44. Liu Y, Cao X (2016) Characteristics and significance of the pre-metastatic niche. Cancer Cell 30(5):668–681
45. Yu M (2019) Metastasis stemming from circulating tumor cell clusters. Trends Cell Biol 29(4): 275–276

46. Soufi A, Garcia MF, Jaroszewicz A, Osman N, Pellegrini M, Zaret KS (2015) Pioneer transcription factors target partial DNA motifs on nucleosomes to initiate reprogramming. Cell 161(3):555–568
47. Ortiz V, Yu M (2018) Analyzing circulating tumor cells one at a time. Trends Cell Biol 28(10): 764–775
48. Gao Y, Bado I, Wang H, Zhang W, Rosen JM, Zhang XH (2019) Metastasis organotropism: redefining the congenial soil. Dev Cell 49(3):375–391
49. Lu X, Kang Y (2007) Organotropism of breast cancer metastasis. J Mammary Gland Biol Neoplasia 12(2–3):153–162
50. Paget S (1989) The distribution of secondary growths in cancer of the breast. Cancer Metastasis Rev 8(2):98–101
51. Wilhelm I, Molnar J, Fazakas C, Hasko J, Krizbai IA (2013) Role of the blood-brain barrier in the formation of brain metastases. Int J Mol Sci 14(1):1383–1411
52. Inoue S, Osmond DG (2001) Basement membrane of mouse bone marrow sinusoids shows distinctive structure and proteoglycan composition: a high resolution ultrastructural study. Anat Rec 264(3):294–304
53. Chen W, Hoffmann AD, Liu H, Liu X (2018) Organotropism: new insights into molecular mechanisms of breast cancer metastasis. NPJ Precis Oncol 2(1):4
54. Greten FR, Grivennikov SI (2019) Inflammation and cancer: triggers, mechanisms, and consequences. Immunity 51(1):27–41
55. Gonzalez H, Hagerling C, Werb Z (2018) Roles of the immune system in cancer: from tumor initiation to metastatic progression. Genes Dev 32(19–20):1267–1284
56. Shi M, Liu D, Yang Z, Guo N (2013) Central and peripheral nervous systems: master controllers in cancer metastasis. Cancer Metastasis Rev 32(3–4):603–621
57. Cole SW, Nagaraja AS, Lutgendorf SK, Green PA, Sood AK (2015) Sympathetic nervous system regulation of the tumour microenvironment. Nat Rev Cancer 15(9):563–572
58. Zahalka AH, Arnal-Estapé A, Maryanovich M, Nakahara F, Cruz CD, Finley LWS et al (2017) Adrenergic nerves activate an angio-metabolic switch in prostate cancer. Science (New York, NY) 358(6361):321–326
59. Colon-Echevarria CB, Lamboy-Caraballo R, Aquino-Acevedo AN, Armaiz-Pena GN (2019) Neuroendocrine regulation of tumor-associated immune cells. Front Oncol 9:1077
60. Shin KJ, Lee YJ, Yang YR, Park S, Suh PG, Follo MY et al (2016) Molecular mechanisms underlying psychological stress and cancer. Curr Pharm Des 22(16):2389–2402
61. Holden RJ, Pakula IS, Mooney PA (1998) An immunological model connecting the pathogenesis of stress, depression and carcinoma. Med Hypotheses 51(4):309–314
62. Reiche EM, Nunes SO, Morimoto HK (2004) Stress, depression, the immune system, and cancer. Lancet Oncol 5(10):617–625
63. Thaker PH, Han LY, Kamat AA, Arevalo JM, Takahashi R, Lu C et al (2006) Chronic stress promotes tumor growth and angiogenesis in a mouse model of ovarian carcinoma. Nat Med 12(8):939–944
64. Renz BW, Tanaka T, Sunagawa M, Takahashi R, Jiang Z, Macchini M et al (2018) Cholinergic signaling via muscarinic receptors directly and indirectly suppresses pancreatic tumorigenesis and cancer stemness. Cancer Discov 8(11):1458–1473
65. Mancino M, Ametller E, Gascon P, Almendro V (2011) The neuronal influence on tumor progression. Biochim Biophys Acta 1816(2):105–118
66. Chen F, Zhuang X, Lin L, Yu P, Wang Y, Shi Y et al (2015) New horizons in tumor microenvironment biology: challenges and opportunities. BMC Med 13:45
67. Wang Y, Wang L, Chen C, Chu X (2018) New insights into the regulatory role of microRNA in tumor angiogenesis and clinical implications. Mol Cancer 17(1):22
68. Saloman JL, Albers KM, Li D, Hartman DJ, Crawford HC, Muha EA et al (2016) Ablation of sensory neurons in a genetic model of pancreatic ductal adenocarcinoma slows initiation and progression of cancer. Proc Natl Acad Sci U S A 113(11):3078–3083

69. Kamiya A, Hayama Y, Kato S, Shimomura A, Shimomura T, Irie K et al (2019) Genetic manipulation of autonomic nerve fiber innervation and activity and its effect on breast cancer progression. Nat Neurosci 22(8):1289–1305

70. Amit M, Takahashi H, Dragomir MP, Lindemann A, Gleber-Netto FO, Pickering CR et al (2020) Loss of p53 drives neuron reprogramming in head and neck cancer. Nature 578(7795): 449–454

71. Magnon C, Hall SJ, Lin J, Xue X, Gerber L, Freedland SJ et al (2013) Autonomic nerve development contributes to prostate cancer progression. Science 341(6142):1236361

72. Tan X, Sivakumar S, Bednarsch J, Wiltberger G, Kather JN, Niehues J et al (2021) Nerve fibers in the tumor microenvironment in neurotropic cancer-pancreatic cancer and cholangiocarcinoma. Oncogene 40(5):899–908

73. Wang H, Zheng Q, Lu Z, Wang L, Ding L, Xia L et al (2021) Role of the nervous system in cancers: a review. Cell Death Discov 7(1):76

74. Pavlova NN, Thompson CB (2016) The emerging hallmarks of cancer metabolism. Cell Metab 23(1):27–47

75. Patra KC, Wang Q, Bhaskar PT, Miller L, Wang Z, Wheaton W et al (2013) Hexokinase 2 is required for tumor initiation and maintenance and its systemic deletion is therapeutic in mouse models of cancer. Cancer Cell 24(2):213–228

76. Shroff EH, Eberlin LS, Dang VM, Gouw AM, Gabay M, Adam SJ et al (2015) MYC oncogene overexpression drives renal cell carcinoma in a mouse model through glutamine metabolism. Proc Natl Acad Sci U S A 112(21):6539–6544

77. Clavell LA, Gelber RD, Cohen HJ, Hitchcock-Bryan S, Cassady JR, Tarbell NJ et al (1986) Four-agent induction and intensive asparaginase therapy for treatment of childhood acute lymphoblastic leukemia. N Engl J Med 315(11):657–663

78. Yun J, Rago C, Cheong I, Pagliarini R, Angenendt P, Rajagopalan H et al (2009) Glucose deprivation contributes to the development of KRAS pathway mutations in tumor cells. Science 325(5947):1555–1559

79. Loo JM, Scherl A, Nguyen A, Man FY, Weinberg E, Zeng Z et al (2015) Extracellular metabolic energetics can promote cancer progression. Cell 160(3):393–406

80. Piskounova E, Agathocleous M, Murphy MM, Hu Z, Huddlestun SE, Zhao Z et al (2015) Oxidative stress inhibits distant metastasis by human melanoma cells. Nature 527(7577): 186–191

81. DeBerardinis RJ, Chandel NS (2016) Fundamentals of cancer metabolism. Sci Adv 2(5): e1600200

82. Parkin DM (2006) The global health burden of infection-associated cancers in the year 2002. Int J Cancer 118(12):3030–3044

83. Butel JS (2000) Viral carcinogenesis: revelation of molecular mechanisms and etiology of human disease. Carcinogenesis 21(3):405–426

84. Elgui de Oliveira D (2007) DNA viruses in human cancer: an integrated overview on fundamental mechanisms of viral carcinogenesis. Cancer Lett 247(2):182–196

85. Watanapa P, Watanapa WB (2002) Liver fluke-associated cholangiocarcinoma. Br J Surg 89(8):962–970

86. Yoshida M, Miyoshi I, Hinuma Y (1982) Isolation and characterization of retrovirus from cell lines of human adult T-cell leukemia and its implication in the disease. Proc Natl Acad Sci U S A 79(6):2031–2035

87. Schiffman M, Castle PE, Jeronimo J, Rodriguez AC, Wacholder S (2007) Human papilloma-virus and cervical cancer. Lancet 370(9590):890–907

88. Peek RM Jr, Blaser MJ (2002) Helicobacter pylori and gastrointestinal tract adenocarcinomas. Nat Rev Cancer 2(1):28–37

89. Raza SA, Clifford GM, Franceschi S (2007) Worldwide variation in the relative importance of hepatitis B and hepatitis C viruses in hepatocellular carcinoma: a systematic review. Br J Cancer 96(7):1127–1134

90. Schiller JT, Lowy DR (2014) Virus infection and human cancer: an overview. Recent Results Cancer Res 193:1–10
91. Rous P (1973) Transmission of a malignant new growth by means of a cell-free filtrate. Conn Med 37(10):526
92. Rous P (1983) Landmark article (JAMA 1911;56:198). Transmission of a malignant new growth by means of a cell-free filtrate. By Peyton Rous. JAMA 250(11):1445–1449
93. Blaser MJ (2006) Who are we? Indigenous microbes and the ecology of human diseases. EMBO Rep 7(10):956–960
94. Blaser MJ, Kirschner D (2007) The equilibria that allow bacterial persistence in human hosts. Nature 449(7164):843–849
95. Turnbaugh PJ, Ley RE, Mahowald MA, Magrini V, Mardis ER, Gordon JI (2006) An obesity-associated gut microbiome with increased capacity for energy harvest. Nature 444(7122): 1027–1031
96. Dethlefsen L, McFall-Ngai M, Relman DA (2007) An ecological and evolutionary perspective on human-microbe mutualism and disease. Nature 449(7164):811–818
97. Blaser MJ, Atherton JC (2004) Helicobacter pylori persistence: biology and disease. J Clin Invest 113(3):321–333
98. Tikkanen MJ, Adlercreutz H, Pulkkinen MO (1973) Effects of antibiotics on oestrogen metabolism. Br Med J 2(5862):369
99. Adlercreutz H, Pulkkinen MO, Hamalainen EK, Korpela JT (1984) Studies on the role of intestinal bacteria in metabolism of synthetic and natural steroid hormones. J Steroid Biochem 20(1):217–229
100. Blaser MJ (2008) Understanding microbe-induced cancers. Cancer Prev Res 1(1):15–20
101. Feng H, Shuda M, Chang Y, Moore PS (2008) Clonal integration of a polyomavirus in human Merkel cell carcinoma. Science 319(5866):1096–1100
102. Seliger B (2005) Strategies of tumor immune evasion. BioDrugs 19(6):347–354
103. Uhr JW, Scheuermann RH, Street NE, Vitetta ES (1997) Cancer dormancy: opportunities for new therapeutic approaches. Nat Med 3(5):505–509
104. Mantovani A, Allavena P, Sica A, Balkwill F (2008) Cancer-related inflammation. Nature 454(7203):436–444
105. de Visser KE, Eichten A, Coussens LM (2006) Paradoxical roles of the immune system during cancer development. Nat Rev Cancer 6(1):24–37
106. Coussens LM, Werb Z (2002) Inflammation and cancer. Nature 420(6917):860–867
107. Grimshaw MJ, Balkwill FR (2001) Inhibition of monocyte and macrophage chemotaxis by hypoxia and inflammation--a potential mechanism. Eur J Immunol 31(2):480–489
108. Ruffell B, DeNardo DG, Affara NI, Coussens LM (2010) Lymphocytes in cancer development: polarization towards pro-tumor immunity. Cytokine Growth Factor Rev 21(1):3–10
109. Johansson M, Denardo DG, Coussens LM (2008) Polarized immune responses differentially regulate cancer development. Immunol Rev 222:145–154
110. Theoret MR, Cohen CJ, Nahvi AV, Ngo LT, Suri KB, Powell DJ Jr et al (2008) Relationship of p53 overexpression on cancers and recognition by anti-p53 T cell receptor-transduced T cells. Hum Gene Ther 19(11):1219–1232
111. Vogelstein B, Lane D, Levine AJ (2000) Surfing the p53 network. Nature 408(6810):307–310
112. Theobald M, Biggs J, Dittmer D, Levine AJ, Sherman LA (1995) Targeting p53 as a general tumor antigen. Proc Natl Acad Sci U S A 92(26):11993–11997
113. Algarra I, Garcia-Lora A, Cabrera T, Ruiz-Cabello F, Garrido F (2004) The selection of tumor variants with altered expression of classical and nonclassical MHC class I molecules: implications for tumor immune escape. Cancer Immunol Immunothers 53(10):904–910
114. Garcia-Lora A, Martinez M, Algarra I, Gaforio JJ, Garrido F (2003) MHC class I-deficient metastatic tumor variants immunoselected by T lymphocytes originate from the coordinated downregulation of APM components. Int J Cancer 106(4):521–527
115. Bubenik J (2004) MHC class I down-regulation: tumour escape from immune surveillance? (review). Int J Oncol 25(2):487–491

116. Maleno I, Aptsiauri N, Cabrera T, Gallego A, Paschen A, Lopez-Nevot MA et al (2011) Frequent loss of heterozygosity in the beta2-microglobulin region of chromosome 15 in primary human tumors. Immunogenetics 63(2):65–71
117. Cabrera T, Lopez-Nevot MA, Gaforio JJ, Ruiz-Cabello F, Garrido F (2003) Analysis of HLA expression in human tumor tissues. Cancer Immunol Immunother 52(1):1–9
118. Mandelboim O, Pazmany L, Davis DM, Vales-Gomez M, Reyburn HT, Rybalov B et al (1997) Multiple receptors for HLA-G on human natural killer cells. Proc Natl Acad Sci U S A 94(26):14666–14670
119. Moretta A, Bottino C, Vitale M, Pende D, Biassoni R, Mingari MC et al (1996) Receptors for HLA class-I molecules in human natural killer cells. Annu Rev Immunol 14:619–648
120. Castriconi R, Carrega P, Dondero A, Bellora F, Casu B, Regis S et al (2018) Molecular mechanisms directing migration and retention of natural killer cells in human tissues. Front Immunol 9:2324
121. Sivori S, Della Chiesa M, Carlomagno S, Quatrini L, Munari E, Vacca P et al (2020) Inhibitory receptors and checkpoints in human NK cells, implications for the immunotherapy of cancer. Front Immunol 11:2156
122. Freud AG, Mundy-Bosse BL, Yu J, Caligiuri MA (2017) The broad spectrum of human natural killer cell diversity. Immunity 47(5):820–833
123. Colonna M, Navarro F, Bellon T, Llano M, Garcia P, Samaridis J et al (1997) A common inhibitory receptor for major histocompatibility complex class I molecules on human lymphoid and myelomonocytic cells. J Exp Med 186(11):1809–1818
124. Moretta A, Vitale M, Sivori S, Bottino C, Morelli L, Augugliaro R et al (1994) Human natural killer cell receptors for HLA-class I molecules. Evidence that the Kp43 (CD94) molecule functions as receptor for HLA-B alleles. J Exp Med 180(2):545–555
125. Speiser DE, Pittet MJ, Valmori D, Dunbar R, Rimoldi D, Lienard D et al (1999) In vivo expression of natural killer cell inhibitory receptors by human melanoma-specific cytolytic T lymphocytes. J Exp Med 190(6):775–782
126. Du Toit A (2013) Cell death: balance through a bivalent regulator. Nat Rev Mol Cell Biol 14(9):546
127. Mohammad RM, Muqbil I, Lowe L, Yedjou C, Hsu HY, Lin LT et al (2015) Broad targeting of resistance to apoptosis in cancer. Semin Cancer Biol 35(Suppl):S78–S103
128. Korsmeyer SJ, Shutter JR, Veis DJ, Merry DE, Oltvai ZN (1993) Bcl-2/Bax: a rheostat that regulates an anti-oxidant pathway and cell death. Semin Cancer Biol 4(6):327–332
129. Morin PJ (2003) Drug resistance and the microenvironment: nature and nurture. Drug Resist Updat 6(4):169–172
130. Chen Q, Daniel V, Maher DW, Hersey P (1994) Production of IL-10 by melanoma cells: examination of its role in immunosuppression mediated by melanoma. Int J Cancer 56(5): 755–760
131. Tada T, Ohzeki S, Utsumi K, Takiuchi H, Muramatsu M, Li XF et al (1991) Transforming growth factor-beta-induced inhibition of T cell function. Susceptibility difference in T cells of various phenotypes and functions and its relevance to immunosuppression in the tumor-bearing state. J Immunol 146(3):1077–1082
132. Gorelik L, Flavell RA (2001) Immune-mediated eradication of tumors through the blockade of transforming growth factor-beta signaling in T cells. Nat Med 7(10):1118–1122
133. Zeidler R, Eissner G, Meissner P, Uebel S, Tampe R, Lazis S et al (1997) Downregulation of TAP1 in B lymphocytes by cellular and Epstein-Barr virus-encoded interleukin-10. Blood 90(6):2390–2397
134. Strand S, Hofmann WJ, Hug H, Muller M, Otto G, Strand D et al (1996) Lymphocyte apoptosis induced by CD95 (APO-1/Fas) ligand-expressing tumor cells--a mechanism of immune evasion? Nat Med 2(12):1361–1366
135. Heppner GH, Miller FR (1998) The cellular basis of tumor progression. Int Rev Cytol 177:1–56
136. Miller BE, Miller FR, Leith J, Heppner GH (1980) Growth interaction in vivo between tumor subpopulations derived from a single mouse mammary tumor. Cancer Res 40(11):3977–3981

137. Jouanneau J, Moens G, Bourgeois Y, Poupon MF, Thiery JP (1994) A minority of carcinoma cells producing acidic fibroblast growth factor induces a community effect for tumor progression. Proc Natl Acad Sci U S A 91(1):286–290
138. Axelrod R, Axelrod DE, Pienta KJ (2006) Evolution of cooperation among tumor cells. Proc Natl Acad Sci U S A 103(36):13474–13479
139. Mueller MM, Fusenig NE (2004) Friends or foes - bipolar effects of the tumour stroma in cancer. Nat Rev Cancer 4(11):839–849
140. Shao ZM, Nguyen M, Barsky SH (2000) Human breast carcinoma desmoplasia is PDGF initiated. Oncogene 19(38):4337–4345
141. Tlsty TD (2001) Stromal cells can contribute oncogenic signals. Semin Cancer Biol 11(2): 97–104
142. Fukino K, Shen L, Matsumoto S, Morrison CD, Mutter GL, Eng C (2004) Combined total genome loss of heterozygosity scan of breast cancer stroma and epithelium reveals multiplicity of stromal targets. Cancer Res 64(20):7231–7236
143. Paterson RF, Ulbright TM, MacLennan GT, Zhang S, Pan C-X, Sweeney CJ et al (2003) Molecular genetic alterations in the laser-capture–microdissected stroma adjacent to bladder carcinoma. Cancer 98(9):1830–1836
144. Ishiguro K, Yoshida T, Yagishita H, Numata Y, Okayasu T (2006) Epithelial and stromal genetic instability contributes to genesis of colorectal adenomas. Gut 55(5):695–702
145. Al-Zoughbi W, Hoefler G (2020) Tumor macroenvironment: an update. Pathobiology 87(2): 58–60
146. Hanahan D, Folkman J (1996) Patterns and emerging mechanisms of the angiogenic switch during tumorigenesis. Cell 86(3):353–364
147. Kalas W, Yu JL, Milsom C, Rosenfeld J, Benezra R, Bornstein P et al (2005) Oncogenes and angiogenesis: down-regulation of thrombospondin-1 in normal fibroblasts exposed to factors from cancer cells harboring mutant ras. Cancer Res 65(19):8878–8886
148. Liotta LA, Kohn EC (2001) The microenvironment of the tumour-host interface. Nature 411(6835):375–379
149. Klein CA (2005) Single cell amplification methods for the study of cancer and cellular ageing. Mech Ageing Dev 126(1):147–151
150. Weaver VM, Gilbert P (2004) Watch thy neighbor: cancer is a communal affair. J Cell Sci 117 (Pt 8):1287–1290
151. Chu GC, Chung LWK, Gururajan M, Hsieh CL, Josson S, Nandana S et al (2019) Regulatory signaling network in the tumor microenvironment of prostate cancer bone and visceral organ metastases and the development of novel therapeutics. Asian J Urol 6(1):65–81
152. de Jong JS, van Diest PJ, van der Valk P, Baak JP (1998) Expression of growth factors, growth-inhibiting factors, and their receptors in invasive breast cancer. II: correlations with proliferation and angiogenesis. J Pathol 184(1):53–57
153. Royuela M, Ricote M, Parsons MS, Garcia-Tunon I, Paniagua R, de Miguel MP (2004) Immunohistochemical analysis of the IL-6 family of cytokines and their receptors in benign, hyperplasic, and malignant human prostate. J Pathol 202(1):41–49
154. Rio MC (2005) From a unique cell to metastasis is a long way to go: clues to stromelysin-3 participation. Biochimie 87(3–4):299–306
155. Guba M, Cernaianu G, Koehl G, Geissler EK, Jauch K-W, Anthuber M et al (2001) A primary tumor promotes dormancy of solitary tumor cells before inhibiting angiogenesis. Cancer Res 61(14):5575–5579
156. Caignard A, Martin MS, Michel MF, Martin F (1985) Interaction between two cellular subpopulations of a rat colonic carcinoma when inoculated to the syngeneic host. Int J Cancer 36(2):273–279
157. Gatenby RA, Vincent TL (2003) Application of quantitative models from population biology and evolutionary game theory to tumor therapeutic strategies. Mol Cancer Ther 2(9):919–927
158. Nagy JD (2004) Competition and natural selection in a mathematical model of cancer. Bull Math Biol 66(4):663–687

159. Rundhaug JE (2005) Matrix metalloproteinases and angiogenesis. J Cell Mol Med 9(2): 267–285
160. Tisdale MJ (2009) Mechanisms of cancer cachexia. Physiol Rev 89(2):381–410
161. Zhou L, Yang K, Andl T, Wickett RR, Zhang Y (2015) Perspective of targeting cancer-associated fibroblasts in melanoma. J Cancer 6(8):717–726
162. Richmond A, Yang J, Su Y (2009) The good and the bad of chemokines/chemokine receptors in melanoma. Pigment Cell Melanoma Res 22(2):175–186
163. Mishra P, Banerjee D, Ben-Baruch A (2011) Chemokines at the crossroads of tumor-fibroblast interactions that promote malignancy. J Leukoc Biol 89(1):31–39
164. Augsten M, Hagglof C, Olsson E, Stolz C, Tsagozis P, Levchenko T et al (2009) CXCL14 is an autocrine growth factor for fibroblasts and acts as a multi-modal stimulator of prostate tumor growth. Proc Natl Acad Sci U S A 106(9):3414–3419
165. Casey TM, Eneman J, Crocker A, White J, Tessitore J, Stanley M et al (2008) Cancer associated fibroblasts stimulated by transforming growth factor beta1 (TGF-beta 1) increase invasion rate of tumor cells: a population study. Breast Cancer Res Treat 110(1):39–49
166. Villanueva J, Herlyn M (2008) Melanoma and the tumor microenvironment. Curr Oncol Rep 10(5):439–446
167. Halaban R, Rubin JS, White W (1993) met and HGF-SF in normal melanocytes and melanoma cells. EXS 65:329–339
168. Gaggioli C, Deckert M, Robert G, Abbe P, Batoz M, Ehrengruber MU et al (2005) HGF induces fibronectin matrix synthesis in melanoma cells through MAP kinase-dependent signaling pathway and induction of Egr-1. Oncogene 24(8):1423–1433
169. Koefinger P, Wels C, Joshi S, Damm S, Steinbauer E, Beham-Schmid C et al (2011) The cadherin switch in melanoma instigated by HGF is mediated through epithelial-mesenchymal transition regulators. Pigment Cell Melanoma Res 24(2):382–385
170. Poser I, Dominguez D, de Herreros AG, Varnai A, Buettner R, Bosserhoff AK (2001) Loss of E-cadherin expression in melanoma cells involves up-regulation of the transcriptional repressor snail. J Biol Chem 276(27):24661–24666
171. Francia G, Emmenegger U, Kerbel RS (2009) Tumor-associated fibroblasts as "Trojan Horse" mediators of resistance to anti-VEGF therapy. Cancer Cell 15(1):3–5
172. Comito G, Giannoni E, Di Gennaro P, Segura CP, Gerlini G, Chiarugi P (2012) Stromal fibroblasts synergize with hypoxic oxidative stress to enhance melanoma aggressiveness. Cancer Lett 324(1):31–41
173. Taddei ML, Giannoni E, Raugei G, Scacco S, Sardanelli AM, Papa S et al (2012) Mitochondrial oxidative stress due to complex I dysfunction promotes fibroblast activation and melanoma cell invasiveness. J Sig Transduct 2012:684592
174. Liekens S, De Clercq E, Neyts J (2001) Angiogenesis: regulators and clinical applications. Biochem Pharmacol 61(3):253–270
175. Stamenkovic I (2003) Extracellular matrix remodelling: the role of matrix metalloproteinases. J Pathol 200(4):448–464
176. Stetler-Stevenson WG (1999) Matrix metalloproteinases in angiogenesis: a moving target for therapeutic intervention. J Clin Invest 103(9):1237–1241
177. McCawley LJ, Matrisian LM (2001) Matrix metalloproteinases: they're not just for matrix anymore! Curr Opin Cell Biol 13(5):534–540
178. Opdenakker G, Van den Steen PE, Van Damme J (2001) Gelatinase B: a tuner and amplifier of immune functions. Trends Immunol 22(10):571–579

Chapter 2
Interactions in the Local *Onco-Sphere*: An Overview

Phei Er Saw and Erwei Song

Abstract Cancer thrives in the microenvironment due to co-operative crosstalks with host immune, inflammatory, stromal cells, among others. All these interactions create a pro-tumoral environment that favors cancer growth and survival. In the local onco-sphere, cancer cells could modify their environment to be hypoxic, leading to physiological changes (i.e. angiogenesis, lymphangiogenesis), biochemical changes (i.e. acidosis, redox imbalance, lipid and amino acid synthesis dysregulation), mechanical changes (i.e. integrin signaling, fibrin and collagen overexpression). In the first part of this book, we will outline these changes in the local onco-sphere to gain deeper insights on their roles in cancer growth.

Introduction

Tumor environment (TME) was conceptualized when Paget's theory of "seed and soil" emerged in 1889, followed by the elucidation of inter-connected relationship between inflammation and cancer [1–3]. Hanahan and Weinberg, in 2000 and 2011, increased their comprehension of cancer and managed to expand the proposed

P. E. Saw
Guangdong Provincial Key Laboratory of Malignant Tumor Epigenetics and Gene Regulation, Guangdong-Hong Kong Joint Laboratory for RNA Medicine, Medical Research Center, Sun Yat-sen Memorial Hospital, Sun Yat-sen University, Guangzhou, China

Nanhai Translational Innovation Center of Precision Immunology, Sun Yat-sen Memorial Hospital, Sun Yat-sen University, Foshan, China

E. Song (✉)
Guangdong Provincial Key Laboratory of Malignant Tumor Epigenetics and Gene Regulation, Guangdong-Hong Kong Joint Laboratory for RNA Medicine, Medical Research Center, Sun Yat-sen Memorial Hospital, Sun Yat-sen University, Guangzhou, China

Nanhai Translational Innovation Center of Precision Immunology, Sun Yat-sen Memorial Hospital, Sun Yat-sen University, Foshan, China

Breast Tumor Center, Sun Yat-sen Memorial Hospital, Sun Yat-sen University, Guangzhou, China
e-mail: songew@mail.sysu.edu.cn

E. Song (ed.), *Tumor Ecosystem*, https://doi.org/10.1007/978-981-99-1183-7_2

characteristics of cancer from six to ten in accordance with the great advancement over the last ten decades [4, 5]. In 2021, 10-year update, they also acknowledged the increased involvement of TME and inclusion of host involvement in cancer development; as they titled this review as "new dimensions" [6]. Indeed, cancer is a complex disease—it spreads through vessels and lymph nodes, not to mention that is also innervated by nerves and involves the entire organism (host). Thus, one should not look at tumor as a stand-alone entity. In other words, TME is insufficient to reflect actual situations to be an effective target for cancer treatment [7], as TME only represents the local *onco-sphere*, not taking into account the inter-onco-spheric interactions with multiple organs (distal *onco-sphere*) and with the host system (systemic *onco-sphere*). However, one often overlooked the importance of the connectivity and the interactions within the local *onco-sphere* and how these interactions influence the distal and the systemic *onco-spheres*.

Cancer initiation is caused by the oncogenic mutations of malignant cells in the local *onco-sphere*. When changes to the tumor cells occur, they send out molecular cues (i.e., cytokines, chemokines, growth factors, proteins, exosomes, etc.) to the surrounding non-transformed cells, including other normal cells and stromal cells. Upon receiving these cues, immune cells and stromal cells are recruited and adapted, further releasing various potent communicators (cytokines, chemokines, exosomes, and vesicles) to create a favorable ecosystem for the survival of the tumor [8]. In short, the local *onco-sphere* could orchestrate changes within the local ecosystem to interfere with distal and systemic *onco-spheres*. For example, oncogenic signaling is activated by chronic inflammation or wound-healing process to foster tumorigenesis [9–11]. Likewise, cancer cells also trigger changes in the local *onco-sphere* that assist with the survival of cells and migration. It is now known that there are specific changes in the local *onco-sphere* that are favorable toward cancer cell survival. Among them, the most prominent changes in the local *onco-sphere* are: (1) metabolic environment, [12, 13] (2) acidic niche as a result of acidosis, [14–16] (3) innervated niche [17–20], (4) mechanical niche [21–24], and (5) inflammatory-immune environment [25–27] (Fig. 2.1). Apart from this, spatial arrangement of the different types of cells is being hauled as the next hallmark of local *onco-sphere*. In this chapter, we will summarize each of these changes and discuss how this affects the tumor ecosystem as a whole. In latter chapters, we will look closely into the molecular changes that lead to the presentation of these hallmarks. It is important to note, however, these environments in the local *onco-sphere* are constantly changing, leading researchers to elucidate on why these changes occur through different stages of cancer and how this affects the current therapeutic modality in cancer.

Ecosystem Concept in Local *Onco-Sphere*: Overview

A "niche" in an ecosystem is a specialized environment, in which the interaction between an organism and its environment could be different in this niche as compared to another one. Similarly, in cancer, tumor ecosystem depicts the detailed interaction between tumor and its local cellular counterparts (local *onco-sphere*),

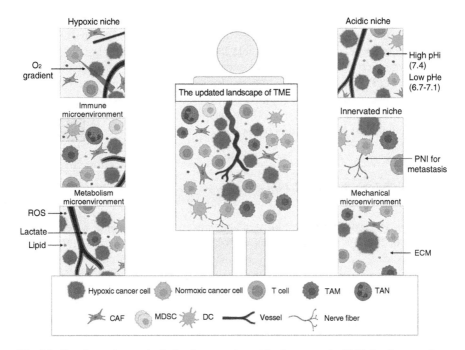

Fig. 2.1 Prominent changes in the local *onco-sphere*. Also known as the TME, local *onco-sphere* is made up of cancer cells, recruited immune cells, reprogrammed stromal cells, new formation of blood vessels, innervation of nerve fibers, ECMs, and other associated acellular components. At a different angle, these *onco-spheres* could be summarized as: (1) hypoxic niche (2) acidic niche, (3) immune microenvironment, (4) innervated niche, (5) metabolic microenvironment, and (6) mechanical microenvironment. Focus should be given to the interconnectivity and relationship regarding interactions within the local *onco-sphere*, interactions between these components with the distal *onco-sphere*s, and how this dictates the changes in the systemic *onco-sphere*s (host)

interaction between disseminated tumors cells with their new metastatic organs (distal *onco-sphere*), and the interaction of tumor with their host (systemic *onco-sphere*). As creatures evolve and adapt into their new environment to survive, cancer cells dramatically and constantly modify their environments, as a result, creating an environment or niche that favors their own growth. For example, tumor cells change their environments' geography via deposition and proteolytic cleavage and clearance of extracellular matrix components [28]. MMP-2 and -9 (key components of the ECM) are proteolytic enzymes that are associated with poorer clinical outcomes in many types of cancer [29–31]. Mechanistically, these proteases change the stiffness of matrix [32], facilitate migration by making room [33], and enhance pro-survival signaling [34]. Cancer cells not only remodel their geography, they also remodel the source of their nutrients. This is seen in the utilization of lactate metabolic pathway as compared to glycolysis used in normal cells. Cancer cells also ensure that pro-angiogenic factors such as VEGF, FGF, EGF, and PDGF are constantly expressed, as these growth factors mediate new vasculature formation, leading to an increment of nutrient source [35]. In addition, within the tumor's environment, tumor cells put pressure on other cell types (i.e., immune cells and stromal cells). For example, cancer cells can release soluble factors that cause fibroblasts to adapt to tumor permissive phenotype [36]. Cancer cells express immune checkpoints PD-L1 and CTLA4 [37] that allow them to escape immune predators or via production of soluble factors, such as TGF-β [38], IL-10 [39], and soluble WNTs [40], which are known to be immunosuppressive. These interactions will be summarized in this chapter and further highlighted in the upcoming chapters.

Hypoxic Niche in Local *Onco-Sphere*

The Nobel Prize in Physiology or Medicine was granted to Kaelin, Ratcliffe, and Semenza in 2019 for their outstanding work in cellular adaptation to oxygen, a work that introduces the importance of the concept of hypoxia in cancer. In normal condition, cells have ample amount of oxygen, a normoxic condition. However, during the fast-paced growth of cancer cells, they need unparallel amount of oxygen supply. When oxygen does not meet the cell's demand, a low oxygen environment is created, known as hypoxia. This stress leads the cells to secrete hypoxia-inducible factors (HIFs). Hypoxia is not only a common condition for malignant and stromal cells, it is now a constant, as elevated hypoxia is usually associated with the progression of many cancers and is usually associated with poor prognosis [41]. Mechanistically, hypoxia activates endothelial cells (ECs), mainly the vascular ECs, to upregulate the transcription of the infamous vascular endothelial growth factor (VEGF) transcription, the key player that enhances angiogenesis [42, 43]. In this hypoxic *onco-sphere*, elevation of hypoxia has been found to correlate with higher mutational load of oncogenes and tumor suppressors (i.e., PTEN, Myc, and p53) [44, 45]. Therefore, in hypoxic environment in the local *onco-sphere*, cancer cells were then cued to respond in various ways, including increased cancer progression, stemness, dormancy, and resistance [41]. Currently, the Buffa signature, a list of 15 hypoxia-associated genes, is considered the standard for hypoxia assessment [46]. In a large-scale clinical assessment, hypoxia in cancer was investigated in various cancer types ($n = 38$), in 2658 subtypes of cancers; and they were subjected to whole-genome sequencing [47]. Interestingly, data revealed that not only hypoxia has intra- and inter-heterogeneity among various cancer types, but they also differ among different patients with similar cancer type. Moreover, tumors with higher genetic diversity tend to have elevated hypoxic signaling and higher expression of hypoxia-associated genes, which are associated with a poorer OS and PFS [48]. This again reinforces the need of personalized therapeutic modality, as patient-to-patient variation might be huge. The detailed summary of the mechanism and pathway of angiogenesis is discussed in Chap. 6.

Biochemical Changes in Local *Onco-Sphere*

In homeostasis, all cells function under an intricate control in their respective biochemical pathways. However, during cancer progression, many of the cellular behaviors are modified or triggered due to biological, mechanical, or physical stress. Herein, we summarize the biochemical changes that might be seen during cancer progression, namely acidosis, redox imbalance, lipid synthesis dysregulation, and amino acid dysregulation.

Acidosis

Cancer cell has dysregulated pH. Under normal circumstances, the pH of intracellular compartment (pHi) of a cell is around pH 7.2, and an extracellular pHe of ~pH 7.4. Cancer cells, however, tend to have a higher pHi ~7.4 but a lower pHe ~6.7–7.1. Therefore, it is common for the referral of the tumor cells as "acidic." This is an interesting phenomenon as higher pHi is favorable for cancer cell survival, proliferation, migration, and invasion, while hindering apoptosis, and the same is true for lower pHe [49]. It was found that acidic niche is vital for epithelial–mesenchymal transition (EMT), oxidative phosphorylation, and invasiveness of melanoma, breast, and neuroblastoma cells [50, 51]. Similar to hypoxic niche, acidic niche generation is also driven by oncogene activation (e.g., Ras and Myc) and inactivation of tumor suppressors (e.g., p. 53) [52]. Acidic niche is a product of lactate metabolic process, a pathway known as Warburg effect, commonly used by cancer cells [16]. Proton (H^+) accumulation due to hypoxia (mentioned above) is also a factor to increase acidic niche [52]. Monocarboxylate transporters (MCTs) are an important component in metabolic pathway. MCT4 exports lactate, while MCT1 synergistically co-transport of H^+ imports it into cancer cells, exemplifying a co-operative symbiotic relationship within the local *onco-sphere* [53]. In turn, the acidic niche now is favorable for lactate metabolism, a highly supportive environment for cancer development [53]. Under acidic condition, in order to transfer waste and excess acid, cancer cells also increase their secretion of extracellular vesicle (EV) and exosome [54, 55], which are two potent communicators of the tumor ecosystem (detailed in Chap. 13). Interestingly, acidosis shows different regulative effects immune and stromal cells in the local *onco-sphere*. For example, acidic niche favors M2-like pro-tumoral phenotype and impedes the TILs cytotoxicity activity [56]. Acidic niche promotes ECM remodeling and localized invasion of stromal fibroblast. These cancer-associated fibroblasts (CAFs) then release inflammatory cytokines that in turn lead to the release of cathepsins and the reorganization of collagen [57]. These findings also reinforce the concept of a constantly communicating local *onco-sphere*. We will discuss the intra-onco-spherical relationship with immune and stromal cells within the local *onco-sphere*s in Chaps. 3 and 4, respectively.

Redox Imbalance

Emerging data are showing that there is significant elevation in redox imbalance in cancer, which is caused by oxidation. Interestingly, these increments are related to aggressive behavior in cancer, as benign hyperplasia was shown to have lower redox imbalance compared to their malignant counterparts. Since redox imbalance can lead to altered gene expression and posttranslational modification of the protein may also alter protein stability, all these could impact the normal running of the biochemical cellular programs in the cell [58]. There are usually standard methods in identifying increased ROS/oxidative stress in the cells (by fluorescent dye analysis or Fenton assay), while biochemical analysis of the stoichiometry is commonly used to measure redox imbalance. For example, the coupling of NAD/NADH, NADP/NADPH calculating the H^+ ions; glutathione (GSH)/glutathione disulfide, thioredoxin (TRX)/thioredoxin disulfide calculating the S-S bonding. Other methods include identifying the posttranslational modification of metabolites or macromolecules that are directly involved in the redox imbalance pathway. The in-depth mechanism of the biochemical changes in redox imbalance will be discussed in Chap. 8: biochemical changes in the local *onco-sphere*.

Lipid Synthesis Dysregulation

The most important function in lipids is mostly seen intertwined in metabolic changes in the local *onco-sphere*. Lipids are very diverse, with many classes, varying in compositions and functions (i.e., fatty acyls, glycerophospholipids, and sphingolipids to sterol and prenol lipids), which are all vital in biochemical pathways in the cellular metabolism [59, 60]. These lipids are also the reservoir for future energy use in cell growth and proliferation [61, 62]. Changes in lipid biosynthesis are crucial as this is fundamental in cell signaling and metabolism and even named as one of the hallmarks of cancer [63, 64]. Especially, in cancer cells, phospholipids (the main constituents of the cell membrane) are critical for cell proliferation. Apart from that, by circulating free fatty acids (FFAs) and other lipid molecules are important for cell signaling and cell growth [65, 66]. In tumors, tumors have dense ECM, therefore experiencing desmoplasia, and the local *onco-sphere* is usually deficient in nutrient. This is prominent in pancreatic ductal adenocarcinoma (PDAC), where cancer cells can use CAF-secreted lysophosphatidylcholine (LPC) and lysophosphatidic acid (LPA) to be used as their own nutrient, a classic example of competition in the ecology concept [67]. More details on lipid dysregulation are also discussed in Chap. 8.

Amino Acid Synthesis Dysregulation

As we mentioned above, in the local *onco-sphere*, the changes in how the cancer cells respirate change the core metabolic behavior. Warburg effect is the main difference where the cancer uses a different metabolic pathway to induce biochemical changes in the cell. This also leads to the changes in amino acids (both in intra-extracellular condition), which can have significant effect, not only on the cell metabolism but also on the overall development of the tumor. Some vital alterations are seen in glutamine, sarcosine, methionine, cysteine, sarcosine, and arginine, among others [68]. Arginine especially has been linked to the cross talk in TAMs' phenotypical changes and is able to skew the TAM into M2-like pro-tumoral phenotype, indicating the intricate cross talk between each component in the local *onco-sphere*. Namely, alterations in the metabolism of amino acids glutamine, sarcosine, aspartate, methionine, and cysteine have been previously connected to the tumor progression and aggressivity of cancer. The details on amino acid changes are also detailed in Chap. 8.

Immune and Stromal Cells in the Local *Onco-Sphere*

In a solid tumor, there is an infiltration of a plethora of both innate and adaptive immune cells. Innate immune cells include natural killer (NK) cells, dendritic cells (DCs), tumor-associated macrophages (TAMs), tumor-associated neutrophils (TANs), myeloid-derived suppressor cells (MDSCs), and mast cells, while adaptive immune cells include T cells of various subsets and B cells [69]. Stromal cells such as fibroblasts (cancer associated fibroblasts, CAFs), adipocytes, pericytes, and endothelial cells are also main regulators of the tumor environment. To date, the prognosis of cancer is defined with the infiltration of immune cells [69–71]. Most immune checkpoint blockade (ICB) therapies are judged to be effective by the amount of CD8$^+$ T cells infiltration, as the abundant infiltration of CD3$^+$ or CD8$^+$ T cells was interpreted as a sign of a positive response toward ICB therapy [72]. However, most tumors evade surveillance to progress and metastasize. The overexpression of PD-1, PD-2 on T cells and PD-L1, PD-L2 on tumor cells are one example of tumor-immune cell interactions in the local *onco-sphere* that ultimately leads to immune escape.

Within the local *onco-sphere*, tumors are presented with the concurrent occurrence of both immune-enhancing CD8$^+$ and CD4$^+$ T cells and with immune-inhibiting or regulatory cells (i.e., Tregs, Bregs, TAMs, TANs, and MDSCs). For example, high amount of Tregs indicated immunosuppressive phenotype [73], although their roles in cancer progression are yet to be fully understood [74]. B cells are reported to have opposite effects. Some have reported its anti-tumor role in melanoma mouse models by enhancing T cell functionality [75], and in human cancers, CD20$^+$ B cells are associated with good prognosis [76, 77]. In opposite views, in a murine mouse model, B cells have been reported to negatively regulate anti-tumor immunity [78]. Interestingly, macrophage-secreted chemokine CXCL13 recruits B cells to secrete lymphotoxin and in turn promotes the progression of castrate-resistant prostate cancer (CRPC) [79]. In a T cell-B cell cross talk, the removal of plasmacytes (an immunosuppressive B cell subtype) is required to enhance PD-L1 therapy. These plasmacytes expressed IgA, IL-10, and PD-L1, which are strongly connected to CD8 T cell exhaustion, and suppressed CTL responses [80]. However, the intricate cross talks between each component of the tumor, immune, and stromal cells, including their secreted cytokines, chemokines, and extracellular vesicles are crucial in the concept of tumor ecosystem. These immunosuppressive cells, including stromal cells, could hinder lymphocyte infiltration and modulate their trafficking in multiple areas. For example, VEGF secreted by cancer cells due to hypoxia leads to creation of abnormal neovasculature, which in turn reduces adhesion of immune cells, downregulates chemotactic signals from tumor endothelium [81], and again signifies the concept of cooperative symbiotic relationship within the local *onco-sphere*. The interactions of the immune-tumor cells in the local *onco-sphere* are detailed in Chap. 3, while the interactions of stromal-tumor cells are detailed in Chap. 4.

Innervated Niche in the Local *Onco-Sphere*

Innervated niche is defined as "the communications between nerve and cancer mediated by nerve-derived neurotransmitters or neuropeptides." Innervated niche includes: (1) nerve–tumor cell physical contact via peripheral nerve (these includes sensory, sympathetic, and parasympathetic nerves) or (2) indirect communication of nerve located nearby tumor cells. Indirect communication includes the innervation of stromal and cancer cells via the release of neurotransmitters or neuropeptides (i.e., acetylcholine, catecholamine, and dopamine) [17]. For example, gastric cancer cells secrete neurotrophins, a neuropeptide that encourages nerve infiltration into the local *onco-sphere* [82]. In high-grade glioma, active neurons secrete neuroligin-3 (NLGN3), which activates PI3K-mTOR pathway to promote tumor growth [83]. In hematological cancers, the innervation of sympathetic nervous system (SNS) induces stem cells motility from bone marrow to the tumor site [84], indicating a close-knit communication between the host neuronal system and the local *onco-sphere*. Furthermore, primary brain tumors and metastasis are closely associated with innervation. However, it is important to note that the innervation of cancers is dissimilar from innervation of normal organs [82, 85–87].

The nervous system has been found to intervene and affect cancer therapy through multiple pathways: (1) electrochemical interaction within to tumor (local), (2) paracrine interactions (local, distal, and systemic) and (3) neural cancer interactions (systemic) [88]. This further solidifies our concept of systemic *onco-sphere*, as the cross talk between tumor and host nervous system creates a different local ecosystem for solid tumor. This is especially obvious in breast cancer metastasis. In this process, a "pseudo-tripartite synapse," a breast-to-brain metastasis, is created through formation of synapse and innervation between cancer cells and neurons. These synapses activated N-methyl-D-aspartate receptor-mediated colonization of the metastatic breast cancer cells, resulting in a more supportive innervated niche at the distal *onco-sphere* (in this case, the brain), favoring the cancer cell survival in this new soil. In another form of indirect communication, oral squamous cell carcinoma (OSCC) cells with p53 mutation use the signal transduction of EVs to reprogram tumor-associated neurons to adrenergic phenotype to favor tumor progression. The detailed mechanism of host–tumor innervation will be discussed in detail in Chap. 23.

Metabolic Environment in Local *Onco-Sphere*

One of the major hallmarks of cancer is the alteration in its metabolic reprogramming. Cancer is often associated with the increased metabolism of multiple pathways, namely glucose uptake pathway, lipid reprogramming, glutamine, amino acids, lactate accumulation, and ROS increment [32–34]. As mentioned above, in normal cells, energy is usually obtained through oxidative phosphorylation, and glycolysis is hindered under normoxic condition, while cancer cells favor elevated lactate metabolism and enhanced glycolysis rather than oxidative phosphorylation, known as the Warburg effect [89]. Subsequently, Warburg stated that regardless of oxygen content, cancer cells favor glycolysis over oxidative phosphorylation [90]. Thenceforth, researchers have been intrigued and focused on the following: [1] why glycolysis is preferred over oxidative phosphorylation in cancer cells, although the latter provides more energy; [2] ways lactate metabolism is utilized in cancer cells; and [3] the inherent ability to treat cancer by target lactate metabolism pathways.

Over the past decades, we have achieved great advancement even though these issues remain unaddressed. Both malignant and stromal cells have the involvement of lactate metabolism. However, recently, the "cause and effect" structure has been questioned as emerging evidence shows that lactate may be a metabolite able to provide a positive feedback mechanism to rewire stromal, immune, and cancer cells. In a high lactate environment, macrophages are repolarized into pro-tumoral (M2-like) phenotypes [14, 91]. Foxp3 expression on Treg suppressed glycolysis, producing a conducive immunosuppressive environment for cancer cells [92]. Lactate stimulates an acidic environment, increases the survival of hypoxic cells, which then stimulates angiogenesis, to provide a positive feedback mechanism that promotes tumor growth [93]. We will discuss the effect of host metabolic changes to cancer progression in Chap. 25.

Mechanical and Physical Stress in Local *Onco-Sphere*

In cancer therapeutic, the physical and mechanical microenvironment in the local *onco-sphere* is often overlooked [21, 22]. Since the involvement of stromal cells is beginning to emerge, we now acknowledge the importance of these stromal cells (CAFs, extracellular matrix) and their intracellular components (actin filament, vimentin, and neurofilaments), intercellular signaling (integrin), and other extracellular components (fibrin and collagen) in cancer progression [94]. CAFs produce MMPs such as MMP-2, -3, -9, in which the elevation of these components leads to ECM degradation and remodeling and increased EMT [95, 96]. Mechanical environment depicts the functions and behavior of various factors in oncogenesis: cell morphology, oncogenes, tumor suppressors, and therapeutic responses [97]. In a breast cancer lung metastasis model, the colonization of cancer cells is via platelet recruitment through HSP 47/COL1 axis by tumor cell-produced ECM [98]. Lysyl oxidase (Lox) production is promoted by HIF1 to increase integrin signaling and enhance stiffness of the tumor-matrix [99]. In an interesting study, it was found that cancer cells' stiffness encourages them to maintain a high metabolism, further clarifying the heterogeneous specialized niches in the local *onco-sphere* [21]. Interesting insights on the function of ECM in the modulation of cancer have been discussed in detail elsewhere [100, 101]. We will discuss the details of mechanical and physical stress in the maintenance of local *onco-sphere* in Chap. 9.

Box 2.1 Spatial Arrangement of Cells in Local Onco-Sphere
In 1944, Harold Samuel quoted this famous line "location, location, location." Although this quotation is true in real estate development, now, emerging data are indicative of the importance of the location of cells within the local *onco-sphere*. Given the fact that most, if not all, inter-*onco spherical* relationships are dependent on either cell-to-cell contact or indirect paracrine manner, the 3D spatial relationships in these solid tumors could provide a framework for deeper understanding of the tumor microenvironment. This is exemplified in an experiment done on Oxi4503, a vascular disrupting agent. Although this agent successfully eliminates 90% of tumor, a thin rim of viable cells could be seen at the tumor periphery, which in time leads to recurrence [102]. The researchers then found a significant difference of (1) mature vessels, (2) accumulation of immune cells, (3) growth factor, (4) level of hypoxia, and (5) EMT between the tumor periphery and core. OXi4503 treatment only resulted in vessel collapse of vessels in the tumor center and not tumor periphery. Interestingly, even tumor apoptosis and proliferation level were differentially modulated between center and periphery following Oxi4503 treatment [102]. Therefore, this result hinted that there is molecular difference in "where" the cells are and "when" is the appropriate time for treatment. In spatial analysis, not only the location is important, we also need to factor in

(continued)

The Constantly Changing Local *Onco-Sphere*

Tumor microenvironment (TME) is a very convoluted system containing multiple stromal cells and noncellular ECM imbedded by these cells. Tumor cells, as well as the local habitat in which they arise, are referred to as primary *onco-sphere*. Dysregulated tumor–stroma interplays stand out among the other aberrant biological events that define cancer hallmarks [4–6]. Constant communication between cancer cells and their stromal counterparts is enabled by cytokine shuttling, exosome transmission, and direct cell–cell contact. This elicits a variety of malignant cell behaviors [104]. Cancer-derived growth factors recruit, stimulate, or educate stromal cells, endowing them with tumor-promoting phenotypes that encourage angiogenesis, inflammation, and invasion, resulting in commensal behaviors. Conditions and alterations in the tumor microenvironment drastically affect cancer development [105]. For instance, when teratocarcinoma cells are implanted into blastocysts of mice, the carcinogenicity of it is inhibited [70]. Metastasis may be inhibited by inoculating a metastatic cell line into a heterotopic site [71]. A microenvironment with overexpressed growth signals level, on the other hand, can promote the

Fig. 2.2 An example of spatial analysis from a single cell, tissue structure, and whole tumor. In each level, the proximity of each cell, the distance of cell–cell variation in intra-tumoral area vs. peritumoral area, and the level of tumor-immune (or tumor cells with other cells in the *onco-sphere*) could be clearly analyzed [103]. Permission is not needed as this work is published under creativecommons.org/licenses/by-nc/4.0/

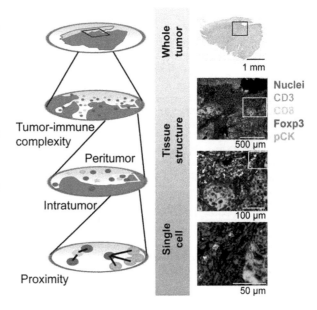

development of cancer. At a site highly saturated with HGF and/or TGFβ1, normal epithelial cells may turn into invasive carcinomas [106]. Studies involving mice showed that fibroblasts produce increased level of HGF and/or stromal cell derived factor 1 (SDF1). This contributes to epithelial neoplasms' formation [107]. The examples above proposed that by changing the tumor microenvironment, the development of cancer can be managed. Too much modification, however, may not only eliminate cancer cells, but normal cells as well. On the other hand, inadequate modification may increase the "survival of the fittest" effect that can cause cells with less advantageous qualities to die off. For that reason, having a steady and moderate amount of change may promote heterogeneity and growth [108]. It is likely that repeated injury or damage promotes carcinogenesis by generating a variety of growth-promoting microenvironments throughout the healing process.

Conclusion

In this chapter, we summarized the overview of interactions of different cellular components (immune cells, stromal cells) and other molecular components in the local *onco-spheres*. As we will see in the latter chapter of this book, distant sites can be remodeled by the signaling factors produced by cancer cells from the local *onco-sphere* for successful metastasis. Therefore, as far as the cancer cell is concern, the ecosystem of the local oncosphere is vital for its growth, progression, and metastasis and cancer cell will try to orchestrate the environment to be pro-tumoral. Therefore, understanding the molecular mechanism underlying each factor of the establishment of local *onco-sphere* is crucial for the development of precise personalized cancer therapeutics.

References

1. Paget S (1989) The distribution of secondary growths in cancer of the breast. 1889. Cancer Metastasis Rev 8(2):98–101
2. Maman S, Witz IP (2018) A history of exploring cancer in context. Nat Rev Cancer 18(6): 359–376
3. Kalluri R, LeBleu VS (2020) The biology, function, and biomedical applications of exosomes. Science 367(6478):eaau6977
4. Hanahan D, Weinberg RA (2011) Hallmarks of cancer: the next generation. Cell 144(5): 646–674
5. Hanahan D, Weinberg RA (2000) The hallmarks of cancer. Cell 100(1):57–70
6. Hanahan D (2022) Hallmarks of cancer: new dimensions. Cancer Discov 12(1):31–46
7. Laplane L, Duluc D, Bikfalvi A, Larmonier N, Pradeu T (2019) Beyond the tumour microenvironment. Int J Cancer 145(10):2611–2618
8. Balkwill FR, Capasso M, Hagemann T (2012) The tumor microenvironment at a glance. J Cell Sci 125(Pt 23):5591–5596

9. Khosravi N, Caetano MS, Cumpian AM, Unver N, De la Garza Ramos C, Noble O et al (2018) IL22 promotes kras-mutant lung cancer by induction of a protumor immune response and protection of stemness properties. Cancer Immunol Res 6(7):788–797

10. Todoric J, Karin M (2019) The fire within: cell-autonomous mechanisms in inflammation-driven cancer. Cancer Cell 35(5):714–720

11. Deng S, Clowers MJ, Velasco WV, Ramos-Castaneda M, Moghaddam SJ (2019) Understanding the complexity of the tumor microenvironment in K-ras mutant lung cancer: finding an alternative path to prevention and treatment. Front Oncol 9:1556

12. Montenegro F, Indraccolo S (2020) Metabolism in the tumor microenvironment. Adv Exp Med Biol 1263:1–11

13. Garcia-Canaveras JC, Chen L, Rabinowitz JD (2019) The tumor metabolic microenvironment: lessons from lactate. Cancer Res 79(13):3155–3162

14. Paolini L, Adam C, Beauvillain C, Preisser L, Blanchard S, Pignon P et al (2020) Lactic acidosis together with GM-CSF and M-CSF induces human macrophages toward an inflammatory protumor phenotype. Cancer Immunol Res 8(3):383–395

15. Boedtkjer E, Pedersen SF (2020) The acidic tumor microenvironment as a driver of cancer. Annu Rev Physiol 82:103–126

16. Corbet C, Feron O (2017) Tumour acidosis: from the passenger to the driver's seat. Nat Rev Cancer 17(10):577–593

17. Shurin MR, Shurin GV, Zlotnikov SB, Bunimovich YL (2020) The neuroimmune axis in the tumor microenvironment. J Immunol (Baltimore, Md: 1950) 204(2):280–285

18. Zahalka AH, Frenette PS (2020) Nerves in cancer. Nat Rev Cancer 20(3):143–157

19. Cole SW, Nagaraja AS, Lutgendorf SK, Green PA, Sood AK (2015) Sympathetic nervous system regulation of the tumour microenvironment. Nat Rev Cancer 15(9):563–572

20. Faulkner S, Jobling P, March B, Jiang CC, Hondermarck H (2019) Tumor neurobiology and the war of nerves in cancer. Cancer Discov 9(6):702–710

21. Ayad NME, Weaver VM (2020) Tension in tumour cells keeps metabolism high. Nature 578(7796):517–518

22. Liu Y, Lv J, Liang X, Yin X, Zhang L, Chen D et al (2018) Fibrin stiffness mediates dormancy of tumor-repopulating cells via a Cdc42-driven Tet2 epigenetic program. Cancer Res 78(14): 3926–3937

23. Park JS, Burckhardt CJ, Lazcano R, Solis LM, Isogai T, Li L et al (2020) Mechanical regulation of glycolysis via cytoskeleton architecture. Nature 578(7796):621–626

24. Wisdom KM, Adebowale K, Chang J, Lee JY, Nam S, Desai R et al (2018) Matrix mechanical plasticity regulates cancer cell migration through confining microenvironments. Nat Commun 9(1):4144

25. Coussens LM, Werb Z (2002) Inflammation and cancer. Nature 420(6917):860–867

26. Balkwill F, Mantovani A (2001) Inflammation and cancer: back to Virchow? Lancet 357(9255):539–545

27. Zhao H, Wu L, Yan G, Chen Y, Zhou M, Wu Y et al (2021) Inflammation and tumor progression: signaling pathways and targeted intervention. Signal Transduct Target Ther 6(1):263

28. Lavin Y, Kobayashi S, Leader A, Amir ED, Elefant N, Bigenwald C et al (2017) Innate immune landscape in early lung adenocarcinoma by paired single-cell analyses. Cell 169(4): 750–65.e17

29. Fischer GM, Jalali A, Kircher DA, Lee WC, McQuade JL, Haydu LE et al (2019) Molecular profiling reveals unique immune and metabolic features of melanoma brain metastases. Cancer Discov 9(5):628–645

30. Friebel E, Kapolou K, Unger S, Núñez NG, Utz S, Rushing EJ et al (2020) Single-cell mapping of human brain cancer reveals tumor-specific instruction of tissue-invading leukocytes. Cell 181(7):1626–42.e20

31. Wang L, Dai J, Han R-R, Dong L, Feng D, Zhu G, et al. Single-cell map of diverse immune phenotypes in the metastatic brain tumor microenvironment of non small cell lung cancer. 2019:2019.12.30.890517.
32. Mao XY, Jin MZ, Chen JF, Zhou HH, Jin WL (2018) Live or let die: neuroprotective and anti-cancer effects of nutraceutical antioxidants. Pharmacol Ther 183:137–151
33. Parks SK, Mueller-Klieser W, Pouysségur J (2020) Lactate and acidity in the cancer microenvironment. Ann Rev Cancer Biol 4(1):141–158
34. Peck B, Schulze A (2019) Lipid metabolism at the nexus of diet and tumor microenvironment. Trends Cancer 5(11):693–703
35. Vaupel P, Kallinowski F, Okunieff P (1989) Blood flow, oxygen and nutrient supply, and metabolic microenvironment of human tumors: a review. Cancer Res 49(23):6449–6465
36. Alkasalias T, Moyano-Galceran L, Arsenian-Henriksson M, Lehti K (2018) Fibroblasts in the tumor microenvironment: shield or spear? Int J Mol Sci 19(5):1532
37. Pardoll DM (2012) The blockade of immune checkpoints in cancer immunotherapy. Nat Rev Cancer 12(4):252–264
38. Wojtowicz-Praga S (2003) Reversal of tumor-induced immunosuppression by TGF-beta inhibitors. Investig New Drugs 21(1):21–32
39. Kim R, Emi M, Tanabe K, Arihiro K (2006) Tumor-driven evolution of immunosuppressive networks during malignant progression. Cancer Res 66(11):5527–5536
40. Liang X, Fu C, Cui W, Ober-Blobaum JL, Zahner SP, Shrikant PA et al (2014) Beta-catenin mediates tumor-induced immunosuppression by inhibiting cross-priming of CD8(+) T cells. J Leukoc Biol 95(1):179–190
41. Qiu GZ, Jin MZ, Dai JX, Sun W, Feng JH, Jin WL (2017) Reprogramming of the tumor in the hypoxic niche: the emerging concept and associated therapeutic strategies. Trends Pharmacol Sci 38(8):669–686
42. Palazon A, Tyrakis PA, Macias D, Veliça P, Rundqvist H, Fitzpatrick S et al (2017) An HIF-1α/VEGF-A axis in cytotoxic T cells regulates tumor progression. Cancer Cell 32(5): 669–83.e5
43. Ribatti D (2016) Tumor refractoriness to anti-VEGF therapy. Oncotarget 7(29):46668–46677
44. Bhandari V, Li CH, Bristow RG, Boutros PC, PCAWG Consortium (2020) Divergent mutational processes distinguish hypoxic and normoxic tumours. Nat Commun 11(1):737
45. Bhandari V, Hoey C, Liu LY, Lalonde E, Ray J, Livingstone J et al (2019) Molecular landmarks of tumor hypoxia across cancer types. Nat Genet 51(2):308–318
46. Buffa FM, Harris AL, West CM, Miller CJ (2010) Large meta-analysis of multiple cancers reveals a common, compact and highly prognostic hypoxia metagene. Br J Cancer 102(2): 428–435
47. Bhandari V, Li CH, Bristow RG, Boutros PC (2020) Divergent mutational processes distinguish hypoxic and normoxic tumours. Nat Commun 11(1):737
48. Ma L, Hernandez MO, Zhao Y, Mehta M, Tran B, Kelly M et al (2019) Tumor cell biodiversity drives microenvironmental reprogramming in liver cancer. Cancer Cell 36(4): 418–30.e6
49. Webb BA, Chimenti M, Jacobson MP, Barber DL (2011) Dysregulated pH: a perfect storm for cancer progression. Nat Rev Cancer 11(9):671–677
50. Peppicelli S, Toti A, Giannoni E, Bianchini F, Margheri F, Del Rosso M et al (2016) Metformin is also effective on lactic acidosis-exposed melanoma cells switched to oxidative phosphorylation. Cell Cycle (Georgetown, Tex) 15(14):1908–1918
51. Lamonte G, Tang X, Chen JL, Wu J, Ding CK, Keenan MM et al (2013) Acidosis induces reprogramming of cellular metabolism to mitigate oxidative stress. Cancer Metab 1(1):23
52. Chiche J, Brahimi-Horn MC, Pouysségur J (2010) Tumour hypoxia induces a metabolic shift causing acidosis: a common feature in cancer. J Cell Mol Med 14(4):771–794
53. Sonveaux P, Vegran F, Schroeder T, Wergin MC, Verrax J, Rabbani ZN et al (2008) Targeting lactate-fueled respiration selectively kills hypoxic tumor cells in mice. J Clin Invest 118(12): 3930–3942

54. Parolini I, Federici C, Raggi C, Lugini L, Palleschi S, De Milito A et al (2009) Microenvironmental pH is a key factor for exosome traffic in tumor cells. J Biol Chem 284(49): 34211–34222
55. Yáñez-Mó M, Siljander PR, Andreu Z, Zavec AB, Borràs FE, Buzas EI et al (2015) Biological properties of extracellular vesicles and their physiological functions. J Extracell Vesicles 4: 27066
56. Gillies RJ, Pilot C, Marunaka Y, Fais S (2019) Targeting acidity in cancer and diabetes. Biochim Biophys Acta Rev Cancer 1871(2):273–280
57. Damaghi M, Tafreshi NK, Lloyd MC, Sprung R, Estrella V, Wojtkowiak JW et al (2015) Chronic acidosis in the tumour microenvironment selects for overexpression of LAMP2 in the plasma membrane. Nat Commun 6:8752
58. Jorgenson TC, Zhong W, Oberley TD (2013) Redox imbalance and biochemical changes in cancer. Cancer Res 73(20):6118–6123
59. Hopperton KE, Duncan RE, Bazinet RP, Archer MC (2014) Fatty acid synthase plays a role in cancer metabolism beyond providing fatty acids for phospholipid synthesis or sustaining elevations in glycolytic activity. Exp Cell Res 320(2):302–310
60. Yao CH, Fowle-Grider R, Mahieu NG, Liu GY, Chen YJ, Wang R et al (2016) Exogenous fatty acids are the preferred source of membrane lipids in proliferating fibroblasts. Cell Chem Biol 23(4):483–493
61. Wen YA, Xing X, Harris JW, Zaytseva YY, Mitov MI, Napier DL et al (2017) Adipocytes activate mitochondrial fatty acid oxidation and autophagy to promote tumor growth in colon cancer. Cell Death Dis 8(2):e2593
62. Lin H, Patel S, Affleck VS, Wilson I, Turnbull DM, Joshi AR et al (2017) Fatty acid oxidation is required for the respiration and proliferation of malignant glioma cells. Neuro-Oncology 19(1):43–54
63. Seyfried TN, Flores RE, Poff AM, D'Agostino DP (2014) Cancer as a metabolic disease: implications for novel therapeutics. Carcinogenesis 35(3):515–527
64. Hsu PP, Sabatini DM (2008) Cancer cell metabolism: Warburg and beyond. Cell 134(5): 703–707
65. Jensen MD, Haymond MW, Rizza RA, Cryer PE, Miles JM (1989) Influence of body fat distribution on free fatty acid metabolism in obesity. J Clin Invest 83(4):1168–1173
66. Boden G, Shulman GI (2002) Free fatty acids in obesity and type 2 diabetes: defining their role in the development of insulin resistance and beta-cell dysfunction. Eur J Clin Investig 32 (Suppl 3):14–23
67. Auciello FR, Bulusu V, Oon C, Tait-Mulder J, Berry M, Bhattacharyya S et al (2019) A stromal lysolipid-autotaxin signaling axis promotes pancreatic tumor progression. Cancer Discov 9(5):617–627
68. Stepka P, Vsiansky V, Raudenska M, Gumulec J, Adam V, Masarik M (2021) Metabolic and amino acid alterations of the tumor microenvironment. Curr Med Chem 28(7):1270–1289
69. Fridman WH, Pages F, Sautes-Fridman C, Galon J (2012) The immune contexture in human tumours: impact on clinical outcome. Nat Rev Cancer 12(4):298–306
70. Chang DZ, Ma Y, Ji B, Wang H, Deng D, Liu Y et al (2011) Mast cells in tumor microenvironment promotes the in vivo growth of pancreatic ductal adenocarcinoma. Clin Cancer Res 17(22):7015–7023
71. Sahai E, Astsaturov I, Cukierman E, DeNardo DG, Egeblad M, Evans RM et al (2020) A framework for advancing our understanding of cancer-associated fibroblasts. Nat Rev Cancer 20(3):174–186
72. Tumeh PC, Harview CL, Yearley JH, Shintaku IP, Taylor EJ, Robert L et al (2014) PD-1 blockade induces responses by inhibiting adaptive immune resistance. Nature 515(7528): 568–571
73. Pacella I, Piconese S (2019) Immunometabolic checkpoints of treg dynamics: adaptation to microenvironmental opportunities and challenges. Front Immunol 10:1889

74. Zhang Y, Lazarus J, Steele NG, Yan W, Lee H-J, Nwosu ZC et al (2020) Regulatory T-cell depletion alters the tumor microenvironment and accelerates pancreatic carcinogenesis. Cancer Discov 10(3):422–439
75. DiLillo DJ, Yanaba K, Tedder TF (2010) B cells are required for optimal CD4+ and CD8+ T cell tumor immunity: therapeutic B cell depletion enhances B16 melanoma growth in mice. J Immunol 184(7):4006–4016
76. Nielsen JS, Sahota RA, Milne K, Kost SE, Nesslinger NJ, Watson PH et al (2012) CD20+ tumor-infiltrating lymphocytes have an atypical CD27- memory phenotype and together with CD8+ T cells promote favorable prognosis in ovarian cancer. Clin Cancer Res 18(12): 3281–3292
77. Svensson MC, Warfvinge CF, Fristedt R, Hedner C, Borg D, Eberhard J et al (2017) The integrative clinical impact of tumor-infiltrating T lymphocytes and NK cells in relation to B lymphocyte and plasma cell density in esophageal and gastric adenocarcinoma. Oncotarget 8(42):72108–72126
78. de Visser KE, Korets LV, Coussens LM (2005) De novo carcinogenesis promoted by chronic inflammation is B lymphocyte dependent. Cancer Cell 7(5):411–423
79. Ammirante M, Luo JL, Grivennikov S, Nedospasov S, Karin M (2010) B-cell-derived lymphotoxin promotes castration-resistant prostate cancer. Nature 464(7286):302–305
80. Shalapour S, Font-Burgada J, Di Caro G, Zhong Z, Sanchez-Lopez E, Dhar D et al (2015) Immunosuppressive plasma cells impede T-cell-dependent immunogenic chemotherapy. Nature 521(7550):94–98
81. Johansson-Percival A, He B, Ganss R (2018) Immunomodulation of tumor vessels: it takes two to tango. Trends Immunol 39(10):801–814
82. Gillespie S, Monje M (2020) The neural regulation of cancer. Ann Rev Cancer Biol 4:371–390
83. Venkatesh HS, Johung TB, Caretti V, Noll A, Tang Y, Nagaraja S et al (2015) Neuronal activity promotes glioma growth through neuroligin-3 secretion. Cell 161(4):803–816
84. Katayama Y, Battista M, Kao WM, Hidalgo A, Peired AJ, Thomas SA et al (2006) Signals from the sympathetic nervous system regulate hematopoietic stem cell egress from bone marrow. Cell 124(2):407–421
85. Venkataramani V, Tanev DI, Strahle C, Studier-Fischer A, Fankhauser L, Kessler T et al (2019) Glutamatergic synaptic input to glioma cells drives brain tumour progression. Nature 573(7775):532–538
86. Venkatesh HS, Morishita W, Geraghty AC, Silverbush D, Gillespie SM, Arzt M et al (2019) Electrical and synaptic integration of glioma into neural circuits. Nature 573(7775):539–545
87. Zeng Q, Michael IP, Zhang P, Saghafinia S, Knott G, Jiao W et al (2019) Synaptic proximity enables NMDAR signalling to promote brain metastasis. Nature 573(7775):526–531
88. Monje M, Borniger JC, D'Silva NJ, Deneen B, Dirks PB, Fattahi F et al (2020) Roadmap for the emerging field of cancer neuroscience. Cell 181(2):219–222
89. Romero-Garcia S, Moreno-Altamirano MM, Prado-Garcia H, Sánchez-García FJ (2016) Lactate contribution to the tumor microenvironment: mechanisms, effects on immune cells and therapeutic relevance. Front Immunol 7:52
90. Warburg O (1956) On the origin of cancer cells. Science 123(3191):309–314
91. Colegio OR, Chu NQ, Szabo AL, Chu T, Rhebergen AM, Jairam V et al (2014) Functional polarization of tumour-associated macrophages by tumour-derived lactic acid. Nature 513(7519):559–563
92. Angelin A, Gil-de-Gómez L, Dahiya S, Jiao J, Guo L, Levine MH et al (2017) Foxp3 reprograms T cell metabolism to function in low-glucose, high-lactate environments. Cell Metab 25(6):1282–93.e7
93. Hunt TK, Aslam RS, Beckert S, Wagner S, Ghani QP, Hussain MZ et al (2007) Aerobically derived lactate stimulates revascularization and tissue repair via redox mechanisms. Antioxid Redox Signal 9(8):1115–1124
94. Nagelkerke A, Bussink J, Rowan AE, Span PN (2015) The mechanical microenvironment in cancer: how physics affects tumours. Semin Cancer Biol 35:62–70

95. Panciera T, Azzolin L, Cordenonsi M, Piccolo S (2017) Mechanobiology of YAP and TAZ in physiology and disease. Nat Rev Mol Cell Biol 18(12):758–770

96. Plaks V, Kong N, Werb Z (2015) The cancer stem cell niche: how essential is the niche in regulating stemness of tumor cells? Cell Stem Cell 16(3):225–238

97. Ulrich TA, de Juan Pardo EM, Kumar S (2009) The mechanical rigidity of the extracellular matrix regulates the structure, motility, and proliferation of glioma cells. Cancer Res 69(10):4167–4174

98. Xiong G, Chen J, Zhang G, Wang S, Kawasaki K, Zhu J et al (2020) Hsp47 promotes cancer metastasis by enhancing collagen-dependent cancer cell-platelet interaction. Proc Natl Acad Sci U S A 117(7):3748–3758

99. Cooper J, Giancotti FG (2019) Integrin signaling in cancer: mechanotransduction, stemness, epithelial plasticity, and therapeutic resistance. Cancer Cell 35(3):347–367

100. Leight JL, Drain AP, Weaver VM (2017) Extracellular matrix remodeling and stiffening modulate tumor phenotype and treatment response. Ann Rev Cancer Biol 1(1):313–334

101. Lu P, Weaver VM, Werb Z (2012) The extracellular matrix: a dynamic niche in cancer progression. J Cell Biol 196(4):395–406

102. Nguyen L, Fifis T, Malcontenti-Wilson C, Chan LS, Costa PN, Nikfarjam M et al (2012) Spatial morphological and molecular differences within solid tumors may contribute to the failure of vascular disruptive agent treatments. BMC Cancer 12:522

103. Tsujikawa T, Mitsuda J, Ogi H, Miyagawa-Hayashino A, Konishi E, Itoh K et al (2020) Prognostic significance of spatial immune profiles in human solid cancers. Cancer Sci 111(10):3426–3434

104. Ribatti D, Ennas MG, Vacca A, Ferreli F, Nico B, Orru S et al (2003) Tumor vascularity and tryptase-positive mast cells correlate with a poor prognosis in melanoma. Eur J Clin Investig 33(5):420–425

105. Ribatti D, Crivellato E (2009) The controversial role of mast cells in tumor growth. Int Rev Cell Mol Biol 275:89–131

106. Gupta GP, Massagué J (2006) Cancer metastasis: building a framework. Cell 127(4):679–695

107. Pan C, Schoppe O, Parra-Damas A, Cai R, Todorov MI, Gondi G et al (2019) Deep learning reveals cancer metastasis and therapeutic antibody targeting in the entire body. Cell 179(7):1661–76.e19

108. Valiente M, Ahluwalia MS, Boire A, Brastianos PK, Goldberg SB, Lee EQ et al (2018) The evolving landscape of brain metastasis. Trends Cancer 4(3):176–196

Chapter 3
Local *Onco-Sphere:* Tumor–Immune Cells Interactions

Phei Er Saw and Erwei Song

Abstract In the local onco-sphere, tumor cells are constantly communicating with their surrounding environment, including immune cells, stromal cells and other biochemical cues. In this chapter, we will only focus on the tumor-immune interactions, summarizing the importance of host immune cells (both innate and adaptive immunity) in changing the landscape of the local onco-sphere.

Introduction

Rather than being understood as a mass of transformed cells, cancers refer to a newly developed organ that consists of different nonmalignant cells, making up a major part of the tumor, collectively failing to persist in dialogue that supports the balance of the tissue architecture [1]. In the local *onco-sphere*, among these nonmalignant cells, immune cells play a major role in modulating the environment that favors tumor progression [2]. Similar to the process of organogenesis, tumor and stromal cells undergo an evolution in specific relation to each other; the interactions between

P. E. Saw
Guangdong Provincial Key Laboratory of Malignant Tumor Epigenetics and Gene Regulation, Guangdong-Hong Kong Joint Laboratory for RNA Medicine, Medical Research Center, Sun Yat-sen Memorial Hospital, Sun Yat-sen University, Guangzhou, China

Nanhai Translational Innovation Center of Precision Immunology, Sun Yat-sen Memorial Hospital, Sun Yat-sen University, Foshan, China

E. Song (✉)
Guangdong Provincial Key Laboratory of Malignant Tumor Epigenetics and Gene Regulation, Guangdong-Hong Kong Joint Laboratory for RNA Medicine, Medical Research Center, Sun Yat-sen Memorial Hospital, Sun Yat-sen University, Guangzhou, China

Nanhai Translational Innovation Center of Precision Immunology, Sun Yat-sen Memorial Hospital, Sun Yat-sen University, Foshan, China

Breast Tumor Center, Sun Yat-sen Memorial Hospital, Sun Yat-sen University, Guangzhou, China
e-mail: songew@mail.sysu.edu.cn

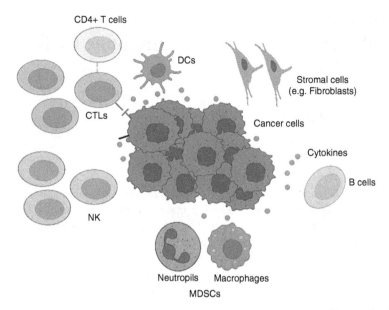

Fig. 3.1 Immune cells in the local *onco-sphere*: a close-knit connection. In the local *onco-sphere*, tumor environment is made up of various kinds of non-tumoral cells, including stromal cells and infiltrating immune cells. Here, we will discuss the communication between tumor cells and immune cells in the local *onco-sphere*, while in Chap. 4, we will discuss the interactions between tumor cells and its surrounding stromal cells. Infiltrated immune cells include innate immune cells, such as neutrophils, macrophages, MDSCs, and NK cells, while adaptive immune cells include T cells and B cells. The constant communication between cancer cells and these immune cells is not only through direct contact but also through indirect contact via secretions of growth factors (GFs), cytokines, chemokines, and also extracellular vehicles (including exosomes). All of these interactions are crucial in determining the fate of the immune cell phenotype after infiltration to the tumor, and this in turn determines the fate of the cancer cells

the varying parts result in a persisting functional and phenotypic plasticity. Junctions, receptors, and a host of signals generated by the abovementioned cell types within a ECM act as the conductor for dynamic cross talks between the cells in the local *onco-sphere*. Tumor–stromal and tumor–secretome interaction will be detailed in subsequent chapters. Here, we will discuss the changes in the infiltrated immune cells and how these immune and tumor cells have a bidirectional communication to promote tumor growth (Figs. 3.1 and 3.3).

Due to the interference in tissue homeostasis, the cellular metabolism and functionality of immune and stromal cells undergo various dynamic alterations [3]. These alterations are mostly pro-tumoral, a classic ecological behavior as the tumor cells turn immune cells from "foes to friends," thereby re-educating these immune cells to secrete pro-tumoral growth factors, cytokines and chemokines, to aid in cancer growth and metastasis. In turn, these tumor cells also secrete these factors or overexpressing ligands that could skew the phenotype changes in immune cells into pro-tumoral phenotypes (i.e., M2-like macrophages, Tregs, Bregs), known as a symbiotic relationship. In other cases, tumor cells can lead to the exhaustion or anergy of effector T cells, which does not bring any benefit to the immune cells; a relationship known as commensalism. In this chapter, we will discuss two major immune cell type, the innate and adaptive immune cell infiltration to the local *onco-sphere*, and how they interact with tumors, and how their bidirectional relationship can lead to cancer cell growth and metastasis.

Innate Immune Cells

Neutrophils

Neutrophils, also known as polymorphonuclear (PMN) leukocytes, are the most prevalent forms of white blood cells and are descended from the myeloid lineage. The most active form of an innate immune cell, neutrophils are created in the bone marrow and have a daily production rate of almost 10^{11} neutrophils [4, 5]. As the first defense against acute inflammation, neutrophils undergo phagocytosis, degranulation, and the creation of neutrophil extracellular traps (NETs) to confine invading bacteria [5]. Up until recently, neutrophils were thought to only have three functions: host defense, immunological regulation, and tissue injury [6]. However, it has been noted that neutrophils work in a more complex manner than just eliminating microbes. More evidences are pointing toward neutrophils as being transcriptionally active cells that exhibit phenotypic variability and functional diversity and are responsive to numerous signals by generating a variety of inflammatory cytokines and immune system-regulating factors [7, 8]. Therefore, it is clear that in homeostasis, neutrophils are vital for keeping the host safe from external pathogens. However, this is not the case in the local *onco-sphere*.

An interesting fact is that neutrophil is not originally found in tumor. Neutrophil has to undergo mobilization from the bone marrow to tumor sites. This can happen via chemoattractants secreted by the tumor cells. Once the neutrophils receive the cue to mobilize to tumor, they have to first mature in the bone marrow, then intravasate into blood circulation through attachment of blood vessel endothelial cells (ECs), follow the concentration gradient of the chemoattractant (i.e., GM-CSF), and finally extravasate to the tumor vicinity, in a process called leukocyte rolling, similar to the activation of wound healing process, which we will discuss further in latter chapters.

When neutrophils arrive at the tumor, they are called tumor-associated neutrophils (TANs). These TANs could be polarized into N1-type or N2-type according to the cues given by the tumor cells. TANs are generally divided into two phenotypes (N1 and N2), according to whether they are pro- or anti-tumoral. This is very similar to the polarization of tumor-associated macrophages (TAMs), where they are also divided according to their pro- and anti-tumoral phenotype (discussed in detail below). N1 phenotype is caused by an elevated production of TNF-α, ICAM-1, and FAS in cancer cells. In tumor-bearing mice, deactivation of TGFβ also showed

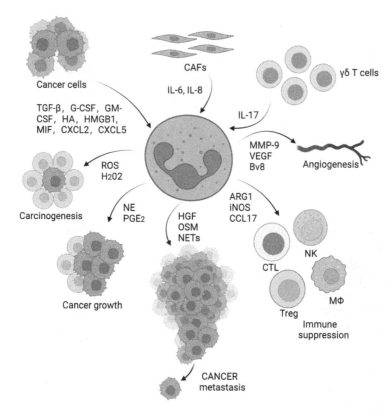

Fig. 3.2 Cross talk between neutrophils and the local *onco-sphere*. Interactions between neutrophils and the tumor, immune cells, and secretome in the progression of the tumor. Neutrophil not only have a bidirectional relationship with the tumor cells, they are also constantly in communication with other cells in the local onco-sphere, including CAFs and T cells. Through the secretion of soluble factors of neutrophil, they can also direct changes in the local onco-sphere. For example, neutrophil-secreted MMP-9, VEGF, and Bv8 can trigger angiogenesis process, while secretion of ARG1 iNOS and CCL17 can inhibit effector T-cell activation, while high levels of ROS, hydrogen peroxide, HGF, and NETs could induce carcinogenesis and cancer metastasis. Likewise, tumor cell-derived TGF-β, GM-CSF, chemokines can induce N2-like pro-tumoral phenotypes. IL-17 secreted by γδ-T cells also elevates the N2-like phenotype in TANs. Therefore, all the multidirectional continuous cues are working in favor of the tumor to keep the neutrophil in a pro-tumoral phenotype

an increment in N1 phenotype [9]. An N1-specific phenotype is a hyper-segmented nucleus, which could clearly distinguish them from N2 TANs [9]. On the contrary, N2 TANs are pro-tumoral, and they are distinguished by a unique circular nucleus. An elevated amount of N2 TANs could induce high expression of arginase (which reduces T-cell cytotoxicity) and pro-tumoral chemokines (CCL2, CCL5) and other factors (cathepsin G, neutrophil elastase) [8]. It was speculated that the environment in the local *onco-sphere* could stimulate neutrophils toward different, phenotype, which is not surprising, as the communications within the local *onco-sphere* are more often than not, a bidirectional communication (Fig. 3.2).

Biochemical Changes in Neutrophils in the Local *Onco-Sphere*

During an immune response, neutrophils act as the first responder, to get rid of infection at the site of inflammation [6]. One of the major killing methods of neutrophil is phagocytosis [10]. The pathogen is engulfed by neutrophils, which then create phagosomes and merge them with lysosomes [11]. In order to kill the pathogen, neutrophils' granules produce NADPH oxidase, which alters the pH of the phagosome and lysosome, causing higher ROS and respiratory burst [12]. Higher ROS not only could lead to DNA damage, which ultimately brings upon mutation [13, 14], but also cause epithelial injury and infection inside the tumor [15], while increasing cellular proliferation, suppressing immune cells infiltration [16], increasing chemoresistance [17] and also EMT in many cancers [18]. Hydrogen peroxide functions as a secondary messenger to control many cell-signaling pathways critical to cellular biology, including the PI3K/Akt, IKK/NF-kB, and MAPK/Erk1/2 pathways. Nevertheless, study results have been contradicting. It was shown that one of the methods for getting rid of tumor cells is thought to be the neutrophils' creation of hydrogen peroxide [19]. In particular, after coming into contact with cancer cells physically, neutrophils can release hydrogen peroxide, which causes tumor cells to die due to Ca^{2+} influx through the TRPM2 Ca^{2+} pathway [20]. Likewise, in TANs, nitric oxide was released to kill the tumor cells when the Met receptor binds to hepatocyte growth factor (HGF) [21]. Therefore, neutrophils' pro- or anti-tumor behavior is highlight dependent on the amount of ROS/RNS [22].

In response to external stimuli in the local *onco-sphere*, neutrophils can secrete many different cytokines and chemokines [23, 24]. They not only influence other tumor-associated stromal cells' pro- or anti-tumor responses, but these factors could also act in an autocrine manner to polarize neutrophils into N1 or N2 TANs [9, 22]. Studies revealed that the cytokines and chemokines released by neutrophils are skewed in favor of pro-tumoral behavior. For example, a study found that co-culturing human breast cancer cells with neutrophils leads to an increased secretion of VEGF, which promotes angiogenesis [25]. In another breast cancer research, neutrophil-released TGF-β increases EMT phenotype in cancer cells [26]. Neutrophil-secreted IL17 can accelerate tumor growth of pancreatic cancer cells and encourages these cells to develop stem-cell-like characteristics [27]. Not only that, IL17 increases CXCR2 ligand expression to facilitate neutrophil recruitment, indirectly causing tumor growth [28]. In a zebrafish model, inflammation-induced CXCL8 is responsible for neutrophil recruitment [29], suggesting a cross talk between inflammation, immune cells infiltration, and tumor progression [30]. Generally, neutrophils can release ample CC ligands and CXC chemokines, which act as immune cells chemoattractants, to attract Treg cells, monocytes, and other immune cells [31, 32].

Several cytoplasmic granules found inside a mature neutrophil are responsible for the diverse functions of neutrophils, and these granules can be released by membrane-bound organelles during activation [33]. There are three main types of granules, specific to their functions. Primary granules are linked to microbicidal action, while secondary and tertiary granules are linked to ECM remodeling. For example, during EMT, cathepsin G (CG), neutrophil elastase (NE), proteinase 3 (PR3), and MMP-9 are all proteases derived from neutrophil granules, which enhance metastasis. Recent research suggests that NE can activate the PI3K and EGFR/MEK/ERK signaling pathways, to stimulate cancer cells progression [34]. In patients with metastatic breast cancer, NE expression level has a direct correlation to a poorer response to tamoxifen therapy [35]. Interestingly, in cancer cells that do not produce NE, they can still express neuropilin receptor to induce extracellular NE uptake [36], indicating that NE could potentially be used a marker in cancer prognosis, especially in breast, colorectal, and gastric cancers [37].

MMP-9 is uniquely stored in the neutrophil granules [38], and its catalytic activity depends on zinc as a cofactor [39]. The ECM can be modified by an active MMP-9 by degrading extracellular proteins [39] and activating pro-tumoral cytokines and other growth factors, including TGF-β [40]. Neutrophil's release of MMP9 is dependent on TNF-α, TGF-β, and VEGF [41]. MMP-9 expression level has been associated with sunitinib resistance. MMP-9 is highly expressed in breast cancers, with enhanced angiogenesis, and predicts poor survival [42]. MMP-8 (collagenase-2) is released by neutrophils, which is crucial for neutrophil mobilization [40]. There have been contradictory research studies on MMP-8 as anti-tumoral and pro-tumoral. In breast cancer cohort study, MMP-8 expression was inversely correlated with metastasis, especially metastasis to lymph nodes [43]. However, in a more recent study, MMP-8 expression elevates the expression IL-6 and IL-8, suggesting a pro-tumoral activity [44]. In another cohort study, patients have a lower survival rate when MMP-8 level in their serum is elevated [45].

When neutrophil is triggered by any stimuli, NETosis can occur. NETosis is the formation of neutrophil extracellular nets (NETs), which could be released to the extracellular space, without causing neutrophil death. The NET is full of granules, bactericidal proteins that could "trap" these pathogens. NETosis is a new way of killing found in neutrophils, in addition to the usual phagocytosis or degranulation [46]. NETs were once thought to kill pathogens by rupturing the cytoplasmic membrane in response to stimuli such as CXCL8 or lipopolysaccharide (LPS), which also cause NADPH oxidase to produce ROS [47]. Due to the release of mitochondrial DNA, neutrophils can avoid cell death while forming NETs [47, 48]. Compared to healthy controls, the cancer patients' blood plasma level of NETs is found to be significantly increased [49, 50]. Since NET levels are higher in Ewing's sarcoma patients who have metastasized [51], NETs may be useful as a diagnostic marker. In recent work, we found that NET-DNA could be a chemotactic factor to draw cancer cells and that NET-dependent metastasis is mediated by the transmembrane DNA receptor CCDC25 [52].

Macrophages in the Local *Onco-Sphere*

Macrophages are able to secrete a large number of cytokines and other factors that can modulate the immune environment in the local *onco-sphere*. In an indirect mechanism, macrophage can activate the complement system, resulting in inflammation, which in turn leads to cancer progression. Macrophages can be broadly divided into two groups, known as classically activated macrophages (M1) and alternatively activated macrophages (M2) (Fig. 3.3), with distinct roles. Both of these groups are capable of changing into one another in response to changes in the internal environment [53]. While there are disagreements over the exact classification of TAMs, we will concentrate on their broad M1- and M2-like characteristics in the context of the local *onco-sphere* in this chapter.

Alteration of TAMs Signaling Pathways in the Local *Onco-Sphere*

PD-1/PD-L1 Signaling Known as "programmed cell death protein" (PD-1), PD-1 is a member of the CD28 superfamily, a transmembrane protein of 40 kDa. PD-1 is an immunosuppressive molecule. In normal condition, PD-1 ligand, PD-L1, is expressed by antigen-presenting cells (APCs). When bound to PD-1 expressed on T cells, T cells will not be activated, therefore not initiating an attack on healthy host [54]. In tumor cells, they can upregulate PD-L1 as a decoy or APC-mimicking process, therefore, inhibiting T-cell activity when they bind to PD-L1 on tumor, recognizing these tumor cells as "friends" rather than "foe" [55]. In the immune system cross talk, TAMs also produce PD-1. TAMs expression of PD-1 increases with time and with disease stage. The overexpression of PD-1 in TAM has a negative correlation with their phagocytic potency toward cancer cells. Apart from that, overexpression of PD-1 on TAMs also leads to the dysfunctional regulation of other immune cells, such as reducing the efficacy of effector T cells, NK cells, and DCs in their antigen presentation [56] (Fig. 3.4).

CD47-SIRPα Signaling CD47 is a transmembrane immunoreceptor tyrosine-based inhibitory motif receptor, highly expressed on tumor cells, while its ligand, SIRPα, is mostly produced on macrophages. The cytosolic tyrosine phosphatases SHP-1 and SHP-2 on CD47 are attracted to and activated by the interaction of the ITIM motif's NH_2 terminal domain. As a result, this connection can dephosphorylate a variety of substrates, control signaling cascades downstream, and eventually prevent macrophages from phagocytosing healthy cells. CD47 is hence frequently known as the "do-not-eat-me" signal [57]. There is a balance between these two molecules, and their interaction can result in a number of physiological processes. The equilibrium is broken when the amount of CD47 expressed on a cell surface rises as CD47 prevents phagocytosis by sending the "do-not-eat-me" signal, thereby leading to an escape from cell death and encouraging tumor growth.

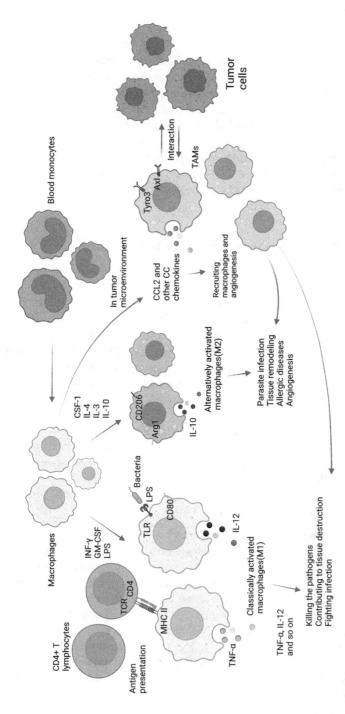

Fig. 3.3 Multiple pathways of macrophage activation. Generally, macrophages are classified into M1 and M2 phenotype. M1-like macrophages are activated by pro-inflammatory factors such as IFNγ, GM-CSF, and play a significant role in upregulation of inflammation in tumor cells, inducing a constant inflammation-like tumor environment. M2-like macrophages are activated by CSF-1, IL-4, IL-13, IL-10; are involved in angiogenesis and pro-tumoral activities. In the local onco-sphere, high levels of CSF-1, IL-3, IL-4, and IL-10 leads to a skewing of phenotype toward the M2-like phenotype, favoring pro-tumoral progression

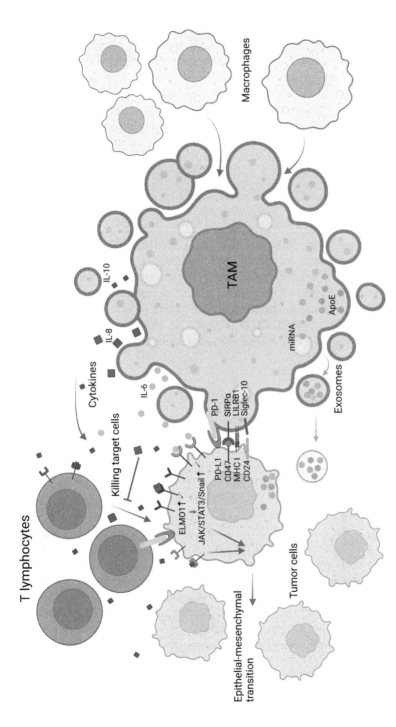

Fig. 3.4 Various pathways of TAMs in inhibiting immunotherapy to promote tumor progression. TAMs are capable of secreting cytokines such as IL-6, IL-8, and IL-10 that support the growth of tumors. Additionally, numerous molecular pathways could be activated by TAMs, having an impact on immunosuppression. The probability of tumor immune escape is encouraged by the PD-1/L1 signaling pathway since it can prevent macrophages from performing their usual functions. The "do-not-eat-me" signal is associated with the SIRPα/CD47 pathway, and tumor cells that express CD47 could be misidentified as self. β2-microglobulin, an important component of LILRB1/MHC class I, is another important tumor escape pathway. Siglec-10 can interact with CD24 on tumor cells to facilitate immune escape in cases of breast and ovarian cancer

MHC-I β2-Microglobulin/Immunoglobulin-Like Receptor Subfamily B Member 1 (LILRB1) Signaling Recently, Weissman and associates discovered that tumor cells and macrophages have a different recognition system that shields cancer cells from macrophages: the MHC class I component β2-microglobulin [58]. When β2-microglobulin on MHC-1 is inhibited or silenced, tumor-bearing mice showed a significant 70% longer life span, as macrophages are now activated to enhance phagocytosis of tumor cells. In another related pathway, it was shown that silencing LILRB1 on macrophage surface, tumor growth is inhibited. Interestingly, simultaneous inhibition of LILRB1 protein and supplementation of anti-CD47 monoclonal antibodies could boost macrophage phagocytosis ability in vivo, indicating the feasibility of using this pathway for future immunotherapy ICBs [58].

CD24-Siglec-10 Signaling CD 24 is a prominent innate immune checkpoint and a viable target for immunotherapy in female cancers (i.e., ovarian and breast cancer). Current findings showed that TAM-expressed sialic acid-binding Ig-like lectin 10 (Siglec-10, an inhibitory molecule) that could bind to CD24 expressed on tumor cells to enhance immune escape. Not surprisingly, further research has revealed that Siglec-10 is highly expressed in TAMs, while CD24 is overexpressed in a variety of cancers. TAMs activity against all human cancers expressing CD24 can be improved by either using monoclonal antibodies to block CD24/Siglec-10 interaction or by silencing either of CD24 or Siglec-10. These data merit additional investigation and suggest a novel strategy for tumor immunotherapy [59].

Myeloid-Derived Suppressor Cells (MDSCs)

The two main subsets of mouse MDSCs—polymorphonuclear $Ly6G^+Ly6C^{lo}$ (PMN) and monocytic $Ly6GLy6C^{hi}$ (M) cells—express CD11b and Gr1 markers [60–62]. In humans, the same two subsets can be characterized as $Lin^-HLA-DR^-/loCD33^+$ or $Lin^-HLA-DR^-/_{lo}CD11b^+CD14^-CD15^+CD33^+$ for PMN-MDSCs and $CD14^+HLA-DR_{neg}/_{lo}$ or $Lin^-HLA-DR_{neg}/loCD11b^+CD14^+CD15^-$ for M-MDSCs [63, 64]. MDSCs develop from bone marrow hematopoietic precursor cells, and they demonstrate significant immunosuppressive and tumorigenic activities, such as (1) lack arginine and cysteine (crucial for effector T-cell activity); (2) production of NO and ROS, which inhibits TCR and chemokines crucial for T-cell migration or induce the apoptosis of T cells and NK cells; (3) an increased secretion of pro-tumoral cytokines (IL-10 and TGF-β); (4) an upregulated assertion of PD-L1 to suppress T-cell activity; (5) a decrease in the expression of the TCR ζ-chain, inhibiting TCR-mediated antigen recognition coupling to various signal transduction pathways; (6) the increment of angiogenic factors production to promote tumor neovascularization, and (7) the generation of multiple MMPs, cytokines, chemokines, GFs; to promote tumor growth and skew immune responses toward the Th2 phenotype and activate Tregs [62, 65–72].

Dendritic Cells (DCs)

Dendritic cells (DCs) are the main class of antigen-presenting cells (APCs) in human. DCs are capable to capturing antigens after these antigens were processed by the MHC complex. DCs then act as a "delivery man" to transport these peptide sequences (antigens) to T cells [73]. Originated from a myeloid cell population, DCs population varies, depending on their morphological, ontogenetic, and immunological characteristics, and most importantly, their location. Some of the famous DCs subset are Langerhans cell (in skin, pancreas), stellate cells (in the liver), among others. Various subsets of DCs might vary in their specific immunological process. For example, (1) epidermal Langerhans cells prime CD8$^+$ T-cell immunity and interstitial/dermal (CD14$^+$) DCs could trigger humoral immunity; and (2) plasmacytoid (pDCs) cells secrete high levels of Type I IFN [74].

Adaptive Immune Cells in the Local *Onco-Sphere*

T Cells

Undoubtedly, T cells are the key of adaptive immune responders. The cytotoxic CD8$^+$ T-cell population is fully responsible to eradicate tumors, while being supported by Th1-subtype of CD4$^+$ T helper T cells, which could generate IL2 and IFNγ (both anti-tumoral cytokines). Studies have indicated that high CD8$^+$ T cell and Th1 population are directly proportional to a better prognosis in cancer patients [75, 76]. However, the local *onco-sphere* is always skewed toward a pro-tumoral T-cell phenotype due to the constant inflammatory environment. Under constant inflammation, different T cell subsets are encouraged such as the CD4+ T-cell subsets Th2 and Th17. Another CD4$^+$ T cells, Tregs have high expression of CD25 and FOXP3, infamously known for regulating peripheral immunological tolerance [77]. Treg cells often prevent effector T cells from activating, proliferating, and surviving by releasing immunosuppressive chemicals such as TGF-β and IL-10 [78, 79]. In fact, they also upregulate TNF receptor superfamily members, as well as markers linked to T-cell malfunction or trafficking such as CCR4, CD39, and CD73 [80–82]. Tregs are frequently found in large numbers in the TME, and their primary function is to stifle the anti-tumor response.

T cells are primarily responsible for controlling the progression of cancers; however, they must first infiltrate the tumors. In a recent immune checkpoint blockades (ICBs) study, multiple factors should be considered when regarding T cells in immunotherapy; including but not limited to (1) the amount of T- cell infiltration, (2) T-cell functionality, and (3) T-cell spatiotemporal distribution in the tumor [83, 84]. Currently, T-cell abundance and activities are one of the main characteristics in dividing the solid tumors into three phenotypes: inflamed (where most of the inhibitory cell subsets are present in the tumor core), immune-excluded

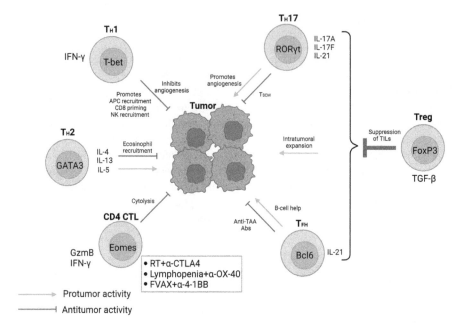

Fig. 3.5 A summary of the interaction between different types of T lymphocyte subsets with the tumor within the local *onco-sphere*

(most inhibitory cells are present, but excluded at the tumor periphery), and immune-desert (where the tumor has minimal immune cell infiltration) phenotypes [85, 86] (Fig. 3.5).

T-Cell Dysfunction in the Local *Onco-Sphere*

Chronic antigen exposure impairs T-cell function, which is known as T-cell dysfunction, in chronic infections and tumors [78, 87]. Earlier research has shown a correlation between the level of antigen stimulation and the severity of dysfunction [88, 89]. Additionally, it has been demonstrated that particular TCR-dependent pathways, such as those controlled by Nuclear Factor of Activated T cells (NFAT) and Sprouty Homolog 2 (SPRY2), are implicated in T-cell dysfunction, which is consistent with the results of persistent TCR activation [90, 91]. Likewise, NFAT cytoplasmic 1 (NFATc1) continues to express PD-1 in response to repeated antigen stimulation [92]. PD-1 may also control the amount of TCR signaling [93, 94]. As a result, the intensity and duration of antigenic stimulation seem to be key elements that contribute to T-cell dysfunction and are linked to how severe the dysfunction is.

T-cell dysfunction is exemplified by T-cell exhaustion. Exhausted T cells (T_{ex}) are distinct from anergic T cells and senescent T cells, among other defective T cells

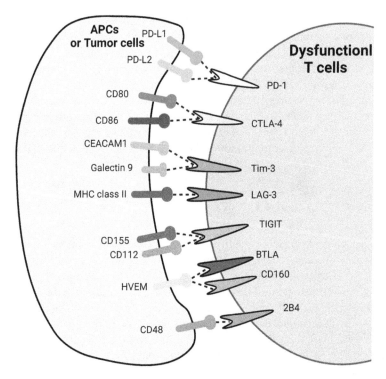

Fig. 3.6 IRs presented on T cells that leads to T-cell dysfunction. Dysfunctional T lymphocytes express a variety of IRs. These ligands bind to respective ligands, which are expressed in high quantity in tumor cells or APCs. Once binding occurs, T cells are led into exhaustion, leading to a dysfunctional T cell, unable to exert their tumor killing effect

[95, 96]. T-cell anergy is brought upon by suboptimal stimulation, whereas recurrent stimulation leads to the terminal differentiation T-cells senescence, which also leads to telomerase shortening and cell cycle arrest. In dysfunctional T cells, co-expression of two or more inhibitory receptors (IRs; such as PD-1, CTLA-4. Tim-3, LAG3, TIGIT; Fig. 3.6) is all positively related [97, 98]. Interestingly, in both mouse and human studies, dysfunction CD8$^+$ T cells could simultaneously upregulate many IRs, which ultimately leads to severe T-cell exhaustion [99, 100]. It is interesting to note, however, IRs have different outcomes in T-cell immunology. For instance, in healthy control, circulating PD-1$^+$CD8$^+$ T cells are indicative of effector memory T cells and not dysfunctional T cells [101]. Also, cancerous environment differs from infection [102]. The B- and T-lymphocyte attenuator (BTLA) is elevated in cancerous dysfunctional CD8$^+$ T cells but is not present in lymphocytic choriomeningitis virus (LCMV) dysfunctional CD8$^+$ T cells [100]. This study suggests that there may be some differences between cancer and chronic infections in the molecular pathways that result in IR overexpression and T-cell dysfunction. One of the possible

reasons is that in cancer, IRs need to interact with their respective ligands (usually only expressed by tumor cells, or other tumor-related stromal and immune cells, to be able to influence T-cell dysfunction (Fig. 3.6). Therefore, the presence and quantity of ligands in the local *onco-sphere* are essential for IR to exert a negative regulatory effect on CD8$^+$ T cells. For example, the binding of PD1/PD-L1 is dependent upon exposures of inflammatory cytokines [103]. In melanoma cells, they continually express CD112 and CD155 (ligands of TIGIT) to provide a constant environment to trigger T cells exhaustion [98]. Tim-3 also binds to Galectin-9 and CEACAM1 overexpressed on tumor or APCs, inhibiting T-cell activity [104, 105].

B Lymphocytes in the Local *Onco-Sphere*

Although T cells are always thought as the major contributor to induce tumor death and improve clinical outcome, recent publications are pointing toward an indispensable role of B cells in anti-cancer immune function. B cells are activated in the tertiary lymphoid structures (TLSs) and could exert their anti-tumor activity via two potent mechanisms: (1) by presenting tumor-associated antigen (TAA) to T cells, in order for T cell to recognize these tumor antigens and exert their cytotoxic activities or (2) produce antibodies specific to these TAAs, increasing the probability of being recognized by T cells. Either way, both could achieve beneficial clinical outcome [106].

Antigen Presentation

The B-cell receptor (BCR) is used by B cells to identify and ingest native proteins and glycoproteins. The immunotyrosine activation sequence of the CD79α and β signaling chains linked to the antigen-recognizing Ig inside the BCR causes them to internalize the proteins. The proteins are then processed in the cytoplasm, allowing the antigenic peptide to link with MHC-II molecules, which could be presented to CD4 T helper cells and CD8 T cells [107, 108]. Antigen transfer to DCs and effective antigen demonstration to T cells require direct contact with BCR-bound antigen [109]. During breast cancer chemotherapy, dying tumor cells can activate the complement system. Complement systems can also activate B cells as the complement cleavage C3b binds to CR2 receptor on B cells, inducing the development of ICOS-L$^+$ B-cell fraction. ICOS-L$^+$ B cell could increase the infiltration of CD8 T cells, and Th1/Treg ratio, leading to neoadjuvant chemotherapy therapeutic efficacy in breast cancer, notably in triple-negative cancers, where patient survival is significantly prolonged [110, 111].

Antibody Production

Antibodies are generated by plasma cells in TLS GCs. These antibodies can perform effector roles in addition to enhancing T-cell immunity through antigen presentation. Clinically, in NSCLC patients, supernatants taken from tumor-infiltrating B cells indicated that about half the cohort possess TAA-specific antibodies, such as LAGE-1, MAGE antigens, and NY-ESO-1 [112]. Similarly, in a breast cancer study, antibodies against the gangliosides GD3, CEA, MUC1, and FN1 have been found [107, 113]. These antibodies may also be effective in anti-tumor responses even though they are tumor-associated instead of cancer-specific (i.e., RAS-mutated cancers), as TAAs could be shared and recognized by B cells [114]. Due to their unique morphology, antibodies can active NK cells to kill tumor cells via antibody-dependent cell death (ADCC), where the Fc region of the antibodies attached to the FC receptors on NK cells ADCC is a potent mechanism and is effective in killing tumor cells even when the antigen load is modest. However, ADCC may not be highly effective in solid tumors with few and anergic NK cells [115]. To overcome this problem, B cells can also activate macrophages, through antibody-dependent cell phagocytosis [116]. Even so, macrophages can counter this ADCP by increasing PD-L1 and IDO production [117]. Macrophages could also secrete VEGF and TGF-β, encouraging immunosuppressive phenotypes [118]. Furthermore, IgG immune complexes can promote prolonged inflammation [119, 120], angiogenesis, and immunosuppression by activating macrophages, all of which promote tumor growth.

Tertiary Lymphoid Structures (TLSs) and B-Cells Activation

As mentioned above, B cells were primarily found in TLSs. TLSs are lymphoid organs that are ectopically expressed in or near the inflamed tissue, as a result of persistent antigen stimulation. Ironically, chemotherapy or radiotherapy, the main treatments for cancer, can also bring on pro-immunogenic inflammation, which leads to the development of TLSs [110, 121, 122]. TLSs begin to develop in inflamed areas when stromal cell secretes high level of IL-7, which comes into contact with monocytic cells, Th17 cells, or B cells in an environment that is high in CXCL13 [123–125]. CXCL13 and CCL19, along with adhesion molecules, control how the developing TLSs are structurally organized, whereas CCL21 and CXCL12 contribute to the activation of lymphocytes [126]. In a lymphotoxin α-deficient mouse model, TLSs serve as locations for the development of immunological responses to antigens, even when lymph node is absent [127]. Similar to a lymph node, mature TLSs consist of a T-cell zone, where fully developed DCs introduce antigen to T cells, and a notable B-cell zone structured in a germinal center (GC), which is surrounded by high endothelial venules (HEVs) and contains proliferating B cells and follicular DCs (fDCs). These B cells also express activation-induced deaminase and BCL-6, which allow these B cells to switch and mature toward antibody-producing plasma cells [128].

The presence of TLSs in a tumor has been correlated with favorable prognosis [129]; as TLS GCs stimulated B cells, causing them to multiply and develop into plasma cells that produce antibodies against TAAs. In NSCLC, a high B-cell follicle density was associated with longer PFS and OS [112]. Numerous cancer forms have been documented to include TLSs, including melanoma, bladder, colorectal, gastric, ovarian, liver, pancreatic cancers, among others [130–139]. In fact, TLSs discovered in high-grade dysplastic and initial HCC nodules were immature, taking the shape of lymphoid aggregates lacking a fully developed GC, during the premalignant early stages of HCC. They were connected with indicators of immunological depletion, immunosuppression, and inflammation, which may favor the development of HCC [140]. In a mouse model of HCC, another finding suggests that TLSs may act as habitats that protect tumor cells [141]. All things considered, these results show that TLSs may form immunity that fights cancer and that B cells, as well as their location within the local *onco-sphere*, are significant and may have an impact on clinical results. A significant predictor of a good prognosis is CXCL13 [106]. In melanoma, the CXCL13 signature was clearly correlated to a good prognosis [142]. In an interesting study, a robust B-cell signature was significantly linked with prolonged OS in soft tissue sarcoma; however, there was no association among T-cell signatures and OS [143]. However, there is a correlation between T follicular helper cells and B-cell activation in breast cancer and head and neck carcinomas [144, 145]; and further supports a role for B cells in cancer protection. Studies also indicates that the intra-tumoral density of B cells are directly linked toward a favorable prognosis in many cancers, including breast cancer, colorectal cancers, ovarian cancer, melanoma, hepatocellular carcinoma, among others [112, 146–152].

In an in vitro study of NSCLS and ovarian cancer, intra-tumoral B cells could undergo isotypic switching to generate IgA and IgG specific to TAAs. Fc receptor of B cells is activated depending on B-cell isotype, similar to the complement activation. In the case of IgG antibodies, IgG may be actively involved in local and systemic anti-tumor activity, through NK cells activation (via antibody-dependent cellular cytotoxicity; ADCC) and macrophage stimulation (via antibody-dependent cellular phagocytosis; ADCP) [116]. This has been proven in the positive impact shown by circulating anti-MUC1 IgG, which has been directly elevated prognosis on breast, gastric and pancreatic cancers [153, 154]. However, B-cell plasma activation is not always linked to good prognosis. Since tumor-bound IgG is able to active classical complement system in situ, this could cause chronic inflammation and lead to a poor prognosis, as seen in clear cell renal cell carcinoma. Mechanistically, tumor-associated IgG antibodies could interact with complement component C1q on macrophages, which then recruits other complement components, such as C1r, C1s, C2, C3, C4, and C5, which could be all generated by tumor cells [155]. In another mechanism, B cells are seen to induce a pro-tumorigenic function in SCC cells through the deposition of immune complexes containing IgG that promote myeloid cell activation that is FcγR-dependent and promotes inflammation. Activation of the classical path in NSCLC is partially IgM-dependent [156] and is associated with a

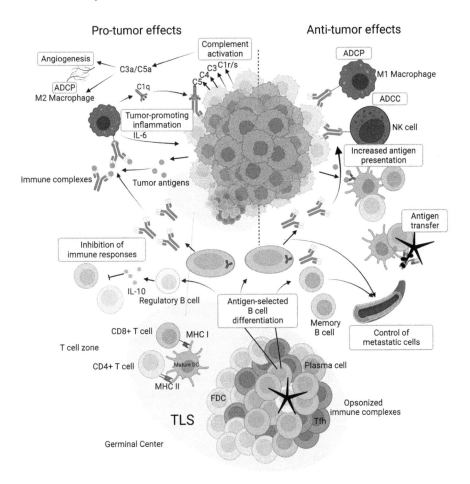

Fig. 3.7 B cells in the local *onco-sphere*. In tumor, B cells are produced and activated in the TLS. They multiply and differentiate into memory B cells and plasma cells with the aid of T follicular helper (Tfh) cells. CD4 and CD8 T cells receive antigens from B cells. IgG antibodies, which are made by plasma cells, enhance antigen presentation to T cells. These antibodies could also induce the activity of NK cells and macrophages through ADCC and ADCP mechanism, respectively. However, as we discussed above, there are both sides of B cells and B-cell derived plasma and soluble factors in cancer. By activating the complement system, B cells can indirectly enhance tumor growth as the complement factors C3a and C5 could induce angiogenesis

poor prognosis [157]. Furthermore, IgA/IgGH transcripts in melanoma and bladder cancer reveal that anticancer IgA antibodies have a negative effect on patient prognosis [158, 159]. IgA$^+$ B cells in HCC suppress cytotoxic T-cell reactions that stop hepatocarcinogenesis in the diseased liver [160]. Therefore, the effect of B lymphocytes may be a double-edged sword that depends on the tumor environment (Fig. 3.7).

Conclusion

In this chapter, we discussed the close-knit communication in the local *onco-sphere* where the role of infiltrating immune cells is closely related by the local *onco-sphere*. Interestingly, although most immune cells are immuno-stimulating, once infiltrated into the local *onco-sphere*, their phenotype could be skewed or reversed; forces researchers to think deeply on the underlying mechanism that leads to the immuno-suppressive behavior of these immune cells, which if not curbed, could promote tumor progression and stimulate tumor development, creating a pre-metastatic environment favoring the expansion of local to distal *onco-sphere*.

References

1. Bissell MJ, Radisky D (2001) Putting tumours in context. Nat Rev Cancer 1(1):46–54
2. Hanahan D, Coussens LM (2012) Accessories to the crime: functions of cells recruited to the tumor microenvironment. Cancer Cell 21(3):309–322
3. Galli F, Aguilera JV, Palermo B, Markovic SN, Nistico P, Signore A (2020) Relevance of immune cell and tumor microenvironment imaging in the new era of immunotherapy. J Exp Clin Cancer Res 39(1):89
4. Wu L, Saxena S, Singh RK (2020) Neutrophils in the tumor microenvironment. Adv Exp Med Biol 1224:1–20
5. Selders GS, Fetz AE, Radic MZ, Bowlin GL (2017) An overview of the role of neutrophils in innate immunity, inflammation and host-biomaterial integration. Regen Biomat 4(1):55–68
6. Kruger P, Saffarzadeh M, Weber AN, Rieber N, Radsak M, von Bernuth H et al (2015) Neutrophils: between host defence, immune modulation, and tissue injury. PLoS Pathog 11(3):e1004651
7. Rosales C (2018) Neutrophil: a cell with many roles in inflammation or several cell types? Front Physiol 9:113
8. Mollinedo F (2019) Neutrophil degranulation, plasticity, and cancer metastasis. Trends Immunol 40(3):228–242
9. Fridlender ZG, Sun J, Kim S, Kapoor V, Cheng G, Ling L et al (2009) Polarization of tumor-associated neutrophil phenotype by TGF-beta: "N1" versus "N2" TAN. Cancer Cell 16(3): 183–194
10. Dale DC, Boxer L, Liles WC (2008) The phagocytes: neutrophils and monocytes. Blood 112(4):935–945
11. Peyron P, Maridonneau-Parini I, Stegmann T (2001) Fusion of human neutrophil phagosomes with lysosomes in vitro: involvement of tyrosine kinases of the Src family and inhibition by mycobacteria. J Biol Chem 276(38):35512–35517
12. Winterbourn CC, Kettle AJ, Hampton MB (2016) Reactive oxygen species and neutrophil function. Annu Rev Biochem 85:765–792
13. Cadet J, Wagner JR (2013) DNA base damage by reactive oxygen species, oxidizing agents, and UV radiation. Cold Spring Harb Perspect Biol 5(2):a012559
14. Cooke MS, Evans MD, Dizdaroglu M, Lunec J (2003) Oxidative DNA damage: mechanisms, mutation, and disease. FASEB J 17(10):1195–1214
15. Coffelt SB, Wellenstein MD, de Visser KE (2016) Neutrophils in cancer: neutral no more. Nat Rev Cancer 16(7):431–446
16. Uribe-Querol E, Rosales C (2015) Neutrophils in cancer: two sides of the same coin. J Immunol Res 2015:983698

17. Parekh A, Das S, Parida S, Das CK, Dutta D, Mallick SK et al (2018) Multi-nucleated cells use ROS to induce breast cancer chemo-resistance in vitro and in vivo. Oncogene 37(33): 4546–4561
18. Liou GY, Storz P (2010) Reactive oxygen species in cancer. Free Radic Res 44(5):479–496
19. Dallegri F, Ottonello L, Ballestrero A, Dapino P, Ferrando F, Patrone F et al (1991) Tumor cell lysis by activated human neutrophils: analysis of neutrophil-delivered oxidative attack and role of leukocyte function-associated antigen 1. Inflammation 15(1):15–30
20. Gershkovitz M, Fainsod-Levi T, Zelter T, Sionov RV, Granot Z (2019) TRPM2 modulates neutrophil attraction to murine tumor cells by regulating CXCL2 expression. Cancer Immunol Immunother 68(1):33–43
21. Finisguerra V, Di Conza G, Di Matteo M, Serneels J, Costa S, Thompson AA et al (2015) MET is required for the recruitment of anti-tumoural neutrophils. Nature 522(7556):349–353
22. Wu L, Saxena S, Awaji M, Singh RK (2019) Tumor-associated neutrophils in cancer: going pro. Cancers 11(4):564
23. Powell DR, Huttenlocher A (2016) Neutrophils in the tumor microenvironment. Trends Immunol 37(1):41–52
24. Scapini P, Lapinet-Vera JA, Gasperini S, Calzetti F, Bazzoni F, Cassatella MA (2000) The neutrophil as a cellular source of chemokines. Immunol Rev 177:195–203
25. Queen MM, Ryan RE, Holzer RG, Keller-Peck CR, Jorcyk CL (2005) Breast cancer cells stimulate neutrophils to produce oncostatin M: potential implications for tumor progression. Cancer Res 65(19):8896–8904
26. Elaskalani O, Razak NB, Falasca M, Metharom P (2017) Epithelial-mesenchymal transition as a therapeutic target for overcoming chemoresistance in pancreatic cancer. World J Gastrointest Oncol 9(1):37–41
27. Zhang H, Chen J (2018) Current status and future directions of cancer immunotherapy. J Cancer 9(10):1773–1781
28. Li TJ, Jiang YM, Hu YF, Huang L, Yu J, Zhao LY et al (2017) Interleukin-17-producing neutrophils link inflammatory stimuli to disease progression by promoting angiogenesis in gastric cancer. Clin Cancer Res 23(6):1575–1585
29. de Oliveira S, Reyes-Aldasoro CC, Candel S, Renshaw SA, Mulero V, Calado A (2013) Cxcl8 (IL-8) mediates neutrophil recruitment and behavior in the zebrafish inflammatory response. J Immunol (Baltimore, Md: 1950) 190(8):4349–4359
30. Dumitru CA, Fechner MK, Hoffmann TK, Lang S, Brandau S (2012) A novel p38-MAPK signaling axis modulates neutrophil biology in head and neck cancer. J Leukoc Biol 91(4): 591–598
31. Mishalian I, Bayuh R, Eruslanov E, Michaeli J, Levy L, Zolotarov L et al (2014) Neutrophils recruit regulatory T-cells into tumors via secretion of CCL17--a new mechanism of impaired antitumor immunity. Int J Cancer 135(5):1178–1186
32. Sokol CL, Luster AD (2015) The chemokine system in innate immunity. Cold Spring Harb Perspect Biol 7(5):a016303
33. Borregaard N, Cowland JB (1997) Granules of the human neutrophilic polymorphonuclear leukocyte. Blood 89(10):3503–3521
34. Lerman I, Hammes SR (2018) Neutrophil elastase in the tumor microenvironment. Steroids 133:96–101
35. Foekens JA, Ries C, Look MP, Gippner-Steppert C, Klijn JG, Jochum M (2003) Elevated expression of polymorphonuclear leukocyte elastase in breast cancer tissue is associated with tamoxifen failure in patients with advanced disease. Br J Cancer 88(7):1084–1090
36. Kerros C, Tripathi SC, Zha D, Mehrens JM, Sergeeva A, Philips AV et al (2017) Neuropilin-1 mediates neutrophil elastase uptake and cross-presentation in breast cancer cells. J Biol Chem 292(24):10295–10305
37. Akizuki M, Fukutomi T, Takasugi M, Takahashi S, Sato T, Harao M et al (2007) Prognostic significance of immunoreactive neutrophil elastase in human breast cancer: long-term follow-up results in 313 patients. Neoplasia (New York, NY) 9(3):260–264

38. Chakrabarti S, Zee JM, Patel KD (2006) Regulation of matrix metalloproteinase-9 (MMP-9) in TNF-stimulated neutrophils: novel pathways for tertiary granule release. J Leukoc Biol 79(1): 214–222

39. Nagase H, Visse R, Murphy G (2006) Structure and function of matrix metalloproteinases and TIMPs. Cardiovasc Res 69(3):562–573

40. Lin M, Jackson P, Tester AM, Diaconu E, Overall CM, Blalock JE et al (2008) Matrix metalloproteinase-8 facilitates neutrophil migration through the corneal stromal matrix by collagen degradation and production of the chemotactic peptide Pro-Gly-Pro. Am J Pathol 173(1):144–153

41. Gordon GM, Ledee DR, Feuer WJ, Fini ME (2009) Cytokines and signaling pathways regulating matrix metalloproteinase-9 (MMP-9) expression in corneal epithelial cells. J Cell Physiol 221(2):402–411

42. Finke J, Ko J, Rini B, Rayman P, Ireland J, Cohen P (2011) MDSC as a mechanism of tumor escape from sunitinib mediated anti-angiogenic therapy. Int Immunopharmacol 11(7): 856–861

43. Gutiérrez-Fernández A, Fueyo A, Folgueras AR, Garabaya C, Pennington CJ, Pilgrim S et al (2008) Matrix metalloproteinase-8 functions as a metastasis suppressor through modulation of tumor cell adhesion and invasion. Cancer Res 68(8):2755–2763

44. Thirkettle S, Decock J, Arnold H, Pennington CJ, Jaworski DM, Edwards DR (2013) Matrix metalloproteinase 8 (collagenase 2) induces the expression of interleukins 6 and 8 in breast cancer cells. J Biol Chem 288(23):16282–16294

45. Böckelman C, Beilmann-Lehtonen I, Kaprio T, Koskensalo S, Tervahartiala T, Mustonen H et al (2018) Serum MMP-8 and TIMP-1 predict prognosis in colorectal cancer. BMC Cancer 18(1):679

46. Brinkmann V, Reichard U, Goosmann C, Fauler B, Uhlemann Y, Weiss DS et al (2004) Neutrophil extracellular traps kill bacteria. Science (New York, NY) 303(5663):1532–1535

47. Erpenbeck L, Schön MP (2017) Neutrophil extracellular traps: protagonists of cancer progression? Oncogene 36(18):2483–2490

48. Pilsczek FH, Salina D, Poon KK, Fahey C, Yipp BG, Sibley CD et al (2010) A novel mechanism of rapid nuclear neutrophil extracellular trap formation in response to Staphylococcus aureus. J Immunol (Baltimore, Md: 1950) 185(12):7413–7425

49. Oklu R, Sheth RA, Wong KHK, Jahromi AH, Albadawi H (2017) Neutrophil extracellular traps are increased in cancer patients but does not associate with venous thrombosis. Cardiovas Diagn Ther 7(Suppl 3):S140–S1s9

50. Richardson JJR, Hendrickse C, Gao-Smith F, Thickett DR (2017) Neutrophil extracellular trap production in patients with colorectal cancer in vitro. Int J Inflamm 2017:4915062

51. Berger-Achituv S, Brinkmann V, Abed UA, Kühn LI, Ben-Ezra J, Elhasid R et al (2013) A proposed role for neutrophil extracellular traps in cancer immunoediting. Front Immunol 4:48

52. Yang L, Liu Q, Zhang X, Liu X, Zhou B, Chen J et al (2020) DNA of neutrophil extracellular traps promotes cancer metastasis via CCDC25. Nature 583(7814):133–138

53. Zhou J, Tang Z, Gao S, Li C, Feng Y, Zhou X (2020) Tumor-associated macrophages: recent insights and therapies. Front Oncol 10:188

54. Boussiotis VA, Chatterjee P, Li L (2014) Biochemical signaling of PD-1 on T cells and its functional implications. Cancer J 20(4):265–271

55. Yu GT, Bu LL, Huang CF, Zhang WF, Chen WJ, Gutkind JS et al (2015) PD-1 blockade attenuates immunosuppressive myeloid cells due to inhibition of CD47/SIRPα axis in HPV negative head and neck squamous cell carcinoma. Oncotarget 6(39):42067–42080

56. Katsuya Y, Horinouchi H, Asao T, Kitahara S, Goto Y, Kanda S et al (2016) Expression of programmed death 1 (PD-1) and its ligand (PD-L1) in thymic epithelial tumors: impact on treatment efficacy and alteration in expression after chemotherapy. Lung Cancer 99:4–10

57. Chao MP, Weissman IL, Majeti R (2012) The CD47-SIRPα pathway in cancer immune evasion and potential therapeutic implications. Curr Opin Immunol 24(2):225–232

58. Barkal AA, Weiskopf K, Kao KS, Gordon SR, Rosental B, Yiu YY et al (2018) Engagement of MHC class I by the inhibitory receptor LILRB1 suppresses macrophages and is a target of cancer immunotherapy. Nat Immunol 19(1):76–84
59. Barkal AA, Brewer RE, Markovic M, Kowarsky M, Barkal SA, Zaro BW et al (2019) CD24 signalling through macrophage Siglec-10 is a target for cancer immunotherapy. Nature 572(7769):392–396
60. Bronte V, Brandau S, Chen SH, Colombo MP, Frey AB, Greten TF et al (2016) Recommendations for myeloid-derived suppressor cell nomenclature and characterization standards. Nat Commun 7:12150
61. De Sanctis F, Solito S, Ugel S, Molon B, Bronte V, Marigo I (2016) MDSCs in cancer: conceiving new prognostic and therapeutic targets. Biochim Biophys Acta 1865(1):35–48
62. Kumar V, Patel S, Tcyganov E, Gabrilovich DI (2016) The nature of myeloid-derived suppressor cells in the tumor microenvironment. Trends Immunol 37(3):208–220
63. Solito S, Marigo I, Pinton L, Damuzzo V, Mandruzzato S, Bronte V (2014) Myeloid-derived suppressor cell heterogeneity in human cancers. Ann N Y Acad Sci 1319:47–65
64. Filipazzi P, Huber V, Rivoltini L (2012) Phenotype, function and clinical implications of myeloid-derived suppressor cells in cancer patients. Cancer Immunol Immunother 61(2): 255–263
65. Gabrilovich DI, Ostrand-Rosenberg S, Bronte V (2012) Coordinated regulation of myeloid cells by tumours. Nat Rev Immunol 12(4):253–268
66. Parker KH, Beury DW, Ostrand-Rosenberg S (2015) Myeloid-derived suppressor cells: critical cells driving immune suppression in the tumor microenvironment. Adv Cancer Res 128:95–139
67. Ostrand-Rosenberg S (2010) Myeloid-derived suppressor cells: more mechanisms for inhibiting antitumor immunity. Cancer Immunol Immunother 59(10):1593–1600
68. Pickup M, Novitskiy S, Moses HL (2013) The roles of TGFβ in the tumour microenvironment. Nat Rev Cancer 13(11):788–799
69. Meirow Y, Kanterman J, Baniyash M (2015) Paving the road to tumor development and spreading: myeloid-derived suppressor cells are ruling the fate. Front Immunol 6:523
70. Umansky V, Sevko A (2012) Melanoma-induced immunosuppression and its neutralization. Semin Cancer Biol 22(4):319–326
71. Qu P, Yan C, Du H (2011) Matrix metalloproteinase 12 overexpression in myeloid lineage cells plays a key role in modulating myelopoiesis, immune suppression, and lung tumorigenesis. Blood 117(17):4476–4489
72. Pan PY, Ma G, Weber KJ, Ozao-Choy J, Wang G, Yin B et al (2010) Immune stimulatory receptor CD40 is required for T-cell suppression and T regulatory cell activation mediated by myeloid-derived suppressor cells in cancer. Cancer Res 70(1):99–108
73. Klechevsky E, Morita R, Liu M, Cao Y, Coquery S, Thompson-Snipes L et al (2008) Functional specializations of human epidermal Langerhans cells and CD14+ dermal dendritic cells. Immunity 29(3):497–510
74. Palucka K, Ueno H, Zurawski G, Fay J, Banchereau J (2010) Building on dendritic cell subsets to improve cancer vaccines. Curr Opin Immunol 22(2):258–263
75. Fridman WH, Pages F, Sautes-Fridman C, Galon J (2012) The immune contexture in human tumours: impact on clinical outcome. Nat Rev Cancer 12(4):298–306
76. Fridman WH, Zitvogel L, Sautes-Fridman C, Kroemer G (2017) The immune contexture in cancer prognosis and treatment. Nat Rev Clin Oncol 14(12):717–734
77. Josefowicz SZ, Lu LF, Rudensky AY (2012) Regulatory T cells: mechanisms of differentiation and function. Annu Rev Immunol 30:531–564
78. Wherry EJ, Kurachi M (2015) Molecular and cellular insights into T cell exhaustion. Nat Rev Immunol 15(8):486–499
79. Kurtulus S, Sakuishi K, Ngiow SF, Joller N, Tan DJ, Teng MW et al (2015) TIGIT predominantly regulates the immune response via regulatory T cells. J Clin Invest 125(11):4053–4062

80. Turk MJ, Guevara-Patiño JA, Rizzuto GA, Engelhorn ME, Sakaguchi S, Houghton AN (2004) Concomitant tumor immunity to a poorly immunogenic melanoma is prevented by regulatory T cells. J Exp Med 200(6):771–782

81. Sugiyama D, Nishikawa H, Maeda Y, Nishioka M, Tanemura A, Katayama I et al (2013) Anti-CCR4 mAb selectively depletes effector-type FoxP3+CD4+ regulatory T cells, evoking antitumor immune responses in humans. Proc Natl Acad Sci U S A 110(44):17945–17950

82. Bulliard Y, Jolicoeur R, Zhang J, Dranoff G, Wilson NS, Brogdon JL (2014) OX40 engagement depletes intratumoral Tregs via activating FcγRs, leading to antitumor efficacy. Immunol Cell Biol 92(6):475–480

83. Sharma P, Allison JP (2015) The future of immune checkpoint therapy. Science 348(6230): 56–61

84. Binnewies M, Roberts EW, Kersten K, Chan V, Fearon DF, Merad M et al (2018) Understanding the tumor immune microenvironment (TIME) for effective therapy. Nat Med 24(5): 541–550

85. Chen DS, Mellman I (2017) Elements of cancer immunity and the cancer-immune set point. Nature 541(7637):321–330

86. Jiang P, Gu S, Pan D, Fu J, Sahu A, Hu X et al (2018) Signatures of T cell dysfunction and exclusion predict cancer immunotherapy response. Nat Med 24(10):1550–1558

87. Schietinger A, Philip M, Krisnawan VE, Chiu EY, Delrow JJ, Basom RS et al (2016) Tumor-specific T cell dysfunction is a dynamic antigen-driven differentiation program initiated early during tumorigenesis. Immunity 45(2):389–401

88. Bucks CM, Norton JA, Boesteanu AC, Mueller YM, Katsikis PD (2009) Chronic antigen stimulation alone is sufficient to drive CD8+ T cell exhaustion. J Immunol 182(11):6697–6708

89. Blackburn SD, Shin H, Haining WN, Zou T, Workman CJ, Polley A et al (2009) Coregulation of CD8+ T cell exhaustion by multiple inhibitory receptors during chronic viral infection. Nat Immunol 10(1):29–37

90. Chiu YL, Shan L, Huang H, Haupt C, Bessell C, Canaday DH et al (2014) Sprouty-2 regulates HIV-specific T cell polyfunctionality. J Clin Invest 124(1):198–208

91. Martinez GJ, Pereira RM, Aijo T, Kim EY, Marangoni F, Pipkin ME et al (2015) The transcription factor NFAT promotes exhaustion of activated CD8(+) T cells. Immunity 42(2):265–278

92. Oestreich KJ, Yoon H, Ahmed R, Boss JM (2008) NFATc1 regulates PD-1 expression upon T cell activation. J Immunol 181(7):4832–4839

93. Honda T, Egen JG, Lammermann T, Kastenmuller W, Torabi-Parizi P, Germain RN (2014) Tuning of antigen sensitivity by T cell receptor-dependent negative feedback controls T cell effector function in inflamed tissues. Immunity 40(2):235–247

94. Okazaki T, Chikuma S, Iwai Y, Fagarasan S, Honjo T (2013) A rheostat for immune responses: the unique properties of PD-1 and their advantages for clinical application. Nat Immunol 14(12):1212–1218

95. Wherry EJ (2011) T cell exhaustion. Nat Immunol 12(6):492–499

96. Schietinger A, Greenberg PD (2014) Tolerance and exhaustion: defining mechanisms of T cell dysfunction. Trends Immunol 35(2):51–60

97. Johnston RJ, Comps-Agrar L, Hackney J, Yu X, Huseni M, Yang Y et al (2014) The immunoreceptor TIGIT regulates antitumor and antiviral CD8(+) T cell effector function. Cancer Cell 26(6):923–937

98. Chauvin JM, Pagliano O, Fourcade J, Sun Z, Wang H, Sander C et al (2015) TIGIT and PD-1 impair tumor antigen-specific CD8(+) T cells in melanoma patients. J Clin Invest 125(5): 2046–2058

99. Fourcade J, Sun Z, Benallaoua M, Guillaume P, Luescher IF, Sander C et al (2010) Upregulation of Tim-3 and PD-1 expression is associated with tumor antigen-specific CD8+ T cell dysfunction in melanoma patients. J Exp Med 207(10):2175–2186

100. Fourcade J, Sun Z, Pagliano O, Guillaume P, Luescher IF, Sander C et al (2012) CD8(+) T cells specific for tumor antigens can be rendered dysfunctional by the tumor microenvironment through upregulation of the inhibitory receptors BTLA and PD-1. Cancer Res 72(4):887–896
101. Duraiswamy J, Ibegbu CC, Masopust D, Miller JD, Araki K, Doho GH et al (2011) Phenotype, function, and gene expression profiles of programmed death-1(hi) CD8 T cells in healthy human adults. J Immunol 186(7):4200–4212
102. Baitsch L, Baumgaertner P, Devevre E, Raghav SK, Legat A, Barba L et al (2011) Exhaustion of tumor-specific CD8(+) T cells in metastases from melanoma patients. J Clin Invest 121(6): 2350–2360
103. Taube JM, Anders RA, Young GD, Xu H, Sharma R, McMiller TL et al (2012) Colocalization of inflammatory response with B7-h1 expression in human melanocytic lesions supports an adaptive resistance mechanism of immune escape. Sci Transl Med 4(127):127ra37
104. Huang YH, Zhu C, Kondo Y, Anderson AC, Gandhi A, Russell A et al (2015) CEACAM1 regulates TIM-3-mediated tolerance and exhaustion. Nature 517(7534):386–390
105. Zhu C, Anderson AC, Schubart A, Xiong H, Imitola J, Khoury SJ et al (2005) The Tim-3 ligand galectin-9 negatively regulates T helper type 1 immunity. Nat Immunol 6(12): 1245–1252
106. Fridman WH, Petitprez F, Meylan M, Chen TW, Sun CM, Roumenina LT et al (2021) B cells and cancer: to B or not to B? J Exp Med 218(1):e20200851
107. Garaud S, Buisseret L, Solinas C, Gu-Trantien C, de Wind A, Van den Eynden G et al (2019) Tumor infiltrating B-cells signal functional humoral immune responses in breast cancer. JCI Insight 5(18):e129641
108. Wouters MCA, Nelson BH (2018) Prognostic significance of tumor-infiltrating B cells and plasma cells in human cancer. Clin Cancer Res 24(24):6125–6135
109. Harvey BP, Raycroft MT, Quan TE, Rudenga BJ, Roman RM, Craft J et al (2014) Transfer of antigen from human B cells to dendritic cells. Mol Immunol 58(1):56–65
110. Lu Y, Zhao Q, Liao JY, Song E, Xia Q, Pan J et al (2020) Complement signals determine opposite effects of B cells in chemotherapy-induced immunity. Cell 180(6):1081–97.e24
111. Sautès-Fridman C, Roumenina LT (2020) B cells and complement at the forefront of chemo- therapy. Nat Rev Clin Oncol 17(7):393–394
112. Germain C, Gnjatic S, Tamzalit F, Knockaert S, Remark R, Goc J et al (2014) Presence of B cells in tertiary lymphoid structures is associated with a protective immunity in patients with lung cancer. Am J Respir Crit Care Med 189(7):832–844
113. Montfort A, Pearce O, Maniati E, Vincent BG, Bixby L, Böhm S et al (2017) A strong B-cell response is part of the immune landscape in human high-grade serous ovarian metastases. Clin Cancer Res 23(1):250–262
114. Heesters BA, van der Poel CE, Das A, Carroll MC (2016) Antigen presentation to B cells. Trends Immunol 37(12):844–854
115. Platonova S, Cherfils-Vicini J, Damotte D, Crozet L, Vieillard V, Validire P et al (2011) Profound coordinated alterations of intratumoral NK cell phenotype and function in lung carcinoma. Cancer Res 71(16):5412–5422
116. Gül N, van Egmond M (2015) Antibody-dependent phagocytosis of tumor cells by macro- phages: a potent effector mechanism of monoclonal antibody therapy of cancer. Cancer Res 75(23):5008–5013
117. Su S, Zhao J, Xing Y, Zhang X, Liu J, Ouyang Q et al (2018) Immune checkpoint inhibition overcomes ADCP-induced immunosuppression by macrophages. Cell 175(2):442–57.e23
118. Campa MJ, Gottlin EB, Bushey RT, Patz EF Jr (2015) Complement factor H antibodies from lung cancer patients induce complement-dependent lysis of tumor cells, suggesting a novel immunotherapeutic strategy. Cancer Immunol Res 3(12):1325–1332
119. Clynes R, Ravetch JV (1995) Cytotoxic antibodies trigger inflammation through Fc receptors. Immunity 3(1):21–26

120. Sylvestre D, Clynes R, Ma M, Warren H, Carroll MC, Ravetch JV (1996) Immunoglobulin G-mediated inflammatory responses develop normally in complement-deficient mice. J Exp Med 184(6):2385–2392
121. Kuwabara S, Tsuchikawa T, Nakamura T, Hatanaka Y, Hatanaka KC, Sasaki K et al (2019) Prognostic relevance of tertiary lymphoid organs following neoadjuvant chemoradiotherapy in pancreatic ductal adenocarcinoma. Cancer Sci 110(6):1853–1862
122. Boivin G, Kalambaden P, Faget J, Rusakiewicz S, Montay-Gruel P, Meylan E et al (2018) Cellular composition and contribution of tertiary lymphoid structures to tumor immune infiltration and modulation by radiation therapy. Front Oncol 8:256
123. Nayar S, Campos J, Chung MM, Navarro-Núñez L, Chachlani M, Steinthal N et al (2016) Bimodal expansion of the lymphatic vessels is regulated by the sequential expression of IL-7 and lymphotoxin α1β2 in newly formed tertiary lymphoid structures. J Immunol (Baltimore, Md: 1950) 197(5):1957–1967
124. Barone F, Gardner DH, Nayar S, Steinthal N, Buckley CD, Luther SA (2016) Stromal fibroblasts in tertiary lymphoid structures: a novel target in chronic inflammation. Front Immunol 7:477
125. Jones GW, Hill DG, Jones SA (2016) Understanding immune cells in tertiary lymphoid organ development: it is all starting to come together. Front Immunol 7:401
126. Pitzalis C, Jones GW, Bombardieri M, Jones SA (2014) Ectopic lymphoid-like structures in infection, cancer and autoimmunity. Nat Rev Immunol 14(7):447–462
127. Moyron-Quiroz JE, Rangel-Moreno J, Hartson L, Kusser K, Tighe MP, Klonowski KD et al (2006) Persistence and responsiveness of immunologic memory in the absence of secondary lymphoid organs. Immunity 25(4):643–654
128. Ager A (2017) High endothelial venules and other blood vessels: critical regulators of lymphoid organ development and function. Front Immunol 8:45
129. Dieu-Nosjean MC, Antoine M, Danel C, Heudes D, Wislez M, Poulot V et al (2008) Long-term survival for patients with non-small-cell lung cancer with intratumoral lymphoid structures. J Clin Oncol Off J Am Soc Clin Oncol 26(27):4410–4417
130. Ladányi A, Kiss J, Somlai B, Gilde K, Fejos Z, Mohos A et al (2007) Density of DC-LAMP(+) mature dendritic cells in combination with activated T lymphocytes infiltrating primary cutaneous melanoma is a strong independent prognostic factor. Cancer Immunol Immunother 56(9):1459–1469
131. Zirakzadeh AA, Sherif A, Rosenblatt R, Ahlén Bergman E, Winerdal M, Yang D et al (2020) Tumour-associated B cells in urothelial urinary bladder cancer. Scand J Immunol 91(2): e12830
132. Posch F, Silina K, Leibl S, Mündlein A, Moch H, Siebenhüner A et al (2018) Maturation of tertiary lymphoid structures and recurrence of stage II and III colorectal cancer. Onco Targets Ther 7(2):e1378844
133. Yamakoshi Y, Tanaka H, Sakimura C, Deguchi S, Mori T, Tamura T et al (2020) Immuno-logical potential of tertiary lymphoid structures surrounding the primary tumor in gastric cancer. Int J Oncol 57(1):171–182
134. Lin Q, Tao P, Wang J, Ma L, Jiang Q, Li J et al (2020) Tumor-associated tertiary lymphoid structure predicts postoperative outcomes in patients with primary gastrointestinal stromal tumors. Onco Targets Ther 9(1):1747339
135. Li H, Wang J, Liu H, Lan T, Xu L, Wang G et al (2020) Existence of intratumoral tertiary lymphoid structures is associated with immune cells infiltration and predicts better prognosis in early-stage hepatocellular carcinoma. Aging 12(4):3451–3472
136. Calderaro J, Petitprez F, Becht E, Laurent A, Hirsch TZ, Rousseau B et al (2019) Intra-tumoral tertiary lymphoid structures are associated with a low risk of early recurrence of hepatocellular carcinoma. J Hepatol 70(1):58–65
137. Kroeger DR, Milne K, Nelson BH (2016) Tumor-infiltrating plasma cells are associated with tertiary lymphoid structures, cytolytic T-cell responses, and superior prognosis in ovarian cancer. Clin Cancer Res 22(12):3005–3015

138. Li K, Guo Q, Zhang X, Dong X, Liu W, Zhang A et al (2020) Oral cancer-associated tertiary lymphoid structures: gene expression profile and prognostic value. Clin Exp Immunol 199(2): 172–181
139. Siliņa K, Soltermann A, Attar FM, Casanova R, Uckeley ZM, Thut H et al (2018) Germinal centers determine the prognostic relevance of tertiary lymphoid structures and are impaired by corticosteroids in lung squamous cell carcinoma. Cancer Res 78(5):1308–1320
140. Meylan M, Petitprez F, Lacroix L, Di Tommaso L, Roncalli M, Bougoüin A et al (2020) Early hepatic lesions display immature tertiary lymphoid structures and show elevated expression of immune inhibitory and immunosuppressive molecules. Clin Cancer Res 26(16):4381–4389
141. Finkin S, Yuan D, Stein I, Taniguchi K, Weber A, Unger K et al (2015) Ectopic lymphoid structures function as microniches for tumor progenitor cells in hepatocellular carcinoma. Nat Immunol 16(12):1235–1244
142. Helmink BA, Reddy SM, Gao J, Zhang S, Basar R, Thakur R et al (2020) B cells and tertiary lymphoid structures promote immunotherapy response. Nature 577(7791):549–555
143. Petitprez F, de Reyniès A, Keung EZ, Chen TW, Sun CM, Calderaro J et al (2020) B cells are associated with survival and immunotherapy response in sarcoma. Nature 577(7791):556–560
144. Gu-Trantien C, Migliori E, Buisseret L, de Wind A, Brohée S, Garaud S et al (2017) CXCL13-producing TFH cells link immune suppression and adaptive memory in human breast cancer. JCI Insight 2(11):e91487
145. Cillo AR, Kürten CHL, Tabib T, Qi Z, Onkar S, Wang T et al (2020) Immune landscape of viral- and carcinogen-driven head and neck cancer. Immunity 52(1):183–99.e9
146. Edin S, Kaprio T, Hagström J, Larsson P, Mustonen H, Böckelman C et al (2019) The prognostic importance of CD20(+) B lymphocytes in colorectal cancer and the relation to other immune cell subsets. Sci Rep 9(1):19997
147. Berntsson J, Eberhard J, Nodin B, Leandersson K, Larsson AH, Jirström K (2018) Expression of programmed cell death protein 1 (PD-1) and its ligand PD-L1 in colorectal cancer: relationship with sidedness and prognosis. Onco Targets Ther 7(8):e1465165
148. van Herpen CM, van der Voort R, van der Laak JA, Klasen IS, de Graaf AO, van Kempen LC et al (2008) Intratumoral rhIL-12 administration in head and neck squamous cell carcinoma patients induces B cell activation. Int J Cancer 123(10):2354–2361
149. Santoiemma PP, Reyes C, Wang LP, McLane MW, Feldman MD, Tanyi JL et al (2016) Systematic evaluation of multiple immune markers reveals prognostic factors in ovarian cancer. Gynecol Oncol 143(1):120–127
150. Goeppert B, Frauenschuh L, Zucknick M, Stenzinger A, Andrulis M, Klauschen F et al (2013) Prognostic impact of tumour-infiltrating immune cells on biliary tract cancer. Br J Cancer 109(10):2665–2674
151. Garg K, Maurer M, Griss J, Brüggen MC, Wolf IH, Wagner C et al (2016) Tumor-associated B cells in cutaneous primary melanoma and improved clinical outcome. Hum Pathol 54:157–164
152. Garnelo M, Tan A, Her Z, Yeong J, Lim CJ, Chen J et al (2017) Interaction between tumour-infiltrating B cells and T cells controls the progression of hepatocellular carcinoma. Gut 66(2): 342–351
153. Kurtenkov O, Klaamas K, Mensdorff-Pouilly S, Miljukhina L, Shljapnikova L, Chuzmarov V (2007) Humoral immune response to MUC1 and to the Thomsen-Friedenreich (TF) glycotope in patients with gastric cancer: relation to survival. Acta Oncol (Stockholm, Sweden) 46(3): 316–323
154. Fremd C, Stefanovic S, Beckhove P, Pritsch M, Lim H, Wallwiener M et al (2016) Mucin 1-specific B cell immune responses and their impact on overall survival in breast cancer patients. Onco Targets Ther 5(1):e1057387
155. Roumenina LT, Daugan MV, Noé R, Petitprez F, Vano YA, Sanchez-Salas R et al (2019) Tumor cells hijack macrophage-produced complement C1q to promote tumor growth. Cancer Immunol Res 7(7):1091–1105

156. Kwak JW, Laskowski J, Li HY, McSharry MV, Sippel TR, Bullock BL et al (2018) Complement activation via a c3a receptor pathway alters CD4(+) T lymphocytes and mediates lung cancer progression. Cancer Res 78(1):143–156
157. Ajona D, Pajares MJ, Corrales L, Perez-Gracia JL, Agorreta J, Lozano MD et al (2013) Investigation of complement activation product c4d as a diagnostic and prognostic biomarker for lung cancer. J Natl Cancer Inst 105(18):1385–1393
158. Bosisio FM, Wilmott JS, Volders N, Mercier M, Wouters J, Stas M et al (2016) Plasma cells in primary melanoma. Prognostic significance and possible role of IgA. Mod Pathol 29(4): 347–358
159. Welinder C, Jirström K, Lehn S, Nodin B, Marko-Varga G, Blixt O et al (2016) Intra-tumour IgA1 is common in cancer and is correlated with poor prognosis in bladder cancer. Heliyon 2(8):e00143
160. Shalapour S, Lin XJ, Bastian IN, Brain J, Burt AD, Aksenov AA et al (2017) Inflammation-induced IgA+ cells dismantle anti-liver cancer immunity. Nature 551(7680):340–345

Chapter 4
Local *Onco-Sphere*: Tumor–Stroma Interaction

Phei Er Saw and Erwei Song

Abstract The stroma is a major component of tissues. In a homeostatic condition, stroma of healthy tissues regulates tissue growth, function, and reactivity to external agents by elaborating and modifying the extracellular matrix (ECM), which then transmits signals to surrounding epithelial cells. In a dysfunctional condition, cancer cells interact reciprocally with stroma component (i.e. fibroblasts, adipocytes, etc.), creating a symbiotic relationship that leads to a phenotypical change in tumor-associated stromal components that favors tumor growth. In this chapter, we will focus on summarizing these tumor-stroma interactions in order to understand the close-knit interactions between tumor and stroma in the local onco-sphere.

Introduction

The relevance of cellular interplay is widely understood in developmental biology research [1–4]. These interplays promote organogenesis and maintain homeostasis in normal tissues. The stroma is a major component of tissues, which constitutes of

P. E. Saw
Guangdong Provincial Key Laboratory of Malignant Tumor Epigenetics and Gene Regulation, Guangdong-Hong Kong Joint Laboratory for RNA Medicine, Medical Research Center, Sun Yat-sen Memorial Hospital, Sun Yat-sen University, Guangzhou, China

Nanhai Translational Innovation Center of Precision Immunology, Sun Yat-sen Memorial Hospital, Sun Yat-sen University, Foshan, China

E. Song (✉)
Guangdong Provincial Key Laboratory of Malignant Tumor Epigenetics and Gene Regulation, Guangdong-Hong Kong Joint Laboratory for RNA Medicine, Medical Research Center, Sun Yat-sen Memorial Hospital, Sun Yat-sen University, Guangzhou, China

Nanhai Translational Innovation Center of Precision Immunology, Sun Yat-sen Memorial Hospital, Sun Yat-sen University, Foshan, China

Breast Tumor Center, Sun Yat-sen Memorial Hospital, Sun Yat-sen University, Guangzhou, China
e-mail: songew@mail.sysu.edu.cn

healthy tissues that regulate tissue growth, function, and reactivity to external agents by elaborating and modifying the extracellular matrix (ECM), which then transmits signals to surrounding epithelial cells. Injuries and other pathological settings induce basic alterations in the stroma that are critical for optimal tissue responsiveness [5]. The fibroblast is the primary cell in the stroma, which triggers the production of the majority of connective tissue constituents such as various collagens, proteolytic enzymes, their inhibitory agents, growth regulators, and intercellular adhesion determinants [5]. Due to every tissue's unique needs, fibroblasts from various organs exhibit distinct variants of the abovementioned fundamental molecular types. Additionally, the stroma's fibroblasts alter in response to various physiological cues, including both normal and pathologic [6]. The stromal features of neoplastic tumors, as well as stroma's contribution to carcinogenic processes, will be the focus in this chapter.

Cancer Cell and Stroma Component: A Symbiotic Relationship in the Local *Onco-Sphere*

As the main focus of this book, we focus on the communication in the tumor as an ecosystem. More evidences are pointing toward an evolving cross talk between cancer cells and its surrounding stroma. Prior to this, stromal cells were originally thought to be have a mechanistic or supportive role, regarding as a by-stander rather than an active contributor to cancer malignancy. The tumor stroma is now seen as a specific framework of interconnected communication, including immune cells, fibroblasts, inflammatory cells, pericytes, adipocytes, etc. This network closely resembles the granulation tissue, which was formed during wound healing and therefore was termed as "a wound that never heals" by Hal Dvorak [7]. Tumor cell and its surrounding stroma have a symbiotic relationship where both generate a supportive environment, favoring the growth of the other. For example, cancer cells produce stromal-modulating growth factors (GFs), namely VEGF, PDGF, bFGF, TGF-β, interleukins, cytokines, and chemokines [8]. These factors then act in a paracrine manner to include pro-tumoral stromal reactions, including angiogenesis and inflammatory response; disrupting normal tissue homeostasis. Furthermore, these secreted factors further activate surrounding stromal cells, including fibroblasts, adipocytes, pericytes among others; inducing these cells to secrete additional GFs and proteases (i.e., MMPs, TIMP), forming a positive feedback mechanism that favors cancer cell growth and ultimately leads to tumor progression [9]. The proteases secreted by the stromal cells are capable of degrading ECM molecules to generate new molecule fragments or cryptic peptide/protein that could have pro-angiogenic and pro-migratory function.

Changes in Stroma Components in Cancer Progression

Initially, pathologists noticed the stromal alterations that occur in conjunction with cancer cell development. The firmness of the carcinogenic tumor was related to increased collagen levels and fibroblasts, which were frequently observed around neoplastic development. Desmoplasia was named after the multiplication of fibroblasts, the unique production of α-smooth muscle actin, and the increased prevalence of collagen in the proximity of cancer cells, which signified a shift from the resting [10]. The desmoplastic response is a typical feature of several solid tumors, such as the breast, prostate, colon, and lung cancer, and is sometimes coupled with the induction of inflammatory cells [11]. Early research found an increment in production of stromal cell-associated protein, such as α-smooth muscle actin, vimentin, smooth muscle myosin, calponin, tenascin, and desmin [12]. As myofibroblasts coordinate the healing response, the proteins listed above are frequently produced in response to tissue regeneration or inflammation [5]. Furthermore, the expression level of laminin, an adhesion protein necessary for the structural integrity of the ECM, is either minimally expressed or phenotypically changed in fibroblasts detected in the malignant cells, also known as Cancer-Associated Fibroblasts (CAFs). Recent researchers also found significant changes in other molecules such as dipeptidyl peptidase IV, MMPs, metalloproteinase inhibitors, growth regulators, and collagens [13], and these molecules are also dysregulated (either upregulated or downregulated), to be pro-tumoral. In tumor stroma, fibroblasts exhibit distinct phenotypic characteristics. Many features of fibroblasts in the proximity of tumors have undergone changes. In fibroblasts derived from human malignancies, collagen yield was increased, and hyaluronate synthesis was stimulated [14, 15]. Similarly, multiple in vitro investigations revealed that fibroblasts derived from tumorigenic lesions had irregular growth patterns, uncontrolled multiplication, and altered proliferation capacity (immortality) [11]. Surprisingly, phenotypic alterations in fibroblasts have been observed extrinsically to the lesion's immediate proximity, indicating that fibroblast could also be programmed to influence nearby cells to promote tumor growth (Fig. 4.1) (Box 4.1).

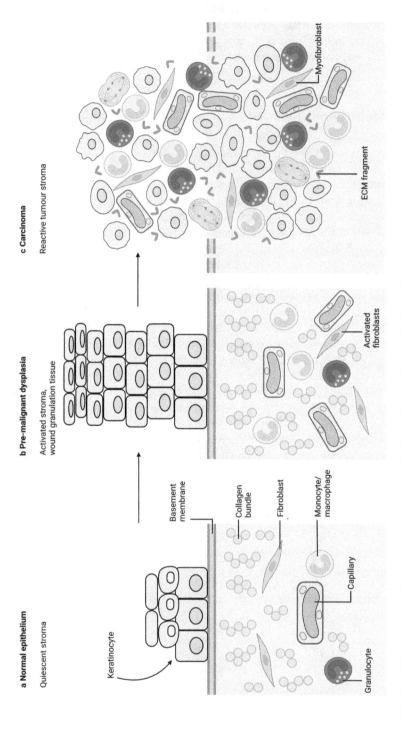

Fig. 4.1 Different stages of stromal activation. (**a**) A typical well-distinguished stratified epithelium is composed of keratinocytes in the epidermis layer and is segregated from the dermal or stromal division by a well-defined basement membrane. This stromal segment is generally made up of collagen comprises resting fibroblasts, mature unbroken blood vessels surrounded by fully functioned capillaries, with few local leukocytes (monocytes and macrophages). (**b**) The

Box 4.1 Does the Aberrant Stroma Play a Functional Role in the Carcinogenic Process?

The short answer is "yes." Multiple experiments, including transplantation of different fibroblasts in conjunction with epithelial cells, were done to specifically address a vital role for stromal fibroblasts in the cancer [16]. Recent research looked at the influence of fibroblasts on nontumorigenic cells as an alternate method [6, 16]. When implanted into host animals singly, each of the four groups of human cells was found to be nontumorigenic. Transplanting carcinoma-associated fibroblasts with human prostatic epithelial cells led to clear alterations in particular phenotypes of the epithelial cells. When regular human prostatic epithelial cells were combined with CAFs, they grew slowly but produced ductal formations resembling Prostatic Intraepithelial Neoplasia (PIN). These grafts demonstrate that the CAFs signals could be received by regular prostatic epithelial cells, but the intercellular interplay does not lead to full-scale tumorigenicity. Transplantation of immortalized human epithelial cells with CAFs yielded the most striking impact. The resultant tumors might weigh 5 g more in a wet state, easily outweighing the mass of control transplants by 500 times. The histopathological study of these tumors revealed that they were malignant. Surprisingly, isolating human epithelial cell populations from these malignant tumors and thereafter transplanting them into another host mice successfully produced tumor of their own. In conclusion, oncogenic cues from the CAF aided in the transformation of a nontumorigenic cell pool into a tumorigenic one. These cells' metamorphosis was associated with non-randomized chromosomal alterations. CAFs stimulated epithelial cells, causing increased cell proliferation, decreased cell death, increased angiogenesis, modified epithelial cells' adhesion characteristics, and, lastly, elevated genomic instability [6].

Fig. 4.1 (continued) differentiation of epithelial cells is disrupted during the progression to pre-malignant dysplasia, leading to the formation of a hyperplastic epithelium (indicated as blue cells). The basement membrane stays undisturbed. Fibroblasts, on the other hand, are activated at this point, and the number of macrophages rises. Angiogenesis occurs, vasculature is matured. (**c**) In carcinoma progression, epithelial cell growth is connected to formation of active tumor stroma. Because of the higher turnover ECM elements like collagen bundles are destroyed in this circumstance. Inflammatory cells increase, fibroblasts develop into myofibroblasts, inducing the production of growth hormones, matrix components, and protease-degrading enzymes. Sustainable angiogenesis leads to the creation of a large number of tumor arteries having leakage. Angiogenesis is sustained so that tumor cell invasion can commence through the damaged basement membrane

Main Stromal Components in Local *Onco-Sphere*

Cancer-Associated Fibroblasts (CAFs)

CAFs are the most abundant stromal cells in the local environment of a solid tumor and are considered the conductor of cross-communications between various cells and their components within the tumor stroma. CAFs are highly heterogeneous, which could be presented as different subtypes, with both pro- and anti-tumoral functions. The origin of CAFs is numerous, and each tumor could comprise a mixture of activated fibroblasts that can originate from quiet resident fibroblasts, bone-marrow-derived mesenchymal stem cells (BM-MSCs), tumor cells, endothelial cells, adipocytes, and stellate cells [17]. TGF-β and PDGF are growth factors released by tumor cells that are interconnected with the activation of CAFs [18] However, the precise role of TGF-β in tumor growth remains debatable. At one end, blocking TGF-β signaling in stromal fibroblasts by blocking TGFβ receptor II has been demonstrated to cause cancer development in epithelial cells [19]. Aberrant expression of TGFβ in skin papilloma of a transgenic rodent model, in contrast, relates to advancement in metastatic tumors, which might be driven by both autocrine and paracrine signaling [20]. TGF-β, in conjunction with PDGF, was demonstrated to be the primary activator of desmoplasia by impacting stromal fibroblasts [21].

CAFs are recognized by an immunocytochemical technique using a mix of markers such as α-smooth muscle actin, vimentin, desmin, and fibroblast activation protein expression (FAP) [22, 23]. FAP is a serine protease available on cell surfaces of reactive tumor stromal fibroblasts identified in granulation tissue during the process of healing injuries [24]. CAFs have been found in the active tumor stroma of numerous cancers, including breast cancer [25], prostate cancer [16], and skin cancer [26]. It has been postulated that their existence predates the initiation of attack and contributes to tumor development and advancement [18]. An in vivo mixture of healthy human prostatic epithelial cells and CAFs constrained the growth of the tumor, corresponding to prostatic intraepithelial neoplasia, whereas grafting CAFs with immortalized non-cancerous prostatic epithelial cells expressing the SV40T antigen led to the development of cancerous tumors [27]. As a result, oncogenic impulses from CAFs appear to promote the development of a nontumorigenic group of epithelial cells in a tumorigenic pool. Research has found that stromal fibroblasts have an identical tumor-inducing function in human SCCs of the skin. Transfecting the nontumorigenic immortalized human keratinocytes (HaCaT) with a vector overexpressing PDGF expression followed by transplantation into mice leads to the production of transitory stromal activation, causing benign tumor development, though non-PDGF-expressing cells continued to be nontumorigenic [26]. Other research has revealed that PDGF-stimulated stromal amplification is facilitated by the transformation of normal dermal fibroblasts into active SMA⁺ fibroblasts that with an identical phenotype to CAFs, which then produce a variety of pro-stroma growth inducers including VEGF and proteases [28]. CAF activation might accelerate tumor growth in multiple ways. They release tenascin and other pro-migratory ECM substances [29]. CAF increases the production of serine proteases and MMPs (i.e. urokinase plasminogen activator (uPA)), where the latter is a mandatory protease required for plasminogen activation to plasmin, a molecule responsible for breakdown and rebuilding of the ECM [30].

Anti-Tumorigenic Role of CAFs

As mentioned above, CAFs are made up of various subsets, in which each has a different and non-connecting role with the others. Therefore, the pro-/anti-tumoral role of CAFs is restricted to specific subtypes. For example, Meflin$^+$ CAFs were shown to be associated with good prognosis in PDAC patients, signifying its anti-tumoral role [31]. Also in PDAC mouse model, deletion of α-SMA$^+$ CAFs increases CD4$^+$ FOXp3$^+$ Treg population in tumor, indicating the importance of α-SMA$^+$ CAFs as having anti-tumoral property [32]. In ER$^+$ breast cancer, CD146 expression is responsible for maintaining ER expression, estrogen responsiveness, and sensitivity toward tamoxifen [33]. VACN$^-$ CAFs promote murine fibrosarcoma growth and angiogenesis, as the loss of VCAN resulted in inhibition of collagen biosynthesis and fibroblast proliferation, which in turn reduces collagen stiffness [34].

Pro-tumorigenic Role of CAFs

On the other hand, CAFs are more famously known to be pro-tumorigenic, as most CAF subsets are prone toward pro-tumoral. CAFs promote cancer development, progression and metastasis, enhanced cell proliferation, inducing migration of cancer cells and increasing therapeutic resistance. TGF-β is one of the most prominent cytokines secreted by CAFs. TGF-β promotes tumor growth and metastasis in various cancers, while promoting EMT via both TGF-β/SMAD and non-SMAD pathways [35]. Furthermore, TGF-β can act as an autocrine that causes positive feedback to prolong constant CAF activation [36]. In hypoxic condition, CAF-secreted VEGF, increases NCBP2-AS2/HIAR axis to promote endothelial sprouting in for new vessel formation [37]. Other CAF-mediated pro-angiogenic factors include FGFs, MMPs, angiopoietin-1, -2, and WNT2 [38].

Immunosuppressive Activity of CAFs

In immunosuppression, CAF-derived cytokines such as TGF-β, IL-6, CXCL5, CXCL12, and SDF-1 are among the important cytokines that suppress immune activity of multiple cell types in the local *onco-sphere*. For example, CAF-derived IL6, SDF-1, and M-CSF are reported to promote the polarization of macrophage toward the M2-like phenotypes that promote EMT and invasion of cancer cells

[39]. Furthermore, CAF-derived PD-1, PD-2, CXCL5, and PGE2 could suppress T cells and NK cells function, leading to an immunosuppressive environment [40, 41].

Metabolic Activity Modulation of CAFs

CAFs can also modulate cancer cells through interference with the metabolic pathways. Under metabolic reprogramming and increment of aerobic glycolysis, CAFs could communicate with proximal cancer cells by the secretion of metabolites (i.e., pyruvate, lactate), thereby increases cancer cell's ATP production, which in turn increases cell proliferation and tumor growth [42–44]. For example, CAFs deprived of Caveolin-1 (CAV-1) have been associated with the increased of glycolytic enzyme's expression, which directly promotes tumor growth and angiogenesis [45, 46]. Furthermore, CCL5, IL6, and CXCL-10 and derived by CAFs and ECM-secreted molecules such as proline were involved in different metabolic signaling pathway to regulate cancer cells [47, 48] (Box 4.2).

Box 4.2 Is CAF Subsets Important in Determining Their Phenotype?

Since CAFs are implicated in all aspects of carcinogenesis, more and more studies are now trying to elucidate the importance of CAF subsets, which are unique in each type of cancer. Apart from the generally accepted categorization using FAP or α-SMA, identifying the pro- or anti-tumoral phenotype of CAF is crucial as there are no specific categorization of CAFs using definite subset identification. Many different biomarkers based on the unique receptors found on CAFs and are currently under preclinical and clinical studies (i.e., LRRC15$^+$, CD10$^+$GPR77$^+$, Netrin G1, Neuregulin 1, CD105, Gli1$^+$, among others). A comprehensive review has been done before in [17]. These subsets have a distinct and usually opposite functions with their counterparts. For example, CD105$^+$ CAFs (found in pancreatic cancer) are pro-tumoral, while CD105− CAFs indicated anti-tumor activity by activating host immune system. This not only affirm the importance of targeting CAF subset specifically; this also indicates a strong relationship between tumor stroma and host immune system [49]. In another example, specific to breast cancer, four subsets have been reported in both the primary tumor and lymph nodes (CAF-S1 to CAF-S4). Among these subsets, CAF-S1 could secrete CXCL12 to recruit CD4$^+$CD25$^+$ Treg cells (an indication of immuno-suppressive phenotype). In the metastatic lymph node, only CAF-S4$^+$ CAFs were more susceptible to distant metastasis [50]. In drug resistance mechanism, NRG1$^+$ CAFs in HER2$^+$ breast cancer patients are indicative of trastuzumab resistance via HER3/AKT pathway [51]. Recently, we also elucidated a unique CD10$^+$GPR77$^+$ CAF subtype in breast cancer and lung cancer that could sustain cancer stem cell renewal ability through activation of NK-kB pathway

(continued)

Box 4.2 (continued)
that results in chemoresistance [52]. In the most recent publication in Cell, our collaborator has identified a novel CD16$^+$ CAFs that are resistant toward trastuzumab treatment. Mechanistically, CD16$^+$ CAF could activate SYK/VAV2/MLC2/MRTF-A axis to increase the collagen expression and α-SMA upregulation, leading a denser and stiff stromal environment, leading to a pro-tumoral environment [53].

Extracellular Matrix (ECM)

The ECM, as a noncellular element, not only offers structural and functional support to cells but also functions as a vast repository of regulators engaged in many cellular functions [54]. Similar with stromal cells, malignant cancer cells may also deposit, degrade, and modify the ECM. By producing multiple ECM proteins such as collagens, fibronectins, laminins, and proteolytic enzymes, cancer cells can now regulate the aberrant behaviors of these ECM components [55]. CAF-secreted VEGF-A could also alter the biochemical composition of the ECM, leading to hydroxylation or enzymatic cross-bonding, increasing their dispersion and permeability across the local *onco-sphere* [56]. Furthermore, as mentioned in the previous chapter, the physical features of ECM, such as stiffness, density, rigidity, and tension, change the environment of the tumor and have a critical impact on the aggressive phenotype (invasion, metastasis) of tumor cells [57]. Matrix breakdown and replacement, as a crucial driver of tissue homeostasis, are controlled by the MMP family members, allowing enhanced angiogenesis, leading to new blood vessel production, which ultimately leads to tumor invasion [58]. As the tumor proliferates, malignant cells fight with neighboring tissues for space and metabolic advantages, leading to the formation of a niche that is simultaneously hypoxic, acidic, and nutrient-deficient, which is favorable in support of the natural selection of cancer cells, as "the survival of the fittest"—only cancer cells with extremely aggressive behavior could survive and proliferate, a major phenomenon seen in the concept of tumor ecosystem.

Major components of ECM such as integrin, thrombospondin-1 (TSP1), fibronectin, and collagen type IV deliver pro- as well as anti-angiogenic cues on the basis of their structural strength and composition. ECM signaling tends to increase the expression of integrin to mediate the adherence of various signaling molecules, to stimulate the malignant phenotype of certain breast carcinomas and SCCs [9]. Both fibronectin and collagen type IV have been proven to possess pro-angiogenic properties due to their binding capacity with 51-integrin and 11-integrin (fibronectin), as well as 21-integrin (collagen type IV) [59], although these are much dependent on different subtypes.

In malignancy, components of the ECM change significantly. As a major component of the ECM, fibronectin is important not only for structural support but also as an anchor for cell-to-cell interactions with integrin, fibrin, and other molecules [60]. Fibronectin is made up of various domains (i.e., Extra-domain A, Extra-domain B and, C), in which some are closely linked to cancer malignancy. In liver cancer, it was found that the strong expression of EDA could be found in neovasculature of liver metastases [61]. In brain glioblastoma cells, the level of malignancy increases as the amount of fibronectin Extra-domain B (EDB) fragment increases [62]. Therefore, we proposed that EDB could be an alternative prognostic biomarker for malignant glioma [63]. The same is true for Tenascin-C, where its overexpression leads to pediatric brainstem glioma tumor progression [64]. As a balancing mechanism, cells also secretes MMPs to degrade the basement-membrane proteins, which in turn limits signaling through these integrins and hence suppresses angiogenesis [65].

Important ECM Constituents

TSP1 a protein generally detected transiently in a wound matrix. In tumor stroma, TSP1 acts as an angiogenesis inhibitory agent. TSP1 overproduction by a carcinogenic and invading human skin SCC cell line restricts the in vivo entry of blood vessels into these tumors, leading to a temporary delay in tumor progression. Although angiogenesis was not originally blocked, the deposition of overproduced TSP1 in a layer encapsulating the tumor hindered the prevention of blood vessel infiltration into the tumor, thus enabling blood vessels to accumulate in the surrounding stroma. Blood-vessel penetration leading to tumor invasion and growth might be restored by inhibiting TSP1 synthesis with antisense oligonucleotides [66]. The latest research suggests that TSP1's anti-angiogenic action is also driven by integrins [67] and maybe inhibited by the breakdown of the TSP1 network by MMPs.

Plasminogen activator inhibitor 1 is an intrinsic protease inhibitor that inhibits plasminogen excitation by urokinase Plasminogen Activator (uPA). In the stroma of skin transplantation animal model, the equilibrium of PAI1 and uPA pushed the balance toward an active protease that may have created anti-angiogenic ECM breakdown products. As a result, tumor vascularization was stopped, and the transplanted mouse skin cancer cells were unable to enter the stroma of the PAI1-deficient host. As a rescue experiment, tumor vascularization and invasion were reinstated, indicating that the vascular deficit occurred due to the lack of PAI1 [68].

Protease function reveals or unlocks cryptic sites that regulate endothelial cells' proliferation, migration, and death [9]. Some of the major proteases in tumor stroma are summarized here. (1) Angiostatin is an amino-terminal component of plasminogen produced by multiple breakdowns of MMP family, including MMP-3, -7, -9, and -12 [69]. As a proteolytic component, angiostatin's major function is to prevent endothelial cell growth and angiogenesis. (2) Endostatin (a proteolytic fragment of type XVIII collagen) suppresses endothelial cell growth and migration as a response to VEGF [70], (3) tumstatin (derived from collagen type IV) has been found to trigger apoptosis in growing endothelial cells [71]. (4) Alternatively, overproduction of membrane-type 1 MMP (MT1-MMP) found in the membrane of melanoma cells is related to enhanced tumor vascularization and tumor development. MT1-MMP promotes tumor angiogenesis by a variety of methods, including $\alpha v \beta 3$—integrin activation (which shields endothelial cells from death), fibrinolytic action, MMP2 activation, and transcriptional control of VEGF expression [72]. In summary, proteases are a double-edged sword. In equilibrium, they can promote angiogenesis by producing reactive ECM components and stimulating angiogenic growth regulators, including VEGF, bFGF, and others [73], but in an imbalanced manner, protease production can offer anti-angiogenic signals, such as the generation of angiogenesis inhibitors by proteolytic alteration of ECM constituents (Fig. 4.2).

CAF-Derived Exosomes: A Potent Communicator

As mentioned above, CAFs can remodel the ECM through autocrine and paracrine factors, namely via cytokines and exosomes. Exosomes (30–150 nm), are a type of natural extracellular vesicles (EVs) [74], usually loaded with proteins, non-coding RNAs, lipids, etc., that could be excreted by the cells to be transferred to another cell, thereby activating or deactivating certain signaling pathways [75]. CAF-derived exosomes are associated with many hallmarks of cancer and therefore are a key communicator between CAF and the other cells in the local *onco-sphere*. We summarized some recent publications on CAFs-derived exosomes in their cross talks with various cells in the local *onco-sphere* (Table 4.1).

As summarized below in Table 4.1, when comparing with normal fibroblast, significant differential expression of cargo could be found in the exosomes of CAF. Since exosomes are packed with proteins, ncRNA, GFs, chemokines, and cytokines, the exosomes can regulate crucial signaling pathway, not only by transferring the exosomes to recipient cells (cancer cells, immune cells, or other stromal cells) in the local *onco-sphere*, they can also act through paracrine manner by releasing these cytokines or chemokines in the tumor vicinity, leading to a cascade of changes in tumor growth, progression, invasion, and metastasis. Nevertheless, exosomes are potentially useful in their clinical translation for cancer therapeutics. Since the cargoes in CAF-exosomes are distinctly different from normal fibroblasts, these can be developed into specific biomarkers in various cancers to detect early prognosis of cancer, while providing an extra layer of personalized therapeutic regimens for individual patient [96]. As a naturally occurring nanosized vehicle, exosomes are non-toxic, fully compatible with minimal adverse effect in patients [97]. Furthermore, exosomes are easily modified or engineered with additional modification to carry specific targeting ligands to increase therapeutic efficacy [98].

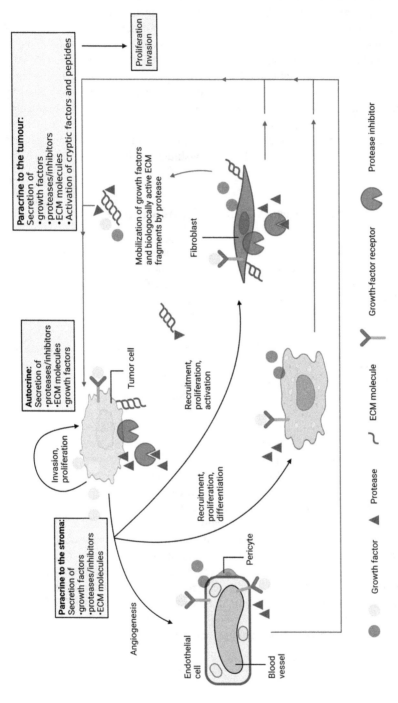

Fig. 4.2 Cross talk between tumor cells and their ECM environment. Tumor cells stimulate their surroundings by producing growth factors and proteases in the stroma. These GF and proteases can either function in autocrine or paracrine manner. The imbalanced (asymmetry) ratio between proteases and their inhibitors results in the degradation of ECM. In paracrine manner, these GFs, proteases, and ECM fragments then stimulate angiogenesis, actively recruit and activate stromal and immune cells. As the main cell type of the stroma, CAFs produce additional growth agents and proteases to augment these signals, resulting in the formation of positive feedback mechanism that favors tumor development

Table 4.1 CAF-derived exosomes in cancer

Function	Cells in local *onco-sphere*	Cargo	Cargo type	Cancer type	Mechanism of action	Ref
Promote EMT and decrease sorafenib sensitivity	Cancer cell	Gremlin-1	Protein	Hepatocellular carcinoma	Regulation of Wnt/β-catenin and BMP signaling pathways	[76]
Promote proliferation and migration	Cancer cell	Sonic Hedgehog (SHH)	Protein	Esophageal squamous cell carcinoma	CAF-exosome transferred SHH to cancer cells	[77]
Promote cell motility	Cancer cells	ADAM metallopeptidase domain 10 (ADAM10)	Protein	Breast cancer	(1) increases ALDH expression through Notch receptor activation	[78]
Increase stem cell marker					(2) enhances motility through RhoA GTPase	
Cell growth and migration	Cancer cells	MFAP5	Protein	oral tongue squamous cell carcinoma (OTSCC)	Through activation of MAPK and AKT pathways	[79]
Cell proliferation and invasion	Macrophages	miRNA-320a	miRNA	Pancreatic cancer	Macrophage polarization to M2 phenotype through PTEN/PI3Kγ signaling	[80]
Promotes gemcitabine resistance	Cancer cells	miR-106b	miRNA	Pancreatic cancer	directly targeting TP53INP1	[81]
Increased survival of drug-resistant cancer cells	Cancer cell	microRNA-146a	miRNA	Epithelial cancer cell	Mi146-a is overexpressed in gemcitabine-treated CAFs (also overexpressing SNAI1).	[82]
Proliferation and metastasis	Cancer cell	miR-34a-5p	miRNA	Oral squamous cell carcinoma	The miR-34a-5p/AXL axis: (1) induce EMT via AKT/GSK-3β/β-catenin signaling pathway (2) enhanced nuclear translocation of β-catenin, induces SNAI1 upregulation, and activate MMP-2 and MMP-9.	[83]

(continued)

Table 4.1 (continued)

Function	Cells in local *onco-sphere*	Cargo	Cargo type	Cancer type	Mechanism of action	Ref
Inhibit proliferation, invasion, migration, and EMT; facilitated apoptosis	Cancer cell	miR-181d-5p	miRNA	Breast cancer	Effective through downregulation of CDX2 and HOXA5	[84]
Proliferation and metastasis	Cancer cell	miR-500a-5p	miRNA	Breast cancer	target and reduces the expression of ubiquitin-specific peptidase 28 (USP28)	[85]
Proliferation, promotes apoptosis	Cancer cells / Infiltrated immune ells	miRNA-92	miRNA	Breast cancer	LATS2 interacts directly with YAP1 to enhance YAP1 nuclear translocation, bind to the enhancer region of PD-L1	[86]
Therapeutic resistance	Cancer cells	miR-22	miRNA	Breast cancer	target estrogen receptor 1 (ESR1) and PTEN; suppressed both expression	[87]
Therapeutic resistance	Cancer cells	miR-423-5p	miRNA	Prostate cancer	Promote taxanes resistance via GREM2 targeting and enhances TGF-β signaling	[88]
Radio resistance	Cancer cells	miR-590-3p	miRNA	Colorectal cancer	Positively regulates the CLCA4-dependent PI3K/Akt signaling pathway	[89]
Enhance cancer stem cell plasticity	CD44+ cancer cells	circHIF1A	circRNA	Breast cancer	decrease the level of miR-580-5p through sponging mechanism, targets CD44 mRNA to downregulate CD44 protein	[90]
Proliferation and invasion	Cancer cell	circEIF3K	circRNA	Colorectal cancer	Targeting miR-214/PD-L1 axis in hypoxic condition	[91]
cell proliferation, migration, invasion and EMT progression	Cancer cells	LINC00659	lncRNA	Colorectal cancer	Direct interaction with miR-342-3p, and increases Annexin A2 (ANXA2) expression	[92]
Promote EMT	Cancer cells	LINC01410	lncRNA			[93]

Multiple metabolic pathways: inhibit mitochondrial oxidative phosphorylation, increase glycolysis carboxylation	Cancer cells	lncRNA SNHG3	lncRNA	Esophageal squamous cell carcinoma	miR-122–5p sponging to increase PKM2 level
				Breast cancer	SNHG3 acts as a miR-330-5p sponge to positively regulate PKM expression	[94]
reprogram the metabolic machinery	Cancer cells	Full CAF-derived exosomes (CDEs) analysis	—	Prostate and pancreatic cancer	Increasing mitochondrial oxidative phosphorylation, increasing glycolysis and glutamine-dependent reductive carboxylation	[95]

Cross talk: Host Systemic *Onco-Sphere* Induces Pro-tumoral Stroma Growth

We are exposed to external carcinogens every second of our lives. Direct exposure to all types of physical carcinogens leads to detrimental effect to the host and induces stromal changes that leads to tumor growth. For example, physical carcinogen (i.e., UV light), chemical carcinogens (i.e., nitroamines), and viral carcinogen (i.e. HPV) were proved to potentially alter cell stroma to stimulate carcinogenesis [6]. Here, we summarize the inherent/internal changes in the systemic *onco-sphere* (the host) that should be taken into consideration, as they might have similar pro-tumorigenic effects. Aging is accompanied by increased collagen as a natural programming system when fibroblast enters senescence. This process also increases the amount of MMPs. Although not much is known about how the increments of collagen and MMPs could contribute to tumor growth, some has suggested that these changes can modulate carcinogenesis [99]. Secondly, the effect of hormone imbalance might be influencing tumor growth. Although no data were shown in human, in rat model, exposure to hormones dramatically changes stromal–tumor cell interaction, leading to the growth of adenocarcinoma. Interestingly, as the sex hormones were elevated, so does the expression of VEGF, TGF-β, and IGF-1, indicating the stimulation of both tumor–stroma interactions to induce tumor growth [100]. Thirdly, inherent congenital or acquired mutation in host cells could generate abnormal phenotypes of cells. For example, when fibroblast-containing congenital mutations are exposed to cancers, these cells were reported to alter tumor–stromal interactions, as seen in a genetic disease, juvenile polyposis of the colon [101]. Taken together, the above factors could be potentially influence carcinogenesis and therefore are equally important and should be taken into consideration in rationalizing cancer treatments (Box 4.3).

Box 4.3 Normalizing the Stroma: A Rational Approach
There is ample evidence to show that an aberrant stromal environment helps in tumor initiation and spread. As a result, "normalization" of the stromal milieu should have the potential for delaying or even reversing tumor growth. Illmensee and Mintz were the first to demonstrate the ability of a normal setting for suppressing a tumorigenic phenotype. They had also revealed that malignant mouse teratocarcinoma cells, cultivated as in vivo ascites tumors through multiple transplant generations, had the ability to develop as normal tissues and produce normal ice upon being injected into blastocysts under development [102]. Others discovered that the existence of a reconstructed physiological basement membrane stops the growth of pre-malignant breast epithelial cells that form polarized alveolar architectures [103]. This normalization is partially achieved by integrins since blocking signals by β1-integrin

---

(continued)

Box 4.3 (continued)
causes regression of carcinogenesis despite the presence of genetic defects in epithelial cells [104]. Similarly, inducing granulation-tissue production in nude mice by implanting a hyaluronan-produced scaffold prior to implanting malignant keratinocytes led to the creation of a fibrotic-rich stroma that could the growth of tumors. This suppression was associated with a dearth of tumor vascularization and was likely induced by the re-creation of a near normal ECM and basement membrane components. Finally, inhibiting angiogenesis is an additional method of regulating the tumor milieu, which can lead to a phenotypic reversal of a cancerous and invasive tumor to a non-invasive pre-malignant tumor phenotype. Collectively, these findings suggest that the tumor microenvironment might be a good therapeutic target. One advantage of attacking the stroma is that the genetic instability of these cells makes them less prone to acquire drug resistance. There are already some remarkable successful anecdotes in tumor stroma's therapeutic targeting. Inhibiting inflammatory cells and cytokines using nonsteroidal anti-inflammatory drugs (NSAIDs) has been found to reduce the likelihood of colon and breast cancer and may help in deterring other cancers as well [105].

Conclusion

It is clear that CAFs are a key stromal component that acts both in favor of and against tumor formation and advancement via a variety of substances secreted by these cells. Other stromal cells and their components are also vital to the creation of a pro-tumoral *onco-sphere*. Although stroma–tumor interaction is vital in the local *onco-sphere*, the intercommunication and cross talk with the systemic *onco-sphere* are crucial when looking at the global effect of the local onco-spheric changes (immune cells, stroma, TME components, etc.) in cancer growth progression. Furthermore, GFs, hormones, EVs, and exosomes generated by either cancer or stromal cells in the local *onco-sphere* can impact biological activities that control malignant growth, tumor response to medicines, and the building of chemoresistance. As we slowly decipher the importance of each component of local, distal, and systemic *onco-sphere*, we will slowly understand the ecological view of cancer.

References

1. Sakakura T, Nishizuka Y, Dawe CJ (1976) Mesenchyme-dependent morphogenesis and epithelium-specific cytodifferentiation in mouse mammary gland. Science 194(4272): 1439–1441

2. Cunha GR, Fujii H, Neubauer BL, Shannon JM, Sawyer L, Reese BA (1983) Epithelial-mesenchymal interactions in prostatic development. I. morphological observations of prostatic induction by urogenital sinus mesenchyme in epithelium of the adult rodent urinary bladder. J Cell Biol 96(6):1662–1670

3. Hayward SW, Cunha GR, Dahiya R (1996) Normal development and carcinogenesis of the prostate. A unifying hypothesis. Ann N Y Acad Sci 784:50–62

4. Johnson RL, Tabin CJ (1997) Molecular models for vertebrate limb development. Cell 90(6): 979–990

5. Sappino AP, Schürch W, Gabbiani G (1990) Differentiation repertoire of fibroblastic cells: expression of cytoskeletal proteins as marker of phenotypic modulations. Lab Investig 63(2): 144–161

6. Tlsty TD (2001) Stromal cells can contribute oncogenic signals. Semin Cancer Biol 11(2): 97–104

7. Dvorak HF, Senger DR, Dvorak AM (1983) Fibrin as a component of the tumor stroma: origins and biological significance. Cancer Metastasis Rev 2(1):41–73

8. Werner S, Grose R (2003) Regulation of wound healing by growth factors and cytokines. Physiol Rev 83(3):835–870

9. Kalluri R (2003) Basement membranes: structure, assembly and role in tumour angiogenesis. Nat Rev Cancer 3(6):422–433

10. Wilis R (1967) Pathology of tumors, 4th edn. Butterworth and Company, London

11. van den Hooff A (1988) Stromal involvement in malignant growth. Adv Cancer Res 50:159–196

12. Mackie EJ, Chiquet-Ehrismann R, Pearson CA, Inaguma Y, Taya K, Kawarada Y et al (1987) Tenascin is a stromal marker for epithelial malignancy in the mammary gland. Proc Natl Acad Sci U S A 84(13):4621–4625

13. Rasmussen AA, Cullen KJ (1998) Paracrine/autocrine regulation of breast cancer by the insulin-like growth factors. Breast Cancer Res Treat 47(3):219–233

14. Bauer EA, Uitto J, Walters RC, Eisen AZ (1979) Enhanced collagenase production by fibroblasts derived from human basal cell carcinomas. Cancer Res 39(11):4594–4599

15. Knudson W, Biswas C, Toole BP (1984) Interactions between human tumor cells and fibroblasts stimulate hyaluronate synthesis. Proc Natl Acad Sci U S A 81(21):6767–6771

16. Olumi AF, Grossfeld GD, Hayward SW, Carroll PR, Tlsty TD, Cunha GR (1999) Carcinoma-associated fibroblasts direct tumor progression of initiated human prostatic epithelium. Cancer Res 59(19):5002–5011

17. Saw PE, Chen J, Song E (2022) Targeting CAFs to overcome anticancer therapeutic resistance. Trends Cancer 8(7):527–555

18. De Wever O, Mareel M (2003) Role of tissue stroma in cancer cell invasion. J Pathol 200(4): 429–447

19. Bhowmick NA, Chytil A, Plieth D, Gorska AE, Dumont N, Shappell S et al (2004) TGF-beta signaling in fibroblasts modulates the oncogenic potential of adjacent epithelia. Science 303(5659):848–851

20. Weeks BH, He W, Olson KL, Wang XJ (2001) Inducible expression of transforming growth factor beta1 in papillomas causes rapid metastasis. Cancer Res 61(20):7435–7443

21. Löhr M, Schmidt C, Ringel J, Kluth M, Müller P, Nizze H et al (2001) Transforming growth factor-beta1 induces desmoplasia in an experimental model of human pancreatic carcinoma. Cancer Res 61(2):550–555

22. Garin-Chesa P, Old LJ, Rettig WJ (1990) Cell surface glycoprotein of reactive stromal fibroblasts as a potential antibody target in human epithelial cancers. Proc Natl Acad Sci U S A 87(18):7235–7239

23. Lazard D, Sastre X, Frid MG, Glukhova MA, Thiery JP, Koteliansky VE (1993) Expression of smooth muscle-specific proteins in myoepithelium and stromal myofibroblasts of normal and malignant human breast tissue. Proc Natl Acad Sci U S A 90(3):999–1003

24. Park JE, Lenter MC, Zimmermann RN, Garin-Chesa P, Old LJ, Rettig WJ (1999) Fibroblast activation protein, a dual specificity serine protease expressed in reactive human tumor stromal fibroblasts. J Biol Chem 274(51):36505–36512
25. Chauhan H, Abraham A, Phillips JR, Pringle JH, Walker RA, Jones JL (2003) There is more than one kind of myofibroblast: analysis of CD34 expression in benign, in situ, and invasive breast lesions. J Clin Pathol 56(4):271–276
26. Skobe M, Fusenig NE (1998) Tumorigenic conversion of immortal human keratinocytes through stromal cell activation. Proc Natl Acad Sci U S A 95(3):1050–1055
27. Cunha GR, Hayward SW, Wang YZ, Ricke WA (2003) Role of the stromal microenvironment in carcinogenesis of the prostate. Int J Cancer 107(1):1–10
28. Fusenig NE, Skobe M, Vosseler S, Hansen M, Lederle W, Airola K et al (2002) Tissue models to study tumor-stroma interactions. In: Foidart JM, Muschel RJ (eds) Proteases and their inhibitors in cancer metastasis. Cancer metastasis — biology and treatment, vol 4. Springer, Dordrecht
29. De Wever O, Nguyen QD, Van Hoorde L, Bracke M, Bruyneel E, Gespach C et al (2004) Tenascin-C and SF/HGF produced by myofibroblasts in vitro provide convergent pro-invasive signals to human colon cancer cells through RhoA and Rac. FASEB J 18(9):1016–1018
30. Sato T, Sakai T, Noguchi Y, Takita M, Hirakawa S, Ito A (2004) Tumor-stromal cell contact promotes invasion of human uterine cervical carcinoma cells by augmenting the expression and activation of stromal matrix metalloproteinases. Gynecol Oncol 92(1):47–56
31. Mizutani Y, Kobayashi H, Iida T, Asai N, Masamune A, Hara A et al (2019) Meflin-positive cancer-associated fibroblasts inhibit pancreatic carcinogenesis. Cancer Res 79(20):5367–5381
32. Ozdemir BC, Pentcheva-Hoang T, Carstens JL, Zheng X, Wu CC, Simpson TR et al (2015) Depletion of carcinoma-associated fibroblasts and fibrosis induces immunosuppression and accelerates pancreas cancer with reduced survival. Cancer Cell 28(6):831–833
33. Brechbuhl HM, Finlay-Schultz J, Yamamoto TM, Gillen AE, Cittelly DM, Tan AC et al (2017) Fibroblast subtypes regulate responsiveness of luminal breast cancer to estrogen. Clin Cancer Res 23(7):1710–1721
34. Fanhchaksai K, Okada F, Nagai N, Pothacharoen P, Kongtawelert P, Hatano S et al (2016) Host stromal versican is essential for cancer-associated fibroblast function to inhibit cancer growth. Int J Cancer 138(3):630–641
35. Yu Y, Xiao CH, Tan LD, Wang QS, Li XQ, Feng YM (2014) Cancer-associated fibroblasts induce epithelial-mesenchymal transition of breast cancer cells through paracrine TGF-beta signalling. Br J Cancer 110(3):724–732
36. Fiori ME, Di Franco S, Villanova L, Bianca P, Stassi G, De Maria R (2019) Cancer-associated fibroblasts as abettors of tumor progression at the crossroads of EMT and therapy resistance. Mol Cancer 18(1):70
37. Kugeratski FG, Atkinson SJ, Neilson LJ, Lilla S, Knight JRP, Serneels J et al (2019) Hypoxic cancer-associated fibroblasts increase NCBP2-AS2/HIAR to promote endothelial sprouting through enhanced VEGF signaling. Sci Signal 12(567):eaan8247
38. Unterleuthner D, Neuhold P, Schwarz K, Janker L, Neuditschko B, Nivarthi H et al (2020) Cancer-associated fibroblast-derived WNT2 increases tumor angiogenesis in colon cancer. Angiogenesis 23(2):159–177
39. Comito G, Giannoni E, Segura CP, Barcellos-de-Souza P, Raspollini MR, Baroni G et al (2014) Cancer-associated fibroblasts and M2-polarized macrophages synergize during prostate carcinoma progression. Oncogene 33(19):2423–2431
40. Pinchuk IV, Saada JI, Beswick EJ, Boya G, Qiu SM, Mifflin RC et al (2008) PD-1 ligand expression by human colonic myofibroblasts/fibroblasts regulates CD4+ T-cell activity. Gastroenterology 135(4):1228–1237, 37.e1-2.
41. Li T, Yang Y, Hua X, Wang G, Liu W, Jia C et al (2012) Hepatocellular carcinoma-associated fibroblasts trigger NK cell dysfunction via PGE2 and IDO. Cancer Lett 318(2):154–161

42. Pavlides S, Whitaker-Menezes D, Castello-Cros R, Flomenberg N, Witkiewicz AK, Frank PG et al (2009) The reverse Warburg effect: aerobic glycolysis in cancer associated fibroblasts and the tumor stroma. Cell Cycle 8(23):3984–4001

43. Gentric G, Mechta-Grigoriou F (2021) Tumor cells and cancer-associated fibroblasts: an updated metabolic perspective. Cancers 13(3):399

44. Wilde L, Roche M, Domingo-Vidal M, Tanson K, Philp N, Curry J et al (2017) Metabolic coupling and the Reverse Warburg Effect in cancer: implications for novel biomarker and anticancer agent development. Semin Oncol 44(3):198–203

45. Shen XJ, Zhang H, Tang GS, Wang XD, Zheng R, Wang Y et al (2015) Caveolin-1 is a modulator of fibroblast activation and a potential biomarker for gastric cancer. Int J Biol Sci 11(4):370–379

46. Simpkins SA, Hanby AM, Holliday DL, Speirs V (2012) Clinical and functional significance of loss of caveolin-1 expression in breast cancer-associated fibroblasts. J Pathol 227(4): 490–498

47. Olivares O, Mayers JR, Gouirand V, Torrence ME, Gicquel T, Borge L et al (2017) Collagen-derived proline promotes pancreatic ductal adenocarcinoma cell survival under nutrient limited conditions. Nat Commun 8:16031

48. Curtis M, Kenny HA, Ashcroft B, Mukherjee A, Johnson A, Zhang Y et al (2019) Fibroblasts mobilize tumor cell glycogen to promote proliferation and metastasis. Cell Metab 29(1): 141–55.e9

49. Hutton C, Heider F, Blanco-Gomez A, Banyard A, Kononov A, Zhang X et al (2021) Single-cell analysis defines a pancreatic fibroblast lineage that supports anti-tumor immunity. Cancer Cell 39(9):1227–44.e20

50. Pelon F, Bourachot B, Kieffer Y, Magagna I, Mermet-Meillon F, Bonnet I et al (2020) Cancer-associated fibroblast heterogeneity in axillary lymph nodes drives metastases in breast cancer through complementary mechanisms. Nat Commun 11(1):404

51. Guardia C, Bianchini G, Arpi LO, Menendez S, Casadevall D, Galbardi B et al (2021) Preclinical and clinical characterization of fibroblast-derived neuregulin-1 on trastuzumab and pertuzumab activity in HER2-positive breast cancer. Clin Cancer Res 27(18):5096–5108

52. Su S, Chen J, Yao H, Liu J, Yu S, Lao L et al (2018) CD10(+)GPR77(+) Cancer-associated fibroblasts promote cancer formation and chemoresistance by sustaining cancer stemness. Cell 172(4):841–56.e16

53. Liu X, Lu Y, Huang J, Xing Y, Dai H, Zhu L et al (2022) CD16(+) fibroblasts foster a trastuzumab-refractory microenvironment that is reversed by VAV2 inhibition. Cancer Cell 40(11):1341–57.e13

54. Cox TR (2021) The matrix in cancer. Nat Rev Cancer 21:217

55. Mohan V, Das A, Sagi I (2020) Emerging roles of ECM remodeling processes in cancer. Semin Cancer Biol 62:192–200

56. Lee S, Jilani SM, Nikolova GV, Carpizo D, Iruela-Arispe ML (2005) Processing of VEGF-A by matrix metalloproteinases regulates bioavailability and vascular patterning in tumors. J Cell Biol 169(4):681–691

57. Wu JS, Sheng SR, Liang XH, Tang YL (2017) The role of tumor microenvironment in collective tumor cell invasion. Fut Oncol 13(11):991–1002

58. Giraudo E, Inoue M, Hanahan D (2004) An amino-bisphosphonate targets MMP-9-expressing macrophages and angiogenesis to impair cervical carcinogenesis. J Clin Invest 114(5): 623–633

59. Jain RK (2003) Molecular regulation of vessel maturation. Nat Med 9(6):685–693

60. Proctor RA (1987) Fibronectin: a brief overview of its structure, function, and physiology. Rev Infect Dis 9(Suppl 4):S317–S321

61. Rybak J-N, Roesli C, Kaspar M, Villa A, Neri D (2007) The extra-domain a of fibronectin is a vascular marker of solid tumors and metastases. Cancer Res 67(22):10948–10957

62. Hooper AT, Marquette K, Chang CB, Golas J, Jain S, Lam MH et al (2022) Anti-extra domain B splice variant of fibronectin antibody-drug conjugate eliminates tumors with enhanced efficacy when combined with checkpoint blockade. Mol Cancer Ther 21(9):1462–1472
63. Saw PE, Xu X, Kang BR, Lee J, Lee YS, Kim C et al (2021) Extra-domain B of fibronectin as an alternative target for drug delivery and a cancer diagnostic and prognostic biomarker for malignant glioma. Theranostics 11(2):941–957
64. Qi J, Esfahani DR, Huang T, Ozark P, Bartom E, Hashizume R et al (2019) Tenascin-C expression contributes to pediatric brainstem glioma tumor phenotype and represents a novel biomarker of disease. Acta Neuropathol Commun 7(1):75
65. Yang C, Zeisberg M, Lively JC, Nyberg P, Afdhal N, Kalluri R (2003) Integrin alpha1beta1 and alpha2beta1 are the key regulators of hepatocarcinoma cell invasion across the fibrotic matrix microenvironment. Cancer Res 63(23):8312–8317
66. Bleuel K, Popp S, Fusenig NE, Stanbridge EJ, Boukamp P (1999) Tumor suppression in human skin carcinoma cells by chromosome 15 transfer or thrombospondin-1 overexpression through halted tumor vascularization. Proc Natl Acad Sci U S A 96(5):2065–2070
67. Lawler J (2000) The functions of thrombospondin-1 and-2. Curr Opin Cell Biol 12(5):634–640
68. Bajou K, Noel A, Gerard RD, Masson V, Brunner N, Holst-Hansen C et al (1998) Absence of host plasminogen activator inhibitor 1 prevents cancer invasion and vascularization. Nat Med 4(8):923–928
69. Dong Z, Kumar R, Yang X, Fidler IJ (1997) Macrophage-derived metalloelastase is responsible for the generation of angiostatin in Lewis lung carcinoma. Cell 88(6):801–810
70. Joki T, Machluf M, Atala A, Zhu J, Seyfried NT, Dunn IF et al (2001) Continuous release of endostatin from microencapsulated engineered cells for tumor therapy. Nat Biotechnol 19(1):35–39
71. Maeshima Y, Colorado PC, Torre A, Holthaus KA, Grunkemeyer JA, Ericksen MB et al (2000) Distinct antitumor properties of a type IV collagen domain derived from basement membrane. J Biol Chem 275(28):21340–21348
72. Sounni NE, Janssen M, Foidart JM, Noel A (2003) Membrane type-1 matrix metalloproteinase and TIMP-2 in tumor angiogenesis. Matrix Biol 22(1):55–61
73. Coussens LM, Werb Z (2002) Inflammation and cancer. Nature 420(6917):860–867
74. Hoshino A, Kim HS, Bojmar L, Gyan KE, Cioffi M, Hernandez J et al (2020) Extracellular vesicle and particle biomarkers define multiple human cancers. Cell 182(4):1044–61.e18
75. Gurunathan S, Kang MH, Jeyaraj M, Qasim M, Kim JH (2019) Review of the isolation, characterization, biological function, and multifarious therapeutic approaches of exosomes. Cells 8(4):307
76. Qin W, Wang L, Tian H, Wu X, Xiao C, Pan Y et al (2022) CAF-derived exosomes transmitted Gremlin-1 promotes cancer progression and decreases the sensitivity of hepatoma cells to sorafenib. Mol Carcinog 61(8):764–775
77. Zhao G, Li H, Guo Q, Zhou A, Wang X, Li P et al (2020) Exosomal Sonic Hedgehog derived from cancer-associated fibroblasts promotes proliferation and migration of esophageal squamous cell carcinoma. Cancer Med 9(7):2500–2513
78. Shimoda M, Principe S, Jackson HW, Luga V, Fang H, Molyneux SD et al (2014) Loss of the Timp gene family is sufficient for the acquisition of the CAF-like cell state. Nat Cell Biol 16(9):889–901
79. Principe S, Mejia-Guerrero S, Ignatchenko V, Sinha A, Ignatchenko A, Shi W et al (2018) Proteomic analysis of cancer-associated fibroblasts reveals a paracrine role for MFAP5 in human oral tongue squamous cell carcinoma. J Proteome Res 17(6):2045–2059
80. Zhao M, Zhuang A, Fang Y (2022) Cancer-associated fibroblast-derived exosomal miRNA-320a promotes macrophage M2 polarization in vitro by regulating PTEN/PI3Kgamma signaling in pancreatic cancer. J Oncol 2022:9514697

81. Fang Y, Zhou W, Rong Y, Kuang T, Xu X, Wu W et al (2019) Exosomal miRNA-106b from cancer-associated fibroblast promotes gemcitabine resistance in pancreatic cancer. Exp Cell Res 383(1):111543

82. Richards KE, Zeleniak AE, Fishel ML, Wu J, Littlepage LE, Hill R (2017) Cancer-associated fibroblast exosomes regulate survival and proliferation of pancreatic cancer cells. Oncogene 36(13):1770–1778

83. Li YY, Tao YW, Gao S, Li P, Zheng JM, Zhang SE et al (2018) Cancer-associated fibroblasts contribute to oral cancer cells proliferation and metastasis via exosome-mediated paracrine miR-34a-5p. EBioMedicine 36:209–220

84. Wang H, Wei H, Wang J, Li L, Chen A, Li Z (2020) MicroRNA-181d-5p-containing exosomes derived from CAFs promote EMT by regulating CDX2/HOXA5 in breast cancer. Mol Ther Nucl Acids 19:654–667

85. Chen B, Sang Y, Song X, Zhang D, Wang L, Zhao W et al (2021) Exosomal miR-500a-5p derived from cancer-associated fibroblasts promotes breast cancer cell proliferation and metastasis through targeting USP28. Theranostics 11(8):3932–3947

86. Dou D, Ren X, Han M, Xu X, Ge X, Gu Y et al (2020) Cancer-associated fibroblasts-derived exosomes suppress immune cell function in breast cancer via the miR-92/PD-L1 pathway. Front Immunol 11:2026

87. Gao Y, Li X, Zeng C, Liu C, Hao Q, Li W et al (2020) CD63(+) Cancer-associated fibroblasts confer tamoxifen resistance to breast cancer cells through exosomal miR-22. Adv Sci 7(21): 2002518

88. Shan G, Gu J, Zhou D, Li L, Cheng W, Wang Y et al (2020) Cancer-associated fibroblast-secreted exosomal miR-423-5p promotes chemotherapy resistance in prostate cancer by targeting GREM2 through the TGF-beta signaling pathway. Exp Mol Med 52(11):1809–1822

89. Chen X, Liu Y, Zhang Q, Liu B, Cheng Y, Zhang Y et al (2021) Exosomal miR-590-3p derived from cancer-associated fibroblasts confers radioresistance in colorectal cancer. Mol Ther Nucl Acids 24:113–126

90. Zhan Y, Du J, Min Z, Ma L, Zhang W, Zhu W et al (2021) Carcinoma-associated fibroblasts derived exosomes modulate breast cancer cell stemness through exonic circHIF1A by miR-580-5p in hypoxic stress. Cell Death Dis 7(1):141

91. Yang K, Zhang J, Bao C (2021) Exosomal circEIF3K from cancer-associated fibroblast promotes colorectal cancer (CRC) progression via miR-214/PD-L1 axis. BMC Cancer 21(1):933

92. Zhou L, Li J, Tang Y, Yang M (2021) Exosomal LncRNA LINC00659 transferred from cancer-associated fibroblasts promotes colorectal cancer cell progression via miR-342-3p/ ANXA2 axis. J Transl Med 19(1):8

93. Shi Z, Jiang T, Cao B, Sun X, Liu J (2022) CAF-derived exosomes deliver LINC01410 to promote epithelial-mesenchymal transition of esophageal squamous cell carcinoma. Exp Cell Res 412(2):113033

94. Li Y, Zhao Z, Liu W, Li X (2020) SNHG3 functions as miRNA sponge to promote breast cancer cells growth through the metabolic reprogramming. Appl Biochem Biotechnol 191(3): 1084–1099

95. Zhao H, Yang L, Baddour J, Achreja A, Bernard V, Moss T et al (2016) Tumor microenvironment derived exosomes pleiotropically modulate cancer cell metabolism. elife 5:e10250

96. LeBleu VS, Kalluri R (2020) Exosomes as a multicomponent biomarker platform in cancer. Trends Cancer 6(9):767–774

97. Popowski K, Lutz H, Hu S, George A, Dinh PU, Cheng K (2020) Exosome therapeutics for lung regenerative medicine. J Extracell Vesic 9(1):1785161

98. Luan X, Sansanaphongpricha K, Myers I, Chen H, Yuan H, Sun D (2017) Engineering exosomes as refined biological nanoplatforms for drug delivery. Acta Pharmacol Sin 38(6): 754–763

99. McCullough KD, Coleman WB, Smith GJ, Grishan JW (1994) Age-dependent regulation of the tumorigenic potential of neoplastically transformed rat liver epithelial cells by the liver microenvironment. Cancer Res 54(14):3668–3671

100. Wang YZ, Wong YC (1998) Sex hormone-induced prostatic carcinogenesis in the noble rat: the role of insulin-like growth factor-I (IGF-I) and vascular endothelial growth factor (VEGF) in the development of prostate cancer. Prostate 35(3):165–177

101. Jacoby RF, Schlack S, Cole CE, Skarbek M, Harris C, Meisner LF (1997) A juvenile polyposis tumor suppressor locus at 10q22 is deleted from nonepithelial cells in the lamina propria. Gastroenterology 112(4):1398–1403

102. Illmensee K, Mintz B (1976) Totipotency and normal differentiation of single teratocarcinoma cells cloned by injection into blastocysts. Proc Natl Acad Sci U S A 73(2):549–553

103. Roskelley CD, Bissell MJ (2002) The dominance of the microenvironment in breast and ovarian cancer. Semin Cancer Biol 12(2):97–104

104. Weaver VM, Petersen OW, Wang F, Larabell CA, Briand P, Damsky C et al (1997) Reversion of the malignant phenotype of human breast cells in three-dimensional culture and in vivo by integrin blocking antibodies. J Cell Biol 137(1):231–245

105. Mueller MM, Fusenig NE (2004) Friends or foes — bipolar effects of the tumour stroma in cancer. Nat Rev Cancer 4(11):839–849

Chapter 5
Local *Onco-Sphere*: Tumor–Secretome Interaction

Phei Er Saw and Erwei Song

Abstract In a tissue, cells secrete proteins, soluble factors, cytokines, chemokines, and metabolites to build up a reservoir, also known as the secretome. In normal physiological condition, the secretome is crucial in controlling the cell-to-cell interaction in a tissue. However, this homeostasis is dysfunctional in cancer condition, as cancer cells could be induced to secrete pro-tumoral juxtracrine and metabolites that favors their growth and survival, while influencing their neighboring cancer, immune and stromal cells into pro-tumoral phenotype. In this chapter, we will discuss about the importance of the interaction between tumor cells and the secretome in the local onco-sphere.

Introduction

The secretome is a reservoir of proteins, soluble factors, cytokines, chemokines, and metabolites that are secreted by a cell. The secretome is crucial in controlling the cell-to-cell relations that are necessary for the local *onco-sphere's* normal physiological functioning (Fig. 5.1). Cancerous secretome changes, which are crucial

P. E. Saw
Guangdong Provincial Key Laboratory of Malignant Tumor Epigenetics and Gene Regulation, Guangdong-Hong Kong Joint Laboratory for RNA Medicine, Medical Research Center, Sun Yat-sen Memorial Hospital, Sun Yat-sen University, Guangzhou, China

Nanhai Translational Innovation Center of Precision Immunology, Sun Yat-sen Memorial Hospital, Sun Yat-sen University, Foshan, China

E. Song (✉)
Guangdong Provincial Key Laboratory of Malignant Tumor Epigenetics and Gene Regulation, Guangdong-Hong Kong Joint Laboratory for RNA Medicine, Medical Research Center, Sun Yat-sen Memorial Hospital, Sun Yat-sen University, Guangzhou, China

Nanhai Translational Innovation Center of Precision Immunology, Sun Yat-sen Memorial Hospital, Sun Yat-sen University, Foshan, China

Breast Tumor Center, Sun Yat-sen Memorial Hospital, Sun Yat-sen University, Guangzhou, China
e-mail: songew@mail.sysu.edu.cn

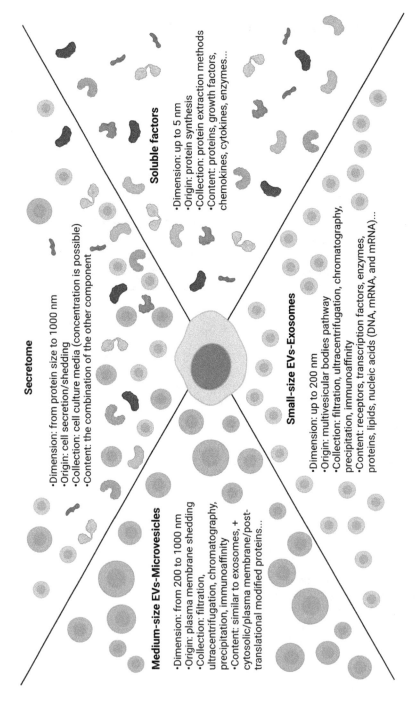

Fig. 5.1 Secretome and their components. Proteins and other soluble components are included in the formulation of a secretome. These include cytokines, chemokines, and biologics such as non-coding RNAs, microvesicles, and small-sized exosomes, without being limited to them

indicators of cancer growth and metastasis, are evident in cancers. Certain bio-markers that have been found through secretome analysis in cancer could be employed therapeutically to treat the disease. Secretome research has also helped researchers understand the molecular basis that cause cancer and, from these knowledge, develop cutting-edge therapeutic approaches [1, 2]. In particular, mutations that promote cancer growth can result in a change in protein expression, dysregulation of cytokines, chemokines, or metabolites, in which all these changes could be easily detected in the serum, providing an easy platform for early diagnosis and treatment response [3]. Herein, we have discussed the significance of these alterations in impacting the distal and systemic *onco-spheres* in this chapter and provided the changes in the local *onco-sphere's* secretome.

Secretome in Cancer

For decades, cancer was thought to be cell-specific, a stand-alone process. The carcinogenesis idea was centered cells being transformed genetically to develop into malignancies [4]. Cancer cells, however, do not behave isolated as they develop into malignant cells, as is becoming increasingly clear. To create a pro-tumoral environment, cancer cells do enlist help from their neighboring cells in the local *onco-sphere*. In a solid tumor, the cancer cell is surrounded by stromal cells (*i.e.,* ECs, fibroblasts, adipocytes) and infiltrated immune cells. In all cases, all these cells would be activated via autocrine or paracrine methods to aid tumor progression [4, 5]. As we learnt in the previous chapter, tumor stroma act as 3D-scaffolds, which are rich in fibronectin, laminins, collagens proteoglycans, providing strong support for tumor tissue [6]. In addition to these structural supports, the non-cellular secretome also serves as a biomolecular scaffold, giving the tumor cell a constant communication with their environment [5]. Some examples of secretome are: cytokines, chemokines, proteins (including hormones), and non-coding RNAs [7, 8].

The heterotypic secretome is a solid proof that the components of a tumor secretome do not originate solely from the tumor cell itself, but rather from its surrounding stromal cells and infiltrated immune cells. This further emphasizes the significance of considering cancer as an ecological system, which was initially put forth in our publication [9], and is extensively covered in this book. Being the center of the *onco-sphere*, tumor cell is a unit that is too small to sustain its own niche. Therefore, it is vital to recruit help from other resident in the niche to create a dynamic, multidirectional communication, which could favor the tumor cell growth, conquering them, turning them from foes to friends. These changes occur dynamically as the tumor grow and progress into malignancy and metastasis, which ultimately changes the normal architecture of a healthy cell's secretome to a site where its high in inflammation, low oxygen, low pH, with dire need for angiogenesis [1, 10].

Genetic mutations and non-mutational alterations that affect gene expression are responsible for changes in secretome composition throughout tumor formation and progression. For example, C-MYC, a transcriptional activator, can activate TGF-β to increase cell proliferation. C-MYC can also activate p53, a secreted factor that promotes cancer cell invasion. PTEN (tumor suppressor protein) loss is also known to lead to an aggressive stromal phenotype, which is also the cause of tumor metastasis [1]. In Ewing sarcoma, Wnt signaling activation leads to an increment in proteases, leading to the degradation/remodeling of ECM [11], which may have an impact on the communication between cancer cells and its surrounding, consequently, the progression of tumors.

Components of the Cancer Secretome

Chemokines

Chemokines are a family of low-molecular-weight soluble proteins (8–15 kDa), which were first discovered as leukocyte trafficking regulators and mediators of the inflammatory process [12, 13]. In addition to their critical roles in angiogenesis, homeostasis, and development, chemokines also play essential roles in autoimmune disorders, tumor-related inflammation, immunology, and tumor growth and metastasis [14, 15]. Chemokines are divided into four major families, which are matching to their receptors; namely CXC, CX3C, CC and C; with their corresponding receptors; CXCR, CX3CR, CCR, and XCR, respectively.

Chemokines and Tumor Growth

Among the chemokines, members of the CXC families, namely CXCL9, CXCL10, and CXCL11, could be stimulated by both classes of interferons: type I (IFN-α and IFN-β) and type II (IFN-γ) IFNs. These chemokines have shown to possess anti-angiogenic activity of CXCR3R-overexpressing ECs, which directly prevents their growth and invasion [16, 17]. These chemokines can also suppress tumor growth by encouraging infiltration on anti-tumoral immune cells into the local *onco-sphere*. CXCL10 and IFN-γ are required for NK cell expansion in tumors, while high levels of stromal cell-secreted CXCR3 and CXCL9 enhance the infiltration of tumor-infiltrating lymphocytes (TILs) [18]. Notably, the release of IFN-γ by tumor cells increases the synthesis of CXC chemokines, further limiting angiogenesis (a phenomenon known as "immuno-angiostasis"). Through this mechanism, chemokines attract more TILs including Th1 CD4+ T cells and CD8+ T cells and also NK cells to the local *onco-sphere* [19]. Not all chemokines are angiostatic, and even non-angiostatic chemokines, such as CXCL16 and CX3CL1, can also promote the activity of T and NKT cells [20]. In renal cancer patients, CXCL16 is produced as a result of radiation therapy and is associated with a better prognosis [21], while in neuroblastoma and colon cancer patients, CX3CL1 expression is correlated with better prognosis.

Tumor and stromal derived-CCL3, CCL4, and CCL5 are crucial for attracting anti-tumoral immune cells to the local *onco-sphere*. In Ewing sarcoma, the expression CXCL9, CXCL10, and CCL5 was associated favorably with the number of CD8$^+$ T cells infiltration, which negatively correlates with tumor growth [22]. In TILs (CD4$^+$ and CD8$^+$ T cells), CCR5 expression is vital for binding to CCL5 on tumor to activate an anti-tumoral response. In addition, CD4$^+$ T cells-activated CCR5 could lead to an overexpression of CD40L on APC, which in turn improves the cross-priming of CD8$^+$ T cell [23]. In an ovarian cancer mouse model, tumor-primed CD4$^+$ T cells could express elevated levels of CCL5, which attract CCR5$^+$ DCs to tumor sites via CD40/CD40L pathway [24]. Clinical data have revealed that CCL20 and CCL17 are important to induce tumoral infiltration of DCs, and therefore, are feasible prognostic markers for early pancreatic cancer diagnosis.

When CCL17 is applied locally to established colon carcinoma lesions, CD4$^+$ and CD8$^+$ T cells (particularly epidermal T cells) are attracted to the skin site and encourage anti-tumoral immunity. Moreover, chemokine and cytokine cocktails, including CCL17, CCL19, CCL21, CCL22, CXCL13, and IL6, can work together to create a functional TLS, which is favorable toward lung cancer patients' survival [25]. TLS may serve as an activation site for tumor-specific T lymphocytes due to the presence of HEVs. When TLS is created, infiltrated DCs in these TLS could interact with memory CD4$^+$ T cells and CD8$^+$ T cells, to reactivate these cells, when necessary [25]. B cells are also one of the major cells presented in the TLS. B cells could secrete CCL4 and CCL22 to attract T cells and then activate these T cells through CD27/CD70 interaction [26]. CXCL10 and CCL21 cause Th1 polarization, whereas CXCL10 and CXCR4 operate as co-stimulators on T cells [27, 28]. There is growing evidence that chemokines released by senescent cells, such as IL-8, cause an innate immune response that clears senescent lesions and regulates benign and preneoplastic lesions [29].

Chemokines and Tumor Progression

By expressing CXCR4, tumor cells can directly bind chemokines that are needed to metastasize [30]. As tumor progresses, to aid in their growth, tumors can alter the local chemokine microenvironment to their favor (Fig. 5.2). For instance, to increase angiogenesis, tumor can secrete CXCL1 and CXCL8 [31, 32]. Additionally, tumors may release various chemokines that attract CD4$^+$CD25$^+$FoxP3$^+$ Tregs, F4/80$^+$ TAMs, and CD11b$^+$Gr-1$^+$ MDSCs immune-suppressive cells. The accumulation of this suppressive infiltration maintains the tolerogenic milieu that promotes tumor growth while undermining antitumor immunity. HIF1α upregulates the intracellular synthesis of CCL28 in ovarian cancer, luring Tregs that then create local immunosuppression, secrete VEGFA, and encourage an increase in the density of the intracellular microvasculature [33]. Tumor-induced immune evasion is promoted by Treg confinement at tumor sites [34], particularly if this is accompanied by a decline in CD8$^+$ T cells [34]. CCL22, a substance released by both cancer cells and TAMs, was also linked to Treg activation in ovarian cancers [35]; however in LLC,

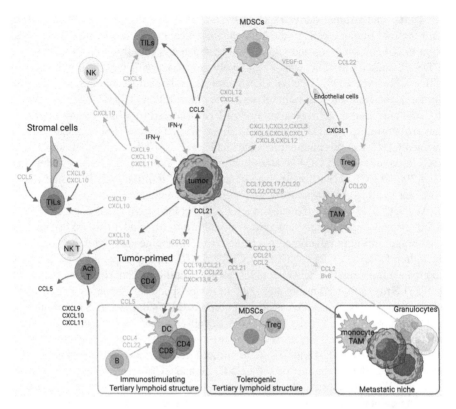

Fig. 5.2 Chemokines, immunity, and cancer progression. Chemokines can be secreted by tumors to have dual effects. They could be anti-tumoral (green) or pro-tumoral (red). In all these signaling pathways, it is clear that chemokines are working closely with various immune cells in the local *onco-sphere*. For example, chemokines could attract the infiltration of immune cells to create a second wave of chemokines (similar with cytokines) that could act in an autocrine or paracrine manner in regulating the tumor growth

this connection is regulated by MDSCs and NK cells [36]. CCL20 was discovered to control CCR6$^+$ Treg migration into colorectal cancer tissues [37]. Additionally, it was discovered that CCL1, CCL17, and CCL22 control the recruitment of Tregs that express CCR4 and CCR8, and they also direct tumorigenic M2-phenotype of macrophage formation [38, 39]. CCL2 also supported the creation of a good milieu for bone marrow metastasis in prostate cancer [40]. Furthermore, in patients with human breast and colorectal cancer, elevated CCL2 was associated with increased TAMs, which leads to lymph node metastases [41, 42].

Although tumor-secreted CCL21 can improve tumor inhibition effect, it also causes lymphangiogenesis. These new lymphoid structures are infiltrated with inhibitory Tregs and MDSCs, creating a tolerogenic environment, indicating a reciprocal relationship that could cancel out the anti-tumoral effect of chemokines although it is currently unclear how the same chemokine could have both pro-tumoral and anti-tumoral effects. One possible reason is the feedback mechanism by the tumor cell per se, which counteracts the functions of chemokines. For example, tumor-secreted TGFβ can suppress $CD8^+$ T cells by polarizing intra-tumoral granulocytes toward an N2 phenotype [43]. The liver X receptor (LXR) oxysterol ligands, among other substances secreted by tumors, can hinder CCR7 expression in DCs, preventing them from moving to lymph nodes and activating T cells that are specific for the tumor. Cancer cells can also overexpress G-CSF, which could increase MDSC mobilization, creating a favorable homing environment for CTCs in a PMN [44, 45].

In various human cancers and mouse tumor studies, the CCL2-CCR2 axis has been shown to be vital in the migration of myeloid cells to the tumor [46]. The build-up of MDSCs in tumors promotes immune evasion and speeds up the development of cancer [47]. In metastatic breast tumor models, the stroma and tumor cells both release CCL2 to stimulate recruitment of inflammatory monocytes ($CD11b^+CD115^+Gr1^+Ly6C^+CCR2^+$) to the lung [48]. The presence of CCR2-expressing MDSCs in melanomas limits the effectiveness of cancer immunotherapy by preventing tumor infiltration of $CD8^+$ T cells [49], and CCR2 deficiency resulted in a considerable reduction of $CD11b^+Gr-1^{int}Ly-6C^{hi}$ monocytic MDSCs and the increment of $CD11b^+Gr-1^{hi}Ly-6C^{int}$ granulocytic MDSCs [50]. The CXCL12/CXCR4 and CXCL5/CXCR2 axes are involved in MDSC infiltration to tumor tissues [51].

Findings from a mammary cancer model, however, bring into question the pro-metastatic function of granulocytes since G-CSF secretion attracts granulocytes to the lungs before any metastatic colonization [52]. Granulocytes, in this instance, displayed a net antimetastatic action by generating hydrogen peroxide, which killed tumor cells. CCL2 was essential in this process for chemoattraction as well as the activation of granulocytes' anticancer activity [52]. B cells may be drawn to tumors by intra0tumoral CXCL13 production, which may have immunosuppressive effects [53], and they may also advance tumors through a variety of mechanisms, such as IgG generation and initiation of Fcγ receptors on myeloid cells. As summarized in Fig. 5.2, we can understand the complexity of tumor-derived chemokines and their multidirectional effect toward other cells (i.e., stromal cells, infiltrated immune cells) in a paracrine manner could also induce feedback favoring the cancer cell growth.

Cytokines in Cancer Secretome

In the local *onco-sphere*, cytokines are important mediators of cell communication [54]. Although cytokines such as IL-2, IFNα, and IFNγ can aid in the TME's antitumor responses, dysregulated cytokine production by cancerous cells, immune cells, and stromal cells plays a role in all stages of carcinogenesis as well as the body's reaction to treatment [55]. Consequently, there is therapeutic value both in utilizing cytokines' immune-stimulating activities and in mitigating their actions when they are dysregulated [56]. Some cytokines are significantly linked to the initiation, growth, and spread of tumors [56, 57] (Fig. 5.3), and aberrant production

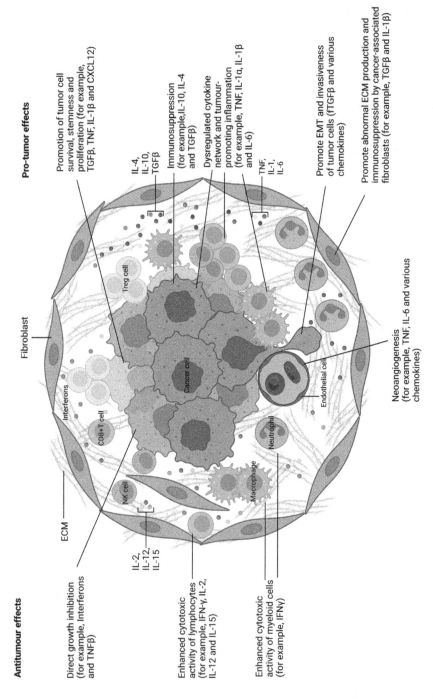

Fig. 5.3 Actions of cytokines in the local *onco-sphere*. The major cell types present in the TME are summarized in this diagram (local *onco-sphere*). The red and green rectangles, which represent tumor-promoting and antitumor actions, respectively, of the cytokines that have been tested in clinical studies on cancer patients, indicate the cytokines' effects on different cell types. Depending on the situation, some cytokines, such as TGF-β, can either have anti-tumoral (LEFT) or pro-tumoral (RIGHT) activity

of inflammatory cytokines is frequently a result of oncogenic alterations in a cell that would otherwise not be malignant. For instance, the exogenous expression of the RET/PTC1 oncogene in non-malignant thyroid cells causes a network of pro-inflammatory cytokines that are equivalent to those conveyed in human thyroid tumors [58]. This oncogene was created through the chromosomal rearrangement of CCDC6 and RET, which is required for the advancement of papillary thyroid cancer. Another illustration is the activation of the Myc proto-oncogene in the setting of murine pancreatic intraepithelial neoplasia, which results in the eventual release of a variety of cytokines that primarily program the progress of a TME with features similar to those of human pancreatic cancer [59]. Ras, Vhl, and Src are examples of common oncogenes and tumor suppressor genes that have yielded similar outcomes [38]. The release of tumor-promoting cytokines during cancer development might also trigger an inflammatory shift in the local *onco-sphere*, despite the fact that it is predicted that 10–25% of all malignancies develop as a result of chronic inflammatory diseases [60, 61].

Six distinct immune subtypes were identified by a meta-analysis of The Cancer Genome Atlas (TCGA) data from over 10,000 tumors representing 33 different cancer types: wound healing, IFN-dominant, inflammatory, lymphocyte deficient, immunologically passive, and TGFβ-dominant [62]. These subgroups often span histology, cell, and origin classifications, while particular driver mutations were connected to variations in immune-cell infiltration in the distal *onco-sphere* (for instance, lower and higher leukocyte densities were associated with the NRAS and BRAF mutations, respectively.). Varied cytokine, chemokine, and their receptor mRNA expression profiles helped to establish the immunological subtypes, and there was also evidence of different cytokine gene methylation, deletion, and amplification patterns [62]. Importantly, the selection of cytokine or cytokine antagonist therapy may be influenced by the classification of tumor subtypes based on cytokine and chemokine signaling networks. In conclusion, numerous solid tumor types share the intricate networks of cytokines and their regulatory pathways found in all TMEs examined to date, while the makeup of these networks can change depending on the immunological environment of a particular lesion (Fig. 5.3).

Exosomes as a Communicator in the Local *Onco-Sphere*

As mentioned briefly in the previous chapter, exosomes may be crucial for cell signaling in the local and systemic *onco-spheres*, according to recently existing research [63]. Exosomes are endocytic-derived, tiny membrane vesicles that range in size from 40 to 100 nm. They include proteins, messenger RNAs (mRNA), DNA fragments, and microRNAs (miRNAs). A donor cell can transfer exosomes to receiving cells [64, 65]. Exosomes from cancer may help recruit the tumor microenvironment and reprogram it to create a pro-tumorigenic setting, according to growing evidence (Fig. 5.4). Generally, exosomal proteins consist of: (1) Annexin, Rab-GTPase (Ras-related protein GTPase Rab), and heat shock proteins (HSPs),

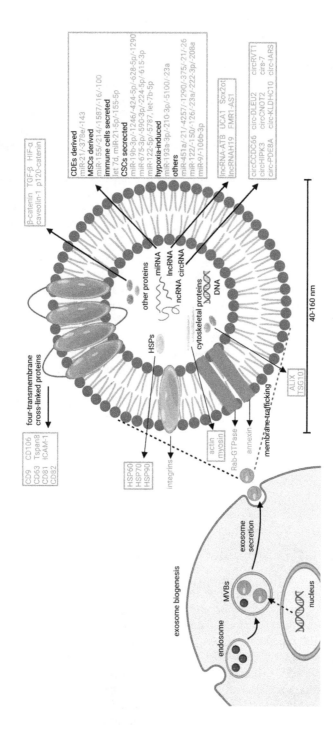

Fig. 5.4 Exosome biogenesis in the local *onco-sphere*. Exosomes are secreted vesicles, which are packed with various biologics, such as proteins, peptides, RNAs, cytokines, chemokines, among others. Research is showing the exosome and their encapsulated materials are crucial to the growth of tumors

such as Hsp60, Hsp70, and Hsp90, which are associated to membrane transport and fusion; (2) Tetraspanins (including CD9, CD63, CD81, CD82, Tspan8, ICAM; (3) MVBs-related proteins include, for example, ALIX and TSG101 (the prototypical exosome biomarker); (4) other proteins, such as integrins, actin, and myosin. The functions of these proteins are reviewed in detail elsewhere [66–68]. Herein, we focus on the recent findings of non-coding RNAs and their functions in tumor-derived exosomes.

Exosomal Noncoding RNAs

miRNA. miRNAs are essential members of small non-coding RNAs with lengths between 20 and 22 nucleotides, mediating posttranscriptional gene silencing of the target mRNA [69, 70]. miRNAs found in exosomes may act as possible biomarkers for cancer prediction and/or grading during the developmental processes of the disease. In NSCLC patients, exosomal miR-451a, miR-21, and miR-4257 were shown to be significantly higher and are associated with tumor growth, relapse, and poor prognosis [71, 72]. In prostate cancer patients, a reduction was seen in Let-7a-5p isolated from plasma EVs. Also in prostate cancer patients, miR-1290 and miR-375 are predictive of the OS of CRPC patients. Data also revealed that patients having consistently high levels of both miR-1290 and miR-375 are predictive of mortality; as this group of patients had a mortality rate of 80%, compared to only 10% of low miRNA-expressing patients [73]. In a series of studies, researchers discovered in the exosomes of CSCs, that there are five miRNAs (miR-224-5p, let-7b-5p, miR-615-3p, miR-122-5p, and miR-5787) that are constantly downregulated, while six signature miRNAs (miR-1246, miR-424-5p, miR-628-5p, miR-1290, miR-675-3p, and miR-590-3p) were upregulated [74–76], indicating the feasibility of the utilization of exosomal miRNA as a potential diagnostic biomarker for CSC detection. Exosomal miRNAs may be advantageous as noninvasive new biomarkers because they can be found in exosomes extracted from body fluids (such as saliva, blood, or serum) [77]. In cholangiocarcinoma, miR-21, miR-26, miR-122, and miR-150 have been used as biomarkers to assess the severity of the disease [78]. In a lung cancer cohort, exosomal miR-126 was shown to be consistently upregulated, while minimally expressed in healthy controls, indicating that exosomal miR-126 is an excellent diagnostic biomarker for lung cancer [79]. Apart from that, serum level of miR-23a has also been found to be overexpressed in lung cancer patients, and miR-23a has been associated with angiogenesis [80]. Interestingly, exosomal miR-222-3p and exosomal miR-208a could also be used to predict gemcitabine sensitivity or radiation responses [81]. Nevertheless, exosomal miRNAs may also aid in the development of tumors in a number of different ways, by communicating with various cells in the local *onco-sphere*. In TNBC cells, exosomal-miR-9 increases the conversion of normal fibroblasts to CAFs by inhibiting E-cadherin secretion, to accelerate tumor migration [82]. Reciprocally, MSCs or CAFs could also secrete exosomes containing miRNAs to be taken up by the tumor cells, initiating tumor growth cascades, leading to drug resistance in gastric cancers, colorectal cancers, and multiple myeloma [83–85].

lncRNA. Over 200 nucleotides in length, long non-coding RNA (lncRNA) lacks crucial coding sequences. lncRNAs have been implicated in many biological functions, especially in cancer [86]. It is a newly discovered that lncRNA has a regulatory role and could be incorporated into exosomes. lncRNAs have been found to modulate various cellular molecular and biological functions such as angiogenesis, metastasis, and tumor growth while also capable of reshaping the local *onco-sphere* [87, 88]. In prostate cancer patients, urine level of exosomal lncRNA-p21 was found to accurately distinguish cancer and benign growth [89]. In colorectal cancer, the cancer cell-derived exosomal lncRNA SNHG10 was found to upregulate inhibin subunit beta C (INHBC), triggering TGF-β pathway to suppress NK cell's function. This study proves that exosomal RNAs could be involved in the immune escape mechanism in colorectal cancer [90]. Furthermore, lncRNAs-ATB promoted tumorigenesis and development primarily by competitively binding to miR-200 family to stimulate EMT in multiple cancers [91]. In liver cancer, CAF-derived exosome carries lncRNA TUG1 to regulate the miR-524-5p/SIX1 axis in cancer cell, leading to dysregulation of glycolysis pathways to promote cancer growth, progression, and metastasis [92]. Additionally, lncRNA is also crucial in cancer resistance [93]. In bladder cancer, by boosting the expression of Wnt6, the lncRNA UCA1 stimulated the Wnt signaling pathway and increases cisplatin resistance [94].

circRNA. Reverse splicing is a unique process for alternative splicing that results in the production of circular RNA (circRNA). It belongs to a unique class of noncoding RNAs that lack polyadenylation tails and the cyclic structure of $5'$-$3'$ polarity and is intrinsically resistant to enzymes that break down nucleic acids by targeting their $5'$ and $3'$ ends [95, 96]. Because of their distinctive circularity, circRNAs are highly stable and can be detected noninvasively in bodily fluids [97]. circRNAs have been demonstrated to bind to endogenous miRNA to prevent miRNA from targeting mRNA and exerting their function [98]. Numerous circRNAs, including circCCDC66, circHIPK3, circPVT1, and cirs-7, are upregulated in cancer, functioning as miRNA competitive inhibitors [99]. circRNAs perform a variety of tasks by controlling the production of genes and microRNAs. They can also influence a number of biological actions that occur during the course of cancer. For example, in prostate cancer patients, circ-IARS were elevated in their plasma exosomes. The increment of circ-IARS resulted in a cascade of events. First, the levels of miR-122 and ZO-1 were dramatically reduced, indicating a sponging mechanism of this circ-IARS, increasing the expression of RhoA and F-actin, which ultimately leads to accelerated tumor growth [100]. The level of serum exosomal-circ-KLDHC10 is indicative of colon cancer [101].

Emerging Player: Cell-Free DNA (cfDNA)

Cell-free DNA (cfDNA) was first found in the serum of a cancer patient in 1977 [102]. Since then, many studies are pointing toward the utilization of cfRNAs either as a diagnostic or as a prognostic biomarker for cancer, as cancer patients in general would always have higher count of total circulating DNA compared to healthy individuals [102, 103]. Furthermore, benign lesion or early-stage cancers have low cfDNAs compared to advanced tumors [104, 105]. cfDNA generated by tumors varied at different stages of cancer; as a result, may represent how the microenvironment and the tumor interact or the distinct metabolic characteristics of developing cancer [106, 107]. For instance, cfDNA levels were found to be linked with metabolic illness in melanoma patients, as determined by ^{18}F-labeled fluorodeoxyglucose PET imaging [108, 109]. The cfDNA level was not just related to tumor volume or the quantity of dying cells, but rather was a complicated reflection of tumor biology. This result implied that cfDNA readings may be more pertinent to disease progression and less pertinent to precancerous lesions. However, the combination of various marker types (such as cfDNA and tumor-related glycoproteins) and the use of multianalyte tools (such as CancerSEEK) indicate potential methods for early tumor diagnosis [110]. Different cfRNAs fragments could contribute to different clinical value. Even the length of cfDNA is important in cancer diagnosis. In a cell-based study, it was revealed that cfDNA is more well-preserved in healthy people [111, 112]. High cfDNA integrity is related to tumor aggressiveness and explained by increased levels of necrotic death in large tumors at late stages [111, 113]. cfDNA could originate from many cellular compartments, such as nucleus. Nuclear DNA is released by neutrophils that have been activated by various stimuli. Such DNA creates neutrophil extracellular traps (NETs). NETosis was formerly thought to just affect neutrophils, but it has since been discovered to also affect mast cells, basophils, and macrophages [114]. These NETs were coated with layers of antibacterial proteins, ECMs, and others that make into a fibrous shape of nets (as the name implies) [114–118]. On the contrary, a different subset of polymorphonuclear leukocytes has the ability to quickly excrete vesicular NETs, allowing them to respond to bacteria in an efficient and timely manner. The residual anuclear neutrophils are not lysed and continue to have the ability to go across NETosis to ingest bacteria [115, 118] (Box 5.1).

Box 5.1 NETosis in Cancer

NETs are observed in tumors at locations where neutrophils have accumulated, in addition to their function in antibacterial defense. These NETs may affect the cancer microenvironment, encourage cancer progression, and help create a pre-metastatic niche, according to certain theories [119]. DNA released by NETosis is activated by a contact channel, which strongly promotes the clotting process. After treatment, this reaction was seen in women

---

(continued)

Box 5.1 (continued)

with breast cancer [120]. It has been demonstrated that the accumulation of NETs in the microvasculature helps to capture and immobilize tumor cells, shields them physically, or produces thrombi that promote tumor growth [118, 121]. NETosis may support the establishment of metastatic niches and enhance metastases. Surgical stress and increased NET development were linked to a fourfold decrease in DFS of liver and colorectal cancer patients [122]. Additionally, even in the lack of infection, cancer cells can cause neutrophils to develop NETs that facilitate metastasis [123]. Certain NET components, including MMP9, may also stimulate ECM remodeling and an promoting angiogenesis to promote metastasis [124]. It has recently been demonstrated that NETs may encourage the development of cancer cells that are currently latent [125]. A hypoxic microenvironment and tumor-derived exosomes can both promote NETosis. In cancer patients, elevated plasma levels of G-CSF, IL-8, and TGF-β can trigger neutrophils to induce NETosis [121, 124, 126]. Potential therapeutic approaches may be suggested by comprehending the part NETs play in the development of tumors. NET-induced vascular dysfunction was reduced by blocking G-CSF and IL-8 production [118, 121, 127]. Vascular function was restored, inflammation was restrained, and tumor cell invasion and metastasis were decreased after NETs were degraded by DNase [123, 128]. P-selectin glycoprotein ligand 1 (PSGL-1), which is involved in the contacts between neutrophils and platelets, can be blocked by antibodies. PAD4, which is connected to the NETosis marker histone citrullination, can also be inhibited. These methods can be viewed as appealing interventional choices for disorders connected to NETs [121, 127–131].

Our group has recently identified a crucial function of NETs in metastasis through activation of ILK/β-parvin/CDC42/Rac1 axis. In this work, we observed an abundance of NETs in breast cancer and colon cancer patients having liver metastasis. In these patients, NET is an independent risk factor for the liver metastasis occurrence, especially in patients with early-stage breast cancer. In the distal *onco-sphere* (in this case, liver), NET-DNA not only functions as a "trap" due to its net-like morphology to immobilize the cancer cells, it also functions as a potent chemotactic factor that could use this chemokine gradient to attract the voluntary movement of these cancer cells toward this new distal *onco-sphere*. Herein, we presented a novel mechanism of an active participation of NET-DNA in the process of distal *onco-sphere* preconditioning (Fig. 5.5).

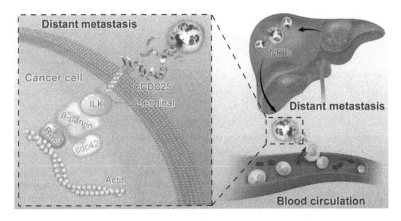

Fig. 5.5 An overall schematic representation of how the NET-DNA binds to a transmembrane protein CCDC25 to activate a cascade of ILK pathway, leading to cancer cell metastasis. Figure reproduced with permission [132]

Cross talk with the Systemic *Onco-Sphere*: Secretome Components and Angiogenesis

In the next chapter, we will look at the physiological changes in the local *oncosphere*, focusing on angiogenesis. Here, we discuss on how the secretome in the local oncosphere could affect angiogenesis, an example of a symbiotic relationship, where constant bidirectional communication is evident. Growth factor regulators, such as HIF1-α, growth factors (*i.e.,* VEGF, FGF, PDGF, and EGF), lysophosphatidic acid (LPA) are the main contributors to angiogenesis [133, 134]. The tumor cells, stromal cells, or infiltrated immune cells may emit these pro- and anti-angiogenic substances [133]. Research found that co-culturing stromal and lung cancer cells encouraged a secretome that boosted stromal cell migration, activated the creation of endothelial tubes, and stimulated cell proliferation [135]. Glioblastoma cells could secrete IL-8, while bone marrow stem cells could produce hepatoma-derived growth factor (HDGF), both are important in angiogenesis [136]. EVs from metastatic cells carry CD276 (or B7-H3), immunoregulator and cell surface tumor endothelial antigen, which has been known to increase micro-vessel density [137]. Tumor-derived RalA-binding protein 1 (also known as RalBP1) is overexpressed in many malignancies. RalBP1 functions through upregulating VEGF secretion and activating HIF-1α transcriptional activity to induce EC proliferation and migration [138, 139]. Additionally, it has been discovered that nonsteroidal anti-inflammatory medicines are successful in preventing tumors. Their primary modes of action are promoting apoptosis and blocking angiogenesis, which prevent the malignant transformation of cells and reduce proliferation.

Cross talk with Systemic *Onco-Sphere*: Secretome Components and Immunomodulation

Damage-associated molecular patterns (DAMPs), which are molecules generated as a result of cell death or damage, mediate the effects that have an immunosuppressive nature. The active release of DNA can have proinflammatory consequences (for example, in vital NETosis). Leukocytes can endocytotically take up this released cfDNA and deposit it in the cytoplasm. Intrinsic DNA, which is released from the nucleus or mitochondria into the cytoplasm following DNA damage or during changes in genes that regulate DNA-damage repair, can also have pro-inflammatory effects. Nucleosomes, unprotected cfDNA, and extracellular histones all have different cytotoxic and pro-inflammatory effects [114]. TNF-α, IL-6, IL-10, and MPO are produced as a result of histones' ability to activate toll-like receptors (TLR2/4), which promote proinflammatory signaling. Additionally, histones show TLR-independent cytotoxicity [140, 141]. They can also cause the development of NETs, which releases additional histones. Histones can cause renal failure, macro- and microvascular thrombosis, and endothelial cytotoxicity [141]. Histone antibodies reduced mortality in multiple sepsis-related mouse models [141]. Contrarily, histones have cytotoxic effects, whereas nucleosomes promote several inflammatory pathways instead [114]. Immune cells identify mtDNA, which resembles bacterial DNA, as a DAMP. However, mtDNA does not have the same properties as bacterial DNA. But unlike bacterial DNA, mtDNA does not promote the creation of IL-6 [142–144]. However, the procoagulant and platelet-stimulating potentials of cfDNAs derived from bacterial, nuclear, and mitochondrial sources are identical [144].

White blood cells, such as neutrophils and DCs, are activated by extracellular mtDNA via TLR9 [142–145]. Pro-inflammatory cytokines are released as a result of TLR9 activation, and AIM2 and NLRP3 inflammasome activation also triggers an immunological interferon response [117, 146]. Tumor-associated inflammation is thought to be caused by cytokines that are released as a result of cfDNATLR9 activation. These signals draw in monocytes and trigger the development of pro-tumorigenic M2 macrophages [147, 148]. The cGAS-STING-IRF3 or the STING-NF-kB pathway detects oxidized mtDNAs or defective nuclear DNA that seeps into the cytosol [145, 149]. STING then stimulates the production of chemokines and cytokines that play a role in the growth of tumors. The IFN-I response can also be activated by DNA via the cGAS-STING pathway. An immunological synapse, for example, can allow DNA to be transmitted from T cells to DCs. The transfer of mtDNA is a component of a system that makes dendritic cells more resistant to viral infection by activating the IFN-I pathway [150]. The activation of STING also causes the expression of PD-L1 to increase [151–153]. Immunosuppression can be caused by upregulating PD-L1, including the PD-L1 molecules found on exosomes, as a result of DNA repair errors or DNA-damaging treatment [151, 154–156].

Conclusion

Cancer is indeed an ecosystem; secretome is the base where all the nutrients, communications are provided, in direct or indirect access to the cancer cell. Cancer secretome is both a rich source of cancer biomarkers and a niche for efficient intra-*onco-spherical* communication. By better understanding the inter-and intra-onco-spherical communication (tumor–stroma, tumor–immune, and tumor–secretome interactions), we can identify potential biomarkers therapies, and therapeutic response predictors through in-depth screening of the tumor stroma, which could pave a way for personalized therapy in the near future.

References

1. Paltridge JL, Belle L, Khew-Goodall Y (2013) The secretome in cancer progression. Biochim Biophys Acta 1834(11):2233–2241
2. Xue H, Lu B, Lai M (2008) The cancer secretome: a reservoir of biomarkers. J Transl Med 6: 52
3. Schaaij-Visser TB, de Wit M, Lam SW, Jiménez CR (2013) The cancer secretome, current status and opportunities in the lung, breast and colorectal cancer context. Biochim Biophys Acta 1834(11):2242–2258
4. Mueller MM, Fusenig NE (2004) Friends or foes - bipolar effects of the tumour stroma in cancer. Nat Rev Cancer 4(11):839–849
5. Hanash S, Schliekelman M (2014) Proteomic profiling of the tumor microenvironment: recent insights and the search for biomarkers. Genome Med 6(2):12
6. Mouw JK, Ou G, Weaver VM (2014) Extracellular matrix assembly: a multiscale deconstruction. Nat Rev Mol Cell Biol 15(12):771–785
7. Nasser MW, Elbaz M, Ahirwar DK, Ganju RK (2015) Conditioning solid tumor microenvironment through inflammatory chemokines and S100 family proteins. Cancer Lett 365(1): 11–22
8. Kohlhapp FJ, Mitra AK, Lengyel E, Peter ME (2015) MicroRNAs as mediators and communicators between cancer cells and the tumor microenvironment. Oncogene 34(48):5857–5868
9. Chen X, Song E (2022) The theory of tumor ecosystem. Cancer Commun 42(7):587–608
10. Zeng X, Yang P, Chen B, Jin X, Liu Y, Zhao X et al (2013) Quantitative secretome analysis reveals the interactions between epithelia and tumor cells by in vitro modulating colon cancer microenvironment. J Proteomics 89:51–70
11. Hawkins AG, Basrur V, da Veiga LF, Pedersen E, Sperring C, Nesvizhskii AI et al (2018) The Ewing Sarcoma secretome and its response to activation of Wnt/beta-catenin signaling. Mol Cell Proteomics 17(5):901–912
12. Moser B, Loetscher P (2001) Lymphocyte traffic control by chemokines. Nat Immunol 2(2): 123–128
13. Moser B, Wolf M, Walz A, Loetscher P (2004) Chemokines: multiple levels of leukocyte migration control. Trends Immunol 25(2):75–84
14. Raman D, Sobolik-Delmaire T, Richmond A (2011) Chemokines in health and disease. Exp Cell Res 317(5):575–589
15. Zlotnik A, Yoshie O (2012) The chemokine superfamily revisited. Immunity 36(5):705–716
16. Romagnani P, Annunziato F, Lasagni L, Lazzeri E, Beltrame C, Francalanci M et al (2001) Cell cycle-dependent expression of CXC chemokine receptor 3 by endothelial cells mediates angiostatic activity. J Clin Invest 107(1):53–63

17. Andreu P, Johansson M, Affara NI, Pucci F, Tan T, Junankar S et al (2010) FcRgamma activation regulates inflammation-associated squamous carcinogenesis. Cancer Cell 17(2): 121–134

18. Ohtani H, Jin Z, Takegawa S, Nakayama T, Yoshie O (2009) Abundant expression of CXCL9 (MIG) by stromal cells that include dendritic cells and accumulation of CXCR3+ T cells in lymphocyte-rich gastric carcinoma. J Pathol 217(1):21–31

19. Strieter RM, Burdick MD, Mestas J, Gomperts B, Keane MP, Belperio JA (2006) Cancer CXC chemokine networks and tumour angiogenesis. Eur J Cancer 42(6):768–778

20. Matsumura S, Wang B, Kawashima N, Braunstein S, Badura M, Cameron TO et al (2008) Radiation-induced CXCL16 release by breast cancer cells attracts effector T cells. J Immunol 181(5):3099–3107

21. Gutwein P, Schramme A, Sinke N, Abdel-Bakky MS, Voss B, Obermüller N et al (2009) Tumoural CXCL16 expression is a novel prognostic marker of longer survival times in renal cell cancer patients. Eur J Cancer 45(3):478–489

22. Berghuis D, Santos SJ, Baelde HJ, Taminiau AH, Egeler RM, Schilham MW et al (2011) Pro-inflammatory chemokine-chemokine receptor interactions within the Ewing sarcoma microenvironment determine CD8(+) T-lymphocyte infiltration and affect tumour progression. J Pathol 223(3):347–357

23. González-Martín A, Gómez L, Lustgarten J, Mira E, Mañes S (2011) Maximal T cell-mediated antitumor responses rely upon CCR5 expression in both CD4(+) and CD8(+) T cells. Cancer Res 71(16):5455–5466

24. Nesbeth YC, Martinez DG, Toraya S, Scarlett UK, Cubillos-Ruiz JR, Rutkowski MR et al (2010) CD4+ T cells elicit host immune responses to MHC class II-negative ovarian cancer through CCL5 secretion and CD40-mediated licensing of dendritic cells. J Immunol 184(10): 5654–5662

25. Dieu-Nosjean MC, Antoine M, Danel C, Heudes D, Wislez M, Poulot V et al (2008) Long-term survival for patients with non-small-cell lung cancer with intratumoral lymphoid structures. J Clin Oncol 26(27):4410–4417

26. Deola S, Panelli MC, Maric D, Selleri S, Dmitrieva NI, Voss CY et al (2008) Helper B cells promote cytotoxic T cell survival and proliferation independently of antigen presentation through CD27/CD70 interactions. J Immunol 180(3):1362–1372

27. Salomon I, Netzer N, Wildbaum G, Schif-Zuck S, Maor G, Karin N (2002) Targeting the function of IFN-gamma-inducible protein 10 suppresses ongoing adjuvant arthritis. J Immunol 169(5):2685–2693

28. Flanagan K, Moroziewicz D, Kwak H, Hörig H, Kaufman HL (2004) The lymphoid chemokine CCL21 costimulates naive T cell expansion and Th1 polarization of non-regulatory CD4+ T cells. Cell Immunol 231(1–2):75–84

29. Acosta JC, Gil J (2009) A role for CXCR2 in senescence, but what about in cancer? Cancer Res 69(6):2167–2170

30. Zlotnik A, Burkhardt AM, Homey B (2011) Homeostatic chemokine receptors and organ-specific metastasis. Nat Rev Immunol 11(9):597–606

31. Gálvez BG, Genís L, Matías-Román S, Oblander SA, Tryggvason K, Apte SS et al (2005) Membrane type 1-matrix metalloproteinase is regulated by chemokines monocyte-chemoattractant protein-1/ccl2 and interleukin-8/CXCL8 in endothelial cells during angiogenesis. J Biol Chem 280(2):1292–1298

32. Singh S, Wu S, Varney M, Singh AP, Singh RK (2011) CXCR1 and CXCR2 silencing modulates CXCL8-dependent endothelial cell proliferation, migration and capillary-like structure formation. Microvasc Res 82(3):318–325

33. Facciabene A, Peng X, Hagemann IS, Balint K, Barchetti A, Wang LP et al (2011) Tumour hypoxia promotes tolerance and angiogenesis via CCL28 and T(reg) cells. Nature 475(7355): 226–230

34. Jacobs JF, Nierkens S, Figdor CG, de Vries IJ, Adema GJ (2012) Regulatory T cells in melanoma: the final hurdle towards effective immunotherapy? Lancet Oncol 13(1):e32–e42

35. Curiel TJ, Coukos G, Zou L, Alvarez X, Cheng P, Mottram P et al (2004) Specific recruitment of regulatory T cells in ovarian carcinoma fosters immune privilege and predicts reduced survival. Nat Med 10(9):942–949
36. Mailloux AW, Clark AM, Young MR (2010) NK depletion results in increased CCL22 secretion and Treg levels in Lewis lung carcinoma via the accumulation of CCL22-secreting CD11b+CD11c+ cells. Int J Cancer 127(11):2598–2611
37. Liu J, Zhang N, Li Q, Zhang W, Ke F, Leng Q et al (2011) Tumor-associated macrophages recruit CCR6+ regulatory T cells and promote the development of colorectal cancer via enhancing CCL20 production in mice. PloS One 6(4):e19495
38. Balkwill FR, Mantovani A (2012) Cancer-related inflammation: common themes and therapeutic opportunities. Semin Cancer Biol 22(1):33–40
39. Roca H, Varsos ZS, Sud S, Craig MJ, Ying C, Pienta KJ (2009) CCL2 and interleukin-6 promote survival of human CD11b+ peripheral blood mononuclear cells and induce M2-type macrophage polarization. J Biol Chem 284(49):34342–34354
40. Loberg RD, Day LL, Harwood J, Ying C, St John LN, Giles R et al (2006) CCL2 is a potent regulator of prostate cancer cell migration and proliferation. Neoplasia 8(7):578–586
41. Bailey C, Negus R, Morris A, Ziprin P, Goldin R, Allavena P et al (2007) Chemokine expression is associated with the accumulation of tumour associated macrophages (TAMs) and progression in human colorectal cancer. Clin Exp Metastasis 24(2):121–130
42. Ueno T, Toi M, Saji H, Muta M, Bando H, Kuroi K et al (2000) Significance of macrophage chemoattractant protein-1 in macrophage recruitment, angiogenesis, and survival in human breast cancer. Clin Cancer Res 6(8):3282–3289
43. Shields JD, Kourtis IC, Tomei AA, Roberts JM, Swartz MA (2010) Induction of lymphoidlike stroma and immune escape by tumors that express the chemokine CCL21. Science 328(5979): 749–752
44. Shojaei F, Wu X, Zhong C, Yu L, Liang XH, Yao J et al (2007) Bv8 regulates myeloid-cell-dependent tumour angiogenesis. Nature 450(7171):825–831
45. Kowanetz M, Wu X, Lee J, Tan M, Hagenbeek T, Qu X et al (2010) Granulocyte-colony stimulating factor promotes lung metastasis through mobilization of Ly6G+Ly6C+ granulocytes. Proc Natl Acad Sci U S A 107(50):21248–21255
46. Huang B, Lei Z, Zhao J, Gong W, Liu J, Chen Z et al (2007) CCL2/CCR2 pathway mediates recruitment of myeloid suppressor cells to cancers. Cancer Lett 252(1):86–92
47. Chioda M, Peranzoni E, Desantis G, Papalini F, Falisi E, Solito S et al (2011) Myeloid cell diversification and complexity: an old concept with new turns in oncology. Cancer Metastasis Rev 30(1):27–43
48. Qian BZ, Li J, Zhang H, Kitamura T, Zhang J, Campion LR et al (2011) CCL2 recruits inflammatory monocytes to facilitate breast-tumour metastasis. Nature 475(7355):222–225
49. Lesokhin AM, Hohl TM, Kitano S, Cortez C, Hirschhorn-Cymerman D, Avogadri F et al (2012) Monocytic CCR2(+) myeloid-derived suppressor cells promote immune escape by limiting activated CD8 T-cell infiltration into the tumor microenvironment. Cancer Res 72(4): 876–886
50. Sawanobori Y, Ueha S, Kurachi M, Shimaoka T, Talmadge JE, Abe J et al (2008) Chemokine-mediated rapid turnover of myeloid-derived suppressor cells in tumor-bearing mice. Blood 111(12):5457–5466
51. Yang L, Huang J, Ren X, Gorska AE, Chytil A, Aakre M et al (2008) Abrogation of TGF beta signaling in mammary carcinomas recruits Gr-1+CD11b+ myeloid cells that promote metastasis. Cancer Cell 13(1):23–35
52. Granot Z, Henke E, Comen EA, King TA, Norton L, Benezra R (2011) Tumor entrained neutrophils inhibit seeding in the premetastatic lung. Cancer Cell 20(3):300–314
53. Qin Z, Richter G, Schüler T, Ibe S, Cao X, Blankenstein T (1998) B cells inhibit induction of T cell-dependent tumor immunity. Nat Med 4(5):627–630
54. Propper DJ, Balkwill FR (2022) Harnessing cytokines and chemokines for cancer therapy. Nat Rev Clin Oncol 19(4):237–253

55. Shalapour S, Karin M (2019) Pas de Deux: control of anti-tumor immunity by cancer-associated inflammation. Immunity 51(1):15–26
56. Waldmann TA (2018) Cytokines in cancer immunotherapy. Cold Spring Harb Perspect Biol 10(12):a028472
57. Berraondo P, Sanmamed MF, Ochoa MC, Etxeberria I, Aznar MA, Pérez-Gracia JL et al (2019) Cytokines in clinical cancer immunotherapy. Br J Cancer 120(1):6–15
58. Borrello MG, Alberti L, Fischer A, Degl'innocenti D, Ferrario C, Gariboldi M et al (2005) Induction of a proinflammatory program in normal human thyrocytes by the RET/PTC1 oncogene. Proc Natl Acad Sci U S A 102(41):14825–14830
59. Sodir NM, Kortlever RM, Barthet VJA, Campos T, Pellegrinet L, Kupczak S et al (2020) MYC instructs and maintains pancreatic adenocarcinoma phenotype. Cancer Discov 10(4): 588–607
60. Diakos CI, Charles KA, McMillan DC, Clarke SJ (2014) Cancer-related inflammation and treatment effectiveness. Lancet Oncol 15(11):e493–e503
61. Mouasni S, Tourneur L (2018) FADD at the crossroads between cancer and inflammation. Trends Immunol 39(12):1036–1053
62. Thorsson V, Gibbs DL, Brown SD, Wolf D, Bortone DS, Ou Yang TH et al (2018) The immune landscape of cancer. Immunity 48(4):812–30.e14
63. Kahlert C, Kalluri R (2013) Exosomes in tumor microenvironment influence cancer progression and metastasis. J Mol Med 91(4):431–437
64. Balaj L, Lessard R, Dai L, Cho YJ, Pomeroy SL, Breakefield XO et al (2011) Tumour microvesicles contain retrotransposon elements and amplified oncogene sequences. Nat Commun 2:180
65. Valadi H, Ekström K, Bossios A, Sjöstrand M, Lee JJ, Lötvall JO (2007) Exosome-mediated transfer of mRNAs and microRNAs is a novel mechanism of genetic exchange between cells. Nat Cell Biol 9(6):654–659
66. Xu J, Liao K, Zhou W (2018) Exosomes regulate the transformation of cancer cells in cancer stem cell homeostasis. Stem Cells Int 2018:4837370
67. Segura E, Nicco C, Lombard B, Véron P, Raposo G, Batteux F et al (2005) ICAM-1 on exosomes from mature dendritic cells is critical for efficient naive T-cell priming. Blood 106(1):216–223
68. Milane L, Singh A, Mattheolabakis G, Suresh M, Amiji MM (2015) Exosome mediated communication within the tumor microenvironment. J Control Release 219:278–294
69. Yang F, Ning Z, Ma L, Liu W, Shao C, Shu Y et al (2017) Exosomal miRNAs and miRNA dysregulation in cancer-associated fibroblasts. Mol Cancer 16(1):148
70. Treiber T, Treiber N, Meister G (2019) Regulation of microRNA biogenesis and its crosstalk with other cellular pathways. Nat Rev Mol Cell Biol 20(1):5–20
71. Kanaoka R, Iinuma H, Dejima H, Sakai T, Uehara H, Matsutani N et al (2018) Usefulness of plasma exosomal microRNA-451a as a noninvasive biomarker for early prediction of recurrence and prognosis of non-small cell lung cancer. Oncology 94(5):311–323
72. Fortunato O, Gasparini P, Boeri M, Sozzi G (2019) Exo-miRNAs as a new tool for liquid biopsy in lung cancer. Cancer 11(6):888
73. Huang X, Yuan T, Liang M, Du M, Xia S, Dittmar R et al (2015) Exosomal miR-1290 and miR-375 as prognostic markers in castration-resistant prostate cancer. Eur Urol 67(1):33–41
74. Sun ZP, Li AQ, Jia WH, Ye S, Van Eps G, Yu JM et al (2017) MicroRNA expression profiling in exosomes derived from gastric cancer stem-like cells. Oncotarget 8(55):93839–93855
75. Shi Y, Wang Z, Zhu X, Chen L, Ma Y, Wang J et al (2020) Exosomal miR-1246 in serum as a potential biomarker for early diagnosis of gastric cancer. Int J Clin Oncol 25(1):89–99
76. Huang J, Shen M, Yan M, Cui Y, Gao Z, Meng X (2019) Exosome-mediated transfer of miR-1290 promotes cell proliferation and invasion in gastric cancer via NKD1. Acta Biochim Biophys Sin 51(9):900–907

77. Nedaeinia R, Manian M, Jazayeri MH, Ranjbar M, Salehi R, Sharifi M et al (2017) Circulating exosomes and exosomal microRNAs as biomarkers in gastrointestinal cancer. Cancer Gene Ther 24(2):48–56

78. Puik JR, Meijer LL, Le Large TY, Prado MM, Frampton AE, Kazemier G et al (2017) miRNA profiling for diagnosis, prognosis and stratification of cancer treatment in cholangiocarcinoma. Pharmacogenomics 18(14):1343–1358

79. Grimolizzi F, Monaco F, Leoni F, Bracci M, Staffolani S, Bersaglieri C et al (2017) Exosomal miR-126 as a circulating biomarker in non-small-cell lung cancer regulating cancer progression. Sci Rep 7(1):15277

80. Hsu YL, Hung JY, Chang WA, Lin YS, Pan YC, Tsai PH et al (2017) Hypoxic lung cancer-secreted exosomal miR-23a increased angiogenesis and vascular permeability by targeting prolyl hydroxylase and tight junction protein ZO-1. Oncogene 36(34):4929–4942

81. Tang Y, Cui Y, Li Z, Jiao Z, Zhang Y, He Y et al (2016) Radiation-induced miR-208a increases the proliferation and radioresistance by targeting p21 in human lung cancer cells. J Exp Clin Cancer Res 35:7

82. Baroni S, Romero-Cordoba S, Plantamura I, Dugo M, D'Ippolito E, Cataldo A et al (2016) Exosome-mediated delivery of miR-9 induces cancer-associated fibroblast-like properties in human breast fibroblasts. Cell Death Dis 7(7):e2312

83. Roccaro AM, Sacco A, Maiso P, Azab AK, Tai YT, Reagan M et al (2013) BM mesenchymal stromal cell-derived exosomes facilitate multiple myeloma progression. J Clin Invest 123(4):1542–1555

84. Wang J, Hendrix A, Hernot S, Lemaire M, De Bruyne E, Van Valckenborgh E et al (2014) Bone marrow stromal cell-derived exosomes as communicators in drug resistance in multiple myeloma cells. Blood 124(4):555–566

85. Hu Y, Yan C, Mu L, Huang K, Li X, Tao D et al (2015) Fibroblast-derived exosomes contribute to chemoresistance through priming cancer stem cells in colorectal cancer. PloS One 10(5):e0125625

86. Saw PE, Xu X, Chen J, Song EW (2021) Non-coding RNAs: the new central dogma of cancer biology. Sci China Life Sci 64(1):22–50

87. Hewson C, Morris KV (2016) Form and function of exosome-associated long non-coding RNAs in cancer. Curr Top Microbiol Immunol 394:41–56

88. Wang M, Zhou L, Yu F, Zhang Y, Li P, Wang K (2019) The functional roles of exosomal long non-coding RNAs in cancer. Cell Mol Life Sci 76(11):2059–2076

89. Isin M, Uysaler E, Ozgur E, Koseoglu H, Sanli O, Yucel OB et al (2015) Exosomal lncRNA-p21 levels may help to distinguish prostate cancer from benign disease. Front Genet 6:168

90. Huang Y, Luo Y, Ou W, Wang Y, Dong D, Peng X et al (2021) Exosomal lncRNA SNHG10 derived from colorectal cancer cells suppresses natural killer cell cytotoxicity by upregulating INHBC. Cancer Cell Int 21(1):528

91. Li J, Li Z, Zheng W, Li X, Wang Z, Cui Y et al (2017) LncRNA-ATB: An indispensable cancer-related long noncoding RNA. Cell Prolif 50(6):e12381

92. Lu L, Huang J, Mo J, Da X, Li Q, Fan M et al (2022) Exosomal lncRNA TUG1 from cancer-associated fibroblasts promotes liver cancer cell migration, invasion, and glycolysis by regulating the miR-524-5p/SIX1 axis. Cell Mol Biol Lett 27(1):17

93. Deng H, Zhang J, Shi J, Guo Z, He C, Ding L et al (2016) Role of long non-coding RNA in tumor drug resistance. Tumour Biol 37(9):11623–11631

94. Chen QN, Wei CC, Wang ZX, Sun M (2017) Long non-coding RNAs in anti-cancer drug resistance. Oncotarget 8(1):1925–1936

95. Fanale D, Taverna S, Russo A, Bazan V (2018) Circular RNA in exosomes. Adv Exp Med Biol 1087:109–117

96. Bao C, Lyu D, Huang S (2016) Circular RNA expands its territory. Mol Cell Oncol 3(2):e1084443

97. Kristensen LS, Andersen MS, Stagsted LVW, Ebbesen KK, Hansen TB, Kjems J (2019) The biogenesis, biology and characterization of circular RNAs. Nat Rev Genet 20(11):675–691

98. Cheng X, Zhang L, Zhang K, Zhang G, Hu Y, Sun X et al (2018) Circular RNA VMA21 protects against intervertebral disc degeneration through targeting miR-200c and X linked inhibitor-of-apoptosis protein. Ann Rheum Dis 77(5):770–779

99. Zhou R, Chen KK, Zhang J, Xiao B, Huang Z, Ju C et al (2018) The decade of exosomal long RNA species: an emerging cancer antagonist. Mol Cancer 17(1):75

100. Li J, Li Z, Jiang P, Peng M, Zhang X, Chen K et al (2018) Circular RNA IARS (circ-IARS) secreted by pancreatic cancer cells and located within exosomes regulates endothelial mono-layer permeability to promote tumor metastasis. J Exp Clin Cancer Res 37(1):177

101. Li Y, Zheng Q, Bao C, Li S, Guo W, Zhao J et al (2015) Circular RNA is enriched and stable in exosomes: a promising biomarker for cancer diagnosis. Cell Res 25(8):981–984

102. Leon SA, Shapiro B, Sklaroff DM, Yaros MJ (1977) Free DNA in the serum of cancer patients and the effect of therapy. Cancer Res 37(3):646–650

103. Zhu YJ, Zhang HB, Liu YH, Zhang FL, Zhu YZ, Li Y et al (2017) Quantitative cell-free circulating EGFR mutation concentration is correlated with tumor burden in advanced NSCLC patients. Lung Cancer 109:124–127

104. Thierry AR, El Messaoudi S, Gahan PB, Anker P, Stroun M (2016) Origins, structures, and functions of circulating DNA in oncology. Cancer Metastasis Rev 35(3):347–376

105. Myint NNM, Verma AM, Fernandez-Garcia D, Sarmah P, Tarpey PS, Al-Aqbi SS et al (2018) Circulating tumor DNA in patients with colorectal adenomas: assessment of detectability and genetic heterogeneity. Cell Death Dis 9(9):894

106. Diehl F, Li M, Dressman D, He Y, Shen D, Szabo S et al (2005) Detection and quantification of mutations in the plasma of patients with colorectal tumors. Proc Natl Acad Sci U S A 102(45):16368–16373

107. Xia L, Li Z, Zhou B, Tian G, Zeng L, Dai H et al (2017) Statistical analysis of mutant allele frequency level of circulating cell-free DNA and blood cells in healthy individuals. Sci Rep 7(1):7526

108. Wong SQ, Raleigh JM, Callahan J, Vergara IA, Ftouni S, Hatzimihalis A et al (2017) Circulating tumor DNA analysis and functional imaging provide complementary approaches for comprehensive disease monitoring in metastatic melanoma. JCO Precis Oncol 1:1–14

109. McEvoy AC, Warburton L, Al-Ogaili Z, Celliers L, Calapre L, Pereira MR et al (2018) Correlation between circulating tumour DNA and metabolic tumour burden in metastatic melanoma patients. BMC Cancer 18(1):726

110. Cohen JD, Li L, Wang Y, Thoburn C, Afsari B, Danilova L et al (2018) Detection and localization of surgically resectable cancers with a multi-analyte blood test. Science 359(6378):926–930

111. Chen H, Sun LY, Zheng HQ, Zhang QF, Jin XM (2012) Total serum DNA and DNA integrity: diagnostic value in patients with hepatitis B virus-related hepatocellular carcinoma. Pathology 44(4):318–324

112. Gang F, Guorong L, An Z, Anne GP, Christian G, Jacques T (2010) Prediction of clear cell renal cell carcinoma by integrity of cell-free DNA in serum. Urology 75(2):262–265

113. Agostini M, Pucciarelli S, Enzo MV, Del Bianco P, Briarava M, Bedin C et al (2011) Circulating cell-free DNA: a promising marker of pathologic tumor response in rectal cancer patients receiving preoperative chemoradiotherapy. Ann Surg Oncol 18(9):2461–2468

114. Marsman G, Zeerleder S, Luken BM (2016) Extracellular histones, cell-free DNA, or nucle-osomes: differences in immunostimulation. Cell Death Dis 7(12):e2518

115. Yipp BG, Petri B, Salina D, Jenne CN, Scott BN, Zbytnuik LD et al (2012) Infection-induced NETosis is a dynamic process involving neutrophil multitasking in vivo. Nat Med 18(9): 1386–1393

116. Sansone P, Savini C, Kurelac I, Chang Q, Amato LB, Strillacci A et al (2017) Packaging and transfer of mitochondrial DNA via exosomes regulate escape from dormancy in hormonal therapy-resistant breast cancer. Proc Natl Acad Sci U S A 114(43):E9066–E9e75

117. Ingelsson B, Söderberg D, Strid T, Söderberg A, Bergh AC, Loitto V et al (2018) Lymphocytes eject interferogenic mitochondrial DNA webs in response to CpG and non-CpG oligodeoxynucleotides of class C. Proc Natl Acad Sci U S A 115(3):E478–Ee87
118. Demers M, Wagner DD (2014) NETosis: a new factor in tumor progression and cancer-associated thrombosis. Semin Thromb Hemost 40(3):277–283
119. Demers M, Wong SL, Martinod K, Gallant M, Cabral JE, Wang Y et al (2016) Priming of neutrophils toward NETosis promotes tumor growth. Oncoimmunology 5(5):e1134073
120. Swystun LL, Mukherjee S, Liaw PC (2011) Breast cancer chemotherapy induces the release of cell-free DNA, a novel procoagulant stimulus. J Thromb Haemost 9(11):2313–2321
121. Olsson AK, Cedervall J (2016) NETosis in cancer - platelet-neutrophil crosstalk promotes tumor-associated pathology. Front Immunol 7:373
122. Tohme S, Yazdani HO, Al-Khafaji AB, Chidi AP, Loughran P, Mowen K et al (2016) Neutrophil extracellular traps promote the development and progression of liver metastases after surgical stress. Cancer Res 76(6):1367–1380
123. Park J, Wysocki RW, Amoozgar Z, Maiorino L, Fein MR, Jorns J et al (2016) Cancer cells induce metastasis-supporting neutrophil extracellular DNA traps. Sci Transl Med 8(361): 361ra138
124. Erpenbeck L, Schön MP (2017) Neutrophil extracellular traps: protagonists of cancer progression? Oncogene 36(18):2483–2490
125. Albrengues J, Shields MA, Ng D, Park CG, Ambrico A, Poindexter ME et al (2018) Neutrophil extracellular traps produced during inflammation awaken dormant cancer cells in mice. Science 361(6409):eaao4227
126. Mouchemore KA, Anderson RL, Hamilton JA (2018) Neutrophils, G-CSF and their contribution to breast cancer metastasis. FEBS J 285(4):665–679
127. Kazzaz NM, Sule G, Knight JS (2016) Intercellular interactions as regulators of NETosis. Front Immunol 7:453
128. Cedervall J, Olsson AK (2015) NETosis in cancer. Oncoscience 2(11):900–901
129. Etulain J, Martinod K, Wong SL, Cifuni SM, Schattner M, Wagner DD (2015) P-selectin promotes neutrophil extracellular trap formation in mice. Blood 126(2):242–246
130. Pfeiler S, Stark K, Massberg S, Engelmann B (2017) Propagation of thrombosis by neutrophils and extracellular nucleosome networks. Haematologica 102(2):206–213
131. Kustanovich A, Schwartz R, Peretz T, Grinshpun A (2019) Life and death of circulating cell-free DNA. Cancer Biol Ther 20(8):1057–1067
132. Yang L, Liu Q, Zhang X, Liu X, Zhou B, Chen J et al (2020) DNA of neutrophil extracellular traps promotes cancer metastasis via CCDC25. Nature 583(7814):133–138
133. Gerling M, Büller NV, Kirn LM, Joost S, Frings O, Englert B et al (2016) Stromal Hedgehog signalling is downregulated in colon cancer and its restoration restrains tumour growth. Nat Commun 7:12321
134. Shin K, Lim A, Zhao C, Sahoo D, Pan Y, Spiekerkoetter E et al (2014) Hedgehog signaling restrains bladder cancer progression by eliciting stromal production of urothelial differentiation factors. Cancer Cell 26(4):521–533
135. Pallangyo CK, Ziegler PK, Greten FR (2015) IKKβ acts as a tumor suppressor in cancer-associated fibroblasts during intestinal tumorigenesis. J Exp Med 212(13):2253–2266
136. Harper J, Sainson RC (2014) Regulation of the anti-tumour immune response by cancer-associated fibroblasts. Semin Cancer Biol 25:69–77
137. Ueshima E, Fujimori M, Kodama H, Felsen D, Chen J, Durack JC et al (2019) Macrophage-secreted TGF-β(1) contributes to fibroblast activation and ureteral stricture after ablation injury. Am J Physiol Renal Physiol 317(7):F52–f64
138. Shiga K, Hara M, Nagasaki T, Sato T, Takahashi H, Takeyama H (2015) Cancer-associated fibroblasts: their characteristics and their roles in tumor growth. Cancer 7(4):2443–2458
139. Mantovani A, Sica A, Sozzani S, Allavena P, Vecchi A, Locati M (2004) The chemokine system in diverse forms of macrophage activation and polarization. Trends Immunol 25(12): 677–686

140. Abrams ST, Zhang N, Manson J, Liu T, Dart C, Baluwa F et al (2013) Circulating histones are mediators of trauma-associated lung injury. Am J Respir Crit Care Med 187(2):160–169

141. Xu J, Zhang X, Pelayo R, Monestier M, Ammollo CT, Semeraro F et al (2009) Extracellular histones are major mediators of death in sepsis. Nat Med 15(11):1318–1321

142. Zhang Q, Raoof M, Chen Y, Sumi Y, Sursal T, Junger W et al (2010) Circulating mitochondrial DAMPs cause inflammatory responses to injury. Nature 464(7285):104–107

143. Paunel-Görgülü A, Wacker M, El Aita M, Hassan S, Schlachtenberger G, Deppe A et al (2017) cfDNA correlates with endothelial damage after cardiac surgery with prolonged cardiopulmonary bypass and amplifies NETosis in an intracellular TLR9-independent manner. Sci Rep 7(1):17421

144. Bhagirath VC, Dwivedi DJ, Liaw PC (2015) Comparison of the proinflammatory and procoagulant properties of nuclear, mitochondrial, and bacterial DNA. Shock 44(3):265–271

145. Xu MM, Pu Y, Han D, Shi Y, Cao X, Liang H et al (2017) Dendritic cells but not macrophages sense tumor mitochondrial DNA for cross-priming through signal regulatory protein α signaling. Immunity 47(2):363–73.e5

146. Yang H, Biermann MH, Brauner JM, Liu Y, Zhao Y, Herrmann M (2016) New insights into neutrophil extracellular traps: mechanisms of formation and role in inflammation. Front Immunol 7:302

147. Nishimoto S, Fukuda D, Higashikuni Y, Tanaka K, Hirata Y, Murata C et al (2016) Obesity-induced DNA released from adipocytes stimulates chronic adipose tissue inflammation and insulin resistance. Sci Adv 2(3):e1501332

148. Corrêa LH, Corrêa R, Farinasso CM, de Sant'Ana Dourado LP, Magalhães KG (2017) Adipocytes and macrophages interplay in the orchestration of tumor microenvironment: new implications in cancer progression. Front Immunol 8:1129

149. Dunphy G, Flannery SM, Almine JF, Connolly DJ, Paulus C, Jønsson KL et al (2018) Non-canonical activation of the DNA sensing adaptor STING by ATM and IFI16 mediates NF-κB signaling after nuclear DNA damage. Mol Cell 71(5):745–60.e5

150. Torralba D, Baixauli F, Villarroya-Beltri C, Fernández-Delgado I, Latorre-Pellicer A, Acín-Pérez R et al (2018) Priming of dendritic cells by DNA-containing extracellular vesicles from activated T cells through antigen-driven contacts. Nat Commun 9(1):2658

151. Parkes EE, Walker SM, Taggart LE, McCabe N, Knight LA, Wilkinson R et al (2017) Activation of STING-dependent innate immune signaling by S-phase-specific DNA damage in breast cancer. J Natl Cancer Inst 109(1):djw199

152. Ahn J, Xia T, Konno H, Konno K, Ruiz P, Barber GN (2014) Inflammation-driven carcinogenesis is mediated through STING. Nat Commun 5:5166

153. Härtlova A, Erttmann SF, Raffi FA, Schmalz AM, Resch U, Anugula S et al (2015) DNA damage primes the type I interferon system via the cytosolic DNA sensor STING to promote anti-microbial innate immunity. Immunity 42(2):332–343

154. Chen G, Huang AC, Zhang W, Zhang G, Wu M, Xu W et al (2018) Exosomal PD-L1 contributes to immunosuppression and is associated with anti-PD-1 response. Nature 560(7718):382–386

155. Theodoraki MN, Yerneni SS, Hoffmann TK, Gooding WE, Whiteside TL (2018) Clinical significance of PD-L1(+) exosomes in plasma of head and neck cancer patients. Clin Cancer Res 24(4):896–905

156. Yang Y, Li CW, Chan LC, Wei Y, Hsu JM, Xia W et al (2018) Exosomal PD-L1 harbors active defense function to suppress T cell killing of breast cancer cells and promote tumor growth. Cell Res 28(8):862–864

Chapter 6
Physiological Changes in the Local
Onco-Sphere: Angiogenesis

Phei Er Saw and Erwei Song

Abstract Angiogenesis plays a critical role in the growth of cancer as tumors consistently require ample blood supply, especially during their exponential growth phase. Tumors will activate angiogenesis pathways through secretion of chemokines and cytokines if they are to grow beyond a few millimeters in size. In this chapter, we will focus on the importance of tumor in initiating angiogenesis in the local onco-sphere, and how angiogenesis also encourages cancer metastasis.

Introduction

The definition of angiogenesis is "the emergence of new blood vessels which occurs from the endothelium of the pre-existing vasculature." This process is essential in the progression, growth, and metastasis of a tumor [1]. Tumor cells receive oxygen and exchange metabolites via this wide network of blood vessels. Aside from the growth of the primary tumor, metastasis of the tumor relies on neovascularzation, whereby the metastatic cells first exit the primary tumor via the blood vessels, and when it

P. E. Saw
Guangdong Provincial Key Laboratory of Malignant Tumor Epigenetics and Gene Regulation, Guangdong-Hong Kong Joint Laboratory for RNA Medicine, Medical Research Center, Sun Yat-sen Memorial Hospital, Sun Yat-sen University, Guangzhou, China

Nanhai Translational Innovation Center of Precision Immunology, Sun Yat-sen Memorial Hospital, Sun Yat-sen University, Foshan, China

E. Song (✉)
Guangdong Provincial Key Laboratory of Malignant Tumor Epigenetics and Gene Regulation, Guangdong-Hong Kong Joint Laboratory for RNA Medicine, Medical Research Center, Sun Yat-sen Memorial Hospital, Sun Yat-sen University, Guangzhou, China

Nanhai Translational Innovation Center of Precision Immunology, Sun Yat-sen Memorial Hospital, Sun Yat-sen University, Foshan, China

Breast Tumor Center, Sun Yat-sen Memorial Hospital, Sun Yat-sen University, Guangzhou, China
e-mail: songew@mail.sysu.edu.cn

arrives at distant organs, angiogenesis is induced from the metastatic cells to promote the growth of the metastasized tumor to a considerable size. Folkman was the first to state the hypothesis where a tumor could be restricted from growing or even be reduced in size by targeting the inhibition of blood vessel formation [2]. However, the limitations to this hypothesis were that the tumor could not be in an avascular state nor exceed a size of $1–2 \ mm^3$. Henceforth, intensive research on the molecular mechanisms of tumor angiogenesis was started and has proven to be successful in the future. Since cancer cells are highly proliferative in nature, tumors are required to develop a network of blood supply to support it. However, blood vessels formed by tumors are immature, and this impairs their functionality [1]. These immature blood vessels are the products of abnormal secretion of VEGF by both tumor and stromal cells, PDGFβ, members of angiopoietins, and TGF-β families [3]. The defective blood vessels that are formed can cause hypoxia, increased risks of metastatic dissemination, and decreased immune cell infiltration and activity, which are profound implications for the local *onco-sphere* [3].

Angiogenesis: Initiation of Tumor Vascularization in the Local *Onco-Sphere*

The "Angiogenic Switch"

In the early stages of cancer progression of multistage carcinoma, in both genetically engineered mouse models and human tissue, the lack of active formation of blood vessels can be frequently observed in small dormant tumors [4]. Homeostasis in the vascular system is regulated by both anti- and pro-angiogenic factors. The vascular system is kept in a quiescent state when endothelial cells are non-proliferative and GFs are balanced. When the balance is tipped (i.e., when pro-angiogenic signaling is overpowering), new vessel formation is initiated in the process called the "angiogenic switch" [5]. Tumors were woken up from their dormant state, activated, and induce rapid growth and proliferation of malignant cells in response to these neo-blood vessels. In Hanahan's laboratory, a genetically engineered mouse model, the RIP1-Tag2 model of pancreatic insulinoma, which expresses the Simian Virus 40 large T (SV40T) oncogene, was developed and widely used as the standard model for studying angiogenic switch [6]. It was observed in this model that mice carrying the trans-gene sequentially developed tumors, which initially started as non-angiogenic dysplastic cell clusters from which a portion subsequently developed into tumor islets that were angiogenic, then further progressed into sizable, highly vascularized tumors, which finally metastasized to the lungs. This observation further supports the notion of the existence of a wide range of cellular mechanisms as well as factors that enable the initiation of blood vessel formation in tumors [7]. Activation of the angiogenic switch can also lead to cross-communication with many factors within the local *onco-sphere*, resulting in tumor-associated inflammation, recruitment of immune cells, hypoxia, increased proliferation, and constant expression of pro-angiogenic factors [2].

Neo-Blood Vessel Formation in the Local *Onco-Sphere*

The blood circulatory system consists of the aorta, branching out into arteries, then into smaller capillaries, then converges back into veins, which is essential in transporting blood throughout the body. The main components in circulation system include arteries, veins, and capillaries. Arteries are vessels that carry oxygenated blood from the heart to the tissues. The arteries will further branch into smaller capillaries as it reaches the targeted tissues, in which the thin walls of capillaries enable the exchange of gases between blood and tissues. The blood facilitates the release of oxygen into the cell and carbon dioxide out of the cell to the bloodstream. The carbon dioxide is then transported via the veins back to the heart. Post-capillary venules play a role in the transmigration of immune cells into the tissues. Angiogenesis typically starts at the capillaries and is an essential part in the maintenance, growth, and metastasis of a tumor.

Sprouting Angiogenesis

Sprouting angiogenesis is a multistep process where new capillaries can bud from parental vessels: The sprout formation process consists of: (a) Tip cell selection: One of the cells from the parent vessel is selected to be the migratory leading cell, and it initiates lateral inhibition process to prevent its neighboring cells from becoming a tip cell. (b) Sprout extension: the selected tip cell, followed by trailing stalk cells, migrates along the chemotactic path, thus extending itself. (c) Lumen formation: connection occurs between the developing sprout and other vessels through anastomosis. In normal circumstances, endothelial cells are usually quiescent. However, sprouting and angiogenesis can be initiated by VEGF, which is a pro-angiogenic factor. The relation of tip and stalk cell selection is kept in balance through the signaling between DLL4/Notch pathways and VEGF [8]. Tip cell will produce PDGFβ, VEGFR-3/Flt-4, and VEGFR-2 as a response to VEGF [9–11]. Notch signaling is blocked by VEGF, and this results in an elevated activity of sprouting, migratory capacity, branching, and filopodia formation in tip cells [12]. DLL4 produced by tip cells will activate Notch signaling in its neighboring endothelial cells, which inhibits VEGFR2 and VEGFR3 expression, resulting in suppression of the formation of tip cells in them, as well as enhancing the expression of VEGFR1 (decoy for VEGF) [13–16]. Numerous filopodia are extended from tip cells where they acquire motility and invasive properties, inducing formation of new blood vessels toward the VEGF gradient via secretion of matrix degrading proteins [17]. A type of non-tyrosine kinase receptor known as neuropilins enhances VEGFR2 and VEGFR3 signaling, which promotes tip cell function [18, 19]. Stalk cells follow the tip cells, establish junctional connections and vascular lumen to the forming sprout by branching out from the existing vessel. As compared to tips cells, stalk cells have fewer filopodia and are more proliferative, in which Notch-regulated ankyrin repeat protein is responsible for fine-tuning [20] (Fig. 6.1a).

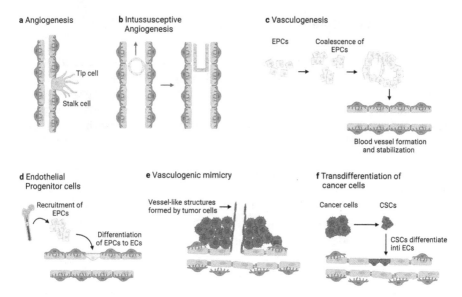

Fig. 6.1 Different mechanisms of various types of angiogenesis in the local onco-sphere. (**a**) Sprouting angiogenesis: Sprouts (tips cells) form and extend to fuse with either an existing vessel or a newly formed spout. (**b**) Intussusceptive angiogenesis: new vasculature is formed at the site where a preexisting vessel diverges into two. (**c**) Vasculogenesis: A process where EPCs multiply, forming new lumens, and develop into new blood vessels. (**d**) Recruitment of EPCs to the tumor site for enhancing new vessel formation. (**e**) Vascular mimicry: tumors mimicking the formation of blood vessel via a network consisting of matrix-embedded fluid-conducting meshwork. (**f**) Transdifferentiation of CSCs: Differentiation of tumor CSCs into ECs from CSCs initiates neovascularization

Intussusceptive Angiogenesis

"Intussusception" develops inside vessels that are already formed and subsequently fuses with the parental vessel. Throughout this process, the vascular plexus is remodeled. This type of neo-angiogenesis could be seen in lung capillary remodeling [21, 22]. Few studies ventured into intussusceptive angiogenesis; therefore, their molecular mechanisms are yet to be fully understood. However, GFs such as VEGF, PDGF, and erythropoietin are still the key players [23–25]. Interestingly, various tumors exhibit intussusceptive angiogenesis, such as breast tumors, melanoma, glioma, and colorectal cancer [26–29]. For example, in melanoma, intussusceptive angiogenesis and intraluminal tissue folds occurrence are closely related to VEGF expression [26]. Intussusceptive angiogenesis is observed to be utilized in tumors from xenografts of human adenocarcinoma [28] (Fig. 6.1b).

Vasculogenesis

Vasculogenesis is a process in which blood vessels are formed through the association and differentiation of endothelial progenitor cells (EPCs), and this is especially seen in de novo blood vessel formation in embryos [30, 31]. In human, vasculogenesis is also observed in adults when capillaries are formed post-ischemia [32] or in tumors where the increasing need for nutrients and oxygen supply induces this process for neo-vascularization [33]. As observed in preclinical glioma models, in glioma recurrence after irradiation, the revascularization process that occurs is seen to be primarily mediated by vasculogenesis and not typical angiogenesis [34]. In tumor, this vasculogenesis process is mediated by recruitment of BMDCs or EPCs [35, 36]. EPCs are unipotent adult stem cells, having the capabilities of self-renewal, proliferation, and taking part in the repair of endothelial tissue and neovascularization [37, 38]. In tumors, vasculogenesis is mediated by the signaling between EPCs in the bone marrow and tumor cells, revealing a long-distance communication between the local and systemic onco-sphere. Interestingly, VEGFR2 and EPCs from the bone marrow are mobilized by the signal of VEGF from the local onco-sphere [39–41]. Furthermore, tumor-secreted CCL2 and CCL5, adiponectin [42–44], CXCL 12 (also known as SDF-1, 42), have the ability to mobilize EPCs from the bone marrow to the tumor bed, again revealing the importance of the inter-onco-spherical communication (Fig. 6.1c, d).

Vascular Mimicry

Tumor cells that are aggressively growing have the capability to create "vessel-like structures." Even without the contribution of endothelial cells, these structures can be formed as an alternate pathway to source sufficient nutrients and blood supply to meet the demands of growing tumor cells. Vascular mimicry is now observed in various tumor types. Initially, there was a debate in the field on the existence and relative important of vascular mimicry [45], but evidence from several findings in various research groups has been found to support it [46]. Tumor samples with IHC using Periodic acid-Schiff (PAS) and CD31 as markers have been found to exhibit structures formed via vascular mimicry [47]. These endothelial-mimicking tumor cells can secrete factors that aid in the formation of tubular structure and its stabilization (i.e., collagens, proteoglycans, laminin, heparin sulfate, and tissue transglutaminase antigen 2, among others) [48]. In uveal melanoma, it was found that tumor cells that underwent vascular mimicry expressed CD271 and had multipotent, stem cell-like phenotypes [49]. Vascular mimicry can contribute to tumor progression via multiple mechanisms. As seen in melanoma, activation of Met proto-oncogene occurs under hypoxia conditions via mitochondrial reactive oxygen species, which then promotes vascular mimicry, resulting in tumor cell motility, invasion, and metastasis [50]. However, in an interesting turn of events, it was found that increased vascular mimicry activity was the result of anti-angiogenic therapy in glioma [51]. This suggests that there may be an adaptive neovascularization process, a viable alternative that allows the tumor cells to survive (Fig. 6.1e).

Cancer Stem Cells (CSCs) Trans-Differentiation into Vasculatures

In several tumor types, trans-differentiation to vascular smooth muscle-like cells and endothelial cells from cancer cells, which gave rise to neovascularization, was observed [52–56]. In an in vitro culture of glioma CSCs using an endothelial promoting media, these CSCs expresses pan endothelial markers such as CD31, CD34, and vWF, as well as an increased level of LDL and formation of tubular structures [52, 57]. There was evidence of the development of tumor vessels with ECs, which expressed human endothelial proteins VEGFR2, CD34, and CD144. The disruption of vasculature and eradication of the tumor are possible by targeting Tie-2 overexpressing cells [52]. However, since there were no reports regarding endothelial cells in human glioblastoma harboring genetic alteration in other studies, the results were deemed controversial [58, 59]. In another study, it was reported that glioma CSCs possessed the capability to differentiate into pericytes to halt tumor growth through inhibition of tumor vessels [60] (Fig. 6.1f).

Vessel Co-Option: Hijacking Host Vascular System

All tumors are the winners of "survival of the fittest" game. They are capable of producing, modifying, and mimicking host vascular structures in order for them to receive more oxygen and nutrients as much as possible at a short period of time. There is a method that tumor cells can use (different from all the angiogenic types mentioned above and in Fig. 6.1) that is called vessel co-option. Vessel co-option has been identified recently, as one of the most efficient ways for a tumor to grow, without having to produce their own blood vessels; in another words, tumor cells "hijack" the existing normal vasculature of the host in the surrounding tissues that are non-cancerous [61]; or known as "parasitism" in the ecological definition. The repercussion of this is twofold: (1) cancer cells do not need to go the extra mile to make new blood vessels, which leads to a more vigorous growth; (2) anti-angiogenic drugs that are targeting cancerous angiogenic factor are rendered useless in this mechanism. The major differences between common angiogenesis and vessel co-option are listed in Table 6.1 below.

Table 6.1 Major difference in the local onco-sphere in angiogenesis-based blood vessel formation vs. through vessel co-option

Characteristics	Angiogenesis	Vessel co-option
Specific shape (contour)	Regular	Irregular
Stromal architecture	New desmoplastic stroma is formed	Host stroma is preserved
Stromal environment	Hypoxic and necrotic	Minimally hypoxic or necrotic
Tumor-stroma ratio	Lower	Higher
Vessel architecture	Chaotic, insufficient vasculature	Orderly
Destruction of host tissue	Yes	No
Blood vessel density	Formation of vascular hotspots (low vessel density area exist)	High density at periphery, low at tumor core
Endothelial cells	Proliferative, angiogenic phenotype	May undergo phenotypical changes, but usually retain normal characteristics
Epithelial cells	No normal epithelial cell	Host normal epithelial cells could be found
Tumor-epithelial cell contact	No contact	In contact
Arrangement of cancer cells	Confined to the tumor	Can be sparsely distant from each clone
Tumor type	Generally, well-differentiated tumors	Generally, less-differentiated tumors
Inflammation at tumor site	Yes	Less likely

Adapted from [62]

Currently, not much is known on the exact mechanism of vessel co-option. However, the pattern of vessel co-option is entirely non-angiogenic, which makes it very different from the host response in desmoplasia or inflammation. Vessel co-option has been identified in organs that are highly dependent on vasculature, for example, the lung and liver [63]. Under normal circumstances, the endothelial cells in both organs will enhance the secretion of angiocrine factors through immature pneumocytes hepatocytes, respectively. Therefore, some had suspected that the tumors could hijack these programs [64]. The question is why some tumors activate their own angiogenesis and not vessel co-option and vice versa. Many studies had linked vessel co-option with bad prognosis in many cancers, indicating that vessel co-option could be a much more aggressive option for a tumor to grow and metastasize. Besides, the vessels in co-option are irregular, which increases the mobility of cancer cells, therefore supporting the notion of "self-metastasis," without the need of making their own blood vessels [65].

Blood Vessels in the Local *Onco-Sphere*: Mechanism and Function

In normal physiological condition, for example, development, wound healing, or menstrual cycle, blood vessel formation is a tightly regulated process. Under these circumstances, when the need of blood vessel ceases, the process halt. However, in tumor, this process is unregulated, due to the consistently high expression of pro-angiogenic factors in the local onco-sphere. However, under constant pro-angiogenic signaling in tumors, newly formed blood vessels may fail to mature [66, 67]. As a result, there is uneven blood flow and inconsistent blood vessel in the tumor parenchyma, leading to areas of intermittent or persisting hypoxia [68, 69]. In tumor vessels, the endothelial junctions are disrupted, causing increased interstitial fluid pressure due to its enhanced permeability [70]. This contributes to the reduction of efficacy of cancer therapy due to poor vascular perfusion and compression of tumor vessels, which hampers drug delivery [71]. Pericytes in tumor vessels are generally partially detached from the endothelial cells, as well as having an unevenly distributed basement membrane, which may lead to an increase risk of hemorrhage due to the fragility of these vessels [72–74].

Besides functional and structural defects, the tumor blood vessels are responsive to environmental cues via transcriptional regulation of gene expression [75–83]. Depending on the anatomical location, malignancy grade, and tumor type, transcriptional signatures of tumor ECs vary. However, the subsets of genes that are typically upregulated by tumor vessels (e.g., TIE1, TIE2, and VEGFR2) are those that are transcriptionally active during development and physiological angiogenesis [84]. However, increased permeability was associated with CD-93 deficiency, while metastatic dissemination and intravasation of tumor cells are promoted by endosialin expression in pericytes, indicating their opposite roles in the regulation of vascular integrity [85, 86]. The endothelial barrier is further strengthened by the upregulation of FASL in tumor vessels and induces apoptosis of cytotoxic T-lymphocytes, which results in the suppression of the immune system [87]. Similarly, T-cell homing was observed to be decreased in ovarian cancer where tumor vessels express endothelin B [88]. The changes induced by the tumor microenvironment in endothelial gene expression may be beneficial for therapy, especially in brain tumors [89]. Therefore, understanding the molecular signature underlying angiogenesis could lead to possible emergence of new targets for therapy from the alteration of vascular function by proteins that are upregulated in tumor vessels, which we will discuss further in the following section. We have also summarized the major effectors of angiogenesis, including cytokines, chemokines, and GFs in Table 6.2 below.

Table 6.2 Angiogenesis-related cytokines, chemokines, and GFs in the local *onco-sphere*

Cytokines	Functions	Ref
VEGF family VEGF-A, VEGF-B, VEGF-C, VEGF-D, including activation of VEGF-receptors	• VEGFR-2 expressed by ECs induces VEGF to from active blood vessels, via activation of rho GTPases and PI3K stimulation • Increases ECs survival and proliferation via ERK and PI3K/Akt pathways • Increased MMP-2, −9, uPA to degrade stromal ECM and basal membrane, allowing ECs migration and formation of capillary sprouts • Increasing vascular permeability through (a) induction of fenestrae, (b) junctional remodeling, and (c) vesiculo-vascular organelles (VVOs) • Increases interstitial fluid pressure (IFP) and impaired therapeutic delivery, facilitate membrane leakage, encouraging tumor cell dissemination into bloodstream to establish metastasis is a suitable distal *onco-sphere* • Activates NFAT in ECs via PLCγ/calcineurin, increase IL-1β-like expression to increase vascular inflammation • Activate Akt/NF-κB pathway, resulting in the increased leukocytes infiltration and contributes to angiogenesis	[90–96]
Placental growth factors (PlGF)	• Dual/controversial role in angiogenesis • Enhances pathological angiogenesis via the initiation of a cross-talk between VEGFR-1 and VEGFR-2	[97, 98]
Platelet derived growth factor (PDGF) family Namely A, B, C, and D; signaling occurs through PDGFRα and PDGFRβ	• Promoting vessel maturation, inducing upregulation of VEGF and recruiting pericytes • Mice deprived of PDGF-B/PDGFRβ pathway demonstrated increased lethality, including increased vessel leakage and the presence of micro-hemorrhages • In a glioma model, PDGF-B increases VEGF expression stimulation in the tumor ECs	[99–101]
Fibroblast growth factor (FGF) family; signaling through FGFR Comprises of 22 molecules, of which 18 interact with high affinity to tyrosine kinase receptors such as FGFR1, FGFR2, FGFR3, and FGFR4	• FGF-2 exerts a paracrine signaling to affect ECs. • FGF-2 coordinates with VEGF to promote angiogenesis through inducing the secretion of MMPs, collagenases, and uPA, which are responsible for the organization and degradation of the ECM • FGF signaling modulates	[102–104]

(continued)

Table 6.2 (continued)

Cytokines	Functions	Ref
	MYC-dependent glycolysis to increase ECs sprouting and proliferation	
Ephrin and ephrin receptors Superfamily of tyrosine kinase receptors, includes 14 human type 1 transmembrane protein members. Two subgroups of the Eph proteins (EphA and EphB), based on their sequence homologies and their ability to bind their ligands	• EphA2 and EphA1 were detected in the vasculature of pre-clinical models of Kaposi's sarcoma and breast carcinoma, which enhanced tumor angiogenesis and blood vessel growth • EphB4-ephB2 signaling increases tumor angiogenesis and resistance to anti-angiogenic therapy • In a glioma model, overexpression of EphB4 leads to a shift in vascular morphogenesis and pericyte coverage, causing resistance to therapy • In glioblastoma stem-like cells study, EphB2 was identified as a regulator of perivascular invasion • EphB2 could induce the VEGF signaling to internalize VEGFR2 and VEGFR3 to regulate angiogenesis and lymphangiogenesis during tumor progression	[105–117]
Angiopoietins (ANGPTs) and ANGPT-1, ANGPT-2, and ANGPT-4; mediated by endothelial receptor tyrosine kinase TIE-1 and TIE-2	• ANGPT-1 promotes maturation of vessels through the Akt/Survivin pathway • ANGPT-2 induces vessel destabilisation, vessel sprouting, pericytes detachment, and angiogenesis • ANGPT-2 expression is elevated in ECs in tumor-associated vessels • ANGPT-2 is an autocrine modulator of ECs inflammatory response, sensitizes ECs towards TNFα, and upregulates adhesion molecules • In a glioblastoma model, upregulation of ANGPT-2 increased resistance • In many cancer models, ANGPT-2/VEGFR2 inhibition certainly impairs the growth of tumors, prolonging vessel normalization, and blocks the recruitment of macrophages	[118–124]
Apelin/APLNR pathway endogenous peptide-ligand of APJ (APLNR), a G protein-coupled receptor	• In tumors, Apelin is modulated by hypoxia, to stimulate tumor cell proliferation, migration, and metastasis through angiogenic pathways • Apelin enhances microvascular proliferation and neo-angiogenesis within the tumor • In breast and lung cancer model,	[125–131]

(continued)

Table 6.2 (continued)

Cytokines	Functions	Ref
	targeting Apelin has been shown to reduce tumor growth and metastasis, where improvement in vessel function prevented resistance associated with anti-angiogenic therapy • In glioma mouse model, the combination of co-targeting VEGFR2 and Apelin has shown an improvement in mice survival • Clinically, high APLNR expression was found to be negatively correlated with tumor PD-L1 expression	

Chemokines CC, CXC, XC, and CX3X	Functions	Ref
CXCR2	• In a PDAC murine model, inhibition of CXCR2 decreases tumor growth and angiogenesis • In human ovarian carcinoma mouse model, activation of CXCR2 enhances VEGF expression, increases angiogenesis • CXCR2 on neutrophils leads to leukocytes arrest	[132–134]
CXCR4	• Tip cells (major step in angiogenesis) are enriched with CXCR4 and are highly expressed in tumor vessels • CXCL12/SDF1 binds to CXCR4 to exert pro-angiogenic and chemotactic activity	[135]
CXCL8	• Induce the release of pro-angiogenic factors such as VEGF, MMP-2, and MMP-9 • Support ECs survival • Attracts neutrophils and it induces neutrophil respiratory burst	[136–140]
CXCL12	• CXCL12 is upregulated in hypoxic region a result of hypoxic-induced stabilization of HIF1α • recruits CXCR4-expressing EPCs from the bone marrow during vasculogenesis • CXCL12/CXCR4 is involved in the trafficking of leucocytes to the tumor as well as in vessel co-option • Tumor-expressed CCL2 interacts with CCR2 on tumor ECs to modulate the permeability of ECs and promoting metastasis • CCL2 is a necessity for the mobilization of EPCs	[141–143]

Other pro-angiogenic factors	Functions	Ref
MMPs	• Remodeling of ECM to promote tumor angiogenesis, progression and metastasis • The secretion of MMP-2 and MMP-9 activates TGF-β to promote angiogenesis and tumor invasion	[144]
TGF-β	• Important modulators of neovascularization in tumors • Promoting angiogenesis by stimulating pro-angiogenic factors (i.e., VEGF)	[145]

(continued)

Table 6.2 (continued)

Other pro-angiogenic factors	Functions	Ref
TNFα	• VEGFR2 expression could induce anti-angiogenic effects	[146]
Pleiotrophin (PTN)	• PTN level was found in several types of cancer, leading to increase tumor growth either thorough (1) stimulation of angiogenesis, direct effects on tumor cells, or remodeling of the TME • In astrocytoma patients, higher level of PTN is indicative vascular abnormalities leading to poor survival • In murine glioma models, PTN is shown to stimulate tumor vasculature and enhance tumor growth	[147–149]
Nogo, Nogo-A, Nogo-B, and Nogo-C), belongs to the reticulon 4 (RTN4) protein family	• Nogo-B is essential in vascular remodeling. • In Nogo-A/B deficient mice, arteriogenesis angiogenesis is reduced due to impaired macrophage infiltration • In hepatocellular carcinoma, Nogo-B expression was upregulated, correlates with the density of tumor vessels and leads to increased tumor growth and metastasis	[150–152]

Intra-*Onco Spherical* Cross Talks: Contributions of Immune Cells to Tumor Angiogenesis

The tumor milieu is made up of a diverse range of cells, such as stromal cells, endothelial cells, immune cells, and inflammatory cells, as discussed in Chap. 3. The continuous interaction between the cells constituting the tumor microenvironment and the malignant cells induces a strong tumor-provoking condition [153]. The endothelial and immune cells have an intense collaborative interaction. The synthesis of adhesive molecules on endothelial cell lining depends on immune cells for extravasating into tumor cells; wherein immune cells demonstrate anti-tumor activities [154–156].

Tumor-Associated Macrophages (TAMs)

TAMs tend to promote and modify angiogenesis, wherein depletion of TAMs inhibits tumor angiogenesis, but TAM restoration promotes angiogenesis in murine samples of cancer [157, 158]. Hypoxia inside the tumor milieu promotes TAMs' metabolic adaptability and pro-angiogenic properties. TAMs predominantly stimulate angiogenesis by producing several pro-angiogenic elements that promote endothelial cellular proliferation, budding, tube creation, and development of new blood vessels. The pro-angiogenic elements synthesized by TAMs are VEGFA, VEGFC, VEGFD, EGF, FGF2, chemokines (CXCL8, CXCL12, TNFα, and MCP-1), adrenomedullin, and thymidine phosphorylase [159–161]. TAMs produce a variety of angiogenesis-regulating chemicals, including enzymes (COX-2, iNOS), MMPs-1, 2, 3, 9, and 12, cathepsin proteases and plasmin, urokinase plasminogen activating agent [162]. These substances work together to erode the basement membrane and extracellular matrix, disrupt the vasculature, and promote endothelial cellular movement and proliferation.

Myeloid-Derived Suppressor Cells (MDSCs)

Considering the lack of a definitive set of indicators for distinguishing G-MDSCs from neutrophils, the link and identification of these two cell types remain under controversy and uncertainty in the industry [163]. MDSC adhesion to tumors can be triggered by a variety of stimuli, including CSF3, IL-1β, and IL-6, which activate STAT3, making them pro-angiogenic and immunosuppressive [164]. MDSCs are comparable to M2-like TAMs in their ability to regulate and sustain tumor angiogenesis mainly by secreting MMPs. MMP-9 is popular as a tumor neovascularization and angiogenesis stimulating agent by enhancing accessibility to VEGF [165]. As a result, VEGF can further promote MDSC activation, resulting in the creation of a cascaded loop [166]. The proportion of intra-tumoral VEGF is connected to MDSC reserves in the tumor with the advancement of the illness [167]. The availability of VEGF enables MDSCs to maintain a pro-angiogenic microenvironment in the tumor by releasing angiogenic elements such as CCL2, CXCL2, CXCL8, ANGPT1, ANGPT2, IL-1β, and GM-CSF [168, 169]. These chemokines increase the aggregation of MDSCs in the tumor, thus enhancing the malignancy. Bv8 commonly referred to as prokineticin 2, is also synthesized, which impacts MDSC-controlled angiogenesis [170]. The build-up of MDSCs in the tumor tissues makes them more resistant to anti-angiogenic therapy, whereas MDSC removal has been demonstrated to generate collaborative benefits with anti-VEGF/VEGFR treatment [166, 171].

Neutrophils

Neutrophils, the most prevalent kind of leukocytes, form the body's foremost defense system against intruding microorganisms [172] and possess a high volume of soluble antimicrobial agents, including peptides, cytokines, reactive oxygen species (ROS), and enzymes. Neutrophils are a major generator of VEGF, which is a significant factor in angiogenesis under specific physiological circumstances such as endometrial angiogenesis during menstruation [173, 174]. Additional investigations have shown that neutrophil reduction impacts the neovascularization process in model organisms of angiogenesis [175, 176]. Analytical assessment of the RIP1-Tag2 multifarious pancreatic carcinogenesis murine model has yielded compelling proof of the role played by neutrophils in tumor angiogenesis. Furthermore, there are two kinds of neutrophils: TGFβ—independent type 1 (N1), possessing antimicrobial capabilities, and TGFβ—dependent tumor-associated neutrophils (N2, TANs), with pro-tumor and pro-angiogenic properties, as described at least in mouse tumor models [177, 178]. The stimulation of STAT3 signaling by CSF3-CSF3R is required for neutrophil growth and viability in malignancies. MMP9-producing TANs also aid in the onset of angiogenesis and the advancement of carcinogenesis [179]. In contrast to TIMP1/MMP9 aggregates synthesizing cells, the absence of tissue inhibitors of metalloproteinases (TIMP1) in TANs increases their proclivity to angiogenesis [180].

Lymphocytes (T Cells, B Cells, and NK Cells)

T Cells

T cells release angiogenesis-promoting substances such as FGF-2 and heparin-binding epidermal growth factor (HB-EGF) [181]. TNFα, TGFβ, and IFNs are the most significant T-cell-produced factors having anti-angiogenic capabilities [182–184]. TNF and IFNs prevent the development of capillary-like substances by inhibiting collagen production and extracellular matrix formation in vitro [185, 186]. IFN-γ has been shown to prevent neovascularization and promote cell death in endothelial cells of mouse glioma models [182]. Synthesis of IFNγ is stimulated by Type-I polarized T lymphocytes (Th1), whose existence in the tumor milieu has been linked to superior clinical results [187]. Interferon-cajoled CXC family chemokines limit tumor development by inhibiting endothelial cell growth and promoting infiltration of Th1 type T cell, NK, and DC cells [188–190].

B Cells

The capacity of B lymphocytes to control tumor angiogenesis depends on STAT3 stimulation. $Rag1^{-/-}$ mice with STAT3- producing B cells experienced an accelerated rate of tumor development and angiogenesis [191]. B lymphocytes also promote tumor angiogenesis by activating Fcγ receptors with the help of antibodies on TAMs, which promotes the release of IL-1 and boosts the infiltration of myofibroblasts to enhance angiogenesis [192].

NK Cells

In the gestational phase, a subpopulation of NK cells (CD56^{bright}CD16$^-$KIR$^+$, dNK cells) having low cytotoxicity and pro-angiogenic ability is observed in the decidua. Factors including Placental Growth Factor (PlGF), VEGF, IL10, IFNγ, and CXCL8 are all secreted by these NK cells, which are necessary for vascularizing the decidua and development of the spiral artery [193, 194]. Normally functioning donor NK cells can produce PlGF and VEGF at a higher rate due to TGFβ-driven dNK cell polarization [195, 196]. TGFβ initiates the transformation of NK cells to Type-1 innate lymphoid cells, resulting in the avoidance of immune response and the inefficiency of regulating tumor development and metastasis [197].

Conclusion

In this chapter, we looked at the molecular mechanism of angiogenesis in local *onco-sphere* and how the process is intertwined with the cross talk with various factors in the local *onco-sphere* (i.e., cytokines, chemokines, immune cells, stromal cells). Although angiogenesis is one of the important hallmarks of cancer, single-agent targeting angiogenesis has proven to be ineffective, as with other types of cancer therapeutics. Several recent investigations have increased our comprehension and awareness regarding molecular processes that regulate tumor lymph production, including the participation of different GFs, chemokines, and signaling cascades. Therefore, one should look at angiogenic process at various levels, to understand the role of each component in the local onco-sphere in affecting tumor angiogenesis, and how the host could interfere in this process.

References

1. Folkman J (1971) Tumor angiogenesis: therapeutic implications. N Engl J Med 285(21): 1182–1186
2. Cao Y, Arbiser J, D'Amato RJ, D'Amore PA, Ingber DE, Kerbel R et al (2011) Forty-year journey of angiogenesis translational research. Sci Transl Med 3(114):114rv3
3. Folkman J, Merler E, Abernathy C, Williams G (1971) Isolation of a tumor factor responsible for angiogenesis. J Exp Med 133(2):275–288
4. Lugano R, Ramachandran M, Dimberg A (2020) Tumor angiogenesis: causes, consequences, challenges and opportunities. Cell Mol Life Sci 77(9):1745–1770
5. Hanahan D, Folkman J (1996) Patterns and emerging mechanisms of the angiogenic switch during tumorigenesis. Cell 86(3):353–364
6. Hanahan D (1985) Heritable formation of pancreatic beta-cell tumours in transgenic mice expressing recombinant insulin/simian virus 40 oncogenes. Nature 315(6015):115–122
7. Nowak-Sliwinska P, Alitalo K, Allen E, Anisimov A, Aplin AC, Auerbach R et al (2018) Consensus guidelines for the use and interpretation of angiogenesis assays. Angiogenesis 21(3):425–532

8. Jakobsson L, Bentley K, Gerhardt H (2009) VEGFRs and notch: a dynamic collaboration in vascular patterning. Biochem Soc Trans 37(Pt 6):1233–1236
9. Tammela T, Zarkada G, Wallgard E, Murtomäki A, Suchting S, Wirzenius M et al (2008) Blocking VEGFR-3 suppresses angiogenic sprouting and vascular network formation. Nature 454(7204):656–660
10. Strasser GA, Kaminker JS, Tessier-Lavigne M (2010) Microarray analysis of retinal endothelial tip cells identifies CXCR4 as a mediator of tip cell morphology and branching. Blood 115(24):5102–5110
11. Shawber CJ, Funahashi Y, Francisco E, Vorontchikhina M, Kitamura Y, Stowell SA et al (2007) Notch alters VEGF responsiveness in human and murine endothelial cells by direct regulation of VEGFR-3 expression. J Clin Invest 117(11):3369–3382
12. Jakobsson L, Franco CA, Bentley K, Collins RT, Ponsioen B, Aspalter IM et al (2010) Endothelial cells dynamically compete for the tip cell position during angiogenic sprouting. Nat Cell Biol 12(10):943–953
13. Hellström M, Phng LK, Hofmann JJ, Wallgard E, Coultas L, Lindblom P et al (2007) Dll4 signalling through Notch1 regulates formation of tip cells during angiogenesis. Nature 445(7129):776–780
14. Lobov IB, Renard RA, Papadopoulos N, Gale NW, Thurston G, Yancopoulos GD et al (2007) Delta-like ligand 4 (Dll4) is induced by VEGF as a negative regulator of angiogenic sprouting. Proc Natl Acad Sci U S A 104(9):3219–3224
15. Harrington LS, Sainson RC, Williams CK, Taylor JM, Shi W, Li JL et al (2008) Regulation of multiple angiogenic pathways by Dll4 and notch in human umbilical vein endothelial cells. Microvasc Res 75(2):144–154
16. Funahashi Y, Shawber CJ, Vorontchikhina M, Sharma A, Outtz HH, Kitajewski J (2010) Notch regulates the angiogenic response via induction of VEGFR-1. J Angiogenes Res 2(1):3
17. Gerhardt H, Golding M, Fruttiger M, Ruhrberg C, Lundkvist A, Abramsson A et al (2003) VEGF guides angiogenic sprouting utilizing endothelial tip cell filopodia. J Cell Biol 161(6):1163–1177
18. Fantin A, Vieira JM, Plein A, Denti L, Fruttiger M, Pollard JW et al (2013) NRP1 acts cell autonomously in endothelium to promote tip cell function during sprouting angiogenesis. Blood 121(12):2352–2362
19. Segarra M, Ohnuki H, Maric D, Salvucci O, Hou X, Kumar A et al (2012) Semaphorin 6A regulates angiogenesis by modulating VEGF signaling. Blood 120(19):4104–4115
20. Phng LK, Potente M, Leslie JD, Babbage J, Nyqvist D, Lobov I et al (2009) Nrarp coordinates endothelial notch and Wnt signaling to control vessel density in angiogenesis. Dev Cell 16(1):70–82
21. Patan S, Alvarez MJ, Schittny JC, Burri PH (1992) Intussusceptive microvascular growth: a common alternative to capillary sprouting. Arch Histol Cytol 55(Suppl):65–75
22. Burri PH, Tarek MR (1990) A novel mechanism of capillary growth in the rat pulmonary microcirculation. Anat Rec 228(1):35–45
23. Hellström M, Kalén M, Lindahl P, Abramsson A, Betsholtz C (1999) Role of PDGF-B and PDGFR-beta in recruitment of vascular smooth muscle cells and pericytes during embryonic blood vessel formation in the mouse. Development 126(14):3047–3055
24. Wilting J, Birkenhäger R, Eichmann A, Kurz H, Martiny-Baron G, Marmé D et al (1996) VEGF121 induces proliferation of vascular endothelial cells and expression of flk-1 without affecting lymphatic vessels of chorioallantoic membrane. Dev Biol 176(1):76–85
25. Crivellato E, Nico B, Vacca A, Djonov V, Presta M, Ribatti D (2004) Recombinant human erythropoietin induces intussusceptive microvascular growth in vivo. Leukemia 18(2):331–336
26. Ribatti D, Nico B, Floris C, Mangieri D, Piras F, Ennas MG et al (2005) Microvascular density, vascular endothelial growth factor immunoreactivity in tumor cells, vessel diameter and intussusceptive microvascular growth in primary melanoma. Oncol Rep 14(1):81–84

27. Nico B, Crivellato E, Guidolin D, Annese T, Longo V, Finato N et al (2010) Intussusceptive microvascular growth in human glioma. Clin Exp Med 10(2):93–98
28. Patan S, Munn LL, Jain RK (1996) Intussusceptive microvascular growth in a human colon adenocarcinoma xenograft: a novel mechanism of tumor angiogenesis. Microvasc Res 51(2): 260–272
29. Djonov V, Högger K, Sedlacek R, Laissue J, Draeger A (2001) MMP-19: cellular localization of a novel metalloproteinase within normal breast tissue and mammary gland tumours. J Pathol 195(2):147–155
30. Risau W, Sariola H, Zerwes HG, Sasse J, Ekblom P, Kemler R et al (1988) Vasculogenesis and angiogenesis in embryonic-stem-cell-derived embryoid bodies. Development 102(3):471–478
31. Risau W, Lemmon V (1988) Changes in the vascular extracellular matrix during embryonic vasculogenesis and angiogenesis. Dev Biol 125(2):441–450
32. Asahara T, Murohara T, Sullivan A, Silver M, van der Zee R, Li T et al (1997) Isolation of putative progenitor endothelial cells for angiogenesis. Science 275(5302):964–967
33. Bussolati B, Grange C, Camussi G (2011) Tumor exploits alternative strategies to achieve vascularization. FASEB J 25(9):2874–2882
34. Kioi M, Vogel H, Schultz G, Hoffman RM, Harsh GR, Brown JM (2010) Inhibition of vasculogenesis, but not angiogenesis, prevents the recurrence of glioblastoma after irradiation in mice. J Clin Invest 120(3):694–705
35. Ahn JB, Rha SY, Shin SJ, Jeung HC, Kim TS, Zhang X et al (2010) Circulating endothelial progenitor cells (EPC) for tumor vasculogenesis in gastric cancer patients. Cancer Lett 288(1): 124–132
36. Greenfield JP, Cobb WS, Lyden D (2010) Resisting arrest: a switch from angiogenesis to vasculogenesis in recurrent malignant gliomas. J Clin Invest 120(3):663–667
37. Chopra H, Hung MK, Kwong DL, Zhang CF, Pow EHN (2018) Insights into endothelial progenitor cells: origin, classification, potentials, and prospects. Stem Cells Int 2018:9847015
38. Schmidt A, Brixius K, Bloch W (2007) Endothelial precursor cell migration during vasculogenesis. Circ Res 101(2):125–136
39. Asahara T, Takahashi T, Masuda H, Kalka C, Chen D, Iwaguro H et al (1999) VEGF contributes to postnatal neovascularization by mobilizing bone marrow-derived endothelial progenitor cells. EMBO J 18(14):3964–3972
40. Hattori K, Dias S, Heissig B, Hackett NR, Lyden D, Tateno M et al (2001) Vascular endothelial growth factor and angiopoietin-1 stimulate postnatal hematopoiesis by recruitment of vasculogenic and hematopoietic stem cells. J Exp Med 193(9):1005–1014
41. Kopp HG, Ramos CA, Rafii S (2006) Contribution of endothelial progenitors and proangiogenic hematopoietic cells to vascularization of tumor and ischemic tissue. Curr Opin Hematol 13(3):175–181
42. Chang EI, Chang EI, Thangarajah H, Hamou C, Gurtner GC (2007) Hypoxia, hormones, and endothelial progenitor cells in hemangioma. Lymphat Res Biol 5(4):237–243
43. Spring H, Schüler T, Arnold B, Hämmerling GJ, Ganss R (2005) Chemokines direct endothelial progenitors into tumor neovessels. Proc Natl Acad Sci U S A 102(50):18111–18116
44. Nakamura N, Naruse K, Matsuki T, Hamada Y, Nakashima E, Kamiya H et al (2009) Adiponectin promotes migration activities of endothelial progenitor cells via Cdc42/Rac1. FEBS Lett 583(15):2457–2463
45. Fausto N (2000) Vasculogenic mimicry in tumors. Fact or artifact? Am J Pathol 156(2):359
46. Seftor RE, Hess AR, Seftor EA, Kirschmann DA, Hardy KM, Margaryan NV et al (2012) Tumor cell vasculogenic mimicry: from controversy to therapeutic promise. Am J Pathol 181(4):1115–1125
47. Folberg R, Maniotis AJ (2004) Vasculogenic mimicry. APMIS: acta pathologica, microbiologica, et immunologica. Scandinavica 112(7–8):508–525
48. Angara K, Borin TF, Arbab AS (2017) Vascular mimicry: a novel neovascularization mechanism driving anti-Angiogenic therapy (AAT) resistance in glioblastoma. Transl Oncol 10(4): 650–660

49. Valyi-Nagy K, Kormos B, Ali M, Shukla D, Valyi-Nagy T (2012) Stem cell marker CD271 is expressed by vasculogenic mimicry-forming uveal melanoma cells in three-dimensional cultures. Mol Vis 18:588–592

50. Comito G, Calvani M, Giannoni E, Bianchini F, Calorini L, Torre E et al (2011) HIF-1α stabilization by mitochondrial ROS promotes met-dependent invasive growth and vasculogenic mimicry in melanoma cells. Free Radic Biol Med 51(4):893–904

51. Angara K, Rashid MH, Shankar A, Ara R, Iskander A, Borin TF et al (2017) Vascular mimicry in glioblastoma following anti-angiogenic and anti-20-HETE therapies. Histol Histopathol 32(9):917–928

52. Ricci-Vitiani L, Pallini R, Biffoni M, Todaro M, Invernici G, Cenci T et al (2010) Tumour vascularization via endothelial differentiation of glioblastoma stem-like cells. Nature 468(7325):824–828

53. Wang R, Chadalavada K, Wilshire J, Kowalik U, Hovinga KE, Geber A et al (2010) Glioblastoma stem-like cells give rise to tumour endothelium. Nature 468(7325):829–833

54. Mei X, Chen YS, Chen FR, Xi SY, Chen ZP (2017) Glioblastoma stem cell differentiation into endothelial cells evidenced through live-cell imaging. Neuro-Oncology 19(8):1109–1118

55. Bussolati B, Grange C, Sapino A, Camussi G (2009) Endothelial cell differentiation of human breast tumour stem/progenitor cells. J Cell Mol Med 13(2):309–319

56. Alvero AB, Fu HH, Holmberg J, Visintin I, Mor L, Marquina CC et al (2009) Stem-like ovarian cancer cells can serve as tumor vascular progenitors. Stem Cells 27(10):2405–2413

57. Zhao Y, Dong J, Huang Q, Lou M, Wang A, Lan Q (2010) Endothelial cell transdifferentiation of human glioma stem progenitor cells in vitro. Brain Res Bull 82(5–6):308–312

58. Kulla A, Burkhardt K, Meyer-Puttlitz B, Teesalu T, Asser T, Wiestler OD et al (2003) Analysis of the TP53 gene in laser-microdissected glioblastoma vasculature. Acta Neuropathol 105(4):328–332

59. Rodriguez FJ, Orr BA, Ligon KL, Eberhart CG (2012) Neoplastic cells are a rare component in human glioblastoma microvasculature. Oncotarget 3(1):98–106

60. Cheng L, Huang Z, Zhou W, Wu Q, Donnola S, Liu JK et al (2013) Glioblastoma stem cells generate vascular pericytes to support vessel function and tumor growth. Cell 153(1):139–152

61. Kuczynski EA, Vermeulen PB, Pezzella F, Kerbel RS, Reynolds AR (2019) Vessel co-option in cancer. Nat Rev Clin Oncol 16(8):469–493

62. Latacz E, Caspani E, Barnhill R, Lugassy C, Verhoef C, Grunhagen D et al (2020) Pathological features of vessel co-option versus sprouting angiogenesis. Angiogenesis 23(1):43–54

63. Matsumoto K, Yoshitomi H, Rossant J, Zaret KS (2001) Liver organogenesis promoted by endothelial cells prior to vascular function. Science 294(5542):559–563

64. Bentolila LA, Prakash R, Mihic-Probst D, Wadehra M, Kleinman HK, Carmichael TS et al (2016) Imaging of Angiotropism/vascular co-option in a murine model of brain melanoma: implications for melanoma progression along extravascular pathways. Sci Rep 6:23834

65. Enderling H, Hlatky L, Hahnfeldt P (2009) Migration rules: tumours are conglomerates of self-metastases. Br J Cancer 100(12):1917–1925

66. Baluk P, Hashizume H, McDonald DM (2005) Cellular abnormalities of blood vessels as targets in cancer. Curr Opin Genet Dev 15(1):102–111

67. McDonald DM, Baluk P (2005) Imaging of angiogenesis in inflamed airways and tumors: newly formed blood vessels are not alike and may be wildly abnormal: Parker B Francis lecture. Chest 128(6 Suppl):602s–608s

68. Kimura H, Braun RD, Ong ET, Hsu R, Secomb TW, Papahadjopoulos D et al (1996) Fluctuations in red cell flux in tumor microvessels can lead to transient hypoxia and reoxygenation in tumor parenchyma. Cancer Res 56(23):5522–5528

69. Bennewith KL, Durand RE (2004) Quantifying transient hypoxia in human tumor xenografts by flow cytometry. Cancer Res 64(17):6183–6189

70. Hashizume H, Baluk P, Morikawa S, McLean JW, Thurston G, Roberge S et al (2000) Openings between defective endothelial cells explain tumor vessel leakiness. Am J Pathol 156(4):1363–1380

71. Padera TP, Stoll BR, Tooredman JB, Capen D, di Tomaso E, Jain RK (2004) Pathology: cancer cells compress intratumour vessels. Nature 427(6976):695
72. Abramsson A, Berlin O, Papayan H, Paulin D, Shani M, Betsholtz C (2002) Analysis of mural cell recruitment to tumor vessels. Circulation 105(1):112–117
73. Morikawa S, Baluk P, Kaidoh T, Haskell A, Jain RK, McDonald DM (2002) Abnormalities in pericytes on blood vessels and endothelial sprouts in tumors. Am J Pathol 160(3):985–1000
74. Baluk P, Morikawa S, Haskell A, Mancuso M, McDonald DM (2003) Abnormalities of basement membrane on blood vessels and endothelial sprouts in tumors. Am J Pathol 163(5):1801–1815
75. St Croix B, Rago C, Velculescu V, Traverso G, Romans KE, Montgomery E et al (2000) Genes expressed in human tumor endothelium. Science 289(5482):1197–1202
76. Zhang L, Yang N, Park JW, Katsaros D, Fracchioli S, Cao G et al (2003) Tumor-derived vascular endothelial growth factor up-regulates angiopoietin-2 in host endothelium and destabilizes host vasculature, supporting angiogenesis in ovarian cancer. Cancer Res 63(12): 3403–3412
77. Carson-Walter EB, Watkins DN, Nanda A, Vogelstein B, Kinzler KW, St CB (2001) Cell surface tumor endothelial markers are conserved in mice and humans. Cancer Res 61(18): 6649–6655
78. Huang X, Bai X, Cao Y, Wu J, Huang M, Tang D et al (2010) Lymphoma endothelium preferentially expresses Tim-3 and facilitates the progression of lymphoma by mediating immune evasion. J Exp Med 207(3):505–520
79. Dieterich LC, Mellberg S, Langenkamp E, Zhang L, Zieba A, Salomäki H et al (2012) Transcriptional profiling of human glioblastoma vessels indicates a key role of VEGF-A and TGFβ2 in vascular abnormalization. J Pathol 228(3):378–390
80. Roudnicky F, Poyet C, Wild P, Krampitz S, Negrini F, Huggenberger R et al (2013) Endocan is upregulated on tumor vessels in invasive bladder cancer where it mediates VEGF-a-induced angiogenesis. Cancer Res 73(3):1097–1106
81. Zhao Q, Eichten A, Parveen A, Adler C, Huang Y, Wang W et al (2018) Single-cell transcriptome analyses reveal endothelial cell heterogeneity in Tumors and changes following antiangiogenic treatment. Cancer Res 78(9):2370–2382
82. Buckanovich RJ, Sasaroli D, O'Brien-Jenkins A, Botbyl J, Hammond R, Katsaros D et al (2007) Tumor vascular proteins as biomarkers in ovarian cancer. J Clin Oncol 25(7):852–861
83. Zhang L, He L, Lugano R, Roodakker K, Bergqvist M, Smits A et al (2018) IDH mutation status is associated with distinct vascular gene expression signatures in lower-grade gliomas. Neuro Oncol 20(11):1505–1516
84. Masiero M, Simões FC, Han HD, Snell C, Peterkin T, Bridges E et al (2013) A core human primary tumor angiogenesis signature identifies the endothelial orphan receptor ELTD1 as a key regulator of angiogenesis. Cancer Cell 24(2):229–241
85. Langenkamp E, Zhang L, Lugano R, Huang H, Elhassan TE, Georganaki M et al (2015) Elevated expression of the C-type lectin CD93 in the glioblastoma vasculature regulates cytoskeletal rearrangements that enhance vessel function and reduce host survival. Cancer Res 75(21):4504–4516
86. Viski C, König C, Kijewska M, Mogler C, Isacke CM, Augustin HG (2016) Endosialin-expressing pericytes promote metastatic dissemination. Cancer Res 76(18):5313–5325
87. Motz GT, Santoro SP, Wang LP, Garrabrant T, Lastra RR, Hagemann IS et al (2014) Tumor endothelium FasL establishes a selective immune barrier promoting tolerance in tumors. Nat Med 20(6):607–615
88. Buckanovich RJ, Facciabene A, Kim S, Benencia F, Sasaroli D, Balint K et al (2008) Endothelin B receptor mediates the endothelial barrier to T cell homing to tumors and disables immune therapy. Nat Med 14(1):28–36
89. Phoenix TN, Patmore DM, Boop S, Boulos N, Jacus MO, Patel YT et al (2016) Medulloblastoma genotype dictates blood brain barrier phenotype. Cancer Cell 29(4):508–522

90. Apte RS, Chen DS, Ferrara N (2019) VEGF in signaling and disease: beyond discovery and development. Cell 176(6):1248–1264

91. Claesson-Welsh L, Welsh M (2013) VEGFA and tumour angiogenesis. J Intern Med 273(2): 114–127

92. Jiang BH, Liu LZ (2009) PI3K/PTEN signaling in angiogenesis and tumorigenesis. Adv Cancer Res 102:19–65

93. Lamalice L, Le Boeuf F, Huot J (2007) Endothelial cell migration during angiogenesis. Circ Res 100(6):782–794

94. van Hinsbergh VW, Koolwijk P (2008) Endothelial sprouting and angiogenesis: matrix metalloproteinases in the lead. Cardiovasc Res 78(2):203–212

95. Azzi S, Hebda JK, Gavard J (2013) Vascular permeability and drug delivery in cancers. Front Oncol 3:211

96. Hofer E, Schweighofer B (2007) Signal transduction induced in endothelial cells by growth factor receptors involved in angiogenesis. Thromb Haemost 97(3):355–363

97. Autiero M, Waltenberger J, Communi D, Kranz A, Moons L, Lambrechts D et al (2003) Role of PlGF in the intra- and intermolecular cross talk between the VEGF receptors Flt1 and Flk1. Nat Med 9(7):936–943

98. Schomber T, Kopfstein L, Djonov V, Albrecht I, Baeriswyl V, Strittmatter K et al (2007) Placental growth factor-1 attenuates vascular endothelial growth factor-A-dependent tumor angiogenesis during beta cell carcinogenesis. Cancer Res 67(22):10840–10848

99. Franco M, Roswall P, Cortez E, Hanahan D, Pietras K (2011) Pericytes promote endothelial cell survival through induction of autocrine VEGF-A signaling and Bcl-w expression. Blood 118(10):2906–2917

100. Betsholtz C (2004) Insight into the physiological functions of PDGF through genetic studies in mice. Cytokine Growth Factor Rev 15(4):215–228

101. Guo P, Hu B, Gu W, Xu L, Wang D, Huang HJ et al (2003) Platelet-derived growth factor-B enhances glioma angiogenesis by stimulating vascular endothelial growth factor expression in tumor endothelia and by promoting pericyte recruitment. Am J Pathol 162(4):1083–1093

102. Turner N, Grose R (2010) Fibroblast growth factor signalling: from development to cancer. Nat Rev Cancer 10(2):116–129

103. Yu P, Wilhelm K, Dubrac A, Tung JK, Alves TC, Fang JS et al (2017) FGF-dependent metabolic control of vascular development. Nature 545(7653):224–228

104. Incio J, Ligibel JA, McManus DT, Suboj P, Jung K, Kawaguchi K et al (2018) Obesity promotes resistance to anti-VEGF therapy in breast cancer by up-regulating IL-6 and potentially FGF-2. Sci Transl Med 10(432):eaag0945

105. Surawska H, Ma PC, Salgia R (2004) The role of ephrins and Eph receptors in cancer. Cytokine Growth Factor Rev 15(6):419–433

106. Dodelet VC, Pasquale EB (2000) Eph receptors and ephrin ligands: embryogenesis to tumorigenesis. Oncogene 19(49):5614–5619

107. Dong Y, Wang J, Sheng Z, Li G, Ma H, Wang X et al (2009) Downregulation of EphA1 in colorectal carcinomas correlates with invasion and metastasis. Mod Pathol 22(1):151–160

108. Hafner C, Bataille F, Meyer S, Becker B, Roesch A, Landthaler M et al (2003) Loss of EphB6 expression in metastatic melanoma. Int J Oncol 23(6):1553–1559

109. Ogawa K, Pasqualini R, Lindberg RA, Kain R, Freeman AL, Pasquale EB (2000) The ephrin-A1 ligand and its receptor, EphA2, are expressed during tumor neovascularization. Oncogene 19(52):6043–6052

110. Dobrzanski P, Hunter K, Jones-Bolin S, Chang H, Robinson C, Pritchard S et al (2004) Antiangiogenic and antitumor efficacy of EphA2 receptor antagonist. Cancer Res 64(3): 910–919

111. Brantley DM, Cheng N, Thompson EJ, Lin Q, Brekken RA, Thorpe PE et al (2002) Soluble Eph a receptors inhibit tumor angiogenesis and progression in vivo. Oncogene 21(46): 7011–7026

112. Cheng N, Brantley D, Fang WB, Liu H, Fanslow W, Cerretti DP et al (2003) Inhibition of VEGF-dependent multistage carcinogenesis by soluble EphA receptors. Neoplasia 5(5): 445–456
113. Noren NK, Lu M, Freeman AL, Koolpe M, Pasquale EB (2004) Interplay between EphB4 on tumor cells and vascular ephrin-B2 regulates tumor growth. Proc Natl Acad Sci U S A 101(15):5583–5588
114. Uhl C, Markel M, Broggini T, Nieminen M, Kremenetskaia I, Vajkoczy P et al (2018) EphB4 mediates resistance to antiangiogenic therapy in experimental glioma. Angiogenesis 21(4): 873–881
115. Krusche B, Ottone C, Clements MP, Johnstone ER, Goetsch K, Lieven H et al (2016) EphrinB2 drives perivascular invasion and proliferation of glioblastoma stem-like cells. Elife 5:e14845
116. Wang Y, Nakayama M, Pitulescu ME, Schmidt TS, Bochenek ML, Sakakibara A et al (2010) Ephrin-B2 controls VEGF-induced angiogenesis and lymphangiogenesis. Nature 465(7297): 483–486
117. Sawamiphak S, Seidel S, Essmann CL, Wilkinson GA, Pitulescu ME, Acker T et al (2010) Ephrin-B2 regulates VEGFR2 function in developmental and tumour angiogenesis. Nature 465(7297):487–491
118. Reiss Y, Knedla A, Tal AO, Schmidt MHH, Jugold M, Kiessling F et al (2009) Switching of vascular phenotypes within a murine breast cancer model induced by angiopoietin-2. J Pathol 217(4):571–580
119. Shim WS, Ho IA, Wong PE (2007) Angiopoietin: a TIE(d) balance in tumor angiogenesis. Mol Cancer Res 5(7):655–665
120. Fiedler U, Reiss Y, Scharpfenecker M, Grunow V, Koidl S, Thurston G et al (2006) Angiopoietin-2 sensitizes endothelial cells to TNF-alpha and has a crucial role in the induction of inflammation. Nat Med 12(2):235–239
121. Chae SS, Kamoun WS, Farrar CT, Kirkpatrick ND, Niemeyer E, de Graaf AM et al (2010) Angiopoietin-2 interferes with anti-VEGFR2-induced vessel normalization and survival benefit in mice bearing gliomas. Clin Cancer Res 16(14):3618–3627
122. Peterson TE, Kirkpatrick ND, Huang Y, Farrar CT, Marijt KA, Kloepper J et al (2016) Dual inhibition of Ang-2 and VEGF receptors normalizes tumor vasculature and prolongs survival in glioblastoma by altering macrophages. Proc Natl Acad Sci U S A 113(16):4470–4475
123. Kloepper J, Riedemann L, Amoozgar Z, Seano G, Susek K, Yu V et al (2016) Ang-2/VEGF bispecific antibody reprograms macrophages and resident microglia to anti-tumor phenotype and prolongs glioblastoma survival. Proc Natl Acad Sci U S A 113(16):4476–4481
124. Wu FT, Man S, Xu P, Chow A, Paez-Ribes M, Lee CR et al (2016) Efficacy of Cotargeting Angiopoietin-2 and the VEGF pathway in the adjuvant postsurgical setting for early breast, colorectal, and renal cancers. Cancer Res 76(23):6988–7000
125. Kälin RE, Kretz MP, Meyer AM, Kispert A, Heppner FL, Brändli AW (2007) Paracrine and autocrine mechanisms of apelin signaling govern embryonic and tumor angiogenesis. Dev Biol 305(2):599–614
126. Berta J, Kenessey I, Dobos J, Tovari J, Klepetko W, Jan Ankersmit H et al (2010) Apelin expression in human non-small cell lung cancer: role in angiogenesis and prognosis. J Thorac Oncol 5(8):1120–1129
127. Tolkach Y, Ellinger J, Kremer A, Esser L, Müller SC, Stephan C et al (2019) Apelin and apelin receptor expression in renal cell carcinoma. Br J Cancer 120(6):633–639
128. Seaman S, Stevens J, Yang MY, Logsdon D, Graff-Cherry C, St Croix B (2007) Genes that distinguish physiological and pathological angiogenesis. Cancer Cell 11(6):539–554
129. Macaluso NJ, Pitkin SL, Maguire JJ, Davenport AP, Glen RC (2011) Discovery of a competitive apelin receptor (APJ) antagonist. ChemMedChem 6(6):1017–1023
130. Uribesalgo I, Hoffmann D, Zhang Y, Kavirayani A, Lazovic J, Berta J et al (2019) Apelin inhibition prevents resistance and metastasis associated with anti-angiogenic therapy. EMBO Mol Med 11(8):e9266

131. Mastrella G, Hou M, Li M, Stoecklein VM, Zdouc N, Volmar MNM et al (2019) Targeting APLN/APLNR improves antiangiogenic efficiency and blunts proinvasive side effects of VEGFA/VEGFR2 blockade in glioblastoma. Cancer Res 79(9):2298–2313
132. Ijichi H, Chytil A, Gorska AE, Aakre ME, Bierie B, Tada M et al (2011) Inhibiting Cxcr2 disrupts tumor-stromal interactions and improves survival in a mouse model of pancreatic ductal adenocarcinoma. J Clin Invest 121(10):4106–4117
133. Yang G, Rosen DG, Liu G, Yang F, Guo X, Xiao X et al (2010) CXCR2 promotes ovarian cancer growth through dysregulated cell cycle, diminished apoptosis, and enhanced angiogenesis. Clin Cancer Res 16(15):3875–3886
134. Smith ML, Olson TS, Ley K (2004) CXCR2- and E-selectin-induced neutrophil arrest during inflammation in vivo. J Exp Med 200(7):935–939
135. Xu J, Liang J, Meng YM, Yan J, Yu XJ, Liu CQ et al (2017) Vascular CXCR4 expression promotes vessel sprouting and sensitivity to Sorafenib treatment in hepatocellular carcinoma. Clin Cancer Res 23(15):4482–4492
136. Martin D, Galisteo R, Gutkind JS (2009) CXCL8/IL8 stimulates vascular endothelial growth factor (VEGF) expression and the autocrine activation of VEGFR2 in endothelial cells by activating NFkappaB through the CBM (Carma3/Bcl10/Malt1) complex. J Biol Chem 284(10):6038–6042
137. Scapini P, Morini M, Tecchio C, Minghelli S, Di Carlo E, Tanghetti E et al (2004) CXCL1/macrophage inflammatory protein-2-induced angiogenesis in vivo is mediated by neutrophil-derived vascular endothelial growth factor-A. J Immunol 172(8):5034–5040
138. Zhao X, Town JR, Li F, Zhang X, Cockcroft DW, Gordon JR (2009) ELR-CXC chemokine receptor antagonism targets inflammatory responses at multiple levels. J Immunol 182(5): 3213–3222
139. Li A, Varney ML, Valasek J, Godfrey M, Dave BJ, Singh RK (2005) Autocrine role of interleukin-8 in induction of endothelial cell proliferation, survival, migration and MMP-2 production and angiogenesis. Angiogenesis 8(1):63–71
140. Kobayashi Y (2008) The role of chemokines in neutrophil biology. Front Biosci 13:2400–2407
141. Ceradini DJ, Kulkarni AR, Callaghan MJ, Tepper OM, Bastidas N, Kleinman ME et al (2004) Progenitor cell trafficking is regulated by hypoxic gradients through HIF-1 induction of SDF-1. Nat Med 10(8):858–864
142. Wolf MJ, Hoos A, Bauer J, Boettcher S, Knust M, Weber A et al (2012) Endothelial CCR2 signaling induced by colon carcinoma cells enables extravasation via the JAK2-Stat5 and p38MAPK pathway. Cancer Cell 22(1):91–105
143. Chen X, Wang Y, Nelson D, Tian S, Mulvey E, Patel B et al (2016) CCL2/CCR2 regulates the tumor microenvironment in HER-2/neu-driven mammary carcinomas in mice. PLoS One 11(11):e0165595
144. Yu Q, Stamenkovic I (2000) Cell surface-localized matrix metalloproteinase-9 proteolytically activates TGF-beta and promotes tumor invasion and angiogenesis. Genes Dev 14(2):163–176
145. Gupta MK, Qin RY (2003) Mechanism and its regulation of tumor-induced angiogenesis. World J Gastroenterol 9(6):1144–1155
146. Sainson RC, Johnston DA, Chu HC, Holderfield MT, Nakatsu MN, Crampton SP et al (2008) TNF primes endothelial cells for angiogenic sprouting by inducing a tip cell phenotype. Blood 111(10):4997–5007
147. Lu KV, Jong KA, Kim GY, Singh J, Dia EQ, Yoshimoto K et al (2005) Differential induction of glioblastoma migration and growth by two forms of pleiotrophin. J Biol Chem 280(29): 26953–26964
148. Chen H, Campbell RA, Chang Y, Li M, Wang CS, Li J et al (2009) Pleiotrophin produced by multiple myeloma induces transdifferentiation of monocytes into vascular endothelial cells: a novel mechanism of tumor-induced vasculogenesis. Blood 113(9):1992–2002

149. Zhang L, Kundu S, Feenstra T, Li X, Jin C, Laaniste L et al (2015) Pleiotrophin promotes vascular abnormalization in gliomas and correlates with poor survival in patients with astrocytomas. Sci Signal 8(406):ra125
150. Acevedo L, Yu J, Erdjument-Bromage H, Miao RQ, Kim JE, Fulton D et al (2004) A new role for Nogo as a regulator of vascular remodeling. Nat Med 10(4):382–388
151. Zhu B, Chen S, Hu X, Jin X, Le Y, Cao L et al (2017) Knockout of the Nogo-B gene attenuates tumor growth and metastasis in hepatocellular carcinoma. Neoplasia 19(7):583–593
152. Cai H, Saiyin H, Liu X, Han D, Ji G, Qin B et al (2018) Nogo-B promotes tumor angiogenesis and provides a potential therapeutic target in hepatocellular carcinoma. Mol Oncol 12(12): 2042–2054
153. Hanahan D, Coussens LM (2012) Accessories to the crime: functions of cells recruited to the tumor microenvironment. Cancer Cell 21(3):309–322
154. de Visser KE, Coussens LM (2006) The inflammatory tumor microenvironment and its impact on cancer development. Contrib Microbiol 13:118–137
155. Benelli R, Lorusso G, Albini A, Noonan DM (2006) Cytokines and chemokines as regulators of angiogenesis in health and disease. Curr Pharm Des 12(24):3101–3115
156. Albini A, Bruno A, Noonan DM, Mortara L (2018) Contribution to tumor angiogenesis from innate immune cells within the tumor microenvironment: implications for immunotherapy. Front Immunol 9:527
157. Lin EY, Li JF, Gnatovskiy L, Deng Y, Zhu L, Grzesik DA et al (2006) Macrophages regulate the angiogenic switch in a mouse model of breast cancer. Cancer Res 66(23):11238–11246
158. Zhang W, Zhu XD, Sun HC, Xiong YQ, Zhuang PY, Xu HX et al (2010) Depletion of tumor-associated macrophages enhances the effect of sorafenib in metastatic liver cancer models by antimetastatic and antiangiogenic effects. Clin Cancer Res 16(13):3420–3430
159. Mantovani A, Sica A (2010) Macrophages, innate immunity and cancer: balance, tolerance, and diversity. Curr Opin Immunol 22(2):231–237
160. Špirić Z, Eri Ž, Erić M (2015) Significance of vascular endothelial growth factor (VEGF)-C and VEGF-D in the progression of cutaneous melanoma. Int J Surg Pathol 23(8):629–637
161. Cejudo-Martín P, Morales-Ruiz M, Ros J, Navasa M, Fernández-Varo G, Fuster J et al (2002) Hypoxia is an inducer of vasodilator agents in peritoneal macrophages of cirrhotic patients. Hepatology 36(5):1172–1179
162. Zhang J, Sud S, Mizutani K, Gyetko MR, Pienta KJ (2011) Activation of urokinase plasminogen activator and its receptor axis is essential for macrophage infiltration in a prostate cancer mouse model. Neoplasia 13(1):23–30
163. Coffelt SB, Wellenstein MD, de Visser KE (2016) Neutrophils in cancer: neutral no more. Nat Rev Cancer 16(7):431–446
164. Kumar V, Patel S, Tcyganov E, Gabrilovich DI (2016) The nature of myeloid-derived suppressor cells in the tumor microenvironment. Trends Immunol 37(3):208–220
165. Jacob A, Prekeris R (2015) The regulation of MMP targeting to invadopodia during cancer metastasis. Front Cell Dev Biol 3:4
166. Horikawa N, Abiko K, Matsumura N, Hamanishi J, Baba T, Yamaguchi K et al (2017) Expression of vascular endothelial growth factor in ovarian cancer inhibits tumor immunity through the accumulation of myeloid-derived suppressor cells. Clin Cancer Res 23(2): 587–599
167. Karakhanova S, Link J, Heinrich M, Shevchenko I, Yang Y, Hassenpflug M et al (2015) Characterization of myeloid leukocytes and soluble mediators in pancreatic cancer: importance of myeloid-derived suppressor cells. Onco Targets Ther 4(4):e998519
168. Chun E, Lavoie S, Michaud M, Gallini CA, Kim J, Soucy G et al (2015) CCL2 promotes colorectal carcinogenesis by enhancing Polymorphonuclear myeloid-derived suppressor cell population and function. Cell Rep 12(2):244–257
169. Obermajer N, Muthuswamy R, Odunsi K, Edwards RP, Kalinski P (2011) PGE(2)-induced CXCL12 production and CXCR4 expression controls the accumulation of human MDSCs in ovarian cancer environment. Cancer Res 71(24):7463–7470

170. Shojaei F, Wu X, Zhong C, Yu L, Liang XH, Yao J et al (2007) Bv8 regulates myeloid-cell-dependent tumour angiogenesis. Nature 450(7171):825–831
171. van Hooren L, Georganaki M, Huang H, Mangsbo SM, Dimberg A (2016) Sunitinib enhances the antitumor responses of agonistic CD40-antibody by reducing MDSCs and synergistically improving endothelial activation and T-cell recruitment. Oncotarget 7(31):50277–50289
172. Tecchio C, Scapini P, Pizzolo G, Cassatella MA (2013) On the cytokines produced by human neutrophils in tumors. Semin Cancer Biol 23(3):159–170
173. Mueller MD, Lebovic DI, Garrett E, Taylor RN (2000) Neutrophils infiltrating the endometrium express vascular endothelial growth factor: potential role in endometrial angiogenesis. Fertil Steril 74(1):107–112
174. Heryanto B, Girling JE, Rogers PA (2004) Intravascular neutrophils partially mediate the endometrial endothelial cell proliferative response to oestrogen in ovariectomised mice. Reproduction 127(5):613–620
175. Shaw JP, Chuang N, Yee H, Shamamian P (2003) Polymorphonuclear neutrophils promote rFGF-2-induced angiogenesis in vivo. J Surg Res 109(1):37–42
176. Benelli R, Morini M, Carrozzino F, Ferrari N, Minghelli S, Santi L et al (2002) Neutrophils as a key cellular target for angiostatin: implications for regulation of angiogenesis and inflammation. FASEB J 16(2):267–269
177. Shaul ME, Fridlender ZG (2017) Neutrophils as active regulators of the immune system in the tumor microenvironment. J Leukoc Biol 102(2):343–349
178. Fridlender ZG, Sun J, Kim S, Kapoor V, Cheng G, Ling L et al (2009) Polarization of tumor-associated neutrophil phenotype by TGF-beta: "N1" versus "N2" TAN. Cancer Cell 16(3):183–194
179. Nozawa H, Chiu C, Hanahan D (2006) Infiltrating neutrophils mediate the initial angiogenic switch in a mouse model of multistage carcinogenesis. Proc Natl Acad Sci U S A 103(33):12493–12498
180. Ardi VC, Kupriyanova TA, Deryugina EI, Quigley JP (2007) Human neutrophils uniquely release TIMP-free MMP-9 to provide a potent catalytic stimulator of angiogenesis. Proc Natl Acad Sci U S A 104(51):20262–20267
181. Blotnick S, Peoples GE, Freeman MR, Eberlein TJ, Klagsbrun M (1994) T lymphocytes synthesize and export heparin-binding epidermal growth factor-like growth factor and basic fibroblast growth factor, mitogens for vascular cells and fibroblasts: differential production and release by CD4+ and CD8+ T cells. Proc Natl Acad Sci U S A 91(8):2890–2894
182. Fathallah-Shaykh HM, Zhao LJ, Kafrouni AI, Smith GM, Forman J (2000) Gene transfer of IFN-gamma into established brain tumors represses growth by antiangiogenesis. J Immunol 164(1):217–222
183. Friesel R, Komoriya A, Maciag T (1987) Inhibition of endothelial cell proliferation by gamma-interferon. J Cell Biol 104(3):689–696
184. Madri JA, Pratt BM, Tucker AM (1988) Phenotypic modulation of endothelial cells by transforming growth factor-beta depends upon the composition and organization of the extracellular matrix. J Cell Biol 106(4):1375–1384
185. Sato N, Nariuchi H, Tsuruoka N, Nishihara T, Beitz JG, Calabresi P et al (1990) Actions of TNF and IFN-gamma on angiogenesis in vitro. J Invest Dermatol 95(6 Suppl):85s–89s
186. Maheshwari RK, Srikantan V, Bhartiya D, Kleinman HK, Grant DS (1991) Differential effects of interferon gamma and alpha on in vitro model of angiogenesis. J Cell Physiol 146(1):164–169
187. Fridman WH, Pages F, Sautes-Fridman C, Galon J (2012) The immune contexture in human tumours: impact on clinical outcome. Nat Rev Cancer 12(4):298–306
188. Strieter RM, Burdick MD, Gomperts BN, Belperio JA, Keane MP (2005) CXC chemokines in angiogenesis. Cytokine Growth Factor Rev 16(6):593–609
189. Burdick MD, Murray LA, Keane MP, Xue YY, Zisman DA, Belperio JA et al (2005) CXCL11 attenuates bleomycin-induced pulmonary fibrosis via inhibition of vascular remodeling. Am J Respir Crit Care Med 171(3):261–268

190. Lasagni L, Francalanci M, Annunziato F, Lazzeri E, Giannini S, Cosmi L et al (2003) An alternatively spliced variant of CXCR3 mediates the inhibition of endothelial cell growth induced by IP-10, Mig, and I-TAC, and acts as functional receptor for platelet factor 4. J Exp Med 197(11):1537–1549
191. Yang C, Lee H, Pal S, Jove V, Deng J, Zhang W et al (2013) B cells promote tumor progression via STAT3 regulated-angiogenesis. PLoS One 8(5):e64159
192. Andreu P, Johansson M, Affara NI, Pucci F, Tan T, Junankar S et al (2010) FcRgamma activation regulates inflammation-associated squamous carcinogenesis. Cancer Cell 17(2): 121–134
193. Hanna J, Goldman-Wohl D, Hamani Y, Avraham I, Greenfield C, Natanson-Yaron S et al (2006) Decidual NK cells regulate key developmental processes at the human fetal-maternal interface. Nat Med 12(9):1065–1074
194. Blois SM, Klapp BF, Barrientos G (2011) Decidualization and angiogenesis in early pregnancy: unravelling the functions of DC and NK cells. J Reprod Immunol 88(2):86–92
195. Keskin DB, Allan DS, Rybalov B, Andzelm MM, Stern JN, Kopcow HD et al (2007) TGFbeta promotes conversion of CD16+ peripheral blood NK cells into CD16- NK cells with similarities to decidual NK cells. Proc Natl Acad Sci U S A 104(9):3378–3383
196. Bruno A, Focaccetti C, Pagani A, Imperatori AS, Spagnoletti M, Rotolo N et al (2013) The proangiogenic phenotype of natural killer cells in patients with non-small cell lung cancer. Neoplasia 15(2):133–142
197. Gao Y, Souza-Fonseca-Guimaraes F, Bald T, Ng SS, Young A, Ngiow SF et al (2017) Tumor immunoevasion by the conversion of effector NK cells into type 1 innate lymphoid cells. Nat Immunol 18(9):1004–1015

Chapter 7
Physiological Changes in Local *Onco-Sphere:* Lymphangiogenesis

Phei Er Saw and Erwei Song

Abstract Lymphangiogenesis is the process of formation of new lymphatic vessels from already existing lymphatic capillaries. This process is especially important in cancer metastasis as lymphangiogenesis is the major pathway of cancer cells metastasizing to the regional lymph nodes. Therefore, the mechanism underlying lymphangiogenesis in the local onco-sphere is crucial in determining the metastatic potential of a solid tumor. In this chapter, we will summarize the detailed mechanism and function of cancer lymphangiogenesis. We will also outline the various tumor-derived chemokines that drives activation of lymphangiogenesis, that ultimately leads to cancer metastasis in the regional and distal onco-sphere.

Introduction

The lymphatic system is primarily a highway, with constant fluid exchange to maintain tissue fluid homeostasis, collecting and trapping antigens and macromolecules from proximal neighboring tissues. However, the most important function of a lymphatic system, including lymph nodes, is to transport various immune cells,

P. E. Saw
Guangdong Provincial Key Laboratory of Malignant Tumor Epigenetics and Gene Regulation, Guangdong-Hong Kong Joint Laboratory for RNA Medicine, Medical Research Center, Sun Yat-sen Memorial Hospital, Sun Yat-sen University, Guangzhou, China

Nanhai Translational Innovation Center of Precision Immunology, Sun Yat-sen Memorial Hospital, Sun Yat-sen University, Foshan, China

E. Song (✉)
Guangdong Provincial Key Laboratory of Malignant Tumor Epigenetics and Gene Regulation, Guangdong-Hong Kong Joint Laboratory for RNA Medicine, Medical Research Center, Sun Yat-sen Memorial Hospital, Sun Yat-sen University, Guangzhou, China

Nanhai Translational Innovation Center of Precision Immunology, Sun Yat-sen Memorial Hospital, Sun Yat-sen University, Foshan, China

Breast Tumor Center, Sun Yat-sen Memorial Hospital, Sun Yat-sen University, Guangzhou, China
e-mail: songew@mail.sysu.edu.cn

particularly APCs such as DCs, from adjacent tumor cells to lymph nodes [1–4]. The lymphatic system's vasculature is a one-way transportation mechanism without having a central pump as the blood circulatory system, which makes lymph transport dependent on respiratory activities and skeletal muscle compression. The absence of the central pump in the lymphatic system prompts a cellular transportation system with less shear stress and enhanced cell viability [5]. Furthermore, the lymphatic system's vasculature consists of blind-ended thin-walled capillaries in the peripheral tissues with a physically ideal capacity to absorb or ingest proteins, fluids, and cells. Furthermore, lymphatic capillaries are bordered by a layer of sequentially arranged single-celled endothelial cells having an uneven basal layer, whereas blood vessels are encircled by smooth muscle cells or pericytes. Furthermore, tightly adherent synapses between lymphatic endothelial cells are uncommon since most cellular interactions involving endothelial cells are mediated by particular "button-like" junctions. These intersections impart considerable permeability to peripheral lymphatic vessels to ingest interstitial fluids and proteins, thus increasing immune cell transmigration [6].

The anchoring strands present between lymphatic vessels and surrounding tissues act as connectors that extend deeply into the adjacent tissues to securely adhere to the lymphatic endothelial cells (LECs) through ECM. These ECM-overexpressing fibers ensure the exact opening time of the vessels, which otherwise remain closed in normal conditions. During cancer progression, tissue pressure is raised (also discussed in detail in Chap. 9), allowing lymph fluid (containing proteins, cytokines, chemokines, GFs, etc.) and immune cells to enter the lymphatic vasculature [7–9]. Lymph penetrating through the peripheral lymphatic capillaries empties into lymphatic vessels that eventually connect with the bigger lymphatic vessels surrounded by the basal layer and smooth muscle cells, stimulating lymph circulation. These valves' one-way passage also tends to prevent any backward flow of the lymph [8, 10].

The lymph transport process is as follows: (1) All lymph is first pushed toward the lymphatic vessel due to the increased pressure (IFP) in the local *onco-sphere*, (2) pressure induces a one-way flow of lymph into the lymphatic vessel, (3) lymph is delivered by lymphatic vessels traversing through many sequential lymph nodes, (4) lymph is re-absorbed by the thoracic duct and (5) to be reintroduced into the circulation system, and (6) gathers at the venous circulatory node of the jugular and subclavian veins (Fig. 7.1). As a result, the lymphatic system's distinct morphology facilitates tissue fluid absorption as well as immune cell movement. Nonetheless, tumor cells can use the transportation system to their advantage by leveraging conjoint synapses of endothelial cells as well as the uneven basal layer of lymphatic capillaries to ensure their viability. This aspect is evident in lymphangiogenesis, where new lymphatic vessels are actively created at the local *onco-sphere* (discussed in detail in Chap. 10 on the regional *onco-sphere*: development of metastatic lymph nodes) [11–13].

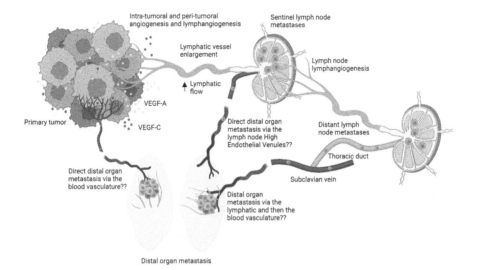

Fig. 7.1 Lymphangiogenesis induced by tumor supports metastasis. VEGF-A and -C, growth factors vital in lymphangiogenesis GFs could promote tumoral lymphangiogenesis. Both GFs also promote the formation of lymph within the tumor-releasing lymph node prior to the progression of the metastatic tumor, which is subsequently aided by the invasion of the metastatic cells. VEGF-induced lymphangiogenesis results in an increase in lymphatic flow into the lymph nodes, as a result, increases metastasis to distant organs, a mechanism often seen via the thoracic duct. However, the mechanisms through which metastatic cells reach the bloodstream remain unknown

Lymphangiogenic Factors

Adults can only experience lymphangiogenesis under particular pathological situations such as inflammation, tissue healing, or malignancies [2, 3, 14]. In the event of certain pathological disorders, new lymphatic vessels proliferate and sprout from preexisting lymphatic vessels [11, 12]. Regardless of this, the precise link between new vasculature and circulating endothelial progenitor cells remains unknown [13]. The latest research found multiple key lymphatic molecular indicators and features that promote the formation of lymphatic vessels, broadening our understanding of the significance of lymphatic morphology in healthy and diseased conditions.

The initial and most widely studied factors were VEGF-C and -D, which are both connected to a tyrosine kinase receptor, namely VEGFR3, found on the lymphatic endothelium [15–18]. The presence of VEGFR-2 in the lymphatic system, as well as on the blood endothelium, supports both lymphangiogenic and angiogenic responses of GFs [19, 20]. The pro-lymphangiogenic features of VEGF-A in mouse models linked with VEGFR-2 but not VEGFR-3 suggest the active role of VEGFR-2 in aiding lymphangiogenesis [21–23]. Neuropilin receptor-2, first discovered during nervous system development, also functions as a co-receptor for VEGF-A, VEGF-C, and VEGF-D. Because of extremely small intracellular domains, they are not thought to aid signaling pathway activation or enzymatic function. Furthermore,

Nrps predominantly promote VEGF receptor signaling by increasing the adherence of VEGF ligands to the receptors [24, 25]. Furthermore, a recent study has shown that Nrps can work independently in the absence of VEGF receptors during the regulation of endothelial cell motility [26, 27]. Additionally, neuropilin-2-deficient mice had poor lymphatic maturation indicated by aberrant patterning, as well as a decreased number of tiny lymphatic capillaries and vessels [28]. Several other elements depicting pro-lymphangiogenic activity have recently been identified, including HGF, which facilitates binding with the C-Met receptor, Angiopoietin-1 and its endothelial cell-specific receptor Tie-2, FGF-1 and -2, PDGF from platelets, IGF-1 and -2, adrenomedullin, and endothelin-1 [29–36]. Herein, we summarized the major factors in lymphangiogenesis in Table 7.1.

Lymphangiogenesis in the Local *Onco-Spheres*

Tumor initiation by lymphangiogenesis is mediated by lymph GFs released and controlled by the tumor cells, stromal cells, tumor-infiltrating macrophages, or active platelets [58–61]. Upregulation of VEGF-C or VEGF-D has significantly aided tumor-linked lymphatic vessel formation and increased the likelihood of lymph node metastases [38, 40, 62]. Alternatively, blocking VEGFR-3 signaling by soluble VEGFR-3 recombinant proteins diminishes tumor lymphangiogenesis and lymphatic metastasis [38, 63–65]. When administered with a skin cancer model, transgenic mouse models that overproduced VEGF-A on their skin demonstrated an enhancement in local tumor lymphangiogenesis by secretion of VEGFs, which in turn leads to an increase in metastasis to the lymph nodes and other organs [37]. Furthermore, lymphogenic growth elements operate to stretch and broaden lymphatic vessels in order to increase the thickness of lymphatic vessels [66–68]. Interestingly, VEGFR-2, a key mediator for vascularization, could also bind to VEGFR-3, which is highly important for lymphangiogenic budding [69], indicating the close relationship between vasculogenesis and lymphangiogenesis. Neuropilin-2 (NRP-2) is a transmembrane glycoprotein. There are many functions of NRP-2, including serving as a receptor for semaphorins during angiogenesis, while in axonogenesis, NRP2 helps guiding axonal growth; indicating the constant cross talk between the *oncospheres*. NRP2 has been found to be highly expressed in tumor-linked lymphatic vessels in both murine and human tumor models [70, 71]. Inhibiting neuropilin-2 with a neutralizing antibody was crucially discovered to restrict lymphatic endothelial cell migration barring its growth, reduce tumor-initiated lymphangiogenesis, and defer its spread to sentinel lymph nodes [70]. The presence of neuropilin-2 on tumor-based lymphatic vessels rather than on healthy preestablished lymphatic vessels suggests the likely use of their receptor as a potential target for suppressing lymph node metastases via lymphatic vessels [70]. Furthermore, preclinical tumor specimens have demonstrated that tumor-initiated lymphangiogenesis improves lymphatic structures, which is driven by pro-lymphangiogenic drugs, and corresponds with increased metastatic rate to lymph nodes and, most likely, even to distant organs [72].

Table 7.1 Major lymphangiogenic factors and their respective functions

Factors	Receptors	Function	Ref
VEGF-A	VEGFR-2	Induce tumor lymphangiogenesis	[37]
		Induce tumor metastasis to regional *onco-sphere* (regional lymph node)	
VEGF-C	VEGFR-2	Tumor-induced VEGF-C induces lymphangiogenesis	[11, 38, 39]
	VEGFR-3	Dilate lymphatics	
		Increases lymph node metastasis	
		Binds VEGFR2 to induce tumor angiogenesis	
VEGF-D	VEGFR-2	Stimulate tumor lymphangiogenesis	[40–43]
	VEGFR-3	Binds VEGFR2 to induce tumor angiogenesis	
Fibroblast growth factor -2 (FGF-2)	FGFR-3	Regulating VEGF-C and D to induce angiogenesis and lymphangiogenesis	[31, 44]
		FGF-2 is correlated with lymphatic metastasis	
Insulin-like growth factor (IGF-1, -2)	IGFR	Induce lymphangiogenesis (in murine model)	[34, 45]
		In gastric cancer cell line, IGF-1R can modulate the expression of VEGF to induce angiogenesis and lymphangiogenesis.	
Hepatocyte growth factor (HGF)	c-met	Overexpression of HGF induces lymphatic vessel hyperplasia and lymphatic metastasis	[46, 47]
		Activates VEGFR3 to stimulate outgrowth of peritumor lymphatic vessels	
Angiopoietin (Ang-1, -2)	Tie-2	Overexpression of Ang-1 induces lymphatic sprouting and hyperplasia in murine model	[48, 49]
		Ang-2 is secreted by ECs, associated with melanoma progression	
Ephrin B2 (Eph)	EphR	Ephrin B2 needs to interact with PDZ for lymphatic vasculature remodeling	[50, 51]
		Ephrin B silencing leads to inhibition of glioma angiogenesis	
PDGF-BB	PDGFR-α, -β	In fibrosarcoma, PDGF-BB expression induce intratumoral lymphangiogenesis and also aggravate lymphatic metastasis.	[33]
Fibronectin	Integrin α4β1	Tumor lymphatic endothelium has high expression of Integrin α4β1	[52]
Growth hormone (GH)	Growth hormone receptor	In tissue granulation during wound formation, GH promotes lymphangiogenesis.	[53, 54]
		Recently, GH has been found in breast cancer and pancreatic cancer tissues	
Endothelin-1 (ET-1)	Endothelin A and B receptor	ET(A)R and ET(B)R can trigger ET-1 overexpression in breast cancer	[36, 55, 56]
		Both ET-Et(A)R and Et(B)R are correlated with lymphatic invasion of breast cancer	
		Enhances VEGF-A, -C, VEGFR-3 expression, directly induce lymphatic vessel formation	
		In metastatic LECs, ET-1 is highly expressed	
	Unknown		[57]

(continued)

Table 7.1 (continued)

Factors	Receptors	Function	Ref
Netrin 4 (secreted by ECs)		In breast cancer, Netrin 4 is highly expressed in tumor lymph nodes and blood vessels	
		Overexpression of Netrin 4 induces lymph node and lung metastasis	
		Mechanistically, Netrin-4 activates GTPase and Src family kinase/FAK to stimulate lymphatic permeability.	

The Function of Tumor-Induced Lymphatic Vessels in the Local *Onco-Sphere*

Lymphangiogenesis can occur at the tumor cells' peripheral lining or inside the tumor cell mass. Although peritumoral lymphangiogenic vessels persist in tumor cell metastasis, it is unclear whether this stands true for intra-tumoral veins also. The majority of intra-tumoral vessels are occluded by invading malignant cells and are most probably non-operative [73]. Furthermore, approximately 40% of peritumoral vasculatures, including or excluding intra-tumoral vessels, were shown to be operational after using transplanted B16F10 melanomas that overproduce VEGF-C [74]. The subsequent investigations, which would likewise use B16F10, reveal the increased flow of lymph into draining lymph nodes as compared to tumor-free subjects [75, 76]. On the one side, fibrosarcoma is involved in the overproduction of VEGF-C and exhibited enhanced volumes of lymphatic flow, which was associated with tumor cell dissemination and lymph node metastases [77]. Inhibiting VEGF-C, on the other side, reduced lymphatic hyperplasia, lymph flow, and lymph node metastases [72, 78] (Box 7.1).

> **Box 7.1 Inter-*Onco Spheric* Interactions Toward Regional *Onco-Sphere*: Distant Lymphangiogenesis**
> At present, studies have identified a specialized pathway for tumor-mediated lymphatic metastasis, where the transport of the tumor cells from local *onco-sphere* to the lymph node prior to metastasis has been elucidated [39]. Overexpression of VEGF-A or VEGF-C is sufficient to aggravate a significant increase in lymphangiogenesis in primary tumor, as evidenced in a carcinogenesis mouse model experiment. Surprisingly, the occurrence of lymphangiogenesis inside the lymph node was observed prior to the arrival of metastatic cells. Tumor cells in the local *onco-sphere* could overexpress VEGF-C and VEGF-A, and these tumor cells are then transported to the lymph nodes. Here, the GFs are responsible for lymphangiogenesis progression. The main observation of lymphangiogenesis would be a significant

(continued)

Box 7.1 (continued)

increase in lymphatic flow and the induction of lymphangiogenesis in distally located nodes. Significantly, the findings of this model suggest that VEGF-C promotes metastasis to both draining lymph nodes and distal organs [39]. Furthermore, the absence of lymph node metastases resulted in the failure to detect metastases in distal organs, demonstrating the importance of lymphatic metastasis in tumor cell dissemination. In another study, results indicated that compared to normal controls, patients with breast cancer reveal a significant alteration in their axillary lymph nodes, and these changes are closely linked to the probability of metastasis. The above results again suggest an inter-onco-spherical cross talk where tumor-derived lymphangiogenic GFs and other factors may facilitate the preparation of a premetastatic setting, to create a PMN that favors the establishment of secondary tumors. The remote lymphangiogenic properties controlled by VEGF-C prior to metastasis demonstrate the systemic transformations induced by lymphangiogenic growth factors in tissue stroma in the primary tumor as well as in draining lymph nodes, secondary lymphoid organs, and other distantly located metastatic sites. As a result, these findings have crucial implications for discovering bigger, more diversified, and more powerful locations for lymphangiogenic variables in the spread of metastatic cancers in comparison to previous assumption [72]. These mechanisms will be discussed in detail in Chap. 12.

Tumor-Derived Chemokines in Lymphangiogenesis

The movement of host immune cells from peripheral organs to the lymph nodes for initiating adaptive immune responses is the key circulatory task of the lymphatic system. Tumor cells can secrete various chemokines, along with their receptors as an autocrine mechanism, or a paracrine factor that can leverage the lymphatic transport system's function to control the entrance into the lymphatic vascular network as well as to enable metastases in lymph nodes and distant organs [79]. The tumor-secreted chemokines have distinctly different functions in normal physiological setting, compared to in cancer [80, 81].

CXCR4 and CXCL12 (SDF-1)

The CXCR4/CXCL12 chemokine axis was observed to increase the lymphatic movement of dendritic cells in diseased mice skin, typically indicating the inclusion of dendritic cells in lymphatic channels via CXCL12 expression [82]. CXCR4 production has also been reported by several diverse kinds of tumor cells located in varying tissues [83]. Though the methods by which tumor cells stimulate the production of functional CXCR4 are unknown, several studies have speculated its occurrence due to CXCR4 upregulation induced by hypoxia, implying cross-communication across distinct oncospheres. Tumor cells involved in the expression of CXCR4 exhibit targeted metastasis into CXCL12-producing organs [84]. Highly concentrated CXCL12 in the lymph nodes, as well as the accompanying gradient inside lymphatic arteries, can significantly entice tumor cells, thus enhancing metastatic rate to the nodes (Fig. 7.2) [85–87]. Tumor-associated lymphatic vessels produce high CXCL12 levels, indicating that the tumor-linked lymphatic endothelium is actively involved in the spread of metastatic malignancies [71]. Furthermore, it has been demonstrated that a CXCL12 gradient controls the spreading of metastases to distant tissues located remotely to the draining lymph node. Tissues with a high rate of CXCL12 production, such as the lung, liver, and bone tissues, are preferential metastatic sites [79, 88, 89]. The CXCR4/CXCL12 axis also serves an important role in the metastatic spread of melanoma, resulting in enhanced tolerance to chemotherapy [90]. Presently, the activated CXCR4/CXCL12 axis is being recognized as a major factor for lymphatic infiltration as well as tumor cell metastasis in individuals with extramammary Paget disease [71]. The invasive cells under observation exhibit enhanced production of CXCR4, while CXCL12 production increased in subcapsular lymphatic endothelial cells and macrophages prior to the arrival of metastatic cells in tumor-draining nodes [71].

CCL19 and CCL21: Ligands of CCR7

CCL19 and CCL21 play primary and proactive roles in the metastatic lymphatic dissemination of tumor cells. A couple of these chemokines are the sole CCR7 ligands, and they trigger the movement of CCR7[+] T and B cells, along with DCs, to the lymph nodes under specific physiological circumstances. The fibroblast reticular cells and high endothelial venules from secondary lymph nodes both release CCL21, whereas the CCL19 is released only from the fibroblast reticular cells inside the lymph node [91, 92]. CCR7 production in tissues of various cancer cells is linked to lymph node metastases [79, 93–96]. CCR7[+] tumor cells migrate chemotactically to reach CCL21-deficient lymphatic ECs [83] and promote metastasis to tumor-draining lymph nodes (Fig. 7.3) [97]. Furthermore, inhibiting CCL21 with the integration of a soluble inhibitor has been shown to decrease in vivo metastatic movement [98]. Tumor cells can recognize chemotactic gradients collected in lymphatic ECs, as well as arrange autologous gradients inside the ECM with the help of CCL19 and CCL21 [99]. Surprisingly, CCL21 is vital for inducing lymphoid structure formation, as it triggers the activation of lymphoid tissue inducer (LTi) cells, indicating its fundamental involvement in neo-lymphoid formation [100]. In CCL21 overepxressed melanoma cells, new lymphoid-like reticular stromal cells were observed, especially in the peritumoral regions of the tumor. Furthermore, CCL21 can also promote an anti-tumoral immunosuppressive environment by increasing the Treg phenotype and enhance MDSC infiltration, which in turn results in an immunosuppressive cytokine setting (Fig. 7.3). Furthermore, in a melanoma

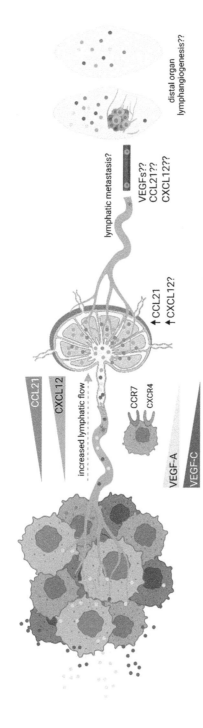

Fig. 7.2 The intervention of chemokines through the lymphatic vasculature. In the tumor, many chemokines are produced. These tumor-secreted chemokines, along with their receptors can have an autocrine or paracrine function to activate lymphangiogenesis. For example, CCR7 and their ligands CCL19/21; and CXCR4 and their ligands CXCL12 are crucial in this process. Due to lymphatic flow, these chemokines can flow toward the lymph nodes to activate LECs, which in turn drives these chemokine-expressing cells into the lymphatic channels, into the sentinel-draining lymph nodes. At the same time, cytokines such as VEGF-C may also upregulate the chemokines production, favoring the positive feedback mechanism to aid metastatic progression. Moreover, the elevated levels of CXCL12 in tissues of the preferable metastatic locations tend to induce chemokines to help metastatic cells reach remote organs

cell lines, as compared to CCL21$^+$ B16F10 cells, CCL21$^-$B16F10 cells demonstrated a lower tumor development rate [101]. CCL19 synthesis, in conjunction with higher interstitial fluid pressure (IFP), may drive tumor cells toward additional lymphatic channels [99]. The flow-mediated elevation of CCL21 increased DC transmigration, showing the significance of flow-controlled chemotactic augmentation for the rapid transit of CCR7$^+$ metastatic cells into the lymphatic vessels [75, 76]. Interestingly, co-expression or simultaneous increase in cytokines and chemokine level in the local *onco-sphere* is also important. For example, in the interactions involving the simultaneous production of VEGF-C and CCL21, the co-upregulation of both is important in driving tumor cells along the chemotaxis flow to the lymphatic vessels [102]. Similarly, the production of VEGF-C and CCR7 on tumor cells was revealed to enhance synergistic tumor cell infiltration into the lymphatic system, again affirming the concept of tumor ecosystem where the process of lymphangiogenesis is closely related to chemokines produced by metastatic cells.

Inter-*Onco Spherical* Cross Talk: Lymphangiogenesis and Tumor Immunity

In cancer patients, the immune system could be suppressed by various mechanism, namely high intra-tumoral and circulating suppressor myeloid cells, expression of Tregs, cytokine polarization (from a cytotoxic Th1 to Th2 phenotype), and low expression of tumor-derived antigens. The sentinel lymph node, being the location of direct tumor outflow, is greatly influenced by tumor-derived substances. Sentinel lymph nodes act as an essential site of connection for antigens produced from malignant as well as immune cells and are therefore studied for initial immunological alterations aiding tumor growth.

Dendritic Cells (DCs)

VEGFs may support tumor-immune system monitoring by influencing the development and recruitment of DCs. Tumor-generated VEGF-A can influence DC differentiation directly [103]. Additionally, recombinant VEGF-A administration to mouse models inhibited DC growth and raised the ratio of MDSCs to reduce antitumor immunity [104, 105]. Large numbers of immature DCs (iDCs) were seen in areas with high levels of VEGF-A. T cells exhibit an immunosuppressive behavior while co-cultured with these iDCs. Upon co-culture, these T cells are overexpressing CTLA-4 (in immune inhibitory checkpoint) and CD25 expression, while inducing tumor-promoting cytokines and interleukins such as TGFβ, VEGF-A, and IL-10 [106]. However, inhibiting VEGF-A during the use of a neutral antibody was able to restore DC functioning in mice [107]. Moreover, IHC labeling of cancer tissues in gastric cancer patients revealed a negative connection between

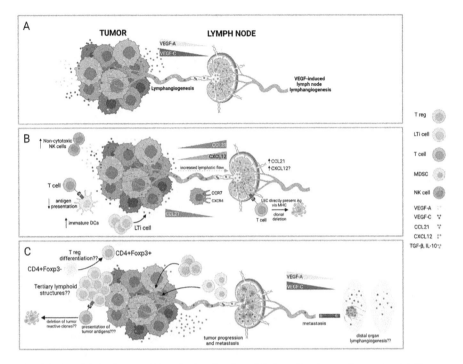

Fig. 7.3 Possible pathways of lymphatic-related modulation of antitumor immunity. (**a**) Tumor-derived VEGFs enhance lymphangiogenesis by expanding the lymphatic vasculature inside tumor-releasing lymph nodes. CCL21 levels are elevated in tumor-associated lymphatic structures, either directly as a result of VEGF-C or because of increased lymphatic flow. The production of VEGF-A and VEGF-C inside the local oncosphere reduces the number of mature DCs, reducing antigen expression to effector T cells and inhibiting their antitumor cytotoxicity (**b**) Innate immunity via NK cells is involved in lymphangiogenesis. Tumor-related lymphatic ECs that produce CCL21 increasingly may use lymphoid tissue inducer (LTi) cells to generate a milieu for immunosuppressive Tregs and MDSCs. (**c**) Enhanced synthesis of tumor-related VEGF and CCL21 may also produce a tolerogenic milieu defined by increased TGF-β and IL-10 production, enabling tumor dissemination to drain lymph nodes and boosting metastasis to distant organs

DC penetration and VEGF-A production [108]. Tumor-produced VEGF-C has been discovered to have a considerable impact on DC infiltration into gastric cancer. An elevated level of VEGF-C presentation was adversely linked with the quantity of DC infiltration in the tumor, pointing toward the deleterious impact of VEGF-C on DC movement [109].

T cell

T-cell activities are highly modulated by cytokines, especially the VEGF family. VEGFs have been shown to modulate the propagation, phenotypic attributes, and activities of T cells. Knockdown of VEGF-C, particularly, leads to a dramatic decrease in the proportion of CD4$^+$ T and CD8$^+$ cell population, whereas the immature form of CD11b-CD11c$^+$ DCs exhibited an increased concentration, demonstrating the ability of VEGF-A to govern and modulate T cell activity. In vitro proliferative tests in an ovarian cancer model revealed that migrating T cells had elevated levels of VEGF-A, which inhibits T-cell growth [110]. VEGF has the ability to switch the phenotypic traits of peripheral T cells from a Th1 to a Th2 [111]. Since Th1 cells may produce the proinflammatory cytokine IFN-γ, which is required for their viability and proliferation, along with the effector role of cytotoxic T cells, Th1 phenotype is unfavorable for tumor growth and progression. Therefore, by polarizing T cells to the immunosuppressive IL-4-generating Th2 phenotype may provide a favorable milieu for tumor cell development and metastasis [112]. VEGF-A is also linked to the induction and maintenance of Treg cells [113, 114]. Overexpression of tumor-derived VEGF-A expanded the proportion of Tregs in melanoma and colon carcinoma mouse models, whereas co-culture of overproduced VEGF-A colon cancer with PBMC cells also enhanced the Treg cell count [113, 114]. Tregs from cancer patients exhibited expression of VEGFR-2, especially in a subpopulation with substantial Foxp3 production and an immunosuppressive profile [115]. Collectively, these findings indicate that VEGF-A or the VEGFR-clan is a viable immunotherapeutic benchmark for the depletion of this enhanced suppressive cell subgroup and that inhibiting either of these might lower intratumoral Tregs, allowing anticancer immunotherapies to be more effective [113, 116]. Remarkably, lymphatic ECs in peripheral lymph nodes (draining to skin) were discovered to provide an epitope of the melanocyte-linked tyrosinase protein to tyrosinase-linked CD8$^+$ T lymphocytes, triggering clonal elimination and promoting immuno-resistance. According to the latest research, CCL21 also controls T cells in the peripheral lymphoid tissues to form a CD4$^+$Foxp3$^-$ T reg population. These progenitor cells could differentiate into CD4$^+$Foxp3$^-$ Treg cells and had potent immunosuppressive properties. As a result, structures comparable to VEGF-derived lymphoid can provide a stromal milieu for the differentiation of these regulatory progenitor cells into Foxp3$^+$ Treg cells [117].

Natural Killer Cells (NK)

Natural Killer (NK) cells exhibit crucial involvement in innate antitumor immunity. The influence of lymphangiogenesis on NK cells has not been researched extensively, but a recent study discovered VEGF-C to be the principal regulatory agent of NK cell cytotoxicity that plays an important role in controlling and facilitating immunological resistance. Non-cytotoxic NK cells lining the uterine walls were shown to produce high volumes of VEGF-C than their cytotoxic NK cell equivalents [118]. Mechanistically VEGF-C was primarily related to increased target cell production of TAP-1, an essential molecule for assembling MHC class I (MHC-I) [119].

Conclusion

Several recent investigations have increased our comprehension and awareness regarding molecular processes that regulate tumor lymph production, including the participation of different GFs, chemokines, and signaling cascades. Despite significant progress made in comprehending lymphangiogenesis and its involvement in cancer development and metastasis, many elements remain a mystery. When evaluating a therapy technique that targets lymphangiogenesis or its associated components, the holistic view of the association between angiogenesis, host inflammation, immunology, and other variables should be considered.

References

1. Tammela T, Alitalo K (2010) Lymphangiogenesis: molecular mechanisms and future promise. Cell 140(4):460–476
2. Cueni LN, Detmar M (2006) New insights into the molecular control of the lymphatic vascular system and its role in disease. J Investig Dermatol 126(10):2167–2177
3. Wang Y, Oliver G (2010) Current views on the function of the lymphatic vasculature in health and disease. Genes Dev 24(19):2115–2126
4. Swartz MA, Skobe M (2001) Lymphatic function, lymphangiogenesis, and cancer metastasis. Microsc Res Tech 55(2):92–99
5. Ran S, Volk L, Hall K, Flister MJ (2010) Lymphangiogenesis and lymphatic metastasis in breast cancer. Pathophysiology 17(4):229–251
6. Baluk P, Fuxe J, Hashizume H, Romano T, Lashnits E, Butz S et al (2007) Functionally specialized junctions between endothelial cells of lymphatic vessels. J Exp Med 204(10): 2349–2362
7. Gerli R, Solito R, Weber E, Aglianó M (2000) Specific adhesion molecules bind anchoring filaments and endothelial cells in human skin initial lymphatics. Lymphology 33(4):148–157
8. Aukland K, Reed RK (1993) Interstitial-lymphatic mechanisms in the control of extracellular fluid volume. Physiol Rev 73(1):1–78
9. Aukland K, Nicolaysen G (1981) Interstitial fluid volume: local regulatory mechanisms. Physiol Rev 61(3):556–643
10. Schmid-Schönbein GW (1990) Microlymphatics and lymph flow. Physiol Rev 70(4): 987–1028
11. Skobe M, Hawighorst T, Jackson DG, Prevo R, Janes L, Velasco P et al (2001) Induction of tumor lymphangiogenesis by VEGF-C promotes breast cancer metastasis. Nat Med 7(2): 192–198
12. He Y, Rajantie I, Ilmonen M, Makinen T, Karkkainen MJ, Haiko P et al (2004) Preexisting lymphatic endothelium but not endothelial progenitor cells are essential for tumor lymphangiogenesis and lymphatic metastasis. Cancer Res 64(11):3737–3740
13. Salven P, Mustjoki S, Alitalo R, Alitalo K, Rafii S (2003) VEGFR-3 and CD133 identify a population of CD34+ lymphatic/vascular endothelial precursor cells. Blood 101(1):168–172
14. Cueni LN, Detmar M (2008) The lymphatic system in health and disease. Lymphat Res Biol 6(3–4):109–122
15. Joukov V, Pajusola K, Kaipainen A, Chilov D, Lahtinen I, Kukk E et al (1996) A novel vascular endothelial growth factor, VEGF-C, is a ligand for the Flt4 (VEGFR-3) and KDR (VEGFR-2) receptor tyrosine kinases. EMBO J 15(2):290–298

16. Orlandini M, Marconcini L, Ferruzzi R, Oliviero S (1996) Identification of a c-fos-induced gene that is related to the platelet-derived growth factor/vascular endothelial growth factor family. Proc Natl Acad Sci U S A 93(21):11675–11680

17. Yamada Y, Nezu J, Shimane M, Hirata Y (1997) Molecular cloning of a novel vascular endothelial growth factor, VEGF-D. Genomics 42(3):483–488

18. Achen MG, Jeltsch M, Kukk E, Mäkinen T, Vitali A, Wilks AF et al (1998) Vascular endothelial growth factor D (VEGF-D) is a ligand for the tyrosine kinases VEGF receptor 2 (Flk1) and VEGF receptor 3 (Flt4). Proc Natl Acad Sci U S A 95(2):548–553

19. Cao Y, Linden P, Farnebo J, Cao R, Eriksson A, Kumar V et al (1998) Vascular endothelial growth factor C induces angiogenesis in vivo. Proc Natl Acad Sci U S A 95(24):14389–14394

20. Marconcini L, Marchio S, Morbidelli L, Cartocci E, Albini A, Ziche M et al (1999) c-fos-induced growth factor/vascular endothelial growth factor D induces angiogenesis in vivo and in vitro. Proc Natl Acad Sci U S A 96(17):9671–9676

21. Nagy JA, Vasile E, Feng D, Sundberg C, Brown LF, Detmar MJ et al (2002) Vascular permeability factor/vascular endothelial growth factor induces lymphangiogenesis as well as angiogenesis. J Exp Med 196(11):1497–1506

22. Hirakawa S, Hong YK, Harvey N, Schacht V, Matsuda K, Libermann T et al (2003) Identification of vascular lineage-specific genes by transcriptional profiling of isolated blood vascular and lymphatic endothelial cells. Am J Pathol 162(2):575–586

23. Hong YK, Lange-Asschenfeldt B, Velasco P, Hirakawa S, Kunstfeld R, Brown LF et al (2004) VEGF-A promotes tissue repair-associated lymphatic vessel formation via VEGFR-2 and the alpha1beta1 and alpha2beta1 integrins. FASEB J 18(10):1111–1113

24. Favier B, Alam A, Barron P, Bonnin J, Laboudie P, Fons P et al (2006) Neuropilin-2 interacts with VEGFR-2 and VEGFR-3 and promotes human endothelial cell survival and migration. Blood 108(4):1243–1250

25. Soker S, Miao HQ, Nomi M, Takashima S, Klagsbrun M (2002) VEGF165 mediates formation of complexes containing VEGFR-2 and neuropilin-1 that enhance VEGF165-receptor binding. J Cell Biochem 85(2):357–368

26. Pan Q, Chanthery Y, Liang WC, Stawicki S, Mak J, Rathore N et al (2007) Blocking neuropilin-1 function has an additive effect with anti-VEGF to inhibit tumor growth. Cancer Cell 11(1):53–67

27. Wang L, Zeng H, Wang P, Soker S, Mukhopadhyay D (2003) Neuropilin-1-mediated vascular permeability factor/vascular endothelial growth factor-dependent endothelial cell migration. J Biol Chem 278(49):48848–48860

28. Yuan L, Moyon D, Pardanaud L, Bréant C, Karkkainen MJ, Alitalo K et al (2002) Abnormal lymphatic vessel development in neuropilin 2 mutant mice. Development 129(20):4797–4806

29. Morisada T, Oike Y, Yamada Y, Urano T, Akao M, Kubota Y et al (2005) Angiopoietin-1 promotes LYVE-1-positive lymphatic vessel formation. Blood 105(12):4649–4656

30. Tammela T, Saaristo A, Lohela M, Morisada T, Tornberg J, Norrmén C et al (2005) Angiopoietin-1 promotes lymphatic sprouting and hyperplasia. Blood 105(12):4642–4648

31. Kubo H, Cao R, Brakenhielm E, Mäkinen T, Cao Y, Alitalo K (2002) Blockade of vascular endothelial growth factor receptor-3 signaling inhibits fibroblast growth factor-2-induced lymphangiogenesis in mouse cornea. Proc Natl Acad Sci U S A 99(13):8868–8873

32. Shin JW, Min M, Larrieu-Lahargue F, Canron X, Kunstfeld R, Nguyen L et al (2006) Prox1 promotes lineage-specific expression of fibroblast growth factor (FGF) receptor-3 in lymphatic endothelium: a role for FGF signaling in lymphangiogenesis. Mol Biol Cell 17(2):576–584

33. Cao R, Bjorndahl MA, Religa P, Clasper S, Garvin S, Galter D et al (2004) PDGF-BB induces intratumoral lymphangiogenesis and promotes lymphatic metastasis. Cancer Cell 6(4): 333–345

34. Björndahl MA, Cao R, Burton JB, Brakenhielm E, Religa P, Galter D et al (2005) Vascular endothelial growth factor-a promotes peritumoral lymphangiogenesis and lymphatic metastasis. Cancer Res 65(20):9261–9268

35. Fritz-Six KL, Dunworth WP, Li M, Caron KM (2008) Adrenomedullin signaling is necessary for murine lymphatic vascular development. J Clin Invest 118(1):40–50
36. Spinella F, Garrafa E, Di Castro V, Rosano L, Nicotra MR, Caruso A et al (2009) Endothelin-1 stimulates lymphatic endothelial cells and lymphatic vessels to grow and invade. Cancer Res 69(6):2669–2676
37. Hirakawa S, Kodama S, Kunstfeld R, Kajiya K, Brown LF, Detmar M (2005) VEGF-A induces tumor and sentinel lymph node lymphangiogenesis and promotes lymphatic metastasis. J Exp Med 201(7):1089–1099
38. Karpanen T, Egeblad M, Karkkainen MJ, Kubo H, Yla-Herttuala S, Jaattela M et al (2001) Vascular endothelial growth factor C promotes tumor lymphangiogenesis and intralymphatic tumor growth. Cancer Res 61(5):1786–1790
39. Hirakawa S, Brown LF, Kodama S, Paavonen K, Alitalo K, Detmar M (2007) VEGF-C-induced lymphangiogenesis in sentinel lymph nodes promotes tumor metastasis to distant sites. Blood 109(3):1010–1017
40. Stacker SA, Caesar C, Baldwin ME, Thornton GE, Williams RA, Prevo R et al (2001) VEGF-D promotes the metastatic spread of tumor cells via the lymphatics. Nat Med 7(2):186–191
41. Von Marschall Z, Scholz A, Stacker SA, Achen MG, Jackson DG, Alves F et al (2005) Vascular endothelial growth factor-D induces lymphangiogenesis and lymphatic metastasis in models of ductal pancreatic cancer. Int J Oncol 27(3):669–679
42. Koch M, Dettori D, Van Nuffelen A, Souffreau J, Marconcini L, Wallays G et al (2009) VEGF-D deficiency in mice does not affect embryonic or postnatal lymphangiogenesis but reduces lymphatic metastasis. J Pathol 219(3):356–364
43. Rissanen TT, Markkanen JE, Gruchala M, Heikura T, Puranen A, Kettunen MI et al (2003) VEGF-D is the strongest angiogenic and lymphangiogenic effector among VEGFs delivered into skeletal muscle via adenoviruses. Circ Res 92(10):1098–1106
44. Chang LK, Garcia-Cardena G, Farnebo F, Fannon M, Chen EJ, Butterfield C et al (2004) Dose-dependent response of FGF-2 for lymphangiogenesis. Proc Natl Acad Sci U S A 101(32):11658–11663
45. Li H, Adachi Y, Yamamoto H, Min Y, Ohashi H, Ii M et al (2011) Insulin-like growth factor-I receptor blockade reduces tumor angiogenesis and enhances the effects of bevacizumab for a human gastric cancer cell line, MKN45. Cancer 117(14):3135–3147
46. Kajiya K, Hirakawa S, Ma B, Drinnenberg I, Detmar M (2005) Hepatocyte growth factor promotes lymphatic vessel formation and function. EMBO J 24(16):2885–2895
47. Cao R, Bjorndahl MA, Gallego MI, Chen S, Religa P, Hansen AJ et al (2006) Hepatocyte growth factor is a lymphangiogenic factor with an indirect mechanism of action. Blood 107(9): 3531–3536
48. Augustin HG, Koh GY, Thurston G, Alitalo K (2009) Control of vascular morphogenesis and homeostasis through the angiopoietin-Tie system. Nat Rev Mol Cell Biol 10(3):165–177
49. Helfrich I, Edler L, Sucker A, Thomas M, Christian S, Schadendorf D et al (2009) Angiopoietin-2 levels are associated with disease progression in metastatic malignant melanoma. Clin Cancer Res 15(4):1384–1392
50. Sawamiphak S, Seidel S, Essmann CL, Wilkinson GA, Pitulescu ME, Acker T et al (2010) Ephrin-B2 regulates VEGFR2 function in developmental and tumour angiogenesis. Nature 465(7297):487–491
51. Makinen T, Adams RH, Bailey J, Lu Q, Ziemiecki A, Alitalo K et al (2005) PDZ interaction site in ephrinB2 is required for the remodeling of lymphatic vasculature. Genes Dev 19(3): 397–410
52. Garmy-Susini B, Makale M, Fuster M, Varner JA (2007) Methods to study lymphatic vessel integrins. Methods Enzymol 426:415–438
53. Stoll BA (1997) Breast cancer: further metabolic-endocrine risk markers? Br J Cancer 76(12): 1652–1654
54. Ezzat S, Ezrin C, Yamashita S, Melmed S (1993) Recurrent acromegaly resulting from ectopic growth hormone gene expression by a metastatic pancreatic tumor. Cancer 71(1):66–70

55. Wulfing P, Diallo R, Kersting C, Wulfing C, Poremba C, Rody A et al (2003) Expression of endothelin-1, endothelin-A, and endothelin-B receptor in human breast cancer and correlation with long-term follow-up. Clin Cancer Res 9(11):4125–4131

56. Clasper S, Royston D, Baban D, Cao Y, Ewers S, Butz S et al (2008) A novel gene expression profile in lymphatics associated with tumor growth and nodal metastasis. Cancer Res 68(18): 7293–7303

57. Larrieu-Lahargue F, Welm AL, Thomas KR, Li DY (2010) Netrin-4 induces lymphangiogenesis in vivo. Blood 115(26):5418–5426

58. Neuchrist C, Erovic BM, Handisurya A, Fischer MB, Steiner GE, Hollemann D et al (2003) Vascular endothelial growth factor C and vascular endothelial growth factor receptor 3 expression in squamous cell carcinomas of the head and neck. Head Neck 25(6):464–474

59. Mohammed RA, Green A, El-Shikh S, Paish EC, Ellis IO, Martin SG (2007) Prognostic significance of vascular endothelial cell growth factors -A, -C and -D in breast cancer and their relationship with angio- and lymphangiogenesis. Br J Cancer 96(7):1092–1100

60. Schoppmann SF, Fenzl A, Nagy K, Unger S, Bayer G, Geleff S et al (2006) VEGF-C expressing tumor-associated macrophages in lymph node positive breast cancer: impact on lymphangiogenesis and survival. Surgery 139(6):839–846

61. Wartiovaara U, Salven P, Mikkola H, Lassila R, Kaukonen J, Joukov V et al (1998) Peripheral blood platelets express VEGF-C and VEGF which are released during platelet activation. Thromb Haemost 80(1):171–175

62. Mandriota SJ, Jussila L, Jeltsch M, Compagni A, Baetens D, Prevo R et al (2001) Vascular endothelial growth factor-C-mediated lymphangiogenesis promotes tumour metastasis. EMBO J 20(4):672–682

63. Lin J, Lalani AS, Harding TC, Gonzalez M, Wu WW, Luan B et al (2005) Inhibition of lymphogenous metastasis using adeno-associated virus-mediated gene transfer of a soluble VEGFR-3 decoy receptor. Cancer Res 65(15):6901–6909

64. Shimizu K, Kubo H, Yamaguchi K, Kawashima K, Ueda Y, Matsuo K et al (2004) Suppression of VEGFR-3 signaling inhibits lymph node metastasis in gastric cancer. Cancer Sci 95(4): 328–333

65. Roberts N, Kloos B, Cassella M, Podgrabinska S, Persaud K, Wu Y et al (2006) Inhibition of VEGFR-3 activation with the antagonistic antibody more potently suppresses lymph node and distant metastases than inactivation of VEGFR-2. Cancer Res 66(5):2650–2657

66. He Y, Rajantie I, Pajusola K, Jeltsch M, Holopainen T, Yla-Herttuala S et al (2005) Vascular endothelial cell growth factor receptor 3-mediated activation of lymphatic endothelium is crucial for tumor cell entry and spread via lymphatic vessels. Cancer Res 65(11):4739–4746

67. Liang P, Hong JW, Ubukata H, Liu HR, Watanabe Y, Katano M et al (2006) Increased density and diameter of lymphatic microvessels correlate with lymph node metastasis in early stage invasive colorectal carcinoma. Virchows Arch 448(5):570–575

68. Dadras SS, Paul T, Bertoncini J, Brown LF, Muzikansky A, Jackson DG et al (2003) Tumor lymphangiogenesis: a novel prognostic indicator for cutaneous melanoma metastasis and survival. Am J Pathol 162(6):1951–1960

69. Wirzenius M, Tammela T, Uutela M, He Y, Odorisio T, Zambruno G et al (2007) Distinct vascular endothelial growth factor signals for lymphatic vessel enlargement and sprouting. J Exp Med 204(6):1431–1440

70. Caunt M, Mak J, Liang WC, Stawicki S, Pan Q, Tong RK et al (2008) Blocking neuropilin-2 function inhibits tumor cell metastasis. Cancer Cell 13(4):331–342

71. Hirakawa S, Detmar M, Kerjaschki D, Nagamatsu S, Matsuo K, Tanemura A et al (2009) Nodal lymphangiogenesis and metastasis: role of tumor-induced lymphatic vessel activation in extramammary Paget's disease. Am J Pathol 175(5):2235–2248

72. Christiansen A, Detmar M (2011) Lymphangiogenesis and cancer. Genes Cancer 2(12): 1146–1158

73. Padera TP, Kadambi A, di Tomaso E, Carreira CM, Brown EB, Boucher Y et al (2002) Lymphatic metastasis in the absence of functional intratumor lymphatics. Science 296(5574): 1883–1886
74. Isaka N, Padera TP, Hagendoorn J, Fukumura D, Jain RK (2004) Peritumor lymphatics induced by vascular endothelial growth factor-C exhibit abnormal function. Cancer Res 64(13):4400–4404
75. Harrell MI, Iritani BM, Ruddell A (2007) Tumor-induced sentinel lymph node lymphangiogenesis and increased lymph flow precede melanoma metastasis. Am J Pathol 170(2):774–786
76. Proulx ST, Luciani P, Derzsi S, Rinderknecht M, Mumprecht V, Leroux JC et al (2010) Quantitative imaging of lymphatic function with liposomal indocyanine green. Cancer Res 70(18):7053–7062
77. Ben-Baruch A (2003) Host microenvironment in breast cancer development: inflammatory cells, cytokines and chemokines in breast cancer progression: reciprocal tumor-microenvironment interactions. Breast Cancer Res 5(1):31–36
78. Padera TP, Kuo AH, Hoshida T, Liao S, Lobo J, Kozak KR et al (2008) Differential response of primary tumor versus lymphatic metastasis to VEGFR-2 and VEGFR-3 kinase inhibitors cediranib and vandetanib. Mol Cancer Ther 7(8):2272–2279
79. Müller A, Homey B, Soto H, Ge N, Catron D, Buchanan ME et al (2001) Involvement of chemokine receptors in breast cancer metastasis. Nature 410(6824):50–56
80. Zlotnik A, Yoshie O (2000) Chemokines: a new classification system and their role in immunity. Immunity 12(2):121–127
81. Campbell JJ, Butcher EC (2000) Chemokines in tissue-specific and microenvironment-specific lymphocyte homing. Curr Opin Immunol 12(3):336–341
82. Kabashima K, Shiraishi N, Sugita K, Mori T, Onoue A, Kobayashi M et al (2007) CXCL12-CXCR4 engagement is required for migration of cutaneous dendritic cells. Am J Pathol 171(4):1249–1257
83. Balkwill F (2004) The significance of cancer cell expression of the chemokine receptor CXCR4. Semin Cancer Biol 14(3):171–179
84. Cardones AR, Murakami T, Hwang ST (2003) CXCR4 enhances adhesion of B16 tumor cells to endothelial cells in vitro and in vivo via beta(1) integrin. Cancer Res 63(20):6751–6757
85. Zhang JP, Lu WG, Ye F, Chen HZ, Zhou CY, Xie X (2007) Study on CXCR4/SDF-1alpha axis in lymph node metastasis of cervical squamous cell carcinoma. Int J Gynecol Cancer 17(2):478–483
86. Kaifi JT, Yekebas EF, Schurr P, Obonyo D, Wachowiak R, Busch P et al (2005) Tumor-cell homing to lymph nodes and bone marrow and CXCR4 expression in esophageal cancer. J Natl Cancer Inst 97(24):1840–1847
87. Yoshitake N, Fukui H, Yamagishi H, Sekikawa A, Fujii S, Tomita S et al (2008) Expression of SDF-1 alpha and nuclear CXCR4 predicts lymph node metastasis in colorectal cancer. Br J Cancer 98(10):1682–1689
88. Li YM, Pan Y, Wei Y, Cheng X, Zhou BP, Tan M et al (2004) Upregulation of CXCR4 is essential for HER2-mediated tumor metastasis. Cancer Cell 6(5):459–469
89. Phillips RJ, Burdick MD, Lutz M, Belperio JA, Keane MP, Strieter RM (2003) The stromal derived factor-1/CXCL12-CXC chemokine receptor 4 biological axis in non-small cell lung cancer metastases. Am J Respir Crit Care Med 167(12):1676–1686
90. Kim M, Koh YJ, Kim KE, Koh BI, Nam DH, Alitalo K et al (2010) CXCR4 signaling regulates metastasis of chemoresistant melanoma cells by a lymphatic metastatic niche. Cancer Res 70(24):10411–10421
91. Carlsen HS, Haraldsen G, Brandtzaeg P, Baekkevold ES (2005) Disparate lymphoid chemokine expression in mice and men: no evidence of CCL21 synthesis by human high endothelial venules. Blood 106(2):444–446

92. Link A, Vogt TK, Favre S, Britschgi MR, Acha-Orbea H, Hinz B et al (2007) Fibroblastic reticular cells in lymph nodes regulate the homeostasis of naive T cells. Nat Immunol 8(11): 1255–1265

93. Günther K, Leier J, Henning G, Dimmler A, Weissbach R, Hohenberger W et al (2005) Prediction of lymph node metastasis in colorectal carcinoma by expression of chemokine receptor CCR7. Int J Cancer 116(5):726–733

94. Takanami I (2003) Overexpression of CCR7 mRNA in nonsmall cell lung cancer: correlation with lymph node metastasis. Int J Cancer 105(2):186–189

95. Mashino K, Sadanaga N, Yamaguchi H, Tanaka F, Ohta M, Shibuta K et al (2002) Expression of chemokine receptor CCR7 is associated with lymph node metastasis of gastric carcinoma. Cancer Res 62(10):2937–2941

96. Koizumi K, Kozawa Y, Ohashi Y, Nakamura ES, Aozuka Y, Sakurai H et al (2007) CCL21 promotes the migration and adhesion of highly lymph node metastatic human non-small cell lung cancer Lu-99 in vitro. Oncol Rep 17(6):1511–1516

97. Wiley HE, Gonzalez EB, Maki W, Wu MT, Hwang ST (2001) Expression of CC chemokine receptor-7 and regional lymph node metastasis of B16 murine melanoma. J Natl Cancer Inst 93(21):1638–1643

98. Lanati S, Dunn DB, Roussigné M, Emmett MS, Carriere V, Jullien D et al (2010) Chemotrap-1: an engineered soluble receptor that blocks chemokine-induced migration of metastatic cancer cells in vivo. Cancer Res 70(20):8138–8148

99. Shields JD, Fleury ME, Yong C, Tomei AA, Randolph GJ, Swartz MA (2007) Autologous chemotaxis as a mechanism of tumor cell homing to lymphatics via interstitial flow and autocrine CCR7 signaling. Cancer Cell 11(6):526–538

100. Randall TD, Carragher DM, Rangel-Moreno J (2008) Development of secondary lymphoid organs. Annu Rev Immunol 26:627–650

101. Shields JD, Kourtis IC, Tomei AA, Roberts JM, Swartz MA (2010) Induction of lymphoid like stroma and immune escape by tumors that express the chemokine CCL21. Science (New York, NY) 328(5979):749–752

102. Issa A, Le TX, Shoushtari AN, Shields JD, Swartz MA (2009) Vascular endothelial growth factor-C and C-C chemokine receptor 7 in tumor cell-lymphatic cross-talk promote invasive phenotype. Cancer Res 69(1):349–357

103. Gabrilovich DI, Chen HL, Girgis KR, Cunningham HT, Meny GM, Nadaf S et al (1996) Production of vascular endothelial growth factor by human tumors inhibits the functional maturation of dendritic cells. Nat Med 2(10):1096–1103

104. Gabrilovich D, Ishida T, Oyama T, Ran S, Kravtsov V, Nadaf S et al (1998) Vascular endothelial growth factor inhibits the development of dendritic cells and dramatically affects the differentiation of multiple hematopoietic lineages in vivo. Blood 92(11):4150–4166

105. Gabrilovich DI, Nagaraj S (2009) Myeloid-derived suppressor cells as regulators of the immune system. Nat Rev Immunol 9(3):162–174

106. Strauss L, Volland D, Kunkel M, Reichert TE (2005) Dual role of VEGF family members in the pathogenesis of head and neck cancer (HNSCC): possible link between angiogenesis and immune tolerance. Med Sci Monit 11(8):Br280–Br292

107. Ishida T, Oyama T, Carbone DP, Gabrilovich DI (1998) Defective function of Langerhans cells in tumor-bearing animals is the result of defective maturation from hemopoietic progenitors. J Immunol 161(9):4842–4851

108. Saito H, Tsujitani S, Ikeguchi M, Maeta M, Kaibara N (1998) Relationship between the expression of vascular endothelial growth factor and the density of dendritic cells in gastric adenocarcinoma tissue. Br J Cancer 78(12):1573–1577

109. Takahashi A, Kono K, Itakura J, Amemiya H, Feng Tang R, Iizuka H et al (2002) Correlation of vascular endothelial growth factor-C expression with tumor-infiltrating dendritic cells in gastric cancer. Oncology 62(2):121–127

110. Ziogas AC, Gavalas NG, Tsiatas M, Tsitsilonis O, Politi E, Terpos E et al (2012) VEGF directly suppresses activation of T cells from ovarian cancer patients and healthy individuals via VEGF receptor Type 2. Int J Cancer 130(4):857–864
111. Nevala WK, Vachon CM, Leontovich AA, Scott CG, Thompson MA, Markovic SN (2009) Evidence of systemic Th2-driven chronic inflammation in patients with metastatic melanoma. Clin Cancer Res 15(6):1931–1939
112. van Sandick JW, Boermeester MA, Gisbertz SS, ten Berge IJ, Out TA, van der Pouw Kraan TC et al (2003) Lymphocyte subsets and T(h)1/T(h)2 immune responses in patients with adenocarcinoma of the oesophagus or oesophagogastric junction: relation to pTNM stage and clinical outcome. Cancer Immunol Immunother 52(10):617–624
113. Li B, Lalani AS, Harding TC, Luan B, Koprivnikar K, Huan Tu G et al (2006) Vascular endothelial growth factor blockade reduces intratumoral regulatory T cells and enhances the efficacy of a GM-CSF-secreting cancer immunotherapy. Clin Cancer Res 12(22):6808–6816
114. Wada J, Suzuki H, Fuchino R, Yamasaki A, Nagai S, Yanai K et al (2009) The contribution of vascular endothelial growth factor to the induction of regulatory T-cells in malignant effusions. Anticancer Res 29(3):881–888
115. Suzuki H, Onishi H, Wada J, Yamasaki A, Tanaka H, Nakano K et al (2010) VEGFR2 is selectively expressed by FOXP3high CD4+ Treg. Eur J Immunol 40(1):197–203
116. Manning EA, Ullman JG, Leatherman JM, Asquith JM, Hansen TR, Armstrong TD et al (2007) A vascular endothelial growth factor receptor-2 inhibitor enhances antitumor immunity through an immune-based mechanism. Clin Cancer Res 13(13):3951–3959
117. Schallenberg S, Tsai PY, Riewaldt J, Kretschmer K (2010) Identification of an immediate Foxp3(-) precursor to Foxp3(+) regulatory T cells in peripheral lymphoid organs of nonmanipulated mice. J Exp Med 207(7):1393–1407
118. Kalkunte SS, Mselle TF, Norris WE, Wira CR, Sentman CL, Sharma S (2009) Vascular endothelial growth factor C facilitates immune tolerance and endovascular activity of human uterine NK cells at the maternal-fetal interface. J Immunol 182(7):4085–4092
119. Ayalon O, Hughes EA, Cresswell P, Lee J, O'Donnell L, Pardi R et al (1998) Induction of transporter associated with antigen processing by interferon gamma confers endothelial cell cytoprotection against natural killer-mediated lysis. Proc Natl Acad Sci U S A 95(5): 2435–2440

Chapter 8
Biochemical Changes in the Local *Onco-Sphere*

Phei Er Saw and Erwei Song

Abstract The biochemical local onco-sphere changes as cancer grows, especially in the metabolic pathways of cancer cells. In cancer, formation and elimination of metabolically-active substances that favors the development of a pro-tumoral micro-environment could also induce a local onco-sphere that is fundamentally different from a normal cell (*i.e.* increased acidosis, amino acid and lipid metabolism). Metabolic alterations also cause redox imbalance, a major contributor to cancer growth. In this chapter, we discuss the major biochemical changes in the local onco-sphere and the important crosstalks between tumor cells and its surrounding metabolic substances in the creation of a pro-tumoral local onco-sphere.

Introduction

In the previous chapters, we have discussed the physiological changes that are acquired by the tumor cells in the local onco-sphere: angiogenesis and lymphangiogenesis. In this chapter, we will look at the major biochemical changes

P. E. Saw
Guangdong Provincial Key Laboratory of Malignant Tumor Epigenetics and Gene Regulation, Guangdong-Hong Kong Joint Laboratory for RNA Medicine, Medical Research Center, Sun Yat-sen Memorial Hospital, Sun Yat-sen University, Guangzhou, China

Nanhai Translational Innovation Center of Precision Immunology, Sun Yat-sen Memorial Hospital, Sun Yat-sen University, Foshan, China

E. Song (✉)
Guangdong Provincial Key Laboratory of Malignant Tumor Epigenetics and Gene Regulation, Guangdong-Hong Kong Joint Laboratory for RNA Medicine, Medical Research Center, Sun Yat-sen Memorial Hospital, Sun Yat-sen University, Guangzhou, China

Nanhai Translational Innovation Center of Precision Immunology, Sun Yat-sen Memorial Hospital, Sun Yat-sen University, Foshan, China

Breast Tumor Center, Sun Yat-sen Memorial Hospital, Sun Yat-sen University, Guangzhou, China
e-mail: songew@mail.sysu.edu.cn

that occur in the local onco-sphere that could be the cause of tumor inherent genetic and metabolic changes. These changes can also be brought on by the changes of the tumor stroma or infiltrated immune cells. These changes, namely the changes of pH that leads to lower intracellular pH (also known as acidosis), are closely related to the Warburg effect as a specialized fermentative glycolysis utilized by the tumor cell. Since cancer cells have high metabolic demand, this leads to various metabolic changes that are based on amino acid and lipid synthesis, two main core functions in cellular maintenance and cell growth. Dysregulation of amino acid and lipid not only changes the core metabolic pathway in cancer cells, they also are closely linked toward the communication with other components in the local *onco-sphere*, which can synergistically enhance cancer growth. In this chapter, we will decipher the important molecular mechanism and changes behind the biochemical changes, an important anatomical change in the local *onco-sphere* that has major effect in tumor growth, progression, and metastasis, affecting the distal and systemic *onco-sphere*.

Acidosis in the Local *Onco-Sphere*

Varying characteristics of perfusion across a range of differing microenvironments emerge as a result of the increased level of tumor heterogeneity across several aspects, owing to the abnormal vasculature of tumors [1, 2]. Glucose, oxygen, and amino acids, among other substrates and nutrients, may suffer from significant shortages due to the deficiency in perfusion. For instance, fermentative glycolysis is essential for satisfying the energy demands of hypoxic environments that are deficient in oxygen. Cells are bound to expire due to necrosis since the combined deprivation of glucose and oxygen may not be rectified. Significant deficits in perfusion have been linked to necrotic cores, frequently observed across the radiographs of clinical cancer [3, 4]. Regardless, due to "pseudohypoxia," HIF-1 (and/or HIF-2) is hardwired into remaining stable and allows fermentative metabolism to take place despite the conditions being sufficiently oxygenated in the context of malignant cancers [5].

Since tumor ecosystem is a "survival of the fittest," the metabolic condition mentioned above is indeed an increased benefit, which is crucial phenotype to be selected by early carcinogenesis [6, 7]. Although the underlying causes of this phenomenon (aerobic glycolysis), as well as the fitness advantages of the pseudo-hypoxic phenotype, remain unknown, significant levels of lactic acids are produced while high levels of glucose are consumed by tumors that demonstrate a Warburg effect. In recent studies, FDG PET imaging and CEST MRI [8] were employed to identify a robust link between the uptake of glucose and acidosis, the latter of which has been found to be further facilitated by deficient perfusion, since there is a notable reduction in pH when the distance from the blood vessels is greater; this phenomenon results in an acidic tumor pHe with low pH values of ~6.5 [9–12].

Other stromal or cancer cells in the tumor may consider the high levels of lactate as a source of nutrients, which are taken up by monocarboxylate transporter 4 (MCT-4), which is generally assumed responsible for lactate efflux, or MCT-1, which has been linked with lactate influx; both of which are non-electrogenic permeases and monocarboxylate transporters that respond to the immediate concentrations of H^+ and lactate on either side of the membrane. Eventually, the lactate is adopted in the process of oxidative metabolism to produce energy [13]. With its uptake mediated by MCT-1, lactate produced in a particular region of a lung tumor was found to operate as a major source of fuel for other cells therein—this was identified in a recent work of research that employed ^{13}C-labeled precursors in human tumors [14]. With the use of dynamic nuclear hyperpolarized MRI, the conversion to ^{13}C lactate from ^{13}C pyruvate (or conversely, pyruvate to lactate) can be observed in patients [15]. A significant level of acidity is observed in regions close to the cell membrane due to the production of acid from the fermentative cells. Within 20 nM from the plasma membrane of the tumor cells, a severely low pH value was discovered to be reliant upon NHE using Raman spectroscopy with gold nanoparticles, characterizing one of the many works that would contribute to the design and development of drugs that are dependent on pH levels [16].

Acidosis has recently been considered vital to the regulation of the progression of tumors across contemporary empirical research in the field. Furthermore, pH alterations in the cytosolic compartment of tumor cells that cannot resist acidification, due to the reliance on intracellular enzymatic machinery, initially result in H^+ ion accumulation in the ECM, which causes tumor acidosis. The functions of certain residues of amino acids may be modified as a result of these ions, resulting in the death of the cells in case the excess is not extracted; this characterizes the metabolic preferences of cancer cells in a tumor area as inducing differing phenotypic adaptations that simultaneously determine the cancer cell behavior in the acidic extracellular environment and sustain the pHi in an optimal range. Further, the careful balance shared by pHe and pHi is highlighted as well (Fig. 8.1) [1].

Cancer Constantly Maintains Acidic Environment in the Local *Onco-Sphere*

While the accumulation of lactic acid in the extracellular environment, as well as tumor hypoxia, has been linked to tumor acidity, further deliberation is required with regard to this relationship [17]. There are certain considerations to be made in this context: (1) Rather than being understood as lactic acid, H^+ ions, and the lactate must be regarded separately; (2) the pHi of the tumor is typically alkaline to a slight extent when the pHe is acidic—a feature that is infrequent in healthy tissues; (3) finally, the acidification of tumor regions that are oxygenated can result in CO_2 derived from respiration [1].

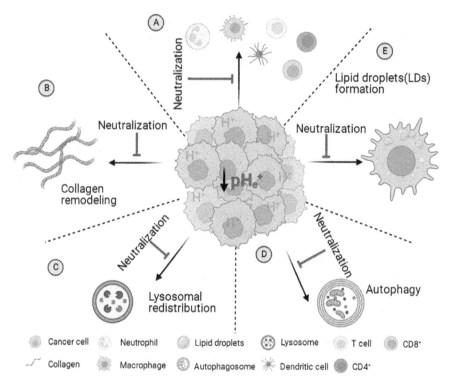

Fig. 8.1 Schematic diagram of tumor acidosis and its effect to the local *onco-sphere*. Adaptive mechanisms that may be impeded by the process of neutralization are improved by tumor-cell-generated acidosis

Glycolysis and H⁺ Ions

Due to intense perfusion of the tumor as well as limited O_2 consumption and diffusion, low partial pO_2 results in various tumor areas, which are collectively characterized as tumor hypoxia [18]. Tumor tissues beyond the 80–150 μm (wherein capillaries supply oxygen in a periodic manner that results in cycles of moderate and deep hypoxia) are considered hypoxic [19, 20]. The proliferation is sustained in the hostile environment by the tumor metabolism, which resists cell death; moreover, perfusion is increased by new blood vessels [18]. The adoption of glucose by cancer cells is significantly altered by the metabolic adaptation in response to hypoxia. The expression of different glycolytic enzymes and glucose transporters that play a role in the glucose-pyruvate conversion is significantly increased by HIF1α, a master transcription factor that emerges as a consequence of hypoxia. In cases where the availability of oxygen is restrained, a significant level of biosynthetic intermediates and a rich source of energy are offered to tumor cells by such metabolic reprogramming. During hypoxia, an increased glycolytic flux is facilitated by the genes coded for MCT4 and LDHA (lactate dehydrogenase A), whose upregulation is mediated by HIF1α [21]. While the passive release of lactate and its concentration gradient is favored by MCT4, LDHA ensures NAD^+ regeneration by converting pyruvate into lactate [22] (Fig. 8.2). The efflux of H^+ ions from cancer cells that are hypoxic is facilitated by MCT4, which is a symporter of lactate/H^+ [23]. Nevertheless, the cytosolic source of H^+ ions was found not to be the terminal production of lactate. Whereas the production of H^+ ions is caused by the consumption of ATP derived from glycolysis by various kinases and ATPases, pyruvate is reduced into lactate for NAD^+ regeneration when the H^+ ions, which are generated during the glucose-pyruvate conversion, are consumed; while ATP phosphorylation cascades facilitate oncogenic signaling, the production of biomass is underpinned by specific reactions that receive energy from ATP hydrolysis [23]. Hence, while H^+ and lactate are independently expressed during hypoxia, lactic acid is formed by the combination of limited amounts of each. This is due to the fact that the pHe, as well as the cytosolic pH, is higher than the pKa (~3.9) for the disassociation of carboxyl hydrogen. Moreover, although the pyruvate derived from glucose is generally converted into lactate, the hypoxic context wherein glucose is fully reduced to $2H^+$ ions and lactate molecules each is purely theoretical [2].

Intracellular pH and H^+ and HCO_3^- Transporters

Typically, a reversed pH gradient is observed among the membranes of cancer cells due to the pHi of normal cells being lower than that of cancer cells (pHi >7.4/pHi ~7.2), thereby contributing to the prevention of apoptosis and the facilitation of cell proliferation [3]. Moreover, the high pH 1 also contributed to the increase in different H^+ transporters, including MCTs [3, 4]. When the concentration of lactate is high in the extracellular TME, the rate of proton efflux demonstrates relatively low efficiency through transport that relies upon MCT, due to its passive nature. H^+ ions are actively transported against their gradient owing to the energy stores in the Na^+ gradient or ATP hydrolysis, adopted by Na^+/H^+ exchangers (NHEs) and H^+-ATPases, which are examples of various H^+ extruders. The excess intracellular H+ ions are titrated by the bicarbonate produced by Na^+/HCO_3^- co-transporters, which are independent of hypoxia and help to maintain a satisfactory level of pHi at a mildly alkaline level, regardless of the status of oxygenation [5].

It is under significantly restrained access to oxygen that the following two processes occur: the metabolic use of TCA (tricarboxylic acid), oxidative phosphorylation, and the transition toward the mitochondrial oxidation of pyruvates (Fig. 8.2). In the context of moderate hypoxia, respiration is improved in an efficient manner due to the remodeling of mitochondrial cristae and the isoform switch to COX4I2 from COX4I1 [6, 7]. The production of CO_2 leads to oxidative cancer cells producing more acidity; carbonic anhydrases employ extracellularly positioned CAXII and CAIX to hydrate carbon dioxide into H^+ and HCO_3^- ions (Fig. 8.2). Further, the decarboxylation of metabolic intermediates mediates the production of carbon dioxide, which is enhanced by glutaminolysis and PPP. Although the transport systems involved in deep hypoxia for cancer cells can regulate the movement of

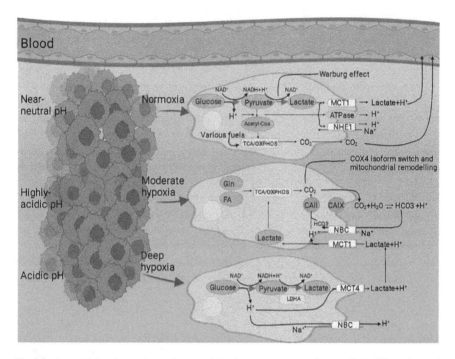

Fig 8.2 A model that demonstrates the association between sources of extracellular H$^+$ venting and levels of oxygen in the local *onco-sphere*. Mediated by MCT4, cancer cells that are significantly reliant upon glycolysis, secrete H$^+$ and lactate in areas of hypoxia where there is a reduction in the availability of substrate and prevention of oxidative phosphorylation (OXPHOS). Specific H$^+$ transporters, such as Na$^+$/H$^+$ exchanger 1 (NHE1), can also export H$^+$. The TCA cycle and OXPHOS may be fueled by a variety of substrates, such as lactate, fatty acids, and glutamine, in a moderately hypoxic environment, producing CO$_2$. It should be noted, however, that under a low partial pressure of oxygen (pO$_2$), the process of respiration is optimized by a switch in COX4 as well as the remodeling of the mitochondrial cristae. HCO$_3^-$ and H$^+$ are produced through the operation of carbonic anhydrase, which hydrates CO$_2$ following the diffusion of the membrane, governed by pO$_2$ levels

H$^+$ ions in oxidative cancer cells, the pHi shall remain unaltered due to the direct diffusion of CO$_2$ out of the cell, as far as the transmembrane CO$_2$ gradient remains favorable. Due to the coefficient of the high lipid–water partition, the lipid bilayer of the plasma membrane can be crossed freely by non-polar carbon dioxide. Aquaporins [10], among other gas channels, can encourage such permeability; however, this remains a subject of debate across empirical studies [1, 11].

Extracellular H$^+$ Venting

The minimization of accumulating cytosolic acid considers essential for the venting of lactate, H$^+$, HCO$_3^-$ and/or CO$_2$, which, when built up extracellularly, can complicate the intracellular removal of H$^+$ due to an activity induced by limited tumor blood perfusion. Acid dissipation may operate with the support of carbon dioxide and its role in the venting of H^+ ions that emerge from respiration and glycolysis, since, relative to lactic acid, CO_2 is more diffusible and weaker acid. The control of pHe was found to have involved CAIX, as supported by research that recapitulates three-dimensional tumor organization with the implementation of in vitro spheroids [15]. pHe is bound to increase when HCO_3^- titrates H^+ ions that were released in the extracellular medium, as seen in Fig. 8.2, where it is indicated that while oxygen levels may be sufficiently low in certain areas of the tumor, thereby inducing CAIX expression, this level is ideal for the sustained activity of the mitochondrial respiratory chain. H^+ can be reproduced intracellularly when CO_2 that is generated via the intracellular titration of H^+ or respiration diffuses out of the cell and is hydrated. In the context of transport metabolons, the function of transporting membrane proteins that carry H^+ and HCO_3^- may be improved by the presence of CAs [16, 24–26].

The absence of a relationship between different markers of hypoxia and the production of CAIX supports the faulty superimposition of the gradients of acidosis and hypoxia; this is also proven by the spatial heterogeneity revealed by the evaluation of intratumoral pH and pO_2 [27–31]. Similarly, the capacity to convert the extracellular environment into an acidic one is sustained by tumor cell lines that are deficient in LDH or glycolysis-impaired [32–34]. Moreover, it was recently identified that the respiratory production of carbon dioxide is a significant determinant of acid output in different lines of cancer cells [35]. The extracellular medium is bypassed by acidosis, induced by hypoxia, and mediated by syncytium. The intercellular transport of released H^+ ions is directly communicated through gap junctions between stromal cells; this allows for venting to a distance further from the area of hypoxia [1] (Box 8.1).

Box 8.1 Adaptation of Cancer Cells to Acidosis in the Local
Onco-Sphere
Generally, the pHe of normal tissues is alkaline (7.2–7.4), as compared to the high acidic quality of solid tumors, where the pH ranges between 6.5 and 6.9 [36–38]. Interestingly, the acid that solid tumor releases into the parenchyma actually causes cell death of surrounding normal cells. This will encourage the surrounding cells to secrete more proteases to breakdown of ECM. However, it is specifically because of this, tumor will take advantage of this loosening to ECM to invade to other tissues [39]. The mechanisms of adaptation, such as chronic autophagy, must improve in order to ensure the survival of cancer cells in such an acidic environment. Cells under stress employ the catabolic system known as autophagy, which has been retained throughout evolution, to maintain homeostasis by self-digestion [40]. While our work has specifically illustrated that chronic autophagy is caused by acid adaptation, the literature has demonstrated that even in conditions of high acidity and starvation,

(continued)

Box 8.1 (continued)

autophagy is upregulated by several tumors, which results in therapeutic vulnerability [41–43]. Thus, certain tumor models may benefit from a therapy that involves the targeting of autophagy, specifically that of both cancer and stromal cells [44]. This was demonstrated in a PDAC model where their stromal cells exhibit autophagy mechanism, whereby releasing elevated levels of alanine. Cancer cells need alanine as an essential source of nutrient. Therefore, targeting PSC cells in the surrounding stroma could be a strategy to prevent the progression of the malignancy [44]. The increase in lysosomal redistribution and turnover characterizes a different mechanism of adaptation. The homeostasis of cellular macromolecular components is supported by lysosomes, which are cellular organelles that contain the enzymes necessary for cell digestion and necessitate an acidic pH for efficient functioning [45].

Chronic acidosis has been shown to promote lysosome and exosome turnover, enable cells to use ATPase proton pumps to pump excess cytoplasmic protons into lysosomes, and regulate the cytoplasmic pH [46–48]. Recently, a lysosomal protein, LAMP-2, has been identified as a potential IHC marker for acidosis. Through proteomics analysis, the study indicated that there was an elevation in the profile of lysosomal proteins after the cells were adapted to the acidic environment. Interestingly, this observation is followed by seeing an active transfer of these proteins from the lysosome to the plasma membrane (similar to sending troupes to protect a country's defense line), leading to successful blocking of external invasion of acid-mediated toxicities. Especially in ductal carcinoma in situ (DCIS) patients, LAMP-2 is highly co-located at the peri-luminal region of the tumor cells [49]. In another example, the mammalian circadian clock can be disabled by prolonged acidosis. For example, it has been shown in chronic acidosis, lysosome can be redistributed. This change leads to the reduced binding of mTOR to Ras homolog enriched in the brain (RHEB), which, in turn, disables the circadian clock [50].

A large rise in adiposomes, intracellular lipid droplets that act as organelles for storing fat and are also implicated in lipid metabolism, cell signaling, inflammation, and cancer, is another often noticeable adaptation [51, 52]. An adaption to acidic or oxidative stress is reflected by LDs [53, 54], which are studies in the etiopathology of fatty liver disease [55, 56]. There is a positive correlation between the LD and the level of aggressiveness, which has been illustrated using various lines of breast cancer cells [57]. Many metabolic enzymes, including GAPDH and its paralog GAPDHS, which catalyze the sixth stage of glycolysis, become important for sustenance as a result of adapting to acidosis by elevating intracellular pH (pHi); in combination with in vitro testing and validation, an approach using silicon systems was used to observe these findings [58]. Thus, many pathways that are probably connected to one another, though the relationships are not yet completely understood, are involved in the adaptation of cells to chronic acidosis.

Amino Acids Metabolic Reprogramming in the Local *Onco-Sphere*

Proliferating tumor cells regulate their own energy metabolism to be able to catch up with their rapid division. Therefore, energy metabolism reprogramming has emerged as an important marker for cancer [59]. At the very core of metabolism is the utilization of amino acids. Amino acids are the building block of peptides and proteins, which account for most, if not all, functional soluble factors, hormones, receptors, and other functional cellular compartments in a cell. Therefore, dysregulation of amino acid could be detrimental for a normal cell. However, this abnormality did not lead to cell death in cancer cells, rather, spur their growth, invasion, and malignancy, indicating the intricacy and the complexity of this amino acid network and their relationship with cancer cell signaling [60]. Herein, we will focus on some major amino acids and their dysbiosis in cancer cell.

Glutamine

Glutamine metabolism is vital for cancer cell survival, and this could be observed in many types of cancer. Although glucose is still their number one choice of energy, glutamine could be a good substitute and is also a favorite choice for the cancer cells. In fact, some cancer cells utilize glutamine as their major energy source. There have been contradictory reports on the cross talk between glucose and glutamine, but not much is known about the mechanistic details. The major difference is that glucose uses glycolysis pathway while glutamine uses glutaminolysis pathway, which could provide cancer cells with a durable supply of nitrogen and carbon [61]. For example, glutamine can provide an amide (γ-nitrogen) group involved in nucleotide synthesis, which is an important rate-limiting factor affecting tumor cells proliferation [62]. Some tumor cells are so glutamine-addicted that they die without exogenous glutamine [63]. In cancer cells, glutamine could be transported into the cytoplasm through specific receptors, namely (e.g., Na^+-coupled neutral amino acid transporters (SNATs), ASC (alanine/serine/cysteine-preferring), or Na^+-dependent transporters). Upon uptake, glutamine is catalyzed by glutaminase (GLS) and be converted to glutamate [64, 65]. Glutamate is then further converted to α-ketoglutarate (α-KG) via transamination by glutamate-linked transaminase or oxidative deamination by glutamate dehydrogenase (GLUD1), which participates in the TCA to produce energy for tumor cells. In pancreatic cancer, K-Ras has been shown to reprogram glutamine metabolism by upregulating aspartate aminotransferase (GOT1) and GLUD1 [66].

Serine

As mentioned above, all amino acids serve as important precursors for the synthesis of proteins, lipids, and nucleic acids associated with cancer proliferation. However, most studies have indicated the importance of serine in carcinogenesis. Many types of cancers exhibit serine import from the extracellular environment and enhanced serine biosynthesis. This is proved by the elevated expression of the phosphoserine phosphatase (PSPH), phosphoserine aminotransferase (PSAT1), slave serine synthases phosphoglycerate dehydrogenase (PHGDH), and serine transporters solute carrier family 1 member 4 and 5 (SLC1A4 and SLC1A5) [67]. In the mitochondria of neuroblastoma and breast cancer cells, serine catabolism hydroxymethyltransferase-2 (SHMT2) and PHGDH (a rate-limiting enzyme for serine biosynthesis) are positively correlated with each other. Furthermore, PHGDH activity inhibits SHMT1 activity to facilitate serine integration into nucleotides via the mitochondrial 1C pathway [68, 69]. Controversy regarding whether exogenous serine could be accomplices toward cancer cell proliferation remains. There has been research that indicated that cancer cells selectively consume exogenous serine, which is transformed into intracellular glycine and single carbon units to structure nucleotides [70]. However, the relationship between serine and glycine remains ambiguous. Also, this phenomenon could be cancer-specific and not a general phenomenon.

Arginine

A study showed that arginine plays an important role in epigenetic regulation. Mechanistically, arginine can modulate the acetylation of histone on the chromosome, increase the OXPHOs gene coding in prostate cancer cells [71]. Arginine also enables transcriptional-enhanced associate domain 4 (TEAD 4) to remain in the nucleus. This collaborates with the increasing OXPHOS, as when OXPHOS is enhanced, they will be recruited via TEAD4 to the enhancer/promoter domain [71]. In glioma cells, the reprogramming of arginine reduced the level of arginine in the local onco-sphere. The decrement of arginine level significantly inhibits T-cell activation and proliferation, leading to an immunosuppressive environment [72]. Arginosuccinate synthetase 1 (ASS-1), a rate-limiting enzyme for arginine de novo synthesis in human cells, is defective in more than 70% of cancer cells [73]. These ASS- 1 low-expressing tumor cells become arginine-nutrient-deficient and heavily addicted on extracellular arginine for survival. Arginine-deficient cancer cells manifest transcriptional reprogramming, mitochondrial dysfunction, and eventual cell death. Given this characteristic of tumor cells, arginine-deprivation therapy using arginine-metabolizing enzymes (e.g., arginase or arginine deiminase) has been used clinically for cancer therapy [74]. In contrast, in high L-arginine-addicted tumors (e.g., breast cancer and hepatocellular carcinoma), we observed the transporter SLC7A1 (CAT-1) was upregulation, and SLC7A1 (CAT-1) knockdown hinders the viability of tumor cells and induces apoptosis [75, 76]. Glycolysis to oxidative phosphorylation metabolism of activated T cells can be reprogrammed by high level of intracellular L-arginine to promote the production of central memory T cells with antitumor activity and increase T-cell viability [77].

Tryptophan

Tryptophan, an important component of protein biosynthesis, and its metabolites have been shown to regulate the activation of Kynurenine (KYN)-related pathways. In some solid tumors (e.g., breast cancer and bladder cancer), alteration in tryptophan metabolism and increment in its metabolites are thought to be key drivers of cancer development [78, 79]. Elevated expression of tryptophan 2 and 3-dioxygenase 2 (TDO2) has been found in prostate cancer patients, and the overexpression of TDO2 promotes tumor tryptophan metabolism [80]. The tryptophan metabolite-KYN promotes nuclear translocation and upregulation of the transcription factor aryl hydrocarbon receptor (AhR) [80]. It also makes it possible to target the IDO1/TDO2-KYN-AhR signaling pathway as a checkpoint for tumor immunotherapy.

In summary, amino acid metabolism reprogramming in tumor cells affects the original metabolic pathways, ultimately making the cells more complex and flexible to evade tumor immunotherapy [81]. In addition to providing tumor cells with the raw materials and energy needed for metabolism, amino acids also affect epigenetic regulation and ROS homeostasis through acetylation, lacylation, sumolyation, and methylation, and all of which can promote tumor aggressiveness. By fully understanding the diversity and flexibility of amino acid metabolism in cancer cells, it is possible to further probe the metabolic-dependent mechanisms for better use in tumor immunotherapy.

Lipid Metabolism in the Local *Onco-Sphere* and Tumor Progression

Apart from the metabolic reprogramming of amino acids, the lipid metabolic reprogramming is also a typical characteristic of malignant tumors. Lipid, the basic structure of cell membranes, contains different components (e.g., glycerophospholipids, fatty acyls, prenol lipids, and sphingolipids) that perform different functions, which play an important role in the growth and survival of cancer cells. In the local onco-sphere, tumor tissues have different levels of lipid metabolism compared to normal cells and often present higher levels of lipid metabolism. As tumor cells are fast growing, the need of synthesizing new membrane, to have more energy synthesis and storage, in addition to increased signaling pathway transmission require constant replenishing of lipid molecules. Among the many lipids, the three major pathways are fatty acid (FA) synthesis and mevalonate (MVA) pathway during lipid metabolism. These pathways have been indicated in cancer cell's differentiation, growth, migration, and invasion of tumor cells [82].

Fatty Acid (FA) Synthesis

FA (bio) synthesis is one of the early changes that are featured in tumor cells. In cancer, FA-pathway-related receptors and transporter proteins are upregulated (i.e., ACC (FA synthesis rate-limiting enzyme), CD36 (FA translocase), SLC27 (FA transporter protein family), and FABPs (plasma membrane FA binding protein)) [83]. In the local onco-sphere, with the help of other factors present, the cross talk of stromal cells and immune cells could enhance the tumor cell uptake of FA. For example, adipocytes and fibroblasts can induce tumor cells to increase the cellular uptake of FA, leading to mitogenic signal generation to maintain tumor cell proliferation [84, 85]. Cytoplasmic acetyl-coenzyme A (acetyl-CoA) is an important substrate for lipid synthesis; Thus, the levels of acetyl-CoA are a key factor in lipid biosynthesis. ATP-citrate lyase (ACLY) catalyzes the conversion of citric acid and CoA to oxaloacetate and acetyl-CoA. In various types of cancer, decreased ACLY expression reduces tumor cells viability and inhibits tumor cells proliferation, invasion, and metastasis [86]. Acetyl-CoA synthase (ACCS) produces acetyl-CoA via acetate linkage to CoA. ACCS2 is transcriptionally upregulated by SREBP and expressed in most tumors, and particularly, it is critical for acetate catalysis in maintaining tumor cells growth under metabolic stress [87]. Additionally, ACC can also catalyze the carboxylation of acetyl-CoA to malonyl-coenzyme A. ACC1 and ACC2 are two isoforms of ACC that are essential for FA synthesis. ACC1 has been proven to be closely involved in cancer, as ACC1 is usually expressed in high concentration in many human cancers, while the depletion of ACC1 leads to a significant reduction in FA biosynthesis, leading to elevated apoptosis in both breast cancer and prostate cancer through fatty acid oxidation (FAO) pathway [88]. ACC2 controls mitochondrial uptake of FA and is also deemed to be highly expressed in cancer. In fact, high ACC2 expression has been correlated with a reduction of 5-year OS in laryngeal cancer [89]. Mechanistically, FA is oxidized by β-oxidation pathways (FAO), which allows the conversion of long-chain FA to acetyl-CoA in mitochondria, which enters the TCA and generates ATP and malic enzyme-dependent NADPH. In multiple cancer types, especially cancer with K-Ras mutations (i.e., lung cancer, triple-negative breast cancer, and glioma), the activity of FAO is exceptionally high, with a significant increment in the protein's expression level in FAO pathways. However, cells are careful not to have an overactive FAO, as this could lead to a detrimental effect in excessive ROS, which leads to apoptosis in glioma cells [90].

Cholesterol Biosynthesis

Numerous studies have depicted the relationship between cholesterol and cancer [91]. In various clinical studies, hypercholesterolemia and high-fat diet can directly affect cancer development (will be detailed in Chap. 18. Mechanistically, extracellular cholesterol could activate HHG pathway, while intracellular cholesterol induces mTORC1 signaling, both crucial pathways in cell growth, metastasis, and stemness-like properties. In lipid raft formation, cholesterol is the single most important component. Lipid rafts are major platforms for cancer regulation pathway signaling; inhibiting or chelation of membrane-bound cholesterol has been proven effective in disrupting lipid raft's function, which is an effective strategy to inhibit cancer growth. Key molecular changes in cholesterol metabolism include mevalonic acid (MVA), isoprenoids, and oxysterols [92].

In cancer cells, cholesterol catabolism and anabolism are often reprogrammed. MVA, an important cholesterol precursor, is synthesized by HMG CoA reductase. Mechanistically, MVA can activate PI3K pathway, activates mTOR and NK-kB pathway, leading to the inhibition of P21 and P27 [93], which ultimately changes the cell metabolism and increases migration of cancer cells [94]. When MVA is elevated, this leads to a large production of isoprenoids (i.e., isopentenyl-diphosphate (IPP), farnesyl-pyrophosphate (FPP), and geranylgeranyl-pyrophosphate (GGPP) [93]. The main function of isoprenoids is the prenylation of small GTPases (i.e., Rho and Ras), leading to their translocation to the cell membrane, leading to cellular pathway activation [95]. Interestingly, many GTPases that are prenylated by isoprenoids are involved in carcinogenesis. In one study, prenylated RhoA enhances P27kip1 degradation, prevents its translocation to the nucleus, leading to concentration imbalance, especially in cancer stem cells, which induces their activation [96]. Oxysterols are sterol precursor and also act as the ligand for Liver X receptors (LXR) [97]. LXR is a sensitive molecule that can act as a sensor in cholesterol homeostasis by disrupting SREBP pathways or accelerating HMGCR degradation [98]. In brain malignant glioblastoma, the cells are dependent on cholesterol. Introduction of LXR agonist induces high cancer cell death [99]. In breast cancer cell lines, the activation of LXR also reduces proliferation significantly [100]. Interestingly, in a combination immunotherapy, LXR activation therapy enhances T-cell activation, which in turn leads to strong anti-tumor response in mice, suggesting the feasibility of utilizing ApoE/LXR axis as a cancer immunotherapy target [101].

Lipogenesis is transcriptionally regulated by the sterol regulatory element-binding proteins (SREBPs) family. SREBP1 mainly regulates the expression of FA synthesis genes and LDLR, while SREBP2 preferentially controls the expression of cholesterol biosynthesis genes [102]. In addition, SREBP activation is regulated by sterol fluctuations in ER. Cholesterol binds to SREBP cleavage-activating protein (SCAP), thereby disrupting the interaction between SCAP and COPII and retaining SREBP in ER. Inhibition of cholesterol acyltransferase (ACAT) accumulates ER cholesterol, reduces lipid droplet formation, and inhibits prostate tumor cells and glioblastoma growth aggressiveness by blocking SREBP1-regulated gene expression [103]. SREBP1 is a crucial bridge between FA metabolism and onco-genic signaling, and its regulation in tumor cells is equally sophisticated [104]. SREBP2 also can activate the MVA pathway in P53-deficient colon cancer cells, altering the metabolic activity and enhancing ubiquinone synthesis of tumor cells [105]. Protein arginine methyltransferase 5 (PRMT5)-induced methylation hinders GSK3β phosphorylation of SREBP1a on S430, resulting to its dissociation from FBXW7 and evasion of degradation via the ubiquitin-proteasome pathway [106]. mSREBP1a methylated by PRMT5 promotes transcription of adipogenic genes and subsequent intracellular lipid synthesis, leading to increased adipogenesis, accelerated tumor cells proliferation, and poor prognosis in hepatocellular carcinoma [106]. It has been shown that leptin can promote breast cancer cells proliferation, invasion, and migration by upregulating ACAT2 through the PI3K/AKT/SREBP2 signaling pathway [107]. Activation of SREBP-related pathway plays an important role in lipid metabolism and promotion of cancer cells proliferation. Thus, targeting this pathway might become one of the new strategies for tumor immunotherapy.

Redox Imbalance and Regulation in the Local *Onco-Sphere*

Influenced by metabolic alterations and tumor-related gene signaling pathways, the redox status of tumor cells is often in an imbalanced state and manifested by abnormally high ROS levels and oxidative stress. The intracellular ROS is mainly derived from mitochondria, followed by ER and peroxisomes [108]. It can be shown that there are different molecular sites of superoxide production inside the mito-chondria via using isolated mitochondria [109]. Normal cells in the presence of oxygen can produce NADH via the TCA cycle, and the generated NADH acts as an electron source within the mitochondria to start electron transfer and produce ATP. In contrast, tumor cells tend to be hypoxic, which causes aberrant electron flow in the electron transport chain (ETC) to produce massive ROS [110]. Simultaneously, abnormalities in mitochondrial structure and function, such as mutations in mito-chondrial DNA (mtDNA), can lead to abnormal electron leakage due to dysfunction of the respiratory chain. Free electrons react with molecular oxygen to generate superoxide anion radicals, which can subsequently be converted to other types of ROS [111]. Alterations in mtDNA accumulated in tumor cells due to ROS produc-tion and aberrant mtDNA repair and mutations or copy number variation in mtDNA result in defects in ATP generation via OXPHOS [112]. Additionally, recent evi-dence suggests that mitochondria-mediated ROS production is closely associated with ferroptosis [113]. Two important biochemical features of ferroptosis are iron accumulation and lipid peroxidation. Intracellular iron can generate massive ROS through the Fenton reaction and thus lead to oxidative damage. The current view-point is that the induction of ferroptosis is associated with GSH metabolism, iron chelation, regulation of system Xc^-, and glutathione peroxidase 4 (GPX4) activity, ultimately leading to an imbalance in ROS homeostasis. It has been shown that ferroptosis suppressor protein 1 (FSP1) inhibits ferroptosis independently via the classical glutathione-based GPX4 pathway, through the non-mitochondrial CoQ10 antioxidant system [114]. NADPH, a metabolic substrate, is essential for many biological processes and depletion of NADPH leads to a decrease in thioredoxin (TXN) and GSH levels, which promotes the accumulation of lipid ROS in biological membranes [115]. Isocitrate dehydrogenase (IDH1/2) is one of the biological enzymes that generate NADPH, and IDH1/2 mutant cells become sensitive to ferroptosis inducers due to reduced NADPH levels [116]. Thus, inhibition of IDH mutants affects ROS levels and has a potential for anticancer therapy.

Tumor cells usually have a high rate of aerobic glycolysis (known as the Warburg effect). Glucose can be used to generate lactate and ATP, while also shifting to anabolic processes, including the pentose phosphate pathway (PPP). Glucose is involved in ATP and lactate production, NADPH generation, and nucleotide biosynthesis in tumor cells, and some of these biosynthetic pathways are determined by the activity of pyruvate kinase. Notably, tumor cells express pyruvate lyase M2 (PKM2, a specific pyruvate kinase subtype) and increased ROS target the specific Cys residues in PKM2 that transfers generated glucose from lactate to PPP, which leads to an increment of NADPH production and thus redox buffering via GSH [117]. Autophagy is also closely related between tumor metabolism and ROS. There is a strong link between intracellular redox status and autophagic flux. Some autophagy inducers elevate intracellular ROS levels, and this oxidative stress subsequently inactivates ATG4 (Cys protease, a negative regulator of autophagosome formation) [118]. The oncogene-TP53 induced apoptosis regulator (TIGAR) inhibits the elevation of ROS to reduce oxidative levels and autophagic flux [119]. In contrast, the lack of normal autophagic flux leads to an increment of ROS levels, which in turn result in increased DNA damage [120].

After acute exposure to ROS, NADPH produced by G6PD plays a crucial role in mitigating oxidative stress. Excessive levels of ROS can lead to oxidative damage to lipids, proteins, and DNA. Within a moderate range, ROS can stimulate MAPK and ERK phosphorylation, cyclin D1 expression and JNK activation, and all signaling molecules associated with tumor growth [121]. It has been shown that a certain level of increased ROS in tumor cells contributes to cell proliferation, survival, differentiation, and migration [122]. In contrast, when ROS is severely elevated beyond the level tolerated by cellular antioxidant mechanisms, it can lead to cellular damage and even death. To prevent the damage caused by ROS, these tumor cells are able to control the level of ROS within the appropriate range through their own regulatory mechanisms. The ability of tumor cells to enhance their oxidative stress is mainly through the high expression of enzymes responsible for scavenging ROS and the production of a series of antioxidant molecules (e.g., GSH, NADPH, and TRX). It has been shown that inducing oxidative stress also promotes the activation of antioxidant mechanisms in tumor cells [123]. Oxidative regulation of tumor cells may involve multiple signaling pathways to activate redox-sensitive transcription factors, such as NRF2, NF-κB, and HIF-1 [124, 125]. Activation of these transcription factors promotes gene expression of antioxidant systems (e.g., superoxide dismutase, peroxisomal enzymes, thioredoxin, and glutathione). For example, the NRF2 pathway is the first line of cellular defense against ROS and regulates cellular metabolism through a series of downstream responses. NRF2 also promotes cellular synthesis and utilization of glutathione, which is known to promote alkylator metabolism and detoxification, and reduced GSH reverses the tumor suppressive effects of 3-bromopyruvate (3-BrPA) [126]. KEAP1 (a negative regulator of NRF2) mutations and NRF2 activation promote tumor cells development by enhancing endogenous antioxidant responses [127]. The KEAP1/NRF2/ARE pathway regulates the response of many antioxidants and activates a range of defense systems to block or reverse cancer development by inhibiting the activation of carcinogens or inducing the detoxification of phase II metabolizing enzymes, and the KEAP1/NRF2/ARE pathway has been shown to be closely related to cancer development in a variety of cancer models [128, 129].

Genomic instability is also another important mechanism of redox adaption and regulation in tumor cells. Genetic instability allows for functional alterations or aberrant expression of the proteins they encode and provides for cellular adaptation to the oxidative stress environment and its survival advantage in the TME [108]. Tumor cells can maintain ROS in a more stable and tolerable range by increasing the capacity of endogenous antioxidant systems and activating cell survival pathways through redox regulation. Upregulated antioxidant systems, such as GSH and NADPH, confer greater antioxidant capacity and enhance DNA repair, thereby reducing apoptosis [130], as summarized in Fig. 8.3 below.

Crosstalk in the Local *Onco-Sphere*: Biochemical Changes and Tumor Metabolism

The extracellular environment may become more acidic as a result of tumor metabolism. Recently, more research studies are showing on how tumor acidity may affect tumor metabolic preferences [8, 131–135]. In the section below, we will discuss in detail how biochemical changes affect tumor growth by modulating tumor metabolism within the local *onco-sphere*.

Ion Changes and Acidosis

There has not yet been any information on a transcriptional H^+-responsive element that might change how genes are expressed. HIF2, however, has so far being identified as the major regulator of metabolic tolerance to acidosis [132, 133, 136, 137], while HIF1α was generally downregulated [132, 138, 139]. Along with opposing changes in HIF isoform abundance, acidosis also increases SIRT1 and SIRT6 activity in an NAD^+-dependent manner, supporting the divergent impacts on the activity of both HIFs [132, 138, 139]. While comparable deacetylation in HIF1 hinders p300 binding and represses HIF1 transcriptional activity, it is linked with

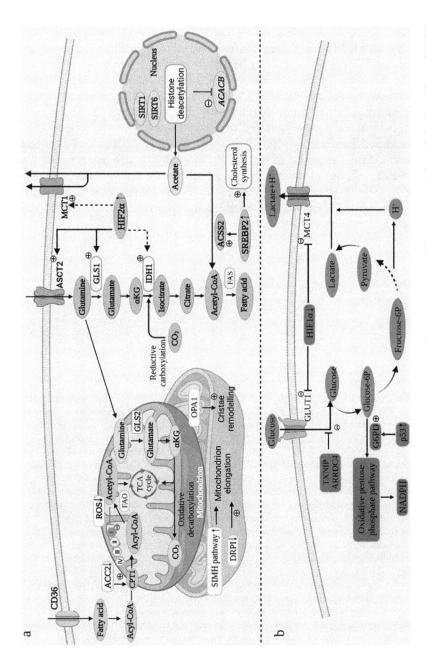

Fig 8.3 A summary of biochemical changes in many pathways of tumor metabolic adaptation. (**a**) Here, the metabolism of stimulated fatty acid is illustrated as a response to acidosis. While the synthesis of fatty acids is maintained by the carboxylation of α-ketoglutarate as derived from glutamine, the canonical TCA cycle is facilitated by mitochondrial oxidative metabolism. The upregulation of GLS1 and ASCT2 is facilitated by the increased activity and production of

enhanced transcriptional regulatory activity in the HIF2 amino-terminal transactivation domain (NTAD) region [140]. HIF2 activation and overexpression in cancer cells of the pharynx, colon, and cervix were demonstrated to promote glutamine metabolism by increasing the expression of the glutamine transporters ASCT2 and GLS1, in place of the preferred glucose metabolism seen at neutral pH [132]. Instead, HIF1 target genes were negatively regulated in acidosis, resulting in substantial reductions in the expression of GLUT1 and MCT4. It is interesting to note that studies contrasting the effects of lactic acidosis and glucose restriction on the transcriptome of breast cancer cells indicated that both stressors cause a starving response, but that some genes were differently regulated [139, 141]. Among these, acidosis-induced induction of TXNIP and its paralogue ARRDC4 and glucose deprivation-induced repression of both were observed. It is also hypothesized that TXNIP would function as a switch to inhibit glycolysis during acidosis because of its capacity to impede glucose absorption [142]. Further research is necessary to determine whether TXNIP may be regarded as a universal switch in different malignancies, notwithstanding this idea.

Hypoxia

In glioblastoma and HEK293 cells, for instance, recent investigations have found that HIF1 is upregulated during acidosis [133, 134]. HIF-mediated transcriptome

---

Fig 8.3 (continued) HIF2α, which supports the former pathway and is linked with the higher secretion of MCT1 and IDH1. Due to the activation of SREBP2, which is motivated by acidosis, the synthesis of cholesterol and fatty acids is increased; moreover, SREB2 supports the increase in production of the cytosolic enzyme, ACSS2, which triggers the activation of acetate into acetyl-CoA, which is generally adopted in the synthesis of lipids. The downregulation of ACC2, which takes place during the deacetylation of ACACB (which encodes ACC2), as mediated by SIRT6 and SIRT1, the concomitant oxidation of fatty acids takes place under acidosis. The partial inhibition of the respiratory chain complex I, in addition to the non-enzymatic acetylation, is responsible for restraining the risky production of mitochondrial reactive oxygen species. Further, through a reduction in the interaction between mitochondrial FIS1 and DRP1, mitochondrial fragmentation, as induced by hypoxia, is prevented by acidosis; further, in a manner that relies upon the SIMH pathway, mitochondrial elongation is improved and facilitated. Resistance to cell death and improved respiration are associated with an increase in the number of cristae and change in their morphology, which occur due to the increase in OPA1 as a result of acidosis. (**b**) Alterations in glucose metabolism under acidosis. The expression of GLUT1, MCT4, and glycolytic enzymes is decreased due to the reduction in the activity and abundance of HIF1α. Through the reduction of glucose absorption in breast cancer cells, upregulation of thioredoxin-interacting protein (TXNIP) and its paralog arrestin domain-containing protein 4 (ARRDC4) under lactic acidosis significantly contributes to the inhibition of tumor glycolytic characteristics. A p53-dependent increase in glucose-6-phosphate dehydrogenase facilitates a rerouting of a portion of the glucose taken in by the cancer cell away from lactate formation and toward the oxidative branch of the pentose phosphate pathway (PPP), an alternate metabolic pathway (G6PD)

alterations may be dynamically influenced by the worsening of tumor hypoxia, which might be caused by increased O_2 consumption under acidosis. Last but not least, it is crucial to note that the rapidly developing area of pH sensors is likely to provide significant new insights into the signaling networks linking extracellular acidosis to gene reprogramming [143]. It has been established that the protonation of histidine residues found in the extracellular region of GPCRs, such as GPR4, GPR65, and GPR68, activates these receptors [144]. Various pathways, such as adenylyl cyclase and PLC, were activated, in addition to the transduction of signals via varying G proteins, which was noted through the observance of the receptors capable of sensing pH [145]. The extracellular acidic pH was also found to be detected by ASIC1 and TRPV1, which have been reported as non-GPCRs [145]. In the context of acidosis-exposed prostate and breast cancer cells, the activation of NF-κB was caused by the opening of the channels, which leads to an influx of calcium [146, 147]. Additionally, pH sensing can directly result from changes in the protonation of certain signaling proteins due to the charged nature of particular residues, such as histidine and arginine [3, 148]. The mutations that modify the activities of critical proteins, in addition to the glycolytic enzymes that engage in activities sensitive to pH, are in support of this finding [3]. For instance, the tumor suppressor protein p53's arginine-to-histidine substitution R337H in the tetramerization domain inhibits DNA binding when the pHi is elevated [149].

Metabolic Adjustment

The production of a lactate gradient, with the greatest amounts detected in the most hypoxic tumor regions, is connected to one of the very early tumor metabolic adjustments to TME acidosis. There are several different kinds of tumor cells that have been described by numerous independent researchers [7, 150–154]; following lactate-to-pyruvate conversion, other cancer cells may take the support of MCT1 to capture and consume the substance, thereby prompting the idea of a metabolic symbiosis, which takes place in solid cancers, between lactate-consuming and -generating cells [22, 155–157]. The neutralization of intracellular H^+ ions is essential for sustaining the lactate shuttle, given that the transportation of lactate and H^+ ions necessitates MCT1 as a pathway. By encouraging the neutralization of H^+ ions and the hydration of CO_2, respectively, intracellular and extracellular CA activities may perform this function.

Lipid metabolism is associated with another very noticeable change in the metabolic preferences of cancer cells under acidosis. It has been demonstrated that fatty acid synthesis (FAS) is facilitated by acidosis-driven reductive carboxylation of glutamine-derived-ketoglutarate by generating acetyl-CoA from citrate [132]. When SREBP2 is activated and ACSS2 is subsequently upregulated, acetate was discovered as a source of acetyl-CoA for fatty acid synthesis in acidosis [135]. Although it was also shown that the two pathways supporting FAS were activated in response to hypoxic stress, the concurrent activation of FAO marks a significant distinction from hypoxic settings. This ability to concurrently utilize FAS and FAO was shown to be increased under acidosis in a variety of cancer cells, including those from the colon, cervical, and oropharyngeal cancers. This was demonstrated by the downregulation of ACC2 [158–161]. A significant increase in the non-enzymatic acetylation of several proteins, including ETC complex members, is also brought on by FAO-derived acetyl-CoA in addition to feeding the TCA cycle [131]. In cancer cells that have acclimated to acidosis, the activity of acetylated ETC complex I has been measured to be inhibited. Although reducing complex I activity has been shown to reduce ROS generation as a result of mitochondrial overfeeding without totally inhibiting OXPHOS, ETC inhibition may seem contradictory given the reported increase in mitochondrial respiration caused by FAO [131]. It was discovered that numerous breast cancer cell lines that had been acutely exposed to acidic conditions for 24 h also exhibited another form of antioxidant activity [162]. When glucose was diverted to the oxidative branch of the PPP, more NADPH was produced, partly due to the transcriptional activation of G6PD that was p53-dependent [162]. Therefore, regardless of a brief or prolonged acidosis exposure, tumor cells generate ROS, which leads to tumor growth and progression.

Intracellular Vs. Extracellular pH Changes

Numerous research works link TME acidity with characteristics of cancer progression, particularly local tumor invasion and distant metastasis [163–165], along with description of insightful mathematical models of acid-mediated invasion [39, 166]. According to these findings, enhanced cancer cell motility in response to a drop in pHe is primarily caused by modifications to the cytoskeletal dynamics that alter cancer cell polarization as well as an increase in the activity of TAMs and fibroblasts' proteases [3]. It was discovered that a slight alkalization of cancer cell pHi promoted cell migration by increasing the activity of numerous actin-binding proteins in a pH-dependent manner, whereas extracellular acidification activated proteases that altered cell–matrix adhesion and cell–cell interactions [167]. Intravital imaging (IVM) was used to track the invasion of HCT-116 colon cancer cells and the peritumoral pHe in a time-dependent manner to confirm this model of acid-mediated tumor invasion [168]. Specifically, tumor areas with the highest local tumor invasion were linked to those with the lowest levels of pHe. It has also been shown that enhanced angiogenesis brought on by matrix breakdown and the subsequent release of imprisoned pro-angiogenic chemicals, such as VEGF, causes acidic pH to accelerate the spread of metastatic disease [169]. The intravital fluorescence imaging of VEGF promoter activity was used to detect a direct increase in VEGF transcription in acidic regions of human glioma cells transplanted in mice under a cranial window [170]. In the same tumor type, acidic circumstances, irrespective of a decrease in O_2 availability, enhanced the expression of glioma stem cell markers, whose capability to cause tumors was supported by the creation of angiogenic factors [171].

Conclusion

In conclusion, biochemical changes in the local *onco-sphere* have multiple effects on the tumor environment, especially in their cross-communication with cancer cell to affect their growth, metabolic rewiring, and metastasis. These biochemical changes are revolved around the metabolic changes in the local onco-sphere, which can be induced not only by the tumor cells but also stromal cells and infiltrated immune cells. All these changes render the cancer cells to have adaptive mechanisms that lead to their enhanced growth and survival, even to increase their stem-cell like properties. However, it is important to note that these biochemical changes are not unique to cancer cells. Normal cells are also highly metabolic, albeit the pathways and some mechanism might differ. Therefore, cancer therapy targeting metabolism or the biochemical changes in the local onco-sphere should be used with extra caution. One approach could be the use of synergistic combination therapy, in which the concept of tumor ecosystem would be helpful in determining the best approach in targeting tumor biochemical changes. Therefore, one should consider looking at tumor as an ecological system, to synergistically target various mechanisms or pathways in local *onco-sphere* for effective cancer therapy.

References

1. Corbet C, Feron O (2017) Tumour acidosis: from the passenger to the driver's seat. Nat Rev Cancer 17(10):577–593
2. Zu XL, Guppy M (2004) Cancer metabolism: facts, fantasy, and fiction. Biochem Biophys Res Commun 313(3):459–465
3. Webb BA, Chimenti M, Jacobson MP, Barber DL (2011) Dysregulated pH: a perfect storm for cancer progression. Nat Rev Cancer 11(9):671–677
4. Lagadic-Gossmann D, Huc L, Lecureur V (2004) Alterations of intracellular pH homeostasis in apoptosis: origins and roles. Cell Death Differ 11(9):953–961
5. Hulikova A, Harris AL, Vaughan-Jones RD, Swietach P (2013) Regulation of intracellular pH in cancer cell lines under normoxia and hypoxia. J Cell Physiol 228(4):743–752
6. Fukuda R, Zhang H, Kim JW, Shimoda L, Dang CV, Semenza GL (2007) HIF-1 regulates cytochrome oxidase subunits to optimize efficiency of respiration in hypoxic cells. Cell 129(1):111–122
7. Boidot R, Végran F, Meulle A, Le Breton A, Dessy C, Sonveaux P et al (2012) Regulation of monocarboxylate transporter MCT1 expression by p53 mediates inward and outward lactate fluxes in tumors. Cancer Res 72(4):939–948
8. Khacho M, Tarabay M, Patten D, Khacho P, MacLaurin JG, Guadagno J et al (2014) Acidosis overrides oxygen deprivation to maintain mitochondrial function and cell survival. Nat Commun 5:3550
9. Supuran CT (2008) Carbonic anhydrases: novel therapeutic applications for inhibitors and activators. Nat Rev Drug Discov 7(2):168–181
10. Musa-Aziz R, Chen LM, Pelletier MF, Boron WF (2009) Relative CO2/NH3 selectivities of AQP1, AQP4, AQP5, AmtB, and RhAG. Proc Natl Acad Sci U S A 106(13):5406–5411
11. Hulikova A, Swietach P (2014) Rapid CO_2 permeation across biological membranes: implications for CO_2 venting from tissue. FASEB J 28(7):2762–2774

12. Svastová E, Hulíková A, Rafajová M, Zat'ovicová M, Gibadulinová A, Casini A et al (2004) Hypoxia activates the capacity of tumor-associated carbonic anhydrase IX to acidify extracellular pH. FEBS Lett 577(3):439–445

13. Swietach P, Vaughan-Jones RD, Harris AL, Hulikova A (2014) The chemistry, physiology and pathology of pH in cancer. Philos Trans R Soc Lond Ser B Biol Sci 369(1638):20130099

14. Hulikova A, Vaughan-Jones RD, Swietach P (2011) Dual role of $CO_2/HCO_3(-)$ buffer in the regulation of intracellular pH of three-dimensional tumor growths. J Biol Chem 286(16): 13815–13826

15. Swietach P, Hulikova A, Vaughan-Jones RD, Harris AL (2010) New insights into the physiological role of carbonic anhydrase IX in tumour pH regulation. Oncogene 29(50): 6509–6521

16. Becker HM, Klier M, Schüler C, McKenna R, Deitmer JW (2011) Intramolecular proton shuttle supports not only catalytic but also noncatalytic function of carbonic anhydrase II. Proc Natl Acad Sci U S A 108(7):3071–3076

17. Neri D, Supuran CT (2011) Interfering with pH regulation in tumours as a therapeutic strategy. Nat Rev Drug Discov 10(10):767–777

18. Michiels C, Tellier C, Feron O (2016) Cycling hypoxia: a key feature of the tumor microenvironment. Biochim Biophys Acta 1866(1):76–86

19. Secomb TW, Dewhirst MW, Pries AR (2012) Structural adaptation of normal and tumour vascular networks. Basic Clin Pharmacol Toxicol 110(1):63–69

20. Vaupel P, Mayer A (2014) Hypoxia in tumors: pathogenesis-related classification, characterization of hypoxia subtypes, and associated biological and clinical implications. Adv Exp Med Biol 812:19–24

21. Corbet C, Feron O (2017) Cancer cell metabolism and mitochondria: nutrient plasticity for TCA cycle fueling. Biochim Biophys Acta Rev Cancer 1868(1):7–15

22. Draoui N, Feron O (2011) Lactate shuttles at a glance: from physiological paradigms to anti-cancer treatments. Dis Model Mech 4(6):727–732

23. Vander Heiden MG, Cantley LC, Thompson CB (2009) Understanding the Warburg effect: the metabolic requirements of cell proliferation. Science 324(5930):1029–1033

24. Deitmer JW, Becker HM (2013) Transport metabolons with carbonic anhydrases. Front Physiol 4:291

25. Klier M, Andes FT, Deitmer JW, Becker HM (2014) Intracellular and extracellular carbonic anhydrases cooperate non-enzymatically to enhance activity of monocarboxylate transporters. J Biol Chem 289(5):2765–2775

26. Jamali S, Klier M, Ames S, Barros LF, McKenna R, Deitmer JW et al (2015) Hypoxia-induced carbonic anhydrase IX facilitates lactate flux in human breast cancer cells by non-catalytic function. Sci Rep 5:13605

27. Helmlinger G, Yuan F, Dellian M, Jain RK (1997) Interstitial pH and pO_2 gradients in solid tumors in vivo: high-resolution measurements reveal a lack of correlation. Nat Med 3(2): 177–182

28. Vaupel PW, Frinak S, Bicher HI (1981) Heterogeneous oxygen partial pressure and pH distribution in C3H mouse mammary adenocarcinoma. Cancer Res 41(5):2008–2013

29. Bittner MI, Wiedenmann N, Bucher S, Hentschel M, Mix M, Rücker G et al (2016) Analysis of relation between hypoxia PET imaging and tissue-based biomarkers during head and neck radiochemotherapy. Acta Oncol 55(11):1299–1304

30. Le QT, Kong C, Lavori PW, O'Byrne K, Erler JT, Huang X et al (2007) Expression and prognostic significance of a panel of tissue hypoxia markers in head-and-neck squamous cell carcinomas. Int J Radiat Oncol Biol Phys 69(1):167–175

31. Rademakers SE, Lok J, van der Kogel AJ, Bussink J, Kaanders JH (2011) Metabolic markers in relation to hypoxia; staining patterns and colocalization of pimonidazole, HIF-1α, CAIX, LDH-5, GLUT-1, MCT1 and MCT4. BMC Cancer 11:167

32. Helmlinger G, Sckell A, Dellian M, Forbes NS, Jain RK (2002) Acid production in glycolysis-impaired tumors provides new insights into tumor metabolism. Clin Cancer Res 8(4): 1284–1291

33. Newell K, Franchi A, Pouysségur J, Tannock I (1993) Studies with glycolysis-deficient cells suggest that production of lactic acid is not the only cause of tumor acidity. Proc Natl Acad Sci U S A 90(3):1127–1131

34. Yamagata M, Hasuda K, Stamato T, Tannock IF (1998) The contribution of lactic acid to acidification of tumours: studies of variant cells lacking lactate dehydrogenase. Br J Cancer 77(11):1726–1731

35. Mookerjee SA, Goncalves RLS, Gerencser AA, Nicholls DG, Brand MD (2015) The contributions of respiration and glycolysis to extracellular acid production. Biochim Biophys Acta 1847(2):171–181

36. Ibrahim-Hashim A, Estrella V (2019) Acidosis and cancer: from mechanism to neutralization. Cancer Metastasis Rev 38(1–2):149–155

37. Gillies RJ, Liu Z, Bhujwalla Z (1994) 31P-MRS measurements of extracellular pH of tumors using 3-aminopropylphosphonate. Am J Phys 267(1 Pt 1):C195–C203

38. Zhang X, Lin Y, Gillies RJ (2010) Tumor pH and its measurement. J Nucl Med 51(8): 1167–1170

39. Gatenby RA, Gawlinski ET, Gmitro AF, Kaylor B, Gillies RJ (2006) Acid-mediated tumor invasion: a multidisciplinary study. Cancer Res 66(10):5216–5223

40. Mizushima N, Klionsky DJ (2007) Protein turnover via autophagy: implications for metabolism. Annu Rev Nutr 27:19–40

41. Marino ML, Pellegrini P, Di Lernia G, Djavaheri-Mergny M, Brnjic S, Zhang X et al (2012) Autophagy is a protective mechanism for human melanoma cells under acidic stress. J Biol Chem 287(36):30664–30676

42. Wojtkowiak JW, Rothberg JM, Kumar V, Schramm KJ, Haller E, Proemsey JB et al (2012) Chronic autophagy is a cellular adaptation to tumor acidic pH microenvironments. Cancer Res 72(16):3938–3947

43. Wojtkowiak JW, Gillies RJ (2012) Autophagy on acid. Autophagy 8(11):1688–1689

44. Pellegrini P, Strambi A, Zipoli C, Hägg-Olofsson M, Buoncervello M, Linder S et al (2014) Acidic extracellular pH neutralizes the autophagy-inhibiting activity of chloroquine: implications for cancer therapies. Autophagy 10(4):562–571

45. Sousa CM, Biancur DE, Wang X, Halbrook CJ, Sherman MH, Zhang L et al (2016) Pancreatic stellate cells support tumour metabolism through autophagic alanine secretion. Nature 536(7617):479–483

46. Glunde K, Guggino SE, Solaiyappan M, Pathak AP, Ichikawa Y, Bhujwalla ZM (2003) Extracellular acidification alters lysosomal trafficking in human breast cancer cells. Neoplasia 5(6):533–545

47. Rozhin J, Sameni M, Ziegler G, Sloane BF (1994) Pericellular pH affects distribution and secretion of cathepsin B in malignant cells. Cancer Res 54(24):6517–6525

48. Steffan JJ, Snider JL, Skalli O, Welbourne T, Cardelli JA (2009) Na+/H+ exchangers and RhoA regulate acidic extracellular pH-induced lysosome trafficking in prostate cancer cells. Traffic 10(6):737–753

49. Damaghi M, Tafreshi NK, Lloyd MC, Sprung R, Estrella V, Wojtkowiak JW et al (2015) Chronic acidosis in the tumour microenvironment selects for overexpression of LAMP2 in the plasma membrane. Nat Commun 6:8752

50. Walton ZE, Patel CH, Brooks RC, Yu Y, Ibrahim-Hashim A, Riddle M et al (2018) Acid suspends the circadian clock in hypoxia through inhibition of mTOR. Cell 174(1):72–87.e32

51. Delikatny EJ, Chawla S, Leung DJ, Poptani H (2011) MR-visible lipids and the tumor microenvironment. NMR Biomed 24(6):592–611

52. Pillai S, Wojtkowiak JW, Damaghi M, Gatenby R, Gillies R (2017) Abstract 3538: enhanced dependence on lipid metabolism is a cellular adaptation to acidic microenvironment. Cancer Res 77(13_Supplement):3538

53. Carr RM, Ahima RS (2016) Pathophysiology of lipid droplet proteins in liver diseases. Exp Cell Res 340(2):187–192
54. Wallstab C, Eleftheriadou D, Schulz T, Damm G, Seehofer D, Borlak J et al (2017) A unifying mathematical model of lipid droplet metabolism reveals key molecular players in the development of hepatic steatosis. FEBS J 284(19):3245–3261
55. Tirinato L, Pagliari F, Limongi T, Marini M, Falqui A, Seco J et al (2017) An overview of lipid droplets in cancer and cancer stem cells. Stem Cells Int 2017:1656053
56. Krahmer N, Farese RV Jr, Walther TC (2013) Balancing the fat: lipid droplets and human disease. EMBO Mol Med 5(7):973–983
57. Antalis CJ, Uchida A, Buhman KK, Siddiqui RA (2011) Migration of MDA-MB-231 breast cancer cells depends on the availability of exogenous lipids and cholesterol esterification. Clin Exp Metastasis 28(8):733–741
58. Persi E, Duran-Frigola M, Damaghi M, Roush WR, Aloy P, Cleveland JL et al (2018) Systems analysis of intracellular pH vulnerabilities for cancer therapy. Nat Commun 9(1):2997
59. Pavlova NN, Thompson CB (2016) The emerging hallmarks of cancer metabolism. Cell Metab 23(1):27–47
60. Li Z, Zhang H (2016) Reprogramming of glucose, fatty acid and amino acid metabolism for cancer progression. Cell Mol Life Sci 73(2):377–392
61. DeBerardinis RJ, Cheng T (2010) Q's next: the diverse functions of glutamine in metabolism, cell biology and cancer. Oncogene 29(3):313–324
62. Cox AG, Hwang KL, Brown KK, Evason K, Beltz S, Tsomides A et al (2016) Yap reprograms glutamine metabolism to increase nucleotide biosynthesis and enable liver growth. Nat Cell Biol 18(8):886–896
63. Still ER, Yuneva MO (2017) Hopefully devoted to Q: targeting glutamine addiction in cancer. Br J Cancer 116(11):1375–1381
64. Kandasamy P, Gyimesi G, Kanai Y, Hediger MA (2018) Amino acid transporters revisited: new views in health and disease. Trends Biochem Sci 43(10):752–789
65. Matés JM, Segura JA, Martín-Rufián M, Campos-Sandoval JA, Alonso FJ, Márquez J (2013) Glutaminase isoenzymes as key regulators in metabolic and oxidative stress against cancer. Curr Mol Med 13(4):514–534
66. Son J, Lyssiotis CA, Ying H, Wang X, Hua S, Ligorio M et al (2013) Glutamine supports pancreatic cancer growth through a KRAS-regulated metabolic pathway. Nature 496(7443): 101–105
67. Li AM, Ye J (2020) Reprogramming of serine, glycine and one-carbon metabolism in cancer. Biochim Biophys Acta Mol basis Dis 1866(10):165841
68. Ye J, Fan J, Venneti S, Wan YW, Pawel BR, Zhang J et al (2014) Serine catabolism regulates mitochondrial redox control during hypoxia. Cancer Discov 4(12):1406–1417
69. Pacold ME, Brimacombe KR, Chan SH, Rohde JM, Lewis CA, Swier LJ et al (2016) A PHGDH inhibitor reveals coordination of serine synthesis and one-carbon unit fate. Nat Chem Biol 12(6):452–458
70. Labuschagne CF, van den Broek NJ, Mackay GM, Vousden KH, Maddocks OD (2014) Serine, but not glycine, supports one-carbon metabolism and proliferation of cancer cells. Cell Rep 7(4):1248–1258
71. Chen CL, Hsu SC, Chung TY, Chu CY, Wang HJ, Hsiao PW et al (2021) Arginine is an epigenetic regulator targeting TEAD4 to modulate OXPHOS in prostate cancer cells. Nat Commun 12(1):2398
72. Hou X, Chen S, Zhang P, Guo D, Wang B (2022) Targeted arginine metabolism therapy: a dilemma in glioma treatment. Front Oncol 12:938847
73. Cheng CT, Qi Y, Wang YC, Chi KK, Chung Y, Ouyang C et al (2018) Arginine starvation kills tumor cells through aspartate exhaustion and mitochondrial dysfunction. Commun Biol 1: 178
74. Feun LG, Kuo MT, Savaraj N (2015) Arginine deprivation in cancer therapy. Curr Opin Clin Nutr Metab Care 18(1):78–82

75. Abdelmagid SA, Rickard JA, McDonald WJ, Thomas LN, Too CK (2011) CAT-1-mediated arginine uptake and regulation of nitric oxide synthases for the survival of human breast cancer cell lines. J Cell Biochem 112(4):1084–1092

76. Kishikawa T, Otsuka M, Tan PS, Ohno M, Sun X, Yoshikawa T et al (2015) Decreased miR122 in hepatocellular carcinoma leads to chemoresistance with increased arginine. Oncotarget 6(10):8339–8352

77. Geiger R, Rieckmann JC, Wolf T, Basso C, Feng Y, Fuhrer T et al (2016) L-arginine modulates T cell metabolism and enhances survival and anti-tumor activity. Cell 167(3): 829–42.e13

78. D'Amato NC, Rogers TJ, Gordon MA, Greene LI, Cochrane DR, Spoelstra NS et al (2015) A TDO2-AhR signaling axis facilitates anoikis resistance and metastasis in triple-negative breast cancer. Cancer Res 75(21):4651–4664

79. Lee SH, Mahendran R, Tham SM, Thamboo TP, Chionh BJ, Lim YX et al (2021) Tryptophan-kynurenine ratio as a biomarker of bladder cancer. BJU Int 127(4):445–453

80. Li F, Zhao Z, Zhang Z, Zhang Y, Guan W (2021) Tryptophan metabolism induced by TDO2 promotes prostatic cancer chemotherapy resistance in a AhR/c-Myc dependent manner. BMC Cancer 21(1):1112

81. Vander Heiden MG, DeBerardinis RJ (2017) Understanding the intersections between metabolism and cancer biology. Cell 168(4):657–669

82. Guo R, Chen Y, Borgard H, Jijiwa M, Nasu M, He M et al (2020) The function and mechanism of lipid molecules and their roles in the diagnosis and prognosis of breast cancer. Molecules 25(20):4864

83. Su X, Abumrad NA (2009) Cellular fatty acid uptake: a pathway under construction. Trends Endocrinol Metab 20(2):72–77

84. Bensaad K, Favaro E, Lewis CA, Peck B, Lord S, Collins JM et al (2014) Fatty acid uptake and lipid storage induced by HIF-1α contribute to cell growth and survival after hypoxia-reoxygenation. Cell Rep 9(1):349–365

85. Auciello FR, Bulusu V, Oon C, Tait-Mulder J, Berry M, Bhattacharyya S et al (2019) A stromal lysolipid-autotaxin signaling axis promotes pancreatic tumor progression. Cancer Discov 9(5):617–627

86. Khwairakpam AD, Banik K, Girisa S, Shabnam B, Shakibaei M, Fan L et al (2020) The vital role of ATP citrate lyase in chronic diseases. J Mol Med (Berl) 98(1):71–95

87. Comerford SA, Huang Z, Du X, Wang Y, Cai L, Witkiewicz AK et al (2014) Acetate dependence of tumors. Cell 159(7):1591–1602

88. Chin K, DeVries S, Fridlyand J, Spellman PT, Roydasgupta R, Kuo WL et al (2006) Genomic and transcriptional aberrations linked to breast cancer pathophysiologies. Cancer Cell 10(6): 529–541

89. German NJ, Yoon H, Yusuf RZ, Murphy JP, Finley LW, Laurent G et al (2016) PHD3 loss in cancer enables metabolic reliance on fatty acid oxidation via deactivation of ACC2. Mol Cell 63(6):1006–1020

90. Cheng X, Geng F, Pan M, Wu X, Zhong Y, Wang C et al (2020) Targeting DGAT1 ameliorates glioblastoma by increasing fat catabolism and oxidative stress. Cell Metab 32(2):229–42.e8

91. King RJ, Singh PK, Mehla K (2022) The cholesterol pathway: impact on immunity and cancer. Trends Immunol 43(1):78–92

92. Ding X, Zhang W, Li S, Yang H (2019) The role of cholesterol metabolism in cancer. Am J Cancer Res 9(2):219–227

93. Yeganeh B, Wiechec E, Ande SR, Sharma P, Moghadam AR, Post M et al (2014) Targeting the mevalonate cascade as a new therapeutic approach in heart disease, cancer and pulmonary disease. Pharmacol Ther 143(1):87–110

94. Tsubaki M, Mashimo K, Takeda T, Kino T, Fujita A, Itoh T et al (2016) Statins inhibited the MIP-1alpha expression via inhibition of Ras/ERK and Ras/Akt pathways in myeloma cells. Biomed Pharmacother 78:23–29

95. Casey PJ, Seabra MC (1996) Protein prenyltransferases. J Biol Chem 271(10):5289–5292
96. Ginestier C, Charafe-Jauffret E, Birnbaum D (2012) p53 and cancer stem cells: the mevalonate connexion. Cell Cycle 11(14):2583–2584
97. Griffiths WJ, Abdel-Khalik J, Hearn T, Yutuc E, Morgan AH, Wang Y (2016) Current trends in oxysterol research. Biochem Soc Trans 44(2):652–658
98. Bovenga F, Sabba C, Moschetta A (2015) Uncoupling nuclear receptor LXR and cholesterol metabolism in cancer. Cell Metab 21(4):517–526
99. Villa GR, Hulce JJ, Zanca C, Bi J, Ikegami S, Cahill GL et al (2016) An LXR-cholesterol axis creates a metabolic co-dependency for brain cancers. Cancer Cell 30(5):683–693
100. Vedin LL, Lewandowski SA, Parini P, Gustafsson JA, Steffensen KR (2009) The oxysterol receptor LXR inhibits proliferation of human breast cancer cells. Carcinogenesis 30(4): 575–579
101. Tavazoie MF, Pollack I, Tanqueco R, Ostendorf BN, Reis BS, Gonsalves FC et al (2018) LXR/ApoE activation restricts innate immune suppression in cancer. Cell 172(4):825–40e18
102. Gouw AM, Margulis K, Liu NS, Raman SJ, Mancuso A, Toal GG et al (2019) The MYC oncogene cooperates with sterol-regulated element-binding protein to regulate lipogenesis essential for neoplastic growth. Cell Metab 30(3):556–72.e5
103. Geng F, Cheng X, Wu X, Yoo JY, Cheng C, Guo JY et al (2016) Inhibition of SOAT1 suppresses glioblastoma growth via blocking SREBP-1-mediated lipogenesis. Clin Cancer Res 22(21):5337–5348
104. Guo D, Bell EH, Mischel P, Chakravarti A (2014) Targeting SREBP-1-driven lipid metabolism to treat cancer. Curr Pharm Des 20(15):2619–2626
105. Kaymak I, Maier CR, Schmitz W, Campbell AD, Dankworth B, Ade CP et al (2020) Mevalonate pathway provides ubiquinone to maintain pyrimidine synthesis and survival in p53-deficient cancer cells exposed to metabolic stress. Cancer Res 80(2):189–203
106. Liu L, Zhao X, Zhao L, Li J, Yang H, Zhu Z et al (2016) Arginine methylation of SREBP1a via PRMT5 promotes De novo lipogenesis and tumor growth. Cancer Res 76(5):1260–1272
107. Huang Y, Jin Q, Su M, Ji F, Wang N, Zhong C et al (2017) Leptin promotes the migration and invasion of breast cancer cells by upregulating ACAT2. Cell Oncol (Dordr) 40(6):537–547
108. Holmström KM, Finkel T (2014) Cellular mechanisms and physiological consequences of redox-dependent signalling. Nat Rev Mol Cell Biol 15(6):411–421
109. Brand MD (2010) The sites and topology of mitochondrial superoxide production. Exp Gerontol 45(7–8):466–472
110. Kung-Chun Chiu D, Pui-Wah Tse A, Law CT, Ming-Jing XI, Lee D, Chen M et al (2019) Hypoxia regulates the mitochondrial activity of hepatocellular carcinoma cells through HIF/HEY1/PINK1 pathway. Cell Death Dis 10(12):934
111. Brandon M, Baldi P, Wallace DC (2006) Mitochondrial mutations in cancer. Oncogene 25(34):4647–4662
112. Yin PH, Lee HC, Chau GY, Wu YT, Li SH, Lui WY et al (2004) Alteration of the copy number and deletion of mitochondrial DNA in human hepatocellular carcinoma. Br J Cancer 90(12):2390–2396
113. Lee H, Zandkarimi F, Zhang Y, Meena JK, Kim J, Zhuang L et al (2020) Energy-stress-mediated AMPK activation inhibits ferroptosis. Nat Cell Biol 22(2):225–234
114. Bersuker K, Hendricks JM, Li Z, Magtanong L, Ford B, Tang PH et al (2019) The CoQ oxidoreductase FSP1 acts parallel to GPX4 to inhibit ferroptosis. Nature 575(7784):688–692
115. Yang L, Wang H, Yang X, Wu Q, An P, Jin X et al (2020) Auranofin mitigates systemic iron overload and induces ferroptosis via distinct mechanisms. Signal Transduct Target Ther 5(1): 138
116. Wang TX, Liang JY, Zhang C, Xiong Y, Guan KL, Yuan HX (2019) The oncometabolite 2-hydroxyglutarate produced by mutant IDH1 sensitizes cells to ferroptosis. Cell Death Dis 10(10):755

117. Anastasiou D, Poulogiannis G, Asara JM, Boxer MB, Jiang JK, Shen M et al (2011) Inhibition of pyruvate kinase M2 by reactive oxygen species contributes to cellular antioxidant responses. Science 334(6060):1278–1283
118. Scherz-Shouval R, Shvets E, Fass E, Shorer H, Gil L, Elazar Z (2007) Reactive oxygen species are essential for autophagy and specifically regulate the activity of Atg4. EMBO J 26(7): 1749–1760
119. Bensaad K, Cheung EC, Vousden KH (2009) Modulation of intracellular ROS levels by TIGAR controls autophagy. EMBO J 28(19):3015–3026
120. Mathew R, Karp CM, Beaudoin B, Vuong N, Chen G, Chen HY et al (2009) Autophagy suppresses tumorigenesis through elimination of p62. Cell 137(6):1062–1075
121. Song JS, Kim EK, Choi YW, Oh WK, Kim YM (2016) Hepatocyte-protective effect of nectandrin B, a nutmeg lignan, against oxidative stress: role of Nrf2 activation through ERK phosphorylation and AMPK-dependent inhibition of GSK-3β. Toxicol Appl Pharmacol 307: 138–149
122. Rhee SG (2006) Cell signaling. H_2O_2, a necessary evil for cell signaling. Science 312(5782): 1882–1883
123. Diehn M, Cho RW, Lobo NA, Kalisky T, Dorie MJ, Kulp AN et al (2009) Association of reactive oxygen species levels and radioresistance in cancer stem cells. Nature 458(7239): 780–783
124. Bartolini D, Dallaglio K, Torquato P, Piroddi M, Galli F (2018) Nrf2-p62 autophagy pathway and its response to oxidative stress in hepatocellular carcinoma. Transl Res 193:54–71
125. Kipp AP, Deubel S, Arnér ESJ, Johansson K (2017) Time- and cell-resolved dynamics of redox-sensitive Nrf2, HIF and NF-κB activities in 3D spheroids enriched for cancer stem cells. Redox Biol 12:403–409
126. Rodrigues-Ferreira C, da Silva AP, Galina A (2012) Effect of the antitumoral alkylating agent 3-bromopyruvate on mitochondrial respiration: role of mitochondrially bound hexokinase. J Bioenerg Biomembr 44(1):39–49
127. DeNicola GM, Karreth FA, Humpton TJ, Gopinathan A, Wei C, Frese K et al (2011) Oncogene-induced Nrf2 transcription promotes ROS detoxification and tumorigenesis. Nature 475(7354):106–109
128. Rajakumar T, Pugalendhi P, Thilagavathi S, Ananthakrishnan D, Gunasekaran K (2018) Allyl isothiocyanate, a potent chemopreventive agent targets AhR/Nrf2 signaling pathway in chemically induced mammary carcinogenesis. Mol Cell Biochem 437(1–2):1–12
129. Choi EJ, Jung BJ, Lee SH, Yoo HS, Shin EA, Ko HJ et al (2017) A clinical drug library screen identifies clobetasol propionate as an NRF2 inhibitor with potential therapeutic efficacy in KEAP1 mutant lung cancer. Oncogene 36(37):5285–5295
130. Hayes JD, Dinkova-Kostova AT, Tew KD (2020) Oxidative stress in cancer. Cancer Cell 38(2):167–197
131. Corbet C, Pinto A, Martherus R, Santiago de Jesus JP, Polet F, Feron O (2016) Acidosis drives the reprogramming of fatty acid metabolism in cancer cells through changes in mitochondrial and histone acetylation. Cell Metab 24(2):311–323
132. Corbet C, Draoui N, Polet F, Pinto A, Drozak X, Riant O et al (2014) The SIRT1/HIF2α axis drives reductive glutamine metabolism under chronic acidosis and alters tumor response to therapy. Cancer Res 74(19):5507–5519
133. Filatova A, Seidel S, Böğürcü N, Gräf S, Garvalov BK, Acker T (2016) Acidosis acts through HSP90 in a PHD/VHL-independent manner to promote HIF function and stem cell maintenance in glioma. Cancer Res 76(19):5845–5856
134. Nadtochiy SM, Schafer X, Fu D, Nehrke K, Munger J, Brookes PS (2016) Acidic pH is a metabolic switch for 2-Hydroxyglutarate generation and signaling. J Biol Chem 291(38): 20188–20197
135. Kondo A, Yamamoto S, Nakaki R, Shimamura T, Hamakubo T, Sakai J et al (2017) Extracellular acidic pH activates the sterol regulatory element-binding protein 2 to promote tumor progression. Cell Rep 18(9):2228–2242

136. Mekhail K, Gunaratnam L, Bonicalzi ME, Lee S (2004) HIF activation by pH-dependent nucleolar sequestration of VHL. Nat Cell Biol 6(7):642–647

137. Hjelmeland AB, Wu Q, Heddleston JM, Choudhary GS, MacSwords J, Lathia JD et al (2011) Acidic stress promotes a glioma stem cell phenotype. Cell Death Differ 18(5):829–840

138. Tang X, Lucas JE, Chen JL, LaMonte G, Wu J, Wang MC et al (2012) Functional interaction between responses to lactic acidosis and hypoxia regulates genomic transcriptional outputs. Cancer Res 72(2):491–502

139. Chen JL, Lucas JE, Schroeder T, Mori S, Wu J, Nevins J et al (2008) The genomic analysis of lactic acidosis and acidosis response in human cancers. PLoS Genet 4(12):e1000293

140. Dioum EM, Chen R, Alexander MS, Zhang Q, Hogg RT, Gerard RD et al (2009) Regulation of hypoxia-inducible factor 2alpha signaling by the stress-responsive deacetylase sirtuin 1. Science 324(5932):1289–1293

141. Chen JL, Merl D, Peterson CW, Wu J, Liu PY, Yin H et al (2010) Lactic acidosis triggers starvation response with paradoxical induction of TXNIP through MondoA. PLoS Genet 6(9): e1001093

142. Parikh H, Carlsson E, Chutkow WA, Johansson LE, Storgaard H, Poulsen P et al (2007) TXNIP regulates peripheral glucose metabolism in humans. PLoS Med 4(5):e158

143. Glitsch M (2011) Protons and Ca2+: ionic allies in tumor progression? Physiology 26(4): 252–265

144. Ludwig MG, Vanek M, Guerini D, Gasser JA, Jones CE, Junker U et al (2003) Proton-sensing G-protein-coupled receptors. Nature 425(6953):93–98

145. Damaghi M, Wojtkowiak JW, Gillies RJ (2013) pH sensing and regulation in cancer. Front Physiol 4:370

146. Gupta SC, Singh R, Pochampally R, Watabe K, Mo YY (2014) Acidosis promotes invasiveness of breast cancer cells through ROS-AKT-NF-κB pathway. Oncotarget 5(23): 12070–12082

147. Chen B, Liu J, Ho TT, Ding X, Mo YY (2016) ERK-mediated NF-κB activation through ASIC1 in response to acidosis. Oncogenesis 5(12):e279

148. Srivastava J, Barber DL, Jacobson MP (2007) Intracellular pH sensors: design principles and functional significance. Physiology 22:30–39

149. DiGiammarino EL, Lee AS, Cadwell C, Zhang W, Bothner B, Ribeiro RC et al (2002) A novel mechanism of tumorigenesis involving pH-dependent destabilization of a mutant p53 tetramer. Nat Struct Biol 9(1):12–16

150. Sonveaux P, Vegran F, Schroeder T, Wergin MC, Verrax J, Rabbani ZN et al (2008) Targeting lactate-fueled respiration selectively kills hypoxic tumor cells in mice. J Clin Invest 118(12): 3930–3942

151. Végran F, Boidot R, Michiels C, Sonveaux P, Feron O (2011) Lactate influx through the endothelial cell monocarboxylate transporter MCT1 supports an NF-κB/IL-8 pathway that drives tumor angiogenesis. Cancer Res 71(7):2550–2560

152. Allen E, Miéville P, Warren CM, Saghafinia S, Li L, Peng MW et al (2016) Metabolic Symbiosis enables adaptive resistance to anti-angiogenic therapy that is dependent on mTOR Signaling. Cell Rep 15(6):1144–1160

153. Jiménez-Valerio G, Martínez-Lozano M, Bassani N, Vidal A, Ochoa-de-Olza M, Suárez C et al (2016) Resistance to antiangiogenic therapies by metabolic symbiosis in renal cell carcinoma PDX models and patients. Cell Rep 15(6):1134–1143

154. Pisarsky L, Bill R, Fagiani E, Dimeloe S, Goosen RW, Hagmann J et al (2016) Targeting metabolic Symbiosis to overcome resistance to anti-angiogenic therapy. Cell Rep 15(6): 1161–1174

155. Feron O (2009) Pyruvate into lactate and back: from the Warburg effect to symbiotic energy fuel exchange in cancer cells. Radiother Oncol 92(3):329–333

156. Doherty JR, Cleveland JL (2013) Targeting lactate metabolism for cancer therapeutics. J Clin Invest 123(9):3685–3692

157. Marchiq I, Pouysségur J (2016) Hypoxia, cancer metabolism and the therapeutic benefit of targeting lactate/H(+) symporters. J Mol Med 94(2):155–171
158. Sun RC, Denko NC (2014) Hypoxic regulation of glutamine metabolism through HIF1 and SIAH2 supports lipid synthesis that is necessary for tumor growth. Cell Metab 19(2):285–292
159. Wise DR, Ward PS, Shay JE, Cross JR, Gruber JJ, Sachdeva UM et al (2011) Hypoxia promotes isocitrate dehydrogenase-dependent carboxylation of α-ketoglutarate to citrate to support cell growth and viability. Proc Natl Acad Sci U S A 108(49):19611–19616
160. Metallo CM, Gameiro PA, Bell EL, Mattaini KR, Yang J, Hiller K et al (2011) Reductive glutamine metabolism by IDH1 mediates lipogenesis under hypoxia. Nature 481(7381): 380–384
161. Schug ZT, Peck B, Jones DT, Zhang Q, Grosskurth S, Alam IS et al (2015) Acetyl-CoA synthetase 2 promotes acetate utilization and maintains cancer cell growth under metabolic stress. Cancer Cell 27(1):57–71
162. Lamonte G, Tang X, Chen JL, Wu J, Ding CK, Keenan MM et al (2013) Acidosis induces reprogramming of cellular metabolism to mitigate oxidative stress. Cancer Metab 1(1):23
163. Peppicelli S, Bianchini F, Calorini L (2014) Extracellular acidity, a "reappreciated" trait of tumor environment driving malignancy: perspectives in diagnosis and therapy. Cancer Metastasis Rev 33(2–3):823–832
164. Parks SK, Chiche J, Pouysségur J (2013) Disrupting proton dynamics and energy metabolism for cancer therapy. Nat Rev Cancer 13(9):611–623
165. Mason SD, Joyce JA (2011) Proteolytic networks in cancer. Trends Cell Biol 21(4):228–237
166. Robertson-Tessi M, Gillies RJ, Gatenby RA, Anderson AR (2015) Impact of metabolic heterogeneity on tumor growth, invasion, and treatment outcomes. Cancer Res 75(8): 1567–1579
167. Mohamed MM, Sloane BF (2006) Cysteine cathepsins: multifunctional enzymes in cancer. Nat Rev Cancer 6(10):764–775
168. Estrella V, Chen T, Lloyd M, Wojtkowiak J, Cornnell HH, Ibrahim-Hashim A et al (2013) Acidity generated by the tumor microenvironment drives local invasion. Cancer Res 73(5): 1524–1535
169. Lee S, Jilani SM, Nikolova GV, Carpizo D, Iruela-Arispe ML (2005) Processing of VEGF-A by matrix metalloproteinases regulates bioavailability and vascular patterning in tumors. J Cell Biol 169(4):681–691
170. Fukumura D, Xu L, Chen Y, Gohongi T, Seed B, Jain RK (2001) Hypoxia and acidosis independently up-regulate vascular endothelial growth factor transcription in brain tumors in vivo. Cancer Res 61(16):6020–6024
171. Avnet S, Di Pompo G, Chano T, Errani C, Ibrahim-Hashim A, Gillies RJ et al (2017) Cancer-associated mesenchymal stroma fosters the stemness of osteosarcoma cells in response to intratumoral acidosis via NF-κB activation. Int J Cancer 140(6):1331–1345

Chapter 9
Biophysical Changes in Local *Onco-Sphere*

Phei Er Saw and Erwei Song

Abstract Although biophysical changes in shaping the cancer ecosystem is important, it is often overlooked. Biophysical changes in the local onco-sphere includes mechanotransduction (mechanical force between cells in creating tissue tension), stiffness (changes in extra-cellular matrix components in response to cancer cell-secreted juxtacrine), and re-organization of cytoskeleton (important factor in epithelial-mesenchymal transition in metastasis). In this chapter, we will summarize major biophysical changes in the local onco-sphere to show that these mechanistic changes in the local onco-sphere is important in cancer growth and metastasis.

Introduction

Mechanotransduction is an important factor that regulates tissue homeostasis and tumor progression. The process is facilitated through intercellular adhesions, cell contractility, and forces created within the cells. Mechanotransduction is influenced by several factors such as the composition, organization, and compliance of the extracellular matrix [1]. The mechanical force generated because of interactions

P. E. Saw
Guangdong Provincial Key Laboratory of Malignant Tumor Epigenetics and Gene Regulation, Guangdong-Hong Kong Joint Laboratory for RNA Medicine, Medical Research Center, Sun Yat-sen Memorial Hospital, Sun Yat-sen University, Guangzhou, China

Nanhai Translational Innovation Center of Precision Immunology, Sun Yat-sen Memorial Hospital, Sun Yat-sen University, Foshan, China

E. Song (✉)
Guangdong Provincial Key Laboratory of Malignant Tumor Epigenetics and Gene Regulation, Guangdong-Hong Kong Joint Laboratory for RNA Medicine, Medical Research Center, Sun Yat-sen Memorial Hospital, Sun Yat-sen University, Guangzhou, China

Nanhai Translational Innovation Center of Precision Immunology, Sun Yat-sen Memorial Hospital, Sun Yat-sen University, Foshan, China

Breast Tumor Center, Sun Yat-sen Memorial Hospital, Sun Yat-sen University, Guangzhou, China
e-mail: songew@mail.sysu.edu.cn

E. Song (ed.), *Tumor Ecosystem*, https://doi.org/10.1007/978-981-99-1183-7_9

between different cells can manipulate tissue tension, thereby functioning as a molecular switch that decides the fate of the cells [2]. In order to counter the extracellular tension, cells create an opposing force; this is known as mechano-reciprocity. During embryo development, these tensile forces influence tissue organization [3]. Similarly, the mammary acinar structure depends on matrix compliance and cell tension [4]. These forces also play an important role in tumor progression and spread, which occurs along the tracks made of fibers of ECM; these tracks are formed by protease and tensile forces. For instance, the reticular collagen fibers around the mammary glands form a protective layer against metastasis; however, the rigidity of the matrix due to mechano-reciprocal induction of Rho-dependent cell contractility, resulting from dense collagen fibers aligning themselves perpendicular to the tumor surface, stimulates the growth and spread of breast cancer [5]. Tumor proliferation and metastasis are also dependent on activated CAFs and mesenchymal stem cells; the mechanism involved is paracrine cytokine signaling [6, 7]. Mechanical forces in the modulation of local *onco-sphere* have not been given much focus. However, more studies are being done to show that mechanistic changes such as stiffness to have a direct role in tumorigenesis and metastasis. Therefore, in this chapter, we unravel the importance of integrating mechanical pathology in the intra-onco-spherical interactions in the local *onco-sphere*.

Types of Extracellular Stress

Mechanical forces cause cells to change their intracellular stress (Fig. 9.1). This is accomplished by harmonized cytoskeletal reorganization and actomyosin constriction. Under the process of mechanotransduction, the cells recognize and react to mechanical cues (such as ECM stiffness, compaction, and tension) by converting these mechanical signs into biochemical impulses. These biochemical indications are interpreted by the cells, which alters their shape, behavior, and functioning. There are three main stresses that cells are enduring constantly, namely solid stress, shear stress, and interstitial fluid pressure, which we will summarize below.

Solid Stress

Uncontrolled cancer cell growth causes accelerated enlargement of tumor mass, compaction of the tumor interior, and extension of the adjacent stromal tissue. Solid stress refers to the stresses imposed by the developing tumor mass as well as the resilience to the deformity of adjacent stromal tissue. Many novel techniques for measuring solid stress in tumors have been proposed in recent years, revealing that type of tumor and its size, along with the features of the adjacent tissues, impact the solid stress in tumors [8]. Pressure and stresses transferred from the tumor to the adjacent stromal tissues can enhance ECM tension and restructuring, as well as distort the shape and size of the tissue around the tumor mass [9]. The increased level

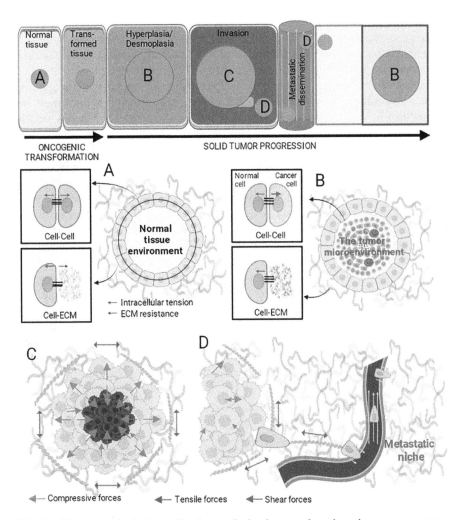

Fig. 9.1 Diverse mechanical stimuli acting on the local *onco-sphere* throughout cancer progression. (**a**) In normal tissues, homeostasis is balanced between cell–cell and cell–ECM communication. (**b**) However, when cancer cells are in abundance, intracellular tension increased, while inducing changes to surrounding ECMs to increasingly stiffened to provide a physical resistance, in addition to an increased activation of stromal cell (i.e., CAFs), and infiltration of immune cells (invaded through cues in the systemic *onco-sphere*, detailed in Part III of this book). (**c**) As the stroma continues to stiffen, interstitial fluid pressure (IFP) is also increased, compressing both tumor and stroma, creating a positive feedback mechanism. (**d**) IFP gradient resulted in a gradual dismissal of cells from the tumor, disseminating cells beyond tumor periphery, promoting the establishment of pre-metastatic niche in the distal *onco-sphere* (detailed in Part II of this book)

of ECM stress in the surrounding tissues may be intensified due to the growth of tumor-linked myofibroblast and penetration of immune cells in the course of desmoplastic and pro-inflammatory stromal reactions. Moreover, modification of the physical attributes of ECM (for example, stiffness induced by accumulation/

restructuring) also tends to augment tumor development and solid stress. Stiffening of collagen strands under strain prevents additional stretching, whereas hyaluronan can retain interstitial fluid and expand because of hydration, preventing compaction and increasing solid stress inside the tumor [9]. The growth of a tumor in terms of size is dependent on its displacement or degradation of adjacent non-malignant tissues. According to mathematical modeling, a solid tumor's rigidity must be greater than 1.5 times in comparison to the adjacent tissues for its continuous growth [10]. On the other hand, topically applied pressures that squeeze or limit the tumor volume may inhibit cancer cell growth, cause apoptotic cell death, boost ECM reorganization, and enhance tumor cells' tendency to invade and metastasize [11]. Cell populations with low growth rates have an increased resistance to therapeutic interventions, whereas compacting the tumor cell may impair the effectiveness of chemotherapeutic drugs [12]. Furthermore, solid stress restricts blood vessels in the core of the tumor, impairing the supply of oxygen and nutrition and momentarily inhibiting cancer development [13]. Solid forces at the tumor's perimeter can adequately compress blood vessels around the tumor, causing the deformation of the vessels in the adjacent healthy tissues to oval structures [14], while compressing the lymphatic vasculature inside the stromal tissues inhibits extravasated fluid outflow [9]. The limited interstitial space and impaired fluid collection owing to blockage in the vessels increase the proclivity of solid stress to generate an enhanced flow of interstitial fluid. In the case of a restricted tumor, like glioblastoma multiforme (GBM), this tension may be exacerbated due to the compression of the brain by the skull. Low blood flow and high interstitial stress, when combined, impede the effective distribution of chemotherapeutics to the tumor and aggravate hypoxia, thus reducing the efficiency of radiotherapy [15]. According to computational modeling, altered collective tension at the tumor stoma junction due to intracellular adhesion can influence tumor morphology, and the reduced tension can enhance migration and metastasis among cell groups [16]. Thus, the solid stress dynamics may influence the pace and direction of migrating tumor cells.

Shear Stress

Tumor cells are exposed to a range of new milieus and pressures throughout the metastatic phase. The exit of tumor cells from the parent tumor and their transition through the circulation expose them to a variety of solid and fluid pressures, most of which induce shear stress. The fluid viscosity and velocity of fluid flow both impact hemodynamic shear stress, which is induced by blood circulation alongside the cellular surface [17]. Solid pressure imposed by endothelial cell interaction can also induce shear stress during intravasation and extravasation of tumor cells from the vasculature. The occurrence of metastasis demands the survival of tumor cells while traveling in the circulation, and presumably, tumor cells have exhibited strong resistance to shear stress in comparison to healthy cells [18]. Interestingly, tumor cell longevity is determined by the length of time tumor cells spend in circulation and the amount of shear stress they endure [19]. Hence, a tumor cell's capacity to endure the multiple dynamic mechanical pressures faced during its exit from the parent tumor and the creation of a new tumor location would necessitate constant biological adaptation. Metastatic locations are not randomly selected. Primary tumors from diverse organ sites prefer colonization into various secondary organs, probably owing to the mix of blood flow rhythm (mechanical theory) and microenvironment preference (seed and soil theory) [17]. Extravasation requires the adherence of circulating tumor cells on the vessel lining. Excessive shear force exacerbates the rate of tumor endothelial cell interaction while impairing these cells' potential to establish permanent cell–cell junctures. For extravasating under high shear stresses, tumor cells must form robust adhesions. As a result, tumor cells frequently extravasate at the transition point or after their confinement in microscopic capillaries. Comparable to the radical cytoskeleton restructuring and deflection undergone by the cells for compressing themselves to traverse through a closely packed ECM matrix, compression of actomyosin-generated cellular stress potentially plays a crucial part in making tumor cells resistant to shear stresses, allowing their viability while circulating and extravasating across ECs [17]. Significantly, hemodynamic pressures influence the phenotypic and functional aspects of endothelial cells that make up the vasculature, influencing cancer growth via this pathway.

Interstitial Fluid Pressure (IFP)

As the tumor progresses, compression due to hypervascularization increases the interstitial hydrodynamic pressure by ten times [20] and causes hypoxia, which facilitates an increased expression of pro-oncogenes, further exacerbating malignancy [9, 21], as well as inhibiting anti-tumoral immune cell functions; this inhibition is achieved through angiogenesis [22–24]. Additionally, IFP can cause the vessels to close up, thereby prohibiting drug supply to the target tissues. A study on mice with pancreatic neuroendocrine tumors showed that interstitial flow induces *N*-methyl-D-aspartate receptor, which induces malignancy [25]. Another in vitro 3D microfluidic assay showed that interstitial flow removes the morphogenetic gradients of VEGF, thereby inducing angiogenesis and vascularization of the growing tumor [26]. Advanced tumors comprise tortuous and disrupted vessels, which decelerate the blood flow [24]. This creates stress, which leads to fiber formation, further aggravating endothelial resistance to hydrodynamic flow. Abnormal blood flow leading to endothelial remodeling induces tumor angiogenesis, probably due to the mechanical induction of the nuclear translocation of the NF-KB leading to PDGF expression [27–30]. Tumor stiffness due to highly fibrous network formation also promotes angiogenesis, possibly due to the overexpression of fibronectin, as well as PKCβII and VEGF 165β anti-angiogenic repression, probably involving the PI3K/AKT mechanosensitive pathway [31]. A study on hepatocarcinoma cell culture showed that these pathways lead to overexpression of angiogenic VEGF [32]. Another in vivo study on rats showed that subcutaneous insertion of polyethylene glycol hydrogel implants increased neovascularization on soft substrates [33], and that treatment using ascorbate and β-aminopropionitrile (BAPN) decreased tumor stiffness, which further impeded tumor vascularization [34]. Overall, mechanical strains generated due to pathological static and dynamic flow promote tumorigenesis.

Mechanotransducive Stiffness Pressure in Advancing Tumor Growth in the Local *Onco-Sphere*

Tumor Cell-Induced Stiffness

Several other characteristic features of tumors use mechanotransduction to facilitate tumor growth. Moreover, corneal cells assume a unique shape and sensitivity to growth factors when cells start becoming stiff [35]. An increase in tumor stiffness is associated with a corresponding increase in substrate stiffness. This promotes epithelial cell–ECM interaction instead of cell–cell interactions, which physically triggers EMT phenotypes [36–39]. Stiffness in tumor cells has the following characteristics: (1) increased motility due to increased association with focal adhesion of kinase (FAK) and PI3K/integrin signaling, (2) increased cell proliferation and cell growth, (3) enhanced feature of EMT to trigger metastatic cascade, and (4) suppressed apoptosis through elevation of TGF-β1–dependent pathway [40–43]. Although the above phenomenon can be generalized, however, not all tumors show stiffness; the following observations were made in different instances: (1) H-RAS-transformed NIH3T3 cells showed poor stiffness, (2) neuroblastoma favors multiplication on softer substrate compared to hard ones; (3) prostate and colon cancer cells undergo EMT in a low-stiffness environment; (4) human tongue squamous carcinoma cells exhibited negligible stiffness per se [44–47].

ECM Substrate Stiffness

Studies have found that cells use cytoskeleton actomyosin-II contractibility to match the ECM stiffness, which creates forces that activate mechanotransduction. For example, in C2C12 mouse myogenic cells, the cytoskeletal organization applies forces that regulate the cadherin-mediated intercellular junctions [48–50]. Notably, cell stiffness activates integrin/FAK signaling pathways, which increase tumor hyperproliferation and motility [51–53]. The stiffness of the matrix then activates the FAK-Src complexes, which then activates downstream Rho/ROCK signaling pathway to activate myosin-mediated contractile force, thereby resulting in metastasis. This is regulated by ERK phosphorylation, which hyperactivates the Ras-MAPK pathway, leading to epithelial cell hyperproliferation [38, 52,

54]. Actomyosin motors exhibit cohesive effects that lead to long-range rigidity among multicellular clusters than individual cells [55]. In squamous cell carcinomas, collective cell migration was guided by fibronectin [56]; moreover, low matrix degradability promoted this migration [57]. Bond dissociation or rearranged scaffold proteins initiate cellular mechano-sensing. For example, Cyclin D1 expression disrupts ECM-integrin bond, which is important in cell proliferation and survival [58, 59]. Similarly, conformation opens the phosphorylation sites of p130Cas for Src, as well as for Talin, which initiates migration, transformation, and invasion [60–63]. A study on a kidney cell culture revealed that a 12pN physiological force stretches the Talin rod domain to reveal its Vinculin binding site that in turn promotes Vinculin binding [62]. Vinculin binds and releases Talin in a continuous circular loop, resulting in the conversion of a mechanical signal into a biochemical one [63]. Further, the link between matrix rigidity and force causes transmission and transduction into the cytoplasm via the actin-Talin-integrin-fibronectin clutch; this helps cells to sense changes in the surroundings [64]. A study on mouse embryonic fibroblasts presented a model describing the unfolding of Talin; the force triggering mechanotransduction is initiated by a stiffness threshold of 5 kPa; if this threshold is crossed, then Talin unfolds and binds to Vinculin, which initiates adhesions and the mitotic YAP factor getting translocated to the nucleus. When the contractibility of actomyosin raises the rigidity levels of tumor cells, these cells get extruded from the epithelial layers. This increases the metastasis of human epithelial colorectal adeno-carcinoma [65], in which N-WASP—it regulated junctional tension by stabilizing F-actin and Myo-II at cell lateral contacts—triggered apical cell extrusion. The increased stiffness of the matrix in the breast cancels cells activates mitotic YAP/TAZ signaling, as well as integrins; this phosphorylates Twist, which initiates metastasis at Tyr107 [66–69]. The Twist protein is anchored to the G3BP2 protein. After phosphorylation, Twist is released and translocated into the nucleus; this initiates the transcriptional events of EMT, invasion, and metastasis.

The Role of CAFs in ECM Stiffening

Tumorigenic hypoxia activates CAFs, which leads to collagen reticulation, thereby favoring metastasis [70, 71]. Fibroblasts secrete TGFβ, which increases ECM stiffening. This promotes the mechano-transductive action of CAF actomyosin contractility of translocating YAP into the nucleus. YAP is one of the factors that regulate CAF activities in regard to ECM remodeling and stiffening, thereby generating a positive tumorigenic feedback loop [72, 73]. CAFs also pull and stretch the basement membranes, leading to gaps in the membrane; this increases tumor invasiveness [74]. Another major action of CAFs is its ability to render radiotherapeutic treatment ineffective due to cell-adhesion-mediated resistance; this is carried out by depositing ECM through β1-integrin binding, also seen in BRAF-mutated melanoma [75, 76]. ICAM-1 is a membrane-bound glycoprotein that belongs to the immunoglobulin superfamily, and it functions as a factor responsible for the contraction of

ECM during inflammation; its expression is controlled by actomyosin contractility. CAFs are also associated with the positive feedback signaling between ICAM-1 and actomyosin contractility. This shows the indirect way in which ICAM-1 enhances the remodeling of the stromal pro-invasive matrix through the action of CAFs, upstream of the Scr/RhoA/ROCK/MLC2-signaling pathway [77]. When the membrane tension increases due to actomyosin constriction induced by stress, caveolae depolymerization occurs at the plasma membrane of the epithelial and stromal cells. This induces changes in tumor progression through mechanotransduction [78].

The Molecular Mechanisms of Mechanotransduction

The process of mechanotransduction involves translating mechanical cues into various cells, resulting in specific changes in intracellular dynamics [79]. As mechanical strength is focused on junctional or cytoskeleton structure, mechanistic changes usually result in a drastic change in a protein 3D structure or inhibiting protein endocytosis [2, 61, 80–83]. The energy exchange during protein conformation or endocytic vesicle formation is about 10 kT [84, 85]. Therefore, even slight physiological or mechanical strain created by biochemical energy can deform them. Deformation of protein structure could expose multiple phosphorylation sites to kinases. In addition, mechanical strain can increase protein binding affinities; for instance, it can enhance the interaction between IL-7 and fibronectin, which can result in IL-7 getting trapped in the ECM [86]. Another effect of the application of mechanical strain is the flattening of membranes, which can inhibit protein endocytosis and degradation, thereby resulting in downstream signaling pathways getting activated. An example of this is the trans-differentiation of myoblast–osteoblast, which is dependent on the mechanical inhibition of BMP2 endocytosis [81]. Membrane flattening also happens as cell's immediate response to mechanical shocks [83]. Tensile forces in the membranes can also open ionic pores as part of neuronal sensation [87, 88]. Mechanistic stiffness can also occur due to an increase in the amine oxidase cross-linking enzyme LOX and actomyosin contractibility induced by Rock [5, 89]. The same findings were reported by a study on cell culture, in which increased matrix stiffness was found to induce EMT [36]. Endogenous LOX activity and actomyosin contractibility can be inhibited through BAPN treatment and ROCK inhibitor LIMKi and the Myo-II inhibitor Y27632, respectively. This is a potentially effective treatment modality that acts by restricting the cell response to stiffness, thereby arresting or slowing down tumor progression [34]. BAPN preventive therapeutic value has been observed in rat models, in which it arrested the growth and spread of prostate tumors [90]. Similarly, LIMKi has been observed to arrest pancreatic tumor growth in rats [91]. Further, studies on hemangiomas in rats have revealed the therapeutic value of Y-27632 in that it was capable of inducing and downregulating p53 and regulated VEGF expression, respectively; this arrested cell proliferation and promoted apoptosis in hemangioma cells [92]. In the section below, we summarize the major pathways of tumor, stromal cells, and their ECM in inducing mechanical stress in the local *onco-sphere*.

Tumor hyperproliferation creates a force on healthy surrounding epithelial tissues. To counter this force, the surrounding tissues also generate pressure. The division of adherent cells at the confluence stops as part of feedback [93, 94]. Mechanical cues induced by pressure also transform healthy cells into pathological cells by activating the β-cat pathway. A study on mouse models revealed that mechanical cues induce the phosphorylation of Y654–β-cat and β-cat nuclear translocation [95]. Another function of β-cat is osteogenesis induction and adipogenesis inhibition [96]. In an in vivo experiment, pressure was applied to mesenchymal cells of the colon by stabilizing ultramagnetic liposomes. It resulted in Y654 phosphorylation and subsequent activation of the β-cat pathway. Consequently, the Myc, Axin, and Zeb-1 tumorigenic target genes were expressed, which play an active role in both hyperproliferation and invasiveness. Anomalous crypts were created as a result of subsequent hyperproliferation. An in vivo study on mouse epidermis showed that an activated tumorigenic β-cat pathway can result in increased stiffness; this happens when ROCK is transgenically overactivated, which stimulates actomyosin [89]. To further explain this, GSK3β was inhibited by ROCK along with integrin through Ser9; this resulted in an increase in cytoplasmic and nuclear β-cat content. As a result of strain generated due to hyperproliferation p-GSK3 Ser9 further promoted Y654–β-cat phosphorylation via a Ret kinase-dependent process [97]. This shows that the force generated due to hyperproliferation aggravates the stiffness-induced tumorigenic effects commonly seen during the advanced stages of tumor progression.

Crosstalk in the Local *Onco-Sphere*: miRNA and Chromatin Deformation

As explained before, through mechanotransduction, mechanical activation of junctional, cytoskeleton, or membrane protein triggers biochemical pathways that induce tumor formation. Several recent studies have reported that microRNA expression also shows a significant effect on regulating tumor growth and malignancy; specifically, this is achieved through the ability to modulate ECM stiffness. Gene expression is regulated by several factors, including miRNAs, which also modulate oncogenes and tumor suppressors [98]. Studies on breast tissues have shown that increased stiffness of the matrix induces miR-18a and promotes PI3K-dependent tumor progression and malignancy; β-cat is activated with the help of integrins, whereas tumor suppressor phosphatase and Tensin homolog are targeted to activate Myc [99]. Another effect of increased ECM density and stiffness of mammary gland tissues is the miR-203 expression getting downregulated. This results in the upregulation of Robo1, a tumor suppressor. When the binding sites in its 3′ UTR are targeted, in order to maintain cell shape and create an anti-metastasis barrier, Rac and FAK get activated [100]. Even in the absence of tumors, shear stress can induce miR-33-5p expression. Osteoblast differentiation is positively promoted by miR-33-5p expression through the inhibition of its target HMGA2. Similarly, suppressed miR-33-5p expression can result in a decrease in osteoblast differentiation; this is commonly observed after clinorotation similar to microgravity [101]. The cytoskeleton is capable of transferring forces to the chromatin from the ECM; this can initiate mechanotransduction being transmitted into the nucleus directly [102]. Factors such as these can cause deformations of the nucleus [103] and activate signaling pathways [104].

Crosstalk in the Local *Onco-Sphere*: Nucleus and the Cytoskeleton

Only recently were the proteins forming links between the cytoskeleton and the nucleus identified. At the cytoplasmic sites of focal adhesions, Nesprin family (Nesprin-1, -2,-3,-4) could transfer these forces from the cytoplasm to the nucleus, through actin filament in "nuclear membrane–cytoskeleton" interactions. The Lamin proteins, as well as chromatin anchored to SUN proteins, regulate the physical characteristics of the nucleus, such as its integrity. Nesprin's Klarsicht-ANC-Syne-homology (KASH) domain is anchored at the outer nuclear membrane; where proteins such as SUN could interact with KASH domain, resulting in subsequent binding to the nuclear lamina and other nucleoplasmic proteins [105]. These linker-nesprins and SUN proteins are known as linkers of nucleoskeleton and cytoskeleton (LINC) complexes; LINC acts as a channel for force transmission through the nuclear envelope to Lamins. The Lamin intermediate filaments are organized into a polymer network in an orderly fashion in the form of several coils stacked parallel to each other. Three different genes are responsible for the expression of the Lamin protein: the LMNA gene is spliced to give Lamin-A and -C, which together are known as "A-type" Lamins; on the other hand, the LMNB1 and LMNB2 genes encode Lamin-B1 and -B2, respectively, which are together known as "B-type" Lamins. Both types of Lamins have functions opposite to each other, that is, while the A-type Lamins are responsible for viscosity, B-type Lamins are responsible for elasticity. When the A-type Lamin content in tissues is dominant, it gives rise to laminopathies, including muscular dystrophies and cardiopathies. The actions of the two types of Lamins can be observed through micropipette aspiration experiments that measure the nuclei deformation rate under pressure [102]. Interactions among proteins within the nucleus facilitate the interactions between Lamins. Notably, the A-type Lamins bind directly to the DNA. In addition, Lamins also bind to nuclear actin polymers and Emerin, a nuclear membrane protein [106, 107].

Nucleoskeleton structures undergo remodeling when subjected to mechanical stress. Within a cell, the nucleus is subjected to mechanical stress from the ECM through integrins at focal adhesion sites, actin filaments and myosin, the LINC complex, including Nesprins attachment to SUN proteins, and Lamin-A and -C. Mechanical stress can cause dephosphorylation of Lamin, thereby decreasing the solubility of A-type Lamin and lamina strengthening. A- and B-type Lamins regulate the physical characteristics of the nucleus, such as shape, elasticity, and the nuclear envelope stiffness. A study on human-derived U251 glioblastoma showed an increase in nuclear stiffness as a result of increased Lamin-A levels due to inhibition of an enzyme responsible for inducing its phosphorylation, solubilization, and degradation [108]. Variation in Lamin organization results in altered kinase interactions, which results in suppressed phosphorylation when the cells experience stress. Further, activation of mechano-sensors increases nuclear stiffness, along with the expression of B-type Lamin [108]. Therefore, the anomalous shape of nuclei in cancer cells can be attributed to misexpression or local aberration in Lamins [109].

When Actin and Nesprin2 in NIH3T3 cells were subjected to fluorescence resonance energy transfer analysis, dynamic interactions were observed that were responsible for keeping the nucleus in a pre-stressed state. When cells get transfected with dominant negative KASH without the Actin–Nesprin2 binding domain, the LINC complex gets disturbed; following this, the apical side of the nucleus sees the appearance of actin stress fibers. This results in nuclear elongation; this could be associated with suppressed cross-linking nuclear structures causing chromatin de-condensation, which leads to the exhibition of downstream transcriptional effects [110]. Substrate stiffness induced by fibrosis regulates nuclear mechano-transductive cues; however, it is unclear if these cues play a role in tumor progression. Further, advanced tumors show increased cell motility and invasiveness. During this stage, the heterogeneous dense tissues are invaded by tumor cells, which deforms the cytoskeleton, as well as the nucleus [111, 112]. To this end, the nucleus tries to prevent cell movements by functioning as an anchor, with A-type Lamin acting as a line of defense against deformation by preventing entry at the defective pores. Studies show that lamina composition is an important factor determining nucleus deformation; an overexpression of Lamin-A limits migration, whereas Lamin-A knock-down facilitates migration [111]. However, it has been observed that high levels of A-type Lamin in nuclei slow down post-deformation recovery, because of which the nuclei retain elongation for a while after emerging from the pores; on the other hand, high levels of elastic B-type Lamin help nuclei reassume their original spheroid shape quickly [113–115].

Several studies on cancer and other diseases have identified discrepancies in the levels of Lamin-A levels; specifically, the levels decreased in malignant carcinomas [109, 116]. Further, migration of cells of osteosarcoma and lung adenocarcinoma across interstitial spaces through ECM constrictions deforms the nucleus and leads to chromatin and lamina contacts formation, which increases gene expression heterogeneity. In addition, it can damage the nuclear envelope integrity and factors responsible for repairing the DNA, which can lead to genetically transmissible mutations [117, 118]. Thus, ironically, it can be said that DNA repair factors can transform into mechanosensitive factors capable of changing DNA sequences [119]. Notably, mutations resulting from cancer seem to be more common in tissues that naturally show more stiffness, such as bone or muscles, than in soft tissue cancers [120]. Altered protein and chromosome conformation, translated transcription factors, and dilated or ruptured nuclear membrane initiate nuclear mechanosensing. Mechanosensory proteins are vital for the growth of the embryo and aging, as well as when a disease attacks the body; this has been proved using omics-based meta-transcriptome and proteome data analysis [121]. Therefore, it can be presumed that diverse mechano-sensors appear in the body owing to the links formed between junks, plasma membrane, and the cytoskeleton and the nuclear membrane and chromatin. It can also be anticipated that the appearance of new mechano-sensors, as well as novel implications for mRNA, would further complicate the regulation of mechanotransduction.

Box 9.1 Reactivation of Mechanotransduction in Cancer: A Response to Pathological Mechanical Strains?

One of the factors controlling angiogenesis is the mechanical strains caused due to hydrodynamic blood flow; the VEGFR2-dependent mechanosensitive pathway is involved in this process. Decreased VE-Cadherin tension is thought to be an important factor responsible for this. When the tissues experience stress, the aorta junctions are downregulated [82, 122]. In addition, p190RhoGAP-dependent mechanical activation of GATA nuclear translocation leads to angiogenic VEG FR2 expression [123]. Stiffness acts as a determinant of embryonic biomechanical morphogenesis [124, 125]. A study on early *Caenorhabditis elegans* embryos showed that, when Myo-II contractibility generates forces, lateral stiffness anisotropies within the fiber-reinforced dorsoventral epidermis cause an anteroposterior elongation [126]. Further, in response to activation of Myo-II, embryonic tissues reacted to shape change and increased stiffness [127–129]. Studies on embryos have observed that gastrulation's morphogenetic movements can deform the endoderm and mesoderm tissues, which can activate their β-cat pathway and lead to downstream differentiation [130–132]. When Y654 gets phosphorylated, a pool of β-cat is released from the junctions formed between its major site of interaction with E-cadherins, into the cytoplasm and nuclei; this activates the β-cat pathway and leads to the transcription of mesoendoderm genes [132]. Thus, it can be hypothesized that the β-cat pathway gets reactivated due to mechanical strains generated by the tumor, which then reactivates the development of endomesoderm within adult colonic tissue. As a result, the homeostatic stability gets disturbed, which further promotes tumor progression through mechanotransduction. Notably, for mechanical induction of tumors, just one copy of APC needs to get mutated [97]. Before nuclear translocation, the APC/GSK3β complex degrades cytoplasmic β-cat. However, in the APC$^{+/-}$ genetic environment, the APC/GSK3β complex loses its efficiency by 50%.

(continued)

Box 9.1 (continued)

Thus, in comparison with WT, in the APC$^{+/-}$ environment, the chances of nuclear translocation of β-cat increase. This explains the role of genetic and microenvironmental biomechanical anomalies in producing a synergistic effect on tumors. This can be exemplified by the most recent evidence of the synergistic effect of smoking fumes and nutrition [133]. Although external environmental factors responsible for causing cancers can be controlled, internal microenvironmental factors cannot be regulated. As mentioned before, the use of Y-27632- and BAPN-mediated treatment modalities is effective in inhibiting tumor progression [5, 34, 89], they can exhibit deleterious effects on the body. Thus, a combination approach using efficient drug-targeting methodologies can prove to be successful in the near future [79]. The changes in external stress toward the cellular's biochemical changes could be seen in Fig. 9.2.

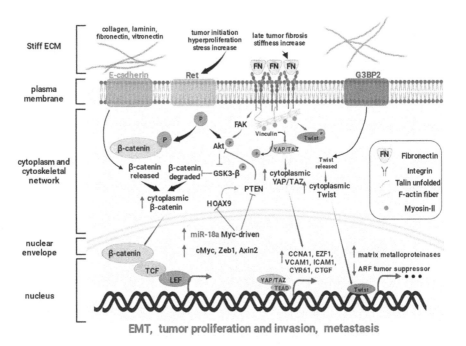

Fig. 9.2 Mechano-induced stress could lead to biochemical changes in the cell that in turn activates gene related to cancer growth, invasion, EMT, and metastasis, in various pathways

Conclusion

Within the local *onco-sphere* (TME), tumor cells are exposed to various mechanical stimuli; stress within the cell compartments, cell–cell interaction, cell–ECM tension, which ultimately leads to compression stress. The cross talk between tumor cells and these stimuli leads to positive feedback loop, leading to the eliciting of specific responses (increased cellular actomyosin contractility and ECM stiffening), which promotes tumor progression, aggression, and metastatic potential. Interestingly, although biophysical changes can be detected in almost all malignancies (especially cancer), interventions targeting these factors are not widely appreciated. Thus, in-depth understanding of the physical interactions between components in the local *onco-sphere* and the molecular mechanisms regulating cellular responses to mechanical inputs within the local *onco-sphere* might be key in the design of effective therapeutics to treat all cancers.

References

1. Goetz JG, Minguet S, Navarro-Lerida I, Lazcano JJ, Samaniego R, Calvo E et al (2011) Biomechanical remodeling of the microenvironment by stromal caveolin-1 favors tumor invasion and metastasis. Cell 146(1):148–163
2. Engler AJ, Sen S, Sweeney HL, Discher DE (2006) Matrix elasticity directs stem cell lineage specification. Cell 126(4):677–689
3. Krieg M, Arboleda-Estudillo Y, Puech PH, Kafer J, Graner F, Muller DJ et al (2008) Tensile forces govern germ-layer organization in zebrafish. Nat Cell Biol 10(4):429–436
4. Ronnov-Jessen L, Bissell MJ (2009) Breast cancer by proxy: can the microenvironment be both the cause and consequence? Trends Mol Med 15(1):5–13
5. Levental KR, Yu H, Kass L, Lakins JN, Egeblad M, Erler JT et al (2009) Matrix crosslinking forces tumor progression by enhancing integrin signaling. Cell 139(5):891–906
6. Karnoub AE, Dash AB, Vo AP, Sullivan A, Brooks MW, Bell GW et al (2007) Mesenchymal stem cells within tumour stroma promote breast cancer metastasis. Nature 449(7162):557–563
7. Orimo A, Gupta PB, Sgroi DC, Arenzana-Seisdedos F, Delaunay T, Naeem R et al (2005) Stromal fibroblasts present in invasive human breast carcinomas promote tumor growth and angiogenesis through elevated SDF-1/CXCL12 secretion. Cell 121(3):335–348
8. Nia HT, Liu H, Seano G, Datta M, Jones D, Rahbari N et al (2016) Solid stress and elastic energy as measures of tumour mechanopathology. Nat Biomed Eng 1:0004
9. Jain RK, Martin JD, Stylianopoulos T (2014) The role of mechanical forces in tumor growth and therapy. Annu Rev Biomed Eng 16:321–346
10. Voutouri C, Mpekris F, Papageorgis P, Odysseos AD, Stylianopoulos T (2014) Role of constitutive behavior and tumor-host mechanical interactions in the state of stress and growth of solid tumors. PLoS One 9(8):e104717
11. Yu H, Mouw JK, Weaver VM (2011) Forcing form and function: biomechanical regulation of tumor evolution. Trends Cell Biol 21(1):47–56
12. Mascheroni P, Stigliano C, Carfagna M, Boso DP, Preziosi L, Decuzzi P et al (2016) Predicting the growth of glioblastoma multiforme spheroids using a multiphase porous media model. Biomech Model Mechanobiol 15(5):1215–1228
13. Padera TP, Stoll BR, Tooredman JB, Capen D, di Tomaso E, Jain RK (2004) Pathology: cancer cells compress intratumour vessels. Nature 427(6976):695

14. Stylianopoulos T, Martin JD, Snuderl M, Mpekris F, Jain SR, Jain RK (2013) Coevolution of solid stress and interstitial fluid pressure in tumors during progression: implications for vascular collapse. Cancer Res 73(13):3833–3841
15. Mpekris F, Angeli S, Pirentis AP, Stylianopoulos T (2015) Stress-mediated progression of solid tumors: effect of mechanical stress on tissue oxygenation, cancer cell proliferation, and drug delivery. Biomech Model Mechanobiol 14(6):1391–1402
16. Katira P, Bonnecaze RT, Zaman MH (2013) Modeling the mechanics of cancer: effect of changes in cellular and extra-cellular mechanical properties. Front Oncol 3:145
17. Wirtz D, Konstantopoulos K, Searson PC (2011) The physics of cancer: the role of physical interactions and mechanical forces in metastasis. Nat Rev Cancer 11(7):512–522
18. Mitchell MJ, Denais C, Chan MF, Wang Z, Lammerding J, King MR (2015) Lamin A/C deficiency reduces circulating tumor cell resistance to fluid shear stress. Am J Physiol Cell Physiol 309(11):C736–C746
19. Fan R, Emery T, Zhang Y, Xia Y, Sun J, Wan J (2016) Circulatory shear flow alters the viability and proliferation of circulating colon cancer cells. Sci Rep 6:27073
20. Boucher Y, Jain RK (1992) Microvascular pressure is the principal driving force for interstitial hypertension in solid tumors: implications for vascular collapse. Cancer Res 52(18): 5110–5114
21. Pennacchietti S, Michieli P, Galluzzo M, Mazzone M, Giordano S, Comoglio PM (2003) Hypoxia promotes invasive growth by transcriptional activation of the met protooncogene. Cancer Cell 3(4):347–361
22. Griffioen AW, Damen CA, Blijham GH, Groenewegen G (1996) Tumor angiogenesis is accompanied by a decreased inflammatory response of tumor-associated endothelium. Blood 88(2):667–673
23. Dirkx AE, oude Egbrink MG, Castermans K, van der Schaft DW, Thijssen VL, Dings RP et al (2006) Anti-angiogenesis therapy can overcome endothelial cell anergy and promote leukocyte-endothelium interactions and infiltration in tumors. FASEB J 20(6):621–630
24. Goel S, Duda DG, Xu L, Munn LL, Boucher Y, Fukumura D et al (2011) Normalization of the vasculature for treatment of cancer and other diseases. Physiol Rev 91(3):1071–1121
25. Li L, Hanahan D (2013) Hijacking the neuronal NMDAR signaling circuit to promote tumor growth and invasion. Cell 153(1):86–100
26. Shirure VS, Lezia A, Tao A, Alonzo LF, George SC (2017) Low levels of physiological interstitial flow eliminate morphogen gradients and guide angiogenesis. Angiogenesis 20(4): 493–504
27. Franke RP, Gräfe M, Schnittler H, Seiffge D, Mittermayer C, Drenckhahn D (1984) Induction of human vascular endothelial stress fibres by fluid shear stress. Nature 307(5952):648–649
28. Ingber DE, Folkman J (1989) Mechanochemical switching between growth and differentiation during fibroblast growth factor-stimulated angiogenesis *in vitro*: role of extracellular matrix. J Cell Biol 109(1):317–330
29. Khachigian LM, Resnick N, Gimbrone MA Jr, Collins T (1995) Nuclear factor-kappa B interacts functionally with the platelet-derived growth factor B-chain shear-stress response element in vascular endothelial cells exposed to fluid shear stress. J Clin Invest 96(2): 1169–1175
30. Hay DC, Beers C, Cameron V, Thomson L, Flitney FW, Hay RT (2003) Activation of NF-kappaB nuclear transcription factor by flow in human endothelial cells. Biochim Biophys Acta 1642(1–2):33–44
31. Bordeleau F, Califano JP, Negrón Abril YL, Mason BN, LaValley DJ, Shin SJ et al (2015) Tissue stiffness regulates serine/arginine-rich protein-mediated splicing of the extra domain B-fibronectin isoform in tumors. Proc Natl Acad Sci U S A 112(27):8314–8319
32. Dong Y, Xie X, Wang Z, Hu C, Zheng Q, Wang Y et al (2014) Increasing matrix stiffness upregulates vascular endothelial growth factor expression in hepatocellular carcinoma cells mediated by integrin β1. Biochem Biophys Res Commun 444(3):427–432

33. Schweller RM, Wu ZJ, Klitzman B, West JL (2017) Stiffness of protease sensitive and cell adhesive PEG hydrogels promotes neovascularization *in vivo*. Ann Biomed Eng 45(6): 1387–1398
34. Bordeleau F, Mason BN, Lollis EM, Mazzola M, Zanotelli MR, Somasegar S et al (2017) Matrix stiffening promotes a tumor vasculature phenotype. Proc Natl Acad Sci U S A 114(3): 492–497
35. Gospodarowicz D, Greenburg G, Birdwell CR (1978) Determination of cellular shape by the extracellular matrix and its correlation with the control of cellular growth. Cancer Res 38(11 Pt 2):4155–4171
36. Weaver VM, Fischer AH, Peterson OW, Bissell MJ (1996) The importance of the microenvironment in breast cancer progression: recapitulation of mammary tumorigenesis using a unique human mammary epithelial cell model and a three-dimensional culture assay. Biochem Cell Biol 74(6):833–851
37. Weaver VM, Petersen OW, Wang F, Larabell CA, Briand P, Damsky C et al (1997) Reversion of the malignant phenotype of human breast cells in three-dimensional culture and *in vivo* by integrin blocking antibodies. J Cell Biol 137(1):231–245
38. Paszek MJ, Zahir N, Johnson KR, Lakins JN, Rozenberg GI, Gefen A et al (2005) Tensional homeostasis and the malignant phenotype. Cancer Cell 8(3):241–254
39. Ghajar CM, Bissell MJ (2008) Extracellular matrix control of mammary gland morphogenesis and tumorigenesis: insights from imaging. Histochem Cell Biol 130(6):1105–1118
40. Hadjipanayi E, Mudera V, Brown RA (2009) Close dependence of fibroblast proliferation on collagen scaffold matrix stiffness. J Tissue Eng Regen Med 3(2):77–84
41. Krndija D, Schmid H, Eismann JL, Lother U, Adler G, Oswald F et al (2010) Substrate stiffness and the receptor-type tyrosine-protein phosphatase alpha regulate spreading of colon cancer cells through cytoskeletal contractility. Oncogene 29(18):2724–2738
42. Leight JL, Wozniak MA, Chen S, Lynch ML, Chen CS (2012) Matrix rigidity regulates a switch between TGF-β1-induced apoptosis and epithelial-mesenchymal transition. Mol Biol Cell 23(5):781–791
43. Yuan Y, Zhong W, Ma G, Zhang B, Tian H (2015) Yes-associated protein regulates the growth of human non-small cell lung cancer in response to matrix stiffness. Mol Med Rep 11(6):4267–4272
44. Wang HB, Dembo M, Wang YL (2000) Substrate flexibility regulates growth and apoptosis of normal but not transformed cells. Am J Physiol Cell Physiol 279(5):C1345–C1350
45. Wong SY, Ulrich TA, Deleyrolle LP, MacKay JL, Lin JM, Martuscello RT et al (2015) Constitutive activation of myosin-dependent contractility sensitizes glioma tumor-initiating cells to mechanical inputs and reduces tissue invasion. Cancer Res 75(6):1113–1122
46. Tang X, Kuhlenschmidt TB, Li Q, Ali S, Lezmi S, Chen H et al (2014) A mechanically-induced colon cancer cell population shows increased metastatic potential. Mol Cancer 13:131
47. Runge J, Reichert TE, Fritsch A, Käs J, Bertolini J, Remmerbach TW (2014) Evaluation of single-cell biomechanics as potential marker for oral squamous cell carcinomas: a pilot study. Oral Dis 20(3):e120–e127
48. Discher DE, Janmey P, Wang YL (2005) Tissue cells feel and respond to the stiffness of their substrate. Science 310(5751):1139–1143
49. Geiger B, Spatz JP, Bershadsky AD (2009) Environmental sensing through focal adhesions. Nat Rev Mol Cell Biol 10(1):21–33
50. Ladoux B, Anon E, Lambert M, Rabodzey A, Hersen P, Buguin A et al (2010) Strength dependence of cadherin-mediated adhesions. Biophys J 98(4):534–542
51. Paszek MJ, Weaver VM (2004) The tension mounts: mechanics meets morphogenesis and malignancy. J Mammary Gland Biol Neoplasia 9(4):325–342
52. Provenzano PP, Inman DR, Eliceiri KW, Keely PJ (2009) Matrix density-induced mechanoregulation of breast cell phenotype, signaling and gene expression through a FAK-ERK linkage. Oncogene 28(49):4326–4343

53. Kopanska KS, Alcheikh Y, Staneva R, Vignjevic D, Betz T (2016) Tensile forces originating from cancer spheroids facilitate tumor invasion. PLoS One 11(6):e0156442
54. Wozniak MA, Desai R, Solski PA, Der CJ, Keely PJ (2003) ROCK-generated contractility regulates breast epithelial cell differentiation in response to the physical properties of a three-dimensional collagen matrix. J Cell Biol 163(3):583–595
55. Sunyer R, Conte V, Escribano J, Elosegui-Artola A, Labernadie A, Valon L et al (2016) Collective cell durotaxis emerges from long-range intercellular force transmission. Science (New York, NY) 353(6304):1157–1161
56. Gopal S, Veracini L, Grall D, Butori C, Schaub S, Audebert S et al (2017) Fibronectin-guided migration of carcinoma collectives. Nat Commun 8:14105
57. Trappmann B, Baker BM, Polacheck WJ, Choi CK, Burdick JA, Chen CS (2017) Matrix degradability controls multicellularity of 3D cell migration. Nat Commun 8(1):371
58. Fournier AK, Campbell LE, Castagnino P, Liu WF, Chung BM, Weaver VM et al (2008) Rac-dependent cyclin D1 gene expression regulated by cadherin- and integrin-mediated adhesion. J Cell Sci 121(Pt 2):226–233
59. Friedland JC, Lee MH, Boettiger D (2009) Mechanically activated integrin switch controls alpha5beta1 function. Science 323(5914):642–644
60. Defilippi P, Di Stefano P, Cabodi S (2006) p130Cas: a versatile scaffold in signaling networks. Trends Cell Biol 16(5):257–263
61. Sawada Y, Tamada M, Dubin-Thaler BJ, Cherniavskaya O, Sakai R, Tanaka S et al (2006) Force sensing by mechanical extension of the Src family kinase substrate p130Cas. Cell 127(5):1015–1026
62. del Rio A, Perez-Jimenez R, Liu R, Roca-Cusachs P, Fernandez JM, Sheetz MP (2009) Stretching single talin rod molecules activates vinculin binding. Science (New York, NY) 323(5914):638–641
63. Margadant F, Chew LL, Hu X, Yu H, Bate N, Zhang X et al (2011) Mechanotransduction *in vivo* by repeated talin stretch-relaxation events depends upon vinculin. PLoS Biol 9(12):e1001223
64. Elosegui-Artola A, Oria R, Chen Y, Kosmalska A, Pérez-González C, Castro N et al (2016) Mechanical regulation of a molecular clutch defines force transmission and transduction in response to matrix rigidity. Nat Cell Biol 18(5):540–548
65. Wu SK, Lagendijk AK, Hogan BM, Gomez GA, Yap AS (2015) Active contractility at E-cadherin junctions and its implications for cell extrusion in cancer. Cell Cycle 14(3):315–322
66. Zhao B, Wei X, Li W, Udan RS, Yang Q, Kim J et al (2007) Inactivation of YAP oncoprotein by the Hippo pathway is involved in cell contact inhibition and tissue growth control. Genes Dev 21(21):2747–2761
67. Zhao B, Li L, Wang L, Wang CY, Yu J, Guan KL (2012) Cell detachment activates the Hippo pathway via cytoskeleton reorganization to induce anoikis. Genes Dev 26(1):54–68
68. Dupont S, Morsut L, Aragona M, Enzo E, Giulitti S, Cordenonsi M et al (2011) Role of YAP/TAZ in mechanotransduction. Nature 474(7350):179–183
69. Wei SC, Fattet L, Tsai JH, Guo Y, Pai VH, Majeski HE et al (2015) Matrix stiffness drives epithelial-mesenchymal transition and tumour metastasis through a TWIST1-G3BP2 mechanotransduction pathway. Nat Cell Biol 17(5):678–688
70. Toullec A, Gerald D, Despouy G, Bourachot B, Cardon M, Lefort S et al (2010) Oxidative stress promotes myofibroblast differentiation and tumour spreading. EMBO Mol Med 2(6):211–230
71. Pankova D, Chen Y, Terajima M, Schliekelman MJ, Baird BN, Fahrenholtz M et al (2016) Cancer-associated fibroblasts induce a collagen cross-link switch in tumor stroma. Mol Cancer Res 14(3):287–295
72. Calvo F, Ege N, Grande-Garcia A, Hooper S, Jenkins RP, Chaudhry SI et al (2013) Mechanotransduction and YAP-dependent matrix remodelling is required for the generation and maintenance of cancer-associated fibroblasts. Nat Cell Biol 15(6):637–646

73. Liu F, Lagares D, Choi KM, Stopfer L, Marinković A, Vrbanac V et al (2015) Mechanosignaling through YAP and TAZ drives fibroblast activation and fibrosis. Am J Physiol Lung Cell Mol Physiol 308(4):L344–L357
74. Glentis A, Oertle P, Mariani P, Chikina A, El Marjou F, Attieh Y et al (2017) Cancer-associated fibroblasts induce metalloprotease-independent cancer cell invasion of the basement membrane. Nat Commun 8(1):924
75. Park CC, Zhang H, Pallavicini M, Gray JW, Baehner F, Park CJ et al (2006) Beta1 integrin inhibitory antibody induces apoptosis of breast cancer cells, inhibits growth, and distinguishes malignant from normal phenotype in three dimensional cultures and *in vivo*. Cancer Res 66(3):1526–1535
76. Picco N, Sahai E, Maini PK, Anderson ARA (2017) Integrating models to quantify environment-mediated drug resistance. Cancer Res 77(19):5409–5418
77. Bonan S, Albrengues J, Grasset E, Kuzet SE, Nottet N, Bourget I et al (2017) Membrane-bound ICAM-1 contributes to the onset of proinvasive tumor stroma by controlling acto-myosin contractility in carcinoma-associated fibroblasts. Oncotarget 8(1):1304–1320
78. Lamaze C, Torrino S (2015) Caveolae and cancer: a new mechanical perspective. Biom J 38(5):367–379
79. Broders-Bondon F, Nguyen Ho-Bouldoires TH, Fernandez-Sanchez ME, Farge E (2018) Mechanotransduction in tumor progression: the dark side of the force. J Cell Biol 217(5):1571–1587
80. Chen CS, Mrksich M, Huang S, Whitesides GM, Ingber DE (1997) Geometric control of cell life and death. Science 276(5317):1425–1428
81. Rauch C, Brunet AC, Deleule J, Farge E (2002) C2C12 myoblast/osteoblast transdifferentiation steps enhanced by epigenetic inhibition of BMP2 endocytosis. Am J Physiol Cell Physiol 283(1):C235–C243
82. Grashoff C, Hoffman BD, Brenner MD, Zhou R, Parsons M, Yang MT et al (2010) Measuring mechanical tension across vinculin reveals regulation of focal adhesion dynamics. Nature 466(7303):263–266
83. Sinha B, Koster D, Ruez R, Gonnord P, Bastiani M, Abankwa D et al (2011) Cells respond to mechanical stress by rapid disassembly of caveolae. Cell 144(3):402–413
84. Jin AJ, Nossal R (2000) Rigidity of triskelion arms and clathrin nets. Biophys J 78(3):1183–1194
85. Brujic J, Hermans RI, Garcia-Manyes S, Walther KA, Fernandez JM (2007) Dwell-time distribution analysis of polyprotein unfolding using force-clamp spectroscopy. Biophys J 92(8):2896–2903
86. Ortiz Franyuti D, Mitsi M, Vogel V (2018) Mechanical stretching of fibronectin fibers upregulates binding of interleukin-7. Nano Lett 18(1):15–25
87. Rudnev VS, Ermishkin LN, Fonina LA, Rovin YG (1981) The dependence of the conductance and lifetime of gramicidin channels on the thickness and tension of lipid bilayers. Biochim Biophys Acta 642(1):196–202
88. Chalfie M (2009) Neurosensory mechanotransduction. Nat Rev Mol Cell Biol 10(1):44–52
89. Samuel MS, Lopez JI, McGhee EJ, Croft DR, Strachan D, Timpson P et al (2011) Actomyosin-mediated cellular tension drives increased tissue stiffness and β-catenin activation to induce epidermal hyperplasia and tumor growth. Cancer Cell 19(6):776–791
90. Nilsson M, Adamo H, Bergh A, Halin BS (2016) Inhibition of lysyl oxidase and lysyl oxidase-like enzymes has tumour-promoting and tumour-suppressing roles in experimental prostate cancer. Sci Rep 6:19608
91. Rak R, Haklai R, Elad-Tzfadia G, Wolfson HJ, Carmeli S, Kloog Y (2014) Novel LIMK2 inhibitor blocks Panc-1 tumor growth in a mouse xenograft model. Onco Targets Ther 1(1):39–48
92. Qiu MK, Wang SQ, Pan C, Wang Y, Quan ZW, Liu YB et al (2017) ROCK inhibition as a potential therapeutic target involved in apoptosis in hemangioma. Oncol Rep 37(5):2987–2993

93. Martz E, Steinberg MS (1972) The role of cell-cell contact in "contact" inhibition of cell division: a review and new evidence. J Cell Physiol 79(2):189–210
94. Ukena TE, Goldman E, Benjamin TL, Karnovsky MJ (1976) Lack of correlation between agglutinability, the surface distribution of con A and post-confluence inhibition of cell division in ten cell lines. Cell 7(2):213–222
95. Whitehead J, Vignjevic D, Fütterer C, Beaurepaire E, Robine S, Farge E (2008) Mechanical factors activate beta-catenin-dependent oncogene expression in APC mouse colon. HFSP J 2(5):286–294
96. Song F, Jiang D, Wang T, Wang Y, Lou Y, Zhang Y et al (2017) Mechanical stress regulates osteogenesis and adipogenesis of rat mesenchymal stem cells through PI3K/Akt/GSK-3β/β-catenin signaling pathway. Biomed Res Int 2017:6027402
97. Fernández-Sánchez ME, Barbier S, Whitehead J, Béalle G, Michel A, Latorre-Ossa H et al (2015) Mechanical induction of the tumorigenic β-catenin pathway by tumour growth pressure. Nature 523(7558):92–95
98. Zhang B, Pan X, Cobb GP, Anderson TA (2007) microRNAs as oncogenes and tumor suppressors. Dev Biol 302(1):1–12
99. Mouw JK, Yui Y, Damiano L, Bainer RO, Lakins JN, Acerbi I et al (2014) Tissue mechanics modulate microRNA-dependent PTEN expression to regulate malignant progression. Nat Med 20(4):360–367
100. Le LT, Cazares O, Mouw JK, Chatterjee S, Macias H, Moran A et al (2016) Loss of miR-203 regulates cell shape and matrix adhesion through ROBO1/Rac/FAK in response to stiffness. J Cell Biol 212(6):707–719
101. Wang H, Sun Z, Wang Y, Hu Z, Zhou H, Zhang L et al (2016) miR-33-5p, a novel mechano-sensitive microRNA promotes osteoblast differentiation by targeting Hmga2. Sci Rep 6:23170
102. Swift J, Discher DE (2014) The nuclear lamina is mechano-responsive to ECM elasticity in mature tissue. J Cell Sci 127(Pt 14):3005–3015
103. Wang N, Tytell JD, Ingber DE (2009) Mechanotransduction at a distance: mechanically coupling the extracellular matrix with the nucleus. Nat Rev Mol Cell Biol 10(1):75–82
104. Belaadi N, Aureille J, Guilluy C (2016) Under pressure: mechanical stress management in the nucleus. Cell 5(2):27
105. Esra Demircioglu F, Cruz VE, Schwartz TU (2016) Purification and structural analysis of SUN and KASH domain proteins. Methods Enzymol 569:63–78
106. Simon DN, Zastrow MS, Wilson KL (2010) Direct actin binding to A- and B-type Lamin tails and actin filament bundling by the Lamin a tail. Nucleus 1(3):264–272
107. Isermann P, Lammerding J (2013) Nuclear mechanics and mechanotransduction in health and disease. Curr Biol 23(24):R1113–R1121
108. Swift J, Ivanovska IL, Buxboim A, Harada T, Dingal PC, Pinter J et al (2013) Nuclear Lamin-a scales with tissue stiffness and enhances matrix-directed differentiation. Science (New York, NY) 341(6149):1240104
109. Foster CR, Przyborski SA, Wilson RG, Hutchison CJ (2010) Lamins as cancer biomarkers. Biochem Soc Trans 38(Pt 1):297–300
110. Kumar A, Shivashankar GV (2016) Dynamic interaction between actin and nesprin2 maintain the cell nucleus in a prestressed state. Methods Appl Fluoresc 4(4):044008
111. Harada T, Swift J, Irianto J, Shin JW, Spinler KR, Athirasala A et al (2014) Nuclear Lamin stiffness is a barrier to 3D migration, but softness can limit survival. J Cell Biol 204(5):669–682
112. Krause M, Wolf K (2015) Cancer cell migration in 3D tissue: negotiating space by proteolysis and nuclear deformability. Cell Adhes Migr 9(5):357–366
113. Wolf K, Te Lindert M, Krause M, Alexander S, Te Riet J, Willis AL et al (2013) Physical limits of cell migration: control by ECM space and nuclear deformation and tuning by proteolysis and traction force. J Cell Biol 201(7):1069–1084
114. Saarinen I, Mirtti T, Seikkula H, Boström PJ, Taimen P (2015) Differential predictive roles of A- and B-type nuclear lamins in prostate cancer progression. PLoS One 10(10):e0140671

115. Kaspi E, Frankel D, Guinde J, Perrin S, Laroumagne S, Robaglia-Schlupp A et al (2017) Low Lamin a expression in lung adenocarcinoma cells from pleural effusions is a pejorative factor associated with high number of metastatic sites and poor performance status. PLoS One 12(8): e0183136

116. Sakthivel KM, Sehgal P (2016) A novel role of lamins from genetic disease to cancer biomarkers. Oncol Rev 10(2):309

117. Denais CM, Gilbert RM, Isermann P, McGregor AL, te Lindert M, Weigelin B et al (2016) Nuclear envelope rupture and repair during cancer cell migration. Science (New York, NY) 352(6283):353–358

118. Irianto J, Xia Y, Pfeifer CR, Athirasala A, Ji J, Alvey C et al (2017) DNA damage follows repair factor depletion and portends genome variation in cancer cells after pore migration. Curr Biol 27(2):210–223

119. Discher DE, Smith L, Cho S, Colasurdo M, García AJ, Safran S (2017) Matrix mechanosensing: from scaling concepts in 'Omics data to mechanisms in the nucleus, regeneration, and cancer. Annu Rev Biophys 46:295–315

120. Pfeifer CR, Alvey CM, Irianto J, Discher DE (2017) Genome variation across cancers scales with tissue stiffness - an invasion-mutation mechanism and implications for immune cell infiltration. Curr Opin Syst Biol 2:103–114

121. Cho S, Irianto J, Discher DE (2017) Mechanosensing by the nucleus: from pathways to scaling relationships. J Cell Biol 216(2):305–315

122. Sugden WW, Meissner R, Aegerter-Wilmsen T, Tsaryk R, Leonard EV, Bussmann J et al (2017) Endoglin controls blood vessel diameter through endothelial cell shape changes in response to haemodynamic cues. Nat Cell Biol 19(6):653–665

123. Mammoto A, Connor KM, Mammoto T, Yung CW, Huh D, Aderman CM et al (2009) A mechanosensitive transcriptional mechanism that controls angiogenesis. Nature 457(7233): 1103–1108

124. Fleury V, Chevalier NR, Furfaro F, Duband JL (2015) Buckling along boundaries of elastic contrast as a mechanism for early vertebrate morphogenesis. Eur Phys J E Soft Matter 38(2):92

125. Serwane F, Mongera A, Rowghanian P, Kealhofer DA, Lucio AA, Hockenbery ZM et al (2017) In vivo quantification of spatially varying mechanical properties in developing tissues. Nat Methods 14(2):181–186

126. Vuong-Brender TT, Ben Amar M, Pontabry J, Labouesse M (2017) The interplay of stiffness and force anisotropies drives embryo elongation. Elife 6:e23866

127. Fernandez-Gonzalez R, Simoes Sde M, Röper JC, Eaton S, Zallen JA (2009) Myosin II dynamics are regulated by tension in intercalating cells. Dev Cell 17(5):736–743

128. Pouille PA, Ahmadi P, Brunet AC, Farge E (2009) Mechanical signals trigger myosin II redistribution and mesoderm invagination in Drosophila embryos. Sci Signal 2(66):ra16

129. Mitrossilis D, Röper JC, Le Roy D, Driquez B, Michel A, Ménager C et al (2017) Mechanotransductive cascade of Myo-II-dependent mesoderm and endoderm invaginations in embryo gastrulation. Nat Commun 8:13883

130. Farge E (2003) Mechanical induction of twist in the drosophila foregut/stomodeal primordium. Curr Biol 13(16):1365–1377

131. Desprat N, Supatto W, Pouille PA, Beaurepaire E, Farge E (2008) Tissue deformation modulates twist expression to determine anterior midgut differentiation in Drosophila embryos. Dev Cell 15(3):470–477

132. Brunet T, Bouclet A, Ahmadi P, Mitrossilis D, Driquez B, Brunet AC et al (2013) Evolutionary conservation of early mesoderm specification by mechanotransduction in Bilateria. Nat Commun 4:2821

133. Jaffee EM, Dang CV, Agus DB, Alexander BM, Anderson KC, Ashworth A et al (2017) Future cancer research priorities in the USA: a Lancet Oncology Commission. Lancet Oncol 18(11):e653–e706

Part II
Regional and Distal *Onco-Sphere*

Chapter 10
Field Cancerization: A Malignant Transformation

Phei Er Saw and Erwei Song

Abstract Mutations in a cell is natural, especially in aging cells. However, among all mutated cells, only a certain subset could clonally expand, leading to cancer. These cells then influence their surrounding cells to acquire cancerous phenotype - a phenomenon known as field cancerization. Field cancerization is both enabled by and causes changes to the tissue microenvironment. In this chapter, we introduce the concept of field cancerization in various human cancers. We also discuss how genetic and epigenetic changes in the local onco-sphere could affect field cancerization.

Introduction

This concept of "field cancerization" was proposed by Slaughter about a decade prior to its use in 1953. Through a comprehensive histopathologic analysis of 783 oral cancer patients, the phrase "field cancerization" was employed to characterize initial genetic alterations in the epithelium induced by a carcinogen leading to the formation

P. E. Saw
Guangdong Provincial Key Laboratory of Malignant Tumor Epigenetics and Gene Regulation, Guangdong-Hong Kong Joint Laboratory for RNA Medicine, Medical Research Center, Sun Yat-sen Memorial Hospital, Sun Yat-sen University, Guangzhou, China

Nanhai Translational Innovation Center of Precision Immunology, Sun Yat-sen Memorial Hospital, Sun Yat-sen University, Foshan, China

E. Song (✉)
Guangdong Provincial Key Laboratory of Malignant Tumor Epigenetics and Gene Regulation, Guangdong-Hong Kong Joint Laboratory for RNA Medicine, Medical Research Center, Sun Yat-sen Memorial Hospital, Sun Yat-sen University, Guangzhou, China

Nanhai Translational Innovation Center of Precision Immunology, Sun Yat-sen Memorial Hospital, Sun Yat-sen University, Foshan, China

Breast Tumor Center, Sun Yat-sen Memorial Hospital, Sun Yat-sen University, Guangzhou, China
e-mail: songew@mail.sysu.edu.cn

of many tumors in diverse locations [1]. Numerous tumor foci neighboring each other tend to merge in certain instances. This is one of the reasons behind the lateral expansion of squamous cell carcinomas. Cells that appeared healthy but located proximally to cancer cells were detected with histological aberrations. This signified their existence as part of the altered cells in a specific tumor field, causing the recurrence of local cancers. These explorations were performed prior to the availability of sophisticated molecular methods after the discovery of the double helix structure of DNA by Watson and Crick. The latest evidence using a range of genetic screenings has proven the correctness of this notion [2, 3].

An essential topic of field cancerization that is yet to be solved is the mechanism of evolution of these cancer fields. (1) Can a single carcinogen generate several crucial changes in their genetic information, simultaneously or consecutively in a number of cells, which could lead to a polyclonal (different mutation in different cells in a clone) in pre-cancerous tumor cells? (2) Is this polyclonality a starting point for multiple tumors? (3) Is it possible for just one mutation to occur to alter the genetic sequence in one cell, through cell proliferation, this cell can grow into a clone, which then spreads laterally to substitute the natural epithelium, resulting in a huge pre-neoplastic field that becomes the growth point of many tumors? (4) Do genetic changes in pre-neoplastic/pre-transformed cells happen concurrently in a group of neighboring cells, causing subsequent genetic modifications to induce carcinogenesis in certain cells? (5) Is it also feasible that certain field modifications occur during organogenesis with the proliferation of a few modified cells to form a vast field of the preconditioned epithelial layer, resulting in numerous malignancies due to subsequent genetic errors in certain cells?

These are all plausible mechanisms for inducing malignancy in a field, but molecular findings from cancer investigations corroborate the clonal growth concept [3–5] (for more details on hypothesis on metastasis, please refer to Chap. 11: Overview and origin of metastasis). This hypothesis might elucidate the cause behind the development of multiple tumors in organs having a single epithelial layer, especially skin (largest epithelial organ in human body), and also including internal organs such as the colon, esophagus, stomach, bladder, cervix, and vulva. An interesting fact is that even exposure to an identical carcinogen is less likely to induce the growth of tumors due to the proliferation of monoclonal cells in glandular organs, such as the lung, breast, ovary, pancreas, and prostate, having discontinuous glandular epithelial arrangement. Despite having similar genetic alterations, polyclonal tumor stem cells are probably the cause of numerous cancers in these organs. Another point that needs to be taken into consideration is the loss of heterozygosity (LOH), which is prevalently seen in primary ductal carcinoma *in situ* (DCIS), and this LOH is different in comparison to different subtypes of cancers of the same tissue (*i.e.,* invasive breast ductal carcinoma vs. triple negative breast cancer). This implies that DCIS and adenocarcinoma in the same tissue could be due to mutations from two or more genetically distinct clones [6]. This concept is further proven clinically by micro-dissections of tumor tissues of breast tissues. When samples were taken from healthy glands, marginal glands near the malignant epithelia and cancerous breast tissue, it was found that only one LOH was identified as similar in the breast cancer tissue compared to the healthy and marginal glands, indicating that there are definitely distinct genetic loci that lead to different LOH in the tumor [7].

Field cancerization research may help us better comprehend the multistage paradigm of how tumors originate rather than an evaluation of how pre-cancerous fields evolve. Significantly, genetic data obtained at various phases of cancer development aid in our understanding of cancer biology and the employment of molecular markers in the therapy. Improvement in laboratory methods, especially for molecular works, has advanced our screening methods, to be able to distinctly detect and evaluate many of these alterations at all genomic levels, and also at their epigenetic level, including gene expressions, epigenetic gene silencing, LOH, single-nucleotide polymorphism (SNPs), and others. Variations in the mitochondrial genome (which also possess mitochondrial DNA) can also be detected by comparing pre-cancerous lesions and their normal adjacent cell counterparts [5–14]. Metabolomics, or a study of metabolic changes, is now being integrated into the study of field cancerization. With this method, the metabolic profile in various tissues can be determined to predict the cancerization in various tissue. It is reasonable to assume that the initial modifications in the genes will be retained by both tumor cells and pre-neoplastic cells belonging to the same organ. If these premature molecular alterations were better studied, their assistance in determining risk, detecting cancer early, and tracking how a disease progresses would have been multifold, along with prioritized prevention of individuals from being ill. As a result, minuscule alterations in the DNA molecule may cause genetic destruction at an early stage, rendering it a far more proactive indicator of field cancerization in comparison to nuclear genomic alterations.

Field Cancerization: A General Phenomenon of Epithelial Tumors

Epithelia's protective effect is an essential element of their physiology. As a result, they have to bear constant exposure to environmental factors such as carcinogens, which can induce a wide range of genetic abnormalities concluding in cancer. Epithelial cells undergo frequent replenishment and might develop inappropriately. Hyperplastic epithelia may endure neoplastic alterations that contribute to the most frequent kinds of cancer in humans. Field cancerization's molecular markers have been discovered in a variety of epithelial tumors, such as the skin, head and neck, esophagus, breast, lungs, stomach, colon, ovary, pancreas, and most recently in prostate cancer [15, 16]. These molecular markers include changes in gene expression (*i.e.,* PSCA gene changes in prostate cancer), protein expression changes (PS2, COX2, p-AKT1, Ki67, p-EGFP, PDGFRβ, EGR-1, FAS, etc.), cytomorphological changes, mitochondrial DNA changes, genomic DNA changes, and epigenetic changes [17]. Since the molecular biology of field cancerization varies in each cancer, in this chapter, we will go through each form of epithelial cancer and the mechanism of field cancerization in each kind of cancer.

Head and Neck Squamous Cell Carcinoma (HNSCC)

Considering the initial observation of field cancerization in oral cancers, conducting significant molecular genetic research on head and neck tumors to find out the reason and mechanism of their occurrence is not strange [2, 18, 19]. Though the clonal tendency of these fields is still under deliberation, experiments employing stringent criteria of clonality (including cytogenetic indicators, microsatellite fragility, and mutation assessment) appear to agree with the notion that most, if not all, HNSCC arises from continuous monoclonal pre-neoplastic areas [5]. Moreover, a field of more than 7 cm in size (from the same clone) has been recorded in these tumors, and comparable remainder clonal fields after resection account for approximately 62.5% of HNSCC second primary tumor relapses [14]. The latest research has shown that individuals with HNSCC have distinct protein profiles in comparison to normal people. The analysis of protein profiles of mucosa gathered from 73 healthy subjects, 113 HNSCC, 99 tumor-distant, and 18 tumor-adjacent specimens revealed evidence of field cancerization among 72% of tumor-adjacent specimens and 27.3% of tumor-distant specimens. Surprisingly, even in the specimens taken from distant tissues, their protein profiles are also altered. These alterations of the proteins are those closely related to cancer recurrence, indicating the importance of examining their proteomic alterations not only in adjacent tissues, but also distant tissues, to look for signs of micrometastases [20]. Exposure to carcinogens appears to cause a substantial molecular alteration in the pre-neoplastic field in the aerodigestive tract's epithelium. The latest study has indicated that genetic alterations in stromal tissues might influence the growth of HNSCC. Tumor epithelial and stromal cells derived from 122 patients were collected via laser-capture microdissection for complete genome LOH and allelic imbalance screening utilizing 366 microsatellite loci. Interestingly, these findings were not fully parallel to the clinicopathological factors at the time of diagnosis. The association of three stromal loci with tumor size and nodal metastases, whereas the relation of two epithelial loci to nodal invasion, demonstrated that genetic alterations in the stroma near the tumor or at adjacent tumor tissue could influence the growth and dissemination of HNSCC.

Mitochondria are a vital organelle in the cell, which provide not only energy but also comprising their own set of mitochondrial DNAs (mtDNA), which are now revealed as one important factor in carcinogenesis. Therefore, recently, mtDNA is studied to be used as a biomarker. One study examined 137 pre-cancerous tumors among 93 individuals and discovered mtDNA alterations in 34 samples. These mutations worsened remarkably with the progression of dysplasia, indicating that alterations to the mitochondrial DNA may cause or reveal the mechanism of worsening of the illness. Healthy mucosa alongside dysplastic lesions was also examined. Around 38% tissues surrounding the lesions bearing mtDNA alterations had almost identical mutations. In total, ~43% of the metachronous lesions still exhibited mutations, whereas 8/18 of the synchronized lesions retained a similar profile of mitochondrial mutations [9]. These findings support the notion that certain head and neck cancer fields are composed of single cells. Another research by the same group discovered that pre-malignant lesions had altered mitochondrial composition, which tended to deteriorate with the progress of the disease [21]. Interestingly, mtDNA collected from saliva could predict the malignancy of this disease, and the concentration of these mtDNA seems to be increased as the malignancy progresses, which indicates that the detection and monitoring of head and neck malignancies could be done noninvasively, through mtDNA markers without requiring surgery. In another large cohort study, quantitative PCR (qPCR) was used to compare 4977 bp mtDNA in laser-capture microdissected tissues from paired oral tumors, pre-cancerous lesions, and the sub-mucosal stroma adjacent to the tumor, all taken during lymph node biopsies. Lesions were more prone to removal than lymphocytes. Pre-cancerous lesions showed a higher rate of deletions in comparison to cancerous tissue, and in either case, the submucosal stroma neighboring the lesions experienced a higher frequency of deletions from the lesions themselves [22]. Hence, with greater frequency of deletion levels in pre-cancerous lesions in the mouth, they tend to decrease as the illness progresses and becomes a malignant tumor.

Lung Cancer

The most common reason for lung cancer is smoking. Tissue samples were extracted from the whole tracheobronchial tree of an individual smoking for 50 pack-years but free from lung cancer to study p53 mutations [23]. Researchers attempted to identify cancer areas associated with smoking. The discovery of a transversion in codon 245 across 7 of 10 locations in both lungs demonstrated the involvement of a carcinogen in initiating a mutation in several locations of this person's lung epithelium [23]. The clone size in the lung epithelium of microdissected tumors and healthy bronchial epithelium surrounding the tumors were measured with the help of 12 microsatellite markers, with each clone included up to 90,000 cells. However, many normal-looking epithelial sites also undergo genetic issues. Although a patient might have similar molecular marker changes throughout various clones in the tumor, other field cancerization markers could be significantly different. For example, LOH, particularly at chromosome 12p12, has lately been discovered in the healthy bronchial epithelium of smokers and deletion points at two chromosomal sites (2q35-q36, 12p12p13) have been discovered in non-small-cell lung cancer (NSCLC) compared to normal healthy bronchial cells [24, 25]. This indicates that LOH is likely to signify a person's predisposition to cancer or the pre-existence of cancer among them. It might also indicate the likelihood of normal-looking pre-- cancerous cells transforming into malignancy [26]. Similar to the aerodigestive tract, carcinogens appear to produce a proactive genetic alteration in the tracheobronchial epithelium, resulting in the formation of numerous malignancies. Because 72% of lung cancers have progressed prior to their detection, if noninvasive sequencing of saliva or sputum could be a reliable indicator for tracheobronchial epithelial cancer, patients could then benefit from this early detection method.

Esophageal Cancer

Barrett's esophagus is a disease that can escalate to esophageal cancer, which renders its utilization as a prototype to examine how tumor clonality affects their development in field cancerization. In a molecular study of this disease, researchers have utilized a generally known protein, p53 mutation, as a clonal indicator to study 213 endoscopic biopsies derived from 58 patients with Barrett's esophagus. Results revealed that 50% were clonal and multiple cancer fields are detected, and each field is between 1 cm and 9 cm [3]. In another study, LOH quantification was used. The esophageal map fields indicated that LOH at 9p21 (p16 locus) and 17p13 (p53 locus) was indicative of field cancerization [27]. Seventy-three percent out of the total 404 samples gathered from 61 patients demonstrated LOH at a single or both loci. The clones varied in size, and a lot of them failed to develop fully, whereby few were 2 cm in size, while others spanned the entire Barrett's section [27]. Another investigation discovered a relationship between clone development and the p16 level. Clones containing $p16^{+/+}$ developed by 1.5 cm, clones containing $p16^{+/-}$ grew until 6 cm, and clones containing $p16^{-/-}$ developed up to 8 cm. In reality, mutant p16 clones can span nearly 17 cm of the esophagus [28]. Scientists investigated and used epigenetics to study how APC, CDH1, ESR1, and p16 genes were switched off in Barrett's esophagus. Vast detection of hypermethylation, interconnected fields demonstrated the occurrence of Barrett's metaplasia due to molecular field cancerization [29]. An analysis of 267 individuals revealed that clone sizes (the number of clones X length of Barrett's section coverage), with the additional factor of p53 LOH were strong determinants of adenocarcinoma [30]. Interestingly, even in clones with p16 mutation, without the presence of p53 LOH, this mutation alone is not a risk factor of malignancy, indicating that the worsening condition of Barrett's esophagus must be accompanied by molecular markers of filed cancerization. Lately, a concept known as "clonal cellular diversity" was proposed to describe this progression. With the employment of ecological and evolutionary principles (the rate of mutation, the size of the population of evolving clones, and the rate of natural selection or clonal expansion), clonal diversity served as a powerful determinant of disease progression, even under the consideration of identifiable risk factors such as p53 LOH [31, 32]. This observation is significant with reference to disease monitoring. Also, in mtDNA profiling, a more sensitive array was built to profile lesions from 14 pre-cancerous lesions in gastrointestinal-related samples. Through this technique, all 14 samples (100%) showed mtDNA mutations at varying degree. Comparing two colon samples, two dysplastic lesions that occur at the same time contained identical genetic alterations, suggesting the likelihood of a field cancerization [13].

Gastric Cancer

Various gastric tumors that occur at the same time are correlated to genes. An examination of the mutational patterns of genetic mutation, including the generally known p53, MCC, and APC; in various cancers among 13 individuals revealed variations between the mutation patterns in these tumors [33]. As a result, the generation of all these lesions can be attributed to distinct genetic processes in an epithelium prevailing in a specific condition. A mutation in the epigenetic level could also cause field cancerization. LIMS1 is a gene that enables cell mobility, and it was found that LIMS1 methylation is switched off in 53% of cases of gastrointestinal tumors due to a process known as CpG island hypermethylation [34]. In normal gastric tissue, LIMS1 is generally methylated, indicating that the silencing of epigenetic methylation is occurring initially in gastric neoplasia. Overexpression of C-Erb was observed in certain tumors and healthy mucosa neighboring the tumor periphery and healthy mucosa are commonly characterized by aneuploidy at an approximate distance of about 3 cm from the tumor lining [35].

Colorectal Cancer

Colorectal cancers (CRCs) play a useful role in researching field cancerization because of the connectivity to the epithelium. The concentration of carcinoembryonic antigen (CEA) labeling in normal colonic mucosa was identical to that of the adjacent tumor, but this altered after 1 cm, and the labeling pattern 5 cm from the tumor border was similar to the mucosa lacking a tumor [36]. As a result, there was a gradation of CEA production in the colon epithelial cells surrounding the tumor. The dissemination of CRC to different areas of the body is demonstrated by O6-methylguanine-DNA methyltransferase (MGMT), a promoter that is required for DNA repair mechanism. This well-structured investigation discovered a relationship between methylation in tumors and methylation in normal mucosa neighboring the lesions. In 10 out of 13 tumors, healthy-looking colonic mucosa located 10 cm distantly from tumors appeared to be methylated [12]. Normal mucosa at a distance of 1 cm from the tumor's periphery had a higher possibility of hypermethylation in comparison to normal mucosa at 10 cm distance. Switching off MGMT through epigenetics creates a genetic field that serves as the ground for the development of colorectal cancers. Indeed, epigenetic occurrences are emerging as potential indicators of the molecular pathway that progresses to colorectal cancer [37]. Additional research discovered the mutation of K-Ras oncogene in 30% of adenomas and switched on in 26% of these. Significantly, overexpression of numerous K-downstream Ras targets in adenomas indicated their usefulness in proactive identification and determination of their hazardous propensity.

Vulval Cancers (Including Cervical Cancers)

In vulval cancer subtypes, Vulval Intraepithelial Neoplasia (VIN) is frequently clonal and closely related to Vulval Squamous Cell Carcinoma (VSCC). This indicates the occurrence of VIN in the form of a lesion prior to VSCC. An examination of 9 samples of VIN with inactivated X-chromosome, 10 samples of VSCC having adjacent VIN, and 11 samples of VSCC with non-adjacent VIN revealed a single clone to be responsible for causing most VIN and VSCC. On the contrary, two instances of VIN with non-adjacent VSCC revealed molecular profiles that indicated their origination from separate clones [38]. In cervical intraepithelial tumors, when microdissected specimen were screened on the chromosome 3p allelotyping to detect three markers, results indicated that microsatellite instability (MSI) was more frequently seen in low-grade lesions, implying the origination of pre-malignant and malignant lesions from a single cell [38].

Skin Cancer

The skin exhibits the highest vulnerability to ultraviolet light (UVR), as we are exposed to this environmental carcinogen daily. UVR's absorption causes gene alteration, which potentially leads to development of skin cancer, which is often malignant and lethal. There have been ample studies on the defining gene mutations and alterations with various subtypes of skin cancers. For example, actinic keratosis (AK) is associated with high p53 mutations and only slight elevation of elevated p16 levels, whereas it is associated with both p53 mutation and p16 overexpression, in addition to activated mitogenic Ras pathway, decreased FasR (CD95-R) synthesis, and elevated FasL production. Mutations in the Sonic Hedgehog pathway (SHH) patch gene (PTCH) correlate with basal cell carcinoma (BCC). The easy connectivity and accessibility of skin make it an excellent organ for understanding the mechanism and reason behind field cancerization. In skin cancer, especially, field cancerization is seen as a communal process, where most neighborhood is impacted. Mutation of p53 is frequently seen and is one of the main indicators of clonal characterization of skin cancer. In a melanoma study, p53 mutation was discovered in both cancerous and also their "normal-looking" adjacent tissues [39]. To determine their mechanistic behavior, researchers further utilized a whole-mount culture to trace time-dependent changes of these p53 mutant keratinocytes and how they are transported from dermal-epidermal interfaces [40]. These clones with altered genes may require additional alterations to their genes in order to properly exhibit the malignant phenotype. In another study, a strong correlation was found between a strong dosage of UVA and psoralens for the treatment of psoriasis. p53 mutations were discovered in 54% of the 69 tumors investigated in research. Multiple varieties of mutant cells were discovered in tumors observed in the same patient, which shows their origination from various somatic clones in cancer originated from UVA and psoralen therapy. In mtDNA testing, UV-driven mtDNA alterations were identified in both tumors and healthy tissue neighboring the tumor in non-melanoma skin cancer. In another investigation, mtDNA lost was discovered in both tumor and their adjacent tissue specimens. However, these margin specimens were seen to have additional deletions compared to the tumor tissue, indicating a continuous mutagenic process during field cancerization [41]. However, not just during carcinogenesis, skin tissue surrounding an injury could exhibit more mutant mtDNA keratinocytes, as reflected with DNA biomarkers [40]. Therefore, this is the bottleneck of using field cancerization biomarker, as it is not specific to cancer. Researchers should take note that, especially in skin cancer, using only histologically healthy peri-lesional skin in NMSC research might be insufficient. This is significant because peri-lesional skin is frequently utilized as a reference tissue while researching nuclear DNA damage and skin cancer or skin disorders.

Box 10.1   UV-Induced Skin Cancer: Cross Talk with Dermal Fibroblast

Excessive exposure to light causes mutations in keratinocyte and melanocyte progenitors, which are well-known inducers of skin cancer. Latest research shows that the sun's damaging radiation can trigger epigenetic changes in dermal fibroblasts, which could have tumor-promoting characteristics, emphasizing the role of tumor–stroma linkages in cancer. Previous research has revealed that this inactivation causes severe developmental abnormalities in a variety of tissues. The histological analysis of mice with mutant skin (due to UV irradiation) is badly deformed. This group of mice presented minimal concentrations of elastin and collagen: the two important constituents of the ECM (usually generated by dermal fibroblasts). These mice are also presented with enhanced transdermal permeability, signifying immature skin barrier formation. In addition, the skin also exhibits extensive hyperproliferation of epidermal keratinocytes that constitute the skin's extrinsic surface. CAF markers, FGF, and MMPs, are also plentiful in the afflicted skin, as is an abundance of Tenascin C and Periostin—two interacting proteins in cell-matrix recognized for creating cancer stem cell environments [42]. Surprisingly, the number of inflammatory cells rises around the epidermal proliferative hotspots. In all these settings above, the mice develop cancerous skin lesions exhibiting a close resemblance to human actinic keratosis (histologically), commonly known as solar keratosis, after extensive exposure to the sun (main source of UV carcinogen). Actinic keratosis is a frequently diagnosed skin disorder that is hypothesized to be the precursor of SCC. As the mice grow, the lesions develop well to moderately distinct characteristics of SCC. Herein, an intricate cross talk was seen in tumor–stroma interaction as Notch signaling in dermal fibroblasts was sufficient to cause cancer in the surrounding tissue, including epidermal layer, which then the epidermis cell reacts by

(continued)

Box 10.1 (continued)

recruiting inflammatory cells to enhance inflammation-triggered carcinogenesis. Notch inhibits AP1-driven transcription of numerous GFs, proteases, and ECMs [43].

The study then investigated the possibility of UV radiation causing Notch inactivation in cutaneous fibroblasts. Sun exposure appears to induce susceptibility of the cutaneous fibroblast to be transformed into actinic keratosis and subsequently SCC by epigenetic suppression of Notch signaling in dermal fibroblasts (Fig. 10.1). Interestingly, this phenomenon is only seen in UVA but not UVB therapy. The broader conclusion of this argument is that the process of field cancerization involving the formation of many primary tumors following exposure to mutagens may be driven by stromal changes. Earlier research has actually hinted on this, as data revealed that stroma-specific genetic modification may cause epithelial cancer in mice. Inactivating TGF-βR in stromal cells, for example, causes neoplastic modification in the surrounding epithelial cells lining the forestomach and prostate gland [44]. Mutant fibroblasts can also be chosen in murine models during epithelial carcinogenesis [45].

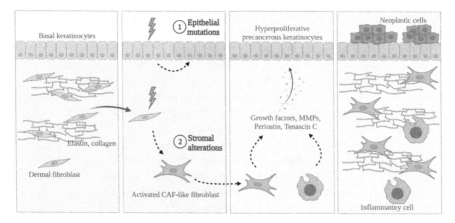

Fig 10.1 UV-Induced SCC: a cross talk with dermal fibroblast. UV irradiation can result in mutations in basal keratinocytes. TP53 mutations lead to actinic keratosis (AK), a pre-cancerous keratinocyte-formed lesion that can evolve into SCC if NOTCH1 and NOTCH2 are also upregulated. UV irradiation can also activate the Notch system in dermal fibroblasts. As a result, the cells adopt a CAF-like phenotype, with decreased elastin and collagen formation and increased release of FGFs and proteases. This causes the surrounding epidermal keratinocytes to proliferate. Epidermal proliferation zones become increasingly concentrated with CD45+ inflammatory cells, which promote keratinocyte proliferation and the formation of actinic keratosis, which can lead to SCCs. This model clearly reflects the interconnected local oncosphere in the tri-directional communication between cancer–stroma–immune cells

Bladder Cancer

The urothelium is continuously subjected to carcinogens as the ultimate place for storage and release of urine, which can be a large reservoir for potential carcinogens. Since bladder is considered a large organ, researchers often need to combine the usage of multiple analysis such as fluorescent in situ hybridization (FISH) with the analysis of LOH and p53 mutation to scan the entire organ's cancer field [46]. In a study, when molecular and histopathologic evidences were compared, it was shown that a single kind of cell is capable of generating multifocal lesions in various regions in bladder cancer [46]. Another research examined 32 tumors affecting six bladders using chromosomal markers, several tumors affecting the same bladder showed the same chromosomal mutations as well as their own modifications, as predicted by the multistep model of carcinogenesis. Therefore, lesions are more likely to occur in genetically altered but otherwise healthy bladder urothelium [47].

Breast Cancer

Breast glandular epithelial cells proliferate cyclically, favoring neoplastic modification. DCIS is a kind of pre-cancerous lesion found in invasive breast cancer. Many studies have found genetic instability in healthy breast lobules in the vicinity of cancer foci, as well as in DCIS. LOH was found in 8/30 instances of healthy breast tissue besides breast cancer, and all had the same missing gene as the primary cancer [11]. By using a fine needle aspiration (FNA) biopsy, LOH was found in two individuals with normal cytology and 14 patients with defective cytology, respectively [48]. These results imply that randomized FNA biopsy sampling of breast tissue might be beneficial in personalized treatment. In a separate investigation, healthy tissue specimens were collected from different breast quadrant of 21 patients with confirmed breast cancer in order to explore LOH and allelic abnormalities [49]. The external breast quadrants exhibited more genomic instability than the internal ones, indicating that an enhanced genomic instability is associated with a higher probability of breast cancer in the external quadrants [49]. LOH was also investigated in samples of women having grade 1 and grade 3 DCIS [6]. Larger losses of grade 3 DCIS were observed at four chromosomal loci (6q, 11p, 17p, and 17q) [6]. Conversely, a recent study utilizing identical LOH assessment suggested that DCIS might advance to invasive ductal carcinoma (IDC). Specimens of seven women having DCIS, eventually developing breast cancer, were studied under this investigation. LOH in DCIS and IDC were consistent at 50 loci, wherein LOH seemed to build up as the illness progressed from DCIS to IDC [50]. Changes in telomeric DNA content and genetic abnormalities were found in healthy breast tissue positioned about 1 cm away from the apparent tumor periphery. As the distance to the primary tumor increases, these alterations diminished. Breast cancer epigenetic gene silencing has also been explored. For example, the methylation of the cyclin D2 promoter, APC methylation, RARβ2, and RASSF1A were detected at higher levels in healthy breast tissues from breast cancer patients; and these epigenetic changes have been known the be related to a higher risk of breast cancer [51]. Although a recent investigation indicated that RASSF1A promoter methylation in breast tissue is higher in primary tumors compared to control, in general, DNA methylation analysis found that surrounding healthy tissues had more methylated genes than specimens of healthy donor [52].

Prostate Cancer

To date, not many studies were conducted on the mechanism of prostate cancer propagation to other areas of the body. Numerous tumors are prevalent in prostate cancer, which is most likely triggered by a carcinogen that alters an organ's DNA. The potential of prostate cancer to spread to other areas of the body has been depicted through genomic instability, changes in gene expression (genetic mutation), and also the changes in the mitochondrial genome (including mtDNA). In prostate cancer, GSTP1 and RARβ2 exhibited methylation not only in the primary tumor but also in their surrounding stroma and healthy glands around the tumor. Interestingly, this phenomenon is not seen in benign prostatic hyperplasia epithelial cells [53]. The altered telomeric composition was discovered in healthy tissues around malignancies. This was discovered to be an excellent predictor of recurring prostate cancer [54]. In an athymic nude mice model, implant of prostate cancer cell lines caused an aberrant change in the originally healthy stromal cell components, indicating that the cancer cells could change their surroundings to fit their own needs to survive (also a sign of survival through an ecosystem concept) [55].

Healthy tissue adjacent to a tumor focal point exhibited gene expression profiles comparable to malignancies but distinct from healthy prostate donor specimens [8, 56]. One of the hints is by the expression of early prostate cancer antigen (EPCA). This antigen is only present in pre-cancerous lesion, so if it is found in healthy tissues around tumors, it is a clue that this region could be a possible field for tumor growth. EPCA was found to be overexpressed in healthy prostate glands of patients who subsequently developed cancer [57, 58]. According to the latest report, multifocal prostate cancer may be constituted of clones. Laser-capture microdissection was used to extract pure glandular epithelial cells from multifocal tumors for studying gene expression. All the single-person-derived specimens revealed the overexpression or no expression of ERG, ETV1, and ETV4. This implies that alterations in these genes may be the initial stages in the progression of prostate cancer [59]. Since prostate cancer is a progressive illness that worsens with age, age-related mechanism should be closely related to field cancerization of this cancer. In aged men, healthy prostate glands adjacent to tumors displayed a prostate cancer DNA phenotype, which was most probably triggered by age-related oxidative DNA damage [60, 61]. This alteration in the structure of cancer DNA most likely occurs initially in the formation of prostate cancer since its occurrence is much before the appearance of tumors [62]. The DNA phenotype of metastatic prostate cancer tumors and the healthy glands surrounding them differed from the initial cancer phenotype

[63]. Few molecular alterations in prostate cancer appear to be particularly valuable as biomarkers for timely identification [64]. Substantial research on mtDNA alterations in prostate tumors hints at the hypothesis of "field cancerization," even if it has not been explicitly challenged [65]. In a comprehensive investigation using laser-capture microdissected tissues from prostatectomies, indicators from the mitochondrial genome were to illustrate certain characteristics of field cancerization [66]. Pure clusters of cells from a malignant focus and healthy-looking cells from two distinct locations, adjacent and distant from the tumor, were collected. The frequency of mtDNA mutations in tumors and glands that appeared healthy remained the same, and they varied considerably from those discovered in cancer-free subjects of the same age [66, 67].

Ovarian Cancer

Serous ovarian cancer, which is the most prevalent kind of ovarian cancer, can occur following serous borderline ovarian tumors (BOTs), which demonstrates the genetic preconditioning of the ovarian epithelium by a carcinogen, prompting tumorigenesis. Furthermore, it was formerly thought that recurring ovarian cancers were formed from the same cells. The evaluation of p53 and K-Ras mutations in eight patients having BOTs that subsequently developed serous carcinomas revealed that the tumors were independent [67]. BOTs and serous carcinomas probably occur by themselves when distinct genetic mutations occur in a preestablished epithelium. An examination of 13 main and equivalent recurring ovarian cancers with four indicators of genomic instability revealed that 10 of the 13 were unique, while the others were identical [68]. Scientists examined the methylation status of the regulators of hMLH1, CDKN2A, and MGMT in ovarian and endometrial malignancies that occurred concurrently without originating from the same site. Both endometrial and ovarian cancers had high frequencies of CDKC2A and MGMT promoter methylation, which implies that epigenetic suppression of these genes may be a preliminary stage in the genesis of both of these malignancies at the same time [69].

Pancreatic Cancer

Numerous intraductal papillary pancreatic cancers are frequent, and ductal hyperplasia can develop pancreatic adenocarcinoma. Mutations in K-Ras occur early in the progression of PDAC, not only in their primary tumor but also non-cancerous pancreatic ductal lesions. Hence, these markers have been utilized in various studies to investigate the evolution of pancreatic cancer with the passage of time. The results of microdissection and analysis of primary tumors of pancreatic cancer and hyperplastic ductal tissue revealed that hyperplasia and pancreatic cancer had distinct genetic issues, especially in X-chromosome and K-Ras mutation. As discovered in this research, early genetic alterations in the epithelium produce polyclonal, multicentric pancreatic tumors [70]. In a cohort study of intraductal papillary-mucinous tumors (IPMT), mutation of K-Ras is significant in peri-tumoral tissue, with statistical data of 66.7%. All IPMT patients having such lesions exhibited at least a single similar mutation in both the tumor and the peritumoral tissue [71]. K-Ras mutation has also been used as a biomarker to detect disease progression, as K-Ras mutation was increased from 16.7% in the healthy epithelium of the pancreas and papillary hyperplasia to 57.1% in high-grade dysplasia, and invasive cancer [72].

Conceptualization of Field Cancerization in Other Non-epithelial Tumors

Hematological Cancers

It has been proposed that extensive injury to the bone marrow can result in the formation of a large number of aberrant clones at the same time. Common bone marrow can be home to cells from many hematological disorders, including severe aplastic anemia, severe promyelocytic leukemia (PML), chronic myeloid leukemia (CML), and myelodysplastic syndrome (MDS). The quicker development of one clone than the others make it outstanding, and it can be utilized to perform a diagnosis. This was referred to as the "field leukemogenic impact" by researchers [16], which could be very similar to field cancerization concept in solid tumor. It will be fascinating to explore if the evolutionary and environmental principles that were used to forecast field cancerization (discussed above) may also be used to study these cancers. One very important early indicator of field cancerization is heteroplasmy, a condition where an individual might have more than one type of mtDNA in one single tissue. The association between MDS to AML with the patterns of mitochondrial genome alterations was observed [73]. The clonal abnormalities of myeloid cells are referred to as MDS, which can transform into AML. In MDS, the worsening of a heteroplasmic mtDNA mutation was also discovered with the progression of the illness till the terminal stage of AML characterized by homoplasmic mutant copies. The restriction digest assessment exposed a positive link between the proportion of mtDNA mutations and the advancement from MDS to AML [73]. These discoveries indicate that heteroplasmy should be a key biomarker to be screened in hematological malignancy.

Neuro-oncology

Gliomatosis Cerebri (GC) is an uncommon kind of brain tumor that often destroys both lobes and, in some cases, the infratentorial areas too. The question arises if this lesion has resulted from a previously injured huge section of brain tissue. In a GC investigation, tissue samples from 24 patients were obtained randomly from various sections of the brain. All samples were checked for chromosomal errors across the whole genome, p53 mutations, and LOH. The p53 gene was mutated in all 24 specimens, while numerous additional tumor specimens revealed chromosomal deletions or abnormalities [15]. In another study, mtDNA was utilized as a clonal indicator to GC. In all but two patients, a continuous reduction of mtDNA was observed, with one of them having p53 mutations [74]. These data reveal that the current findings of field cancerization in epithelial cancers could be used with simple modifications in neuro-oncological cancers, wherever appropriate.

Changes in Local Onco-Sphere That Affect Field Cancerization

As we mentioned above, local *onco-sphere* is made up a plethora of cells, especially stromal cells (*i.e.,* CAFs, ECMs, adipocytes, etc.) reprogramming of stromal cells are playing a crucial role in tumorigenesis [75], and therefore, these changes are equally important in field cancerization. In many cases, changes in the stromal component are already found in pre-malignant tissue. In breast cancer, CAFs are important modulator in the cancer growth and metastasis by directly modulating changes in the epithelial cells or use indirect method (*i.e.,* secretion of cytokines, GFs, exosomes) to induce changes that can lead to field cancerization [76, 77]. This is observable in IBD patients, where severe inflammatory condition in the colon led to a higher risk of CRCs, and inflammation is an independent risk factor for colon cancer [78]. Similarly, in Barrett's Esophagus, changes in gene expression of stromal component can predict malignancy, and these changes are shown to be similar to pre-cancerous GI tracts [79]. In skin cancer, when their mesenchymal cells in the skin is indicative of Notch family signaling loss, epithelial tumorigenesis is induced, again indicating the importance of stromal cell in field cancerization [80]. In colon cancer, changes in BMP pathway variants at multiple loci (GREM1, BMP-2, BMP-4) by stromal cells are found to be the key to modulate cancer risk [81].

There changes in the local *onco-sphere* could indeed alter the genetic and epigenetic changes in epithelial cells, leading to field cancerization. The changes in the local *onco-sphere* could provide the cancer cells a choice to adapt to these pressures, which could lead to a "phenotype adaptation," where cancer cells made appropriate changes in order to survive in the cancerized field. This could happen via changes in genotype (genetic mutation) or phenotype (plasticity of morphology, mimic, camouflage). Among these changes, cancer cells that are adapting on the genome level are important, as these are the changes that would be reflected in future generations, therefore creating stronger "fit" clones that could survive the harsh conditions in the new environment. A model of "fitness landscape" has been proposed for carcinogenesis, with six major barriers that could hinder a malignant phenotype change, a model that represents the intercommunication and cross talk within tumor–stroma–immune cell axis in the local *onco-sphere*. These are: apoptosis, growth retardation, cell senescence, hypoxic condition, high acidic condition, and ischemic condition [82]. We now understand that apart from these factors, the interplay between various cells in the local *onco-sphere*, such as genetic mutations, secretion of various growth factors, cytokines, chemokines, and more recently, the inclusion of nerves, host ecosystem are also very important in cancer outgrowth [83]. Therefore, it is again emphasizing on the importance of observing a cancer and a metastatic clone (field cancerization) as an ecosystem, as these cells are self-sustainable and could easily adapt to produce an especially "fit" close that can survive against anti-tumoral environment.

Box 10.2 Single-Cell Analysis: Spatiotemporal Molecular and Cellular "Atlas" of Field Carcinogenesis

In order to clearly identify the role of each component of the local *onco-sphere* and their contribution toward field carcinogenesis, single-cell-based approaches have been used to screen and identify changes that could be significantly seen among normal, normal-like, pre-malignant, and malignant cells. The dynamic changes during cell's transformation could be extracted and analyzed at the single-cell level, enabling a thorough investigation of cell changes and interactions from the very beginning of hyperplastic and neoplastic progression [84]. Not only that, in-depth study on the cell's interaction with multiple tissues in their proximity could also be identified (Fig. 10.2). Through the addition of -omics platforms (including genomic, transcriptomic, proteomic, and metabolomic profile), we can expect a fully comprehensive understanding of the evolutionary changes that occur in a cell during the pre-malignancy time point, which has not been captured in detail before.

By a deep analysis using single-cell omics approaches, we hope to one day elucidate all the questions raised above, and many others that are related to this field. By the combination of all the -omics approach, one could depict the spatiotemporal molecular and cellular "atlas" of the local *onco-sphere* and keep track of their changes during the process of field cancerization. This includes the landscape of all the tumor cells, stromal cells, immune cells; including various cell subtypes, cell state as well as their interactions that are crucial drivers of field cancerization (Fig. 10.3). Other approaches such as organoid models, organ-on-a-chip, and bioprinting techniques can also be incorporated to this study (detailed in Chap. 30: bioengineering method to mimic cancer ecosystem); as *in vitro* and ex vivo models allow human intervention that could assess the effect of extracellular changes (such as carcinogens, stress, biophysical changes) toward field cancerization [85].

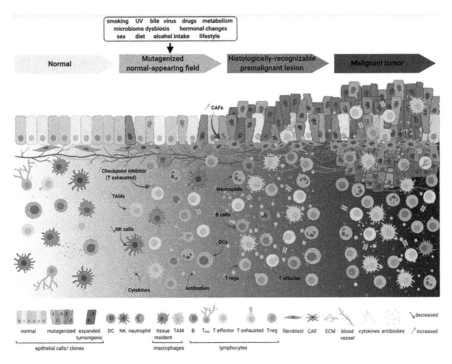

Fig 10.2 A comprehensive summary of how a view of field carcinogenesis would look like in a single-cell analysis. This model clearly depicts the dynamic changes of each cell and their changes into various subtypes and states shortly after the introduction of mutagens or carcinogens, in which the cells are still "normal" in appearance at this stage. Although these changes might not be seen histologically, single-cell changes might be able to pick up the subtle differences. At the third stage of progression, these cells are now entering a phase called "malignant lesion," where distinct morphological changes can be detected in the cells within this field. Single-cell analysis is able to detect not only the changes in each cell type, it can also record phenotypical and genotypical changes, the spatiotemporal changes, their interactions—in short, the dynamic interplay in field cancerization. During this process, the concept of cancer ecosystem is clearly depicted. For example, fibroblast can be modulated to become cancer-associated fibroblasts (CAFs) by the cancer cell, having a pro-tumoral phenotype, which in turn could secrete pro-tumoral soluble factors that support cancer cell growth, a classic symbiotic relationship. These changes are also seen in infiltrated immune cells, where their phenotypes could be skewed toward pro-tumoral (*i.e.*, M2-like TAMs, TANs, Tregs, B regs), which are all favoring cancer progression. Figures are available under Creative Commons license [84]

Clinical Relevance of Assessment of Field Cancerization

Biomarkers observed in tumors but not in adjacent normal cells are considered to aid in the early detection of cancer. These tumor-specific biomarkers are often evaluated and used for testing to identify malignancies that are localized to one organ and have a larger possibility of being cured [86]. Biosensors that demonstrate the origination

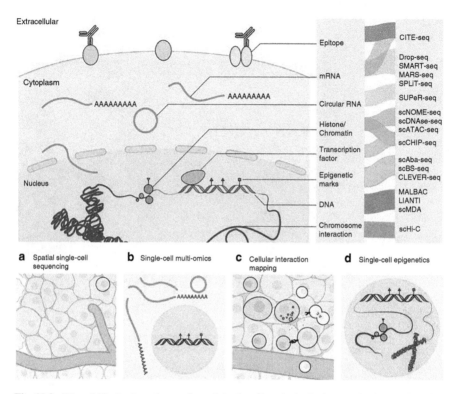

Fig. 10.3 [Upper] The basic understanding of single-cell analysis. Probes can be designed to bind to various extracellular and intracellular molecules. Changes detected in these molecules are a direct reflection of the changes that occur in the cell. [Lower] various approaches in single-cell analysis that could be implicated in the field of carcinogenesis: (**a**) spatial single-cell sequencing, a great tool for identifying the exact location of a cancer cell in relation to the environment; (**b**) single-cell multi-omics, including transcriptomics, proteomics, and metabolomics, a great tool for understanding the functional changes within a cell; (**c**) cellular interaction mapping, important for elucidating the important interactions and network between cancer cells and their surrounding stromal and immune cells; (**d**) single-cell epigenetics, a post-genomic study on how the environment-induced changes in the cell could change the cell's function and communication in the tumor environment. Figures are made available under Creative Commons Attribution 4.0 International License [85]

of an illness, rather than biomarkers of the illness itself, should be the target of future initiatives to develop and evaluate biomarkers. These biosensors may be used to determine how harmful a substance is, detect it early, monitor an illness, and treat it with medications. For instance, LOH in healthy breast epithelial cells was extracted via a random FNA biopsy to determine the likelihood of breast cancer in women having a pre-identified risk of breast cancer [48]. According to the Gail risk model, women lacking LOH had a 16.7% lifetime risk of breast cancer, whereas women having LOH had a 22.9% lifetime risk [48]. Owing to the connection between these indicators and a patient's chance of developing breast cancer, they might be used for its early detection and estimation of the likelihood of its occurrence.

As genetic alteration is usually hidden and not obvious until it has accumulated to a certain threshold, these early genetic alterations should be exploited to identify and stratify individuals with higher cancer risk and probably enlist them for initial chemoprevention. Epigenetic-wise, early indicators in many epithelial cancers include hypermethylation of promoters, transcriptional suppression of anti-tumor related genes. Knowing the mechanism of methylation patterns to evolve into cancer enables us to use drugs that reverse methylation in a regulated manner to prevent cancer from occurring at all. Similarly, relative markers detected in pre-cancerous lesions will be appropriate endpoint measurements or secondary chemoprevention objectives. As an alternative noninvasive method for detecting early signs of field cancerization, biofluids containing cells from a specific organ can be employed as non-harmful or minimally harmful samples for disease monitoring. For instance, nipple aspirate fluids may reveal genetic alterations prior to the development of breast cancer.

Multiphase field cancerization demonstrates two degrees of cancer advancement: molecular progression, involving the accumulation of extra genomic damage in histologically healthy-looking cells with the passage of time, and phenotypic progression, involving the accumulation of additional genetic and phenotypic alterations in a neoplastic cell. Modification of functionally essential channels at the molecular advancement stage must result in effective biosensors for detecting and monitoring cancer at an initial stage. Furthermore, it is generally understood that all pre-cancerous lesions do not develop into malignancies that propagate to other body parts [87]. Thus, early lesions' molecular sequencing is vital, and this can allow researchers to identify crucial pathways or biomarkers that indicate the progression mechanism of a disease. Laser-capture microdissection was employed in ingenious contemporary research to obtain pure cell populations at various phases of prostate cancer development for gene synthesis profiling. Researchers discovered multiple mechanisms and genes that demonstrated the molecular evolution of prostate cancer from benign to cancerous form, beginning with prostatic intraepithelial neoplasia and concluding with prostate cancer, with the help of a novel analytical approach known as the "molecular concept model." Higher expression of genes on 8q that govern the cell cycle has been associated with disease progression [59]. Atypical hyperplasia progresses to adenocarcinoma in approximately 5–20 years. Because of the extended time span, it is feasible to detect early indicators of an activated pre-cancerous epithelial field [87, 88]. Most significantly, field cancerization helps in evaluating pathologic biopsy samples in clinical settings. Histology, the gold standard, is used to look at biopsies to diagnose cancer, and the lack of abnormal cells often rules out a cancer diagnosis. A biopsy specimen that seems healthy but exhibits molecular markers of cancer implies that either the tumor was not detected during the biopsy or that some of the tissue cells are on the verge of turning malignant. These patients at high risk require regular monitoring in order to detect illnesses early.

Tumor Margins and Recurrences

Tumors are prone to frequent recurrence in surgical oncology, and based on the type of tumor, the likelihood of recurrence might be as high as 50% [89]. Local tumor relapses are classified into two types: the ones occurring at the parent site of surgical recurrence (regional or scar recurrence) and the ones occurring in the leftover organ after the removal of the parent tumor *(in situ* recurrences, Second Primary Tumor (SPT), or Second Field Tumors) (SFT)). SFT refers to *in situ* relapses having genetic similarity with the initial tumor, whereas real SPT refers to the relapses having distinct genetic variations from the primary tumor. Field cancerization may result in the recurrence of a huge number of malignancies, for instance, scar recurrence, which is likely to be induced by a surgical resection gap that comprises an area with altered genes. According to this theory, molecular characterization of surgical gaps might help reduce recurrent scars. Considering the presence of several cancer patches in the same organ affected by the same substance, clear molecular margins may fail to stop recurrences in the surviving organ. To illustrate, screening of K-Ras codon 12 mutations in peripheral surgical tissues from 70 individuals suffering from pancreatic cancer yet appearing to be normal histologically might help in determining or conceptualizing how the illness would proceed. In this research, as high as 53% of patients with positive boundaries from molecular screening had a worse OS [90].

Conclusion

Field cancerization is a critical step in cancer infiltration. With the advancement of technology, well-designed research should aid in the discovery of genetic indicators and pathways for future use to treat illnesses. Virtually all investigations based on field cancerization lack sufficient genome-wide analyses to diagnose initial and significant genetic alterations in the evolution of tumors with the passage of time. Several investigations have depended largely on factors that have been related to a certain malignancy. Such tumor indicators may emerge subsequently in the disease cycle and will remain undetected in specimens from the tumor-adjacent fields or pre-cancerous lesions. These pre-cancerous tumors (local metastasis) may give insight into how they differ or are analogous to the metastatic cascade. Field cancerization also prompted us about the significance of each mutagenic/physical alteration in neoplasia and the need for greater attention to be accorded to proactive cancer identification.

References

1. Slaughter D, Southwick H, Smejkal W (1953) Field cancerization in oral stratified squamous epithelium; clinical implications of multicentric origin. Cancer 6(5):963–968
2. Braakhuis BJ, Tabor MP, Kummer JA, Leemans CR, Brakenhoff RH (2003) A genetic explanation of Slaughter's concept of field cancerization: evidence and clinical implications. Cancer Res 63(8):1727–1730
3. Prevo LJ, Sanchez CA, Galipeau PC, Reid BJ (1999) p53-mutant clones and field effects in Barrett's esophagus. Cancer Res 59(19):4784–4787
4. Simon R, Eltze E, Schäfer KL, Bürger H, Semjonow A, Hertle L et al (2001) Cytogenetic analysis of multifocal bladder cancer supports a monoclonal origin and intraepithelial spread of tumor cells. Cancer Res 61(1):355–362
5. Tabor MP, Brakenhoff RH, Ruijter-Schippers HJ, Van Der Wal JE, Snow GB, Leemans CR et al (2002) Multiple head and neck tumors frequently originate from a single preneoplastic lesion. Am J Pathol 161(3):1051–1060
6. Smeds J, Wärnberg F, Norberg T, Nordgren H, Holmberg L, Bergh J (2005) Ductal carcinoma in situ of the breast with different histopathological grades and corresponding new breast tumour events: analysis of loss of heterozygosity. Acta Oncol 44(1):41–49
7. Larson PS, de las Morenas A, Bennett SR, Cupples LA, Rosenberg CL (2002) Loss of heterozygosity or allele imbalance in histologically normal breast epithelium is distinct from loss of heterozygosity or allele imbalance in co-existing carcinomas. Am J Pathol 161(1): 283–290
8. Chandran UR, Dhir R, Ma C, Michalopoulos G, Becich M, Gilbertson J (2005) Differences in gene expression in prostate cancer, normal appearing prostate tissue adjacent to cancer and prostate tissue from cancer free organ donors. BMC Cancer 5:45
9. Ha PK, Tong BC, Westra WH, Sanchez-Cespedes M, Parrella P, Zahurak M et al (2002) Mitochondrial C-tract alteration in premalignant lesions of the head and neck: a marker for progression and clonal proliferation. Clin Cancer Res 8(7):2260–2265
10. Heaphy CM, Bisoffi M, Fordyce CA, Haaland CM, Hines WC, Joste NE et al (2006) Telomere DNA content and allelic imbalance demonstrate field cancerization in histologically normal tissue adjacent to breast tumors. Int J Cancer 119(1):108–116
11. Deng G, Lu Y, Zlotnikov G, Thor AD, Smith HS (1996) Loss of heterozygosity in normal tissue adjacent to breast carcinomas. Science 274(5295):2057–2059
12. Shen L, Kondo Y, Rosner GL, Xiao L, Hernandez NS, Vilaythong J et al (2005) MGMT promoter methylation and field defect in sporadic colorectal cancer. J Natl Cancer Inst 97(18): 1330–1338
13. Sui G, Zhou S, Wang J, Canto M, Lee EE, Eshleman JR et al (2006) Mitochondrial DNA mutations in preneoplastic lesions of the gastrointestinal tract: a biomarker for the early detection of cancer. Mol Cancer 5:73
14. Tabor MP, Brakenhoff RH, Ruijter-Schippers HJ, Kummer JA, Leemans CR, Braakhuis BJ (2004) Genetically altered fields as origin of locally recurrent head and neck cancer: a retrospective study. Clin Cancer Res 10(11):3607–3613
15. Kros JM, Zheng P, Dinjens WN, Alers JC (2002) Genetic aberrations in gliomatosis cerebri support monoclonal tumorigenesis. J Neuropathol Exp Neurol 61(9):806–814
16. Brodsky RA, Jones RJ (2004) Riddle: what do aplastic anemia, acute promyelocytic leukemia, and chronic myeloid leukemia have in common? Leukemia 18(10):1740–1742
17. Trujillo KA, Jones AC, Griffith JK, Bisoffi M (2012) Markers of field cancerization: proposed clinical applications in prostate biopsies. Prostate Cancer 2012:302894
18. van Oijen MG, Slootweg PJ (2000) Oral field cancerization: carcinogen-induced independent events or micrometastatic deposits? Cancer Epidemiol Biomarkers Prev 9(3):249–256
19. Ha PK, Califano JA (2003) The molecular biology of mucosal field cancerization of the head and neck. Crit Rev Oral Biol Med 14(5):363–369

20. Roesch-Ely M, Nees M, Karsai S, Ruess A, Bogumil R, Warnken U et al (2007) Proteomic analysis reveals successive aberrations in protein expression from healthy mucosa to invasive head and neck cancer. Oncogene 26(1):54–64

21. Kim MM, Clinger JD, Masayesva BG, Ha PK, Zahurak ML, Westra WH et al (2004) Mitochondrial DNA quantity increases with histopathologic grade in premalignant and malignant head and neck lesions. Clin Cancer Res 10(24):8512–8515

22. Shieh DB, Chou WP, Wei YH, Wong TY, Jin YT (2004) Mitochondrial DNA 4,977-bp deletion in paired oral cancer and precancerous lesions revealed by laser microdissection and real-time quantitative PCR. Ann N Y Acad Sci 1011:154–167

23. Franklin WA, Gazdar AF, Haney J, Wistuba II, La Rosa FG, Kennedy T et al (1997) Widely dispersed p53 mutation in respiratory epithelium. A novel mechanism for field carcinogenesis. J Clin Invest 100(8):2133–2137

24. Park IW, Wistuba II, Maitra A, Milchgrub S, Virmani AK, Minna JD et al (1999) Multiple clonal abnormalities in the bronchial epithelium of patients with lung cancer. J Natl Cancer Inst 91(21):1863–1868

25. Grepmeier U, Dietmaier W, Merk J, Wild PJ, Obermann EC, Pfeifer M et al (2005) Deletions at chromosome 2q and 12p are early and frequent molecular alterations in bronchial epithelium and NSCLC of long-term smokers. Int J Oncol 27(2):481–488

26. Pan H, Califano J, Ponte JF, Russo AL, Cheng KH, Thiagalingam A et al (2005) Loss of heterozygosity patterns provide fingerprints for genetic heterogeneity in multistep cancer progression of tobacco smoke-induced non-small cell lung cancer. Cancer Res 65(5): 1664–1669

27. Galipeau PC, Prevo LJ, Sanchez CA, Longton GM, Reid BJ (1999) Clonal expansion and loss of heterozygosity at chromosomes 9p and 17p in premalignant esophageal (Barrett's) tissue. J Natl Cancer Inst 91(24):2087–2095

28. Wong DJ, Paulson TG, Prevo LJ, Galipeau PC, Longton G, Blount PL et al (2001) p16(INK4a) lesions are common, early abnormalities that undergo clonal expansion in Barrett's metaplastic epithelium. Cancer Res 61(22):8284–8289

29. Eads CA, Lord RV, Kurumboor SK, Wickramasinghe K, Skinner ML, Long TI et al (2000) Fields of aberrant CpG island hypermethylation in Barrett's esophagus and associated adenocarcinoma. Cancer Res 60(18):5021–5026

30. Maley CC, Galipeau PC, Li X, Sanchez CA, Paulson TG, Blount PL et al (2004) The combination of genetic instability and clonal expansion predicts progression to esophageal adenocarcinoma. Cancer Res 64(20):7629–7633

31. Merlo LM, Pepper JW, Reid BJ, Maley CC (2006) Cancer as an evolutionary and ecological process. Nat Rev Cancer 6(12):924–935

32. Maley CC, Galipeau PC, Finley JC, Wongsurawat VJ, Li X, Sanchez CA et al (2006) Genetic clonal diversity predicts progression to esophageal adenocarcinoma. Nat Genet 38(4):468–473

33. Kang GH, Kim CJ, Kim WH, Kang YK, Kim HO, Kim YI (1997) Genetic evidence for the multicentric origin of synchronous multiple gastric carcinoma. Lab Invest 76(3):407–417

34. Kim SK, Jang HR, Kim JH, Noh SM, Song KS, Kim MR et al (2006) The epigenetic silencing of LIMS2 in gastric cancer and its inhibitory effect on cell migration. Biochem Biophys Res Commun 349(3):1032–1040

35. Kim JY, Cho HJ (2000) DNA ploidy patterns in gastric adenocarcinoma. J Korean Med Sci 15(2):159–166

36. Jothy S, Slesak B, Harłozińska A, Lapińska J, Adamiak J, Rabczyński J (1996) Field effect of human colon carcinoma on normal mucosa: relevance of carcinoembryonic antigen expression. Tumour Biol 17(1):58–64

37. Grady WM (2005) Epigenetic events in the colorectum and in colon cancer. Biochem Soc Trans 33(Pt 4):684–688

38. Rosenthal AN, Ryan A, Hopster D, Jacobs IJ (2002) Molecular evidence of a common clonal origin and subsequent divergent clonal evolution in vulval intraepithelial neoplasia, vulval squamous cell carcinoma and lymph node metastases. Int J Cancer 99(4):549–554

39. Kanjilal S, Strom SS, Clayman GL, Weber RS, el-Naggar AK, Kapur V et al (1995) p53 mutations in nonmelanoma skin cancer of the head and neck: molecular evidence for field cancerization. Cancer Res 55(16):3604–3609
40. Jonason AS, Kunala S, Price GJ, Restifo RJ, Spinelli HM, Persing JA et al (1996) Frequent clones of p53-mutated keratinocytes in normal human skin. Proc Natl Acad Sci U S A 93(24): 14025–14029
41. Eshaghian A, Vleugels RA, Canter JA, McDonald MA, Stasko T, Sligh JE (2006) Mitochondrial DNA deletions serve as biomarkers of aging in the skin, but are typically absent in nonmelanoma skin cancers. J Invest Dermatol 126(2):336–344
42. Oskarsson T, Massagué J (2012) Extracellular matrix players in metastatic niches. EMBO J 31(2):254–256
43. Ratushny V, Gober MD, Hick R, Ridky TW, Seykora JT (2012) From keratinocyte to cancer: the pathogenesis and modeling of cutaneous squamous cell carcinoma. J Clin Invest 122(2): 464–472
44. Bhowmick NA, Chytil A, Plieth D, Gorska AE, Dumont N, Shappell S et al (2004) TGF-beta signaling in fibroblasts modulates the oncogenic potential of adjacent epithelia. Science 303(5659):848–851
45. Hill R, Song Y, Cardiff RD, Van Dyke T (2005) Selective evolution of stromal mesenchyme with p53 loss in response to epithelial tumorigenesis. Cell 123(6):1001–1011
46. Denzinger S, Mohren K, Knuechel R, Wild PJ, Burger M, Wieland WF et al (2006) Improved clonality analysis of multifocal bladder tumors by combination of histopathologic organ mapping, loss of heterozygosity, fluorescence in situ hybridization, and p53 analyses. Hum Pathol 37(2):143–151
47. Höglund M (2007) Bladder cancer, a two phased disease? Semin Cancer Biol 17(3):225–232
48. Euhus DM, Cler L, Shivapurkar N, Milchgrub S, Peters GN, Leitch AM et al (2002) Loss of heterozygosity in benign breast epithelium in relation to breast cancer risk. J Natl Cancer Inst 94(11):858–860
49. Ellsworth DL, Ellsworth RE, Love B, Deyarmin B, Lubert SM, Mittal V et al (2004) Outer breast quadrants demonstrate increased levels of genomic instability. Ann Surg Oncol 11(9): 861–868
50. Amari M, Moriya T, Ishida T, Harada Y, Ohnuki K, Takeda M et al (2003) Loss of heterozygosity analyses of asynchronous lesions of ductal carcinoma in situ and invasive ductal carcinoma of the human breast. Jpn J Clin Oncol 33(11):556–562
51. Lewis CM, Cler LR, Bu DW, Zöchbauer-Müller S, Milchgrub S, Naftalis EZ et al (2005) Promoter hypermethylation in benign breast epithelium in relation to predicted breast cancer risk. Clin Cancer Res 11(1):166–172
52. Yan PS, Venkataramu C, Ibrahim A, Liu JC, Shen RZ, Diaz NM et al (2006) Mapping geographic zones of cancer risk with epigenetic biomarkers in normal breast tissue. Clin Cancer Res 12(22):6626–6636
53. Hanson JA, Gillespie JW, Grover A, Tangrea MA, Chuaqui RF, Emmert-Buck MR et al (2006) Gene promoter methylation in prostate tumor-associated stromal cells. J Natl Cancer Inst 98(4): 255–261
54. Fordyce CA, Heaphy CM, Joste NE, Smith AY, Hunt WC, Griffith JK (2005) Association between cancer-free survival and telomere DNA content in prostate tumors. J Urol 173(2): 610–614
55. Pathak S, Nemeth MA, Multani AS, Thalmann GN, von Eschenbach AC, Chung LW (1997) Can cancer cells transform normal host cells into malignant cells? Br J Cancer 76(9):1134–1138
56. Yu YP, Landsittel D, Jing L, Nelson J, Ren B, Liu L et al (2004) Gene expression alterations in prostate cancer predicting tumor aggression and preceding development of malignancy. J Clin Oncol 22(14):2790–2799
57. Uetsuki H, Tsunemori H, Taoka R, Haba R, Ishikawa M, Kakehi Y (2005) Expression of a novel biomarker, EPCA, in adenocarcinomas and precancerous lesions in the prostate. J Urol 174(2):514–518

58. Dhir R, Vietmeier B, Arlotti J, Acquafondata M, Landsittel D, Masterson R et al (2004) Early identification of individuals with prostate cancer in negative biopsies. J Urol 171(4):1419–1423

59. Tomlins SA, Mehra R, Rhodes DR, Cao X, Wang L, Dhanasekaran SM et al (2007) Integrative molecular concept modeling of prostate cancer progression. Nat Genet 39(1):41–51

60. Malins DC, Gilman NK, Green VM, Wheeler TM, Barker EA, Anderson KM (2005) A cancer DNA phenotype in healthy prostates, conserved in tumors and adjacent normal cells, implies a relationship to carcinogenesis. Proc Natl Acad Sci U S A 102(52):19093–19096

61. Malins DC, Johnson PM, Barker EA, Polissar NL, Wheeler TM, Anderson KM (2003) Cancer-related changes in prostate DNA as men age and early identification of metastasis in primary prostate tumors. Proc Natl Acad Sci U S A 100(9):5401–5406

62. Malins DC, Anderson KM, Gilman NK, Green VM, Barker EA, Hellström KE (2004) Development of a cancer DNA phenotype prior to tumor formation. Proc Natl Acad Sci U S A 101(29):10721–10725

63. Malins DC, Gilman NK, Green VM, Wheeler TM, Barker EA, Vinson MA et al (2004) Metastatic cancer DNA phenotype identified in normal tissues surrounding metastasizing prostate carcinomas. Proc Natl Acad Sci U S A 101(31):11428–11431

64. Perry AS, Foley R, Woodson K, Lawler M (2006) The emerging roles of DNA methylation in the clinical management of prostate cancer. Endocr Relat Cancer 13(2):357–377

65. Jerónimo C, Nomoto S, Caballero OL, Usadel H, Henrique R, Varzim G et al (2001) Mitochondrial mutations in early stage prostate cancer and bodily fluids. Oncogene 20(37):5195–5198

66. Parr RL, Dakubo GD, Crandall KA, Maki J, Reguly B, Aguirre A et al (2006) Somatic mitochondrial DNA mutations in prostate cancer and normal appearing adjacent glands in comparison to age-matched prostate samples without malignant histology. J Mol Diagn 8(3):312–319

67. Ortiz BH, Ailawadi M, Colitti C, Muto MG, Deavers M, Silva EG et al (2001) Second primary or recurrence? Comparative patterns of p53 and K-ras mutations suggest that serous borderline ovarian tumors and subsequent serous carcinomas are unrelated tumors. Cancer Res 61(19):7264–7267

68. Buller RE, Skilling JS, Sood AK, Plaxe S, Baergen RN, Lager DJ (1998) Field cancerization: why late "recurrent" ovarian cancer is not recurrent. Am J Obstet Gynecol 178(4):641–649

69. Furlan D, Carnevali I, Marcomini B, Cerutti R, Dainese E, Capella C et al (2006) The high frequency of de novo promoter methylation in synchronous primary endometrial and ovarian carcinomas. Clin Cancer Res 12(11 pt 1):3329–3336

70. Izawa T, Obara T, Tanno S, Mizukami Y, Yanagawa N, Kohgo Y (2001) Clonality and field cancerization in intraductal papillary-mucinous tumors of the pancreas. Cancer 92(7):1807–1817

71. Kitago M, Ueda M, Aiura K, Suzuki K, Hoshimoto S, Takahashi S et al (2004) Comparison of K-ras point mutation distributions in intraductal papillary-mucinous tumors and ductal adenocarcinoma of the pancreas. Int J Cancer 110(2):177–182

72. Z'Graggen K, Rivera JA, Compton CC, Pins M, Werner J, Fernández-del Castillo C et al (1997) Prevalence of activating K-ras mutations in the evolutionary stages of neoplasia in intraductal papillary mucinous tumors of the pancreas. Ann Surg 226(4):491–498; discussion 498–500

73. Linnartz B, Anglmayer R, Zanssen S (2004) Comprehensive scanning of somatic mitochondrial DNA alterations in acute leukemia developing from myelodysplastic syndromes. Cancer Res 64(6):1966–1971

74. Kirches E, Mawrin C, Schneider-Stock R, Krause G, Scherlach C, Dietzmann K (2003) Mitochondrial DNA as a clonal tumor cell marker: gliomatosis cerebri. J Neurooncol 61(1):1–5

75. Mantovani A, Allavena P, Sica A, Balkwill F (2008) Cancer-related inflammation. Nature 454(7203):436–444

76. Bronisz A, Godlewski J, Wallace JA, Merchant AS, Nowicki MO, Mathsyaraja H et al (2011) Reprogramming of the tumour microenvironment by stromal PTEN-regulated miR-320. Nat Cell Biol 14(2):159–167

77. Quail DF, Joyce JA (2013) Microenvironmental regulation of tumor progression and metastasis. Nat Med 19(11):1423–1437
78. Rutter M, Saunders B, Wilkinson K, Rumbles S, Schofield G, Kamm M et al (2004) Severity of inflammation is a risk factor for colorectal neoplasia in ulcerative colitis. Gastroenterology 126(2):451–459
79. Saadi A, Shannon NB, Lao-Sirieix P, O'Donovan M, Walker E, Clemons NJ et al (2010) Stromal genes discriminate preinvasive from invasive disease, predict outcome, and highlight inflammatory pathways in digestive cancers. Proc Natl Acad Sci U S A 107(5):2177–2182
80. Hu B, Castillo E, Harewood L, Ostano P, Reymond A, Dummer R et al (2012) Multifocal epithelial tumors and field cancerization from loss of mesenchymal CSL signaling. Cell 149(6): 1207–1220
81. Tomlinson IP, Carvajal-Carmona LG, Dobbins SE, Tenesa A, Jones AM, Howarth K et al (2011) Multiple common susceptibility variants near BMP pathway loci GREM1, BMP4, and BMP2 explain part of the missing heritability of colorectal cancer. PLoS Genet 7(6):e1002105
82. Gatenby RA, Gillies RJ (2008) A microenvironmental model of carcinogenesis. Nat Rev Cancer 8(1):56–61
83. Perez-Mancera PA, Young AR, Narita M (2014) Inside and out: the activities of senescence in cancer. Nat Rev Cancer 14(8):547–558
84. Sinjab A, Han G, Wang L, Kadara H (2020) Field carcinogenesis in cancer evolution: what the cell is going on? Cancer Res 80(22):4888–4891
85. Ren X, Kang B, Zhang Z (2018) Understanding tumor ecosystems by single-cell sequencing: promises and limitations. Genome Biol 19(1):211
86. Stemke-Hale K, Hennessy B, Mills GB, Mitra R (2006) Molecular screening for breast cancer prevention, early detection, and treatment planning: combining biomarkers from DNA, RNA, and protein. Curr Oncol Rep 8(6):484–491
87. O'Shaughnessy JA, Kelloff GJ, Gordon GB, Dannenberg AJ, Hong WK, Fabian CJ et al (2002) Treatment and prevention of intraepithelial neoplasia: an important target for accelerated new agent development. Clin Cancer Res 8(2):314–346
88. Vanharanta S, Massague J (2012) Field cancerization: something new under the sun. Cell 149(6):1179–1181
89. Höckel M, Dornhöfer N (2005) The hydra phenomenon of cancer: why tumors recur locally after microscopically complete resection. Cancer Res 65(8):2997–3002
90. Kim J, Reber HA, Dry SM, Elashoff D, Chen SL, Umetani N et al (2006) Unfavourable prognosis associated with K-ras gene mutation in pancreatic cancer surgical margins. Gut 55(11):1598–1605

Chapter 11
Pre-Metastatic Niche: Communication Between Local and Distal *Onco-Spheres*

Phei Er Saw and Erwei Song

Abstract The pre-metastatic niche (PMN) is a complex process of the "seed and soil" compatibility. The PMN microenvironment is formed by the influence of disseminated tumor cells or tumor-derived factors on stromal and immune cells (the seeds) at distal organs (the soil), leading to the creation of a niche suitable for cancer cell growth (a favorable fertile soil for secondary cancer growth). A variety of tumor models have been employed to identify cellular and molecular components that play an important role in the formation of the pre-metastatic niche. Tumor cells, myeloid cells, and stromal cells are capable of secreting these molecular components that promote niches, collaborating with cellular components to initiate, separate, and form pre-metastatic niches in future metastatic organs. In this chapter, we will discuss on the importances of each component in the formation of distal onco-sphere.

P. E. Saw
Guangdong Provincial Key Laboratory of Malignant Tumor Epigenetics and Gene Regulation, Guangdong-Hong Kong Joint Laboratory for RNA Medicine, Medical Research Center, Sun Yat-sen Memorial Hospital, Sun Yat-sen University, Guangzhou, China

Nanhai Translational Innovation Center of Precision Immunology, Sun Yat-sen Memorial Hospital, Sun Yat-sen University, Foshan, China

E. Song (✉)
Guangdong Provincial Key Laboratory of Malignant Tumor Epigenetics and Gene Regulation, Guangdong-Hong Kong Joint Laboratory for RNA Medicine, Medical Research Center, Sun Yat-sen Memorial Hospital, Sun Yat-sen University, Guangzhou, China

Nanhai Translational Innovation Center of Precision Immunology, Sun Yat-sen Memorial Hospital, Sun Yat-sen University, Foshan, China

Breast Tumor Center, Sun Yat-sen Memorial Hospital, Sun Yat-sen University, Guangzhou, China
e-mail: songew@mail.sysu.edu.cn

Introduction

Previously in the second chapter, the local *onco-spheres* were extensively discussed in conjunction with how the local environment of the tumor does not restrict components of niche construction. For the purpose of an environment that is permissive to cancer cells, the pre-metastatic niche is primed by the systemic dissemination of signals [1]. Metastasis may succeed as a result of the remodeling of proximally distant sites due to the secretion of signal factors from cancer cells [2]. The local environment plays a significant role in influencing the production of these factors, subsequently associating the construction of distant niches in pre-metastatic organs with local resource depletion and cell-to-cell cross talk. For example, consider the case of breast cancer mouse models, due to hypoxia, lysyl oxidase expression increased, leading to the recruitment of CD11b$^+$ myeloid cells to the lung, creating a pre-metastatic niche [3]. In a similar fashion, consider preclinical models of melanoma metastasis and lung adenocarcinoma, wherein the recruitment of bone-marrow-derived cells that promote tumor cells was facilitated by the increase of fibronectin secretion in the pre-metastatic niche due to the conditioned media from tumor cells [4]. Similarly, the seeding of tumor cells at premetastatic sites is reinforced by exosomes that carry cargo all across the body and harbor non-coding RNAs, proteins [5, 6], miRNAs [7–9], with notable influences on the ecological niche such as the remodeling of the ECM [10], vascular permeability, and angiogenesis [11], in addition to the recruitment of various immune cell populations [12]. Due to the lack of an ecological approach, several therapies targeting these mechanisms of niche construction have not attained success as intended. Regarding the metastases of tumor cells, first, the cell invades the basal membrane of the blood vessels prior to its intravasation into blood circulation. Following extravasation, the cells finally disseminate in their target organs, remaining dormant at the secondary site for a specific duration before forming observable outgrowth. The occurrence of organotrophic metastasis is directed by a preconditioned niche in the distal organ that supports metastatic seeding and colonization, considering tumor cell-intrinsic metastatic propensities as a prerequisite; these have been titled pre-metastatic niches (PMNs) [1] (Fig. 11.1). A variety of tumor models have been employed to identify cellular and molecular components that play an important role in the formation of the pre-metastatic niche. Tumor cells, myeloid cells, and stromal cells are capable of secreting these molecular components that promote niches, collaborating with cellular components to initiate, separate, and form pre-metastatic niches in future metastatic organs. In this chapter, we will discuss on the importance of each component in the formation of distal *onco-sphere*.

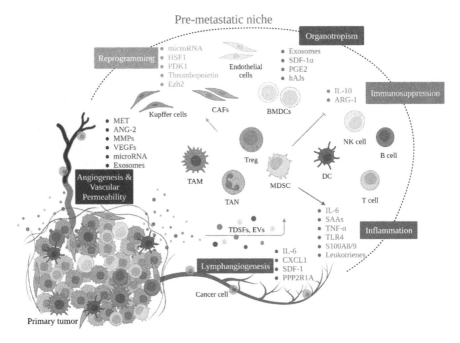

Fig. 11.1 Overview of the outgrowth of local *onco-sphere* toward a pre-metastatic niche. As mentioned in previous chapters, various stimuli can trigger the dissemination of cancer cells to a distal *onco-sphere*; these includes (1) increased angiogenesis and vascular permeability, (2) molecular reprogramming of cells (including immune, stromal, and cancer-associated factors), and (3) lymphangiogenesis. In addition, host factors such as tumor-induced immunosuppression and inflammation should also be taken into account in the process of searching of a pre-metastatic niche as a favorable distal *onco-sphere* for the tumor cell

Pre-Metastatic Niche in the Distal *Onco-Sphere*

Immunosuppression

As a result of immunosurveillance, various steps within the progression of tumors (which include the metastasis of tumors) may become abortive. Without any effect on the growth of the primary tumor, metastasis of the tumor may be prevented by non-"patrolling" monocytes, natural killer cells, and CD8$^+$ T cells [13, 14]. Hence, in order to overcome immunological elimination, tumors and their corresponding metastatic derivatives must establish specific strategies, for instance, by forming an immunosuppressive PMN. Anti-tumor immune responses are potentially suppressed through the induction of pulmonary T-cell subsets: (increasing Treg cells while decreasing effector T-cell responses) [15]. Through ROS and ARG1 production, anti-tumoral T cells may be obstructed by MDSCs accumulated in the PMN [16]. Their pro-metastatic and immunosuppressive functions may be further enforced by Breg cells induced in cancer through TGF-βR1/TGF-βR2 signaling. MDSCs can become even more suppressive to CD8$^+$ T cells in addition to producing more NO and

ROS within the presence of Breg cells [17]. The growth of liver metastasis and the promotion of tumor cell colonization take place as a result of immunosuppression mediated by MDSC as supported by TNFR-2 [18]. Furthermore, by differentiating into MDSCs, immunosuppression within the PMN is enhanced by the activation of hematopoietic progenitor/stem cells [19]. The production of IFN-γ and cytotoxicity of NK cells are suppressed by the recruitment of CD11b$^+$/Ly6C^{med}/Ly6G$^+$ myeloid cells, via monocyte chemotactic protein 1 (MCP1), to the pre-metastatic niche in the lung [20]. Across various types of human cancer, there is a significant expansion of immunosuppressive and Treg cells that promote metastasis in various organs [21]. Through the suppression of anti-tumor T cell responses, an immunosuppressive niche is developed by breast-cancer-preconditioned pulmonary alveolar macrophages, among a variety of tissue-resident cells [22].

Inflammation

In relationships shared by metastasis, inflammation, cancer growth, and regulatory immune cells, there exist several involved signaling pathways and molecular components. To illustrate, further active proliferation and invasion, as well as the death of tumor cells, may take place as a result of the inflammatory responses that take place due to the dysregulation of TLR4 activation and signaling. Such activation (in addition to other innate sensors within immune cells) leads to a type of inflammation that remains unresolved, resulting in its contributions to metastasis and tumor progression [23]. In the promotion of metastasis, inflammatory pre-metastatic niches undertake a similar role. To illustrate, the expression of serum amyloid A (SAA)3, which works to recruit Mac1$^+$ myeloid cells to these sites via TLR4, is induced by S100A9/A8 at pre-metastatic niches in the lung [24]. Tumor metastasis is also enhanced by inflammatory responses enacted by neutrophils accumulated in the PMN. The metastasis of breast cancer cells and colonization of the lung are supported by leukotrienes secreted by neutrophils [25]. Angiogenesis may be stimulated by neutrophilic inflammation driven by TLR4 and MYD88, and these are also responsible for the increase in metastasis of melanoma cells to the lymph nodes and lung [26]. As the expression of Th2 cytokine increases, MMPs increment and IFN-γ production decrement could lead to activation of CD11b$^+$Gr-1$^+$ cells in the lung pre-metastatic niche, where these cells are responsible for converting the niche site into a proliferative and inflammatory proliferative microenvironment [27].

The Spatiotemporal Formation of PMN

Generally, the formation of PMNs is divided into four steps: priming, licensing, initiation, and progression. In this section, we will discuss briefly on the important biological changes in each spatiotemporal formation of the PMN (also summarized in Fig. 11.2 below).

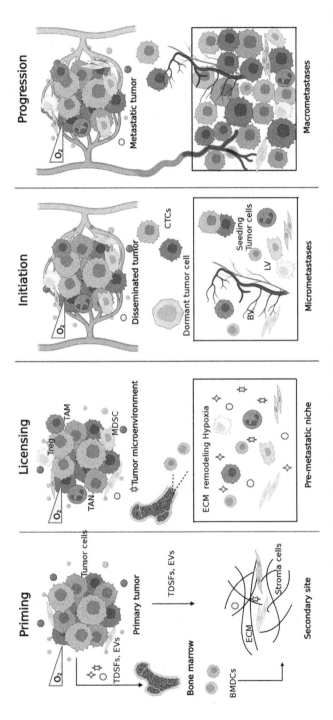

Fig. 11.2 The four steps in PMNs formation. (*Priming*) tumor cells in the local *onco-sphere* produces multiple factors (GFs, EVs, and other biomolecular components) to trigger the PMN in a distal *onco-sphere*. (*Licensing*) In response to the tumor-derived components, immunosuppressive or regulatory immune cells (i.e., BMDCs, Tregs) are mobilized and recruited to the secondary sites of PMN. These sites are nourished and nurtured to prepare for the coming of disseminated tumor cells. (*Initiation*) Here, CTCs will arrive and colonize the "soil," a process called micro-metastasis (detailed in Chap. 12). (*Progression*) PMNs are now fertile and ready for more tumor cells to grow and proliferate

Priming

Without any restraint, primary tumors may proliferate to become inflammatory and hypoxic during the phase of priming, which results in the emergence of various molecular components such as EVs and TDSFs, thereby (1) inducing various immune cells and BMDCs mobilization, (2) reeducating and reprogramming the stromal environment in the distal *onco-sphere*, (3) formation of PMNs in the suitable metastasis site. At this point, however, is the initial step of the whole process. At this phase, the pre-metastatic niche is not sufficiently prepared for the colonization or the seeding of metastatic tumor cells.

Licensing

Licensing is a phase wherein suppressive/immune cells and BMDCs are perpetually recruited and mobilized into secondary sites as a response to tumor cell-secreted EVs and TDSFs. The niche is converted as a mature and fertile site with enriched components that promote tumors in preparation for the CTCs that are incoming as a result of the intensity and duration of the interaction between distant stromal environments and TDSFs/recruited cells. These secondary sites can be predisposed as supportive pre-metastatic niches due to the activation of chemokines and integrins as well as the induction of ECM remodeling. Moreover, EMT (epithelial–mesenchymal transition) of tumor cells may be evoked by ECM remodeling, molecular constituents (e.g., IL-1β) and regulatory immune cells (e.g., MDSCs) [28] in the pre-metastatic niche, thereby promoting invasiveness of tumor cells and endowment of stemness properties. According to recent studies, EMT may not necessarily be considered dispensable for pancreatic cancer metastasis [29, 30]. Further investigation is required for examining the significance of tumor EMT during the formation of pre-metastatic niche in the broader context of tumor metastasis. Regardless, the local microenvironment is significantly modified by the accumulated interactions across host stroma secondary sites, TDSFs, and BMDCs, thereby forming a developed PNMs that prepare the secondary sites for the eventual colonization and seeding of tumor cells.

Initiation

Through the facilitation of extravasating CTCs from the vasculature and attracting colonization of tumor cells into the niche, the initiation of metastasis may be significantly benefited from the primary tumor-educated, mature PNMs. The extravasation and chemotaxis of tumor cells, through the mediation of proangiogenic factors (such as VEGF and PDFG), take place as a result of the increase of HIF-1 in the pre-metastatic niche [31]. Through the act of nudging tumor cells into a state of inertness prior to their reactivation until an ideal niche microenvironment is achieved for outgrowth into metastatic lesions—in this manner, tumor cell dormancy is regulated by the pre-metastatic niche. The induction of tumor cell dormancy is closely linked with chemotherapy, surgery, and anti-tumor response [32]. Through the suppression of the target gene MARCKS, dormancy of breast cancer cells is induced in the pre-metastatic niche as a result of the exosomal transfer of miR-23b from bone marrow MSCs [33]. Tumor cell evades dormancy due to certain pro-metastatic variables in the pre-metastatic niche (such as ECM remodeling and immunosuppression) [34, 35].

Progression

A significant score of tumor cells consistently exists in the aggressive metastatic primary site during this phase. The pathological progression traced from micrometastases to the important micrometastases resulted from the expansion of the tumor mass and the growth of the tumor cell in the metastatic organ owing to components of the PNMs. Through engagement of $\alpha 4\beta 1^+$ integrin receptors, VCAM-1 interacts with osteoclast progenitors to transition from indolent micrometastases to bone metastasis in the bone microenvironment of patients with breast cancer [36]. Tumor dissemination may be further promoted and observable macro-metastases may be expanded in form as a result of established metastatic lesions or the pre-metastatic niche containing the tumor cell.

Crosstalk Between Local *Onco-Sphere* and Metastatic Niche

The Pro-Metastatic Secretome

Taking lung cancer as an example, the first molecules to have demonstrated support for the formation of PMN are pro-angiogenic factors (placenta growth factor and VEGFA) in addition to chemokines and inflammatory cytokines released by primary tumor cells (TNF-α and TGF-β) [24, 37]. Moreover, it was found that out of all the variables that support recruitment of BMDC for potential PMNs, the tumor-secreted G-CSF mimics the microenvironment of the pre-metastatic lung [38]. An additional chemokine that is derived from a tumor and plays an imperative role in the formation of PMNs is the CCL2, a powerful chemoattractant for macrophages, memory T cells, NK cells, and monocytes [39]. The correlation between the overexpression of CCL2 and poor prognosis in various types of primary tumors successfully reflects the significant functionalities of the chemokine in the progression of cancer [39–44]. Following the formation of PMN, the earliest phases of metastatic colonization can be modulated by CCL2 derived from stromal cells and primary breast tumor cells through the recruitment of inflammatory monocytes simplifying the extravasation of CTC in a VEGFA-dependent manner, thereby encouraging the micro-metastasis of the lung in an efficacious manner [45]. In experimental models of both breast cancer and melanoma, CCL2 works to hinder the maturation of NK cells in lung

PMN, potentially reducing their ability to obliterate incoming CTCs [20]. Furthermore, CCL2 works to recruit mature macrophages for the purpose of promoting breast cancer metastasis in the lungs by furthering invasion and early formation of tumor cell clusters; and finally, through the enhancement of osteoclast differentiation as well the "vicious" cycle of bone metastasis [46, 47]. However, neutrophil-mediated cytotoxicity is induced by CCL2 in the pre-metastatic lung in the 4 T1 syngeneic model of breast cancer by elevating levels of G-CSF levels, thereby impeding the seeding process of tumor cells in PMNS; this is proven by the low number of metastatic foci (while there is no reduction in size) [48].

The S100 family of proteins is an important inflammatory mediator, playing critical role in the interactions tumor and stromal cells in the formation of PMNs [49, 50]. It is important to note that these proteins engage in both intracellular and extracellular operations. S100 proteins control the proliferation, differentiation, apoptosis, Ca^{2+} homeostasis, migration, and invasion within cells. Extracellular S100 proteins are demonstrative of paracrine and autocrine effects by activating GPCRs, scavenger receptors, cell surface receptors, N-glycans, and heparan sulfate proteoglycans and N-glycans [50, 51]. The expression of S100A8 and S100A9 is induced by TNF-α, TGF-β, and VEGFA, via ECs and CD11b$^+$ myeloid cells [24, 37, 52]. In mouse models, it was observed that S100 proteins during this process encourage the secretion and expression of serum amyloid A3 (SAA3), thereby recruiting tumor cells and myeloid cells to PMNs; which necessitates the activation of TLR4 via SAA3 in addition to NF-κB signaling [24]. As has been illustrated through preclinical models of breast cancer, PMN formation deems that the activation of HIF1 is highly essential since it is a significant protein that is induced at PMNs [3, 53–55]. Hypoxia responses mediated by HIF1α within the primary tumor potentially bolster the production of EVs and protein factors essential to the metastatic potential and formation of PMN [56]. To illustrate, EV shedding in the lines of breast cancer cells increases due to the expression of the small GTPase RAB22A, which depends on HIF [57]. It is yet uncertain whether vesicle cargo derived from tumors and the subsequent education of stromal cells within distant PMNs are modified by HIF signaling or hypoxia.

EVs are classified based on their origin and size as microvesicles (> 150 nm) and exosomes (30–150 nm); the former develop through a budding mechanism at the surface of the cell while the latter is secreted in the multivesicular and endo-lysosomal compartments to be released externally to the cell [58, 59]. The mechanisms relevant to the release of EVs as well as the fusion and docking involved in the pathological and physiological processes of EVs continue to remain a subject of study. Within the cell, the movement of EVs necessitates associated molecular motors (kinesins and myosins), cytoskeleton (actin and microtubules), molecular switches (small GTPases), and the fusion machinery (SNAREs and tethering factors) [59, 60]. In exosomes, a heightened capability to package and secrete proteins and microRNAs has been associated with metastatic tumor cells [5, 61, 62]. In a similar fashion, the release of exosomes is reinforced by certain stimuli involved in the formation of PMN, such as hypoxia [56]. The need for in vivo microscopy marks a technical limitation in the analysis of PMNs, which has impeded further study on the dynamics of EV in PMNs. EVs derived from tumors can operate separately from plasma and other body fluids to transport genetic material and tumor cell-derived proteins that encourage the progression of diseases [59, 63].

EVs derived from tumor cells combined with resident cells found in PMNs as well as tumors are responsible for the transport of genetic material such as mRNA, miRNA, and DNA; proteins; and metabolites (lipids and small metabolites) [61, 64–68]. According to leading studies, angiogenesis and metastasis can be induced by EVs derived from platelets in lung and breast cancer, particularly by microparticles [69, 70]. Nevertheless, note that the significance of EVs in the context of PMN formation has not been explored in these works of research. However, since this juncture in literature, EVs have been demonstrated as contributing to the transfer and recruitment of material to different types of stromal cells, which include ones that reside in PMNs [63, 71–73]. Target cells that uptake exosomes toward a proinflammatory and pro-metastatic phenotype are educated or reprogrammed by tumor-derived exosomal miRNA and proteins, thereby creating the PMN [5, 61]. The pre-metastatic organ analyzed and the type of cancer determine the education of stromal cells.

The formation of particular microenvironments favoring the exosomes secreted by tumors is enabled by the CD44 variant isoform (CD44v6) produced by pancreatic cancer cells, thereby inducing the formation of PMN and LN [74]. In the context of PMNs in the liver, TGFβ secretion in Kupffer cells is promoted by pancreatic tumor-derived exosomes that express MIF; this, in turn, stimulates the secretion of fibronectin via hepatic stellate cells and reinforces the recruitment of BMDCs [5]. It is interesting to note that miRNAs that compose the genomic content are packaged selectively within EVs, and are participants in the formation of PMN [8, 65, 66, 75]. By transferring miR-122 and obstructing pyruvate kinase, microvesicles derived from tumors are capable of suppressing glucose uptake by stromal cells in the PMNs of the brain, which increases the availability of glucose therein and attracts tumor cells, thereby favoring metastasis of the brain [8]. In a recent study, it was found that RNAs packaged within exosomes derived from tumors are notably involved in the activation of TLR3-dependent signaling in the epithelial cells of lungs; this induces chemokine secretion as well as the reinforcement of PMN formation via recruitment of neutrophils [12]. The abovementioned findings characterize merely the starting point of medical understanding regarding the involvement of tumor-derived EVs in metastasis. Several areas of research remain that require further research. Firstly, researchers must determine the subpopulation of tumor cells that lead to EVs responsible for inducing the formation of PMNs. Secondary, further descriptions of the secreted vesicles and related cargo would inform understanding of the effects of metabolic alterations on the formation of PMN formation. Thirdly, it is important to determine the duration of the EV-mediated education of recipient cells, whether this education can be regressed, and if they can be further reeducated by exposure to new EV content. Finally, the formation of EVs, the adherence, fusion, and education of recipient cells within PMNs require a significant amount of research that would inform the literature on the involvement of EVs in all phases of the formation of PMN.

Crosstalk with Tumor Vasculature

Primary tumor-secreted factors work to remodel the vasculature at PMNs through various mechanisms. In primary breast tumors and distant organs, vascular permeability can be induced by secreted factors such as cyclooxygenase 2 (COX2/PTGS2), EGFR ligand epiregulin, MMP1, and MMP2, thereby allowing the extravasation of CTCs [76]. In the pre-metastatic lung of a melanoma model, blood vessels were synergistically destabilized, due to the upregulation of ANGPT2, MMP-3, and -10 [77]. MMP9 produced by myeloid progenitor cells could also remodel the ECM to form an inflamed PMN in the lung that is both proliferative and immunosuppressive [27]. Altered ECs have been proposed to undertake an active role within the hyperpermeable region of PMNs [77, 78], where the formation of discrete foci was defined by the E-selectin enrichment on the luminal surface of the endothelium [78]. Tumor cell-derived VEGFA-dependent induction of FAK [78] is responsible for mediating E-selectin upregulation, as the impediment of ECs FAK challenges the progress of lung metastasis [79]. In models of breast cancer, the recruitment of monocytes that produce C-C chemokine receptor type 2 (CCR2) is caused by secretion of the stroma and tumor cells, which, in turn, leads to the production of VEGFA. Seeding efficiency and breast cancer experimental metastasis potential are majorly impeded by the monocyte-specific depletion of VEGFA [45]. Specific interactions between tumor cells and endothelial cells in such organs may be demanded by metastatic organotropism [76, 80].

The formation of blood clots is one significant visible alteration at the vascular level associated with PMN. Despite having linked aberrant homeostasis with the progression of cancer and metastasis for over a 100 years and given that VTE (venous thromboembolism) is a leading cause of death among cancer patients, very little research has been expedited on the medical significance of clots in the context of cancer progression and its underpinning mechanisms [81, 82]. During PMN formation, clot formation in the lungs mediated by tissue factors that is responsible for recruiting populations of CD11b, CD68, F4/80, CXCR1-expressing macrophages; this enhances the homing and survival of CTCs [82]. In order to form "early metastatic niches" in the lungs, the swift recruitment of CD11b$^+$MMP9$^+$Ly6G$^+$ granulocytes to tumor must take place, underpinned by platelets; this procedure involves the secretion of CXCL5 and CXCL7 by platelets via contact between varying kinds of tumor cells, thereby promoting metastatic progression and tumor cell seeding within the lungs [83]. The secretion of factors that promote the metastasis of tumors is reinforced by cancer complications such as disseminated intravascular coagulation, wherein hemorrhage and thrombosis take place simultaneously. To develop therapies that may reduce the number of mortalities among cancer patients, it is imperative that both these processes be further defined in the context of PMN biology in addition to determining the role of tumor- and platelet-secreted EVs in cancer-related coagulopathies.

Crosstalk with Stromal Cells (ECM)

In response to the systematic factors secreted from the primary tumor, the ECM at pre-metastatic organ sites goes through highly significant changes at the PMNs [84]. In melanoma and pancreatic cancer mouse models, the stromal fibroblasts activation increases fibronectin deposition in the pre-metastatic liver or lung [4, 47]. Due to the mass increase of fibronectin, BMDCs can easily adhere to the ECMs. Furthermore, in the MMTV-PyMT mouse model of breast cancer, the secretion of periostin from stromal fibroblasts that express α-SMA and vimentin is induced by TGF-β [85]. Type I collagen, fibronectin, BMP1, NOTCH1, and tenascin C have been identified as factors that periostin typically interact with; thus, it involves integrins such as αvβ3 and αvβ5 and encourages motility of cells by operating external to the cell [86]. According to research, periostin was found to upregulate damaged tissue in the wound-healing model of mice to develop a microenvironment similar to PMN and reinforce melanoma cell metastasis toward wound sites [87]. In recent literature concerning the pre-metastatic lung during breast cancer metastasis, it was found that the immunosuppressive capability of MDSCs requires periostin [88]. In the PMN, versican is identified as an ECM proteoglycan with a multitude of operations; for instance, tumor derived was found to activate macrophages via TLR2, thereby developing an inflammatory microenvironment in the pre-metastatic lung of a lung cancer mouse models [89].

In addition to the production of active ECM fragments, vascular integrity is affected by the enzymatic modulation of ECM [3, 90–93]. An increase of MMP2 activity attracts collagen IV peptide to home BMDCs and CTCs to PMNs in the pre-metastatic lung [3]. Stromal fibroblasts, endothelial cells, and BMDCs such as CD11b$^+$ myeloid cells, VEGFR1$^+$ hematopoietic progenitor cells (HPCs), and macrophages are the main sources of such MMPs [3, 4, 37, 94, 95]. The LOX family, which is responsible for the cross-linking of ECM molecules, is a significant class of enzymes that shape the ECM, with collagen as their primary substrate. The expression of LOX in primary breast tumors is significantly controlled by HIF1-α activity [3]. Nevertheless, research still requires further deliberation on the extent to which LOX collagen cross-linking is required for the formation of PMN across varying types of cancer. A modification in physical properties has been considered one of the significant results of ECM remodeling. A series of events involving signal transduction is set off by the tension produced in the ECM, which can operate as a molecular switch in disease progression and development—including metastasis [96–100]. In the ECM, collagen cross-linking also directly increases the tissue stiffness, leading to enhanced tumor cell survival and enhancing metastasis [101]. The limitations in the literature are concerned with the specific functional outcomes of ECM remodeling at the PMN as well as the need to determine whether mechanical tension transduction is the mechanism by which ECM remodeling at PMNs takes place [102].

Crosstalk with Immune Cells

The recruitment of BMDCs is an important and notable characteristic of PMN establishment and evolution. Incoming CTCs are supported by a friendly microenvironment fostered by HPCs that express VLA4 (integrin $\alpha4\beta1$) and VEGFR1 to pre-metastatic organs [4]. The significance of these HPCs during the initiation of PMN is characterized by the reduction in metastasis due to the abrogation of HPC clusters in the pre-metastatic organs either by the depletion of VEGFR1$^+$ BMDCs or the VEGFR1 antibody-mediated blockade [4]. Despite the significance of the upregulation of inhibitor of differentiation 1 gene expression for the mobilization of VEGFR1$^+$ HPC during the formation of PMNs [103], research has not yet determined the tumor-derived factors responsible for ID1 expression and HPC mobilization. Abnormal differentiation and accumulation at PMNs result from the takeover of varying kinds of immune cells by primary tumors responsible for the recruitment of HPCs from the bone marrow. It is important to note that metastasis is promoted and immunosuppression is imposed at PMNs by MDSCs [27, 47, 104–106], which can either be recruited to PMNs or emerge from tissue-resident myeloid populations [27]. This finding implies that the production of a proinflammatory, immunosuppressive PMN via the BMDC recruitment is essential for a successful metastatic progression.

A crucial regulator of ECM remodeling, MMP9, is produced by MDSCs associated with PMN; MMP9 operates as an angiogenic switch that eventually undergirds the formation of metastasis [107, 108]. In metastatic organs, neutrophils at PMNs can expand and mobilized to PMNs through G-CSF, exosomes, or SDF1 [48, 104–106]. Neutrophils are identified as a heterogeneous population characterized by significant functional complexity due to their oversimplification in literature, which marks the need for further immunophenotyping in order to organize and functionally assess immune cells that infiltrate the PMN. According to recent research, only in the absence IFN-I can neutrophil be recruited to PMNs, while reducing their cytotoxic activity [109]. Regardless, due to the multitude of roles attributed to IFNγ, whose tumor-promoting and tumor-suppressive operations typically depend on the microenvironmental, cellular, or molecular context [110]. Studies employing mouse models of breast cancer found neutrophils to have supported the establishment of lung PMNs [25]. Through the isolation of PMN-derived neutrophils, it was found that they are responsible for enhancing metastatic competence by increasing the secretion of leukotrienes, to alter cancer cell biology [25]. The secretion of chemokines and the promotion of neutrophil recruitment take place as a result of the activation of TLR3 in lung epithelial cells due to LLC-derived exosomal RNAs. The role of innate immune cells in supporting the formation of PMNs requires examination. According to recent studies, it is possible that there may be certain other (apart from neutrophils) EV-mediated communication that actively takes place across tumor cells and innate immune cells during the formation of PMNs [111, 112].

Conclusion

The formation and operation of the PMN may be inhibited by a number of potential targets: impeding the secretion of molecular components that promote premetastatic niches, suppression of BMDC recruitment, disruption of cross talk among tumor-immune, tumor-stromal cells in the distal *onco-sphere*, a subversion of the immunosuppressive niche, and the reactivation of anti-tumor immune response. Metastatic cancer treatments may benefit from the integrative targeting of various common cellular and molecular activities responsible for driving the formation of pre-metastatic niches. Furthermore, clinical outcomes may be significantly improved by combining specific regimes of conventional chemotherapy and immunotherapy. The former mode of treatment increases the immunogenicity of malignant cells or inhibits immunosuppression to reinforce anti-tumor responses.

References

1. Peinado H, Zhang H, Matei IR, Costa-Silva B, Hoshino A, Rodrigues G et al (2017) Pre-metastatic niches: organ-specific homes for metastases. Nat Rev Cancer 17(5):302–317
2. Psaila B, Lyden D (2009) The metastatic niche: adapting the foreign soil. Nat Rev Cancer 9(4): 285–293
3. Erler JT, Bennewith KL, Cox TR, Lang G, Bird D, Koong A et al (2009) Hypoxia-induced lysyl oxidase is a critical mediator of bone marrow cell recruitment to form the premetastatic niche. Cancer Cell 15(1):35–44
4. Kaplan RN, Riba RD, Zacharoulis S, Bramley AH, Vincent L, Costa C et al (2005) VEGFR1-positive haematopoietic bone marrow progenitors initiate the pre-metastatic niche. Nature 438(7069):820–827
5. Costa-Silva B, Aiello NM, Ocean AJ, Singh S, Zhang H, Thakur BK et al (2015) Pancreatic cancer exosomes initiate pre-metastatic niche formation in the liver. Nat Cell Biol 17(6): 816–826
6. Hoshino A, Costa-Silva B, Shen TL, Rodrigues G, Hashimoto A, Tesic Mark M et al (2015) Tumour exosome integrins determine organotropic metastasis. Nature 527(7578):329–335
7. Zhou W, Fong MY, Min Y, Somlo G, Liu L, Palomares MR et al (2014) Cancer-secreted miR-105 destroys vascular endothelial barriers to promote metastasis. Cancer Cell 25(4): 501–515
8. Fong MY, Zhou W, Liu L, Alontaga AY, Chandra M, Ashby J et al (2015) Breast-cancer-secreted miR-122 reprograms glucose metabolism in premetastatic niche to promote metastasis. Nat Cell Biol 17(2):183–194
9. Arora S, Rana R, Chhabra A, Jaiswal A, Rani V (2013) miRNA-transcription factor interactions: a combinatorial regulation of gene expression. Mol Gen Genomics 288(3–4):77–87
10. Lu P, Takai K, Weaver VM, Werb Z (2011) Extracellular matrix degradation and remodeling in development and disease. Cold Spring Harb Perspect Biol 3(12):a005058
11. Grange C, Tapparo M, Collino F, Vitillo L, Damasco C, Deregibus MC et al (2011) Microvesicles released from human renal cancer stem cells stimulate angiogenesis and formation of lung premetastatic niche. Cancer Res 71(15):5346–5356
12. Dai L, Liu J, Luo Z, Li M, Cai K (2016) Tumor therapy: targeted drug delivery systems. J Mater Chem B 4(42):6758–6772

13. Bidwell BN, Slaney CY, Withana NP, Forster S, Cao Y, Loi S et al (2012) Silencing of Irf7 pathways in breast cancer cells promotes bone metastasis through immune escape. Nat Med 18(8):1224–1231
14. Hanna RN, Cekic C, Sag D, Tacke R, Thomas GD, Nowyhed H et al (2015) Patrolling monocytes control tumor metastasis to the lung. Science 350(6263):985–990
15. Clever D, Roychoudhuri R, Constantinides MG, Askenase MH, Sukumar M, Klebanoff CA et al (2016) Oxygen sensing by T cells establishes an immunologically tolerant metastatic niche. Cell 166(5):1117–31.e14
16. Tacke RS, Lee HC, Goh C, Courtney J, Polyak SJ, Rosen HR et al (2012) Myeloid suppressor cells induced by hepatitis C virus suppress T-cell responses through the production of reactive oxygen species. Hepatology 55(2):343–353
17. Bodogai M, Moritoh K, Lee-Chang C, Hollander CM, Sherman-Baust CA, Wersto RP et al (2015) Immunosuppressive and prometastatic functions of myeloid-derived suppressive cells rely upon education from tumor-associated B cells. Cancer Res 75(17):3456–3465
18. Ham B, Wang N, D'Costa Z, Fernandez MC, Bourdeau F, Auguste P et al (2015) TNF Receptor-2 facilitates an immunosuppressive microenvironment in the liver to promote the colonization and growth of hepatic metastases. Cancer Res 75(24):5235–5247
19. Giles AJ, Reid CM, Evans JD, Murgai M, Vicioso Y, Highfill SL et al (2016) Activation of hematopoietic stem/progenitor cells promotes immunosuppression within the pre-metastatic niche. Cancer Res 76(6):1335–1347
20. Sceneay J, Chow MT, Chen A, Halse HM, Wong CS, Andrews DM et al (2012) Primary tumor hypoxia recruits CD11b+/Ly6Cmed/Ly6G+ immune suppressor cells and compromises NK cell cytotoxicity in the premetastatic niche. Cancer Res 72(16):3906–3911
21. Lai C, August S, Behar R, Polak M, Ardern-Jones M, Theaker J et al (2015) Characteristics of immunosuppressive regulatory T cells in cutaneous squamous cell carcinomas and role in metastasis. Lancet 385(Suppl 1):S59
22. Sharma SK, Chintala NK, Vadrevu SK, Patel J, Karbowniczek M, Markiewski MM (2015) Pulmonary alveolar macrophages contribute to the premetastatic niche by suppressing antitumor T cell responses in the lungs. J Immunol 194(11):5529–5538
23. Cao X (2016) Self-regulation and cross-regulation of pattern-recognition receptor signalling in health and disease. Nat Rev Immunol 16(1):35–50
24. Hiratsuka S, Watanabe A, Sakurai Y, Akashi-Takamura S, Ishibashi S, Miyake K et al (2008) The S100A8-serum amyloid A3-TLR4 paracrine cascade establishes a pre-metastatic phase. Nat Cell Biol 10(11):1349–1355
25. Wculek SK, Malanchi I (2015) Neutrophils support lung colonization of metastasis-initiating breast cancer cells. Nature 528(7582):413–417
26. Bald T, Quast T, Landsberg J, Rogava M, Glodde N, Lopez-Ramos D et al (2014) Ultraviolet-radiation-induced inflammation promotes angiotropism and metastasis in melanoma. Nature 507(7490):109–113
27. Yan HH, Pickup M, Pang Y, Gorska AE, Li Z, Chytil A et al (2010) Gr-1+CD11b+ myeloid cells tip the balance of immune protection to tumor promotion in the premetastatic lung. Cancer Res 70(15):6139–6149
28. Cui TX, Kryczek I, Zhao L, Zhao E, Kuick R, Roh MH et al (2013) Myeloid-derived suppressor cells enhance stemness of cancer cells by inducing microRNA101 and suppressing the corepressor CtBP2. Immunity 39(3):611–621
29. Fischer KR, Durrans A, Lee S, Sheng J, Li F, Wong ST et al (2015) Epithelial-to-mesenchymal transition is not required for lung metastasis but contributes to chemoresistance. Nature 527(7579):472–476
30. Zheng X, Carstens JL, Kim J, Scheible M, Kaye J, Sugimoto H et al (2015) Epithelial-to-mesenchymal transition is dispensable for metastasis but induces chemoresistance in pancreatic cancer. Nature 527(7579):525–530
31. Unwith S, Zhao H, Hennah L, Ma D (2015) The potential role of HIF on tumour progression and dissemination. Int J Cancer 136(11):2491–2503

32. Romero I, Garrido F, Garcia-Lora AM (2014) Metastases in immune-mediated dormancy: a new opportunity for targeting cancer. Cancer Res 74(23):6750–6757
33. Ono M, Kosaka N, Tominaga N, Yoshioka Y, Takeshita F, Takahashi RU et al (2014) Exosomes from bone marrow mesenchymal stem cells contain a microRNA that promotes dormancy in metastatic breast cancer cells. Sci Signal 7(332):ra63
34. Eyles J, Puaux AL, Wang X, Toh B, Prakash C, Hong M et al (2010) Tumor cells disseminate early, but immunosurveillance limits metastatic outgrowth, in a mouse model of melanoma. J Clin Invest 120(6):2030–2039
35. Kienast Y, von Baumgarten L, Fuhrmann M, Klinkert WE, Goldbrunner R, Herms J et al (2010) Real-time imaging reveals the single steps of brain metastasis formation. Nat Med 16(1):116–122
36. Lu X, Mu E, Wei Y, Riethdorf S, Yang Q, Yuan M et al (2011) VCAM-1 promotes osteolytic expansion of indolent bone micrometastasis of breast cancer by engaging α4β1-positive osteoclast progenitors. Cancer Cell 20(6):701–714
37. Hiratsuka S, Nakamura K, Iwai S, Murakami M, Itoh T, Kijima H et al (2002) MMP9 induction by vascular endothelial growth factor receptor-1 is involved in lung-specific metastasis. Cancer Cell 2(4):289–300
38. Shojaei F, Wu X, Qu X, Kowanetz M, Yu L, Tan M et al (2009) G-CSF-initiated myeloid cell mobilization and angiogenesis mediate tumor refractoriness to anti-VEGF therapy in mouse models. Proc Natl Acad Sci U S A 106(16):6742–6747
39. Melgarejo E, Medina MA, Sánchez-Jiménez F, Urdiales JL (2009) Monocyte chemoattractant protein-1: a key mediator in inflammatory processes. Int J Biochem Cell Biol 41(5):998–1001
40. Lu Y, Cai Z, Galson DL, Xiao G, Liu Y, George DE et al (2006) Monocyte chemotactic protein-1 (MCP-1) acts as a paracrine and autocrine factor for prostate cancer growth and invasion. Prostate 66(12):1311–1318
41. Cai Z, Chen Q, Chen J, Lu Y, Xiao G, Wu Z et al (2009) Monocyte chemotactic protein 1 promotes lung cancer-induced bone resorptive lesions *in vivo*. Neoplasia 11(3):228–236
42. Loberg RD, Ying C, Craig M, Day LL, Sargent E, Neeley C et al (2007) Targeting CCL2 with systemic delivery of neutralizing antibodies induces prostate cancer tumor regression *in vivo*. Cancer Res 67(19):9417–9424
43. Saji H, Koike M, Yamori T, Saji S, Seiki M, Matsushima K et al (2001) Significant correlation of monocyte chemoattractant protein-1 expression with neovascularization and progression of breast carcinoma. Cancer 92(5):1085–1091
44. Lebrecht A, Grimm C, Lantzsch T, Ludwig E, Hefler L, Ulbrich E et al (2004) Monocyte chemoattractant protein-1 serum levels in patients with breast cancer. Tumour Biol 25(1–2): 14–17
45. Qian BZ, Li J, Zhang H, Kitamura T, Zhang J, Campion LR et al (2011) CCL2 recruits inflammatory monocytes to facilitate breast-tumour metastasis. Nature 475(7355):222–225
46. Lu X, Kang Y (2009) Chemokine (C-C motif) ligand 2 engages CCR2+ stromal cells of monocytic origin to promote breast cancer metastasis to lung and bone. J Biol Chem 284(42): 29087–29096
47. Lu X, Kang Y (2007) Organotropism of breast cancer metastasis. J Mammary Gland Biol Neoplasia 12(2–3):153–162
48. Granot Z, Henke E, Comen EA, King TA, Norton L, Benezra R (2011) Tumor entrained neutrophils inhibit seeding in the premetastatic lung. Cancer Cell 20(3):300–314
49. Bresnick AR, Weber DJ, Zimmer DB (2015) S100 proteins in cancer. Nat Rev Cancer 15(2): 96–109
50. Lukanidin E, Sleeman JP (2012) Building the niche: the role of the S100 proteins in metastatic growth. Semin Cancer Biol 22(3):216–225
51. Donato R, Cannon BR, Sorci G, Riuzzi F, Hsu K, Weber DJ et al (2013) Functions of S100 proteins. Curr Mol Med 13(1):24–57

52. Hiratsuka S, Watanabe A, Aburatani H, Maru Y (2006) Tumour-mediated upregulation of chemoattractants and recruitment of myeloid cells predetermines lung metastasis. Nat Cell Biol 8(12):1369–1375
53. Cox TR, Rumney RMH, Schoof EM, Perryman L, Høye AM, Agrawal A et al (2015) The hypoxic cancer secretome induces pre-metastatic bone lesions through lysyl oxidase. Nature 522(7554):106–110
54. Wong CC, Gilkes DM, Zhang H, Chen J, Wei H, Chaturvedi P et al (2011) Hypoxia-inducible factor 1 is a master regulator of breast cancer metastatic niche formation. Proc Natl Acad Sci U S A 108(39):16369–16374
55. Wong CC, Zhang H, Gilkes DM, Chen J, Wei H, Chaturvedi P et al (2012) Inhibitors of hypoxia-inducible factor 1 block breast cancer metastatic niche formation and lung metastasis. J Mol Med (Berl) 90(7):803–815
56. King HW, Michael MZ, Gleadle JM (2012) Hypoxic enhancement of exosome release by breast cancer cells. BMC Cancer 12:421
57. Wang T, Gilkes DM, Takano N, Xiang L, Luo W, Bishop CJ et al (2014) Hypoxia-inducible factors and RAB22A mediate formation of microvesicles that stimulate breast cancer invasion and metastasis. Proc Natl Acad Sci U S A 111(31):E3234–E3242
58. Gould SJ, Raposo G (2013) As we wait: coping with an imperfect nomenclature for extracellular vesicles. J Extracell Vesicles 2:20389. https://doi.org/10.3402/jev.v2i0.20389
59. Colombo M, Raposo G, Théry C (2014) Biogenesis, secretion, and intercellular interactions of exosomes and other extracellular vesicles. Annu Rev Cell Dev Biol 30:255–289
60. Raposo G, Stoorvogel W (2013) Extracellular vesicles: exosomes, microvesicles, and friends. J Cell Biol 200(4):373–383
61. Peinado H, Alečković M, Lavotshkin S, Matei I, Costa-Silva B, Moreno-Bueno G et al (2012) Melanoma exosomes educate bone marrow progenitor cells toward a pro-metastatic phenotype through MET. Nat Med 18(6):883–891
62. Ostenfeld MS, Jeppesen DK, Laurberg JR, Boysen AT, Bramsen JB, Primdal-Bengtson B et al (2014) Cellular disposal of miR23b by RAB27-dependent exosome release is linked to acquisition of metastatic properties. Cancer Res 74(20):5758–5771
63. Peinado H, Lavotshkin S, Lyden D (2011) The secreted factors responsible for pre-metastatic niche formation: old sayings and new thoughts. Semin Cancer Biol 21(2):139–146
64. Balaj L, Lessard R, Dai L, Cho YJ, Pomeroy SL, Breakefield XO et al (2011) Tumour microvesicles contain retrotransposon elements and amplified oncogene sequences. Nat Commun 2:180
65. Valadi H, Ekström K, Bossios A, Sjöstrand M, Lee JJ, Lötvall JO (2007) Exosome-mediated transfer of mRNAs and microRNAs is a novel mechanism of genetic exchange between cells. Nat Cell Biol 9(6):654–659
66. Skog J, Würdinger T, van Rijn S, Meijer DH, Gainche L, Sena-Esteves M et al (2008) Glioblastoma microvesicles transport RNA and proteins that promote tumour growth and provide diagnostic biomarkers. Nat Cell Biol 10(12):1470–1476
67. Al-Nedawi K, Meehan B, Micallef J, Lhotak V, May L, Guha A et al (2008) Intercellular transfer of the oncogenic receptor EGFRvIII by microvesicles derived from tumour cells. Nat Cell Biol 10(5):619–624
68. Ratajczak J, Miekus K, Kucia M, Zhang J, Reca R, Dvorak P et al (2006) Embryonic stem cell-derived microvesicles reprogram hematopoietic progenitors: evidence for horizontal transfer of mRNA and protein delivery. Leukemia 20(5):847–856
69. Janowska-Wieczorek A, Wysoczynski M, Kijowski J, Marquez-Curtis L, Machalinski B, Ratajczak J et al (2005) Microvesicles derived from activated platelets induce metastasis and angiogenesis in lung cancer. Int J Cancer 113(5):752–760
70. Janowska-Wieczorek A, Marquez-Curtis LA, Wysoczynski M, Ratajczak MZ (2006) Enhancing effect of platelet-derived microvesicles on the invasive potential of breast cancer cells. Transfusion 46(7):1199–1209

71. Cocucci E, Racchetti G, Meldolesi J (2009) Shedding microvesicles: artefacts no more. Trends Cell Biol 19(2):43–51
72. Iero M, Valenti R, Huber V, Filipazzi P, Parmiani G, Fais S et al (2008) Tumour-released exosomes and their implications in cancer immunity. Cell Death Differ 15(1):80–88
73. Ratajczak J, Wysoczynski M, Hayek F, Janowska-Wieczorek A, Ratajczak MZ (2006) Membrane-derived microvesicles: important and underappreciated mediators of cell-to-cell communication. Leukemia 20(9):1487–1495
74. Jung T, Castellana D, Klingbeil P, Cuesta Hernández I, Vitacolonna M, Orlicky DJ et al (2009) CD44v6 dependence of premetastatic niche preparation by exosomes. Neoplasia 11(10): 1093–1105
75. Villarroya-Beltri C, Baixauli F, Gutiérrez-Vázquez C, Sánchez-Madrid F, Mittelbrunn M (2014) Sorting it out: regulation of exosome loading. Semin Cancer Biol 28:3–13
76. Gupta GP, Nguyen DX, Chiang AC, Bos PD, Kim JY, Nadal C et al (2007) Mediators of vascular remodelling co-opted for sequential steps in lung metastasis. Nature 446(7137): 765–770
77. Huang Y, Song N, Ding Y, Yuan S, Li X, Cai H et al (2009) Pulmonary vascular destabilization in the premetastatic phase facilitates lung metastasis. Cancer Res 69(19):7529–7537
78. Hiratsuka S, Goel S, Kamoun WS, Maru Y, Fukumura D, Duda DG et al (2011) Endothelial focal adhesion kinase mediates cancer cell homing to discrete regions of the lungs via E-selectin up-regulation. Proc Natl Acad Sci U S A 108(9):3725–3730
79. Jean C, Chen XL, Nam JO, Tancioni I, Uryu S, Lawson C et al (2014) Inhibition of endothelial FAK activity prevents tumor metastasis by enhancing barrier function. J Cell Biol 204(2): 247–263
80. Bos PD, Zhang XH, Nadal C, Shu W, Gomis RR, Nguyen DX et al (2009) Genes that mediate breast cancer metastasis to the brain. Nature 459(7249):1005–1009
81. Gay LJ, Felding-Habermann B (2011) Contribution of platelets to tumour metastasis. Nat Rev Cancer 11(2):123–134
82. Kuderer NM, Ortel TL, Francis CW (2009) Impact of venous thromboembolism and anticoagulation on cancer and cancer survival. J Clin Oncol 27(29):4902–4911
83. Labelle M, Begum S, Hynes RO (2014) Platelets guide the formation of early metastatic niches. Proc Natl Acad Sci U S A 111(30):E3053–E3061
84. Sleeman JP (2012) The metastatic niche and stromal progression. Cancer Metastasis Rev 31(3–4):429–440
85. Malanchi I, Santamaria-Martínez A, Susanto E, Peng H, Lehr HA, Delaloye JF et al (2011) Interactions between cancer stem cells and their niche govern metastatic colonization. Nature 481(7379):85–89
86. Kudo A (2011) Periostin in fibrillogenesis for tissue regeneration: periostin actions inside and outside the cell. Cell Mol Life Sci 68(19):3201–3207
87. Fukuda K, Sugihara E, Ohta S, Izuhara K, Funakoshi T, Amagai M et al (2015) Periostin is a key niche component for wound metastasis of melanoma. PLoS One 10(6):e0129704
88. Wang Z, Xiong S, Mao Y, Chen M, Ma X, Zhou X et al (2016) Periostin promotes immunosuppressive premetastatic niche formation to facilitate breast tumour metastasis. J Pathol 239(4):484–495
89. Kim S, Takahashi H, Lin WW, Descargues P, Grivennikov S, Kim Y et al (2009) Carcinoma-produced factors activate myeloid cells through TLR2 to stimulate metastasis. Nature 457(7225):102–106
90. Egeblad M, Werb Z (2002) New functions for the matrix metalloproteinases in cancer progression. Nat Rev Cancer 2(3):161–174
91. Cameron JD, Skubitz AP, Furcht LT (1991) Type IV collagen and corneal epithelial adhesion and migration. Effects of type IV collagen fragments and synthetic peptides on rabbit corneal epithelial cell adhesion and migration *in vitro*. Invest Ophthalmol Vis Sci 32(10):2766–2773
92. Shahan TA, Fawzi A, Bellon G, Monboisse JC, Kefalides NA (2000) Regulation of tumor cell chemotaxis by type IV collagen is mediated by a ca (2+)-dependent mechanism requiring CD47 and the integrin alpha (V)beta (3). J Biol Chem 275(7):4796–4802

93. Kessenbrock K, Plaks V, Werb Z (2010) Matrix metalloproteinases: regulators of the tumor microenvironment. Cell 141(1):52–67
94. van Deventer HW, O'Connor W Jr, Brickey WJ, Aris RM, Ting JP, Serody JS (2005) C-C chemokine receptor 5 on stromal cells promotes pulmonary metastasis. Cancer Res 65(8): 3374–3379
95. van Deventer HW, Wu QP, Bergstralh DT, Davis BK, O'Connor BP, Ting JP et al (2008) C-C chemokine receptor 5 on pulmonary fibrocytes facilitates migration and promotes metastasis via matrix metalloproteinase 9. Am J Pathol 173(1):253–264
96. Goetz JG, Minguet S, Navarro-Lérida I, Lazcano JJ, Samaniego R, Calvo E et al (2011) Biomechanical remodeling of the microenvironment by stromal caveolin-1 favors tumor invasion and metastasis. Cell 146(1):148–163
97. Engler AJ, Humbert PO, Wehrle-Haller B, Weaver VM (2009) Multiscale modeling of form and function. Science 324(5924):208–212
98. Krieg M, Arboleda-Estudillo Y, Puech PH, Käfer J, Graner F, Müller DJ et al (2008) Tensile forces govern germ-layer organization in zebrafish. Nat Cell Biol 10(4):429–436
99. Rønnov-Jessen L, Bissell MJ (2009) Breast cancer by proxy: can the microenvironment be both the cause and consequence? Trends Mol Med 15(1):5–13
100. Levental KR, Yu H, Kass L, Lakins JN, Egeblad M, Erler JT et al (2009) Matrix crosslinking forces tumor progression by enhancing integrin signaling. Cell 139(5):891–906
101. Cox TR, Bird D, Baker AM, Barker HE, Ho MW, Lang G et al (2013) LOX-mediated collagen crosslinking is responsible for fibrosis-enhanced metastasis. Cancer Res 73(6):1721–1732
102. Aguado BA, Caffe JR, Nanavati D, Rao SS, Bushnell GG, Azarin SM et al (2016) Extracellular matrix mediators of metastatic cell colonization characterized using scaffold mimics of the pre-metastatic niche. Acta Biomater 33:13–24
103. Papaspyridonos M, Matei I, Huang Y, do Rosario Andre M, Brazier-Mitouart H, Waite JC et al (2015) Id1 suppresses anti-tumour immune responses and promotes tumour progression by impairing myeloid cell maturation. Nat Commun 6:6840
104. Kowanetz M, Wu X, Lee J, Tan M, Hagenbeek T, Qu X et al (2010) Granulocyte-colony stimulating factor promotes lung metastasis through mobilization of Ly6G+Ly6C+ granulocytes. Proc Natl Acad Sci U S A 107(50):21248–21255
105. Seubert B, Grünwald B, Kobuch J, Cui H, Schelter F, Schaten S et al (2015) Tissue inhibitor of metalloproteinases (TIMP)-1 creates a premetastatic niche in the liver through SDF-1/CXCR4-dependent neutrophil recruitment in mice. Hepatology 61(1):238–248
106. Casbon AJ, Reynaud D, Park C, Khuc E, Gan DD, Schepers K et al (2015) Invasive breast cancer reprograms early myeloid differentiation in the bone marrow to generate immunosuppressive neutrophils. Proc Natl Acad Sci U S A 112(6):E566–E575
107. Bergers G, Brekken R, McMahon G, Vu TH, Itoh T, Tamaki K et al (2000) Matrix metalloproteinase-9 triggers the angiogenic switch during carcinogenesis. Nat Cell Biol 2(10):737–744
108. Ahn GO, Brown JM (2008) Matrix metalloproteinase-9 is required for tumor vasculogenesis but not for angiogenesis: role of bone marrow-derived myelomonocytic cells. Cancer Cell 13(3):193–205
109. Wu CF, Andzinski L, Kasnitz N, Kröger A, Klawonn F, Lienenklaus S et al (2015) The lack of type I interferon induces neutrophil-mediated pre-metastatic niche formation in the mouse lung. Int J Cancer 137(4):837–847
110. Zaidi MR, Merlino G (2011) The two faces of interferon-γ in cancer. Clin Cancer Res 17(19): 6118–6124
111. Benito-Martin A, Di Giannatale A, Ceder S, Peinado H (2015) The new deal: a potential role for secreted vesicles in innate immunity and tumor progression. Front Immunol 6:66
112. Paget S (1989) The distribution of secondary growths in cancer of the breast. 1889. Cancer Metastasis Rev 8(2):98–101

Chapter 12
Regional *Onco-Sphere*: Lymph Node Metastasis

Phei Er Saw and Erwei Song

Abstract During cancer metastasis, cancer cells spread by dissemination into nearby normal tissue mostly via two major routes (i) lymph nodes and (ii) blood vessels. Cancer cells can travel through lymphatic system or extravasate into blood vessels to other parts of the body and forming new tumors at metastatic sites. In this chapter, we will focus on how vascular remodeling in the local onco-sphere could affect lymph node metastasis. We will also discuss the importance of the crosstalk between tumoral endothelial cells (lymphatic vessels, perivascular cells, endothelial progenitor cells) and tumor cells in lymph node metastasis in the regional onco-sphere.

Introduction

In this chapter, we will look closely at lymph node metastasis, the crucial modulator between local and distal *onco-sphere*. Also termed as a regional *onco-sphere*, lymph node metastasis is caused by angiogenesis and lymphangiogenesis at the local *onco-*

P. E. Saw
Guangdong Provincial Key Laboratory of Malignant Tumor Epigenetics and Gene Regulation, Guangdong-Hong Kong Joint Laboratory for RNA Medicine, Medical Research Center, Sun Yat-sen Memorial Hospital, Sun Yat-sen University, Guangzhou, China

Nanhai Translational Innovation Center of Precision Immunology, Sun Yat-sen Memorial Hospital, Sun Yat-sen University, Foshan, China

E. Song (✉)
Guangdong Provincial Key Laboratory of Malignant Tumor Epigenetics and Gene Regulation, Guangdong-Hong Kong Joint Laboratory for RNA Medicine, Medical Research Center, Sun Yat-sen Memorial Hospital, Sun Yat-sen University, Guangzhou, China

Nanhai Translational Innovation Center of Precision Immunology, Sun Yat-sen Memorial Hospital, Sun Yat-sen University, Foshan, China

Breast Tumor Center, Sun Yat-sen Memorial Hospital, Sun Yat-sen University, Guangzhou, China
e-mail: songew@mail.sysu.edu.cn

sphere. In fact, lymph node is considered a unique organ for circulating/disseminated cancer cells that could be further primed before going to a new distal *onco-sphere*. As researches have shown, lymph node metastasis is indeed a major factor that could predict the prognosis of most human cancers. The inhibition of tumor angiogenesis continues to emerge as a contemporary approach to the treatment of cancer [1, 2]. All forms of therapy that involve such a procedure target are responsible for the migration into the tumor bed as well as the inhibition of endothelial cell proliferation, which is pivotal for the formation of capillaries. Within the context of combination therapy, antiangiogenic agents demonstrate the potential capacity for the enhancement of the therapeutic efficacy and delivery of treatment modalities that directly target cancer cells; for example, monoclonal antibody therapy, chemotherapy, and radiation, among others [3]. The incidence of in situ tumors, especially prostate, thyroid gland, and breast tumors is observed to be substantially higher, relative to the recorded incidence of cancer in general [4], thereby suggesting the comparative lack of frequency of tumor metastases. Recently, the low metastatic activity of in situ tumors has been associated with their inability to acquire an angiogenic phenotype, as both metastasis and the growth of tumors value increased vascularization and a greater expression of angiogenic factors [5–7]. Therefore, the mechanistic study of vasculo-lymphogenic remodeling in the local *onco-sphere* and how this remodel the regional *onco-sphere* is vital for designing personalized cancer therapy.

Vascular Remodeling in the Local *Onco-Sphere*

Embryonic angiogenesis and tumor angiogenesis are similar in some ways, as depicted by their similar mechanisms in the early angiogenic process. The major differences between these two are the fact the tumor angiogenesis is not regulated tightly, and the order of formation is not hierarchically ordered or patterned [8]. In fact, observations of tumor blood vessels allow one to clearly see the differences between a tumor blood vessel and a normal one. Tumor blood vessels are essentially diverse, winding, poorly or sporadically branched, large in circumference, and often hyperpermeable [9–11]. The hyperpermeability of the tumor vasculature leads to an easy diffusion and nutrients, which are supposed to be favoring the tumor growth. However, due to other factors, such as high interstitial fluid pressure (IFPs), the flow of nutrient and oxygen is weakened, thereby leading to a hypoxic and acidic condition, which we covered in the previous chapters [12–15].

In hypoxic condition, HIF-1α is always highly expressed, which in turn induces VEGF-A, a growth factor essential in blood vessel formation and angiogenesis [14]. Furthermore, the acidic and hypoxic condition also increases the tumor cells that are resistance in this condition, which are also apoptosis resistance with enhanced metastatic potentials, while significantly represses chemo-/radiotherapeutic efficacy [16–18]. Leaky tumor blood vessels are essentially characterized typically by their inefficiency in delivering the chemotherapy, in addition to that they also improve the accessibility for the metastasizing of tumor cells [10]. The dysregulated vasculature helps the tumor to thrive. The built of the tumor vasculature can be different from time to time, depending mainly on the type of tumor cells [9, 19]. Angiogenic factors are made up of a family of VEGFs, and different tumors have different indications of angiogenic GFs which can lead to different types of angiogenesis [20–27]. It is interesting that different VEGF-A isoforms can lead to significantly different blood vessel formations. Some examples are as follows: (a) an expression of the $VEGFA_{165}$ isoform in a melanoma model caused a successfully diffused, excellently forked capillary network which is categorized by plentiful intraluminal linking and reinforced by winding exterior vessels, (b) an expression of $VEGF-A_{121}$ isoform produced bigger, more scarce vessels inside malignant tumors [20], and (c) $VEGF-A_{189}$ caused an increase in the vascular area, typically categorized by widened vessels [28]. All these examples depicted different vascular patterning, and this patterning has been associated with tumor growth. Taking human oligodendrogliomas as an example, data has shown that vascular patterning can affect tumor outcome. In grade II tumor that is slow in growth, the tumors had interconnected capillaries at regular intervals, whereas progressive grade III tumors exhibited proliferation of the glomerular endothelium and larger vessels, leading to intestinal. It was suggestive of the growth of invaginated vessels. At this point, there are also new vessel formation by intraluminal fission of larger vessels. In a study on HCC, the classification of vasculatures was done via morphology distinction [20]. Yet, another study in CCRC also indicates that tumor vasculature could be classified by molecular staining, as they possess different expression level and quantity of CD31, α-SMA and CD34, indicating the vascular morphology and patterning should be taken into consideration in future tumor classification. Recently, a study on the morphological classification of vasculature in hepatocellular carcinoma was reported, and the molecular classification of tumor vasculature in clear cell renal carcinoma was also demonstrated by staining with anti-CD34, -CD31, and -αSMA antibodies [29].

Although vasculature patterning could vary among different cancer types, empirical studies have identified common tumor vascular types that have been remodeled [19, 30]. In a study done on "surrogate tumor" model by using ectopically-expressed VEGF-A co-culturing with a tumor tissue, it was observed that (1) the parental vessel, characterized by large-sized, thin-walled, highly permeable, lack of pericyte attachment was first formed. Note that this vessel is derived from pre-existing small vessels; (2) during the detachment of pericytes, the endothelial duct is dilated, cathepsin is then secreted to degrade the basement membrane. Note that the concentration of protease inhibitor will decrease at this point [19]; (3) endothelial tube expansion is induced due to surface expansion and also endothelial cell's proliferation; (4) the regions of the endothelial plasma membrane are enlarged by vesicle-vacuolar organelles, allowing further growth of EC, including EC stretching and thinning [11, 31]; (5) the formation of the parent vessel is transient. It will need to develop into a deformed vasculature, capillary or glomerular microvascular proliferation. In a way, vascular malfunctions look like large veins that are abnormal, with a layer of smooth muscle layer that is irregular. This could be due to pericyte re-attachment during the process [19]. When bridging of a parent vessel of new branch of angiogenesis is formed, capillaries can occur. Glomerular microvascular proliferation resembles renal glomeruli, with a stratified basement membrane and a small endothelium with occasional pericytes that occur over multiple rounds of EC proliferation and intussusception within the parent vessel. Among these three phenotypes, only glomerular microvascular proliferation characteristic has been considered a better prognostic indicator of poor survival [32–34]. It has also been observed that large feeding arteries, outflow veins, capillaries, and vascular malformations identified at late stages of tumor development are relatively insensitive to VEGF. This lack of sensitivity may be related to the lack of inefficiency of certain anti-angiogenic treatments that target the more established tumor vasculature [9].

Crosstalk: Effect on Vascularization on Host Immune Infiltration

Tumor ECs are characterized by a strong inflammatory environment, with reduced expression levels of leukocyte adhesion molecules. For example, E-selectin, CD34, ICAM-1, and VCAM-1, are potent adhesion molecules in normal ECs, are found to be downregulated in tumor ECs. However, tumor ECs also are typically upregulated inflammatory cytokines [35]. In vivo systemic treatment of tumors with anti-angiogenic agents has been shown to restore expression of these adhesion molecules and improve leukocyte infiltration, including cytotoxic CD8$^+$ T cells within tumors [36], indicating the inherent crosstalk between vascularization and host immune system. In swollen ECs in tumor, a specialized venule is formed. This group of blood vessel is called high endothelial venules (HEVs), a specialized post-capillary venule. These HEVs are usually confined in a secondary lymphoid tissue [37–39]. Interestingly, HEVs have also been found in metastatic animal models of lung cancer and melanoma, indicating a possible relationship between HEVs and metastasis [40–42]. In primary tumor, the abundance of HEV has been closely linked to T cell infiltration to the lesion of tertiary lymphoid organs at the tumor site. Due to this, HEVs have been implicated with favorable prognosis in various cancers [43]. Not only that, the presence of HEV largely inhibits the tumor growth and metastasis, as shown in mouse models. In breast cancer patients, HEV is an independent predictor of better prognosis [37]. Recent data indicates that HEV induction in tumor not only supports T cell infiltration to the tumor site but also induces the infiltration of B cells and mature DCs, providing a potent environment for T cell priming and activation, and to elicit a tumor response [40, 41]. As mentioned, lymphangiogenesis is carried out by the activation of lymphotoxin a, LIGHT (TNF superfamily member 14), and lymphotoxin-B receptors, and these are also highly expressed on HEVs [40–43].

Lymphatic Vessels

Lymphatic vessels have also been found to be remodeled in the local *onco-sphere*, as mentioned in Chap. 9 [44]. Not only lymphangiogenesis in the tumors are induced by VEGF-C and -D, lymphangiogenesis around the tumor are also dependent on these growth factors, a feature already confirmed in both mouse and human specimens [45–47] which is also associated with increased metastasis [48, 49]. In fact, similar molecules that are upregulated during vascular remodeling are also interfering with the lymphatic system modulation (i.e., VEGF and angiopoietin), indicating a close relationship between angiogenesis and lymphangiogenesis [50].

Perivascular Cells

Pericytes, especially pericytes, are thought to be essential for vessel stabilization and maturation [51]. Stable pericyte coverage appears to be based on many important molecular pathways, particularly the TGF-β, Ang-1/Tie-2, and PDGFβ/PDGFRβ signaling pathways. Pericyte detachment is essentially the first step of angiogenesis. Only after pericyte detachment, ECs could proliferate and migrate to contribute further to the leakiness phenotype of the unstable tumor blood vessels [52]. Due to the unstable feature of the tumor vessel, in addition to its leakiness, they are much more to anti-angiogenic therapies, while another type of therapy named "vascular normalization" works in reverse: to restore normal function of vessels. The concept of vascular normalization is simple: it is to re-construct a vessel that is near normal, so that the delivery of chemotherapy could be enhanced and therefore leads to an improvement in drug delivery and other kinds of immunotherapeutic [10]. Furthermore, increment in pericyte coverage on tumor vessels can lead to a reduction in metastasis, suggesting a possible mechanical barricade function of pericyte in the blood vessels [53]. Nevertheless, the function of pericytes might be different in the context of specific tumors. Vascular normalization therapy is also detailed in the final chapter of this book, when we discussed on the cancer ecosystem-directed therapeutics.

Endothelial Progenitor Cells (EPCs)

Bone marrow-derived cells (BMDCs) and their role in tumor growth and angiogenesis are increasingly accepted [54–57]. BMDCs are actually the progenitor of many cells described here, such as mesenchymal stromal cells, MDSCs, TAMs, and endothelial progenitor cells (EPC) [56, 58–64]. Although there have been studies depicting the importance of EPCs in their role as anti-angiogenic therapeutics [61, 65–67], the identity and role of BMDC-derived EPCs in tumor angiogenesis remain controversial [68, 69]. This is due to the fact that the differences in EPC levels have been found in many mouse models, and there are no solid evidences that reveals the function of EPCs in the establishment of tumor vessels [70]. However, there is a possibility that the EPC expression level or their involvement in vascular remodeling depends on tumor stage. This is particularly evident in a study where EPCs are clearly identified in about 20% of angiogenic sprouts on tumor vessels, in both transplantation and spontaneous mouse models. Interestingly, targeting these EPCs could inhibit the growth of tumor in a significant manner [71]. Therefore, the hypothesis of the above statement remains true. Furthermore, another study found that EPCs can only be detected in newly-growing blood vessels (emerging vessels), which rapidly falls under undetectable levels during vessel maturation [72]. Thus, vasculo-lytic agents that cause rapid tumor necrosis and hypoxia cause extensive BMDC-derived EPCs recruitment and vascular integration into vasculolytic-resistant tumor margins, suggesting that vasculolytic agent/angiogenesis inhibitor combinations drugs that can combat resistance to both therapies have been suggested [60, 73]. An analysis of a patient who received her BM transplant from a heterosexual donor prior to cancer onset revealed that 4.9% of his tumor vessels had his donor-derived EPCs [74]. In sum, current evidences point towards the involvement of BMDC-derived EPCs in emerging tumor vessels, indicating considerable potential as therapeutic/diagnostic targets. However, the striking lack of distinct EPC surface markers for their unambiguous detection [65, 75–77], coupled with ongoing controversy regarding the extent and timing of EPC involvement, has defined their identity and biology and emphasizes the urgent need for further research.

Lymphangiogenesis in Lymph Nodes

In the context of the carcinogenesis model, draining of the metastasis of lymph nodes is significantly facilitated by the VEGF-A-induced tumor lymphangiogenesis [66, 67]. Note that, relative to mice that were of the wild type, VEGF-A transgenic mice characterized an increased level of distant organ metastases and distant lymph nodes. In the SCC model, VEGF-A induced both angiogenesis and lymphangiogenesis in the tumor and also inside draining lymph nodes [67]. In another SCC metastasis model, metastatic cells were detected in the draining lymph nodes that characterize intranodal lymphangiogenesis [78]. To inhibit cancer metastasis, the theory of lymph node lymphangiogenesis may change clinical care and our comprehension of therapeutic targets. The processes whereby the spreading of tumor from primary local *onco-sphere* to draining/sentinel lymph nodes have been the subject of many studies into tumor development and metastasis. Although local tumors can be eliminated with surgical resection, and the same is true with draining lymph nodes, the existence of distant lymph node or organ metastasis reminds us the local intervention is incomplete. Therefore, it is necessary to determine the mechanism that encourages distant metastases (Fig. 12.1).

Therefore, in the context of tumor metastasis, lymphangiogenesis within regional lymph nodes may be a potential therapeutic target for methods designed to halt the

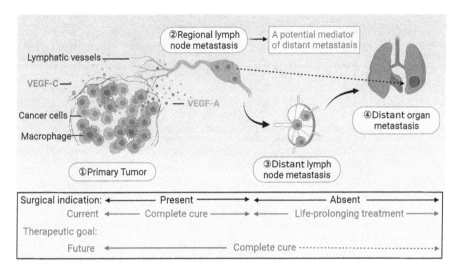

Fig. 12.1 Distant metastasis is significantly mediated by lymph node lymphangiogenesis. Following tumor cell spread to nearby lymph nodes, new lymphatic vessel development is promoted

spread of disease to distant regions, and therefore deserves more attention. In a routine H&E staining on a melanoma tumor, metastasis can be observed not only in the sentinel lymph nodes (characterized by monoclonal antibody HMB-45 for melanoma cells and NZ-1 for podoplanin), but also in the other lymph nodes surrounding the tumor. This is also in line with current clinical characteristics seen in breast cancer patients, where patients with metastasis in regional or axillary lymph nodes are results of lymphangiogenesis [79]. To date, no certainty has been reported on the importance of lymphangiogenesis in distant lymph nodes, and what this means to future cancer therapy, especially those targeting metastasis.

Tumor Metastasis Follows Intranodal Lymphangiogenesis

Within lymph nodes, lymphatic tubes can develop, and the newly created lymphatic endothelium likely encourages the lymphatic dissemination of malignancies. It is not yet apparent, nevertheless, whether nodal lymphangiogenesis transforms the site-specific milieu in lymph nodes from one that functions as an inherent immune system to prevent tumor metastasis to one that serves as a preferred location for metastasis growth. One of the theories indicated that the CSCs could be metastatic due to the lymphovascular niche. In this concept, CSCs can be encouraged to increase in number and to survive better [80–84] (Fig. 12.2). Cutaneous lymphatics arise from thin-walled blunt terminal capillaries that lack a continuous vascular basement membrane. In normal settings, this anatomical feature allows lymphatic capillaries to absorb interstitial tissue fluid, large chemicals, and immune cells.

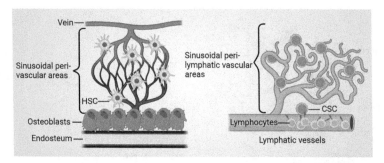

Fig. 12.2 Lymphovascular niche in lymph nodes during tumor metastasis. The specialized sinusoidal endothelium of venous origin (purple) seen in the bone marrow vascular niche (left) creates a milieu for the colonization and maintenance of HSCs. In contrast, tumor-associated lymphangiogenesis inside lymph nodes has led to a striking expansion of the sinusoidal lymphatic endothelium-based lymphatic network (right, green). This particular "lymphovascular niche" in the milieu of the lymph nodes may help to act as a haven for the survival and residency of metastatic CSCs (for interpretation of the references to colour in this figure legend, the reader is referred to the web version of this article)

The lymphatic endothelium of lymph nodes lacks many ECM components and is therefore composed of "sine waves" that are in intimate contact with parenchymal cells. The vascular niche is a specialized environment for the maintenance of hematopoietic stem cells (HSCs), especially bone marrow sinusoidal endothelial cells from stem cell biology [85–87]. The trabecular *endo*-osteosynthesis of the adult bone marrow or sinusoidal perivascular areas is the area where HSCs reside. Thin-walled dendritic venous networks are composed of vascular niche structures that allow venous circulating cells to expand into hematopoietic areas. The inner stellate zone (osteoblastic niche) is expected to promote HSC quiescence, whereas the vascular niche in the bone marrow is thought to promote HSC development, proliferation, and recruitment to the peripheral circulation [88]. Additionally, recent research has demonstrated that CXCL12, which is a ligand for the chemokine receptor CXCR4 produced by HSCs and consequently necessary for colonization in the bone marrow, is secreted at high levels in the bone marrow vascular niche [89, 90]. Lymph nodes produce a lot of CXCL12, whereas metastatic breast cancer cells express high level of its receptor CXCR4, suggesting that a CXCL12-rich microenvironment in lymph nodes may help, forming a lymphovascular niche that attracts and supports a subset of cancer stem cells to metastasize.

Trans Differentiation and Vascular Mimicry

Although blood vessels are constantly present in normal tissue, the formation and differentiation of tumor vasculature is different from the normal process. The tumor could utilize multiple sources of cells in its environment to mimic the ECs, as identified in many cancers, including melanoma [91, 92]. Some even identified the source of the ECs is tissue stem cells in brain, breast, and kidney tumors [93–95]. It has also been reported that CSC-like cells generate endothelium in glioblastoma [96–100]. Although the specific contribution of these findings towards tumor angiogenesis is yet to be elucidated, these findings are clear that tumor will do whatever it takes to keep on surviving, even to circumvent the anti-angiogenic effect of drugs (Box 12.1).

Box 12.1 Regional *Onco-Sphere*: Vascular Remodeling in the Sentinel Lymph Node

In many human cancers, metastatic local lymph node involvement is well established to give rise to oncolytic SLNs. The characteristics of these SLNs are a good reflection of the angiogenic capability of the primary tumor. As reflected by a study, "vascular hotspots" could be identified in SLN, and this phenomenon is correlated with higher metastatic potential of the cancer cells in the SLN [101]. Even in pre-existing lymph node which underwent angiogenesis, HEV represented a major component in these lymph nodes. What is more interesting is that the features of these HEV's characteristics could be modulated by primary tumors via soluble factors, chemokines, cytokines, EVs, etc., indicating a bi-directional relationship between local and the regional *onco-sphere* (Fig. 12.3). This communication is pre-determining the metastatic outcome of the cancer cell, as HEV have been identified to begin their proliferation and expansion even before the arrival of these cancer cells, again indicating a crosstalk between this regional *onco-sphere* to create a favorable new niche for the cancer cells [102–105].

One major change seen in the HEVs prior to metastasis is the loss of CCL21, which is important for lymphocyte homing and adhesion [104]. HEVs can gradually be changed towards erythrocytes-like morphology, eventually losing their peripheral cell's characteristics [102, 106]. In a murine model, it was also observed that BMP-4 was significantly decreased in HEV, and this is a response towards tumor expressing VEGF-D, which also encourages HEV proliferation [107]. Although there has not been a direct evidence that link HEV remodeling towards tumor growth or metastasis, results are indicating that tumor could indeed induce HEV remodeling into capillary-type vessels, which has been known to encourage angiogenesis which in turn increases the rate of metastasis, while simultaneously inducing an *onco-sphere* that is immunosuppressive [103], as lymphocytes could be barred from being trafficked into the SLN [104, 108].

Also, the intercommunication between HEVs and the lymphatic vessels in SLN could also increase the attachment of the CTCs, increasing the probability of these cells being adsorbed into the regional *onco-sphere* [103, 109]. Given the strong connection between HEVs, SLNs, and the immune system, we should consider all these factors when designing a metastatic-targeting drugs [110, 111]. Not only HEVs are modulated by the

(continued)

Box 12.1 (continued)

local *onco-sphere*, but also the lymphatic systems in the SLN are remodeled. Lymphatic network expansion, proliferation, and expansion in tumor deposits generally precedes the arrival of metastatic cells [102, 105, 112, 113] and increases according to metastatic burden [114, 115]. In mouse models, premetastatic LN lymphangiogenesis drains lymphatic flow and increases the next successive LNs [116–118]. Moreover, an association has been established between lymphangiogenesis of involved SLNs, distant LNs, and lung metastases [119, 120]. In Paget's disease and breast cancers, researchers have found a direct link between an increment in SLN lymphangiogenesis, and distant LN metastasis [114, 115, 119, 120]. Soluble factors especially the angiogenic factor VEGF-A have been strongly implicated in LN lymphangiogenesis. In many cancers, the elevated level of VEGF-A is indicative of increased vascular ECs proliferation and is also predictive of LN lymphatic metastasis. Furthermore, in murine models, VEGF-A and -C has been indicated as a direct factor that increases LN lymphangiogenesis in many cancers, including OSCC, lung and breast cancers [105, 112].

Metastatic Vascular Remodeling

Regarding direct evidence of major blood vessels or lymphatic vessels that are involved in metastasis process is limited. This could represent an opportunity for studies and researches that could lead to new potential interventions specifically in this area. However, observations regarding changes in some vessels nearing the tumor site have been studied. For example, arteries and veins that are located in close proximity with a solid tumor are generally tortuous and also dilated [19, 121]. There are also reports on large- sized sample study on lymphatic collections where they indicated that these dilated vessels are induced mostly by lymphangiogenic growth factors (such as VEGFs) or via prostaglandins produced by local ECs, which ultimately enhances the transport of tumor [50, 122].

Although the "seed and soil" hypothesis has been suggested decades ago, the observations remain true today. There is indeed preferential soil that could be prepped for the "welcoming" of the tumor cells. The nurturing of this soil is done by the collaboration of many factors, such as growth factors, cytokines, and chemokines [123]. Another important factor is the local ECs, as their molecular profiles and properties are crucial in deciding the tumor cells dissemination, extravasation, and their survival, ultimately, their metastatic potential [124, 125]. Evidence also suggests that in the blood flow into the metastatic site contains VEGF-A, VEGF-C, and VEGF-D, which could be used by BMDCs VEGFR-1β endothelial precursors to enhance the angiogenesis of blood vessels at the new soil [78, 102, 126, 127]. Furthermore, cancer cell-derived exosomes which contain both DNA and protein components can be secreted and transported in the blood stream. These

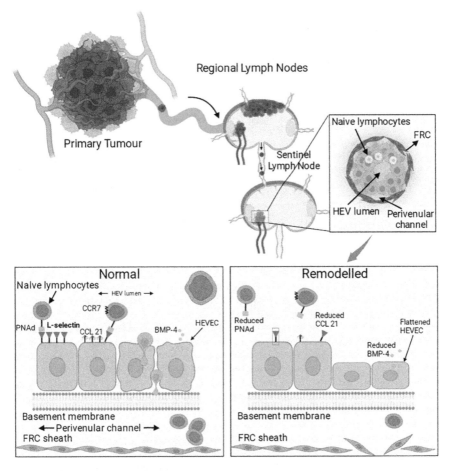

Fig. 12.3 An overview of the cellular and molecular properties of HEV in the SLN and how they are modulated by primary tumors in regional *onco-sphere*. After dissemination, the CTCs reached the regional *onco-sphere* (SLNs) via afferent lymphatics. Prior to this, HEVs had already been pre-conditioned to receive these CTCs, including an increment of "binding" ability of these tumor cells to HEVs to increase their uptake into the SLNs. Difference between HEVs in normal condition vs. in cancer (lower panel)

exosomes are labelled with receptors that could have target organ specificity, as evidenced in a study in renal cancer and melanoma [128, 129].

Over the past 15 years, various antiangiogenic drugs have been developed that target ligands and receptors that regulate tumor angiogenesis, particularly the VEGF-A/VEGFR-2 signaling axis [130]. There are many kinds of drugs within these FDA-approved drugs, including small molecule inhibitors (kinase inhibitors), monoclonal antibodies, or soluble receptor domains. Currently, the top choice among these antiangiogenic drugs is Avastin (Bevacizumab). Avastin is a humanized monoclonal antibody targeting VEGF-A to inhibit angiogenesis. Avastin is currently used in combination with other chemotherapeutic drugs [130–133]. The original

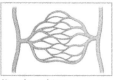

Normal vasculature

- Interaction of arterial and venous circulation
- Capillary bed

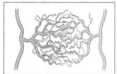

Tumor-induced vasculature

- Vessel remodelling   • Active angiogenesis
- Highly permeable vessels   • Hypoxia is common
- Blood flow is chaotic and slow
- Tumor induction of abnormal vasculature
- Vessel co-option could be used to obtain more blood supply

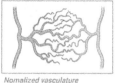

Nomalized vasculature

- Anti-angiogenic therapy can act to normalize the tumor vasculature
- Reduced vascular permeability
- Potentially increased access to chemotherapy
- Reduced tumor bulk

Fig. 12.4 A summary of the differences in normal vs. tumoral blood vessels. "Normal" blood vessels are regular in appearance, with a set arterial and venous segments linked through a capillary bed. The "abnormal" look of the "tumor-induced" vascular bed is seen as dysregulated, where angiogenesis are highly activated. Some of the pathways that are activated includes the following: VEGF-A/VEGFR-2 axis. These are often poorly-formed vessels which show high vascular porousness, and have decreased pericyte coverage. They altogether result in decreased flow of blood and poor tissue perfusion, thus resulting in patches of hypoxia and possibly affected admission for medicines. Inside the tumor, the arterial and the venous side become indistinguishable. In the "normalized" tumor treated with an anti-angiogenic agent, the vasculature looks a lot like its original structure

hypothesis of the usage of anti-angiogenic inhibitor is to create an environment that deplete the tumor's blood vessels and their oxygen and nutrient's supply, leading to a "starvation" environment which ultimately leads to tumor death. However, sub-par clinical and pre-clinical results using these angiogenic inhibitor presented an ugly fact: there are many pathways of angiogenesis in cancer, and one size does not fit all [10, 61]. The above notion of "vascular normalization," however, is proposed based on both preclinical and clinical data [10, 134–136]. According to this concept (Fig. 12.4), tumor's original blood vessels, that are barely functioning, leaky, heterogeneous, and dilated are useless, albeit, did not carry out the normal function of a vessel. Therefore, by re-programming them into their original structure in a non-tumoral environment, these blood vessels may be restored into their "near-normal" structure, with proper functions. In this manner, these tumors could be more receptive towards systemic administration of chemotherapeutics, and these drugs could have better access to the cancer cells.

However, one of the biggest problems with anti-angiogenic drugs is drug resistance. In patients treated with Avastin, patients either stopped responding to the treatment, or slowly developed resistance to the drug after several cycle of treatment [137]. This observation should not come as a surprise, given the diversity of angiogenic pathways present in the tumor, indicating that the tumor could easily switch into another form of angiogenesis for their own survival. This has been summarized in detail in Chap. 6: physiological changes in the local *onco-sphere* (angiogenesis). Furthermore, VEGF family consists of not only VEGF-A (main target of Avastin). When VEGF-A is blocked, tumor will immediately increase their synthesis of VEGF-C and VEGF-D, in which both of these can be proteolytically processed and can activate VEGFR [138–142]. Apart from VEGF family, other ligands/receptor systems (i.e., FGF/FGFR, Ang/Tie-2) could also be the main player for angiogenesis in cancer [143]. In the tumor's crosstalk with the local *onco-sphere*, the hypoxic condition could encourage BMDCs to secrete pro-angiogenic molecules and thus promoting revascularization of the tumor [54, 60, 135]. Another alternative mechanism for improving tumor perfusion during treatment with bevacizumab is resorption of pre-existing blood vessels, or vessel co-option mechanism, also detailed in Chap. 6 [54] (Box 12.2).

Box 12.2 The Theory of Vascular Normalization
The maturation effect on blood vessels has been outlined by vascular normalization as the probable underlying cause of improvements in chemotherapy treatments, when combined with VEGF signaling inhibitors [144]. Insufficient pericyte coverage is represented by immature vessels that are formed due to the increase in VEGF secretion from tumor cells [23]. The active recruitment of pericytes and the reduced permeability by tightening junctions between cells are caused by the restoration of angiogenic signals in tumors, due to the careful dosage administration of VEGF inhibitors, resulting in the increased perfusion among tumors [70]. The activation of Ang-1/Tie2 signaling is partially responsible for the recruitment of pericytes to the blood vessels, which is a consequence of VEGFR2 blockade [71]. Similarly, the facilitation of pericyte maturation and recruitment, in addition to an increase in PDGFRβ signaling, occurs due to VEGF inhibition [23]. The dosage and point in time associated with the administration of VEGF inhibitors to normalize the blood vessels of tumor tend to be narrow and are dependent on the schedule, type of inhibitor, and tumor targeted, thereby posing a challenge to its use [145]. Furthermore, based on the type of the tumor and the kind of drug used, the effect may last up to 4 months, although it is generally not prolonged [72]. Marked vascular regression replaces vascular normalization when VEGF activity is highly neutralized, as demonstrated by long durations of exposition or increased doses; this, in turn, increases the risk of metastatic spread due to higher potential for tumor hypoxia and since the invasive tumor cells are favored in terms of selection [73, 146]. As the therapeutic index of various approaches necessitates the persistence of vascular normalization over longer periods, strategies that effectuate long-term and effective stabilization of the blood vessels of the tumor are in urgent demand [147]. The benefits of

(continued)

Box 12.2 (continued)

treatments against cancer can be enhanced and hypoxia can be alleviated through the vital role of appropriate vascular normalization, as supported by gene expression and imaging studies [74]. The ideal regimen that can be adopted for the achievement of normalization is determined using the functionality of tumor blood vessels following anti-angiogenic treatments, which can be determined using DCE-MRI (dynamic contrast-enhanced magnetic resonance imaging) or radiotracer ^{18}F-MISO, developed for positron emission tomography (PET), both of which are techniques characterized by their non-invasiveness [75, 76]. After treatments that utilize VEGF inhibitors, tracers can be used to supervise the vascular normalization, as exemplified by ^{99m}Tc-RGD, which binds $\alpha v\beta 3$, an integrin secreted during phases of active angiogenesis [65].

Conclusion

The complex nature of the pathways associated with the angiogenesis of tumors is signified by all the above findings and observations. In addition to anti-VEGF treatments, which have proven to enhance the efficiency of systemic chemotherapy, several alternative pathways have been suggested in association with vascular maturation and formation, which may restore a relative more normal tumor vasculature that can enhance the effects of radiotherapy and delivery cytotoxic drugs effectively, all through the controlling of vascular responses in the TME. Further research must be undertaken with regard to the mechanisms that undergird the process of normalization due to the significant heterogeneity in tumor vessels. In addition to identifying and modifying strategies to target varying angiogenesis pathways, predictive biomarkers may be determined to distinguish responders from non-responder groups of patients. Based on their potential response, anti-angiogenic therapies that are personalized to their needs can be offered to patients.

References

1. Tumor JF (2000) Angiogenesis. In: Holland JF, Frei E III, Bast RC Jr et al (eds) Cancer medicine, 5th edn. B.C. Decker, Hamilton, ON, pp 132–152
2. Angiogenesis JF (2001) Harrison's principles of internal medicine. In: Braunwald E, Fauci AS, Kasper DL et al (eds) Harrison's principles of internal medicine, 15th edn. McGraw-Hill, New York, NY, pp 517–530
3. Folkman J (2002) Role of angiogenesis in tumor growth and metastasis. Semin Oncol 29(6 Suppl 16):15–18
4. Black WC, Welch HG (1993) Advances in diagnostic imaging and overestimations of disease prevalence and the benefits of therapy. N Engl J Med 328(17):1237–1243

5. Carmeliet P, Jain RK (2000) Angiogenesis in cancer and other diseases. Nature 407(6801): 249–257
6. Detmar M, Velasco P, Richard L, Claffey KP, Streit M, Riccardi L et al (2000) Expression of vascular endothelial growth factor induces an invasive phenotype in human squamous cell carcinomas. Am J Pathol 156(1):159–167
7. Streit M, Riccardi L, Velasco P, Brown LF, Hawighorst T, Bornstein P et al (1999) Thrombospondin-2: a potent endogenous inhibitor of tumor growth and angiogenesis. Proc Natl Acad Sci U S A 96(26):14888–14893
8. Farnsworth RH, Lackmann M, Achen MG, Stacker SA (2014) Vascular remodeling in cancer. Oncogene 33(27):3496–3505
9. Nagy JA, Dvorak HF (2012) Heterogeneity of the tumor vasculature: the need for new tumor blood vessel type-specific targets. Clin Exp Metastasis 29(7):657–662
10. Carmeliet P, Jain RK (2011) Principles and mechanisms of vessel normalization for cancer and other angiogenic diseases. Nat Rev Drug Discov 10(6):417–427
11. Nagy JA, Feng D, Vasile E, Wong WH, Shih SC, Dvorak AM et al (2006) Permeability properties of tumor surrogate blood vessels induced by VEGF-A. Lab Investig 86(8):767–780
12. Stubbs M, McSheehy PM, Griffiths JR, Bashford CL (2000) Causes and consequences of tumour acidity and implications for treatment. Mol Med Today 6(1):15–19
13. Höckel M, Vaupel P (2001) Biological consequences of tumor hypoxia. Semin Oncol 28(2 Suppl 8):36–41
14. Semenza GL (2001) HIF-1, O (2), and the 3 PHDs: how animal cells signal hypoxia to the nucleus. Cell 107(1):1–3
15. Cardone RA, Casavola V, Reshkin SJ (2005) The role of disturbed pH dynamics and the Na+/ H+ exchanger in metastasis. Nat Rev Cancer 5(10):786–795
16. Sullivan R, Graham CH (2007) Hypoxia-driven selection of the metastatic phenotype. Cancer Metastasis Rev 26(2):319–331
17. Graeber TG, Osmanian C, Jacks T, Housman DE, Koch CJ, Lowe SW et al (1996) Hypoxia-mediated selection of cells with diminished apoptotic potential in solid tumours. Nature 379(6560):88–91
18. Moeller BJ, Richardson RA, Dewhirst MW (2007) Hypoxia and radiotherapy: opportunities for improved outcomes in cancer treatment. Cancer Metastasis Rev 26(2):241–248
19. Nagy JA, Chang SH, Shih SC, Dvorak AM, Dvorak HF (2010) Heterogeneity of the tumor vasculature. Semin Thromb Hemost 36(3):321–331
20. Yu JL, Rak JW, Klement G, Kerbel RS (2002) Vascular endothelial growth factor isoform expression as a determinant of blood vessel patterning in human melanoma xenografts. Cancer Res 62(6):1838–1846
21. Tammela T, He Y, Lyytikkä J, Jeltsch M, Markkanen J, Pajusola K et al (2007) Distinct architecture of lymphatic vessels induced by chimeric vascular endothelial growth factor-C/ vascular endothelial growth factor heparin-binding domain fusion proteins. Circ Res 100(10): 1468–1475
22. Keskitalo S, Tammela T, Lyytikka J, Karpanen T, Jeltsch M, Markkanen J et al (2007) Enhanced capillary formation stimulated by a chimeric vascular endothelial growth factor/ vascular endothelial growth factor-C silk domain fusion protein. Circ Res 100(10):1460–1467
23. Cao R, Eriksson A, Kubo H, Alitalo K, Cao Y, Thyberg J (2004) Comparative evaluation of FGF-2-, VEGF-A-, and VEGF-C-induced angiogenesis, lymphangiogenesis, vascular fenes-trations, and permeability. Circ Res 94(5):664–670
24. Wirzenius M, Tammela T, Uutela M, He Y, Odorisio T, Zambruno G et al (2007) Distinct vascular endothelial growth factor signals for lymphatic vessel enlargement and sprouting. J Exp Med 204(6):1431–1440
25. Woolard J, Bevan HS, Harper SJ, Bates DO (2009) Molecular diversity of VEGF-A as a regulator of its biological activity. Microcirculation 16(7):572–592

26. Konerding MA, Fait E, Dimitropoulou C, Malkusch W, Ferri C, Giavazzi R et al (1998) Impact of fibroblast growth factor-2 on tumor microvascular architecture. A tridimensional morphometric study. Am J Pathol 152(6):1607–1616
27. Konerding MA, Malkusch W, Klapthor B, van Ackern C, Fait E, Hill SA et al (1999) Evidence for characteristic vascular patterns in solid tumours: quantitative studies using corrosion casts. Br J Cancer 80(5–6):724–732
28. Hervé MA, Buteau-Lozano H, Vassy R, Bieche I, Velasco G, Pla M et al (2008) Overexpression of vascular endothelial growth factor 189 in breast cancer cells leads to delayed tumor uptake with dilated intratumoral vessels. Am J Pathol 172(1):167–178
29. Qin L, Bromberg-White JL, Qian CN (2012) Opportunities and challenges in tumor angiogenesis research: back and forth between bench and bed. Adv Cancer Res 113:191–239
30. Paku S, Paweletz N (1991) First steps of tumor-related angiogenesis. Lab Investig 65(3):334–346
31. Dvorak AM, Kohn S, Morgan ES, Fox P, Nagy JA, Dvorak HF (1996) The vesiculo-vacuolar organelle (VVO): a distinct endothelial cell structure that provides a transcellular pathway for macromolecular extravasation. J Leukoc Biol 59(1):100–115
32. Goffin JR, Straume O, Chappuis PO, Brunet JS, Bégin LR, Hamel N et al (2003) Glomeruloid microvascular proliferation is associated with p53 expression, germline BRCA1 mutations and an adverse outcome following breast cancer. Br J Cancer 89(6):1031–1034
33. Straume O, Chappuis PO, Salvesen HB, Halvorsen OJ, Haukaas SA, Goffin JR et al (2002) Prognostic importance of glomeruloid microvascular proliferation indicates an aggressive angiogenic phenotype in human cancers. Cancer Res 62(23):6808–6811
34. Birner P, Piribauer M, Fischer I, Gatterbauer B, Marosi C, Ambros PF et al (2003) Vascular patterns in glioblastoma influence clinical outcome and associate with variable expression of angiogenic proteins: evidence for distinct angiogenic subtypes. Brain Pathol 13(2):133–143
35. Griffioen AW (2008) Anti-angiogenesis: making the tumor vulnerable to the immune system. Cancer Immunol Immunother 57(10):1553–1558
36. Dirkx AE, oude Egbrink MG, Castermans K, van der Schaft DW, Thijssen VL, Dings RP et al (2006) Anti-angiogenesis therapy can overcome endothelial cell anergy and promote leukocyte-endothelium interactions and infiltration in tumors. FASEB J 20(6):621–630
37. Martinet L, Garrido I, Filleron T, Le Guellec S, Bellard E, Fournie JJ et al (2011) Human solid tumors contain high endothelial venules: association with T- and B-lymphocyte infiltration and favorable prognosis in breast cancer. Cancer Res 71(17):5678–5687
38. de Chaisemartin L, Goc J, Damotte D, Validire P, Magdeleinat P, Alifano M et al (2011) Characterization of chemokines and adhesion molecules associated with T cell presence in tertiary lymphoid structures in human lung cancer. Cancer Res 71(20):6391–6399
39. Cipponi A, Mercier M, Seremet T, Baurain JF, Théate I, van den Oord J et al (2012) Neogenesis of lymphoid structures and antibody responses occur in human melanoma metastases. Cancer Res 72(16):3997–4007
40. Hindley JP, Jones E, Smart K, Bridgeman H, Lauder SN, Ondondo B et al (2012) T-cell trafficking facilitated by high endothelial venules is required for tumor control after regulatory T-cell depletion. Cancer Res 72(21):5473–5482
41. Schrama D, thor Straten P, Fischer WH, AD ML, Bröcker EB, Reisfeld RA et al (2001) Targeting of lymphotoxin-alpha to the tumor elicits an efficient immune response associated with induction of peripheral lymphoid-like tissue. Immunity 14(2):111–121
42. Yu P, Lee Y, Liu W, Chin RK, Wang J, Wang Y et al (2004) Priming of naive T cells inside tumors leads to eradication of established tumors. Nat Immunol 5(2):141–149
43. Fridman WH, Galon J, Pagès F, Tartour E, Sautès-Fridman C, Kroemer G (2011) Prognostic and predictive impact of intra- and peritumoral immune infiltrates. Cancer Res 71(17):5601–5605
44. Achen MG, Stacker SA (2008) Molecular control of lymphatic metastasis. Ann N Y Acad Sci 1131:225–234

45. Stacker SA, Caesar C, Baldwin ME, Thornton GE, Williams RA, Prevo R et al (2001) VEGF-D promotes the metastatic spread of tumor cells via the lymphatics. Nat Med 7(2):186–191
46. Skobe M, Hawighorst T, Jackson DG, Prevo R, Janes L, Velasco P et al (2001) Induction of tumor lymphangiogenesis by VEGF-C promotes breast cancer metastasis. Nat Med 7(2):192–198
47. Mandriota SJ, Jussila L, Jeltsch M, Compagni A, Baetens D, Prevo R et al (2001) Vascular endothelial growth factor-C-mediated lymphangiogenesis promotes tumour metastasis. EMBO J 20(4):672–682
48. Achen MG, McColl BK, Stacker SA (2005) Focus on lymphangiogenesis in tumor metastasis. Cancer Cell 7(2):121–127
49. Sleeman JP, Nazarenko I, Thiele W (2011) Do all roads lead to Rome? Routes to metastasis development. Int J Cancer 128(11):2511–2526
50. Karnezis T, Shayan R, Caesar C, Roufail S, Harris NC, Ardipradja K et al (2012) VEGF-D promotes tumor metastasis by regulating prostaglandins produced by the collecting lymphatic endothelium. Cancer Cell 21(2):181–195
51. Armulik A, Abramsson A, Betsholtz C (2005) Endothelial/pericyte interactions. Circ Res 97(6):512–523
52. Raza A, Franklin MJ, Dudek AZ (2010) Pericytes and vessel maturation during tumor angiogenesis and metastasis. Am J Hematol 85(8):593–598
53. Gerhardt H, Semb H (2008) Pericytes: gatekeepers in tumour cell metastasis? J Mol Med (Berl) 86(2):135–144
54. Bergers G, Hanahan D (2008) Modes of resistance to anti-angiogenic therapy. Nat Rev Cancer 8(8):592–603
55. Murdoch C, Muthana M, Coffelt SB, Lewis CE (2008) The role of myeloid cells in the promotion of tumour angiogenesis. Nat Rev Cancer 8(8):618–631
56. Pollard JW (2004) Tumour-educated macrophages promote tumour progression and metastasis. Nat Rev Cancer 4(1):71–78
57. Wels J, Kaplan RN, Rafii S, Lyden D (2008) Migratory neighbors and distant invaders: tumor-associated niche cells. Genes Dev 22(5):559–574
58. Weis SM, Cheresh DA (2011) Tumor angiogenesis: molecular pathways and therapeutic targets. Nat Med 17(11):1359–1370
59. Lyden D, Hattori K, Dias S, Costa C, Blaikie P, Butros L et al (2001) Impaired recruitment of bone-marrow-derived endothelial and hematopoietic precursor cells blocks tumor angiogenesis and growth. Nat Med 7(11):1194–1201
60. Shaked Y, Ciarrocchi A, Franco M, Lee CR, Man S, Cheung AM et al (2006) Therapy-induced acute recruitment of circulating endothelial progenitor cells to tumors. Science 313(5794):1785–1787
61. Carmeliet P, Jain RK (2011) Molecular mechanisms and clinical applications of angiogenesis. Nature 473(7347):298–307
62. McAllister SS, Weinberg RA (2010) Tumor-host interactions: a far-reaching relationship. J Clin Oncol 28(26):4022–4028
63. Yang L, DeBusk LM, Fukuda K, Fingleton B, Green-Jarvis B, Shyr Y et al (2004) Expansion of myeloid immune suppressor gr+CD11b+ cells in tumor-bearing host directly promotes tumor angiogenesis. Cancer Cell 6(4):409–421
64. Gabrilovich DI, Nagaraj S (2009) Myeloid-derived suppressor cells as regulators of the immune system. Nat Rev Immunol 9(3):162–174
65. Mancuso P, Antoniotti P, Quarna J, Calleri A, Rabascio C, Tacchetti C et al (2009) Validation of a standardized method for enumerating circulating endothelial cells and progenitors: flow cytometry and molecular and ultrastructural analyses. Clin Cancer Res 15(1):267–273
66. Hirakawa S (2009) From tumor lymphangiogenesis to lymphvascular niche. Cancer Sci 100(6):983–989

67. Hirakawa S, Kodama S, Kunstfeld R, Kajiya K, Brown LF, Detmar M (2005) VEGF-A induces tumor and sentinel lymph node lymphangiogenesis and promotes lymphatic metastasis. J Exp Med 201(7):1089–1099
68. Yoder MC, Ingram DA (2009) Endothelial progenitor cell: ongoing controversy for defining these cells and their role in neoangiogenesis in the murine system. Curr Opin Hematol 16(4):269–273
69. Patenaude A, Parker J, Karsan A (2010) Involvement of endothelial progenitor cells in tumor vascularization. Microvasc Res 79(3):217–223
70. Purhonen S, Palm J, Rossi D, Kaskenpää N, Rajantie I, Ylä-Herttuala S et al (2008) Bone marrow-derived circulating endothelial precursors do not contribute to vascular endothelium and are not needed for tumor growth. Proc Natl Acad Sci U S A 105(18):6620–6625
71. Nolan DJ, Ciarrocchi A, Mellick AS, Jaggi JS, Bambino K, Gupta S et al (2007) Bone marrow-derived endothelial progenitor cells are a major determinant of nascent tumor neovascularization. Genes Dev 21(12):1546–1558
72. Gao D, Nolan DJ, Mellick AS, Bambino K, McDonnell K, Mittal V (2008) Endothelial progenitor cells control the angiogenic switch in mouse lung metastasis. Science 319(5860):195–198
73. Shaked Y, Henke E, Roodhart JM, Mancuso P, Langenberg MH, Colleoni M et al (2008) Rapid chemotherapy-induced acute endothelial progenitor cell mobilization: implications for antiangiogenic drugs as chemosensitizing agents. Cancer Cell 14(3):263–273
74. Peters BA, Diaz LA, Polyak K, Meszler L, Romans K, Guinan EC et al (2005) Contribution of bone marrow-derived endothelial cells to human tumor vasculature. Nat Med 11(3):261–262
75. Rafii S, Lyden D (2003) Therapeutic stem and progenitor cell transplantation for organ vascularization and regeneration. Nat Med 9(6):702–712
76. Duda DG, Cohen KS, Scadden DT, Jain RK (2007) A protocol for phenotypic detection and enumeration of circulating endothelial cells and circulating progenitor cells in human blood. Nat Protoc 2(4):805–810
77. Bertolini F, Shaked Y, Mancuso P, Kerbel RS (2006) The multifaceted circulating endothelial cell in cancer: towards marker and target identification. Nat Rev Cancer 6(11):835–845
78. Hirakawa S, Brown LF, Kodama S, Paavonen K, Alitalo K, Detmar M (2007) VEGF-C-induced lymphangiogenesis in sentinel lymph nodes promotes tumor metastasis to distant sites. Blood 109(3):1010–1017
79. Van den Eynden GG, Vandenberghe MK, van Dam PJ, Colpaert CG, van Dam P, Dirix LY et al (2007) Increased sentinel lymph node lymphangiogenesis is associated with nonsentinel axillary lymph node involvement in breast cancer patients with a positive sentinel node. Clin Cancer Res 13(18 Pt 1):5391–5397
80. Jordan CT, Guzman ML, Noble M (2006) Cancer stem cells. N Engl J Med 355(12):1253–1261
81. Chiang AC, Massagué J (2008) Molecular basis of metastasis. N Engl J Med 359(26):2814–2823
82. Croker AK, Allan AL (2008) Cancer stem cells: implications for the progression and treatment of metastatic disease. J Cell Mol Med 12(2):374–390
83. Clarke MF, Dick JE, Dirks PB, Eaves CJ, Jamieson CH, Jones DL et al (2006) Cancer stem cells--perspectives on current status and future directions: AACR workshop on cancer stem cells. Cancer Res 66(19):9339–9344
84. Schatton T, Murphy GF, Frank NY, Yamaura K, Waaga-Gasser AM, Gasser M et al (2008) Identification of cells initiating human melanomas. Nature 451(7176):345–349
85. Arai F, Suda T (2007) Maintenance of quiescent hematopoietic stem cells in the osteoblastic niche. Ann N Y Acad Sci 1106:41–53
86. Kopp HG, Avecilla ST, Hooper AT, Rafii S (2005) The bone marrow vascular niche: home of HSC differentiation and mobilization. Physiology (Bethesda) 20:349–356
87. Coultas L, Chawengsaksophak K, Rossant J (2005) Endothelial cells and VEGF in vascular development. Nature 438(7070):937–945

88. Arai F, Hirao A, Ohmura M, Sato H, Matsuoka S, Takubo K et al (2004) Tie2/angiopoietin-1 signaling regulates hematopoietic stem cell quiescence in the bone marrow niche. Cell 118(2): 149–161
89. Sugiyama T, Kohara H, Noda M, Nagasawa T (2006) Maintenance of the hematopoietic stem cell pool by CXCL12-CXCR4 chemokine signaling in bone marrow stromal cell niches. Immunity 25(6):977–988
90. Ara T, Tokoyoda K, Sugiyama T, Egawa T, Kawabata K, Nagasawa T (2003) Long-term hematopoietic stem cells require stromal cell-derived factor-1 for colonizing bone marrow during ontogeny. Immunity 19(2):257–267
91. Maniotis AJ, Folberg R, Hess A, Seftor EA, Gardner LM, Pe'er J et al (1999) Vascular channel formation by human melanoma cells *in vivo* and *in vitro*: vasculogenic mimicry. Am J Pathol 155(3):739–752
92. Rybak SM, Sanovich E, Hollingshead MG, Borgel SD, Newton DL, Melillo G et al (2003) "Vasocrine" formation of tumor cell-lined vascular spaces: implications for rational design of antiangiogenic therapies. Cancer Res 63(11):2812–2819
93. Bruno S, Bussolati B, Grange C, Collino F, Graziano ME, Ferrando U et al (2006) CD133+ renal progenitor cells contribute to tumor angiogenesis. Am J Pathol 169(6):2223–2235
94. Bussolati B, Grange C, Sapino A, Camussi G (2009) Endothelial cell differentiation of human breast tumour stem/progenitor cells. J Cell Mol Med 13(2):309–319
95. Pezzolo A, Parodi F, Corrias MV, Cinti R, Gambini C, Pistoia V (2007) Tumor origin of endothelial cells in human neuroblastoma. J Clin Oncol 25(4):376–383
96. Wang R, Chadalavada K, Wilshire J, Kowalik U, Hovinga KE, Geber A et al (2010) Glioblastoma stem-like cells give rise to tumour endothelium. Nature 468(7325):829–833
97. Ricci-Vitiani L, Pallini R, Biffoni M, Todaro M, Invernici G, Cenci T et al (2010) Tumour vascularization via endothelial differentiation of glioblastoma stem-like cells. Nature 468(7325):824–828
98. Shen R, Ye Y, Chen L, Yan Q, Barsky SH, Gao JX (2008) Precancerous stem cells can serve as tumor vasculogenic progenitors. PLoS One 3(2):e1652
99. Alvero AB, Fu HH, Holmberg J, Visintin I, Mor L, Marquina CC et al (2009) Stem-like ovarian cancer cells can serve as tumor vascular progenitors. Stem Cells 27(10):2405–2413
100. Bussolati B, Bruno S, Grange C, Ferrando U, Camussi G (2008) Identification of a tumor-initiating stem cell population in human renal carcinomas. FASEB J 22(10):3696–3705
101. Guidi AJ, Berry DA, Broadwater G, Perloff M, Norton L, Barcos MP et al (2000) Association of angiogenesis in lymph node metastases with outcome of breast cancer. J Natl Cancer Inst 92(6):486–492
102. Qian CN, Berghuis B, Tsarfaty G, Bruch M, Kort EJ, Ditlev J et al (2006) Preparing the "soil": the primary tumor induces vasculature reorganization in the sentinel lymph node before the arrival of metastatic cancer cells. Cancer Res 66(21):10365–10376
103. Qian CN, Resau JH, Teh BT (2007) Prospects for vasculature reorganization in sentinel lymph nodes. Cell Cycle 6(5):514–517
104. Carrière V, Colisson R, Jiguet-Jiglaire C, Bellard E, Bouche G, Al Saati T et al (2005) Cancer cells regulate lymphocyte recruitment and leukocyte-endothelium interactions in the tumor-draining lymph node. Cancer Res 65(24):11639–11648
105. Chung MK, Do IG, Jung E, Son YI, Jeong HS, Baek CH (2012) Lymphatic vessels and high endothelial venules are increased in the sentinel lymph nodes of patients with oral squamous cell carcinoma before the arrival of tumor cells. Ann Surg Oncol 19(5):1595–1601
106. Lee SY, Qian CN, Ooi AS, Chen P, Tan VK, Chia CS et al (2012) 2011 Young Surgeon's award winner: high endothelial venules: a novel prognostic marker in cancer metastasis and the missing link? Ann Acad Med Singap 41(1):21–28
107. Farnsworth RH, Karnezis T, Shayan R, Matsumoto M, Nowell CJ, Achen MG et al (2011) A role for bone morphogenetic protein-4 in lymph node vascular remodeling and primary tumor growth. Cancer Res 71(20):6547–6557

108. Cochran AJ, Huang RR, Lee J, Itakura E, Leong SP, Essner R (2006) Tumour-induced immune modulation of sentinel lymph nodes. Nat Rev Immunol 6(9):659–670

109. Liao S, Ruddle NH (2006) Synchrony of high endothelial venules and lymphatic vessels revealed by immunization. J Immunol 177(5):3369–3379

110. Girard JP, Moussion C, Förster R (2012) HEVs, lymphatics and homeostatic immune cell trafficking in lymph nodes. Nat Rev Immunol 12(11):762–773

111. Hayasaka H, Taniguchi K, Fukai S, Miyasaka M (2010) Neogenesis and development of the high endothelial venules that mediate lymphocyte trafficking. Cancer Sci 101(11):2302–2308

112. Zhao YC, Ni XJ, Wang MH, Zha XM, Zhao Y, Wang S (2012) Tumor-derived VEGF-C, but not VEGF-D, promotes sentinel lymph node lymphangiogenesis prior to metastasis in breast cancer patients. Med Oncol 29(4):2594–2600

113. Ishii H, Chikamatsu K, Sakakura K, Miyata M, Furuya N, Masuyama K (2010) Primary tumor induces sentinel lymph node lymphangiogenesis in oral squamous cell carcinoma. Oral Oncol 46(5):373–378

114. Kurahara H, Takao S, Shinchi H, Maemura K, Mataki Y, Sakoda M et al (2010) Significance of lymphangiogenesis in primary tumor and draining lymph nodes during lymphatic metastasis of pancreatic head cancer. J Surg Oncol 102(7):809–815

115. Hirakawa S, Detmar M, Kerjaschki D, Nagamatsu S, Matsuo K, Tanemura A et al (2009) Nodal lymphangiogenesis and metastasis: role of tumor-induced lymphatic vessel activation in extramammary Paget's disease. Am J Pathol 175(5):2235–2248

116. Ruddell A, Kelly-Spratt KS, Furuya M, Parghi SS, Kemp CJ (2008) p19/Arf and p53 suppress sentinel lymph node lymphangiogenesis and carcinoma metastasis. Oncogene 27(22): 3145–3155

117. Ruddell A, Mezquita P, Brandvold KA, Farr A, Iritani BM (2003) B lymphocyte-specific c-Myc expression stimulates early and functional expansion of the vasculature and lymphatics during lymphomagenesis. Am J Pathol 163(6):2233–2245

118. Harrell MI, Iritani BM, Ruddell A (2007) Tumor-induced sentinel lymph node lymphangiogenesis and increased lymph flow precede melanoma metastasis. Am J Pathol 170(2):774–786

119. Van den Eynden GG, Van der Auwera I, Van Laere SJ, Huygelen V, Colpaert CG, van Dam P et al (2006) Induction of lymphangiogenesis in and around axillary lymph node metastases of patients with breast cancer. Br J Cancer 95(10):1362–1366

120. Kerjaschki D, Bago-Horvath Z, Rudas M, Sexl V, Schneckenleithner C, Wolbank S et al (2011) Lipoxygenase mediates invasion of intrametastatic lymphatic vessels and propagates lymph node metastasis of human mammary carcinoma xenografts in mouse. J Clin Invest 121(5):2000–2012

121. Yu JL, Rak JW (2003) Host microenvironment in breast cancer development: inflammatory and immune cells in tumour angiogenesis and arteriogenesis. Breast Cancer Res 5(2):83–88

122. Hoshida T, Isaka N, Hagendoorn J, di Tomaso E, Chen YL, Pytowski B et al (2006) Imaging steps of lymphatic metastasis reveals that vascular endothelial growth factor-C increases metastasis by increasing delivery of cancer cells to lymph nodes: therapeutic implications. Cancer Res 66(16):8065–8075

123. Paget S (1889) The distribution of secondary growths in cancer of the breast. Lancet 133(3421):571–573

124. Sleeman JP, Cremers N (2007) New concepts in breast cancer metastasis: tumor initiating cells and the microenvironment. Clin Exp Metastasis 24(8):707–715

125. Psaila B, Lyden D (2009) The metastatic niche: adapting the foreign soil. Nat Rev Cancer 9(4): 285–293

126. Kaplan RN, Riba RD, Zacharoulis S, Bramley AH, Vincent L, Costa C et al (2005) VEGFR1-positive haematopoietic bone marrow progenitors initiate the pre-metastatic niche. Nature 438(7069):820–827

127. Kaplan RN, Rafii S, Lyden D (2006) Preparing the "soil": the premetastatic niche. Cancer Res 66(23):11089–11093

128. Peinado H, Alečković M, Lavotshkin S, Matei I, Costa-Silva B, Moreno-Bueno G et al (2012) Melanoma exosomes educate bone marrow progenitor cells toward a pro-metastatic phenotype through MET. Nat Med 18(6):883–891
129. Grange C, Tapparo M, Collino F, Vitillo L, Damasco C, Deregibus MC et al (2011) Microvesicles released from human renal cancer stem cells stimulate angiogenesis and formation of lung premetastatic niche. Cancer Res 71(15):5346–5356
130. Ferrara N (2002) VEGF and the quest for tumour angiogenesis factors. Nat Rev Cancer 2(10): 795–803
131. Hurwitz H (2004) Integrating the anti-VEGF-A humanized monoclonal antibody bevacizumab with chemotherapy in advanced colorectal cancer. Clin Colorectal Cancer 4 (Suppl 2):S62–S68
132. Hurwitz H, Fehrenbacher L, Novotny W, Cartwright T, Hainsworth J, Heim W et al (2004) Bevacizumab plus irinotecan, fluorouracil, and leucovorin for metastatic colorectal cancer. N Engl J Med 350(23):2335–2342
133. Van Cutsem E, Lambrechts D, Prenen H, Jain RK, Carmeliet P (2011) Lessons from the adjuvant bevacizumab trial on colon cancer: what next? J Clin Oncol 29(1):1–4
134. Jain RK (2005) Normalization of tumor vasculature: an emerging concept in antiangiogenic therapy. Science 307(5706):58–62
135. Batchelor TT, Sorensen AG, di Tomaso E, Zhang WT, Duda DG, Cohen KS et al (2007) AZD2171, a pan-VEGF receptor tyrosine kinase inhibitor, normalizes tumor vasculature and alleviates edema in glioblastoma patients. Cancer Cell 11(1):83–95
136. Hamzah J, Jugold M, Kiessling F, Rigby P, Manzur M, Marti HH et al (2008) Vascular normalization in Rgs5-deficient tumours promotes immune destruction. Nature 453(7193): 410–414
137. Halford MM, Tebbutt NC, Desai J, Achen MG, Stacker SA (2012) Towards the biomarker-guided rational use of antiangiogenic agents in the treatment of metastatic colorectal cancer. Colorectal Cancer 1(2):149–161
138. Joukov V, Pajusola K, Kaipainen A, Chilov D, Lahtinen I, Kukk E et al (1996) A novel vascular endothelial growth factor, VEGF-C, is a ligand for the Flt4 (VEGFR-3) and KDR (VEGFR-2) receptor tyrosine kinases. EMBO J 15(2):290–298
139. Achen MG, Stacker SA (2012) Vascular endothelial growth factor-D: signaling mechanisms, biology, and clinical relevance. Growth Factors 30(5):283–296
140. Achen MG, Jeltsch M, Kukk E, Mäkinen T, Vitali A, Wilks AF et al (1998) Vascular endothelial growth factor D (VEGF-D) is a ligand for the tyrosine kinases VEGF receptor 2 (Flk1) and VEGF receptor 3 (Flt4). Proc Natl Acad Sci U S A 95(2):548–553
141. Stacker SA, Stenvers K, Caesar C, Vitali A, Domagala T, Nice E et al (1999) Biosynthesis of vascular endothelial growth factor-D involves proteolytic processing which generates non-covalent homodimers. J Biol Chem 274(45):32127–32136
142. McColl BK, Paavonen K, Karnezis T, Harris NC, Davydova N, Rothacker J et al (2007) Proprotein convertases promote processing of VEGF-D, a critical step for binding the angiogenic receptor VEGFR-2. FASEB J 21(4):1088–1098
143. Gerald D, Chintharlapalli S, Augustin HG, Benjamin LE (2013) Angiopoietin-2: an attractive target for improved antiangiogenic tumor therapy. Cancer Res 73(6):1649–1657
144. Adams RH, Alitalo K (2007) Molecular regulation of angiogenesis and lymphangiogenesis. Nat Rev Mol Cell Biol 8(6):464–478
145. Alitalo K (2011) The lymphatic vasculature in disease. Nat Med 17(11):1371–1380
146. Reyes M, Dudek A, Jahagirdar B, Koodie L, Marker PH, Verfaillie CM (2002) Origin of endothelial progenitors in human postnatal bone marrow. J Clin Invest 109(3):337–346
147. Aranguren XL, McCue JD, Hendrickx B, Zhu XH, Du F, Chen E et al (2008) Multipotent adult progenitor cells sustain function of ischemic limbs in mice. J Clin Invest 118(2):505–514

Chapter 13
Distal *Onco-Sphere*: The Origin and Overview of Cancer Metastasis

Phei Er Saw and Erwei Song

Abstract In current cancer statistics, most cancer patients died of metastasis and not of primary tumors. Therefore, metastasis could be categorized as a complex and deadly event when occurred in cancer patients. During metastasis, cancer cells spread through growing into nearby normal tissue, moving through lymph nodes or blood vessels, traveling through bloodstream to other parts of the body and forming new tumors in other parts of the body. In this chapter, we will introduce the origin and overview of the mechanistic theory in cancer metastasis. We will also summarize the various theories associated with the development of metastasis. We are dedicating the next few chapters to understand the underlying mechanism and crosstalks between the local and the distal onco-sphere.

Introduction

Metastasis promotes the proliferation of cancer cells from the original tumor to nearby tissues and remote organs, thus being the prime reason for cancer morbidity and mortality. In order to metastasize, cancer cells must first separate from their

P. E. Saw
Guangdong Provincial Key Laboratory of Malignant Tumor Epigenetics and Gene Regulation, Guangdong-Hong Kong Joint Laboratory for RNA Medicine, Medical Research Center, Sun Yat-sen Memorial Hospital, Sun Yat-sen University, Guangzhou, China

Nanhai Translational Innovation Center of Precision Immunology, Sun Yat-sen Memorial Hospital, Sun Yat-sen University, Foshan, China

E. Song (✉)
Guangdong Provincial Key Laboratory of Malignant Tumor Epigenetics and Gene Regulation, Guangdong-Hong Kong Joint Laboratory for RNA Medicine, Medical Research Center, Sun Yat-sen Memorial Hospital, Sun Yat-sen University, Guangzhou, China

Nanhai Translational Innovation Center of Precision Immunology, Sun Yat-sen Memorial Hospital, Sun Yat-sen University, Foshan, China

Breast Tumor Center, Sun Yat-sen Memorial Hospital, Sun Yat-sen University, Guangzhou, China
e-mail: songew@mail.sysu.edu.cn

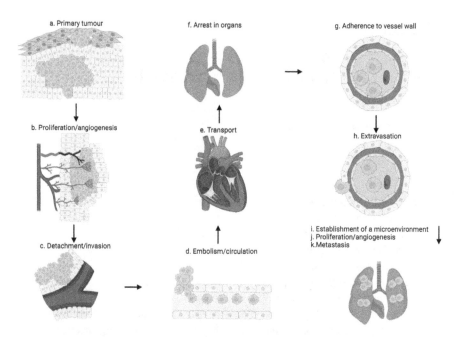

Fig. 13.1 The primary steps in metastasis development. (**a**) Tumor proliferation and cellular metamorphosis. Neoplastic cell growth is gradual, receiving nutrients via simple diffusion. (**b**) Vasculogenesis occurs when tumor's growth expands from 1–2 mm. Angiogenic factor production and secretion from a capillary network from the neighboring host tissue. (**c**) Some tumor cells invade the host stroma regionally by numerous methods. (**d**) Following this, solitary tumor cells or clusters are detached and embolized, and the majority of CTCs are swiftly eliminated. After surviving the circulation, tumor cells get entrapped in the capillary beds of peripheral organs. (**e**) Extravasation follows—most likely by processes identical to those involved during the invasion, but in a reversed manner. (**f**) The metastatic process is completed by proliferation inside the organ parenchyma. For consistent growth, the micro-metastasis must form a vascular network and avoid eradication by host defense mechanisms. (**g**, **h**) Subsequently, the cells can infiltrate blood arteries to enter the bloodstream and cause further metastases [1–6]. (**i**) Establishment of microenvironment in the distal onco-sphere. (**j**) Proliferation and angiogenesis occur at the distal onco-sphere. (**k**) Metastatic niches were developed at the distal onco-sphere

clusters, change their phenotypes (epithelial to mesenchymal transition, EMT), follow molecular clues to intravasate into the vascular and lymphatic systems, avoid the immune response, extravasate at distal blood capillaries, and then infiltrate and propagate in remote organs to conclude the metastatic cycle (Fig. 13.1). Although there are several theories have now been suggested to illustrate the genesis of cancer metastasis, none of these theories are fully comprehensive in explaining the origin of metastasis. These theories include the following: epithelial-mesenchymal shift, an aggregation of mutated stem cells, a macrophage facilitating mechanism, and a macrophage source through metamorphosis or fusion hybridization with neoplastic cells. In this chapter, we decipher the theories behind cancer metastasis and understanding the cross-communication between the tumor, immune and stromal cells in the local *onco-sphere* and the new distal *onco-sphere*.

The Epithelial to Mesenchymal Transition (EMT) Theory

Jean–Paul Thiery presented an in-depth explanation of how EMT may lead to metastasis. The latest research also indicates that misaligned (ectopic) co-expression of just two genes may be the sole requirement for enabling EMT in certain gliomas, despite the complications involved in the process [7]. Nevertheless, the EMT concept of metastasis is fraught with the dispute, as EMT is seldom identified in clinical tumor cultures [8–10]. The EMT is largely thought to be an in vitro occurrence [11]. The existence of an in vivo analog to this in vitro metastatic prototype is quite contentious. The concept of EMT evolved from studies drawing similarities between normal cell behavior during metazoan morphogenesis and malignant cell behavior during tumor growth [12–14]. While the mesenchymal–epithelial transition (MET) is indeed the re-iteration of epithelial features in remote secondary areas and is assumed to entail a reversal of the alterations leading to EMT [12, 14, 15]. There is a lack of studies explaining the mechanism of reversal or suppression of the genomic fragility, multiple-point mutations, and chromosomal reformations that cause the neoplastic mesenchymal phenotype at the time of recapitulation of epithelial phenotype at distant locations [13]. In the case of non-reversal of multiple such genetic modifications, how can they be held primarily responsible for the occurrence of EMT? Interestingly, current findings in the VM mouse model of systemic metastasis indicate that erratic mutations and EMT are not essential for metastatic formation [13, 16]. Close observations have revealed that numerous gene expression patterns found in metastatic malignancies are comparable to those linked with the activity of macrophages or other fusogenic immune cells [11, 17, 18]. Furthermore, numerous gene alterations linked with EMT may be observed in the majority of non-metastatic benign tumors [19, 20]. A large pool of data implies that cancer is not a hereditary illness but instead a metabolic ailment characterized by respiratory inadequacy and remedial fermentation [13]. The genetic volatility observed in tumor cells is a result of the consequent underlying metabolic abnormalities. Reliable cancer metastatic pathways must thus be interpreted in terms of cancer's fundamental nature as a mitochondrial respiratory illness [13]. This has yet to be accomplished by the EMT/MET paradigm.

Communication of Local and Distal *Onco-Sphere*: The "Seeds" Origin

Stem Cells

Many researchers believe in the genesis of metastatic cancer cells originates from tissue stem cells [21–23]. The majority of tissues comprise semi-specialized cells having the potential of substituting dead or destroyed cells because of the routine process of degeneration [13]. Stem cells and cancer cells are frequently characterized by identical gene regulation and biological properties [24]. The notion that embryonic stem cells and tumor cells are both capable of using anaerobic energy (fermentation) for metabolism, accounting for the findings related to the tumor cells' expression of features like undifferentiated stem cells [13]. Usually, tumor cells exhibit a high rate of telomerase activity in comparison to healthy cells, and it is assumed to have connections with fermentation energy [13]. Hence, the interchange of multiple genetic and metabolic characteristics between tumor cells and stem cells is not an unusual feature, considering the usage of fermentation energy by tumor cells for their existence and growth [21, 24, 25]. Despite exhibiting numerous cancer hallmark features, many human-developed xenograft tumor models do not show systemic metastasis when developed in the immune-impaired mouse host [13, 26]. It is possible for metastatic tumors to display features like stem cells, however, exhibiting features like stem cells is not equivalent to the manifestation of remote invasion and metastasis [22].

Macrophages

Macrophages are derived from myeloid descent and have been thought to be the source of human metastatic cancer [16, 27–31]. Macrophages can merge with epithelial cells in an inflammatory milieu, resulting in fusion hybrids that have features of both the epithelial cells and the macrophage [18, 32, 33]. TAMs have the capability of creating the premetastatic position, along with increasing tumor sensitivity and angiogenesis and promote metastatic progression [34–36]. While gene alterations are still assumed to trigger neoplasia according to this paradigm, the functioning of stromal TAMs act as cellular chaperones, and is actually responsible for promoting tumor formation, advancement, and metastatic propagation [24, 34, 37–40]. The stromal TAMs are thought to be an important player in all stages of metastasis, although they are not deemed neoplastic in themselves. Recent data implies that numerous metastatic cancers of humans contain neoplastic cells having macrophage characteristics [13, 16, 41]. Distinguishing neoplastic TAMs from non-neoplastic ones in the inflammatory tumor milieu is difficult since both types have identical gene expression, along with morphological and functional similarities [13, 41, 42].

Myeloid Cells

The myeloid cell genesis of metastasis additionally includes the macrophage fusion concept of metastatic cancer because macrophage features facilitate the metastatic process [28, 43]. Since myeloid cells are already mesenchymal cells, they do not necessitate the complex genetic processes hypothesized for EMT's metastasis. The myeloid cell theory also supports the development of metastatic cancer from hematopoietic stem cells or yolk sac-borne macrophages [44]. Respiratory injury in the homotypic fusion hybrids of these cells can lead to their proliferation uncontrollably [8]. The possibility of production of fusion hybrids between tumor cells and host macrophages cannot be denied; however, this may not result in mitochondrial damage in the macrophages. Neoplastic transformation in humans is a long-term process, as compared to the chronic condition in mice. Murine myeloid cells react abruptly to tumor implantation; however, human myeloid cells in an inflammatory microenvironment exhibit chronic responses to injuries resulting in a tumor. The infrequent existence of extremely metastatic carcinomas in rat tumors in contrast to frequent observation in humans is yet unclear, barring certain exceptions. Under certain conditions, it is feasible to develop chronic situations through repetitive transplants, which can result in fusion hybridizations, eventually concluding in metastasis [45].

Proposed Models of Metastasis: A Hint of Evolution in Tumor Ecosystem

The Progression Model

The progression model has been the most widely recognized model of metastasis (Fig. 13.2a) [46]. Nowell first presented this hypothesis and proposes that a chain of mutational incidents happens either in the original tumor subpopulations or disseminated cells, leading to the acquisition of complete metastatic capability by a tiny portion of cells [47]. This model illustrates the inadequacy of metastasis, considering the low chances of any particular cell inside the original tumor embracing all the changes necessary for the effective application of the metastatic process. Clonal descendants of cell lines have been shown to exhibit distinct metastatic characteristics [48], demonstrating the existence of metastatic subpopulations, at least in vitro. Similar experiments have been conducted in the recent past to indicate that target organ tropism is also caused by genetic changes within cell populations. By using a related cloning and selection technique in a human tumor-derived cell line, others have revealed the existence of separate subpopulations of cells possessing specific patterns of gene expression that make them susceptible to metastasizing to specific organs, probably through a certain type of somatic changes [49–51]. The discovery of metastasis suppressor genes lends credence to the idea that somatic activities play a major role in metastatic development. Metastasis suppressors include genes that inhibit the potential of the cells of metastatic cell lines to develop macroscopic metastases while exhibiting little or no effect on primary tumor progression [52, 53]. Down-regulation of metastatic suppressors in malignancies has been linked to loss of heterozygosity (LOH) [54] or transcriptional silencing [55], which rarely includes mutational inactivation. Despite the mounting evidence in favor of this concept, ambiguities persist, one of which is the occurrence of sufferers with unidentified primary tumor metastatic ailment. According to the stochastically

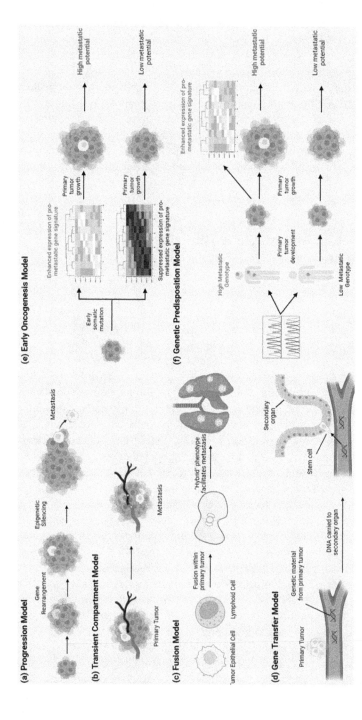

Fig. 13.2 Various models have been proposed as modes of metastasis. (**a**) Progression model: the stochastic accrual of somatic mutations renders a primary tumor with an increasingly more metastatic phenotype. (**b**) Transient compartment model: despite the acquisition of the ability to spread by all living cells in a tumor, positional and/or random epigenetic processes cause only a tiny proportion of them to be qualified to accomplish the process at any particular time. (**c**) Fusion model: to achieve a completely metastatic phenotype, a tumor cell must gain specific lymphoid cell attributes. (**d**) Gene transfer model: the existence of tumor DNA in the bloodstream is a sign of cancer. (**e**) Early oncogenesis model: a primary tumor's metastatic capability is determined early in its history, most likely as a result of somatic mutation. (**f**) Genetic predisposition model: the genetic origin of a primary tumor that emerges influences its metastatic potential, and as a result of constitutional polymorphism, an individual will be potentially vulnerable to tumor proliferation

guided progression model, a primary tumor must have a considerable number of cells to initiate the required series of incidents that cause metastasis. Hence, the unavailability of huge original tumors in patients with unidentified cancer metastatic illness contradicts this hypothesis [56, 57]. As projected by the progression theory, everlasting somatic occurrences that cause metastatic capability would be assumed to be permanently inherited rather than suffering immediate loss.

The Transient Compartment Models

The intention of proposing the dynamic heterogeneity model was to justify the absence of continuous advancement of the metastatic capability of secondary tumors in comparison to original tumors [57]. If the metastatic ability is the result of a chain of hereditary mutational events, as projected by the progression hypothesis, presumably, cells having completed the metastatic cascade successfully should exhibit higher effectiveness at forming new metastatic tumors than the parent tumor. But this was not a consistent finding in a variety of experimental setups [58]. Weiss' transitory metastatic compartment model proposes that all live cells in a tumor develop metastatic capability, but only a few of them are capable of completing the process (Fig. 13.2b) [58]. Studies revealing the methylation inhibitors' potential to modify cell lines' metastatic ability lend support to this notion [59–63]. While global demethylation may resemble some of the postulated epigenetic processes, these agents can generate chromosomal abnormalities [64], raising the likelihood that metastatic potential was modulated by mutational events instead of epigenetic occurrences. Furthermore, genomic instability is a feature of solid tumors, whereas the increased frequency of chromosomal abnormalities is generally associated with an incompetent prognosis [65]. Moreover, the transient compartment model fails to account for metastasis clonality [66–68]. As primary tumors are highly diverse [69], in the case of every cell possessing metastatic capacity that was controlled merely by transitory epigenetic processes, it is improbable that large proportions of secondary cancers would emerge from the clonal origin [48, 70, 71].

The Fusion Model

According to the progression model, de-differentiation caused by the buildup of somatic alterations results in an increasingly embryonic phenotype. However, in a solid tumor, various types of cells are present. This has conceptualized a number of alternate ideas for why tumor-generated epithelial cells develop the potential to metastasis, many of which are based on the notion that metastatic tumor cells obtain lymphoid properties. Tumors can be densely packed with TAMs, prevalently, and is highly related to disease prognosis [72]. The prevalence of a large number of cells possessing leukocytic, phagocytic, and fusogenic attributes in tumors has motivated some researchers to speculate that these cells could act as tumor cell fusion partners, that it is these cells that imbue tumor epithelial cells with multiple properties required to disseminate and populate remote parts [29, 30, 73, 74]. The dilemma related to the frequent occurrence of cell fusion in cancer patients causing metastatic development remains unanswered. Cell fusion in vitro can result in subclones bearing varied metastatic capability [74–76]. As a result, it is uncertain if the transformed metastatic capabilities of such hybrids are actually attributable to fusion or are the result of random subcloning and selection processes, especially given that a few of the cell lines employed in this research were initially generated from metastatic tumors [77]. Currently, there is no clear evidence to prove the substantial part played by cellular fusion in the development of metastatic capability, which may represent the truth that it is not a mechanism of metastatic spread and growth in this period [46] (Fig. 13.2c).

Gene Transfer Models

Horizontal gene transfer is an additional related concept for the development of metastatic capability. The hypothesis of the possible creation of metastatic potential via horizontal transmission of tumor phenotypes was resurrected after multiple years of discovering the presence of circulating tumor DNA (ctDNA) in animal tumor specimens [78] and tumor patients [79]. This notion has recently been reintroduced as the geno-metastasis theory, which is predicated on the fact that horizontal genetic transference has been demonstrated in experimental models in specific conditions [80]. It has especially been proposed that metastases are not caused by circulating cells but by in vivo acquisition of circulating DNA by stem cells at secondary locations [81]. Thus, metastasis would be the result of de novo cancers emerging in cancer patients rather than the offspring of primary tumors. Several observations have dampened excitement for this concept. First, this explanation does not account for metastasis organ specificity [82]. In this geno-metastasis theory, tissue-specific transcription of the oncogenic DNA would be necessary. Although this is theoretically plausible, there is currently no proof supporting this phenomenon in vivo [83–85] (Fig. 13.2d).

Early Oncogenesis Models

Two distinct groups discovered that by utilizing microarrays to measure global gene expression profiles in high volumes of human tumor tissues, it was feasible to create gene signature profiles that may discriminate metastatic from non-metastatic cancers [86, 87]. These findings prompted a rethinking of the progression paradigm, which posits that only a small subset of parent tumor cells will acquire the entire phenotypic nature required for effective colonization of remote organs. Thus, numerous groups have inclined their hypotheses towards the establishment of metastatic proclivity in the early stage of oncogenesis, sometimes performed by the same combinations of activation/inactivation occurrences in the initial tumor, which contradicts the somatic evolution paradigm [87, 88] (Fig. 13.2e). The majority of tumor cells would bear the metastatic gene expression profile if the metastatic state was established early. Furthermore, this approach might describe metastatic illness with an unknown root cause. If the same oncogenic activities generate metastasis, it is easy to see how tiny tumors may instantly begin spreading and colonizing at remote locations. Still, there are drawbacks to this model. First, if metastatic behavior is predominantly governed by initial oncogenic activities, the metastatic ability of maximum tumor epithelial cells becomes predictable, and hence, the distant organs' efficacy to colonize should be substantially higher in comparison to clinical research. Furthermore, the microarray findings do not exclude the existence of uncommon cellular subpopulations inside parent tumors. As the gene expression profiles portray an average of all the cells in the bulk tumor tissue, it is feasible that distinct subpopulations exhibit different elements of the metastatic profile, though it is merely a subset of the whole program. Lastly, this concept is predicated on the assumption that somatic oncogenic actions promote metastatic gene expression patterns. It does not compensate for hereditary polymorphism, which is another important source of genomic diversity reported in human cancer patients.

Genetic Predisposition Model

A mouse model was developed by a highly malignant breast tumor transgenesis that the genetic profile from which the tumor has formed had a major impact on the tumor's capacity to populate the lung effectively [89]. Considering the identical oncogenic source of all tumors, namely transgene activation, findings show that hereditary polymorphism is a substantial component, along with all the metastasis-inducing somatic occurrences in the tumor. Furthermore, because considering the existence of constitutional polymorphisms in all tissues of a person, the impact of metastasis-inducing/reducing polymorphisms may be seen in other tissues rather than the tumor epithelium. It is plausible, for example, that small alterations in lymphocyte activity owing to germline-encoded abnormalities in cell functioning might influence immunosurveillance to a large extent. As a result, the capacity to eliminate disseminated tumor cells at the secondary location may be enhanced or diminished. The gene transcription-altering capacity of hereditary polymorphism has been proven in many studies [90–92], and it serves as the foundation for expression quantitative trait loci evaluation. This research has shown that at least a few genes in a prognostic profile are differently communicated in high vs. low-metastatic genotypes [93]. As a result, it is probable that metastasis anticipatory gene expression profiles are not only a signal of somatic mutations causing propagation but also a gauge of hereditary metastasis vulnerability that runs across the human population. Significantly, the integration of genetic heritage in these models implies that prognosis evaluation using non-tumor tissue should be conceivable, maybe even prior to the evolution of cancer. If a large proportion of metastatic risk is recorded by germline polymorphisms instead of autonomous somatic processes inside the tumor, then its risk should be possibly reflected by any tissue in the body. Although genetic variants may differ throughout tissues, because of the universal fundamental susceptibility polymorphisms, it should theoretically be able to investigate a patient's susceptibility status using any tissue [93]. However, the translatability of this method in human patient warrants further research.

To summarize, none of the suggested hypotheses of metastatic progression can adequately describe all of the clinical characteristics observed during metastasis. However, these models are not compulsorily mutually exclusive. There is a genuine likelihood that many of them are correct within certain points, at least partially, and that there are a variety of methods through which a tumor cell might effectively invade remote organs. Future research should explicitly emphasize the mechanism of interaction, intersection, or sharing commonalities between these multiple putative processes because better knowledge of metastatic illness will be necessary for a remarkable reduction in cancer morbidity and death rates.

Onco-Sphere Crosstalk: Systemic Host Factors Affect Metastatic Outcomes

Metastasis and clinical prognosis have also been linked to underpinning host physiological systems (i.e., metabolic disorders, stress, aging, etc.). Age-related alterations, for example, tend to impact disease development due to the numerous effects of aging on tissue homeostasis that can demonstrate pro- or anti-tumorigenic effects. For instance, senescent fibroblasts release sFRP2, a Wnt inhibitor that triggers the loss of APE1, a redox mediator, in melanoma cells [94]. This deficiency makes melanoma cells more susceptible to oxidative stress, enhances their defiance to targeted treatment, and promotes angiogenesis and metastasis. Age was also found to be a significant predictor of TNBC advancement [95]. According to epidemiological studies, obesity is linked to an increased risk of cancer [96] and a greater prevalence of metastasis [97, 98]. Research on mice mammary tumor models demonstrated that obesity-linked inflammation enhances metastatic development by boosting lung neutrophilia, which is exacerbated by the parent tumor [99]. Enhanced lung neutrophils were associated with greater lung metastases. In both rodent and human specimens, losing weight was adequate to counteract these consequences by lowering circulating GM-CSF and IL-5 levels [99]. Additionally, obesity reduced anti-tumor activity in NK cells of mice and humans by interfering with their cellular metabolism and trafficking [100]. Nevertheless, research has shown that obesity is related to improved results from immunological and targeted treatments [101]. Similarly, subjects of a multi-cohort study having metastatic melanoma who responded to such therapy were abnormally overweight. In another study, obesity also leads to greater efficiency of PD-1/PD-L1 inhibition in both tumor-bearing mice and cancer patients [102]. These results suggest that there could be a difference in patient subset or variation in immune cell signature that leads to controversial findings.

Other variations in lifestyle and ethnicity may influence metastatic development, treatment outcomes, and medication resilience. Diet, for instance, can impact tumor and metastatic development as well as therapy responsiveness [103, 104]. A slight decrease in protein consumption, without any change in carbohydrate intake and total calorie count, the activation of IRE1/RIG1 cascade, which in turn stimulated cytokine secretion to induce cytotoxic T cell activity [104]. Similarly, epidemiological research suggests that a uniform exercise routine may reduce cancer rates and give better results for treatment [103, 105–107]. Exercise may control tumor progression via physical (e.g., enhanced blood flow and shear force on the vasculature) and endocrine (e.g., stress hormones, GFs, and myokines) processes, resulting in enhanced mobility and penetration of innate and cytotoxic immune cells into the tumor milieu [108, 109]. Recent research employing five distinct mice cancer models found that voluntarily exercising boosted NK cell accumulation and stimulation in an epinephrine- and IL-6-dependent fashion, causing a 60% reduction in tumor development [108]. Likewise, daily stretching for 10 min decreased tumor development by 50% in a mouse orthotopic breast cancer model, via the activation of cytotoxic immune function [109].

There is also pre-clinical data to substantiate the hypothesis that systemic alterations linked with pregnancy might influence the formation of incipient breast cancers. In a breast cancer mice models, systemic estrogen signaling assisted in mobilizing and recruiting pro-angiogenic myeloid cells from the bone marrow to remote tumor locations, causing breast cancer growth [110, 111]. Likewise, involution-generated inflammation post-pregnancy in mouse models is marked by a substantially increased immune cell infiltration, comprising immunosuppressive myeloid and FoxP3$^+$ Treg cells [112], as well as a reduction in antigen-specific T cell activation [113]. This involution-based immunity reduction may enhance the involuting mammary gland's tumor-promoting properties and may also have a detrimental influence on the prognosis of individuals diagnosed with breast cancer during the five-year postpartum duration [114]. Similar to the proposal of asthma in lung metastasis, acute inflammation could be an added risk contributor to the development of metastases [115]. In a melanoma mouse model, pulmonary inflammation caused due to allergy made the lungs a target tissue for metastasis via CTC recruitment in a CD4$^+$ T cell-dependent manner [115]. Notably, the prevalence of asthma was greater in breast cancer patients having lung metastases, indicating that treating asthma-related pulmonary inflammation may be feasible for breast cancer patients [116]. All these will be discussed in detail in PART 3 of this book, specifically in Chap. 18: Host response to cancer.

Conclusion

Consideration of cancer as an ecosystem opens doors to innovative approaches to preventing cross-communication of the local *onco-sphere* towards disseminating cancer cells towards distal *onco-sphere*, resulting in metastasis. Three important phases are anticipated to be involved in upcoming metastatic process targeting. In the first step, it will be necessary to discover and define local and systemic variables that promote the creation of a metastatic tumor, as well as devise methods to intervene with them. The second step makes it critical to design effective and repeatable methods for screening individual patients for the likelihood of metastasis. In the third step, the consequences of cancer therapy on the likelihood of metastatic reappearance should be considered. Many malignancies and metastatic recurrences are theoretically avoidable due to the interconnection between certain tumor-promoting systemic effects and changeable variables like chronic inflammation, obesity, and exercise. The subsequent step will incorporate the integration of knowledge regarding the systemic nature of cancer signaling with the continuous development of customized treatment.

References

1. Liotta LA (1986) Tumor invasion and metastases—role of the extracellular matrix: rhoads memorial award lecture. Cancer Res 46(1):1–7
2. Fisher ER, Fisher B (1967) Recent observations on concepts of metastasis. Arch Pathol 83(4): 321–324
3. Fisher B, Fisher ER (1966) The interrelationship of hematogenous and lymphatic tumor cell dissemination. Surg Gynecol Obstet 122(4):791–798
4. Folkman J (1986) How is blood vessel growth regulated in normal and neoplastic tissue? G.H.A. Clowes memorial award lecture. Cancer Res 46(2):467–473
5. Fidler IJ (2003) The pathogenesis of cancer metastasis: the 'seed and soil' hypothesis revisited. Nat Rev Cancer 3(6):453–458
6. Nicolson GL (1988) Cancer metastasis: tumor cell and host organ properties important in metastasis to specific secondary sites. Biochim Biophys Acta 948(2):175–224
7. Carro MS, Lim WK, Alvarez MJ, Bollo RJ, Zhao X, Snyder EY et al (2010) The transcriptional network for mesenchymal transformation of brain tumours. Nature 463(7279):318–325
8. Tarin D (2011) Cell and tissue interactions in carcinogenesis and metastasis and their clinical significance. Semin Cancer Biol 21(2):72–82
9. Hart IR (2009) New evidence for tumour embolism as a mode of metastasis. J Pathol 219(3): 275–276
10. Garber K (2008) Epithelial-to-mesenchymal transition is important to metastasis, but questions remain. J Natl Cancer Inst 100(4):232–233, 9
11. Bacac M, Stamenkovic I (2008) Metastatic cancer cell. Annu Rev Pathol 3:221–247
12. Chaffer CL, Weinberg RA (2011) A perspective on cancer cell metastasis. Science 331(6024): 1559–1564
13. Seyfried T (2012) Cancer as a metabolic disease: on the origin, management, and prevention of cancer. Wiley, Hoboken, NJ, p 432
14. Thiery JP (2002) Epithelial-mesenchymal transitions in tumour progression. Nat Rev Cancer 2(6):442–454

15. Weinberg R (2007) The biology of cancer. Taylor & Francis Group, New York, NY, p 796
16. Huysentruyt LC, Seyfried TN (2010) Perspectives on the mesenchymal origin of metastatic cancer. Cancer Metastasis Rev 29(4):695–707
17. Martin P, Leibovich SJ (2005) Inflammatory cells during wound repair: the good, the bad and the ugly. Trends Cell Biol 15(11):599–607
18. Powell AE, Anderson EC, Davies PS, Silk AD, Pelz C, Impey S et al (2011) Fusion between intestinal epithelial cells and macrophages in a cancer context results in nuclear reprogramming. Cancer Res 71(4):1497–1505
19. Lazebnik Y (2010) What are the hallmarks of cancer? Nat Rev Cancer 10(4):232–233
20. Larue L, Bellacosa A (2005) Epithelial-mesenchymal transition in development and cancer: role of phosphatidylinositol 3′ kinase/AKT pathways. Oncogene 24(50):7443–7454
21. Trosko JE (2009) Review paper: cancer stem cells and cancer nonstem cells: from adult stem cells or from reprogramming of differentiated somatic cells. Vet Pathol 46(2):176–193
22. Reya T, Morrison SJ, Clarke MF, Weissman IL (2001) Stem cells, cancer, and cancer stem cells. Nature 414(6859):105–111
23. Shackleton M, Quintana E, Fearon ER, Morrison SJ (2009) Heterogeneity in cancer: cancer stem cells versus clonal evolution. Cell 138(5):822–829
24. Seyfried TN (2001) Perspectives on brain tumor formation involving macrophages, glia, and neural stem cells. Perspect Biol Med 44(2):263–282
25. Kalluri R (2009) EMT: when epithelial cells decide to become mesenchymal-like cells. J Clin Invest 119(6):1417–1419
26. Hanahan D, Weinberg RA (2011) Hallmarks of cancer: the next generation. Cell 144(5):646–674
27. Pawelek JM (2008) Cancer-cell fusion with migratory bone-marrow-derived cells as an explanation for metastasis: new therapeutic paradigms. Future Oncol 4(4):449–452
28. Pawelek JM (2000) Tumour cell hybridization and metastasis revisited. Melanoma Res 10(6):507–514
29. Munzarová M, Kovařík J (1987) Is cancer a macrophage-mediated autoaggressive disease? Lancet 1(8539):952–954
30. Vignery A (2005) Macrophage fusion: are somatic and cancer cells possible partners? Trends Cell Biol 15(4):188–193
31. Chakraborty AK, de Freitas SJ, Espreafico EM, Pawelek JM (2001) Human monocyte x mouse melanoma fusion hybrids express human gene. Gene 275(1):103–106
32. Van den Bossche J, Bogaert P, van Hengel J, Guérin CJ, Berx G, Movahedi K et al (2009) Alternatively activated macrophages engage in homotypic and heterotypic interactions through IL-4 and polyamine-induced E-cadherin/catenin complexes. Blood 114(21):4664–4674
33. Pawelek JM (2005) Tumour-cell fusion as a source of myeloid traits in cancer. Lancet Oncol 6(12):988–993
34. Qian BZ, Pollard JW (2010) Macrophage diversity enhances tumor progression and metastasis. Cell 141(1):39–51
35. Hanahan D, Coussens LM (2012) Accessories to the crime: functions of cells recruited to the tumor microenvironment. Cancer Cell 21(3):309–322
36. Peinado H, Rafii S, Lyden D (2008) Inflammation joins the "niche". Cancer Cell 14(5):347–349
37. Lewis CE, Pollard JW (2006) Distinct role of macrophages in different tumor microenvironments. Cancer Res 66(2):605–612
38. Pollard JW (2008) Macrophages define the invasive microenvironment in breast cancer. J Leukoc Biol 84(3):623–630
39. Talmadge JE, Donkor M, Scholar E (2007) Inflammatory cell infiltration of tumors: Jekyll or Hyde. Cancer Metastasis Rev 26(3–4):373–400
40. Bingle L, Brown NJ, Lewis CE (2002) The role of tumour-associated macrophages in tumour progression: implications for new anticancer therapies. J Pathol 196(3):254–265

41. Huysentruyt LC, Akgoc Z, Seyfried TN (2011) Hypothesis: are neoplastic macrophages/microglia present in glioblastoma multiforme? ASN Neuro 3(4):e00064
42. Maniecki MB, Etzerodt A, Ulhøi BP, Steiniche T, Borre M, Dyrskjøt L et al (2012) Tumor-promoting macrophages induce the expression of the macrophage-specific receptor CD163 in malignant cells. Int J Cancer 131(10):2320–2331
43. Seyfried TN, Shelton LM, Mukherjee P (2010) Does the existing standard of care increase glioblastoma energy metabolism? Lancet Oncol 11(9):811–813
44. Schulz C, Gomez Perdiguero E, Chorro L, Szabo-Rogers H, Cagnard N, Kierdorf K et al (2012) A lineage of myeloid cells independent of Myb and hematopoietic stem cells. Science 336(6077):86–90
45. Seyfried TN, Huysentruyt LC (2013) On the origin of cancer metastasis. Crit Rev Oncog 18(1–2):43–73
46. Hunter KW, Crawford NP, Alsarraj J (2008) Mechanisms of metastasis. Breast Cancer Res 10 (Suppl 1):S2
47. Nowell PC (1976) The clonal evolution of tumor cell populations. Science 194(4260):23–28
48. Fidler IJ, Kripke ML (1977) Metastasis results from preexisting variant cells within a malignant tumor. Science 197(4306):893–895
49. Kang Y, Siegel PM, Shu W, Drobnjak M, Kakonen SM, Cordón-Cardo C et al (2003) A multigenic program mediating breast cancer metastasis to bone. Cancer Cell 3(6):537–549
50. Minn AJ, Gupta GP, Siegel PM, Bos PD, Shu W, Giri DD et al (2005) Genes that mediate breast cancer metastasis to lung. Nature 436(7050):518–524
51. Minn AJ, Kang Y, Serganova I, Gupta GP, Giri DD, Doubrovin M et al (2005) Distinct organ-specific metastatic potential of individual breast cancer cells and primary tumors. J Clin Invest 115(1):44–55
52. Kauffman EC, Robinson VL, Stadler WM, Sokoloff MH, Rinker-Schaeffer CW (2003) Metastasis suppression: the evolving role of metastasis suppressor genes for regulating cancer cell growth at the secondary site. J Urol 169(3):1122–1133
53. Steeg PS (2003) Metastasis suppressors alter the signal transduction of cancer cells. Nat Rev Cancer 3(1):55–63
54. Wick W, Petersen I, Schmutzler RK, Wolfarth B, Lenartz D, Bierhoff E et al (1996) Evidence for a novel tumor suppressor gene on chromosome 15 associated with progression to a metastatic stage in breast cancer. Oncogene 12(5):973–978
55. Sekita N, Suzuki H, Ichikawa T, Kito H, Akakura K, Igarashi T et al (2001) Epigenetic regulation of the KAI1 metastasis suppressor gene in human prostate cancer cell lines. Jpn J Cancer Res 92(9):947–951
56. Chambers AF, Harris JF, Ling V, Hill RP (1984) Rapid phenotype variation in cells derived from lung metastases of KHT fibrosarcoma. Invasion Metastasis 4(4):225–237
57. Harris JF, Chambers AF, Hill RP, Ling V (1982) Metastatic variants are generated spontaneously at a high rate in mouse KHT tumor. Proc Natl Acad Sci U S A 79(18):5547–5551
58. Weiss L (1990) Metastatic inefficiency. Adv Cancer Res 54:159–211
59. Trainer DL, Kline T, Hensler G, Greig R, Poste G (1988) Clonal analysis of the malignant properties of B16 melanoma cells treated with the DNA hypomethylating agent 5-azacytidine. Clin Exp Metastasis 6(3):185–200
60. Ishikawa M, Okada F, Hamada J, Hosokawa M, Kobayashi H (1987) Changes in the tumorigenic and metastatic properties of tumor cells treated with quercetin or 5-azacytidine. Int J Cancer 39(3):338–342
61. Kerbel RS, Frost P, Liteplo R, Carlow DA, Elliott BE (1984) Possible epigenetic mechanisms of tumor progression: induction of high-frequency heritable but phenotypically unstable changes in the tumorigenic and metastatic properties of tumor cell populations by 5-azacytidine treatment. J Cell Physiol Suppl 3:87–97
62. Olsson L, Forchhammer J (1984) Induction of the metastatic phenotype in a mouse tumor model by 5-azacytidine, and characterization of an antigen associated with metastatic activity. Proc Natl Acad Sci U S A 81(11):3389–3393

63. Stopper H, Pechan R, Schiffmann D (1992) 5-azacytidine induces micronuclei in and morphological transformation of Syrian hamster embryo fibroblasts in the absence of unscheduled DNA synthesis. Mutat Res 283(1):21–28

64. Frost P, Kerbel RS, Hunt B, Man S, Pathak S (1987) Selection of metastatic variants with identifiable karyotypic changes from a nonmetastatic murine tumor after treatment with 2′-deoxy-5-azacytidine or hydroxyurea: implications for the mechanisms of tumor progression. Cancer Res 47(10):2690–2695

65. Ried T, Heselmeyer-Haddad K, Blegen H, Schröck E, Auer G (1999) Genomic changes defining the genesis, progression, and malignancy potential in solid human tumors: a phenotype/genotype correlation. Genes Chromosom Cancer 25(3):195–204

66. Nakayama T, Taback B, Turner R, Morton DL, Hoon DS (2001) Molecular clonality of in-transit melanoma metastasis. Am J Pathol 158(4):1371–1378

67. Chambers AF, Wilson S (1988) Use of NeoR B16F1 murine melanoma cells to assess clonality of experimental metastases in the immune-deficient chick embryo. Clin Exp Metastasis 6(2):171–182

68. Cheung ST, Chen X, Guan XY, Wong SY, Tai LS, Ng IO et al (2002) Identify metastasis-associated genes in hepatocellular carcinoma through clonality delineation for multinodular tumor. Cancer Res 62(16):4711–4721

69. Fidler IJ, Yano S, Zhang RD, Fujimaki T, Bucana CD (2002) The seed and soil hypothesis: vascularisation and brain metastases. Lancet Oncol 3(1):53–57

70. Talmadge JE, Wolman SR, Fidler IJ (1982) Evidence for the clonal origin of spontaneous metastases. Science 217(4557):361–363

71. Fidler IJ, Talmadge JE (1986) Evidence that intravenously derived murine pulmonary melanoma metastases can originate from the expansion of a single tumor cell. Cancer Res 46(10): 5167–5171

72. Pollard JW (2004) Tumour-educated macrophages promote tumour progression and metastasis. Nat Rev Cancer 4(1):71–78

73. Pawelek J, Chakraborty A, Lazova R, Yilmaz Y, Cooper D, Brash D et al (2006) Co-opting macrophage traits in cancer progression: a consequence of tumor cell fusion? Contrib Microbiol 13:138–155

74. Rachkovsky M, Sodi S, Chakraborty A, Avissar Y, Bolognia J, McNiff JM et al (1998) Melanoma x macrophage hybrids with enhanced metastatic potential. Clin Exp Metastasis 16(4):299–312

75. Miller FR, Mohamed AN, McEachern D (1989) Production of a more aggressive tumor cell variant by spontaneous fusion of two mouse tumor subpopulations. Cancer Res 49(15): 4316–4321

76. De Baetselier P, Roos E, Brys L, Remels L, Feldman M (1984) Generation of invasive and metastatic variants of a non-metastatic T-cell lymphoma by *in vivo* fusion with normal host cells. Int J Cancer 34(5):731–738

77. Loustalot P, Algire GH, Legallais FY, Anderson BF (1952) Growth and histopathology of melanotic and amelanotic derivatives of the Cloudman melanoma S91. J Natl Cancer Inst 12(5):1079–1117

78. Bendich A, Wilczok T, Borenfreund E (1965) Circulating DNA as a possible factor in oncogenesis. Science 148(3668):374–376

79. Leon SA, Shapiro B, Sklaroff DM, Yaros MJ (1977) Free DNA in the serum of cancer patients and the effect of therapy. Cancer Res 37(3):646–650

80. Bergsmedh A, Szeles A, Henriksson M, Bratt A, Folkman MJ, Spetz AL et al (2001) Horizontal transfer of oncogenes by uptake of apoptotic bodies. Proc Natl Acad Sci U S A 98(11):6407–6411

81. García-Olmo DC, Ruiz-Piqueras R, García-Olmo D (2004) Circulating nucleic acids in plasma and serum (CNAPS) and its relation to stem cells and cancer metastasis: state of the issue. Histol Histopathol 19(2):575–583

82. Paget S (1889) The distribution of secondary growths in cancer of the breast. Lancet 133(3421):571–573
83. Kramer SA, Farnham R, Glenn JF, Paulson DF (1981) Comparative morphology of primary and secondary deposits of prostatic adenocarcinoma. Cancer 48(2):271–273
84. Johnson DE, Appelt G, Samuels ML, Luna M (1976) Metastases from testicular carcinoma. Study of 78 autopsied cases. Urology 8(3):234–239
85. O'Donnell McGee J (1992) Tumor metastasis. In: O'Donnell McGee J, Isaacson P, Wright N (eds) Oxford textbook of pathology. Oxford University, Oxford, pp 607–633
86. van't Veer LJ, Dai H, van de Vijver MJ, He YD, Hart AA, Mao M et al (2002) Gene expression profiling predicts clinical outcome of breast cancer. Nature 415(6871):530–536
87. Ramaswamy S, Ross KN, Lander ES, Golub TR (2003) A molecular signature of metastasis in primary solid tumors. Nat Genet 33(1):49–54
88. Bernards R, Weinberg RA (2002) A progression puzzle. Nature 418(6900):823
89. Lifsted T, Le Voyer T, Williams M, Muller W, Klein-Szanto A, Buetow KH et al (1998) Identification of inbred mouse strains harboring genetic modifiers of mammary tumor age of onset and metastatic progression. Int J Cancer 77(4):640–644
90. Schadt EE, Monks SA, Drake TA, Lusis AJ, Che N, Colinayo V et al (2003) Genetics of gene expression surveyed in maize, mouse and man. Nature 422(6929):297–302
91. Bystrykh L, Weersing E, Dontje B, Sutton S, Pletcher MT, Wiltshire T et al (2005) Uncovering regulatory pathways that affect hematopoietic stem cell function using 'genetical genomics'. Nat Genet 37(3):225–232
92. Chesler EJ, Lu L, Shou S, Qu Y, Gu J, Wang J et al (2005) Complex trait analysis of gene expression uncovers polygenic and pleiotropic networks that modulate nervous system function. Nat Genet 37(3):233–242
93. Yang H, Crawford N, Lukes L, Finney R, Lancaster M, Hunter KW (2005) Metastasis predictive signature profiles pre-exist in normal tissues. Clin Exp Metastasis 22(7):593–603
94. Kaur A, Webster MR, Marchbank K, Behera R, Ndoye A, Kugel CH 3rd et al (2016) sFRP2 in the aged microenvironment drives melanoma metastasis and therapy resistance. Nature 532(7598):250–254
95. Marsh T, Wong I, Sceneay J, Barakat A, Qin Y, Sjödin A et al (2016) Hematopoietic age at onset of triple-negative breast cancer dictates disease aggressiveness and progression. Cancer Res 76(10):2932–2943
96. Calle EE, Kaaks R (2004) Overweight, obesity and cancer: epidemiological evidence and proposed mechanisms. Nat Rev Cancer 4(8):579–591
97. Ewertz M, Jensen MB, Gunnarsdóttir K, Højris I, Jakobsen EH, Nielsen D et al (2011) Effect of obesity on prognosis after early-stage breast cancer. J Clin Oncol 29(1):25–31
98. Osman MA, Hennessy BT (2015) Obesity correlation with metastases development and response to first-line metastatic chemotherapy in breast cancer. Clin Med Insights Oncol 9:105–112
99. Quail DF, Olson OC, Bhardwaj P, Walsh LA, Akkari L, Quick ML et al (2017) Obesity alters the lung myeloid cell landscape to enhance breast cancer metastasis through IL5 and GM-CSF. Nat Cell Biol 19(8):974–987
100. Michelet X, Dyck L, Hogan A, Loftus RM, Duquette D, Wei K et al (2018) Metabolic reprogramming of natural killer cells in obesity limits antitumor responses. Nat Immunol 19(12):1330–1340
101. McQuade JL, Daniel CR, Hess KR, Mak C, Wang DY, Rai RR et al (2018) Association of body-mass index and outcomes in patients with metastatic melanoma treated with targeted therapy, immunotherapy, or chemotherapy: a retrospective, multicohort analysis. Lancet Oncol 19(3):310–322
102. Wang Z, Aguilar EG, Luna JI, Dunai C, Khuat LT, Le CT et al (2019) Paradoxical effects of obesity on T cell function during tumor progression and PD-1 checkpoint blockade. Nat Med 25(1):141–151

103. Kerr J, Anderson C, Lippman SM (2017) Physical activity, sedentary behaviour, diet, and cancer: an update and emerging new evidence. Lancet Oncol 18(8):e457–ee71
104. Rubio-Patiño C, Bossowski JP, De Donatis GM, Mondragón L, Villa E, Aira LE et al (2018) Low-protein diet induces IRE1α-dependent anticancer immunosurveillance. Cell Metab 27(4): 828–42.e7
105. Hardee JP, Porter RR, Sui X, Archer E, Lee IM, Lavie CJ et al (2014) The effect of resistance exercise on all-cause mortality in cancer survivors. Mayo Clin Proc 89(8):1108–1115
106. Schmid D, Leitzmann MF (2014) Association between physical activity and mortality among breast cancer and colorectal cancer survivors: a systematic review and meta-analysis. Ann Oncol J 25(7):1293–1311
107. Li Y, Gu M, Jing F, Cai S, Bao C, Wang J et al (2016) Association between physical activity and all cancer mortality: dose-response meta-analysis of cohort studies. Int J Cancer 138(4): 818–832
108. Pedersen L, Idorn M, Olofsson GH, Lauenborg B, Nookaew I, Hansen RH et al (2016) Voluntary running suppresses tumor growth through epinephrine- and IL-6-dependent NK cell mobilization and redistribution. Cell Metab 23(3):554–562
109. Berrueta L, Bergholz J, Munoz D, Muskaj I, Badger GJ, Shukla A et al (2018) Stretching reduces tumor growth in a mouse breast cancer model. Sci Rep 8(1):7864
110. Gupta PB, Proia D, Cingoz O, Weremowicz J, Naber SP, Weinberg RA et al (2007) Systemic stromal effects of estrogen promote the growth of estrogen receptor-negative cancers. Cancer Res 67(5):2062–2071
111. Iyer V, Klebba I, McCready J, Arendt LM, Betancur-Boissel M, Wu MF et al (2012) Estrogen promotes ER-negative tumor growth and angiogenesis through mobilization of bone marrow-derived monocytes. Cancer Res 72(11):2705–2713
112. Martinson HA, Jindal S, Durand-Rougely C, Borges VF, Schedin P (2015) Wound healing-like immune program facilitates postpartum mammary gland involution and tumor progression. Int J Cancer 136(8):1803–1813
113. Betts CB, Pennock ND, Caruso BP, Ruffell B, Borges VF, Schedin P (2018) Mucosal immunity in the female murine mammary gland. J Immunol 201(2):734–746
114. Amant F, von Minckwitz G, Han SN, Bontenbal M, Ring AE, Giermek J et al (2013) Prognosis of women with primary breast cancer diagnosed during pregnancy: results from an international collaborative study. J Clin Oncol 31(20):2532–2539
115. Taranova AG, Maldonado D 3rd, Vachon CM, Jacobsen EA, Abdala-Valencia H, McGarry MP et al (2008) Allergic pulmonary inflammation promotes the recruitment of circulating tumor cells to the lung. Cancer Res 68(20):8582–8589
116. Bekaert S, Rocks N, Vanwinge C, Noel A, Cataldo D (2021) Asthma-related inflammation promotes lung metastasis of breast cancer cells through CCL11-CCR3 pathway. Respir Res 22(1):61

Chapter 14
Distal *Onco-Sphere*: Molecular Mechanisms in Metastasis

Phei Er Saw and Erwei Song

Abstract Although there has been some hint in important molecular mechanisms in metastasis, this process is incompletely understood. We now understood the importance of the interactions between cancer cells and its surrounding in the local oncosphere. These interactions in the distal onco-sphere (i.e. cell-cell and cell-matrix adhesion, with the degradation of extracellular matrix, and with the initiation and maintenance of early growth at the new site are also important. In this chapter, we will summarize the molecular drivers of metastasis and the importance of inter-oncospheric communication.

Introduction

Metastasis development is a critical part of cancer, and the molecular basis of this phenomenon has been contested for a long. Although tumor-host interactions determine the preferable organ for dispersion on an epigenetic scale, cancer cells' propensity to spread has a genetic foundation. Encoding of homing receptors, ligands, and extracellular matrix-degenerating proteinases is facilitated by metastatic genes, all of

P. E. Saw
Guangdong Provincial Key Laboratory of Malignant Tumor Epigenetics and Gene Regulation, Guangdong-Hong Kong Joint Laboratory for RNA Medicine, Medical Research Center, Sun Yat-sen Memorial Hospital, Sun Yat-sen University, Guangzhou, China

Nanhai Translational Innovation Center of Precision Immunology, Sun Yat-sen Memorial Hospital, Sun Yat-sen University, Foshan, China

E. Song (✉)
Guangdong Provincial Key Laboratory of Malignant Tumor Epigenetics and Gene Regulation, Guangdong-Hong Kong Joint Laboratory for RNA Medicine, Medical Research Center, Sun Yat-sen Memorial Hospital, Sun Yat-sen University, Guangzhou, China

Nanhai Translational Innovation Center of Precision Immunology, Sun Yat-sen Memorial Hospital, Sun Yat-sen University, Foshan, China

Breast Tumor Center, Sun Yat-sen Memorial Hospital, Sun Yat-sen University, Guangzhou, China
e-mail: songew@mail.sysu.edu.cn

which contribute to infiltration and adherence autonomy. They are unimportant stress response genes liable for physiological governance of immune system cells' homing. Cancer cells' metastatic ability is imparted by abnormal transcription or attachment of these genes. Oncogenes operate upstream of metastasis genes. Oncogenic signaling stimulates different genetic pathways in cancer cells, causing cell cycle advancement and intrusiveness, respectively [1]. Combinations of multi-subunit transcription factors control the activation of metastatic genes. The discovery of genes driving cancer spread suggests that they might be therapeutic targets. Despite its therapeutic benefits, it is still poorly comprehended. In this chapter, we elucidate the molecular drivers of metastasis, the often-overlooked physical interactions within this distal *onco-sphere*, and understanding the inter-onco-spherical communication that leads to the establishment of a distal *onco-sphere*.

Molecular Drivers of Metastasis Towards Distal *Onco-Sphere*

Though cancer cells' inherent features influence their metastatic potential [2], surrounding non-cancerous cells also influence metastatic dissemination and proliferation significantly. Tumor cells' active and constant communication with adjacent stomal cells and infiltrated immune cells, through various cellular and non-cellular elements, assists in the formation of a distal *onco-sphere* with settings that favors metastasis settings, even before the tumor cells arrive at secondary organs [3, 4] (Fig. 14.1). As we mentioned in Chap. 10, the formation of pre-metastatic niche (PNM) is the pre-requisite of a successful metastasis. Therefore, the constant communication between the local *onco-sphere*, especially among tumor-stroma and tumor-immune cells interactions, is crucial. Within these communications, cellular factors such as pro-metastatic cytokines, chemokines, and biologics such as miRNAs, lncRNA, and circRNAs are being transported through the potent communicators: EVs and exosomes [4–6]. Therefore, the development of a PMN in intended organs is a complicated process that involves systemic signaling, cell recruitment, and stimulation, all of which work together to generate a more conducive milieu for circulating tumor cells (CTCs).

For example, exosomes released by cancer cells may control the tissue-selectivity of PMN by preferring fusion with resident cells at their projected location on the basis of integrin expression profiles [7]. For instance, exosomes from the lung undergo fusion with SPC^+ epithelial cells and $S100A4^+$ fibroblasts, whereas exosomes from the liver merge with F4/80 Kupffer cells. This absorption establishes the premetastatic setting for cancer cell entry by upregulating distinct S100 proteins (including S100P and S110A8) in the liver, to favor pro-migratory and pro-inflammatory behaviors at distal *onco-sphere*s. Following active encounters with metastasized cancer cells and continued induction of stromal cells and circulating factors causes the transformation of the pre-metastatic niche into a metastatic niche. CTCs like $CD8^+$ T cells and NK cells must now avoid and decrease cytotoxic leukocyte activities and produce an immunosuppressive milieu [8].

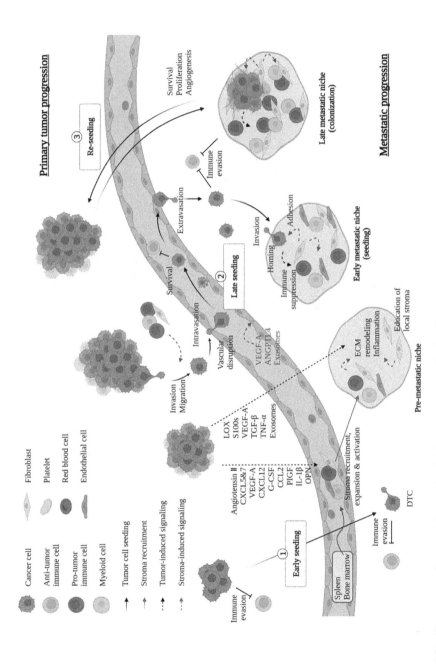

Fig. 14.1 The process of a metastatic cascade. A primary tumor must first be disseminated into the blood circulation, through EMT process. This process can occur very early in the tumor development, in finding a pre-metastasis niche. To aid this process, tumor can secrete factors that activate stromal cells (i.e., CAFs and BMDCs) and other molecular factors and paracrine modulators (i.e., EVs and exosomes), in order to facilitate this process. Throughout this process, immune

Secreted Factors in Metastatic Progression

Cytokines and chemokines derived from tumor cells undergo mobilization and attract stromal cells, including leukocytes, to primary and auxiliary locations. Angiotensin II, CXCL12 (SDF-1α), G-CSF, and OPN, for instance, move bone marrow and spleen-resident cells in the circulatory system, thus promoting tumor growth and metastasis [9]. In the same manner, tumor-derived VEGF-A and PIGF induce the expression of bone marrow-based endothelial progenitors and VEGFR1$^+$ BMCs in the murine cancer models, which later regulate tumor angiogenesis [10] along with the creation of a premetastatic niche by increased MMP9 production in pre-metastatic lung endothelial cells through VEGFR-1/Flt-1 tyrosine kinase indicators or via upregulated production of fibronectin in lung fibroblasts attracting pro-metastatic VEGFR1$^+$ BMCs [11]. VEGF-A, TGF-β, and TNF-α released by tumors also increase S100A8 and S100A9 production in the lung, which attracts circulatory pro-metastatic CD11b$^+$ myeloid cells in a VEGFR1-dependent manner [12]. Likewise, tumor-released LOX deposition attracted bone marrow-produced myeloid cells to pre-metastatic lung niches [13]. Tumor-released compounds also have a significant role in the development of paraneoplastic diseases. While researching a mouse model, IL-6 generated by ovarian cancer increased hepatic TPO synthesis, which in turn infringed megakaryocytes of bone marrow, causing acceleration of platelet creation frequency [14]. Substances secreted by tumor-linked stromal cells have also been aligned with identical systemic impacts. In primary breast cancers, CXCL12 is released by CAFs, and in a xenograft specimen of breast cancer, endothelial precursors, as well as hematopoietic stem and precursor cells, were moved from the bone marrow to respond to fibroblast-derived CXCL12 [15]. Likely, heightened levels of several tumors- and stroma-produced cytokines have been found in primary tumors and plasma of patients suffering from various cancer types, and highly elevated concentrations have been linked to a worse prognosis and greater metastatic load [9]. Prior to their entry into the circulation, several migrated cell groups are enlarged and turned pro-tumorigenic by tumor-produced substances. In a mouse melanoma model, for example, melanoma exosomes guide BMCs in the direction of a pro-metastatic phenotype via MET transfer [16]. Moreover, these exosomes increase capillary permeability in mice lungs, thus increasing melanoma cells' metastatic development [16]. Indeed, COX2, ANGPTL4, and MMPs could also promote metastasis by increasing vascular permeability, which is required for extravasation to body parts like the lung or brain whose vasculature is encased with firmly attached endothelial cells [17]. Cerebrospinal fluid (CSF) was recently discovered that tumor-released Complement component 3 (C3) helps in binding and activating the C3a receptor on choroid plexus epithelial cells, thus breaching the blood-brain obstruction [18]. Plasma mitogens

---

Fig. 14.1 (continued) evasion and angiogenesis are necessary so that the circulating tumor cells (CTCs) can safely reach the new distal *onco-sphere* to begin the process of tumor growth. All the steps mentioned above are closely modulated and regulated by tumor- and stroma-derived factors, indicating the precise crosstalk and communication between a local and distal *onco-sphere*

were permitted to penetrate the CSF and induce metastatic development as a result of this. A correlation between C3 expression in initial tumors of patients having various solid tumors and treatment outcomes was observed, which predicted the leptomeningeal recurrence, showing that inhibition of C3 signaling might be a successful approach for treating leptomeningeal metastasis (Fig. 14.1) [8].

Inter-*Onco Spherical* Interaction: Host Immune System in the Metastatic Cascade

The systemic function of migrated immune cell types in metastasis varies depending on the circumstances. Innate immune cells, such as monocytes and neutrophils, are key players in metastasis. For example, $Gr1^+CD11b^+$ myeloid cells are crucial in mediating immunosuppression in the local *onco-sphere*, leading to an increase in MMPs secretion, disrupting tumor-stroma junction; which leads to an increased tumor cell penetration and metastasis [19]. $Gr1^+CD11b^+$ myeloid cell populations are greatly increased in tumor-bearing mice's bone marrow and spleens [20, 21]. In a breast cancer lung metastasis model, Neutrophil releases CCL2 to stimulate the production of IL-1β in macrophages, which leads to the consistent release of IL-17 by γδT cells, which in turn polarize neutrophil into $CD11b^+Ly6G^+Ly6C^+F4/80$ phenotype [22, 23]. In the complementary scenario, neutralization of CCL2, inhibition of IL-17 or G-CSF, and the exclusion of γδT cells inhibited neutrophil formation, dysregulated the T-cell-inhibitory phenotype, and reduced total pulmonary metastasis. These findings are consistent with previous research in breast cancer models that were characterized by tumor-produced CCL2 recruiting monocytes like macrophages and preosteoclasts to the lung and bones, resulting in enhanced metastasis at these secondary locations [24, 25]. Moreover, in the case of administration of above-specified CCL2 neutralization in the neoadjuvant instead of adjuvant setting, guided by discontinuation of treatment, then suppression of inflammation genuinely led to improved metastasis [23], corresponding to an additional study that adjuvant combined treatment with paclitaxel and an IL-1 IL-1β blocker improved metastatic progression [26].

Furthermore, $CD11b^+/Ly6G^+$ neutrophils activated by G-CSF produced from breast cancer are also capable in blocking NK cell activity [27], dramatically enhancing CTC viability. Neutrophils aided CTC extravasation by releasing IL-1β and MMPs. Significantly, due to the relatively brief half-life and tumor-based proliferation of neutrophils, surgical excision of the main tumor resulted in a rapid decrease of neutrophils in animal models [28]. Additionally, higher levels of plasma G-CSF are linked to acute leukocytosis and a weak prognosis [29, 30], whereas IL-1β secretion has been linked to the development of disease in primary breast tumors [31]. The blood leukocytes of metastatic patients with $HER2^-$ breast cancer comprised an "IL-1 signature" associated with weak prognostic analysis [31], whose mitigation can be done via blocking of IL-1, which indicates the advantages of treatment aiming at IL-1 signaling among patients having IL-1 signature genes.

Similarly, cancer cells generated the development of NETs at parent locations in a mouse model of metastatic breast cancer, thus enhancing CTC metastasis [32].

In contrast, preclinical investigations have indicated that neutrophils bear an anti-metastatic impact by boosting tumor cell death and blocking metastatic development [33]. Compatible to this, a recent study found that early-stage primary breast cancers cause systemic inflammation for mobilizing IL-1-producing neutrophils that penetrate distal metastases and block their continued colonization by keeping them dormant, although this does not succeed in metastatic cell elimination [34]. In accordance, researchers analyzed tumor samples of breast cancer patients having lymph node-positive malignancy and bearing a higher risk of remote metastasis and discovered that elevated IL-1β levels in primary tumors were related to better overall and lifespan devoid of remote metastasis [34]. These numerous results may appear contradictory at an initial look; nevertheless, neutrophils and monocytes are relatively diverse and malleable cell groups having variable morphologies under specific circumstances. The latest research cited above highlighting the mechanisms of metastatic promotion by clonal collaboration in primary tumors in a clinical model of breast cancer provided dramatic support for the role of microenvironment and neutrophil diversity [35].

Stromal Cells

Additional non-inflammatory stromal cells, both from local or systemic *oncosphere*, can be educated and attracted to both primary and secondary tumors. Endothelial progenitor cells (EPCs), for example, can be potentially attracted to tumors to include tumor angiogenesis [10]. TNBC-secreted osteopontin (OPN) stimulates and mobilizes BMCs to primary tumors in tumor-bearing mice as well as to metastatic dormant tumor cells (DTCs) of lungs, where they release GRN. These BMCs are then activated to adopt CAF phenotype and express pro-inflammatory genes and matrix-remodeling genes, which aids tumor growth [36, 37]. Likewise, metastasis is boosted by macrophage-derived granulin in pancreatic cancer models due to stimulation of myofibroblast-induced periostin secretion and liver fibrosis [38]. Recently, single-cell sequencing techniques have uncovered geographically and operationally different subclasses within stromal communities, such as CAFs [39, 40]. Three operationally unique CAF subclasses discovered in a genetically engineered breast tumor mouse model were attributed to several sources, such as the perivascular niche, the mammary fat pad, and the altered epithelium [39]. In clinical samples, gene patterns for each CAF subtype had independent predictive capacity by relating to metastatic cancer. One research discovered four unique CAF subgroups (CAF–S1 to CAF–S4) in human breast cancer, each having its own set of characteristics and degrees of stimulation [40]. These subclasses aggregated differently in juxta-tumor versus tumors, as well as in various breast tumor subtypes. TNBC was surprisingly separated into two subgroups based on CAF–S1 or CAF–S4 abundance. In contrast to CAF–S4, TNBC, having abundant CAF–S1, displayed an immunosuppressive setting with a large concentration of FOXP3$^+$ T cells and a limited invasion of CD8$^+$ T cells. Lastly, unlike CAF–S4, CAF–S1 increased the potential of regulatory T cells to limit T effector growth. Detailed analysis of CAF subsets and their role in cancer resistance could be found in Ref. [41].

Secondary tissue stromal cells are capable of influencing metastatic expansion by reducing or boosting DTC survival and developing them into macro-metastatic tumors. The stromal involvement in metastasis at numerous secondary locations, including the brain, has been studied in preclinical research. For instance, high secretion of CCL2 by metastatic tumor cells of the brain can be attributed to astrocyte-generated PTEN knockdown by exosomal miR-19a, which in turn leads to recruitment of IBA1$^+$ myeloid cells derived from the brain [42]. In turn, the latter stimulated the proliferation of brain metastatic tumor cells. Significantly, PTEN deficiency in brain metastases was associated with increased CCL2 production and IBA1+ myeloid cell activation in cancer patients, confirming the therapeutic relevance.

The latest research on another brain metastasis model of mice explored that a subset of responsive astrocytes around metastatic lesions produced phospho-STAT3 (pSTAT3), which regulated inherent and adaptive dynamic immune reactions, promoting metastatic expansion [43]. Particularly, suppression of CD8$^+$ T cell activation was facilitated by pSTAT3$^+$ astrocytes, whereas they boosted the proliferation of CD74$^+$IBA1$^+$ microglia and macrophage groups. Considering that pSTAT3$^+$ account for over 90% of all brain metastases and are associated with the poorest treatment outcomes [43], this immune reaction may also play a significant role in enhancing brain metastasis among cancer patients. Contrary to the collaborative tumor-stroma interplay observed at the metastatic location, the latest review discovered DTCs from lung and breast cancer samples using L1CAM to propagate on capillaries in the perivascular niche of numerous secondary tissues, replacing native pericytes [44], which undergo perivascular expansion with the aid of L1CAM in normal circumstances. L1CAM triggers the mechanotransduction influencers YAP and MRTF in DTCs, allowing them to proliferate after infiltrating target tissues and emerging from dormancy [8] (Box 14.1).

Box 14.1 Inter-*Onco-Spherical* Crosstalk: CTCs and Host Systemic Circulatory System

As we mentioned in Chap. 9, mechanical stress is vital for the dissemination of a cancer cells, to break through from the local *onco-sphere*, undergoing EMT transition to be sent to through the blood vessel to a new metastatic site (the new distal *onco-sphere*). While tumor cells traverse through the circulatory system, they have to bear hemodynamic pressures, immunological distress and encounters with host cells such as blood cells and endothelial cells lining the vessel wall. All of these pressures may have an impact on cell viability and

(continued)

Box 14.1 (continued)

their propensity to form metastatic foci. Especially CTCs that withstand or even take advantage of fluid shear and immunosurveillance will stick to the vascular endothelial surface of peripheral organs, depart from the circulatory system, and effectively penetrate these tissues [45]. In a normal situation, the diameter of CTC is smaller than the blood vessel; therefore, CTC could pass smoothly ($d_{cell} < d_{vessel}$) [46]. However, as seen in Fig. 14.2, a cell traveling down the wall of a vessel exhibits both longitudinal and vertical (translational and tangential) velocity, not a direct flow as one imagined. A cell's translational velocity always exceeds its surface tangential velocity, causing it to slide relative to the static blood capillary wall. This sliding motion enhances the frequency with which a single receptor on a CTC interacts with the vessel wall ligands [47]. During the rotational movement of a cell, the rotations cause succeeding receptors of the CTC membrane to interact with the vessel wall ligands [48, 49]. These experiments, however, are characterized by linear extrapolation of multiple-bond avidity to measure receptor-ligand attraction, which is an oversimplified process that ignores potential cooperative benefits [50, 51]. Therefore, extensive effort is required for a CTC to reach the distal *onco-sphere* and still being a viable cell.

CTCs and Platelets in the Establishment of a New Distal *Onco-Sphere*: A Symbiotic Relationship

In the process of the establishment of a new distal *onco-sphere*, CTCs must avoid immune detection and enhance their outflow from the circulatory system. In this process, platelets contribution to CTCs in metastasis has been shown in many studies

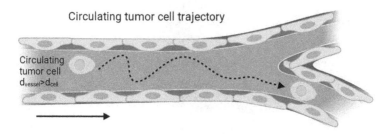

Fig. 14.2 The trajectory of a CTC during metastasis. Tumor cells having a diameter (d_{cell}) smaller than the diameter of the blood vessel wall (d_{vessel}) will travel along a path dictated by the blood vessel surface interactions. Many obstacles are presented to CTCs during their migration: (1) encounter with a blood vessel wall might result in a seizure; (2) tumor cells with a bigger diameter than that of a blood capillary will be trapped; (3) without timely adjustment of cellular receptors, MET would not be possible; and (4) CTCs should acquire neutrophil-like phenotype to adhere and pass through the ECs of a blood vessel

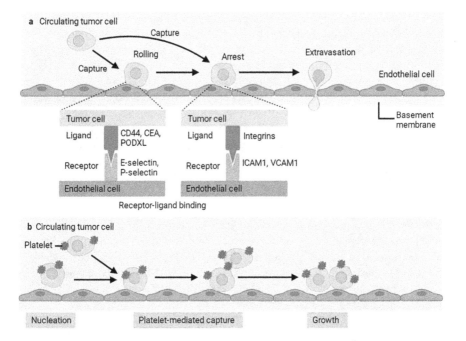

Fig. 14.3 CTCs movement in metastasis. In order to adhere and proliferate in the distal *onco-sphere*, CTCs must first adopt a neutrophil-like adhesion mechanism during the transition into a new environment. (**a**) Because of ligand-receptor linkages, a cell's collision with a vessel wall might result in transitory and/or permanent (strong) adhesion. Transitory adherence is distinguished by weaker connections formed by ligands, including CD44, CEA, or PODXL adhesion to selectin receptors. Permanent adherence occurs after transitory adhesion at an extremely low shear stress level and is caused by interconnections between integrins and their receptors, like ICAM1 and VCAM1. (**b**) Tumor cell interaction with platelets may improve inhibition by platelet-controlled invasion, which is an identical mechanism to nucleation and growth

[52, 53]. In these studies, metastasis was reduced when the amount of platelet decreases, while the opposite is true [54]. Platelets are assumed to disguise and defend CTCs from immune-controlled clearance systems by creating heterotypic adhesive groups with them [55, 56], a classic example of a symbiotic relationship. After their departure from the circulatory system, active platelet-derived substances initiate angiogenesis and spur cell growth at metastatic locations [57]. CTCs may also invade polymorphonuclear leukocytes (PMNs) for detention in remote organ endothelial tissues. CTCs may imitate neutrophil behavior through direct adhesion to the vascular endothelial cells via selectin-regulated tethering and cell rolling succeeded by firm binding (Fig. 14.3) [58, 59]. Moreover, the selectin family (P-, L-, and *E*-selectins) promotes cancer metastasis and cancer cell arrest in the micro-vasculature by governing particular interactions between selectin-producing host cells and tumor cell ligands [60]. Tumor cells are hypothesized to be capable of

forming multicellular aggregates with platelets and leukocytes (through P- and L-selectin-based processes), respectively [61, 62]. These multicellular aggregates then tend to stall in the microvasculature of remote organs before extravasating and establishing metastatic populations. Selectins adhere to sialofucosylated oligosaccharides, for example, Sialyl Lewis X (sLeX) and its isomer sLea, usually found on cell membrane glycoproteins. In colon and pancreatic cancer models, selectins could specifically identify metastatic cell-derived sialofucosylated glycoproteins, including their CD44 variant isoforms, carcinoembryonic antigen (CEA), and podocalyxin (PODXL) [63–65]. CD44v6 and CD44v7, especially, have been causally linked to metastasis, while CEA is a biomarker for cancer progression. Therefore, the overproduction of these compounds on tumor cells is associated with a weak prognosis and tumor growth [66], implying that selectin-controlled adherence to these sialofucosylated protein targets on tumor cells may be a significant predictor of metastatic dissemination. Hence, the intravascular period of the metastatic cascade is a critical stage depicting the effectiveness of medical interventions [67]. Several other molecules, including glycoprotein Iba (GPIba) and GPVI [68, 69], receptors like integrins and their counterparts, ICAM1, and VCAM1, maybe a part of interactions between tumor cells and host cells [66] (Fig. 14.3).

Inter-Onco-Spheric Crosstalk: Exosomes Modulates Key Process in Metastatic Cascade

Regulation of the EMT Process

EMT is a crucial mechanism in the starting phase of metastatic cascade. EMT is notable by the depletion of polarity and losing intracellular adhesive potential cells, changing its physical morphology from an "epithelial" phenotype to a "mesenchymal" phenotype [70, 71]. Tumor-generated exosomes in the local *onco-sphere* can increase metastatic initiation and growth by activating EMT-associated compounds like TGFβ, caveolin-1, HIF-1α, and β-catenin [72]. For example, prostate tumor cells tend to improve stromal cell migration by emanating exosomes containing a lysosomal hyaluronidase, namely, hyaluronidase Hyal-1, implicated in metastatic growth of prostate cancer [73]. Interestingly, exosomes released by highly-metastatic cells are known to enhance the migration capacity of weakly metastatic cells, indicating a co-operative relationship among the cells. Mechanistically, exosomes can typically initiate an EMT cycle through MAPK/ERK activation [74]. Notably, studies have found that under hypoxic condition, tumor cells might discharge exosomes high in miR-21 and MMP-13, resulting in overexpression of vimentin and a decline in E-cadherin to increase EMT cascade and boosting metastasis [75, 76].

Regulation of Angiogenesis

Exosomes can transfer biologically-active chemicals from donor to acceptor cells. In this case, exosomes transferring angiogenesis-related compound (i.e., VEGF, TNF-α) could enhance vascular permeability and thus encourage angiogenesis [77, 78]. For instance, exosomal miR-23a has been demonstrated to increase angiogenesis in nasopharyngeal carcinoma [79]. Hepatoma cells could produce exosomes with having a high concentration of miR-103, which can increase tumor cell mobility by enhancing vascular permeability and attracting different endothelial interface proteins. miR-105 in exosomes can cause increased vascular permeability by particularly disrupting cell-cell tight junctions [80].

Regulation of Immune System

As mentioned before, tumor-derived exosomes are capable of encapsulating various cargoes. However, it is interesting that immune cells in the local *onco-sphere* could also release exosomes to interfere with the metastasis cascade. There are three major mechanisms of how exosomes could be involved.

1. *Inhibition of immune effector cells while increasing the activation of immunosuppressive cells.* For example, exosomes have been implicated with as the driver of CD8$^+$ T cells apoptosis, decreasing NK cells cytotoxicity, while encouraging the expansion of Tregs in multiple solid tumors and also AML [81]. In nasopharyngeal cancer, exosomes derived from the cancer cells are linked with increase in Treg recruitment and differentiation, while inhibiting Th1 and Th17 (antitumorigenic) differentiation. These exosomes also recruited CD4$^+$CD25$^-$T cells and convert these into CD4$^+$CD25$^+$T cells, a highly immunosuppressive Treg subsets [82]. Others have proposed the recruitment of adenosine as a result of enzymatic activation of T cell suppression, brought by the activation of CD39 and CD73 related pathways (highly present on exosomes) [83], while some others proposed that transcriptional regulatory mechanism of immune-related genes could be possible in the recipient cells, leading to a malignant transformation [84].

2. *Employment of decoy mechanism to evade immune recognition.* As we mentioned before, NK cells mainly exert their effect through ADCC. To attenuate this effect, cancer cells can secrete exosomes that could mimic these antibodies, contributing to a "saturation" on tumor cells, that inhibit NK cells to recognize these cells and the proceed with the subsequent ADCC [85]. In another mechanism, the proteins on the surface of exosomes can competitively binds the Abs, leading to a "sink" phenomenon, where the effectiveness of Abs was reduced due to insufficient threshold level in the plasma. This is evident in B cell lymphomas, where CD20 on the surface of exosomes has been shown to bind to anti-CD20 antibody (rituximab), therefore reducing these antibodies binding to the target cancer cells [86].

3. *Converting reactive stromal cells from foes to friends by engaging host inflammation.* In one classic example, hepatic Kupffer cells (liver macrophages) could
uptake high numbers of exosomes derived by pancreatic cancer. These exosomes
are expressing high levels of macrophage inhibitory factors, that they could
activate the pro-inflammatory environment, activating fibronectin production,
which leads to BM-derived macrophages and neutrophil arrest, finally
establishing a pro-metastatic environment [87]. In another example, in a murine
model, when exosome carrying miRNR-21 and miR29-a binds to TLR7, NK-kB
signaling pathway is mediated, pro-inflammatory cytokines (TNFα and IL-6) are
increased, which finally leads to enhanced lung metastasis [88].

Regulation of Metabolic Process

Cancer cells can adapt to a nutrient-deficient environment through metabolic adaptation [89, 90]. As demonstrated by the latest research, tumor cells may change their
metabolic rhythm to fulfill their energy demands in the wake of nutritional restriction, allowing them to penetrate a toxic environment [91, 92]. Exosomes, particularly, act as metabolite transporters to enhance tumor development in nutrient-loaded
microenvironments [93]. Exosomal miRNAs have been demonstrated in several
studies to influence metastasis-related metabolic processes [94, 95]. Exosomes
derived from CD105$^+$ renal cancer stem cells, for instance, contribute to the development of a premetastatic niche by transferring miRNAs [96]. Additionally,
exosomal miR-122 s produced by breast cancer cells can also alter the glucose
uptake of non-tumor cells in the PMNs, thereby promoting metastasis. Exosomes
containing miR-122 can limit glucose intake by downregulating pyruvate kinase,
hence enhancing nutritional supply [97]. Exosomes generated by pancreatic tumor
cells can inhibit the production of GIP and GLP-1 in STC-1 cells in vitro by
activating PCSK1/3, in which a clusters of miRNA were involved (miR-6796-3p,
miR-6763-5p, miR-4750-3p, and miR-197-3p) [98] (Box 14.2).

Box 14.2 Classification of Exosomes
Tumor-derived exosomes. Exosomes carrying Hsp72 are found to increase
MDSCs activation to suppress immunosurveillance [99]. Interestingly, tumor-
derived exosomes with capability to generate tumor antigens have been shown
to promote T cell death while simultaneously suppress T cell activation
[100, 101]. Tumor-produced exosomes releasing FasL could increase lymphocyte death [102]. Furthermore, tumor-produced exosomes can inhibit IL-2-
governed NK cell stimulation and cytotoxic function [103, 104]. Additionally,
tumor-produced exosomes harboring miR-23a may operate as immunosuppressive agents due to the direct downregulation of CD107a production in NK
cells [105]. Surprisingly, TLR3 activation has been shown to play a significant

---

(continued)

Box 14.2 (continued)

role in metastasis but not vital for the primary tumor. Furthermore, researchers verified the activation of TLR3 by tumor-produced exosomal RNAs instead of tumor RNAs, demonstrating the preferential packing of exosomal RNAs [106]. The modification of non-neoplastic tumor cells impacts the recipient cells via the secretion of exosomes that can transmit chemicals essential for metastasis, hence increasing cancer metastasis [107]. Specifically, ovarian cancer cells can generate exosomes harboring oncogenic proteins like STAT3 and FAS that improve tumor cells' motility potential [108]. Pancreatic cancer cells might release exosomes harboring miR-301a-3p, which promotes metastasis by activating macrophage M2 polarization [109].

Stromal-cell derived exosomes. Exosomes also influence how tumor cells and fibroblasts interact, as fibroblasts create exosomes harboring pro-inflammatory cytokines that promote tumor spread. Exosomes carrying miR-1247-3p, for instance, are released by high-metastatic hepatocellular tumor cells and target B4GALT3 for activating β1-integrin-NF-kB signaling in these activated fibroblasts, thus accelerating cancer development by producing pro-inflammatory interleukins that promotes metastasis progression, such as IL-6 and IL-8 [110].

Immune cell-derived exosomes. Exosomes generated by T cells have also been demonstrated to inhibit antitumor immunity by lowering pMHC I transcription in DCs [111]. Additionally, activated T-cell exosomes containing bioactive FasL, belonging to the TNF family, may promote melanoma and lung cancer cell metastasis by boosting MMP9 synthesis [112]. In other examples, the secretion of exosomes by M2-like macrophages that comprise miR-21-5p and miR-155-5p to enhance colorectal cancer metastasis by downregulating BRG1 transcription [113]. Likewise, exosomes released by M2-like macrophages can increase gastric tumor cell dispersion by selective transfer of apolipoprotein E (ApoE), which can modify cytoskeleton-supportive trafficking by stimulating the PI3K-Akt signaling pathway [114].

Conclusion

Metastasis exceedingly complex. Each process, from cancer cell dissemination, EMT transition, circulation in the blood vessels, getting into the pre-formed PMNs, escape from various immunosurveillance, re-transformation of MET, and finally be viable as a new "seed" at the distal *onco-sphere*. We now understand the implication of all components in the local *onco-sphere* towards the metastatic cascade. Through this understanding, we can now design a rational yet personalized therapeutic against metastatic cancer, choosing the synergistic pathways that could work optimally with each other to achieve significant effect in cancer therapeutics.

References

1. Brooks SA, Lomax-Browne HJ, Carter TM, Kinch CE, Hall DM (2010) Molecular interactions in cancer cell metastasis. Acta Histochem 112(1):3–25
2. Lambert AW, Pattabiraman DR, Weinberg RA (2017) Emerging biological principles of metastasis. Cell 168(4):670–691
3. Celià-Terrassa T, Kang Y (2018) Metastatic niche functions and therapeutic opportunities. Nat Cell Biol 20(8):868–877
4. Peinado H, Zhang H, Matei IR, Costa-Silva B, Hoshino A, Rodrigues G et al (2017) Pre-metastatic niches: organ-specific homes for metastases. Nat Rev Cancer 17(5):302–317
5. Quail DF, Joyce JA (2013) Microenvironmental regulation of tumor progression and metastasis. Nat Med 19(11):1423–1437
6. Alečković M, Kang Y (2015) Regulation of cancer metastasis by cell-free miRNAs. Biochim Biophys Acta 1855(1):24–42
7. Hoshino A, Costa-Silva B, Shen TL, Rodrigues G, Hashimoto A, Tesic Mark M et al (2015) Tumour exosome integrins determine organotropic metastasis. Nature 527(7578):329–335
8. Aleckovic M, McAllister SS, Polyak K (2019) Metastasis as a systemic disease: molecular insights and clinical implications. Biochim Biophys Acta Rev Cancer 1872(1):89–102
9. McAllister SS, Weinberg RA (2014) The tumour-induced systemic environment as a critical regulator of cancer progression and metastasis. Nat Cell Biol 16(8):717–727
10. Gao D, Mittal V (2009) The role of bone-marrow-derived cells in tumor growth, metastasis initiation and progression. Trends Mol Med 15(8):333–343
11. Kaplan RN, Riba RD, Zacharoulis S, Bramley AH, Vincent L, Costa C et al (2005) VEGFR1-positive haematopoietic bone marrow progenitors initiate the pre-metastatic niche. Nature 438(7069):820–827
12. Hiratsuka S, Watanabe A, Aburatani H, Maru Y (2006) Tumour-mediated upregulation of chemoattractants and recruitment of myeloid cells predetermines lung metastasis. Nat Cell Biol 8(12):1369–1375
13. Erler JT, Bennewith KL, Nicolau M, Dornhöfer N, Kong C, Le QT et al (2006) Lysyl oxidase is essential for hypoxia-induced metastasis. Nature 440(7088):1222–1226
14. Stone RLA-KV (2013) Causes and consequences of cancer-associated thrombocytosis. Blood 122(21):SCI-33
15. Orimo A, Gupta PB, Sgroi DC, Arenzana-Seisdedos F, Delaunay T, Naeem R et al (2005) Stromal fibroblasts present in invasive human breast carcinomas promote tumor growth and angiogenesis through elevated SDF-1/CXCL12 secretion. Cell 121(3):335–348
16. Peinado H, Alečković M, Lavotshkin S, Matei I, Costa-Silva B, Moreno-Bueno G et al (2012) Melanoma exosomes educate bone marrow progenitor cells toward a pro-metastatic phenotype through MET. Nat Med 18(6):883–891
17. Obenauf AC, Massagué J (2015) Surviving at a distance: organ-specific metastasis. Trends Cancer 1(1):76–91
18. Boire A, Zou Y, Shieh J, Macalinao DG, Pentsova E, Massagué J (2017) Complement component 3 adapts the cerebrospinal fluid for leptomeningeal metastasis. Cell 168(6): 1101–13.e13
19. Yang L, Huang J, Ren X, Gorska AE, Chytil A, Aakre M et al (2008) Abrogation of TGF beta signaling in mammary carcinomas recruits gr-1+CD11b+ myeloid cells that promote metastasis. Cancer Cell 13(1):23–35
20. Serafini P, Borrello I, Bronte V (2006) Myeloid suppressor cells in cancer: recruitment, phenotype, properties, and mechanisms of immune suppression. Semin Cancer Biol 16(1): 53–65
21. Almand B, Clark JI, Nikitina E, van Beynen J, English NR, Knight SC et al (2001) Increased production of immature myeloid cells in cancer patients: a mechanism of immunosuppression in cancer. J Immunol 166(1):678–689

22. Coffelt SB, de Visser KE (2016) Systemic inflammation: cancer's long-distance reach to maximize metastasis. Oncoimmunology 5(2):e1075694
23. Kersten K, Coffelt SB, Hoogstraat M, Verstegen NJM, Vrijland K, Ciampricotti M et al (2017) Mammary tumor-derived CCL2 enhances pro-metastatic systemic inflammation through upregulation of IL1β in tumor-associated macrophages. Oncoimmunology 6(8):e1334744
24. Lu X, Kang Y (2009) Chemokine (C-C motif) ligand 2 engages CCR2+ stromal cells of monocytic origin to promote breast cancer metastasis to lung and bone. J Biol Chem 284(42):29087–29096
25. Qian BZ, Li J, Zhang H, Kitamura T, Zhang J, Campion LR et al (2011) CCL2 recruits inflammatory monocytes to facilitate breast-tumour metastasis. Nature 475(7355):222–225
26. Voloshin T, Alishekevitz D, Kaneti L, Miller V, Isakov E, Kaplanov I et al (2015) Blocking IL1β pathway following paclitaxel chemotherapy slightly inhibits primary tumor growth but promotes spontaneous metastasis. Mol Cancer Ther 14(6):1385–1394
27. Spiegel A, Brooks MW, Houshyar S, Reinhardt F, Ardolino M, Fessler E et al (2016) Neutrophils suppress intraluminal NK cell-mediated tumor cell clearance and enhance extravasation of disseminated carcinoma cells. Cancer Discov 6(6):630–649
28. Coffelt SB, Kersten K, Doornebal CW, Weiden J, Vrijland K, Hau CS et al (2015) IL-17-producing γδ T cells and neutrophils conspire to promote breast cancer metastasis. Nature 522(7556):345–348
29. Hasegawa S, Suda T, Negi K, Hattori Y (2007) Lung large cell carcinoma producing granulocyte-colony-stimulating factor. Ann Thorac Surg 83(1):308–310
30. Granger JM, Kontoyiannis DP (2009) Etiology and outcome of extreme leukocytosis in 758 nonhematologic cancer patients: a retrospective, single-institution study. Cancer 115(17):3919–3923
31. Wu TC, Xu K, Martinek J, Young RR, Banchereau R, George J et al (2018) IL1 receptor antagonist controls transcriptional signature of inflammation in patients with metastatic breast cancer. Cancer Res 78(18):5243–5258
32. Park J, Wysocki RW, Amoozgar Z, Maiorino L, Fein MR, Jorns J et al (2016) Cancer cells induce metastasis-supporting neutrophil extracellular DNA traps. Sci Transl Med 8(361):361ra138
33. Granot Z, Henke E, Comen EA, King TA, Norton L, Benezra R (2011) Tumor entrained neutrophils inhibit seeding in the premetastatic lung. Cancer Cell 20(3):300–314
34. Castaño Z, San Juan BP, Spiegel A, Pant A, DeCristo MJ, Laszewski T et al (2018) IL-1β inflammatory response driven by primary breast cancer prevents metastasis-initiating cell colonization. Nat Cell Biol 20(9):1084–1097
35. Janiszewska M, Tabassum DP, Castaño Z, Cristea S, Yamamoto KN, Kingston NL et al (2019) Subclonal cooperation drives metastasis by modulating local and systemic immune microenvironments. Nat Cell Biol 21(7):879–888
36. McAllister SS, Gifford AM, Greiner AL, Kelleher SP, Saelzler MP, Ince TA et al (2008) Systemic endocrine instigation of indolent tumor growth requires osteopontin. Cell 133(6):994–1005
37. Elkabets M, Gifford AM, Scheel C, Nilsson B, Reinhardt F, Bray MA et al (2011) Human tumors instigate granulin-expressing hematopoietic cells that promote malignancy by activating stromal fibroblasts in mice. J Clin Invest 121(2):784–799
38. Nielsen SR, Quaranta V, Linford A, Emeagi P, Rainer C, Santos A et al (2016) Macrophage-secreted granulin supports pancreatic cancer metastasis by inducing liver fibrosis. Nat Cell Biol 18(5):549–560
39. Bartoschek M, Oskolkov N, Bocci M, Lövrot J, Larsson C, Sommarin M et al (2018) Spatially and functionally distinct subclasses of breast cancer-associated fibroblasts revealed by single cell RNA sequencing. Nat Commun 9(1):5150
40. Costa A, Kieffer Y, Scholer-Dahirel A, Pelon F, Bourachot B, Cardon M et al (2018) Fibroblast heterogeneity and immunosuppressive environment in human breast cancer. Cancer Cell 33(3):463–79.e10

41. Saw PE, Chen J, Song E (2022) Targeting CAFs to overcome anticancer therapeutic resistance. Trends Cancer 8(7):527–555

42. Zhang L, Zhang S, Yao J, Lowery FJ, Zhang Q, Huang WC et al (2015) Microenvironment-induced PTEN loss by exosomal microRNA primes brain metastasis outgrowth. Nature 527(7576):100–104

43. Priego N, Zhu L, Monteiro C, Mulders M, Wasilewski D, Bindeman W et al (2018) STAT3 labels a subpopulation of reactive astrocytes required for brain metastasis. Nat Med 24(7): 1024–1035

44. Er EE, Valiente M, Ganesh K, Zou Y, Agrawal S, Hu J et al (2018) Pericyte-like spreading by disseminated cancer cells activates YAP and MRTF for metastatic colonization. Nat Cell Biol 20(8):966–978

45. Fidler IJ, Yano S, Zhang RD, Fujimaki T, Bucana CD (2002) The seed and soil hypothesis: vascularisation and brain metastases. Lancet Oncol 3(1):53–57

46. Zhu C, Yago T, Lou J, Zarnitsyna VI, McEver RP (2008) Mechanisms for flow-enhanced cell adhesion. Ann Biomed Eng 36(4):604–621

47. Chang KC, Hammer DA (1999) The forward rate of binding of surface-tethered reactants: effect of relative motion between two surfaces. Biophys J 76(3):1280–1292

48. Duguay D, Foty RA, Steinberg MS (2003) Cadherin-mediated cell adhesion and tissue segregation: qualitative and quantitative determinants. Dev Biol 253(2):309–323

49. Niessen CM, Gumbiner BM (2002) Cadherin-mediated cell sorting not determined by binding or adhesion specificity. J Cell Biol 156(2):389–399

50. Huang J, Zarnitsyna VI, Liu B, Edwards LJ, Jiang N, Evavold BD et al (2010) The kinetics of two-dimensional TCR and pMHC interactions determine T-cell responsiveness. Nature 464(7290):932–936

51. Marshall BT, Long M, Piper JW, Yago T, McEver RP, Zhu C (2003) Direct observation of catch bonds involving cell-adhesion molecules. Nature 423(6936):190–193

52. Gasic GJ, Gasic TB, Stewart CC (1968) Antimetastatic effects associated with platelet reduction. Proc Natl Acad Sci U S A 61(1):46–52

53. Camerer E, Qazi AA, Duong DN, Cornelissen I, Advincula R, Coughlin SR (2004) Platelets, protease-activated receptors, and fibrinogen in hematogenous metastasis. Blood 104(2): 397–401

54. Karpatkin S, Pearlstein E, Ambrogio C, Coller BS (1988) Role of adhesive proteins in platelet tumor interaction in vitro and metastasis formation in vivo. J Clin Invest 81(4):1012–1019

55. Nieswandt B, Hafner M, Echtenacher B, Männel DN (1999) Lysis of tumor cells by natural killer cells in mice is impeded by platelets. Cancer Res 59(6):1295–1300

56. Palumbo JS, Talmage KE, Massari JV, La Jeunesse CM, Flick MJ, Kombrinck KW et al (2005) Platelets and fibrin (ogen) increase metastatic potential by impeding natural killer cell-mediated elimination of tumor cells. Blood 105(1):178–185

57. Pinedo HM, Verheul HM, D'Amato RJ, Folkman J (1998) Involvement of platelets in tumour angiogenesis? Lancet 352(9142):1775–1777

58. Burdick MM, JM MC, Kim YS, Bochner BS, Konstantopoulos K (2003) Colon carcinoma cell glycolipids, integrins, and other glycoproteins mediate adhesion to HUVECs under flow. Am J Phys Cell Physiol 284(4):C977–C987

59. Burdick MM, Konstantopoulos K (2004) Platelet-induced enhancement of LS174T colon carcinoma and THP-1 monocytoid cell adhesion to vascular endothelium under flow. Am J Phys Cell Physiol 287(2):C539–C547

60. Borsig L, Wong R, Feramisco J, Nadeau DR, Varki NM, Varki A (2001) Heparin and cancer revisited: mechanistic connections involving platelets, P-selectin, carcinoma mucins, and tumor metastasis. Proc Natl Acad Sci U S A 98(6):3352–3357

61. Jadhav S, Bochner BS, Konstantopoulos K (2001) Hydrodynamic shear regulates the kinetics and receptor specificity of polymorphonuclear leukocyte-colon carcinoma cell adhesive interactions. J Immunol 167(10):5986–5993

62. McCarty OJ, Mousa SA, Bray PF, Konstantopoulos K (2000) Immobilized platelets support human colon carcinoma cell tethering, rolling, and firm adhesion under dynamic flow conditions. Blood 96(5):1789–1797
63. Napier SL, Healy ZR, Schnaar RL, Konstantopoulos K (2007) Selectin ligand expression regulates the initial vascular interactions of colon carcinoma cells: the roles of CD44v and alternative sialofucosylated selectin ligands. J Biol Chem 282(6):3433–3441
64. Thomas SN, Schnaar RL, Konstantopoulos K (2009) Podocalyxin-like protein is an E−/L-selectin ligand on colon carcinoma cells: comparative biochemical properties of selectin ligands in host and tumor cells. Am J Phys Cell Physiol 296(3):C505–C513
65. Thomas SN, Zhu F, Schnaar RL, Alves CS, Konstantopoulos K (2008) Carcinoembryonic antigen and CD44 variant isoforms cooperate to mediate colon carcinoma cell adhesion to E- and L-selectin in shear flow. J Biol Chem 283(23):15647–15655
66. Konstantopoulos K, Thomas SN (2009) Cancer cells in transit: the vascular interactions of tumor cells. Annu Rev Biomed Eng 11:177–202
67. Varki A, Varki NM, Borsig L (2009) Molecular basis of metastasis. N Engl J Med 360(16): 1678–1679; author reply 9-80
68. Jain S, Zuka M, Liu J, Russell S, Dent J, Guerrero JA et al (2007) Platelet glycoprotein Ib alpha supports experimental lung metastasis. Proc Natl Acad Sci U S A 104(21):9024–9028
69. Jain S, Russell S, Ware J (2009) Platelet glycoprotein VI facilitates experimental lung metastasis in syngenic mouse models. J Thromb Haemost 7(10):1713–1717
70. Ye X, Brabletz T, Kang Y, Longmore GD, Nieto MA, Stanger BZ et al (2017) Upholding a role for EMT in breast cancer metastasis. Nature 547(7661):E1–e3
71. Valastyan S, Weinberg RA (2011) Tumor metastasis: molecular insights and evolving paradigms. Cell 147(2):275–292
72. Syn N, Wang L, Sethi G, Thiery JP, Goh BC (2016) Exosome-mediated metastasis: from epithelial-mesenchymal transition to escape from immunosurveillance. Trends Pharmacol Sci 37(7):606–617
73. McAtee CO, Booth C, Elowsky C, Zhao L, Payne J, Fangman T et al (2019) Prostate tumor cell exosomes containing hyaluronidase Hyal1 stimulate prostate stromal cell motility by engagement of FAK-mediated integrin signaling. Matrix Biol 78-79:165–179
74. Chen L, Guo P, He Y, Chen Z, Chen L, Luo Y et al (2018) HCC-derived exosomes elicit HCC progression and recurrence by epithelial-mesenchymal transition through MAPK/ERK signalling pathway. Cell Death Dis 9(5):513
75. Li L, Li C, Wang S, Wang Z, Jiang J, Wang W et al (2016) Exosomes derived from hypoxic Oral squamous cell carcinoma cells deliver miR-21 to normoxic cells to elicit a Prometastatic phenotype. Cancer Res 76(7):1770–1780
76. Shan Y, You B, Shi S, Shi W, Zhang Z, Zhang Q et al (2018) Hypoxia-induced matrix Metalloproteinase-13 expression in exosomes from nasopharyngeal carcinoma enhances metastases. Cell Death Dis 9(3):382
77. Steenbeek SC, Pham TV, de Ligt J, Zomer A, Knol JC, Piersma SR et al (2018) Cancer cells copy migratory behavior and exchange signaling networks via extracellular vesicles. EMBO J 37(15):e98357
78. Kosaka N, Iguchi H, Hagiwara K, Yoshioka Y, Takeshita F, Ochiya T (2013) Neutral sphingomyelinase 2 (nSMase2)-dependent exosomal transfer of angiogenic microRNAs regulate cancer cell metastasis. J Biol Chem 288(15):10849–10859
79. Bao L, You B, Shi S, Shan Y, Zhang Q, Yue H et al (2018) Metastasis-associated miR-23a from nasopharyngeal carcinoma-derived exosomes mediates angiogenesis by repressing a novel target gene TSGA10. Oncogene 37(21):2873–2889
80. Zhou W, Fong MY, Min Y, Somlo G, Liu L, Palomares MR et al (2014) Cancer-secreted miR-105 destroys vascular endothelial barriers to promote metastasis. Cancer Cell 25(4): 501–515
81. Whiteside TL (2013) Immune modulation of T-cell and NK (natural killer) cell activities by TEXs (tumour-derived exosomes). Biochem Soc Trans 41(1):245–251

82. Zhou Y, Xia L, Lin J, Wang H, Oyang L, Tan S et al (2018) Exosomes in nasopharyngeal carcinoma. J Cancer 9(5):767–777
83. Clayton A, Al-Taei S, Webber J, Mason MD, Tabi Z (2011) Cancer exosomes express CD39 and CD73, which suppress T cells through adenosine production. J Immunol 187(2):676–683
84. Olejarz W, Dominiak A, Zolnierzak A, Kubiak-Tomaszewska G, Lorenc T (2020) Tumor-derived exosomes in immunosuppression and immunotherapy. J Immunol Res 2020:6272498
85. Battke C, Ruiss R, Welsch U, Wimberger P, Lang S, Jochum S et al (2011) Tumour exosomes inhibit binding of tumour-reactive antibodies to tumour cells and reduce ADCC. Cancer Immunol Immunother 60(5):639–648
86. Aung T, Chapuy B, Vogel D, Wenzel D, Oppermann M, Lahmann M et al (2011) Exosomal evasion of humoral immunotherapy in aggressive B-cell lymphoma modulated by ATP-binding cassette transporter A3. Proc Natl Acad Sci U S A 108(37):15336–15341
87. Costa-Silva B, Aiello NM, Ocean AJ, Singh S, Zhang H, Thakur BK et al (2015) Pancreatic cancer exosomes initiate pre-metastatic niche formation in the liver. Nat Cell Biol 17(6): 816–826
88. Fabbri M, Paone A, Calore F, Galli R, Gaudio E, Santhanam R et al (2012) MicroRNAs bind to toll-like receptors to induce prometastatic inflammatory response. Proc Natl Acad Sci U S A 109(31):E2110–E2116
89. Payen VL, Porporato PE, Baselet B, Sonveaux P (2016) Metabolic changes associated with tumor metastasis, part 1: tumor pH, glycolysis and the pentose phosphate pathway. Cell Mol Life Sci 73(7):1333–1348
90. Caneba CA, Bellance N, Yang L, Pabst L, Nagrath D (2012) Pyruvate uptake is increased in highly invasive ovarian cancer cells under anoikis conditions for anaplerosis, mitochondrial function, and migration. Am J Physiol Endocrinol Metab 303(8):E1036–E1052
91. Nomura DK, Long JZ, Niessen S, Hoover HS, Ng SW, Cravatt BF (2010) Monoacylglycerol lipase regulates a fatty acid network that promotes cancer pathogenesis. Cell 140(1):49–61
92. Yang L, Moss T, Mangala LS, Marini J, Zhao H, Wahlig S et al (2014) Metabolic shifts toward glutamine regulate tumor growth, invasion and bioenergetics in ovarian cancer. Mol Syst Biol 10(5):728
93. Zhao H, Yang L, Baddour J, Achreja A, Bernard V, Moss T et al (2016) Tumor microenvironment derived exosomes pleiotropically modulate cancer cell metabolism. elife 5:e10250
94. Chau BN, Xin C, Hartner J, Ren S, Castano AP, Linn G et al (2012) MicroRNA-21 promotes fibrosis of the kidney by silencing metabolic pathways. Sci Transl Med 4(121):121ra18
95. Zhu H, Shyh-Chang N, Segrè AV, Shinoda G, Shah SP, Einhorn WS et al (2011) The Lin28/let-7 axis regulates glucose metabolism. Cell 147(1):81–94
96. Grange C, Tapparo M, Collino F, Vitillo L, Damasco C, Deregibus MC et al (2011) Microvesicles released from human renal cancer stem cells stimulate angiogenesis and formation of lung premetastatic niche. Cancer Res 71(15):5346–5356
97. Fong MY, Zhou W, Liu L, Alontaga AY, Chandra M, Ashby J et al (2015) Breast-cancer-secreted miR-122 reprograms glucose metabolism in premetastatic niche to promote metastasis. Nat Cell Biol 17(2):183–194
98. Zhang Y, Huang S, Li P, Chen Q, Li Y, Zhou Y et al (2018) Pancreatic cancer-derived exosomes suppress the production of GIP and GLP-1 from STC-1 cells in vitro by downregulating the PCSK1/3. Cancer Lett 431:190–200
99. Chalmin F, Ladoire S, Mignot G, Vincent J, Bruchard M, Remy-Martin JP et al (2010) Membrane-associated Hsp72 from tumor-derived exosomes mediates STAT3-dependent immunosuppressive function of mouse and human myeloid-derived suppressor cells. J Clin Invest 120(2):457–471
100. Abusamra AJ, Zhong Z, Zheng X, Li M, Ichim TE, Chin JL et al (2005) Tumor exosomes expressing Fas ligand mediate CD8+ T-cell apoptosis. Blood Cells Mol Dis 35(2):169–173
101. Taylor DD, Gerçel-Taylor C (2005) Tumour-derived exosomes and their role in cancer-associated T-cell signalling defects. Br J Cancer 92(2):305–311

102. Andreola G, Rivoltini L, Castelli C, Huber V, Perego P, Deho P et al (2002) Induction of lymphocyte apoptosis by tumor cell secretion of FasL-bearing microvesicles. J Exp Med 195(10):1303–1316
103. Liu C, Yu S, Zinn K, Wang J, Zhang L, Jia Y et al (2006) Murine mammary carcinoma exosomes promote tumor growth by suppression of NK cell function. J Immunol 176(3): 1375–1385
104. Zhang HG, Kim H, Liu C, Yu S, Wang J, Grizzle WE et al (2007) Curcumin reverses breast tumor exosomes mediated immune suppression of NK cell tumor cytotoxicity. Biochim Biophys Acta 1773(7):1116–1123
105. Berchem G, Noman MZ, Bosseler M, Paggetti J, Baconnais S, Le Cam E et al (2016) Hypoxic tumor-derived microvesicles negatively regulate NK cell function by a mechanism involving TGF-β and miR23a transfer. Oncoimmunology 5(4):e1062968
106. Antonopoulos D, Balatsos NAA, Gourgoulianis KI (2017) Cancer's smart bombs: tumor-derived exosomes target lung epithelial cells triggering pre-metastatic niche formation. J Thorac Dis 9(4):969–972
107. Naito Y, Yoshioka Y, Yamamoto Y, Ochiya T (2017) How cancer cells dictate their micro-environment: present roles of extracellular vesicles. Cell Mol Life Sci 74(4):697–713
108. Dorayappan KDP, Wanner R, Wallbillich JJ, Saini U, Zingarelli R, Suarez AA et al (2018) Hypoxia-induced exosomes contribute to a more aggressive and chemoresistant ovarian cancer phenotype: a novel mechanism linking STAT3/Rab proteins. Oncogene 37(28): 3806–3821
109. Wang X, Luo G, Zhang K, Cao J, Huang C, Jiang T et al (2018) Hypoxic tumor-derived Exosomal miR-301a mediates M2 macrophage polarization via PTEN/PI3Kγ to promote pancreatic cancer metastasis. Cancer Res 78(16):4586–4598
110. Fang T, Lv H, Lv G, Li T, Wang C, Han Q et al (2018) Tumor-derived exosomal miR-1247-3p induces cancer-associated fibroblast activation to foster lung metastasis of liver cancer. Nat Commun 9(1):191
111. Xie Y, Zhang H, Li W, Deng Y, Munegowda MA, Chibbar R et al (2010) Dendritic cells recruit T cell exosomes via exosomal LFA-1 leading to inhibition of CD8+ CTL responses through downregulation of peptide/MHC class I and Fas ligand-mediated cytotoxicity. J Immunol 185(9):5268–5278
112. Cai Z, Yang F, Yu L, Yu Z, Jiang L, Wang Q et al (2012) Activated T cell exosomes promote tumor invasion via Fas signaling pathway. J Immunol 188(12):5954–5961
113. Lan J, Sun L, Xu F, Liu L, Hu F, Song D et al (2019) M2 macrophage-derived exosomes promote cell migration and invasion in colon cancer. Cancer Res 79(1):146–158
114. Zheng P, Luo Q, Wang W, Li J, Wang T, Wang P et al (2018) Tumor-associated macrophages-derived exosomes promote the migration of gastric cancer cells by transfer of functional apolipoprotein E. Cell Death Dis 9(4):434

Chapter 15
Distal *Onco-sphere:* Cluster Metastasis

Phei Er Saw and Erwei Song

Abstract In order for cancer cells to metastasize, they need to be disseminated from the local onco-sphere. During this process, cancer cells are known as circulating tumor cells (CTCs) which are now circulating in the blood stream or lymphatic vessels. Cancer cells metastasize easier and faster in a cluster than when they are alone. In fact, it has been proven that clusters that are made of circulating tumor cells (CTCs) had up to 100 times metastatic ability compared to single non-clustered CTCs, leading to the notion "better together". In this chapter, we emphasize on the origin, the various type and the importance of cluster metastasis.

Introduction

Cancer cells metastasize easier and faster in a cluster than when they are alone. In fact, it has been proven that clusters that are made of circulating tumor cells (CTCs) had up to 100 times metastatic ability compared to single non-clustered CTCs [1–4]. The concept of ecosystem is clear in the formation of CTC clusters. Although CTCs can exist as single cells, usually they are found in a group of two or more;

P. E. Saw
Guangdong Provincial Key Laboratory of Malignant Tumor Epigenetics and Gene Regulation, Guangdong-Hong Kong Joint Laboratory for RNA Medicine, Medical Research Center, Sun Yat-sen Memorial Hospital, Sun Yat-sen University, Guangzhou, China

Nanhai Translational Innovation Center of Precision Immunology, Sun Yat-sen Memorial Hospital, Sun Yat-sen University, Foshan, China

E. Song (✉)
Guangdong Provincial Key Laboratory of Malignant Tumor Epigenetics and Gene Regulation, Guangdong-Hong Kong Joint Laboratory for RNA Medicine, Medical Research Center, Sun Yat-sen Memorial Hospital, Sun Yat-sen University, Guangzhou, China

Nanhai Translational Innovation Center of Precision Immunology, Sun Yat-sen Memorial Hospital, Sun Yat-sen University, Foshan, China

Breast Tumor Center, Sun Yat-sen Memorial Hospital, Sun Yat-sen University, Guangzhou, China
e-mail: songew@mail.sysu.edu.cn

hence, the term clusters are used [4]. In ecology, when one wants to survive, they could adopt a "better together" concept, and this rings true for CTCs. Clustering of CTCs is indeed a survival mechanism that has been adapted as these cells navigate the harsh environment in the host, while having the need to find an appropriate distal *onco-sphere* for them to metastasize [4].

CTCs are the key players in the formation of a distal *onco-sphere*. During extravasation, tumor cells are detached from the primary tumor, in order to be able to extravasate from the local *onco-sphere* into the circulation system. Once detached and circulating in blood stream, CTC clusters "seed" then extravasate into suitable metastatic niche "soil" in their quest to conquer their new *onco-sphere*. Therefore, deep understanding of how the CTCs are responsible for the of the metastatic cascade is crucial for determining specific targets that could be used for treating metastasis and its related complications. One of the bottlenecks, however, is to detect and identify these rare CTCs, which could be in the concentration of tens in one liter of blood. Since CTCs have been identified to possess most EMT-like properties and stemness, CTCs are now regarded as the main cell types that are involved in metastatic capacity of a tumor. Interestingly, through harsh conditions in the systemic circulation, only a minute fraction of CTCs remain viable upon reaching the distal *onco-sphere*. However, interestingly, these survived CTCs are able to proliferate in the metastatic site, suggesting an indispensable interaction and modulation between CTCs the host circulatory system, and this interaction is essential for CTC-evoked metastasis from local to distal *onco-sphere*.

Tumor Cell Clusters and Polyclonal Seeding of Metastases

It was discovered in the 1950s that blood samples from cancer patients include both single and clustered tumor cells and that tumor cell clusters may swiftly travel through the lungs in animal models [5, 6]. These findings led to the hypothesis that tumor cell clusters play a role in metastasis. Later studies demonstrated that intravenously injected tumor cell clusters were more effective than single cells at generating metastases in animals [5, 7, 8]. The findings from these early trials are compatible with two quite distinct hypotheses, despite the fact that metastasis is proven to be ineffective [5]. Metastases can emerge either through a less efficient strategy of seeding many single cells or through the process of seeding through rare clusters. Monitoring CTCs and CTC clusters as well as identifying their molecular characteristics across a variety of tumor types has undergone a radical change because of recent technical advancements [1, 2, 9, 10].

A clonal tumor will develop if the metastatic seed is just one cancer cell. The metastasis that results, however, may be polyclonal right from the start of the seed is a CTC cluster. Cancer cell clone evolutionary histories can be recreated during the metastatic progression process using deep sequencing analysis of tumors. You can determine if monoclonal or polyclonal seeding was employed by using these evolutionary histories. One recent research on men with prostate cancer found

Fig. 15.1 Origin of cells are crucial in determining the metastasis outcome. Clusters are always having higher chance of survival and creating a new distal *onco-sphere* compared to a single cell-originated clusters

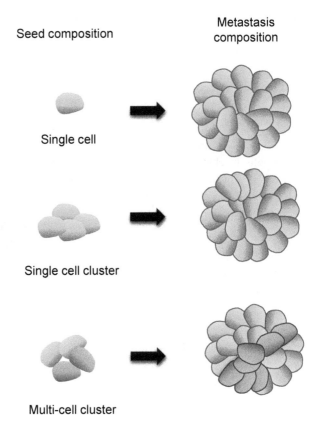

Seed composition

Metastasis composition

Single cell

Single cell cluster

Multi-cell cluster

evidence of frequent polyclonal seeding from the main tumor to secondary locations and the polyclonal spread of existing metastases to new sites in the body [11]. This finding is supported by a growing body of research on the phenotypic and genotypic diversity of primary tumors, as well as a growing understanding of cooperative and competitive dynamics among cancer cell clones [12]. According to such research, the cluster's many clonal combinations may exhibit a wide range of growth and/or therapeutic response characteristics.

Two different processes could result in the development of polyclonal metastases: repeated accumulation of several single cells at a single site or direct seeding with a multicellular cluster. To discriminate between these two systems, mouse models have been helpful. The capacity to create primary tumors that are mixed with cancer cells that display various colored fluorescent proteins is a crucial aspect of these experiments [1, 13, 14]. Single-cell and cell clusters with only one hue will both produce single-colored metastases. Multicolored metastases will emerge from color-rich clusters, which will indicate their polyclonal origin (Fig. 15.1). All three independent research teams that used different mouse models to study this design discovered multi-colored metastases, which is coherent with the notion that poly-clonal metastases can be sparked by tumor cell clusters [1, 13, 14]. In inducing multicolored mammary cancers in mice, the first group regularly found multicolored metastases [1]. When scientists created a single-colored tumor across one side of the mouse and another on the opposite side, the metastases were mainly single-colored [1]. This finding shows that tumor cell clustering within blood or even in a distant organ is ineffective, and that multicolored metastases form because of clusters of tumor cells being seeded [1]. The second group applied lineage analysis to pancreatic cancer demonstrating polyclonal seeding cluster in mice and found significant variations in how far a polyclonal seed developed into a clonal or polyclonal metastasis in various organ sites [13]. A third group examined sporadic breast cancer in rodents and quantitatively linked the degree of clonal mixing within the main tumor with the chance of finding colorful metastases. This led them to believe that over 97 percent of metastases originated from clusters [14]. Additionally, all three investigations directly showed that clusters have greater potential for colony-forming and surviving in both cultures and living organisms. Multi-colored metastases were rarely or never produced in control trials in which different hue tumors were created in various mouse locations or different color tumor cells were administered intravenously at various periods. As a result, evidence from all three investigations supports the idea that a multicellular cluster disperses as a group from the main tumor to distant organs to initiate polyclonal metastases (Fig. 15.1) [1, 13, 14].

Metastatic Seeds' Epithelial Properties

The aforementioned observations give rise to many concerns, such as the manner in which tumor cell clusters find their way from primary tumors as well as their molecular characteristics upon reaching distant sites. The emphasis of this paper will be on breast cancer where significant progress has been made to decipher the tumor cells' properties while entering and traversing across many organs. According to a recent 3D assessment of human breast tumors' stromal borders, there were frequent instances of collective invasions without any proliferation of single cells [15]. Importantly, these invasion strands were likely to expel tiny groups of cancerous cells for getting the metastatic process seeded. Testing for molecular similarities among these cells not only in strands of collective invasion but also during the metastatic spread's later stages is a starting point to get this model validated. These cancerous cells driving collective invasion exhibited overlapping molecular characteristics in breast cancer subtypes in humans and animals [16]. The cancer cells' expression of basal epithelial differentiation molecular markers characterized them, such as p63, K5/K14$^+$, and P-cadherin, among others [17]. K14$^+$ cells were seen during all disseminative spread phases, such as CTC cluster, and collective invasion. However, their presence in macro-metastases and primary tumor was rare [14]. According to these data, different epithelial molecular programs are known to propel the dissemination and growth of tumors. Here, gene expression bears resemblance to the mammary stem cell pertaining to basal phenotype. This, in turn, is in line with metastatic human cancer breast cells' single-cell transcriptomic analysis [14], according to which disseminated cells help the formation of macro-metastases that largely comprise cancer cells of luminal phenotype [18]. It was also shown that alterations when it comes to the epithelial state are accompanied by metastatic dissemination.

Particular complexes of intercellular adhesion denote epithelial cells. Metastasis is seen as something that entails a permanent/temporary erosion of epithelial features via the epithelial-to-mesenchymal transition, or EMT process. Nevertheless, according to recent studies, another model has emerged wherein the role of the aforementioned complexes in metastatic tumor cells becomes important. As per these studies, cells of metastatic breast cancer are able to sustain epithelial cytoskel-etal expression as well as adhesion genes, including P-cadherin/E-cadherin/K14, etc. [14, 17]. Plakoglobin knockdown led to cancerous cells' disaggregation and had their efficiency compromised in the formation of metastasis. On the other hand, K14 loss resulted in the erosion of metastasis-specific genes' larger program like CARD10 and AdamTS1 [14]. Moreover, in a mouse's tumor, improvements were made in invasive cells (K14$^+$) for genes comprising the desmosome, cell-cell adhesion complex (major epithelial), as well as the hemidesmosome. Therefore, it is possible to retain the machinery of epithelial cell adhesion in spreading cell clusters and adding to the process of metastasis. Notably, the epithelial genes' role in metastasis is known to have a context in developmental mechanisms; epithelial cells' migratory clusters are known to utilize mechanical signals via E-cadherin for the purpose of arranging their direction sensing [14]. It is necessary to conduct further studies to ascertain if clusters of cancer cell offer migratory benefits (analo-gous) during the process of metastasis. It could also be the case that improved survival is the rationale behind their better metastatic ability. The epithelial attri-butes' retention within breast cancer clusters is in line with recent studies, as per which cells of breast cancer obviate the need for EMT for achieving metastasis [19]. Even though the data lends credence to the notion of clusters (epithelial-phenotype) being capable of disseminating polyclonal metastases, other ways of metastatic spread cannot be ruled out. Human patients contain CTC clusters, which means that it is possible for the comparative frequency of epithelial-vs. mesenchymal-phenotype to alter with the progression of disease and therapeutic interventions [10].

Metastasis Originating from CTC Clusters

Cancers are known to take over stem cell mechanisms for gaining attributes of 'sternness' promulgating progression or onset of tumors. Most past studies have focused on this stemness' epigenetic/genetic regulation at either metastatic or pri-mary sites wherein CTCs' epigenetic landscapes continue to be underexplored. However, the present study offers key insights relating to the stemness of CTC clusters prone to metastasis, establishing a linkage between this trait's epigenetic regulations and CTCs' phenotypic features (Fig. 15.2). A new field of research has been opened by the revelation that altering cell to cell linkages may rewiring DNA

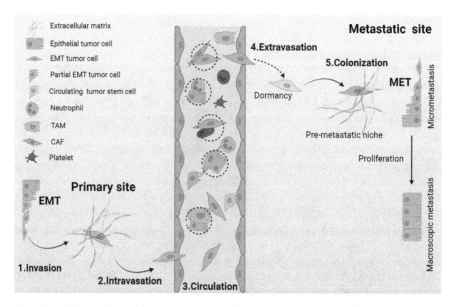

Fig. 15.2 CTCs can form clusters with various cells during metastasis. The process of metastases entails invasion of tumor cells within the primary site, intravasation, and circulation survival in the capacity of CTCs, the interplay involving blood cells, extravasation, and attachment to/from the metastatic site's colonization

methylation whilst blocking stem cell TF binding. As a case in point, it is interesting to determine the least number of cells that are capable of setting up or sustaining epigenetic attributes which promulgate stemness. Notably, it is possible for heterogeneity to be seen across CTC clusters when it comes to cell types as well as size. CTC clusters sometimes also contain other cell types, such as tumor-associated macrophages or TAM, fibroblasts, or leukocytes. Do these heterotypic cell types influence epigenetic status? Furthermore, it remains unknown whether the epigenetic states of the CTC clusters are established prior to shedding or during their journey through circulation? From a mechanistic standpoint, it is unclear if cell-to-cell clustering intervenes in the creation and sustenance of DNA methylation status in regions containing clusters. Certain embryonic stem cell TFs have also been recognized as key factors, like OCT4, which help modulate chromatin's accessibility during the reprogramming process. Hence, it remains to be seen if these TFs catalyze the creation and sustenance of their targets' DNA hypomethylation status to understand the underlying mechanisms of this dynamic regulation and offer insights into therapeutic designs. Properties of cancer stem cells are associated with epithelial mesenchymal transition (or EMT), which cancer frequently hijacks. EMT causes cell–to–cell connection loss and single CTCs that enter the realm of circulation. Stemness seems to regulate via well-defined mechanisms in clustered vs. single CTCs, underscoring the need to develop therapeutic strategies depending on the CTCs' physical state. Interestingly, the class related to cardiac glycosides, which have historically been used for heart diseases, is known to play a role in disturbing the formation of CTC clusters. Recently, benefits of both digitoxin as well as its analogs have been reported in cancer treatments, although there is less clarity on the precise mechanisms that affect cancer cells. Studies have proposed the disruption of cell signaling that gets mediated by not just signalosome but also the genes of cell cycle, but it remains to be seen if the advantages imparted by digitoxin is partially attributed to its ability to prevent cluster formation [5].

CTC Clusters

It is possible for multicellular CTC clusters to comprise tumor-specific cell-to-cell homotypic clusters and blood cell-tumor cell heterotypic clusters involving many functional benefits and mechanisms of formation. While most prior studies refer to 'homotypic CTC clusters' as the default term, recent findings on cell clusters (tumor cell–stromal) in metastasis have been summarized below.

CTC Clusters: Homotypic

Despite their relative rarity, clusters offer 100 time higher metastatic potentiality as compared to single CTCs, which makes them a very clinically pertinent population to explore [11, 14]. Breast cancer patient with at least five CTCs in a single blood draw (7.5-mL) tends to have far worse survival rates [17, 20]. Such prognostic values get even more serious among patients with higher CTC clusters [17]. Conventionally, CTC clusters refer to as tumor cells groups with at least two nuclei capable of shedding as cohesive clusters. They also take place via aggregation of cells on the basis of intravital imaging studies conducted on the formation of homotypic CTC clusters. It is possible to strengthen the mechanism of CTC by arranging cohesive engagements between the cells [15]. Given that CTC clusters have emerged as a vital biomarker to gauge the severity/progression of the disease in many kinds of cancer including lung cancer and breast cancer, it is necessary to unravel the molecular mechanisms underlying clustering [21, 22]. Among patients of breast cancer, it is possible for CD44 homophilic interactions to direct CTCs' homotypic clustering through a recently-found molecule that promotes stemness adhesion, namely, intercellular adhesion molecule 1 (ICAM1) [11, 23, 24]. According to studies typifying CTC clusters, intratumor hypoxia are capable of prompting the formation of clusters and that plakoglobin undergo overexpression in CTC clusters in comparison to single CTCs in cancer patients [15, 25]. Clustering of CTC homotypic improves important stemness genes' DNA hypomethylation, promulgating clustered cells' stemness as well as proliferation [26]. CTC cluster formation may also be promoted by the coordination of several junction/adhesion proteins. Unlike single CTCs, it is also possible for breast cancer CTC clusters to express another marker of stemness, K14. Also, in comparison to single cell CTCs, the cells that express K14 also display higher expression of desmosome and hemidesmosome as well as lower expression of MHC-II genes [14]. K14 reduction lowers cells' metastatic ability *in vivo*, which indicates adhesion involving cytoskeleton as well as a phenotype of immune evasion for cluster formation [14]. According to reports, clustering of tumor cells also induces a mitophagy mediated with hypoxia-inducible factor 1α (HIF1α) as well as hypoxic metabolic switch by clearing reactive oxygen species, or ROS. The enzyme heparanase or HPSE is another interesting candidate that can mediate clustering of homotypic CTC in breast cancer patients [27]. HPSE overexpression is known to cause CTC clustering, thus inducing aggregation predicated on ICAM-1 and FAK [28]. Several preclinical and drug trials have targeted this enzyme. This included one Phase I trial using digoxin, which supposedly suppresses CTC clusters' anoikis and catalyzes their blood stream survival, thus promulgating the formation of metastasis [2]. As per the studies related to CTC clusters' xenograft model of breast cancer, the cells end up creating tumors with lowered ACC1 and heightened BCL2 within primary tumors. This indicates that the survival-enhancing apoptosis pathway is downregulated [29].

Heterotypic CTC Clusters

According to further studies, it is possible for CTC clusters to remain heterogeneous, which implies that CTCs can form clusters with other types of cells, like WBCs. These include suppressor cells derived from myeloid/neutrophils, together with cancer-associated fibroblasts, also referred to as CAFs [30–34]. According to the CTC–WBC clusters' single-cell RNA-sequencing analysis involving breast cancer patients, the majority of these clusters are formed using neutrophils [30]. Importantly, cytoskeletal bridges emerge between tumor and other kinds of cells, which affects heterogeneous cluster formation between blood cells and CTCs with the significant upregulation of VIM/GLU/TUB among patients suffering from metastatic breast cancers [31]. Patients having the aforementioned clusters have considerably aggravated survival prognosis following six months of treatment as compared to patients who lack CTC–WBC clusters in blood at the baseline or specific time points, such as six months [16]. Transcriptomes of CTC–neutrophil clusters are found to be elevated for the progression of cell cycle in comparison to their non-neutrophil counterparts. Platelets also tend to generate aggregates involving tumor cells, offering benefits that protect tumor cells from surveillance of immunity [30, 35]. It is also possible to use satellite platelets of CTC surfaces to isolate CTC. Meanwhile, studies have found CAFs, which help promulgate invasion as well as dissemination of cancer from the primary tumor, with heterotypic CTC clusters when it comes to circulation and migration [32]. According to other studies, close interaction among immune cells helps promulgate immunity evasion and improve CTCs' seeding [36–39]. Cancer cells in these types of heterotypic clusters can utilize their hijacked partner to save/improve dissemination as well as metastatic growth.

At the same time, suppressor cells derived from myeloid are known to help CTC metastatic efficacy by promulgating the survival and proliferation of CTC through the ROS/Notch/Nodal pathway [34] as well as by emerging as a shield that safeguards CTCs from surveillance [33]. It is necessary to carry out further research on how heterotypic CTC clusters function to explicate the benefits imparted to the progression of metastatic. While the technology has advanced in uncovering CTC clustering's molecular drivers, there is a lot more than is yet to be discovered owing to the possibility of many aspects linked to clustering. Molecules affecting clustering tend to differ across cancers. To illustrate, it is possible to define CTC clusters by TTF1 as well as CD56, which had been neglected in standard CTC analysis methodologies depending on EpCAM for the purpose of identification [40].

Box 15.1 Epigenetic Landscape of CTCs

The majority of research has been on the genetic and epigenetic control of the stemness of tumor cells at the original or metastatic sites, whereas the epigenetic settings of CTCs have received little attention. With the help of a relationship between the phenotypic characteristics of CTCs and the epigenetic control of this property, this study offers fascinating fresh perspectives on the stemness clusters of CTCs that are prone to metastasis (Fig. 15.3).

Single-cell analysis is a new toolkit for examining the molecular characteristics of cells. Low coverage plagues several single-cell epigenetic investigations today. For instance, only a small portion of all CpGs is covered by the WGBS. Despite this constraint, single-cell epigenetic investigations have increased the number of cells that are investigated with targeted inquiries, such as the instance of single versus cluster forms of CTCs, helping to reveal important biological features of cells. We anticipate that the rapid advancement of technology will significantly enhance our capacity to delve into interesting biology at the single-cell level in the near future. Due to the connections between these two epigenetic features that are known to exist, it will be fascinating to assess the involvement of histone modifications in forming and sustaining the DNA methylation states of individual CTCs and clusters [41]. CTC clusters are remarkable characteristics of tumor cells in circulation, to sum up. In a new intriguing study, stem cell factors and epigenetics, which give cells the "stemness" to promote metastasis, are linked with CTC clusters.

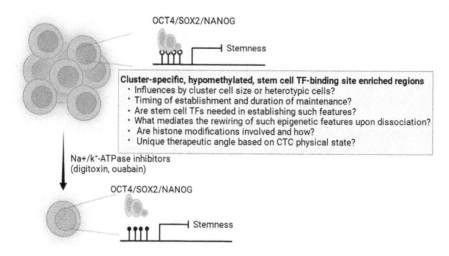

Fig. 15.3 Epigenetic regulation of stemness in circulating tumor cell (CTC) clusters and single CTCs. The authors found that the hypomethylation areas in CTC clusters are associated with embryonic stem cell transcription factor (TF) binding sites (for example, OCT4, SOX2, and NANOG), which corresponded with stemness-related transcriptional pathways and the metastatic phenotype. After Na+/K+-ATPase inhibitors were used to break up CTC clusters into individual CTCs, the hypomethylated areas unique to the cluster underwent methylation and decreased TF accessibility, which suppressed the stemness phenotype

CTC Clusters' Plasticity and Stemness

Plasticity of CTCs

For metastasis to successfully complete, it is important for tumor cell plasticity to change in line with the constantly evolving microenvironment by going through a plethora of reversible alterations when it comes to differentiation status and cellular fate. The cascade of metastasis includes sequence-wise cancer cell detachment steps from the primary tumor, intravasation to the vasculature/surrounding tissue, extravasation, as well as circulation to both distant organs, not to mention secondary colonization [5]. All steps are accompanied by several genetic as well as epigenetic changes in tumor cells regulating myriad processes that include but are not confined to stemness programming based on DNA methylation, EMT during the nascent phases of metastasis, as well as the reverse MET at the final phases that catalyze the progression of cancer [42, 43]. While we have observed spatiotemporal EMT in tumor cells that migrate [43–45], as well as intravasate accompanied by gain of cell motility and loss of cell junctions, MET entails the acquisition of markers of epithelial adhesion such as E-cadherin and EpCAM so that CTCs can colonize [44, 46]. For this reason, dynamic MET/EMT conversions form part of the plastic features to be accompanied or acquired by metastatic tumor cells. Many transcription factors that regulate EMT, including Zeb1, Snail, and Sox9 act in coordination to boost the state of plasticity and stemness in breast cancer [45, 47, 48]. Nevertheless, when clustered cells having enhanced proteins of connective junction shed into broken/leaky vasculature, the need for EMT might diminish.

CTCs' presence involving spatiotemporal mesenchymal attributes has been seen in various carcinomas types and is linked to worsened clinical outcomes and resistance to treatment [10, 49–51]. As per other studies, CTCs that have a mixed epithelial–mesenchymal phenotype are linked to decreased survival rates in patients with metastatic breast cancer and prostate cancer [51, 52]. Such CTCs' relevance is attested to by studies involving mice which demonstrated that cancer cells arrested in mesenchymal states can enter circulation but cannot form distant metastases. Notably, this ability is only acquired after reacquiring epithelial traits via the MET [45, 53–55]. For this reason, it is important to understand the evaluation of CTCs with a mixed epithelial–mesenchymal phenotype for comprehending the underlying process of not only metastatic dissemination but also the progression of tumor in cancer patients. Having said that, the majority of CTC-focused studies place the emphasis solely on epithelial markers, thus leading to underestimating CTCs' prevalence comprising a mixed phenotype. Two studies examining mesenchymal/ epithelial features in CTCs among lung cancer patients showed that CTCs comprising a mixed phenotype signified the peak subpopulation (47%) as compared to those that only express mesenchymal (30%) or epithelial (23%) markers [56, 57]. While these findings were observed in very few patients, it is postulated that this kind of CTC could be more relevant than it was thought to be due to its higher frequency. At the same time, the role of CTC clustering as well as extraneous immune microenvironmental impact in signaling cascades for cycling tumor cells and reprograming DNA methylation must be recognized [26, 30]. The regulation of tumor growth and the accompanying malignancy takes place at level of cell–cell interactions, tissue organization, and extracellular matrix–cell interactions. Extracellular glucose finds out the phenotype of malignant tumor through O-GlcNAc/ EPAC/RAP1 pathways [47, 58]. Several microenvironmental factors modulating stemness/tumor cell plasticity, including iron metabolism, acidic conditions, as well as glucose restriction, could also play a vital role in regulating CTC plasticity [59].

CTC Clusters: Stemness

Metastasizing tumor cells necessitate malignant stem cells' regenerative attributes, which encompasses the ability of potential differentiation, self-renewal, as well as tumorigenicity colonization. Therefore, breast cancer's clinical outcomes can be partly attributed to cancer stem cells' subpopulations, whose plasticity augments recurrence of heterogeneous tumor, metastasis as well as therapeutic resistance. Given that CTCs are required to sustain a certain quantity of plasticity to metastasize and higher metastatic capacity is promulgated by CTC clusters as compared to their single cell counterparts, it is important to ascertain whether CTC clusters regulate or promulgate the requisite signatures of stemness. CTC clustering exhibited a heightened expression of cell adhesion markers related to stemness, including ICAM1/ CD44, in comparison to single CTCs in the blood samples of patients [3, 10,

24]. These findings that indicate elevated plasticity within CTC clusters are congruent with studies which suggest tumor cells associated with a plastic phenotype are more efficacious in generating metastasis when compared with cells impeded in an epithelial state [45, 53–55].

The marker of breast cancer stem cell, CD44, contributes to more than three-fourths of lung metastasis of breast cancer as well as cluster formation (CTC). Notably, CD44 is known to promulgate via its homophilic engagements, thus strengthening stemness pathways through OCT4 and PAK2/FAK signaling. This indicates that CD44 crosstalk within CTC clusters enhances the probability of this cluster surviving during the process of metastasis. Nevertheless, the fact that around 20 percent of CTC clusters as well as 60 percent of single CTCs stain negative for CD44, indicating that CD44-independent mechanisms could also play a role in CTC clustering and plasticity among patients of breast cancer [3]. As per recent studies, ICAM1 is another stemness marker mediating breast CTC clustering as well as tumor cell adhesion to endothelial cells for spreading across to distant organs [3]. Signaling mediated by ICAM1 promulgates self-renewal by upregulating cell cycle kinases [24]. At the same time, within primary tumors, CAFs are known to augment the generation of cell hybrid clusters (CAF–tumor) during migration of tumor cells, which feature hybrid epithelial/mesenchymal or extremely epithelial protein signatures within tumor cells [60]. Previously, CTC clustering and plasticity were examined in a standalone manner, but it is now necessary to comprehend their possible additive and intersecting features of vital receptors mediating the processes [5, 61].

Crosstalk: Interactions of CTCs with Immune and Stromal Cells in Local *Onco-sphere*

Upon entering and undergoing changes in bloodstream, most CTCs face challenging shear stress or end up dying from anoikis, which is a mechanism of cell death caused by cell attachment loss [62, 63]. CTCs could closely interact with neutrophils/platelets/macrophages, as well as myeloid-derived suppressor cells (or MDSCs) to increase survival rates evading the immunity system [64, 65]. According to recent studies, CTCs need to engage with adverse blood microenvironment to facilitate adhesion with tumor metastasis and tissue invasion (Fig. 15.4). We will discuss each CTC interactions, depicted as clusters, with these cells in the section below.

CTCs-Neutrophils Clusters

Neutrophils are the most abundant leukocytes in human body. Recent studies have examined neutrophils to support the progression of cancer [66]. In many cancer types, increased circulation of neutrophils is linked to insufficient prognosis

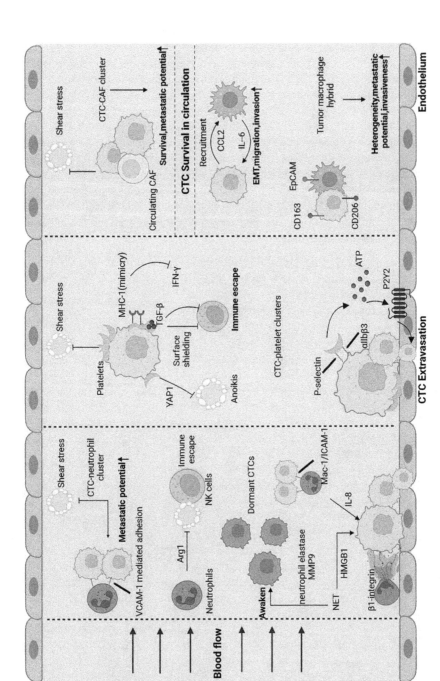

Fig. 15.4 CTC clusters in the blood microenvironment, and their interaction with various immune cells, namely, neutrophils, platelets, CAFs, and TAMs

[67–69]. Previously, the formation of white blood cells clusters was found in the bloodstream [70]. There was a significant correlation between CTCs and neutrophils in both mouse models and in breast cancer patients. A greater potential of metastasis was displayed with higher gene expression involving cell cycle progression when compared with only CTCs [30]. The findings are congruent with prior studies that showed neutrophils' proliferation role within tumor cells. The cell-to-cell junction mediates neutrophil binding and CTC and necessitates the molecule of vascular cell adhesion. Moreover, it is possible for neutrophils to directly comply with CTCs via the interaction between Mac-1 and ICAM-1, thereby promulgating liver metastasis as well as extravasation [71]. Therefore, neutrophils-CTCs clusters end up anchoring to vascular endothelium with regard to extravasation whilst combating shear stress. Many cell adhesion proteins, like integrin, cadherin, as well as glycoprotein of surface mediate the process [72–74]. Neutrophil-induced IL-8 was important to sequestrate neutrophil with the arrested cells of tumor as well as for adjacent tumor cells' extravasation behaviours [75].

Box 15.2 Metastasis Can Also Be Indirectly Induced by Neutrophil-Derived NETs

Neutrophil extracellular traps (or NETs) refer to structures that look like web. They are created by proteins as well as DNA–histone complexes expelled from activated neutrophils, and are capable of impacting CTC biology. According to several studies, NETs successfully captured CTCs in circulating, thus promulgating dissemination of metastasis [76, 77]. In the view of in vitro experiments, β1-integrin mediates CTC's adhesion to neutrophil extracellular traps on cancer cells as well as NET. However, after the administration of DNAse I, this impact was abrogated [77]. The formation of NET expelled high-mobility group Box 15.1 in a surgical stress-based murine model, thus activating TLR9-mediated pathways and expediting liver metastases progression [78]. Furthermore, NETs are capable of promoting metastasis and awakening dormant cancer cell. A recent study showed that a couple of NET-linked proteases concentrate around laminin, promoted its cleavage through the generation of an epitope inducing dormant cancer cell via the activation of integrin activation and FAK/ERK/MLCK/YAP signaling [79]. Tumor-expressed proteins like protease cathepsin lends support to breast cancer's lung metastasis by promulgating the formation of NET in metastatic niches [80]. Coiled-coil domain that comprises a protein expressed on the membrane of cancer cells, namely, Coiled-coil domain-containing protein 25 (CCDC25), is capable of acting as a particular sensor for NETs, thereby inducing tumor cell adhesion and migration [81]. At the same time, NET formation can cause circulating neutrophils to allow CTCs to evade immunity-related surveillance via the suppression of peripheral leukocytes, natural killer cells' function, effector T cells' the antitumor response, and coordination with other immune cells [82–85]. In general, evidence does exist for neutrophils' pro-metastatic role in their CTC interaction, but more details need to be explicated in the future.

CTCs-TAM Clusters

Apart from contributing to metastatic progression in primary tumors, TAMs also promulgate eventual metastasis phases such as CTCs dissemination as well as extravasation [86]. Hamilton et al. attempted to examine the interaction of CTC-macrophage via co-culturing of blood mononuclear cells (peripheral) with the involvement of CTC cell lines derived from patients of lung cancer. According to their findings, CTCs successfully induced monocyte differentiation to TAMs, thereby secreting myriad mediators like MMP9, osteopontin, platelet factor, and chitinase-3-like-1 for promulgating subsequent recruitment, invasion, and migration of leukocytes [87]. A study involving colorectal cancer patients showed that it is necessary to provide the feedback loop between cancer cells and TAMs for the intravasation of the EMT programs of CTCs in the blood. TAM-derived IL6 regulates invasiveness via the STAT3/miR-506-3p/FoxQ1 pathway, thereby increasing tumor cells' CCL2 expression for the purpose of recruiting macrophages [88]. Apparently, TAMs promulgate CTCs' mechanical adhesiveness as well as endurance, which helps them in creating safeguarding cell clusters and resisting the shear stress [89]. The interaction between tumor cells and macrophages could be a possible way of immune invasion/evasion. It was found that macrophage-tumor cell hybrids had both M2-like macrophage phenotypes as well as EpCAM [90, 91]. In addition, they were isolated from the blood of patients suffering from multiple forms of cancer such as melanoma, ovarian, colorectal, and breast [91–93]. Gast et al. conducted a study where they found that fusion hybrids are capable of increasing tumor metastatic behavior and heterogeneity, drawing further correlations with the stage of disease and overall survival rates [94]. At the same time, a linkage was drawn between bigger hybrid sizes and poorer survival rates among cell lung (non-small) cancer patients [95]. Deciphering the mechanism of molecular fusion between macrophages CTC assumes importance to identify therapeutic targets.

CTCs-Platelets Clusters

Cancer progression and metastasis are significantly influenced by platelets' recruitment and activation, thereby facilitating the survival and outgrowth of CTCs across secondary sites [96, 97]. It is also possible for platelets to bind from aggregates with CTCs, with the latter catalyzing aggregation formation via tissue factor expressing or the release of prothrombotic as well as procoagulant micro particles [98, 99]. TGF-β and other mediators released from the platelet speed up the process of EMT in CTCs and end up promulgating metastasis and invasion [100, 101]. In a recent study, it was observed that the heat shock protein's HSP47 expression got activated during EMT, thereby boosting cancer cell–platelet interaction via the secretion of collagen in breast cancer cells [102]. According to prior studies, platelets not only safeguard

CTCs against mechanical stress but also resist anoikis, with the YAP1 pathway activation mediating the latter [103]. Moreover, platelets help CTCs evade from the attack of NK cells via several mechanisms, such as (a) platelet aggregates imparting surface protection to safeguard NK cells' cytolysis impact; (b) normal MHC-I 9 derived from platelets transferred to the tumor cell surface, thereby stymieing the identification of NK cells [104]; (c) downregulation of NKG2D within NK cells by TGF-β and shedding of NKG2D ligands (mediated by platelets), thereby resulting in impeded antitumor cytotoxicity; and (d)TNF-related ligand (induced by glucocorticoid and derived by platelets), thus activating GITR within NK cells and lowering their cytotoxicity levels [105, 106]. At the same time, platelets as well as NK cells are also capable of affecting neutrophils and modulating their immunity. Apart from protecting CTCs in a patient's blood, platelets also help impart adhesion to endothelial cells. Platelet adhesion receptors like integrin αIIbβ3 and P-selectin mediate the attachment of CTCs as well as platelets [107–109], thus imparting support to CTCs' firm adherence with the endothelial wall. In addition, platelets activated by tumor cells expel ATP from dense granules, thereby leading to the endothelial P2Y2 receptor activation and allowing tumor cells' transendothelial migration via heightened permeability [110]. According to a study, the interactions between integrin α6β1 and MMP-9 with their respective receptors, is important to catalyze the cancer cells' extravasation process [111]. Platelets are also capable of enhancing vascular permeability for catalyzing extravasation of tumor cells. According to a preclinical study on lung metastasis, a GPCR, namely tumor cell-associated CD97, is capable of initiating platelet activation and causing granule secretion. This includes the release of ATP as well as lysophosphatidic acid. In a similar manner, a study showed that the interaction between receptor glycoprotein VI as well as its ligand galectin-3 on breast/colon cancer cells promulgated ATP secretion and platelet activation [112]. Consequently, these platelet secretions regulate vascular permeability by favoring the tumor metastasis process.

CTCs-MDSCs Clusters

As a heterogeneous subset belonging to myeloid cells, MDSCs are defined by immunosuppressive properties which promulgate the dissemination of metastasis. Utilizing a standard protocol used to isolate human MDSCs, it was observed in their study that in most types of cancer barring melanoma, there was a significant expansion of polymorphonuclear (PMN)-MDSC in comparison to inflammation and infection [113]. CTC-MDSC clusters escape the T cell response's immune surveillance [33]. Also, a lower circulating MDSCs was linked to a rise in activated OX40⁺PD-1⁻ T cells among patients suffering from large B-cell lymphoma [114]. Correspondingly, in another study, Sprouse et al. showed that CTCs' *in vitro* co-culture obtained from breast cancer patients and melanoma PMN-MDSCs increased the activation of Notch within CTCs via a direct interplay among Jagged1 expressed upon MDSCs as well as the Notch1 receptor whose expression took place on CTCs. Notably, the heightened generation of ROS might upregulate the expression of Notch1 receptor and promulgate the proliferation of CTC [34]. It is still necessary to determine the mechanisms that underlie these CTC-MDSC interactions.

CTCs-CAFs Clusters

CAFs represent one of the most frequently found components in the local *onco-sphere*. Their role assumes great significance in initiating, metastasis and angiogenesis of tumor as well as drug resistance [115]. By remodeling the ECM, CAFs help tumor cells permeate the stroma and interact with cancer cells via the secretion of growth factors, cytokines, as well as chemokines [116]. Nevertheless, there is lack of clarity on how CTCs interact with CAFs. A study showed that in mouse models of lung cancer metastasis, CTCs might transfer CAFs to the metastatic site from the primary tumor [117]. CAFs play a direct role in boosting the survival rates of tumor cells and boosting metastasis formation. At the same time, the depletion of CAFs from lungs causes a substantial reduction in macroscopic metastasis and increase mice survival rate. Furthermore, during the process of dissemination, CAFs are capable of safeguarding CTCs from the fluid shear forces [118]. In a 3D co-culture model, CAFs induced shear resistance for prostrating tumor cells via stable intercellular contact and soluble factors, including CCL2/ CXCL5/CCL7 linked to cell invasion/EMT. Apart from the experimental models, the circulation of CAFs was observed in the peripheral blood sample of metastatic breast cancer patients. However, this was not seen among patients during the nascent stages [119]. Moreover, when a new acoustic microstreaming platform was used for isolation, excellent precision was shown in metastatic diagnosis [120, 121].

Conclusion

CTCs are the key components of cluster metastasis. It is now accepted that cancer cells do not travel alone, and the concept of cluster metastasis is widely accepted. However, the cluster also made the CTCs stronger, and the interactions that these CTC clusters had in the local *onco-sphere* does affect the metastasis process and the environment in the distal *onco-sphere*. The inter-onco-spherical crosstalk with the host factors also represents a major bottleneck of CTC-based therapy. Indeed, CTCs will be a crucial component of "Precision medicine" in the future; however, detailed phenotypic, genotypic, and functional characterization must be done to provide clear indication of metastasis-related therapeutic intervention.

References

1. Aceto N, Bardia A, Miyamoto DT, Donaldson MC, Wittner BS, Spencer JA et al (2014) Circulating tumor cell clusters are oligoclonal precursors of breast cancer metastasis. Cell 158(5):1110–1122
2. Aceto N, Toner M, Maheswaran S, Haber DA (2015) En route to metastasis: circulating tumor cell clusters and epithelial-to-mesenchymal transition. Trends Cancer 1(1):44–52
3. Liu X, Taftaf R, Kawaguchi M, Chang YF, Chen W, Entenberg D et al (2019) Homophilic CD44 interactions mediate tumor cell aggregation and polyclonal metastasis in patient-derived breast cancer models. Cancer Discov 9(1):96–113
4. Massague J, Obenauf AC (2016) Metastatic colonization by circulating tumour cells. Nature 529(7586):298–306
5. Schuster E, Taftaf R, Reduzzi C, Albert MK, Romero-Calvo I, Liu H (2021) Better together: circulating tumor cell clustering in metastatic cancer. Trends Cancer 7(11):1020–1032
6. Zeidman I, Buss J (1952) Transpulmonary passage of tumor cell emboli. Cancer Res 12(10): 731–733
7. Cheung KJ, Ewald AJ (2016) A collective route to metastasis: Seeding by tumor cell clusters. Science 352(6282):167–169
8. Liotta L, Saidel M, Kleinerman J (1976) The significance of hematogenous tumor cell clumps in the metastatic process. Cancer Res 36(3):889–894
9. Hou J, Krebs M, Lancashire L, Sloane R, Backen A, Swain R et al (2012) Clinical significance and molecular characteristics of circulating tumor cells and circulating tumor microemboli in patients with small-cell lung cancer. J Clin Oncol 30(5):525–532
10. Yu M, Bardia A, Wittner B, Stott S, Smas M, Ting D et al (2013) Circulating breast tumor cells exhibit dynamic changes in epithelial and mesenchymal composition. Science 339(6119): 580–584
11. Gundem G, Van Loo P, Kremeyer B, Alexandrov L, Tubio J, Papaemmanuil E et al (2015) The evolutionary history of lethal metastatic prostate cancer. Nature 520(7547):353–357
12. Tabassum D, Polyak K (2015) Tumorigenesis: it takes a village. Nat Rev Cancer 15(8): 473–483
13. Maddipati R, Stanger B (2015) Pancreatic cancer metastases harbor evidence of polyclonality. Cancer Discov 5(10):1086–1097
14. Cheung K, Padmanaban V, Silvestri V, Schipper K, Cohen J, Fairchild A et al (2016) Polyclonal breast cancer metastases arise from collective dissemination of keratin 14-expressing tumor cell clusters. Proc Natl Acad Sci U S A 113(7):E854–E863
15. Yu M (2019) Metastasis stemming from circulating tumor cell clusters. Trends Cell Biol 29(4): 275–276
16. Bronsert P, Enderle-Ammour K, Bader M, Timme S, Kuehs M, Csanadi A et al (2014) Cancer cell invasion and EMT marker expression: a three-dimensional study of the human cancer-host interface. J Pathol 234(3):410–422
17. Cheung K, Gabrielson E, Werb Z, Ewald A (2013) Collective invasion in breast cancer requires a conserved basal epithelial program. Cell 155(7):1639–1651
18. Lawson D, Bhakta N, Kessenbrock K, Prummel K, Yu Y, Takai K et al (2015) Single-cell analysis reveals a stem-cell program in human metastatic breast cancer cells. Nature 526(7571):131–135
19. Cai D, Chen S, Prasad M, He L, Wang X, Choesmel-Cadamuro V et al (2014) Mechanical feedback through E-cadherin promotes direction sensing during collective cell migration. Cell 157(5):1146–1159
20. Cristofanilli M, Budd G, Ellis M, Stopeck A, Matera J, Miller M et al (2004) Circulating tumor cells, disease progression, and survival in metastatic breast cancer. N Engl J Med 351(8): 781–791

21. Murlidhar V, Reddy R, Fouladdel S, Zhao L, Ishikawa M, Grabauskiene S et al (2017) Poor prognosis indicated by venous circulating tumor cell clusters in early-stage lung cancers. Cancer Res 77(18):5194–5206
22. Paoletti C, Li Y, Muñiz M, Kidwell K, Aung K, Thomas D et al (2015) Significance of circulating tumor cells in metastatic triple-negative breast cancer patients within a randomized, Phase II trial: TBCRC 019. Clin Cancer Res 21(12):2771–2779
23. Liu X, Adorno-Cruz V, Chang Y, Jia Y, Kawaguchi M, Dashzeveg N et al (2021) EGFR inhibition blocks cancer stem cell clustering and lung metastasis of triple negative breast cancer. Theranostics 11(13):6632–6643
24. Taftaf R, Liu X, Singh S, Jia Y, Dashzeveg N, Hoffmann A et al (2021) ICAM1 initiates CTC cluster formation and trans-endothelial migration in lung metastasis of breast cancer. Nat Commun 12(1):4867
25. Donato C, Kunz L, Castro-Giner F, Paasinen-Sohns A, Strittmatter K, Szczerba B et al (2020) Hypoxia triggers the intravasation of clustered circulating tumor cells. Cell Rep 32(10): 108105
26. Gkountela S, Castro-Giner F, Szczerba B, Vetter M, Landin J, Scherrer R et al (2019) Circulating tumor cell clustering shapes DNA methylation to enable metastasis seeding. Cell 176:98–112.e14
27. Labuschagne C, Cheung E, Blagih J, Domart M, Vousden K (2019) Cell clustering promotes a metabolic switch that supports metastatic colonization. Cell Metab 30(4):720–34.e5
28. Wei R, Sun D, Yang H, Yan J, Zhang X, Zheng X et al (2018) CTC clusters induced by heparanase enhance breast cancer metastasis. Acta Pharmacol Sin 39(8):1326–1337
29. Thangavel H, De Angelis C, Vasaikar S, Bhat R, Jolly M, Nagi C et al (2019) A CTC-cluster-specific signature derived from OMICS analysis of patient-derived xenograft tumors predicts outcomes in basal-like breast cancer. J Clin Med 8:11
30. Szczerba B, Castro-Giner F, Vetter M, Krol I, Gkountela S, Landin J et al (2019) Neutrophils escort circulating tumour cells to enable cell cycle progression. Nature 566(7745):553–557
31. Kallergi G, Aggouraki D, Zacharopoulou N, Stournaras C, Georgoulias V, Martin S (2018) Evaluation of α-tubulin, detyrosinated α-tubulin, and vimentin in CTCs: identification of the interaction between CTCs and blood cells through cytoskeletal elements. Breast Cancer Res 20(1):67
32. Hurtado P, Martínez-Pena I, Piñeiro R (2020) Dangerous liaisons: circulating tumor cells (CTCs) and cancer-associated fibroblasts (CAFs). Cancer 12:10
33. Liu Q, Liao Q, Zhao Y (2016) Myeloid-derived suppressor cells (MDSC) facilitate distant metastasis of malignancies by shielding circulating tumor cells (CTC) from immune surveillance. Med Hypotheses 87:34–39
34. Sprouse M, Welte T, Boral D, Liu H, Yin W, Vishnoi M et al (2019) PMN-MDSCs enhance CTC metastatic properties through reciprocal interactions via ROS/notch/nodal signaling. Int J Mol Sci 20:8
35. Kanikarla-Marie P, Lam M, Sorokin A, Overman M, Kopetz S, Menter D (2018) Platelet metabolism and other targeted drugs; potential impact on immunotherapy. Front Oncol 8:107
36. Dovas A, Patsialou A, Harney A, Condeelis J, Cox D (2013) Imaging interactions between macrophages and tumour cells that are involved in metastasis in vivo and in vitro. J Microsc 251(3):261–269
37. Harney A, Arwert E, Entenberg D, Wang Y, Guo P, Qian B et al (2015) Real-time imaging reveals local, transient vascular permeability, and tumor cell intravasation stimulated by TIE2hi macrophage-derived VEGFA. Cancer Discov 5(9):932–943
38. Roh-Johnson M, Bravo-Cordero J, Patsialou A, Sharma V, Guo P, Liu H et al (2014) Macrophage contact induces RhoA GTPase signaling to trigger tumor cell intravasation. Oncogene 33(33):4203–4212
39. Wyckoff J, Wang Y, Lin E, Li J, Goswami S, Stanley E et al (2007) Direct visualization of macrophage-assisted tumor cell intravasation in mammary tumors. Cancer Res 67(6): 2649–2656

40. Messaritakis I, Stoltidis D, Kotsakis A, Dermitzaki E, Koinis F, Lagoudaki E et al (2017) TTF-1- and/or CD56-positive circulating tumor cells in patients with small cell lung cancer (SCLC). Sci Rep 7:45351
41. Vasantharajan SS, Eccles MR, Rodger EJ, Pattison S, McCall JL, Gray ES et al (2021) The epigenetic landscape of circulating tumour cells. Biochim Biophys Acta Rev Cancer 1875(2): 188514
42. Nguyen L, Pellacani D, Lefort S, Kannan N, Osako T, Makarem M et al (2015) Barcoding reveals complex clonal dynamics of de novo transformed human mammary cells. Nature 528(7581):267–271
43. Teeuwssen M, Fodde R (2019) Cell heterogeneity and phenotypic plasticity in metastasis formation: the case of colon cancer. Cancer 11:9
44. Luo M, Brooks M, Wicha M (2015) Epithelial-mesenchymal plasticity of breast cancer stem cells: implications for metastasis and therapeutic resistance. Curr Pharm Des 21(10): 1301–1310
45. Tsai J, Donaher J, Murphy D, Chau S, Yang J (2012) Spatiotemporal regulation of epithelial-mesenchymal transition is essential for squamous cell carcinoma metastasis. Cancer Cell 22(6):725–736
46. Padmanaban V, Krol I, Suhail Y, Szczerba B, Aceto N, Bader J et al (2019) E-cadherin is required for metastasis in multiple models of breast cancer. Nature 573(7774):439–444
47. Dashzeveg N, Taftaf R, Ramos E, Torre-Healy L, Chumakova A, Silver D et al (2017) New advances and challenges of targeting cancer stem cells. Cancer Res 77(19):5222–5227
48. Guo W, Keckesova Z, Donaher J, Shibue T, Tischler V, Reinhardt F et al (2012) Slug and Sox9 cooperatively determine the mammary stem cell state. Cell 148(5):1015–1028
49. Satelli A, Brownlee Z, Mitra A, Meng Q, Li S (2015) Circulating tumor cell enumeration with a combination of epithelial cell adhesion molecule- and cell-surface vimentin-based methods for monitoring breast cancer therapeutic response. Clin Chem 61(1):259–266
50. Satelli A, Mitra A, Brownlee Z, Xia X, Bellister S, Overman M et al (2015) Epithelial-mesenchymal transitioned circulating tumor cells capture for detecting tumor progression. Clin Cancer Res 21(4):899–906
51. Xu L, Mao X, Guo T, Chan P, Shaw G, Hines J et al (2017) The novel association of circulating tumor cells and circulating megakaryocytes with prostate cancer prognosis. Clin Cancer Res 23(17):5112–5122
52. Bulfoni M, Gerratana L, Del Ben F, Marzinotto S, Sorrentino M, Turetta M et al (2016) In patients with metastatic breast cancer the identification of circulating tumor cells in epithelial-to-mesenchymal transition is associated with a poor prognosis. Breast Cancer Res 18(1):30
53. Tsuji T, Ibaragi S, Shima K, Hu M, Katsurano M, Sasaki A et al (2008) Epithelial-mesenchymal transition induced by growth suppressor p12CDK2-AP1 promotes tumor cell local invasion but suppresses distant colony growth. Cancer Res 68(24):10377–10386
54. Ocaña O, Córcoles R, Fabra A, Moreno-Bueno G, Acloque H, Vega S et al (2012) Metastatic colonization requires the repression of the epithelial-mesenchymal transition inducer Prrx1. Cancer Cell 22(6):709–724
55. Brabletz T (2012) EMT and MET in metastasis: where are the cancer stem cells? Cancer Cell 22(6):699–701
56. Ku S, Rosario S, Wang Y, Mu P, Seshadri M, Goodrich Z et al (2017) Rb1 and Trp53 cooperate to suppress prostate cancer lineage plasticity, metastasis, and antiandrogen resistance. Science (New York, NY) 355(6320):78–83
57. Mu P, Zhang Z, Benelli M, Karthaus W, Hoover E, Chen C et al (2017) SOX2 promotes lineage plasticity and antiandrogen resistance in TP53- and RB1-deficient prostate cancer. Science (New York, NY) 355(6320):84–88
58. Onodera Y, Nam J, Bissell M (2014) Increased sugar uptake promotes oncogenesis via EPAC/RAP1 and O-GlcNAc pathways. J Clin Invest 124(1):367–384

59. Costa C, Muinelo-Romay L, Cebey-López V, Pereira-Veiga T, Martínez-Pena I, Abreu M et al (2020) Analysis of a real-world cohort of metastatic breast cancer patients shows circulating tumor cell clusters (CTC-clusters) as predictors of patient outcomes. Cancer 12:5

60. Matsumura Y, Ito Y, Mezawa Y, Sulidan K, Daigo Y, Hiraga T et al (2019) Stromal fibroblasts induce metastatic tumor cell clusters via epithelial-mesenchymal plasticity. Life Sci Alliance 2:4

61. Keller L, Pantel K (2019) Unravelling tumour heterogeneity by single-cell profiling of circulating tumour cells. Nat Rev Cancer 19(10):553–567

62. Follain G, Herrmann D, Harlepp S, Hyenne V, Osmani N, Warren S et al (2020) Fluids and their mechanics in tumour transit: shaping metastasis. Nat Rev Cancer 20(2):107–124

63. Strilic B, Offermanns S (2017) Intravascular survival and extravasation of tumor cells. Cancer Cell 32(3):282–293

64. Rejniak K (2016) Circulating tumor cells: when a solid tumor meets a fluid microenvironment. Adv Exp Med Biol 936:93–106

65. Garrido-Navas C, de Miguel-Perez D, Exposito-Hernandez J, Bayarri C, Amezcua V, Ortigosa A et al (2019) Cooperative and escaping mechanisms between circulating tumor cells and blood constituents. Cell 8:11

66. Shaul M, Fridlender Z (2019) Tumour-associated neutrophils in patients with cancer. Nat Rev Clin Oncol 16(10):601–620

67. Aliustaoglu M, Bilici A, Ustaalioglu B, Konya V, Gucun M, Seker M et al (2010) The effect of peripheral blood values on prognosis of patients with locally advanced gastric cancer before treatment. Med Oncol 27(4):1060–1065

68. Hu S, Zou Z, Li H, Zou G, Li Z, Xu J et al (2016) The preoperative peripheral blood monocyte count is associated with liver metastasis and overall survival in colorectal cancer patients. PLoS One 11(6):e0157486

69. Wang Y, Yao R, Zhang D, Chen R, Ren Z, Zhang L (2020) Circulating neutrophils predict poor survival for HCC and promote HCC progression through p53 and STAT3 signaling pathway. J Cancer 11(13):3736–3744

70. Stott S, Hsu C, Tsukrov D, Yu M, Miyamoto D, Waltman B et al (2010) Isolation of circulating tumor cells using a microvortex-generating herringbone-chip. Proc Natl Acad Sci U S A 107(43):18392–18397

71. Spicer J, McDonald B, Cools-Lartigue J, Chow S, Giannias B, Kubes P et al (2012) Neutrophils promote liver metastasis via Mac-1-mediated interactions with circulating tumor cells. Cancer Res 72(16):3919–3927

72. Strell C, Lang K, Niggemann B, Zaenker K, Entschladen F (2007) Surface molecules regulating rolling and adhesion to endothelium of neutrophil granulocytes and MDA-MB-468 breast carcinoma cells and their interaction. Cell Mol Life Sci 64(24):3306–3316

73. Huh S, Liang S, Sharma A, Dong C, Robertson G (2010) Transiently entrapped circulating tumor cells interact with neutrophils to facilitate lung metastasis development. Cancer Res 70(14):6071–6082

74. Rowson-Hodel A, Wald J, Hatakeyama J, O'Neal W, Stonebraker J, VanderVorst K et al (2018) Membrane mucin Muc4 promotes blood cell association with tumor cells and mediates efficient metastasis in a mouse model of breast cancer. Oncogene 37(2):197–207

75. Chen M, Hajal C, Benjamin D, Yu C, Azizgolshani H, Hynes R et al (2018) Inflamed neutrophils sequestered at entrapped tumor cells via chemotactic confinement promote tumor cell extravasation. Proc Natl Acad Sci U S A 115(27):7022–7027

76. Cools-Lartigue J, Spicer J, McDonald B, Gowing S, Chow S, Giannias B et al (2013) Neutrophil extracellular traps sequester circulating tumor cells and promote metastasis. J Clin Invest 123(8):3446–3458

77. Najmeh S, Cools-Lartigue J, Rayes R, Gowing S, Vourtzoumis P, Bourdeau F et al (2017) Neutrophil extracellular traps sequester circulating tumor cells via β1-integrin mediated interactions. Int J Cancer 140(10):2321–2330

78. Tohme S, Yazdani H, Al-Khafaji A, Chidi A, Loughran P, Mowen K et al (2016) Neutrophil extracellular traps promote the development and progression of liver metastases after surgical stress. Cancer Res 76(6):1367–1380
79. Albrengues J, Shields M, Ng D, Park C, Ambrico A, Poindexter M et al (2018) Neutrophil extracellular traps produced during inflammation awaken dormant cancer cells in mice. Science 361:6409
80. Xiao Y, Cong M, Li J, He D, Wu Q, Tian P et al (2021) Cathepsin C promotes breast cancer lung metastasis by modulating neutrophil infiltration and neutrophil extracellular trap formation. Cancer Cell 39(3):423–437
81. Xu Y, Jiang Q, Liu H, Xiao X, Yang D, Saw PE et al (2020) DHX37 impacts prognosis of hepatocellular carcinoma and lung adenocarcinoma through immune infiltration. J Immunol Res 2020:8835393
82. Zhang J, Qiao X, Shi H, Han X, Liu W, Tian X et al (2016) Circulating tumor-associated neutrophils (cTAN) contribute to circulating tumor cell survival by suppressing peripheral leukocyte activation. Tumour Biol 37(4):5397–5404
83. Spiegel A, Brooks M, Houshyar S, Reinhardt F, Ardolino M, Fessler E et al (2016) Neutrophils suppress intraluminal NK cell-mediated tumor cell clearance and enhance extravasation of disseminated carcinoma cells. Cancer Discov 6(6):630–649
84. Kumagai Y, Ohzawa H, Miyato H, Horie H, Hosoya Y, Lefor A et al (2020) Surgical stress increases circulating low-density neutrophils which may promote tumor recurrence. J Surg Res 246:52–61
85. Coffelt S, Kersten K, Doornebal C, Weiden J, Vrijland K, Hau C et al (2015) IL-17-producing γδ T cells and neutrophils conspire to promote breast cancer metastasis. Nature 522(7556): 345–348
86. Doak G, Schwertfeger K, Wood D (2018) Distant relations: macrophage functions in the metastatic niche. Trends Cancer 4(6):445–459
87. Hamilton G, Rath B (2017) Circulating tumor cell interactions with macrophages: implications for biology and treatment. Transl Lung Cancer Res 6(4):418–430
88. Wei C, Yang C, Wang S, Shi D, Zhang C, Lin X et al (2019) Crosstalk between cancer cells and tumor associated macrophages is required for mesenchymal circulating tumor cell-mediated colorectal cancer metastasis. Mol Cancer 18(1):64
89. Osmulski P, Cunsolo A, Chen M, Qian Y, Lin C, Hung C et al (2021) Contacts with macrophages promote an aggressive nanomechanical phenotype of circulating tumor cells in prostate cancer. Cancer Res 81(15):4110–4123
90. Shabo I, Midtbö K, Andersson H, Åkerlund E, Olsson H, Wegman P et al (2015) Macrophage traits in cancer cells are induced by macrophage-cancer cell fusion and cannot be explained by cellular interaction. BMC Cancer 15:922
91. Clawson G, Matters G, Xin P, Imamura-Kawasawa Y, Du Z, Thiboutot D et al (2015) Macrophage-tumor cell fusions from peripheral blood of melanoma patients. PLoS One 10(8):e0134320
92. Clawson G, Matters G, Xin P, McGovern C, Wafula E, dePamphilis C et al (2017) "Stealth dissemination" of macrophage-tumor cell fusions cultured from blood of patients with pancreatic ductal adenocarcinoma. PLoS One 12(9):e0184451
93. Manjunath Y, Porciani D, Mitchem J, Suvilesh K, Avella D, Kimchi E et al (2020) Tumor-cell-macrophage fusion cells as liquid biomarkers and tumor enhancers in cancer. Int J Mol Sci 21: 5
94. Gast C, Silk A, Zarour L, Riegler L, Burkhart J, Gustafson K et al (2018) Cell fusion potentiates tumor heterogeneity and reveals circulating hybrid cells that correlate with stage and survival. Sci Adv 4(9):7828
95. Manjunath Y, Mitchem J, Suvilesh K, Avella D, Kimchi E, Staveley-O'Carroll K et al (2020) Circulating giant tumor-macrophage fusion cells are independent prognosticators in patients with NSCLC. J Thorac Oncol 15(9):1460–1471

96. Schlesinger M (2018) Role of platelets and platelet receptors in cancer metastasis. J Hematol Oncol 11(1):125
97. Gaertner F, Massberg S (2019) Patrolling the vascular borders: platelets in immunity to infection and cancer. Nat Rev Immunol 19(12):747–760
98. Thomas G, Brill A, Mezouar S, Crescence L, Gallant M, Dubois C et al (2015) Tissue factor expressed by circulating cancer cell-derived microparticles drastically increases the incidence of deep vein thrombosis in mice. J Thromb Haemost 13(7):1310–1319
99. Stark K, Schubert I, Joshi U, Kilani B, Hoseinpour P, Thakur M et al (2018) Distinct pathogenesis of pancreatic cancer microvesicle-associated venous thrombosis identifies new antithrombotic targets in vivo. Arterioscler Thromb Vasc Biol 38(4):772–786
100. Labelle M, Begum S, Hynes R (2011) Direct signaling between platelets and cancer cells induces an epithelial-mesenchymal-like transition and promotes metastasis. Cancer Cell 20(5): 576–590
101. Guo Y, Cui W, Pei Y, Xu D (2019) Platelets promote invasion and induce epithelial to mesenchymal transition in ovarian cancer cells by TGF-β signaling pathway. Gynecol Oncol 153(3):639–650
102. Xiong G, Chen J, Zhang G, Wang S, Kawasaki K, Zhu J et al (2020) Hsp47 promotes cancer metastasis by enhancing collagen-dependent cancer cell-platelet interaction. Proc Natl Acad Sci U S A 117(7):3748–3758
103. Haemmerle M, Taylor M, Gutschner T, Pradeep S, Cho M, Sheng J et al (2017) Platelets reduce anoikis and promote metastasis by activating YAP1 signaling. Nat Commun 8(1):310
104. Nieswandt B, Hafner M, Echtenacher B, Männel D (1999) Lysis of tumor cells by natural killer cells in mice is impeded by platelets. Cancer Res 59(6):1295–1300
105. Kopp H, Placke T, Salih H (2009) Platelet-derived transforming growth factor-beta down-regulates NKG2D thereby inhibiting natural killer cell antitumor reactivity. Cancer Res 69(19):7775–7783
106. Maurer S, Kropp K, Klein G, Steinle A, Haen S, Walz J et al (2018) Platelet-mediated shedding of NKG2D ligands impairs NK cell immune-surveillance of tumor cells. Onco Targets Ther 7(2):e1364827
107. Bendas G, Borsig L (2012) Cancer cell adhesion and metastasis: selectins, integrins, and the inhibitory potential of heparins. Int J Cell Biol 2012:676731
108. Lonsdorf A, Krämer B, Fahrleitner M, Schönberger T, Gnerlich S, Ring S et al (2012) Engagement of αIIbβ3 (GPIIb/IIIa) with αvβ3 integrin mediates interaction of melanoma cells with platelets: a connection to hematogenous metastasis. J Biol Chem 287(3):2168–2178
109. Coupland L, Chong B, Parish C (2012) Platelets and P-selectin control tumor cell metastasis in an organ-specific manner and independently of NK cells. Cancer Res 72(18):4662–4671
110. Schumacher D, Strilic B, Sivaraj K, Wettschureck N, Offermanns S (2013) Platelet-derived nucleotides promote tumor-cell transendothelial migration and metastasis via P2Y2 receptor. Cancer Cell 24(1):130–137
111. Jantscheff P, Schlesinger M, Fritzsche J, Taylor L, Graeser R, Kirfel G et al (2011) Lysophosphatidylcholine pretreatment reduces VLA-4 and P-Selectin-mediated b16.f10 melanoma cell adhesion in vitro and inhibits metastasis-like lung invasion in vivo. Mol Cancer Ther 10(1):186–197
112. Mammadova-Bach E, Gil-Pulido J, Sarukhanyan E, Burkard P, Shityakov S, Schonhart C et al (2020) Platelet glycoprotein VI promotes metastasis through interaction with cancer cell-derived galectin-3. Blood 135(14):1146–1160
113. Cassetta L, Bruderek K, Skrzeczynska-Mocznik J, Osiecka O, Hu X, Rundgren I et al (2020) Differential expansion of circulating human MDSC subsets in patients with cancer, infection and inflammation. J Immunother Cancer 8:2
114. Jiménez-Cortegana C, Palazón-Carrión N, Martin Garcia-Sancho A, Nogales-Fernandez E, Carnicero-González F, Ríos-Herranz E et al (2021) Circulating myeloid-derived suppressor cells and regulatory T cells as immunological biomarkers in refractory/relapsed diffuse large

B-cell lymphoma: translational results from the R2-GDP-GOTEL trial. J Immunother Cancer 9:6

115. Chen X, Song E (2019) Turning foes to friends: targeting cancer-associated fibroblasts. Nat Rev Drug Discov 18(2):99–115

116. Gaggioli C, Hooper S, Hidalgo-Carcedo C, Grosse R, Marshall J, Harrington K et al (2007) Fibroblast-led collective invasion of carcinoma cells with differing roles for RhoGTPases in leading and following cells. Nat Cell Biol 9(12):1392–1400

117. Duda D, Duyverman A, Kohno M, Snuderl M, Steller E, Fukumura D et al (2010) Malignant cells facilitate lung metastasis by bringing their own soil. Proc Natl Acad Sci U S A 107(50): 21677–21682

118. Ortiz-Otero N, Clinch A, Hope J, Wang W, Reinhart-King C, King M (2020) Cancer associated fibroblasts confer shear resistance to circulating tumor cells during prostate cancer metastatic progression. Oncotarget 11(12):1037–1050

119. Ao Z, Shah S, Machlin L, Parajuli R, Miller P, Rawal S et al (2015) Identification of cancer-associated fibroblasts in circulating blood from patients with metastatic breast cancer. Cancer Res 75(22):4681–4687

120. Jiang R, Agrawal S, Aghaamoo M, Parajuli R, Agrawal A, Lee A (2021) Rapid isolation of circulating cancer associated fibroblasts by acoustic microstreaming for assessing metastatic propensity of breast cancer patients. Lab Chip 21(5):875–887

121. Lin D, Shen L, Luo M, Zhang K, Li J, Yang Q et al (2021) Circulating tumor cells: biology and clinical significance. Signal Transduct Target Ther 6(1):404

Chapter 16
Distal *Onco-sphere:* Organotrophic Metastasis

Phei Er Saw and Erwei Song

Abstract In order for CTCs to find a suitable soil for its growth, CTCs need to assess the distal onco-sphere for suitability in terms of secreted factors, inflammation, and metabolic changes in the new environment. In this chapter, we discuss on the interesting fact that the tumor cells secrete various factors to create a different distal onco-sphere, leading to predisposition of CTCs to metastasize specifically towards certain organs. We also discuss how to host builds in its protective defense mechanism to counter these organotrophic metastasis events.

Introduction

In the previous chapter, we looked at the early progenitor cells in metastasis: the CTC clusters in starting cell evasion into new distal *onco-spheres*. In reality, metastasis occurs in an orderly pattern across remote organs, which is referred to as "organotropism" or "organ-specific metastasis." Various types and subtypes of tumors exhibit unique organotropisms. Prostate cancer, for instance, preferentially

P. E. Saw
Guangdong Provincial Key Laboratory of Malignant Tumor Epigenetics and Gene Regulation, Guangdong-Hong Kong Joint Laboratory for RNA Medicine, Medical Research Center, Sun Yat-sen Memorial Hospital, Sun Yat-sen University, Guangzhou, China

Nanhai Translational Innovation Center of Precision Immunology, Sun Yat-sen Memorial Hospital, Sun Yat-sen University, Foshan, China

E. Song (✉)
Guangdong Provincial Key Laboratory of Malignant Tumor Epigenetics and Gene Regulation, Guangdong-Hong Kong Joint Laboratory for RNA Medicine, Medical Research Center, Sun Yat-sen Memorial Hospital, Sun Yat-sen University, Guangzhou, China

Nanhai Translational Innovation Center of Precision Immunology, Sun Yat-sen Memorial Hospital, Sun Yat-sen University, Foshan, China

Breast Tumor Center, Sun Yat-sen Memorial Hospital, Sun Yat-sen University, Guangzhou, China
e-mail: songew@mail.sysu.edu.cn

relapses in bone, whereas colonization of uveal melanoma often occurs in the liver [1]. Breast cancer can spread to a variety of places, such as the bone, lung, liver, and brain. Conversely, the luminal subtype is more likely to metastasize to the bone, while triple-negative breast cancer (TNBC) metastases favor visceral body parts [2, 3]. In this chapter, we depict common causes and mechanism of organ-specific distal *onco-spheres* including circulation flow, interactions with tumor-inherent components, and how they communicate with the systemic *onco-sphere* (the host) to influence organotropism [4].

Changes in Local *Onco-sphere* During Organ-Specific Colonization: Genetic Adaption of Tumor Cells

Metastasis is a grueling process for cell survival. After their entrenchment in a capillary, CTCs can either die, extravasate into the organ parenchyma, or spread to produce emboli (cluster of cells) that can break the walls of the capillaries [5]. The successful metastasis window is only less than 72 h, as shown in animal models, where the maximum number of CTCs that penetrate remote organs is significantly reduced within a few days [6–8]. These data show that only a tiny percentage of malignant cells have characteristics that deliberate metastatic colonization capability. However, an interesting investigation indicated, through genome sequencing, that no alterations was found specific to metastatic cells (CTCs) as compared to tumor cells in the local *onco-sphere* [9, 10]. However, clonal predominance for pre-existent mutations identified in primary tumors (i.e., point mutation in RASG13D or BRAFG464V) was observed to be enhanced in metastatic models, which may illustrate the reason for the higher fitness and longevity of metastatic cells in certain organs [11]. Using a metastatic breast cancer model, specific genetic profiles in tumor cells with an improved propensity to infiltrate diverse organs have been found [12–15]. Other organotrophic metastatic gene profiles were identified using the same type of methods [16–18]. CTC viability and motility in the vasculature is affected throughout its journey, including capillary adherence, extravasation, and the migration of stromal elements that might induce organ-specific colonization are all enhanced by genes having these characteristics. Various gene profiles seen in metastatic cells coincide with the colonization obstacles observed in each environment. For instance, effective metastatic bone invasion is ameliorated by proteins (IL11, OPN, CTGF, and FGF5) that enable interactions with stromal elements of the bone milieu to boost bone colonization [13], while genes infused with lung and brain metastasis markers facilitate extravasation or crossing the BBB [12, 14]. The enhancement of genes facilitating oxidative stress and metabolism, such as ALDH1L2, MTHFD1, and CKB, is evident in the liver, which is home to metabolic stress as a prominent component [16, 17]. Surprisingly, several of these organotrophic gene synthesis profiles are shared by cancers of various histology. Like lung-residing breast tumor cells, increased synthesis of SPARC, VCAM1, and

ANGPTL4 in metastatic hepatocellular cancer cells was noticed in lung metastasis [19], implying an identical genetic system guiding metastatic seeding to target organs irrespective of the source of tumor [2].

Metastatic Enhancing Properties of Distal *Onco-spheres*

Secreted Factors

Metastasis growth in diverse organs is also dependent on widespread modifications to physiological circumstances that render some tissues more favorable to metastatic implantation. Secretions like cytokines, growth factors, and extracellular vesicles are frequently engaged in the regulation of such modifications [20, 21]. An initial study to show the systemic organotrophic consequences of tumor-released compounds exposed the diversion of lung cancer cells because of predisposed media from B16 melanoma cells toward melanoma-specific metastatic sites like the spleen, intestine, kidney, and oviduct, that rarely endure metastasis of lung cancer cells [22]. This discovery indicated the contribution of primary tumor components, maybe through a premetastatic niche creation in certain organs, to metastatic tropism. Rather, VEGFA and PlGF released by tumors have been demonstrated to facilitate direct mobilization of cells originated from the bone marrow, including hematopoietic progenitor cells, and matured myeloid cells [22–25] that permit particular organs to create metastatic niches. These juvenile myeloid cells provide a responsive ground for metastatic colonization by rearranging the vascular system and ECM constituents in the local *onco-sphere*. Primary tumor-released cytokines and exosomes have frequently been reported to modify the production of adhesion molecules in stromal components (i.e., fibronectin) in remote distal *onco-sphere*s to increase metastatic tropism, as fibronectin can assist in attracting VLA-4-producing cells [22, 26].

As mentioned in the previous chapter, exosomes are capable of direct contribution to tumor niche development along with substantially affecting immunological reactions, hematopoietic mobilization, and TME reconfiguration [27–30]. Exosome expression of $\alpha6\beta4$ and $\alpha6\beta1$ was correlated to lung metastasis, whereas $\alpha v\beta5$ enhances liver metastasis. Primary tumor exosomes can also transfer c-MET and other substances to the BM via activation and mobilization of stromal cells, causing a modification of metastatic settings [31]. Delivery of TGF-β boosts myofibroblasts activation, and enables the exosomes to modify the PMNs [26, 32]. Exosomes are generated by primary renal cancer cells enhance angiogenesis in the lungs during metastasis [33].

Hypoxia and Inflammation

Primary tumor hypoxia and increased inflammation are critical elements of metastatic niche transformation [34]. The significance of chronic inflammation in tumor metastasis has already been proved and reviewed extensively [35–37]. Th crosstalk between hypoxia and inflammation can be seen when hypoxic tumors induce the secretion of inflammatory mediators that create metastatic niches in the lung and bone. In breast cancer, hypoxia activates the translocation of CD11b[+] myeloid cells from the BM to the lung. In the lung, these CD11b[+] myeloid cells then directly suppress the effects of the anti-tumoral properties of NK cells to promote metastatic cascade [38]. Additionally, hypoxia stimulates the production and built-up of lysyl oxidase (LOX)in lung tissues. LOX fuses with COL4 (collagen IV) proteins in the basal epithelial membranes to generate a viable PMN [39]. Similarly, the adherence of CD11b/Gr1[+] myeloid cells to these fibers in the ECM is coupled with the recruitment of additional BM cells that remodel the distal *onco-sphere* [40].

Organ-Specific Niches

In many cancers, metastasis attacks the lungs most, which may be partly attribut* to the lungs' inflammatory tendency in which cytokines and stromal ce* in particular, the allergy-induction model explains the increased lung me* asis as a consequence of severe inflammation [41]. Likewise, the lungs can suffer from severe inflammation due to bacterial infection, which initiates the occurrence of melanoma and cancer cells in lung, prostate, and colorectal areas via the ubiquitin–CXCR4 axis [42]. Widespread inflammation promotes breast cancer metastasis to spread to the bones and lungs in arthritic mice models [43]. Bones possess numerous highly responsive DTC zones [44, 45]. Unique sub-niches inside the BM are characterized by an abundance of growth factors and cytokines, including CXCL12 and IGF1 that promote DTC spawning and viability [46]. Metastatic prostate cells especially prefer the hematopoietic stem cell niche, overtaking normal hematopoietic stem cells for niche occupancy [47], but breast cancer cells may easily infiltrate the osteogenic niche for effective expansion [48]. Furthermore, inflammatory TGF-β signaling triggers the production of bone-specific genes related to metastasis (i.e., PTHLH, Jagged1, and SPHK1) in tumor cells [49–51]. Significantly, the formation of metastatic lesions in bone causes bone degradation, which in turn produces enormous quantities of TGF-β immersed in the bone matrix that can nurture tumor cells and boost their propensity to spread to bones [52]. As strongly shown by these results, inflammatory cytokines are capable of increasing metastatic spread and survivability in certain organs [53, 54], thus exemplifying the significance of systemic elements in forming multiple organ-specific metastatic niches.

Metabolic Adaptation

When tumor cells enter new habitats [55], they usually face adverse metabolic circumstances such as high amounts of reactive oxygen radicals [56]. Certain tumor cells could regulate their redox signaling to counteract the adverse reactions caused by adverse metabolites. In this way, the cell loves longer and therefore improves metastatic longevity in this organ. Some of the detoxifying enzymes that could be produced by the tumor cells are ALDH1L2 and MTHFD1, both belonging to the folate system. These overexpression of two enzymes have been demonstrated to boost organ-specific metastasis, while simultaneously enhance the viability of cancer cells [17]. For acclimatizing to hazardous conditions, many additional kinds of tumor cells may upregulate certain isoforms of ALDH [57]. For example, ALDH1A3 is overexpressed in human cholangiocarcinoma cells, and their overexpression directly affects cancer prognosis and promoted gemcitabine resistance and influences metastasis [58]. Metastatic cells should find alternative energy sources to fulfil the metabolic needs for existence and development apart from preventing apoptosis in the unfamiliar surroundings of a remote organ. The availability or lack of an exact mix of nutrients and growth agents in distinct tissues will substantially influence the probability of metastasis to certain organs.

Aerobic glycolysis is the predominant source of energy generation for maximum parent tumors, and as DTCs infiltrate external organs, they must embrace alternative energy acquisition strategies, the most prominent being: autophagy, fatty-acid metabolism, peroxide signaling, and mitochondrial oxidative phosphorylation. Detailed review of these pathways is highlighted in References [59–62]. Interruption of the routine glucose absorption cycle is observed in the case of tumor cells' detachment from ECM and extravasate into the blood vessels. The stimulation of metabolic processes engaged in oxidative phosphorylation and peroxide signaling makes up for this [62]. Invasion-prone cancer cells, for instance, enhance PGC1-α transcriptional activity to promote mitochondrial oxygen usage during lung infiltration [59]. Tumor cells may also adopt a latent form in foreign surroundings by activating autophagy channels to satisfy the metabolic needs for dormancy [60]. Metastatic breast cancer cells can come out of the latency phase and resume development in the brain by embracing energy scavenging systems from multiple substrates and channels, such as glycolysis and the tricarboxylic acid cycle, and oxidative phosphorylation [63, 64].

The brain and lungs, on average, offer large quantities of glucose and oxygen [65], whereas the liver contains modest levels of both. Being similar in metabolic pathway, tumor cells derived from original tumors with high aerobic glycolysis will tend to colonize the brain or lungs more easily, while tumor cells residing in the liver must participate in glycolysis to survive. HIF1α-mediated stimulation of PDK1-governed glycolysis is a process that enables breast cancer cells to infiltrate the liver easily [66]. Similarly, colon cancer cells metastasizing to the liver serve as energy scavengers due to the downregulation of miR-483 and miR-551, which enhances CKB (creatine kinase) production and results in extracellular phosphocreatine synthesis from creatine and ATP [16]. Subsequently, tumor cells absorb phosphocreatine to meet their metabolic energy demands. Conversely, the spreading of ovarian cancer cells into abdominal fat regions enables them to metabolize fatty acids generated by adipocytes via FABP4 absorption [61]. Thus, organotropism is considerably influenced by metastatic adaption to various metabolic settings.

Changes in Different Host Distal *Onco-sphere* to Influence Metastatic Colonization

The physiological role of many organs is frequently dependent on unique resident stromal cells, thus making it obvious that stromal cells play critical roles in the genesis of organotrophic metastasis [21, 67, 68]. Herein, we will focus on each distal *onco-sphere* and understand how each distal *onco-sphere* of the host could be strategically modified in favor for the metastasis cascade.

Bone

The functioning of a specifically rich stromal milieu, comprising hematopoietic cells, mesenchymal cells, and resident tissue-specific cells, like osteoclasts and osteoblasts, involved in bone upkeeping, renders bone a considerably recurrent location of metastasis [45, 69]. Secretions of the bone marrow, such as OPN, RANKL, IGF1, and CXCL12, act as a chemotactic origin of recruitment of metastatic cells from primary tumors, which then interact with many stromal groups to foster invasion, sustenance, and expansion [69]. Most prominently, metastatic cells interact with osteoclasts and osteoblasts, causing bone resorption and deterioration, which produces cytokines and feeds back to the metastatic cells, promoting development in a feedback mechanism known as the vicious spiral [70]. Bone metastasis can be classified as osteoblastic, osteolytic, or a combination of these two based on diagnostic characteristics that represent a lack of equilibrium in bone homeostasis [69]. FGF, IGF, VEGF, endothelin-1, and other cytokines activate osteoblasts released by tumor cells, promoting osteoblastic metastasis, which is frequently linked with prostate cancer [71]. The osteolytic lesions often seen in breast and lung malignancies exhibit bone destruction caused due to hyperactive osteoclast [69]. RANKL could be secreted by two pathways: (1) direct secretion by metastatic cells, or (2) indirect secretion by osteoclasts. Regardless of the pathways, this is a result of stimulation by tumor-released PTHLH (parathyroid hormone-like hormone) and IL6, which in turn, boosts osteoclast production and bone degradation [69, 72]. On the other hand, VCAM1 production in CTCs can increase osteoclastogenesis by adhering to integrin $\alpha4\beta1$ on osteoclast progenitor cells, facilitating their migration and maturity [73]. Additionally, increased Jagged-1 transcription in tumor cells activates bone stromal cells via Notch signaling, thus encouraging the development of osteoclasts that release tumor-promoting growth agents, including CTGF and IL-6 [49]. Enhanced SRC–kinase stimulation of AKT assists BM-based DTCs in resisting TRAIL-regulated necrosis because of inherent immune cells [74]. CD4[+] T cells, MDSCs, Tregs, and DCs are among the multiple cells that promote bone metastases. Interestingly, rather than promoting an anticancer immune response, tumor-prone CD4[+] T cells establish a premetastatic niche in the bone by triggering abnormal bone restructuring by releasing RANKL [75]. Prostaglandin E2 released by breast carcinoma cells attracts Tregs that enhance bone

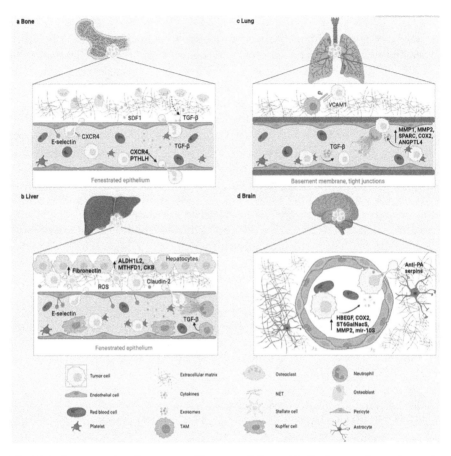

Fig. 16.1 Communications in organotrophic metastasis in specific distal *onco-spheres*. As seen in figure (**a–d**), each organ represents a distinct morphology and different molecular cues that could enhance metastasis potential of cancer cells

metastasis, possibly by effectively building a metastatic bone niche [76]. Similarly, recruitment of MDSCs and Tregs by plasmacytoid DCs to breast tumors causes inhibition of anticancer immune function and promotion of bone metastasis by blocking CD8$^+$ T cell cytotoxicity [77], emphasizing the relevance of immune escape for metastatic tropism (Fig. 16.1).

Liver

Because of the mass prevalence of inherent immune cells, specifically NK cells, in the liver, immunological–stromal interplay, and immune elusion are significant characteristics of liver metastasis. TRAIL is abundantly produced on NK cells in the liver and plays an essential part in the inhibition of tumor metastasis by triggering apoptosis in TRAIL receptive tumor cells [78]. It has been demonstrated that melanoma cells escape immunological response in the liver by releasing FcγRIIb, which prevents B cell identification at the functional level [79]. TGF-β is one of the key players in metastasis enhancement in the liver. In colorectal cancer, tumor-cell secreted TGF-β stimulates stromal fibroblast to synthesize IL-11, which in turn increases STAT3 production to enhance tumor cell viability [80]. Exosomes generated by pancreatic cancer can also trigger liver stromal cells to increase TGF-β secretion, increasing fibronectin transcription on hepatic stellate cells, and enhances macrophage migration, all of which contribute to liver metastasis [81]. TAMs also play a key role in liver tropism by shielding CTCs in the circulatory system and at organ infiltration locations of sinusoids from the immune response. The latest evidence has also discovered a myeloid cell subset (CD11b/Gr1^{mid}) that is driven to the liver by CCL2 to promote colorectal cancer cell metastasis [82].

The retention of CTCs can also be boosted by neutrophils via metastatic propagation in the liver. This trapping is dependent on tumor cell-released CXCL8; this increases αM integrin production in neutrophils, which then interact with ICAM1 on the cancer cells. Tumor cells are constantly interacting with neutrophil through the αM–ICAM1 interplay, and this communication has been demonstrated to be required for lung cancer cells to establish metastases in hepatic sinusoids by enhancing CTC adherence and invasion [83]. It has lately been demonstrated that neutrophils may produce NETs, which supports cancer cell invasion in the liver and lung by enticing CTCs [84]. The functional significance of neutrophils in metastasis remains debated, as neutrophil reduction might, in reality, enhance sporadic breast cancer spread [85]. This indicates the anticancer efficacy of neutrophils in certain settings, and it makes perfect sense that the pro-metastatic neutrophil phenotype is mediated by particular tumor microenvironment stimuli that shift their polarity from N1 to N2 neutrophils [18] (Fig. 16.1b).

Lung

In the lung, CD11b$^+$/Gr1$^+$ MDSCs enhance metastasis by suppression of antitumor effector T and NK cells and blockade of IFN-γ synthesis [86]. MDSCs provide a conducive environment for CTCs by changing the production of binding proteins on resident stromal cells via inflammatory cytokine synthesis and modification of the ECM and vasculature via MMP9 transcription [87]. Similarly, stimulation of S1PR1/STAT3 signaling in MDSCs by melanoma cells is critical for the recruitment and activation of myeloid cells in the premetastatic lung [23]. A substantial role is played by TAMs and monocytes in lung tropism. Both cells are activated in the lungs by tissue factor-assisted thrombosis is a key stage in the establishment of a PMN [88]. CD11b$^+$/LY6C$^+$ monocytes transported to the lung as a consequence of CCL2 increase melanoma metastasis [89], and their elimination by a Ly6G-based antibody inhibits spread and budding [90]. Normally, the breakdown of CSF1 leads to the genetic removal of macrophages which limits the lung metastasis to a considerable extent [91], whereas COX2 inhibitors limit breast cancer lung metastasis via reduction of VEGFA and MMP9 production in TAMs [92]. The significant role of Tregs in the enhancement of lung tropism has also been revealed by reducing the constancy of NK and T cells and anticancer instances. In an in vitro breast cancer model, lung stroma mediated CCL22 production could transfer Tregs to the lung to suppress their immune functions in this metastasis site [93]. Furthermore, tumor cell-derived Galectin 1 governs the Treg polarity and their metastatic potential in the lung [94]. Decreasing the amount of $CD4^+/CD25^+$ Tregs in the original tumor [95], hindering their advancement to the lungs by obstructing TNFα signaling [96], and inactivating immunosuppressive Treg-released agents like β-GBP and TGF-β [93, 97] have all been shown to impede lung metastasis in a significant manner, as evidenced in many solid tumors. Additional stromal components, such as neutrophils, platelets, and fibroblasts, tend to increase lung tropism. Promotion of metastatic initiation in the lungs by neutrophils due to secretion of leukotrienes, in turn, enhances vascular penetrability and extravasation [98], whereas shielding of circulatory CTCs by platelets triggers EMT and engage innate immune cells such as macrophages and granulocytes, to extravasate [88, 99–102]. Fibroblasts could induce and deposit periostin, which promotes Wnt and Notch signaling in CTCs to enhance lung metastasis [103] (Fig. 16.1c).

Brain

The highest degree of therapeutic damage can be reflected by the occurrence of brain metastasis in the majority of cancer patients. This can be attributed to the non-susceptibility of multiple parts of the brain to surgical intervention, as well as the BBB's resistance to several chemotherapies and specialized medications. The interplay between the brain's metastatic cells and stromal cells is also crucial in metastatic spawning. In fact, astrocytes have special features that particularly inhibit metastasis by impeding extravasation, survivability, and expansion. The secretion of plasminogen stimulator by astrocytes in the brain breaks down L1CAM and inhibits extravasation and colonization by preventing metastatic adherence and dissemination on the basal layer of brain capillaries [104]. Furthermore, the synthesis of plasminogen stimulator by astrocytes leads to the breakdown of the active proapoptotic FasL to destroy invading metastatic cells [104]. To avoid astrocyte-governed cell death, metastatic cells release anti-PA serpins, which inhibit the formation of the apoptotic version of FasL, shielding them from outright destruction. Surprisingly, astrocytes also demonstrate the potential to induce metastasis via changes in stromal signals. Tumor cells lack PTEN transcription, especially after spreading to the brain and not to other body parts [105]. PTEN depletion is caused by exosomal microRNAs that target PTEN and are released by resident brain astrocytes. Moreover, PTEN deficiency causes metastatic cells to produce more CCL2, which attracts $IBA1^+$ myeloid cells, thus promoting metastatic development.

Additional stromal interactions in the brain increase the extravasation, survivability, and shielding of metastatic cells from chemotherapeutic interventions. Cathepsin S production in the brain milieu by breast tumor cells as well as macrophages has been demonstrated to facilitate BBB trans-motility and metastatic brain tropism [106]. Indeed, metastatic cells can also choose stromal Notch signals transmitted by astrocytes, which can be degraded by metastatic cells to survive in the brain [107]. Chemotherapeutic tolerance is a characteristic of metastasis in numerous organ locations. Breast tumor and astrocyte interplay in the brain stimulates astrocytes to synthesize endothelin, whose receptors are expressed on cancer cells, and it evidently shields metastatic cells from apoptosis due to chemotherapy [108]. The generation of endothelin was dependent on IL-6 and IL-8 signals produced by metastatic cells, and the shielding impact was also reliant on endothelial cell signals of the brain (Fig. 16.1d).

Host Built-in Protective Defence Mechanism to Counter Organotrophic Metastasis

Host Vasculature

CTCs often follow specific blood flow pathways while disseminating from the source organ to remote tissues, where they get spatially confined in capillary vessels or adhere to endothelial binding proteins. The spread of CTCs may improve the trapping of tumor cells via biochemical or mechanical pathways [109]. Most organs' venous blood flows back toward the lungs, which may partially justify the reason behind the lungs being such a prevalent location of distant metastasis. Similarly, blood from the gastrointestinal system (including stomach, intestines, and colons) initially flushes into the liver, which is typically the primary site of metastasis in gastrointestinal cancers, prevalently, colon cancers [110]. Nevertheless, blood flow rhythm and capillary trapping themselves cannot account for all clinical manifestations of metastatic organotropism. An interesting fact is that most of the major organs (namely, liver, kidneys, and brain) received similar volume of blood flow. However, when it comes to metastatic capacity, the trend as follows are seen: (1) liver has a significantly greater metastatic spawning capacity, (2) the brain has intermediate potency, and (3) the spleen is a comparatively rare destination of metastasis [111]. The design of blood vessel walls and the shape of ECs vary between organs, and these factors can impact the feasibility and probability of CTCs extravasation and colonization [55]. Another important factor is that the sinusoid capillaries of both the liver and bone marrow are fenestrated and contain a fragmented covering of ECs that gives higher permeability in comparison to blood vessels of the lung, where the latter organ has a tighter connections between ECs and basement membrane, rendering transendothelial migration problematic [112]. Disruption of these endothelial synapses via the activities of SPARC, ANGPTL4, and cANGPTL4 enables breast tumor and melanoma cells to promote lung extravasation that leads to enhanced leakage from the blood vessels [113–115]. Over-synthesis of additional agents by metastatic cells governing lung extravasation takes into consideration epiregulin, COX2, MMP1, and MMP2, all of which accelerate breakdown and penetration through the ECM and vascular network [116].

The Blood-Brain Barrier (BBB)

The BBB is the most difficult barrier to penetrate. The original design of the BBB is to protect the brain from lethal infection of viruses, bacteria, and drugs, that could have irreversible effect on the host. Therefore, BBB is a brain-specific barrier to vascular extravasation and provides a unique obstacle for metastatic colonization. To strengthen vessel walls, astrocytes and pericytes create a defensive web surrounding capillaries [112]. Nonetheless, brain metastasis is somehow common in breast cancer and lung cancer. Taking breast cancer as an example, a whooping 15–24% of metastasis occurs in the brain [117], indicating possible changes induced specifically by these tumor cells that changes the BBB structure in the host systemic *onco-sphere* (the vasculature). Mechanistically, tumor cells can penetrate this obstacle by increasing the production of various cytokines, chemokines, biologics, and other stromal-degrading components, such as COX2, MMP2, miR-105, and ST6GalNac5, all of which enhance vascular penetrability in the brain [12, 118, 119]. Lately, Heregulin adherence of HER2–HER3 dimerization on breast tumor cells was demonstrated to boost in vitro degradation of MMPs to enhance transcytosis, proposing a putative alternative method for crossing the BBB in vivo which is characterized by the synthesis of Heregulin in the brain stroma [120].

Regulation of ECs ECM Composition

The composition of ECM is crucial in the local *onco-sphere* as they are vital in the tumor growth process, stimulating a favorable environment for the cancer cell surroundings. In metastasis, however, the degradation, modulation and re-organization of the ECM is equally important. The existence of binding proteins vary by organ surroundings, which may lead to metastatic tropism. For example, the synthesis of E-selectin by endothelial cells in bone marrow has been exemplified to enhance CTC binding and metastasis to the bone [121], along with stimulation of E-selectin production by inflammatory cytokines in the liver, similar to the production of TNFα by tumor-recruited macrophages and Kupffer cells that augments cell binding and liver metastasis [122, 123]. Synthesis of various reserves of binding proteins can be observed in different organs to boost metastatic initiation; for example, N-cadherin [124] and ICAM1 [125], which elevate TEM concentrations, although the involvement of multiple adhesive molecules in the infiltration of target organs is yet ambiguous, similar to the receptors to the CTC ligands, which vary according to the type of cancer [55] (Fig. 16.2).

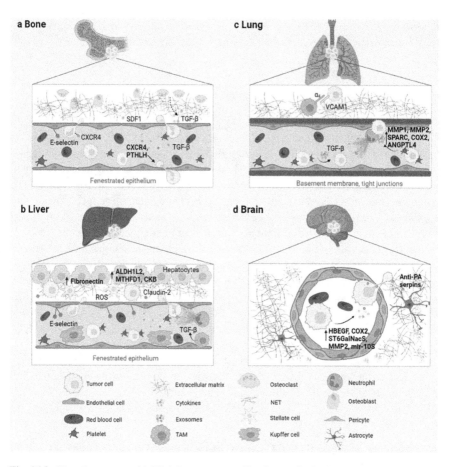

Fig. 16.2 Vascular structure highlighting organ-specific changes in the host systemic vasculature that could obstruct extravasation and metastatic growth. The main barriers to metastatic colonization different organs are presented in a-d specifically. Blood vessels in the bone and liver are made up of a perforated epithelial layer with no intact connections between endothelial cells, allowing for simple colonization; conversely, the lung and brain contain strong endothelial synapses and the basal lamina, making these organs highly resistant to extravasation. Furthermore, astrocytes and pericytes create podia encasing the blood capillaries in the brain, causing the development of the BBB, which obstructs metastasis increasingly. Immune surveillance greatly impairs successful metastatic colonization in every organ, and metastatic cells in the liver must evolve molecular pathways to withstand increased quantities of harmful metabolites. The genes and tumor-released factors involved in organ-specific extravasation and survivability are depicted. Elevated concentrations of ROS and other harmful metabolites in the liver prevent metastatic colonization, and exosomes produced by primary tumor increase stellate cell fibronectin overexpression, which improves CTC adherence. Similarly, Claudin-2 produced by tumor cells serves as an adhesive compound for binding tumor cells with liver stellate cells. Inflammatory cytokines in the liver release E-selectin; for instance, tumor-recruited macrophages and Kupffer cells secrete TNF-α, which promotes adherence and liver metastasis. Neutrophils in the liver and lungs form NETs that entrap CTCs for augmented growth. Furthermore, MMPs and other compounds released by tumor cells gratify ECM to disintegrate and extravasate into the parenchyma. CTCs are also protected in the circulatory pathway and at extravasation sites in the lungs as they interact with TAMs and platelets. Upregulation of multiple factors in the brain, including proteases that break down endothelial intersections along with the ECM and proteins that block astrocyte-produced plasminogen stimulators, is accomplished for traversing the BBB

Conclusion

In this chapter, we understand the molecular changes that was initiated by tumor cells in the local *onco-sphere*, or while searching for a specific distal *onco-sphere*, are crucial for choosing specific sites for metastasis. The host distal *onco-spheres* (*i.e.,* brain, lung, bone, and liver) are major organs for the tumor cell to metastasize. We also saw how the host, under a normal circumstance, would try to protect themselves from being invaded by tumor cells. However, maintaining homeostasis is not easy when tumors have acquired proliferative and metastatic potentials. Therefore, understanding the close connection and constant inter-communication between these local and distal *onco-spheres* will help us dictate better and more effective metastasis-targeting drugs in the near future.

References

1. Nguyen DX, Bos PD, Massagué J (2009) Metastasis: from dissemination to organ-specific colonization. Nat Rev Cancer 9(4):274–284
2. Chen W, Hoffmann AD, Liu H, Liu X (2018) Organotropism: new insights into molecular mechanisms of breast cancer metastasis. NPJ Precis Oncol 2(1):4
3. Wu Q, Li J, Zhu S, Wu J, Chen C, Liu Q et al (2017) Breast cancer subtypes predict the preferential site of distant metastases: a SEER based study. Oncotarget 8(17):27990–27996
4. Gao Y, Bado I, Wang H, Zhang W, Rosen JM, Zhang XH (2019) Metastasis organotropism: redefining the congenial soil. Dev Cell 49(3):375–391
5. Al-Mehdi AB, Tozawa K, Fisher AB, Shientag L, Lee A, Muschel RJ (2000) Intravascular origin of metastasis from the proliferation of endothelium-attached tumor cells: a new model for metastasis. Nat Med 6(1):100–102
6. Fidler IJ (1970) Metastasis: quantitative analysis of distribution and fate of tumor emboli labeled with 125I-5-Iodo-2′-deoxyuridine23. JNCI 45(4):773–782
7. Luzzi KJ, MacDonald IC, Schmidt EE, Kerkvliet N, Morris VL, Chambers AF et al (1998) Multistep nature of metastatic inefficiency: dormancy of solitary cells after successful extravasation and limited survival of early micrometastases. Am J Pathol 153(3):865–873
8. Minn AJ, Kang Y, Serganova I, Gupta GP, Giri DD, Doubrovin M et al (2005) Distinct organ-specific metastatic potential of individual breast cancer cells and primary tumors. J Clin Invest 115(1):44–55
9. Bozic I, Antal T, Ohtsuki H, Carter H, Kim D, Chen S et al (2010) Accumulation of driver and passenger mutations during tumor progression. Proc Natl Acad Sci U S A 107(43): 18545–18550
10. Campbell PJ, Yachida S, Mudie LJ, Stephens PJ, Pleasance ED, Stebbings LA et al (2010) The patterns and dynamics of genomic instability in metastatic pancreatic cancer. Nature 467(7319):1109–1113
11. Jacob LS, Vanharanta S, Obenauf AC, Pirun M, Viale A, Socci ND et al (2015) Metastatic competence can emerge with selection of preexisting oncogenic alleles without a need of new mutations. Cancer Res 75(18):3713–3719
12. Bos PD, Zhang XH, Nadal C, Shu W, Gomis RR, Nguyen DX et al (2009) Genes that mediate breast cancer metastasis to the brain. Nature 459(7249):1005–1009
13. Kang Y, Siegel PM, Shu W, Drobnjak M, Kakonen SM, Cordón-Cardo C et al (2003) A multigenic program mediating breast cancer metastasis to bone. Cancer Cell 3(6):537–549

14. Minn AJ, Gupta GP, Siegel PM, Bos PD, Shu W, Giri DD et al (2005) Genes that mediate breast cancer metastasis to lung. Nature 436(7050):518–524
15. Nguyen DX, Massagué J (2007) Genetic determinants of cancer metastasis. Nat Rev Genet 8(5):341–352
16. Loo JM, Scherl A, Nguyen A, Man FY, Weinberg E, Zeng Z et al (2015) Extracellular metabolic energetics can promote cancer progression. Cell 160(3):393–406
17. Piskounova E, Agathocleous M, Murphy MM, Hu Z, Huddlestun SE, Zhao Z et al (2015) Oxidative stress inhibits distant metastasis by human melanoma cells. Nature 527(7577): 186–191
18. Tabariès S, Dupuy F, Dong Z, Monast A, Annis MG, Spicer J et al (2012) Claudin-2 promotes breast cancer liver metastasis by facilitating tumor cell interactions with hepatocytes. Mol Cell Biol 32(15):2979–2991
19. Wan J, Wen D, Dong L, Tang J, Liu D, Liu Y et al (2015) Establishment of monoclonal HCC cell lines with organ site-specific tropisms. BMC Cancer 15:678
20. Peinado H, Lavotshkin S, Lyden D (2011) The secreted factors responsible for pre-metastatic niche formation: old sayings and new thoughts. Semin Cancer Biol 21(2):139–146
21. Quail DF, Joyce JA (2013) Microenvironmental regulation of tumor progression and metastasis. Nat Med 19(11):1423–1437
22. Kaplan RN, Riba RD, Zacharoulis S, Bramley AH, Vincent L, Costa C et al (2005) VEGFR1-positive haematopoietic bone marrow progenitors initiate the pre-metastatic niche. Nature 438(7069):820–827
23. Deng J, Liu Y, Lee H, Herrmann A, Zhang W, Zhang C et al (2012) S1PR1-STAT3 signaling is crucial for myeloid cell colonization at future metastatic sites. Cancer Cell 21(5):642–654
24. Hiratsuka S, Watanabe A, Aburatani H, Maru Y (2006) Tumour-mediated upregulation of chemoattractants and recruitment of myeloid cells predetermines lung metastasis. Nat Cell Biol 8(12):1369–1375
25. Hiratsuka S, Watanabe A, Sakurai Y, Akashi-Takamura S, Ishibashi S, Miyake K et al (2008) The S100A8-serum amyloid A3-TLR4 paracrine cascade establishes a pre-metastatic phase. Nat Cell Biol 10(11):1349–1355
26. Webber J, Steadman R, Mason MD, Tabi Z, Clayton A (2010) Cancer exosomes trigger fibroblast to myofibroblast differentiation. Cancer Res 70(23):9621–9630
27. Janowska-Wieczorek A, Majka M, Kijowski J, Baj-Krzyworzeka M, Reca R, Turner AR et al (2001) Platelet-derived microparticles bind to hematopoietic stem/progenitor cells and enhance their engraftment. Blood 98(10):3143–3149
28. Janowska-Wieczorek A, Wysoczynski M, Kijowski J, Marquez-Curtis L, Machalinski B, Ratajczak J et al (2005) Microvesicles derived from activated platelets induce metastasis and angiogenesis in lung cancer. Int J Cancer 113(5):752–760
29. Liu Y, Xiang X, Zhuang X, Zhang S, Liu C, Cheng Z et al (2010) Contribution of MyD88 to the tumor exosome-mediated induction of myeloid derived suppressor cells. Am J Pathol 176(5):2490–2499
30. Xiang X, Poliakov A, Liu C, Liu Y, Deng ZB, Wang J et al (2009) Induction of myeloid-derived suppressor cells by tumor exosomes. Int J Cancer 124(11):2621–2633
31. Peinado H, Alečković M, Lavotshkin S, Matei I, Costa-Silva B, Moreno-Bueno G et al (2012) Melanoma exosomes educate bone marrow progenitor cells toward a pro-metastatic phenotype through MET. Nat Med 18(6):883–891
32. Valenti R, Huber V, Filipazzi P, Pilla L, Sovena G, Villa A et al (2006) Human tumor-released microvesicles promote the differentiation of myeloid cells with transforming growth factor-beta-mediated suppressive activity on T lymphocytes. Cancer Res 66(18):9290–9298
33. Grange C, Tapparo M, Collino F, Vitillo L, Damasco C, Deregibus MC et al (2011) Microvesicles released from human renal cancer stem cells stimulate angiogenesis and formation of lung premetastatic niche. Cancer Res 71(15):5346–5356
34. Mantovani A, Allavena P, Sica A, Balkwill F (2008) Cancer-related inflammation. Nature 454(7203):436–444

35. Balkwill F, Mantovani A (2001) Inflammation and cancer: back to Virchow? Lancet 357(9255):539–545
36. de Visser KE, Eichten A, Coussens LM (2006) Paradoxical roles of the immune system during cancer development. Nat Rev Cancer 6(1):24–37
37. Grivennikov SI, Greten FR, Karin M (2010) Immunity, inflammation, and cancer. Cell 140(6): 883–899
38. Sceneay J, Chow MT, Chen A, Halse HM, Wong CS, Andrews DM et al (2012) Primary tumor hypoxia recruits CD11b+/Ly6Cmed/Ly6G+ immune suppressor cells and compromises NK cell cytotoxicity in the premetastatic niche. Cancer Res 72(16):3906–3911
39. Finger EC, Giaccia AJ (2010) Hypoxia, inflammation, and the tumor microenvironment in metastatic disease. Cancer Metastasis Rev 29(2):285–293
40. Cox TR, Rumney RMH, Schoof EM, Perryman L, Høye AM, Agrawal A et al (2015) The hypoxic cancer secretome induces pre-metastatic bone lesions through lysyl oxidase. Nature 522(7554):106–110
41. Taranova AG, Maldonado D, Vachon CM, Jacobsen EA, Abdala-Valencia H, McGarry MP et al (2008) Allergic pulmonary inflammation promotes the recruitment of circulating tumor cells to the lung. Cancer Res 68(20):8582–8589
42. Yan L, Cai Q, Xu Y (2013) The ubiquitin-CXCR4 axis plays an important role in acute lung infection-enhanced lung tumor metastasis. Clin Cancer Res 19(17):4706–4716
43. Roy LD, Ghosh S, Pathangey LB, Tinder TL, Gruber HE, Mukherjee P (2011) Collagen induced arthritis increases secondary metastasis in MMTV-PyV MT mouse model of mammary cancer. BMC Cancer 11:365
44. Esposito M, Kang Y (2014) Targeting tumor-stromal interactions in bone metastasis. Pharmacol Ther 141(2):222–233
45. Ren G, Esposito M, Kang Y (2015) Bone metastasis and the metastatic niche. J Mol Med 93(11):1203–1212
46. Vivanco I, Sawyers CL (2002) The phosphatidylinositol 3-Kinase–AKT pathway in human cancer. Nat Rev Cancer 2(7):489–501
47. Shiozawa Y, Pedersen EA, Havens AM, Jung Y, Mishra A, Joseph J et al (2011) Human prostate cancer metastases target the hematopoietic stem cell niche to establish footholds in mouse bone marrow. J Clin Invest 121(4):1298–1312
48. Wang H, Yu C, Gao X, Welte T, Muscarella AM, Tian L et al (2015) The osteogenic niche promotes early-stage bone colonization of disseminated breast cancer cells. Cancer Cell 27(2): 193–210
49. Sethi N, Dai X, Winter CG, Kang Y (2011) Tumor-derived JAGGED1 promotes osteolytic bone metastasis of breast cancer by engaging notch signaling in bone cells. Cancer Cell 19(2): 192–205
50. Stayrook KR, Mack JK, Cerabona D, Edwards DF, Bui HH, Niewolna M et al (2015) TGFβ-Mediated induction of SphK1 as a potential determinant in human MDA-MB-231 breast cancer cell bone metastasis. BoneKEy Rep 4:719
51. Yin JJ, Selander K, Chirgwin JM, Dallas M, Grubbs BG, Wieser R et al (1999) TGF-beta signaling blockade inhibits PTHrP secretion by breast cancer cells and bone metastases development. J Clin Invest 103(2):197–206
52. Korpal M, Kang Y (2008) The emerging role of miR-200 family of microRNAs in epithelial-mesenchymal transition and cancer metastasis. RNA Biol 5(3):115–119
53. Kim S, Takahashi H, Lin WW, Descargues P, Grivennikov S, Kim Y et al (2009) Carcinoma-produced factors activate myeloid cells through TLR2 to stimulate metastasis. Nature 457(7225):102–106
54. Schelter F, Grandl M, Seubert B, Schaten S, Hauser S, Gerg M et al (2011) Tumor cell-derived Timp-1 is necessary for maintaining metastasis-promoting Met-signaling via inhibition of Adam-10. Clin Exp Metastasis 28(8):793–802
55. Smith HA, Kang Y (2017) Determinants of organotropic metastasis. Ann Rev Cancer Biol 1(1):403–423

56. Pani G, Galeotti T, Chiarugi P (2010) Metastasis: cancer cell's escape from oxidative stress. Cancer Metastasis Rev 29(2):351–378

57. Rodriguez-Torres M, Allan AL (2016) Aldehyde dehydrogenase as a marker and functional mediator of metastasis in solid tumors. Clin Exp Metastasis 33(1):97–113

58. Chen MH, Weng JJ, Cheng CT, Wu RC, Huang SC, Wu CE et al (2016) ALDH1A3, the major aldehyde dehydrogenase isoform in human cholangiocarcinoma cells, affects prognosis and gemcitabine resistance in cholangiocarcinoma patients. Clin Cancer Res 22(16):4225–4235

59. LeBleu VS, O'Connell JT, Gonzalez Herrera KN, Wikman H, Pantel K, Haigis MC et al (2014) PGC-1α mediates mitochondrial biogenesis and oxidative phosphorylation in cancer cells to promote metastasis. Nat Cell Biol 16(10):992–1003

60. Liang J, Shao SH, Xu Z-X, Hennessy B, Ding Z, Larrea M et al (2007) The energy sensing LKB1–AMPK pathway regulates p27kip1 phosphorylation mediating the decision to enter autophagy or apoptosis. Nat Cell Biol 9(2):218–224

61. Nieman KM, Kenny HA, Penicka CV, Ladanyi A, Buell-Gutbrod R, Zillhardt MR et al (2011) Adipocytes promote ovarian cancer metastasis and provide energy for rapid tumor growth. Nat Med 17(11):1498–1503

62. Weber GF (2016) Metabolism in cancer metastasis. Int J Cancer 138(9):2061–2066

63. Chen EI, Hewel J, Krueger JS, Tiraby C, Weber MR, Kralli A et al (2007) Adaptation of energy metabolism in breast cancer brain metastases. Cancer Res 67(4):1472–1486

64. Sansone P, Ceccarelli C, Berishaj M, Chang Q, Rajasekhar VK, Perna F et al (2016) Self-renewal of CD133(hi) cells by IL6/Notch3 signalling regulates endocrine resistance in metastatic breast cancer. Nat Commun 7:10442

65. DeBerardinis RJ, Lum JJ, Hatzivassiliou G, Thompson CB (2008) The biology of cancer: metabolic reprogramming fuels cell growth and proliferation. Cell Metab 7(1):11–20

66. Dupuy F, Tabariès S, Andrzejewski S, Dong Z, Blagih J, Annis Matthew G et al (2015) PDK1-dependent metabolic reprogramming dictates metastatic potential in breast cancer. Cell Metab 22(4):577–589

67. Hanahan D, Coussens LM (2012) Accessories to the crime: functions of cells recruited to the tumor microenvironment. Cancer Cell 21(3):309–322

68. Joyce JA, Pollard JW (2009) Microenvironmental regulation of metastasis. Nat Rev Cancer 9(4):239–252

69. Weilbaecher KN, Guise TA, McCauley LK (2011) Cancer to bone: a fatal attraction. Nat Rev Cancer 11(6):411–425

70. Ell B, Kang Y (2012) SnapShot: bone metastasis. Cell 151(3):690

71. Logothetis CJ, Lin S-H (2005) Osteoblasts in prostate cancer metastasis to bone. Nat Rev Cancer 5(1):21–28

72. Guise TA, Mohammad KS, Clines G, Stebbins EG, Wong DH, Higgins LS et al (2006) Basic mechanisms responsible for osteolytic and osteoblastic bone metastases. Clin Cancer Res 12(20 Pt 2):6213s–6216s

73. Lu X, Mu E, Wei Y, Riethdorf S, Yang Q, Yuan M et al (2011) VCAM-1 promotes osteolytic expansion of indolent bone micrometastasis of breast cancer by engaging α4β1-positive osteoclast progenitors. Cancer Cell 20(6):701–714

74. Zhang XH, Wang Q, Gerald W, Hudis CA, Norton L, Smid M et al (2009) Latent bone metastasis in breast cancer tied to Src-dependent survival signals. Cancer Cell 16(1):67–78

75. Monteiro AC, Leal AC, Gonçalves-Silva T, Mercadante AC, Kestelman F, Chaves SB et al (2013) T cells induce pre-metastatic osteolytic disease and help bone metastases establishment in a mouse model of metastatic breast cancer. PLoS One 8(7):e68171

76. Karavitis J, Hix LM, Shi YH, Schultz RF, Khazaie K, Zhang M (2012) Regulation of COX2 expression in mouse mammary tumor cells controls bone metastasis and PGE2-induction of regulatory T cell migration. PLoS One 7(9):e46342

77. Sawant A, Hensel JA, Chanda D, Harris BA, Siegal GP, Maheshwari A et al (2012) Depletion of plasmacytoid dendritic cells inhibits tumor growth and prevents bone metastasis of breast cancer cells. J Immunol 189(9):4258–4265

78. Takeda K, Hayakawa Y, Smyth MJ, Kayagaki N, Yamaguchi N, Kakuta S et al (2001) Involvement of tumor necrosis factor-related apoptosis-inducing ligand in surveillance of tumor metastasis by liver natural killer cells. Nat Med 7(1):94–100
79. Cohen-Solal JF, Cassard L, Fournier EM, Loncar SM, Fridman WH, Sautès-Fridman C (2010) Metastatic melanomas express inhibitory low affinity fc gamma receptor and escape humoral immunity. Dermatol Res Pract 2010:657406
80. Calon A, Espinet E, Palomo-Ponce S, Tauriello DV, Iglesias M, Céspedes MV et al (2012) Dependency of colorectal cancer on a TGF-β-driven program in stromal cells for metastasis initiation. Cancer Cell 22(5):571–584
81. Costa-Silva B, Aiello NM, Ocean AJ, Singh S, Zhang H, Thakur BK et al (2015) Pancreatic cancer exosomes initiate pre-metastatic niche formation in the liver. Nat Cell Biol 17(6): 816–826
82. Zhao L, Lim SY, Gordon-Weeks AN, Tapmeier TT, Im JH, Cao Y et al (2013) Recruitment of a myeloid cell subset (CD11b/Gr1 mid) via CCL2/CCR2 promotes the development of colorectal cancer liver metastasis. Hepatology 57(2):829–839
83. Spicer JD, McDonald B, Cools-Lartigue JJ, Chow SC, Giannias B, Kubes P et al (2012) Neutrophils promote liver metastasis via Mac-1-mediated interactions with circulating tumor cells. Cancer Res 72(16):3919–3927
84. Cools-Lartigue J, Spicer J, McDonald B, Gowing S, Chow S, Giannias B et al (2013) Neutrophil extracellular traps sequester circulating tumor cells and promote metastasis. J Clin Invest 123(8):3446–3458
85. Granot Z, Henke E, Comen EA, King TA, Norton L, Benezra R (2011) Tumor entrained neutrophils inhibit seeding in the premetastatic lung. Cancer Cell 20(3):300–314
86. Talmadge JE, Gabrilovich DI (2013) History of myeloid-derived suppressor cells. Nat Rev Cancer 13(10):739–752
87. Yan HH, Pickup M, Pang Y, Gorska AE, Li Z, Chytil A et al (2010) Gr-1+CD11b+ myeloid cells tip the balance of immune protection to tumor promotion in the premetastatic lung. Cancer Res 70(15):6139–6149
88. Gil-Bernabé AM, Ferjancic S, Tlalka M, Zhao L, Allen PD, Im JH et al (2012) Recruitment of monocytes/macrophages by tissue factor-mediated coagulation is essential for metastatic cell survival and premetastatic niche establishment in mice. Blood 119(13):3164–3175
89. van Deventer HW, Palmieri DA, Wu QP, McCook EC, Serody JS (2013) Circulating fibrocytes prepare the lung for cancer metastasis by recruiting Ly-6C+ monocytes via CCL2. J Immunol 190(9):4861–4867
90. Toh B, Wang X, Keeble J, Sim WJ, Khoo K, Wong WC et al (2011) Mesenchymal transition and dissemination of cancer cells is driven by myeloid-derived suppressor cells infiltrating the primary tumor. PLoS Biol 9(9):e1001162
91. Lin EY, Nguyen AV, Russell RG, Pollard JW (2001) Colony-stimulating factor 1 promotes progression of mammary tumors to malignancy. J Exp Med 193(6):727–740
92. Kinoshita T, Ishii G, Hiraoka N, Hirayama S, Yamauchi C, Aokage K et al (2013) Forkhead box P3 regulatory T cells coexisting with cancer associated fibroblasts are correlated with a poor outcome in lung adenocarcinoma. Cancer Sci 104(4):409–415
93. Olkhanud PB, Baatar D, Bodogai M, Hakim F, Gress R, Anderson RL et al (2009) Breast cancer lung metastasis requires expression of chemokine receptor CCR4 and regulatory T cells. Cancer Res 69(14):5996–6004
94. Dalotto-Moreno T, Croci DO, Cerliani JP, Martinez-Allo VC, Dergan-Dylon S, Méndez-Huergo SP et al (2013) Targeting galectin-1 overcomes breast cancer-associated immunosuppression and prevents metastatic disease. Cancer Res 73(3):1107–1117
95. Kitamura T, Qian B-Z, Pollard JW (2015) Immune cell promotion of metastasis. Nat Rev Immunol 15(2):73–86
96. Chopra M, Riedel SS, Biehl M, Krieger S, von Krosigk V, Bäuerlein CA et al (2013) Tumor necrosis factor receptor 2-dependent homeostasis of regulatory T cells as a player in TNF-induced experimental metastasis. Carcinogenesis 34(6):1296–1303

97. Smyth MJ, Teng MW, Swann J, Kyparissoudis K, Godfrey DI, Hayakawa Y (2006) CD4+CD25+ T regulatory cells suppress NK cell-mediated immunotherapy of cancer. J Immunol 176(3):1582–1587

98. Wculek SK, Malanchi I (2015) Neutrophils support lung colonization of metastasis-initiating breast cancer cells. Nature 528(7582):413–417

99. Camerer E, Qazi AA, Duong DN, Cornelissen I, Advincula R, Coughlin SR (2004) Platelets, protease-activated receptors, and fibrinogen in hematogenous metastasis. Blood 104(2): 397–401

100. Labelle M, Begum S, Hynes RO (2011) Direct signaling between platelets and cancer cells induces an epithelial-mesenchymal-like transition and promotes metastasis. Cancer Cell 20(5): 576–590

101. Labelle M, Begum S, Hynes RO (2014) Platelets guide the formation of early metastatic niches. Proc Natl Acad Sci U S A 111(30):E3053–E3061

102. Palumbo JS, Talmage KE, Massari JV, La Jeunesse CM, Flick MJ, Kombrinck KW et al (2005) Platelets and fibrin(ogen) increase metastatic potential by impeding natural killer cell-mediated elimination of tumor cells. Blood 105(1):178–185

103. Malanchi I, Santamaria-Martínez A, Susanto E, Peng H, Lehr HA, Delaloye JF et al (2011) Interactions between cancer stem cells and their niche govern metastatic colonization. Nature 481(7379):85–89

104. Valiente M, Obenauf AC, Jin X, Chen Q, Zhang XH, Lee DJ et al (2014) Serpins promote cancer cell survival and vascular co-option in brain metastasis. Cell 156(5):1002–1016

105. Zhang L, Zhang S, Yao J, Lowery FJ, Zhang Q, Huang WC et al (2015) Microenvironment-induced PTEN loss by exosomal microRNA primes brain metastasis outgrowth. Nature 527(7576):100–104

106. Sevenich L, Bowman RL, Mason SD, Quail DF, Rapaport F, Elie BT et al (2014) Analysis of tumour- and stroma-supplied proteolytic networks reveals a brain-metastasis-promoting role for cathepsin S. Nat Cell Biol 16(9):876–888

107. Xing F, Kobayashi A, Okuda H, Watabe M, Pai SK, Pandey PR et al (2013) Reactive astrocytes promote the metastatic growth of breast cancer stem-like cells by activating Notch signalling in brain. EMBO Mol Med 5(3):384–396

108. Kim SW, Choi HJ, Lee HJ, He J, Wu Q, Langley RR et al (2014) Role of the endothelin axis in astrocyte-and endothelial cell-mediated chemoprotection of cancer cells. Neuro-Oncology 16(12):1585–1598

109. Aceto N, Bardia A, Miyamoto DT, Donaldson MC, Wittner BS, Spencer JA et al (2014) Circulating tumor cell clusters are oligoclonal precursors of breast cancer metastasis. Cell 158(5):1110–1122

110. Denève E, Riethdorf S, Ramos J, Nocca D, Coffy A, Daurès JP et al (2013) Capture of viable circulating tumor cells in the liver of colorectal cancer patients. Clin Chem 59(9):1384–1392

111. Budczies J, von Winterfeld M, Klauschen F, Bockmayr M, Lennerz JK, Denkert C et al (2015) The landscape of metastatic progression patterns across major human cancers. Oncotarget 6(1):570–583

112. Aird WC (2007) Phenotypic heterogeneity of the endothelium: I. Structure, function, and mechanisms. Circ Res 100(2):158–173

113. Huang RL, Teo Z, Chong HC, Zhu P, Tan MJ, Tan CK et al (2011) ANGPTL4 modulates vascular junction integrity by integrin signaling and disruption of intercellular VE-cadherin and claudin-5 clusters. Blood 118(14):3990–4002

114. Padua D, Zhang XH, Wang Q, Nadal C, Gerald WL, Gomis RR et al (2008) TGFbeta primes breast tumors for lung metastasis seeding through angiopoietin-like 4. Cell 133(1):66–77

115. Tichet M, Prod'Homme V, Fenouille N, Ambrosetti D, Mallavialle A, Cerezo M et al (2015) Tumour-derived SPARC drives vascular permeability and extravasation through endothelial VCAM1 signalling to promote metastasis. Nat Commun 6:6993

116. Gupta GP, Nguyen DX, Chiang AC, Bos PD, Kim JY, Nadal C et al (2007) Mediators of vascular remodelling co-opted for sequential steps in lung metastasis. Nature 446(7137): 765–770
117. Rostami R, Mittal S, Rostami P, Tavassoli F, Jabbari B (2016) Brain metastasis in breast cancer: a comprehensive literature review. J Neuro-Oncol 127(3):407–414
118. Sevenich L, Joyce JA (2014) Pericellular proteolysis in cancer. Genes Dev 28(21):2331–2347
119. Zhou W, Fong MY, Min Y, Somlo G, Liu L, Palomares MR et al (2014) Cancer-secreted miR-105 destroys vascular endothelial barriers to promote metastasis. Cancer Cell 25(4): 501–515
120. Momeny M, Saunus JM, Marturana F, McCart Reed AE, Black D, Sala G et al (2015) Heregulin-HER3-HER2 signaling promotes matrix metalloproteinase-dependent blood-brain-barrier transendothelial migration of human breast cancer cell lines. Oncotarget 6(6): 3932–3946
121. Barthel SR, Hays DL, Yazawa EM, Opperman M, Walley KC, Nimrichter L et al (2013) Definition of molecular determinants of prostate cancer cell bone extravasation. Cancer Res 73(2):942–952
122. Auguste P, Fallavollita L, Wang N, Burnier J, Bikfalvi A, Brodt P (2007) The host inflammatory response promotes liver metastasis by increasing tumor cell arrest and extravasation. Am J Pathol 170(5):1781–1792
123. Eichbaum C, Meyer AS, Wang N, Bischofs E, Steinborn A, Bruckner T et al (2011) Breast cancer cell-derived cytokines, macrophages and cell adhesion: implications for metastasis. Anticancer Res 31(10):3219–3227
124. Qi J, Chen N, Wang J, Siu CH (2005) Transendothelial migration of melanoma cells involves N-cadherin-mediated adhesion and activation of the beta-catenin signaling pathway. Mol Biol Cell 16(9):4386–4397
125. Rahn JJ, Chow JW, Horne GJ, Mah BK, Emerman JT, Hoffman P et al (2005) MUC1 mediates transendothelial migration *in vitro* by ligating endothelial cell ICAM-1. Clin Exp Metastasis 22(6):475–483

Chapter 17
Cancer Stem Cells (CSCs) in Tumor Ecosystem

Phei Er Saw and Erwei Song

Abstract In cancer, cancer stem cells (CSCs) is a unique cell population that could acquire the stemness ability of a stem cell that enable them to proliferate and grow exponentially. When seen through the perspective of an ecosystem, many different components of the tumor interact with CSCs, in many different directions. These interactions support the complex changes not only in the local and distal onco-sphere, but also dictates the intra-onco-spherical communications, making both onco-spheres constantly changing to grow in the most suitable environment. According to many studies, different from parental tumor cells, CSCs differ in their gene expression, tumor proliferative capacity, immunological interactions, and responsiveness to treatment. In this chapter, we give an overview of the origin and history of CSCs and their reciprocal crosstalks in the local and distal onco-sphere.

P. E. Saw
Guangdong Provincial Key Laboratory of Malignant Tumor Epigenetics and Gene Regulation, Guangdong-Hong Kong Joint Laboratory for RNA Medicine, Medical Research Center, Sun Yat-sen Memorial Hospital, Sun Yat-sen University, Guangzhou, China

Nanhai Translational Innovation Center of Precision Immunology, Sun Yat-sen Memorial Hospital, Sun Yat-sen University, Foshan, China

E. Song (✉)
Guangdong Provincial Key Laboratory of Malignant Tumor Epigenetics and Gene Regulation, Guangdong-Hong Kong Joint Laboratory for RNA Medicine, Medical Research Center, Sun Yat-sen Memorial Hospital, Sun Yat-sen University, Guangzhou, China

Nanhai Translational Innovation Center of Precision Immunology, Sun Yat-sen Memorial Hospital, Sun Yat-sen University, Foshan, China

Breast Tumor Center, Sun Yat-sen Memorial Hospital, Sun Yat-sen University, Guangzhou, China
e-mail: songew@mail.sysu.edu.cn

Introduction

In order to retain a favorable niche, cancer stem cells (CSCs) continuously alter their surroundings. When seen through the perspective of an ecosystem, many different components of the tumor interact with CSCs, in many different directions. These interactions support the complex changes not only in the local and distal *onco-sphere*, but also dictates the intra-onco-spherical communications, making both *onco-spheres* constantly changing to grow in the most suitable environment. According to many studies, different from parental tumor cells, CSCs differ in their gene expression, tumor proliferative capacity, immunological interactions, and responsiveness to treatment [1–6]. Numerous factors may explain these variations, including metabolic and microenvironmental characteristics, genetic and epigenetic clonal variation, and other factors. According to CSC theory, CSCs are in charge of preserving this tumor heterogeneity, which promotes tumor development and therapeutic resistance. In this chapter, we detailed on how CSCs actively shape their milieu and interact with other tumor elements such as immune and stromal cells in the local *onco-sphere*, interactions with specific organs in distal *onco-sphere* to create a suitable pre-metastatic niche and interactions with systemic *onco-sphere* in utilizing host circulatory system and other extracellular signals to create a stable niche in cancer progression and metastasis.

The Origin and History of CSCs

In two back-to-back studies, John E. Dick and his colleagues published on the demonstration of how a few rare cells of AML from mice are sufficient and capable of initiating leukemia in other healthy mice. In their studies, they showed that these cells have exceedingly high capacity of self-renewal (an essential characteristics of stem cells), and these properties are carried down through few generations in successive transplantation [7, 8]. Upon excision, the tumors after transplantation are found to be a mixture of both tumor cells and non-tumoral adjacent cells, which are similar to the composition of initial tumor [8]. This study revolutionizes the way we think about tumor growth. The results indicated the following: (1) tumorigenesis is duplicated and reproduced at each cancer development, even in a new host and new environment, (2) CSCs are capable of producing identical cells at the time of transplantation by self-renewal mechanism, (3) at the same time, CSCs can become differentiated (at various level), and with time, and (4) these CSC-differentiated cells will lose their self-renewal and tumorigenic potential.

The first evidence was demonstrated in breast cancer, where only a few hundred isolated CSCs were able to form tumors in mice, as compared to millions of cells needed for a successful xenograft model using a mixed cell culture in vitro, In this model, a tiny fraction of CD44$^+$/CD24$^-$/Lin$^-$ breast cancer cells was detected and isolated. When CD44$^+$/CD24$^-$/Lin$^-$ cells were transferred to immunocompromised

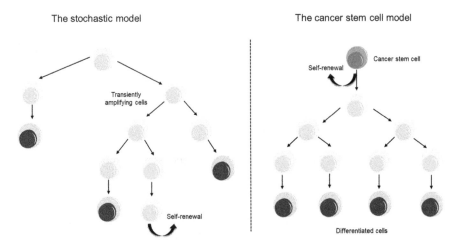

Fig. 17.1 The difference between the cancer stem cell model and the stochastic model. Both of these concepts are thought to contribute to intratumor heterogeneity, and it is now understood that they do not conflict with one another. Nevertheless, there is no solid evidence to proof the absolute correctness of both concepts

animals, tumors can develop from as few as 100 cells, indicating the high stemness properties of this subset [1]. Subsequently, a CD133$^+$ cell population was found in the tumorigenic cells in colon cancer. Although these cells accounts for only ~2.5% of whole tumor population, by injecting only CD133$^+$ cells into mice not only successfully reproduce the original tumor, these tumors can be transplanted for a few generations. Interestingly, in vitro, CD133$^+$ cells can grow exponentially in a spheroid culture for more than a year [4]. Similar result was obtained in human glioma models. Injection of 100 CD133$^+$ cells is sufficient to induce tumor growth in the brain of a SCID mouse model, affirming the stemness of this subset [9]. Since then, CSCs have been identified and characterized in various solid tumors [3, 4, 10, 11] (Fig. 17.1).

Box 17.1 CSCs and Models of Tumor Heterogeneity
Tumor Heterogeneity
Resistance to drug therapy is the main bottleneck in cancer therapy. Most failures in clinical trials are due to the patient's resistance towards continuous and sequential therapy of these drugs. One of the crucial factors in resistance is to acknowledge that a tumor is heterogenous. In a highly heterogenous tumor, a single therapy could not be equally effective in killing all tumor cells [12, 13]. Intratumoral heterogeneity reveals that in one solid tumor, several subpopulations of cancer cells with various morphological and phenotypic differences exists, and these differences might be the polar opposite of each other (i.e., highly metastatic vs. low metastatic phenotype) [14]. Indeed, by

---

(continued)

Box 17.1 (continued)

utilizing massively parallel sequencing (MPS), investigations demonstrate that both spatial and temporal heterogeneity is widespread in malignancies [15]. The stochastic or Darwinian model and the CSC model are the two primary hypotheses used to explain the genesis of cancer heterogeneity.

Stochastic model

This concept is based on Charles Darwin's premise that the fittest creature has the highest chance of surviving, as stated in his book "The Origin of Species." The tumor cells are thought of as an ecosystem, similar to the local *onco-sphere* concept that we are highlighting in this book. In this environment, spontaneous mutations and epigenetic modifications will occur to provide cells a higher fitness. Natural selection will only choose the "fittest" cell population, and therefore, in cancer therapy, the verse "what does not kill you makes you stronger" stands unchallenged. Indeed, tumor will only repopulate with the fittest clone after each therapy. After a few rounds of therapy, the tumor would have selected the fittest cell population, that is the cell clone that is resistant to this therapy [12]. In a statement, stochastic model believes that the tumor growth is random, contributed by the entire tumor population, while only the fittest will survive to become "stem-cell" like.

Cancer stem cell model

This theory describes the presence of a hierarchical structure of cancer cells, similar to the normal stem cell hierarchy in tissues, and assigns heterogeneity to abnormal differentiation programs of CSCs [16]. A tiny number of cells with high self-renewing ability are found at the top of the hierarchy. There are two fates of these cells (1) they may give birth to differentiated cancer cells with a variety of phenotypes, which make up the majority of the tumor and have much lower tumorigenicity, or (2) retain their self-renewal ability and stay on top of the hierarchy. However, in this model, since CSCs are at the top of the hierarchy and is fully responsible to produce other tumor-cells, they could also be the most vulnerable to random mutations and outside stimuli that favor the fittest clones [16]. In a statement, the CSC model believes that certain cells are programmed to be "stem-like" behavior genetically. More researches are pointing towards the fact that CSCs is highly plastic, usually presented as a transient cell state, rather than a specific cell type.

CSCs in the Local *Onco-sphere*

CSCs Resist Cell Death and Increases Resistance

To maintain the viability of a tumor, CSCs needs to have high survival capability, apart from having self-renewal ability. To avoid cell death, highly active DNA damage response mechanisms are seen in CSCs from the breast, glioma, lung, and pancreatic cancers [17, 18]. Although SNAIL family member is responsible for triggering the EMT process during tumor progression, it can also enhance the expression of nucleotide excision repair protein in oral cancer, to induce more repair in DNA damage. This consequently results in cisplatin resistance, a common mechanism seen in oral cancer [19]. In addition to DNA repair mechanisms, CSCs prevent apoptosis by mutating or deactivating genes that control the cell cycle and those that trigger apoptosis [20].

Multidrug resistance (MDR) is a persistent problem in cancer treatment and is most likely the root cause of treatment failure [12, 21]. Numerous studies have shown that CSCs are substantially more likely than differentiated tumor cells to possess innate defences against radiation and chemotherapy [17]. Therefore, the majority of the non-CSC population is eliminated by chemotherapy and radiation but not by CSCs [22]. Compared to CD133$^-$ cells, CSC populations expressing CD133$^+$ cells had lower 5-year OS, with higher resistance towards chemotherapeutics and/or radiotherapeutics in various malignancies [17, 23, 24]. Treatment with chemotherapeutic drugs like cisplatin often resulted in apoptosis resistance. In leukemia and prostate cancer, cisplatin treatment increases the interaction of HDAC and TRIB1, which jointly inactivate p53 to suppress tumor growth [25]. CSC populations in glioblastoma rose two- to fourfold after radiation therapy, most likely as a result of preferential activation of the DNA damage response [26]. In colon, breast, and lung carcinomas, loss of p53 activity will induce the upregulation of SNAIL family, which induced radioresistance and EMT [20]. CD133$^+$ glioma CSCs also upregulate NBS1, a cell cycle checkpoint to increase DNA repair response, which ultimately leads to radioresistance [17].

CSCs Regulates Hypoxic Environment

Solid tumor malignancy and aggressiveness are characterized by hypoxic, acidic, and necrotic areas, which promote CSC maintenance and treatment resistance [27–31]. Acidic stress and nutritional limitation are often present in hypoxic stress situations. Together, these circumstances cause and favor the emergence of a subpopulation of cells with nutrient-restricted survival mechanisms, favoring the transition to aerobic glycolysis and glutamine-mediated fatty acid synthesis [32–36]. The ability of CSCs to survive and grow in these nutrient-poor environments is enhanced, and these environments also favor CSCs re-programming into quiescent and migratory phenotypes [27, 29, 37]. CSCs upregulate immune escape pathways and pathways that maintain the hypoxic niche in response to hypoxia signaling, and they also cause paracrine signaling that encourages vascularization and angiogenesis [38–40].

Hypoxia-inducible factors (HIFs), such as HIF-1 and HIF-2, play a significant role in controlling the consequences of hypoxia. In many organs, acute hypoxia will lead to an overexpression of HIF-1, while in chronic hypoxic condition, HIF-2 is elevated. Since tumor has a constant hypoxic condition, the HIF-2 family is upregulated in hypoxic tumors, leading to the upregulation of Klf4, Sox2, and Oct4, transcription factors vital to stem cell phenotype maintenance, for example in glioblastoma and neuroblastoma [3, 41, 42]. Acidic stress induces HIF2α expression, which supports glioma stemness characteristics [43]. In hypoxia-treated glioblastoma cells, the acute hypoxia increases HIF1 production, which then controls metabolic response to food deprivation and encourages a mesenchymal shift along with the production of pro-survival molecules like ERK and AKT [29, 44]. Additionally, HIF1 can also activate Wnt and Notch signalling pathways [45, 46]. In starvation or glucose restricted environment, HIF1 can induce Nanog, Sox2, and Oct4, key regulators of stem cell to increase cancer stemness [47]. In a breast cancer xenograft model, the hypoxic zones in the tumor reveals functional tumor cells featuring stem cell properties, with specific stem cell markers expression [37]. In an interesting finding, although PI3K/AKT has been identified as a positive regulator of cancer cell stemness, the long-term maintenance of these cells might need additional, epigenetic intervention. Hypoxic induction of stemness characteristics in breast cancer has been demonstrated to vary with estrogen receptor mutation status, underscoring the importance of cell-intrinsic attributes modulating cell-niche interactions and highlighting the difficulty of extrapolating results from model systems [48].

CSC Induces EMT and Metastasis

In the process of EMT, the downregulation of E-cadherin and the upregulation of N-cadherin could be observed, where the epithelial cells would lose their polarity, followed by a morphological change; from an epithelial phenotype into an elongated, fibroblastic-like mesenchymal phenotype [49, 50]. Cells undergoing EMT are mostly regulated by SNAIL, SLUG, ZEB1/2, and TWIST on E-cadherin promoters to inhibit E-cadherin production, thereby enhancing EMT [51]. Numerous studies have been done on the relationship between EMT and CSC phenotypic acquisition [52]. For instance, as mentioned above, TWIST, SNAIL, and also FOXC2 boosted the mesenchymal characteristics of cancer cells in breast cancer. These cells developed the capacity to form mammospheres, and the CD44^{high}/CD24^{low} CSC subpopulation also increased [53, 54]. Prostate cancer cells with the EMT phenotype has increased sphere forming ability, and they expressed elevated percentages of the prostate CSC markers such as NOTCH 1, NANOG, OCT 4, SOX2, OCT4, and LIN28B [55] (Fig. 17.2).

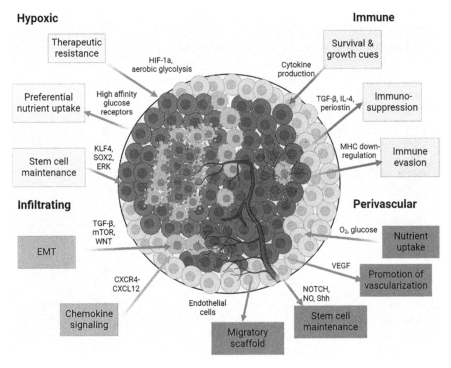

Fig. 17.2 Various functions of CSCs in modulating the tumor ecosystem. CTCs can affect the tumor local and distal *onco-sphere* through regulation of hypoxia, immune system, EMT and metabolic changes. These mechanisms are general, but the key transcription factors modulating these activities in different cancers might vary

Box 17.2 Effect of miRNAs in CSC Phenotype Acquisition

miRNAs have been implicated in cancer development, tumorigenesis, treatment resistance, and possibly the acquisition of CSC traits [56, 57]. One example is miRNA-22, which, in leukemia and myelodysplastic syndrome, where it was shown to be increased, enhances the self-renewal of hematopoietic stem cells by inactivating TET2 [58]. Additionally, it has been shown that the same miRNA promotes metastasis in a mouse model of breast cancer and induces EMT through the TET-miRNA200 axis [59]. Similarly, miRNAs associated with EMT activation has been shown to support CSC phenotype and drug resistance. In an in vitro and in vivo study on pancreatic CSCs, the deletion of the miRNA-200 family boosted the expression of SNAIL, SLUG, ZEB1, and ZEB2, all the transcription factors closely related to EMT [57].

Additionally, hypoxia encourages modifications in the expression profiles of microRNAs, such as the suppression of miR-34a. Under normal condition, miR-34a is overexpressed, and their overexpression is linked to the

(continued)

Box 17.2 (continued)

downregulation of stem cell-regulatory genes and prevents the CSC phenotype [56]. Furthermore, miR-34a could also suppresses the expression of carbonic anhydrase iso-enzyme 9 (CA9). Under hypoxic condition, once miR-34 was suppressed, Slug will then be upregulated, leading to the increased expression of CA9, which eventually, increases the CSCs survival in breast cancer [60, 61]. Importantly, scientists discovered that exosomes, actively secrete miR-34a, suggesting a function for microRNA in the distal *onco-sphere* [61, 62]. Pancreatic cells were driven by hypoxia to produce miRNA-21, which allowed them to undergo EMT and avoid apoptosis [63].

miRNA-27b was shown to be connected to drug resistance. By raising the expression and membrane location of ABCG2, it has been discovered that loss of miRNA-27b increases docetaxel resistance in Luminal A breast-type cancer, and supported CSC phenotype [64]. All of these studies point to the involvement of miRNAs, in several pathways that support the phenotypes of CSCs and the ensuing drug resistance. This opens up possibility of the involvement of other non-coding RNAs, metabolites, chemo-/cytokines in the inter- and intra-onco spherical communication in CSC phenotype acquisition.

Crosstalk: Interactions Between CSCs and Immune and Stromal Cells

CSCs interact with both various components in the local *onco-sphere* in a complex web of reciprocal signaling inside each niche and are exposed to a broad range of external circumstances and signals. Critical mediators of stemness have been shown to be driven by signaling in the chronic hypoxic condition of solid tumors. Solid tumors are characterized by acidic pH, high ROS, low oxygen, and limited nutrition's, as we discussed in previous chapters [3, 18, 43, 47]. However, within this tumor environment, CSCs still can survive and flourish, due to their high adaptive mechanism, for example, using glucose as a source of food. Not only this encourages cellular proliferation and migration, CSCs also triggers multiple pathways that could prove a positive feedback mechanism in the local *onco-sphere*, which in turn increases hypoxia and necrosis, to their favor [29, 47]. Leaky tumor arteries provide a platform for migration and preferential access to nutrients in the perivascular zone, while ECs participate in reciprocal signaling to increase drug resistance [65–67]. Angiogenic factors are then released by CSCs, which aid in neovascularization [68]. Invading CSCs are supported as they move to build an invasive niche by structural and signaling cues from normal tissue, such as CAFs and the ECMs, as well as the physical and structural characteristics of normal tissue architecture [69–71]. Here, we will summarize major crosstalks in the interactions of CSCs with various components in the infiltrated immune cells and stromal cells in the local *onco-sphere*, and how these interactions dictate the CSCs into EMT and metastasis.

Cancer-Associated Fibroblasts (CAFs)

In many malignancies, fibroblasts comprise the most prevalent part of the tumor stroma and are, therefore, the niche. This is particularly true for pancreatic and breast cancer [72, 73]. CAFs are fibroblasts that are prevalent in tumors and are very similar to fibroblasts that actively contribute to wound healing at inflammatory sites [74, 75]. In comparison to normal fibroblasts, CAFs proliferate more, produce more ECM components, and secrete a variety of distinct cytokines, such as SDF1, CXCL12, VEGF, PDGF, and HGF [76, 77]. TGFβ is primarily secreted by CAFs to promote EMT and eventually leads to drug resistance [77]. A cell line originating from invasive breast cancers has been shown to produce EMT in those cells when a high quantity of TGF-β is secreted into the media [78]. Additionally, CAFs supported the stemness of CSCs in breast and gastric cancers. In particular, CAFs increased stemness in gastric cancer by secreting NRG1 and activating NF-kB signaling [79]. In breast cancer cell lines, co-culturing tumor cells with CAFs resulted in a 4.4-fold increase in tamoxifen resistance [80]. Similarly, CAF-derived exosomes could stimulate Wnt signaling to improve colon CSCs' drug resistance to 5-fluorouracil [81]. Similar research demonstrated that exosomes from CAFs stimulated STAT1 in breast cancer cells through the receptor RIG-1; with simultaneous STAT1 stimulation to activate NOTCH3, which enhanced treatment resistance in CSCs [82]. In response to NRG1 released by CAF, which triggered NF-kB signaling [83, 84] producing CSCs traits, gastric, breast, prostate, and glioma cells improved their potential for self-renewal. It is significant to note that CAF increased CSCs' stemness signaling pathways, which contributed to drug resistance, and secreted type I collagen, decreasing drug absorption [85].

Mesenchymal Stem Cells (MSCs)

Adult stem cells (SCs) having the capacity to develop into a range of skeletal tissue cells are known as mesenchymal stem cells (MSCs). MSCs function as immuno-modulators under normal circumstances, but when they are present in the stroma, they trigger the development of CSCs by triggering the NF-kB pathway and secreting a variety of cytokines and chemokines, including chemokines CXCL12, CXCL7, and interleukins IL-6 and IL-8 [26]. These chemokines and interleukins, along with other GFs are also known to contribute to breast cancer therapy resistance via elevation of CSCs [70]. Interestingly, mechanical stress (physical contact) between MSCs and breast cancer stimulates the PI3K/Akt pathway and SRC, a non-receptor tyrosine kinase, which increases resistance to trastuzumab [72]. As epithelial ovarian tumors cells undergo resistance, the acquisition of MDR proteins on tumor cells further enhances the physical interaction with MSCs to promote the resistance to carboplatin and paclitaxel [86].

Tumor-Associated Macrophages (TAMs)

Monocytes and macrophages recruited into tumor tissue are examples of cellular components of inflammation that have been widely examined [87]. Monocytes, which are present in the circulation as $CD34^+$ bone marrow progenitors, give rise to macrophages. They develop into a tissue-specific macrophage after extravasation into tissues [88]. In the tumor, macrophages are presented mostly as the anti-tumoral phenotype or known as tumor-associated macrophages (TAMs, M2-like). TAMs secreted growth factors, cytokines, and chemokines are known to modulate cancer cells into CSCs. TAMs releases TGF-β and TNF-α, the two important GFs in stimulating EMT. These factors are also key modulators of a CSC phenotype in tumors, as seen in the induction of cancer treatment resistance in non-small lung cancer [89, 90]. In $HER2^+$ breast cancer, induction of STAT3/IL-6 signaling pathway increases the production of CSCs, which in turn causing Trastuzumab resistance [91].

Endothelial Cells (ECs)

Endothelial cells (ECs) line the blood arteries. As the main supplier of oxygen and nutrient to the tumor, the vasculature is essential to in the local *onco-sphere*. The idea that the vascular microenvironments in brain tumors enable the development of a self-renewing CSC pool was initially proposed in 2007 [92]. In head and neck squamous cell carcinoma, about 80% of CSCs were found near blood arteries, indicating the importance of ECs in regulating CSC stemness [93]. In head and neck squamous cell carcinoma, colorectal cancer and glioblastoma, the ECs in these tumors were shown to release multiple GFs, including VEGFs, FGFs that promotes and maintenance of CSCs characteristics and promotes EMT [94, 95]. Recent studies in glioma and colorectal cancer have shown that ECs may improve the characteristics of CSCs by activating the Notch signal via, the soluble version of Jagged-1 in glioma and a nitric oxide signaling pathway in colorectal cancer. In breast cancer, the ECs released TNF-α to stimulate the activation of NF-kB signaling pathway in CSCs. Upon activation, these CSCs that secreted various chemokines, including CXCL1 and CXCL, which attracts myeloid cells into the tumor. These myeloid cells then secretes S100A8 and S100A9, chemokines that are responsible for doxorubicin and cyclophosphamide resistance [84]. In an interesting finding, the pathology of the blood vessels, especially the uneven geometry of tumor blood arteries in tumor vicinity, could also reduce the ability of a drug to reach CSCs, creating another method that ECs could use to shield CSCs from therapeutic medicines [96] (Fig. 17.3).

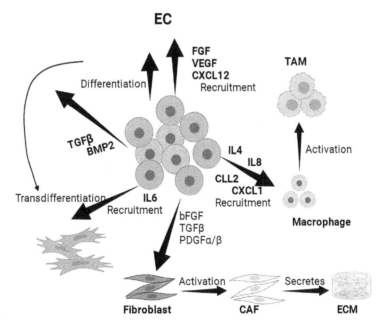

Fig. 17.3 CSC-secreted factors and their respective functions in promoting the recruitment and activation of various cells in the local *onco-spheres*, which in turn promotes stem-cell likeness of CSCs, indicating a bi-directional activity, a common feature of a symbiotic relationship in tumor ecosystem

Extracellular Matrix (ECM)

The majority of the chemicals that make up the extracellular matrix (ECM) are secreted by fibroblasts. Since cancer cells must connect to the ECM in order to develop a tumor, the ECM is essential to the tumor microenvironment. Increased ECM stiffness in solid tumors acts as a physical barrier between treatments and the cells, shielding CSCs from chemotherapeutic drugs [97]. Additionally, a number of proteins in the ECM interact with membrane proteins in CSCs to activate stem and proliferative signaling pathways as well as drug resistance. For instance, the ECM's abundant hyaluronic acid serves as the CD44 receptor's ligand. When there is contact, it mediates the purchase and upkeep of CSC properties [98]. Tenascin C also improves the effectiveness of the Wnt and Notch signaling pathways, stabilizing breast CSCs [99].

Conclusion

Tumor incidence and development are influenced by a variety of factors, including interactions with the tumor microenvironment, which acts as a "fertile soil" for them, and cell-autonomous processes, including genetic and epigenetic modifications. Together, CSCs and their microenvironment interact in a mutually beneficial way to promote tumor growth. Tumor fitness seems to originate from the CSC at the top of the hierarchy due to cellular variety and fast evolutionary potential. Heterogeneity and adaptability within this population, which may then pass on its genetically and epigenetically adaptable features to its descendants, are the currency of treatment resistance. Surgical resistance is made easier by spatial heterogeneity, such as invasion and metastasis. A more comprehensive study of CSC-microenvironment interactions is being facilitated by emerging technology. Profiling of stemness gradients inside tumors is now possible because single-cell genomic and epigenomic technologies and 3D culture techniques also provide new prospects for *in vitro* research on various habitats. *In vivo* dependencies and niche-cell interactions have been the subject of an unprecedented diversity of unique discoveries produced by CRISPR-Cas9 and RNA interference screening approaches. The close-knit connection between CSCs and the local and distal *onco-spheres* indicated the importance of the inter-*onco-spherical* communication in multiple stages of tumor growth, progression, and metastasis.

References

1. Al-Hajj M, Wicha MS, Benito-Hernandez A, Morrison SJ, Clarke MF (2003) Prospective identification of tumorigenic breast cancer cells. Proc Natl Acad Sci U S A 100(7):3983–3988
2. Fang D, Nguyen TK, Leishear K, Finko R, Kulp AN, Hotz S et al (2005) A tumorigenic subpopulation with stem cell properties in melanomas. Cancer Res 65(20):9328–9337
3. Li C, Heidt DG, Dalerba P, Burant CF, Zhang L, Adsay V et al (2007) Identification of pancreatic cancer stem cells. Cancer Res 67(3):1030–1037
4. Ricci-Vitiani L, Lombardi DG, Pilozzi E, Biffoni M, Todaro M, Peschle C et al (2007) Identification and expansion of human colon-cancer-initiating cells. Nature 445(7123):111–115
5. Singh SK, Clarke ID, Terasaki M, Bonn VE, Hawkins C, Squire J et al (2003) Identification of a cancer stem cell in human brain tumors. Cancer Res 63(18):5821–5828
6. Zhang S, Balch C, Chan MW, Lai HC, Matei D, Schilder JM et al (2008) Identification and characterization of ovarian cancer-initiating cells from primary human tumors. Cancer Res 68(11):4311–4320
7. Lapidot T, Sirard C, Vormoor J, Murdoch B, Hoang T, Caceres-Cortes J et al (1994) A cell initiating human acute myeloid leukaemia after transplantation into SCID mice. Nature 367(6464):645–648
8. Bonnet D, Dick JE (1997) Human acute myeloid leukemia is organized as a hierarchy that originates from a primitive hematopoietic cell. Nat Med 3(7):730–737
9. Singh SK, Hawkins C, Clarke ID, Squire JA, Bayani J, Hide T et al (2004) Identification of human brain tumour initiating cells. Nature 432(7015):396–401

10. Patrawala L, Calhoun T, Schneider-Broussard R, Li H, Bhatia B, Tang S et al (2006) Highly purified CD44+ prostate cancer cells from xenograft human tumors are enriched in tumorigenic and metastatic progenitor cells. Oncogene 25(12):1696–1708
11. Hurt EM, Kawasaki BT, Klarmann GJ, Thomas SB, Farrar WL (2008) CD44+ CD24(-) prostate cells are early cancer progenitor/stem cells that provide a model for patients with poor prognosis. Br J Cancer 98(4):756–765
12. Schmidt F, Efferth T (2016) Tumor heterogeneity, single-cell sequencing, and drug resistance, vol 9, Pharmaceuticals, p 2
13. Hanahan D, Weinberg RA (2011) Hallmarks of cancer: the next generation. Cell 144(5): 646–674
14. Nowell PC (1976) The clonal evolution of tumor cell populations. Science 194(4260):23–28
15. Gerlinger M, Rowan AJ, Horswell S, Math M, Larkin J, Endesfelder D et al (2012) Intratumor heterogeneity and branched evolution revealed by multiregion sequencing. N Engl J Med 366(10):883–892
16. Martelotto LG, Ng CK, Piscuoglio S, Weigelt B, Reis-Filho JS (2014) Breast cancer intra-tumor heterogeneity. Breast Cancer Res 16(3):210
17. Bao S, Wu Q, McLendon RE, Hao Y, Shi Q, Hjelmeland AB et al (2006) Glioma stem cells promote radioresistance by preferential activation of the DNA damage response. Nature 444(7120):756–760
18. Diehn M, Cho RW, Lobo NA, Kalisky T, Dorie MJ, Kulp AN et al (2009) Association of reactive oxygen species levels and radioresistance in cancer stem cells. Nature 458(7239): 780–783
19. Tsai L-L, Yu C-C, Lo J-F, Sung W-W, Lee H, Chen S-L et al (2012) Enhanced cisplatin resistance in oral-cancer stem-like cells is correlated with upregulation of excision-repair cross-complementation group 1. J Dent Sci 7(2):111–117
20. Kim NH, Kim HS, Li XY, Lee I, Choi HS, Kang SE et al (2011) A p53/miRNA-34 axis regulates Snail1-dependent cancer cell epithelial-mesenchymal transition. J Cell Biol 195(3): 417–433
21. Yamamoto Y, Yoshioka Y, Minoura K, Takahashi RU, Takeshita F, Taya T et al (2011) An integrative genomic analysis revealed the relevance of microRNA and gene expression for drug-resistance in human breast cancer cells. Mol Cancer 10:135
22. Dallas NA, Xia L, Fan F, Gray MJ, Gaur P, van Buren G et al (2009) Chemoresistant colorectal cancer cells, the cancer stem cell phenotype, and increased sensitivity to insulin-like growth factor-I receptor inhibition. Cancer Res 69(5):1951–1957
23. Bertolini G, Roz L, Perego P, Tortoreto M, Fontanella E, Gatti L et al (2009) Highly tumorigenic lung cancer CD133+ cells display stem-like features and are spared by cisplatin treatment. Proc Natl Acad Sci U S A 106(38):16281–16286
24. Sahlberg SH, Spiegelberg D, Glimelius B, Stenerlöw B, Nestor M (2014) Evaluation of cancer stem cell markers CD133, CD44, CD24: association with AKT isoforms and radiation resistance in colon cancer cells. PLoS One 9(4):e94621
25. Wang L, Liu X, Ren Y, Zhang J, Chen J, Zhou W et al (2017) Cisplatin-enriching cancer stem cells confer multidrug resistance in non-small cell lung cancer via enhancing TRIB1/HDAC activity. Cell Death Dis 8(4):e2746
26. Carnero A, Garcia-Mayea Y, Mir C, Lorente J, Rubio IT, Me LL (2016) The cancer stem-cell signaling network and resistance to therapy. Cancer Treat Rev 49:25–36
27. Carcereri de Prati A, Butturini E, Rigo A, Oppici E, Rossin M, Boriero D et al (2017) Metastatic breast cancer cells enter into dormant state and express cancer stem cells phenotype under chronic hypoxia. J Cell Biochem 118(10):3237–3248
28. Gilchrist KW, Gray R, Fowble B, Tormey DC, Taylor SGt. (1993) Tumor necrosis is a prognostic predictor for early recurrence and death in lymph node-positive breast cancer: a 10-year follow-up study of 728 Eastern Cooperative Oncology Group patients. J Clin Oncol 11(10):1929–1935

29. Siebzehnrubl FA, Silver DJ, Tugertimur B, Deleyrolle LP, Siebzehnrubl D, Sarkisian MR et al (2013) The ZEB1 pathway links glioblastoma initiation, invasion and chemoresistance. EMBO Mol Med 5(8):1196–1212

30. Zhang C, Samanta D, Lu H, Bullen JW, Zhang H, Chen I et al (2016) Hypoxia induces the breast cancer stem cell phenotype by HIF-dependent and ALKBH5-mediated m^6A-demethylation of NANOG mRNA. Proc Natl Acad Sci U S A 113(14):E2047–E2056

31. Zhang H, Lu H, Xiang L, Bullen JW, Zhang C, Samanta D et al (2015) HIF-1 regulates CD47 expression in breast cancer cells to promote evasion of phagocytosis and maintenance of cancer stem cells. Proc Natl Acad Sci U S A 112(45):6215–6223

32. Dong C, Yuan T, Wu Y, Wang Y, Fan TW, Miriyala S et al (2013) Loss of FBP1 by Snail-mediated repression provides metabolic advantages in basal-like breast cancer. Cancer Cell 23(3):316–331

33. Fan J, Kamphorst JJ, Mathew R, Chung MK, White E, Shlomi T et al (2013) Glutamine-driven oxidative phosphorylation is a major ATP source in transformed mammalian cells in both normoxia and hypoxia. Mol Syst Biol 9:712

34. Peng F, Wang JH, Fan WJ, Meng YT, Li MM, Li TT et al (2018) Glycolysis gatekeeper PDK1 reprograms breast cancer stem cells under hypoxia. Oncogene 37(8):1062–1074

35. Warburg O, Wind F, Negelein E (1927) The metabolism of tumors in the body. J Gen Physiol 8(6):519–530

36. Zhang H, Gao P, Fukuda R, Kumar G, Krishnamachary B, Zeller KI et al (2007) HIF-1 inhibits mitochondrial biogenesis and cellular respiration in VHL-deficient renal cell carcinoma by repression of C-MYC activity. Cancer Cell 11(5):407–420

37. Kim H, Lin Q, Glazer PM, Yun Z (2018) The hypoxic tumor microenvironment *in vivo* selects the cancer stem cell fate of breast cancer cells. Breast Cancer Res 20(1):16

38. Conley SJ, Gheordunescu E, Kakarala P, Newman B, Korkaya H, Heath AN et al (2012) Antiangiogenic agents increase breast cancer stem cells via the generation of tumor hypoxia. Proc Natl Acad Sci U S A 109(8):2784–2789

39. Hasmim M, Noman MZ, Messai Y, Bordereaux D, Gros G, Baud V et al (2013) Cutting edge: hypoxia-induced nanog favors the intratumoral infiltration of regulatory T cells and macrophages via direct regulation of TGF-β1. J Immunol 191(12):5802–5806

40. Maxwell PH, Dachs GU, Gleadle JM, Nicholls LG, Harris AL, Stratford IJ et al (1997) Hypoxia-inducible factor-1 modulates gene expression in solid tumors and influences both angiogenesis and tumor growth. Proc Natl Acad Sci U S A 94(15):8104–8109

41. Mathieu J, Zhang Z, Zhou W, Wang AJ, Heddleston JM, Pinna CM et al (2011) HIF induces human embryonic stem cell markers in cancer cells. Cancer Res 71(13):4640–4652

42. Pietras A, Gisselsson D, Ora I, Noguera R, Beckman S, Navarro S et al (2008) High levels of HIF-2alpha highlight an immature neural crest-like neuroblastoma cell cohort located in a perivascular niche. J Pathol 214(4):482–488

43. Hjelmeland AB, Wu Q, Heddleston JM, Choudhary GS, MacSwords J, Lathia JD et al (2011) Acidic stress promotes a glioma stem cell phenotype. Cell Death Differ 18(5):829–840

44. Qiang L, Wu T, Zhang HW, Lu N, Hu R, Wang YJ et al (2012) HIF-1α is critical for hypoxia-mediated maintenance of glioblastoma stem cells by activating notch signaling pathway. Cell Death Differ 19(2):284–294

45. Man J, Yu X, Huang H, Zhou W, Xiang C, Huang H et al (2018) Hypoxic induction of vasorin regulates notch1 turnover to maintain glioma stem-like cells. Cell Stem Cell 22(1):104–118

46. Xu W, Zhou W, Cheng M, Wang J, Liu Z, He S et al (2017) Hypoxia activates Wnt/β-catenin signaling by regulating the expression of BCL9 in human hepatocellular carcinoma. Sci Rep 7: 40446

47. Flavahan WA, Wu Q, Hitomi M, Rahim N, Kim Y, Sloan AE et al (2013) Brain tumor initiating cells adapt to restricted nutrition through preferential glucose uptake. Nat Neurosci 16(10): 1373–1382

48. Harrison H, Rogerson L, Gregson HJ, Brennan KR, Clarke RB, Landberg G (2013) Contrasting hypoxic effects on breast cancer stem cell hierarchy is dependent on ER-α status. Cancer Res 73(4):1420–1433
49. Thiery JP, Sleeman JP (2006) Complex networks orchestrate epithelial-mesenchymal transitions. Nat Rev Mol Cell Biol 7(2):131–142
50. Yang J, Mani SA, Donaher JL, Ramaswamy S, Itzykson RA, Come C et al (2004) Twist, a master regulator of morphogenesis, plays an essential role in tumor metastasis. Cell 117(7): 927–939
51. Peinado H, Portillo F, Cano A (2004) Transcriptional regulation of cadherins during development and carcinogenesis. Int J Dev Biol 48(5-6):365–375
52. Eun K, Ham SW, Kim H (2017) Cancer stem cell heterogeneity: origin and new perspectives on CSC targeting. BMB Rep 50(3):117–125
53. Mani SA, Guo W, Liao MJ, Eaton EN, Ayyanan A, Zhou AY et al (2008) The epithelial-mesenchymal transition generates cells with properties of stem cells. Cell 133(4):704–715
54. Hollier BG, Tinnirello AA, Werden SJ, Evans KW, Taube JH, Sarkar TR et al (2013) FOXC2 expression links epithelial-mesenchymal transition and stem cell properties in breast cancer. Cancer Res 73(6):1981–1992
55. Dembinski JL, Krauss S (2009) Characterization and functional analysis of a slow cycling stem cell-like subpopulation in pancreas adenocarcinoma. Clin Exp Metastasis 26(7):611–623
56. Ji Q, Hao X, Zhang M, Tang W, Yang M, Li L et al (2009) MicroRNA miR-34 inhibits human pancreatic cancer tumor-initiating cells. PLoS One 4(8):e6816
57. Ma C, Ding YC, Yu W, Wang Q, Meng B, Huang T (2015) MicroRNA-200c overexpression plays an inhibitory role in human pancreatic cancer stem cells by regulating epithelial-mesenchymal transition. Minerva Med 106(4):193–202
58. Song SJ, Ito K, Ala U, Kats L, Webster K, Sun SM et al (2013) The oncogenic microRNA miR-22 targets the TET2 tumor suppressor to promote hematopoietic stem cell self-renewal and transformation. Cell Stem Cell 13(1):87–101
59. Song SJ, Poliseno L, Song MS, Ala U, Webster K, Ng C et al (2013) MicroRNA-antagonism regulates breast cancer stemness and metastasis via TET-family-dependent chromatin remodeling. Cell 154(2):311–324
60. De Carolis S, Bertoni S, Nati M, D'Anello L, Papi A, Tesei A et al (2016) Carbonic anhydrase 9 mRNA/microRNA34a interplay in hypoxic human mammospheres. J Cell Physiol 231(7): 1534–1541
61. Papi A, De Carolis S, Bertoni S, Storci G, Sceberras V, Santini D et al (2014) PPARγ and RXR ligands disrupt the inflammatory cross-talk in the hypoxic breast cancer stem cells niche. J Cell Physiol 229(11):1595–1606
62. Taylor DD, Doellgast GJ (1979) Quantitation of peroxidase-antibody binding to membrane fragments using column chromatography. Anal Biochem 98(1):53–59
63. Bao B, Ali S, Ahmad A, Azmi AS, Li Y, Banerjee S et al (2012) Hypoxia-induced aggressiveness of pancreatic cancer cells is due to increased expression of VEGF, IL-6 and miR-21, which can be attenuated by CDF treatment. PLoS One 7(12):e50165
64. Takahashi RU, Miyazaki H, Takeshita F, Yamamoto Y, Minoura K, Ono M et al (2015) Loss of microRNA-27b contributes to breast cancer stem cell generation by activating ENPP1. Nat Commun 6:7318
65. Charles N, Ozawa T, Squatrito M, Bleau AM, Brennan CW, Hambardzumyan D et al (2010) Perivascular nitric oxide activates notch signaling and promotes stem-like character in PDGF-induced glioma cells. Cell Stem Cell 6(2):141–152
66. Lu J, Ye X, Fan F, Xia L, Bhattacharya R, Bellister S et al (2013) Endothelial cells promote the colorectal cancer stem cell phenotype through a soluble form of Jagged-1. Cancer Cell 23(2): 171–185
67. Zhu TS, Costello MA, Talsma CE, Flack CG, Crowley JG, Hamm LL et al (2011) Endothelial cells create a stem cell niche in glioblastoma by providing NOTCH ligands that nurture self-renewal of cancer stem-like cells. Cancer Res 71(18):6061–6072

68. Bao S, Wu Q, Sathornsumetee S, Hao Y, Li Z, Hjelmeland AB et al (2006) Stem cell-like glioma cells promote tumor angiogenesis through vascular endothelial growth factor. Cancer Res 66(16):7843–7848

69. Giannoni E, Bianchini F, Masieri L, Serni S, Torre E, Calorini L et al (2010) Reciprocal activation of prostate cancer cells and cancer-associated fibroblasts stimulates epithelial-mesenchymal transition and cancer stemness. Cancer Res 70(17):6945–6956

70. Liu S, Ginestier C, Ou SJ, Clouthier SG, Patel SH, Monville F et al (2011) Breast cancer stem cells are regulated by mesenchymal stem cells through cytokine networks. Cancer Res 71(2): 614–624

71. Su S, Chen J, Yao H, Liu J, Yu S, Lao L et al (2018) CD10(+)GPR77(+) cancer-associated fibroblasts promote cancer formation and chemoresistance by sustaining cancer stemness. Cell 172(4):841–56 e16

72. Kalluri R, Zeisberg M (2006) Fibroblasts in cancer. Nat Rev Cancer 6(5):392–401

73. Ostman A, Augsten M (2009) Cancer-associated fibroblasts and tumor growth–bystanders turning into key players. Curr Opin Genet Dev 19(1):67–73

74. Dvorak HF (1986) Tumors: wounds that do not heal. Similarities between tumor stroma generation and wound healing. N Engl J Med 315(26):1650–1659

75. Mueller MM, Fusenig NE (2004) Friends or foes - bipolar effects of the tumour stroma in cancer. Nat Rev Cancer 4(11):839–849

76. Orimo A, Gupta PB, Sgroi DC, Arenzana-Seisdedos F, Delaunay T, Naeem R et al (2005) Stromal fibroblasts present in invasive human breast carcinomas promote tumor growth and angiogenesis through elevated SDF-1/CXCL12 secretion. Cell 121(3):335–348

77. Gabbiani G, Ryan GB, Majne G (1971) Presence of modified fibroblasts in granulation tissue and their possible role in wound contraction. Experientia 27(5):549–550

78. Yu Y, Xiao CH, Tan LD, Wang QS, Li XQ, Feng YM (2014) Cancer-associated fibroblasts induce epithelial-mesenchymal transition of breast cancer cells through paracrine TGF-β signalling. Br J Cancer 110(3):724–732

79. Han ME, Kim HJ, Shin DH, Hwang SH, Kang CD, Oh SO (2015) Overexpression of NRG1 promotes progression of gastric cancer by regulating the self-renewal of cancer stem cells. J Gastroenterol 50(6):645–656

80. Martinez-Outschoorn UE, Goldberg A, Lin Z, Ko YH, Flomenberg N, Wang C et al (2011) Anti-estrogen resistance in breast cancer is induced by the tumor microenvironment and can be overcome by inhibiting mitochondrial function in epithelial cancer cells. Cancer Biol Ther 12(10):924–938

81. Hu Y, Yan C, Mu L, Huang K, Li X, Tao D et al (2015) Fibroblast-derived exosomes contribute to chemoresistance through priming cancer stem cells in colorectal cancer. PLoS One 10(5): e0125625

82. Boelens MC, Wu TJ, Nabet BY, Xu B, Qiu Y, Yoon T et al (2014) Exosome transfer from stromal to breast cancer cells regulates therapy resistance pathways. Cell 159(3):499–513

83. Acharyya S, Oskarsson T, Vanharanta S, Malladi S, Kim J, Morris PG et al (2012) A CXCL1 paracrine network links cancer chemoresistance and metastasis. Cell 150(1):165–178

84. Tang DG (2012) Understanding cancer stem cell heterogeneity and plasticity. Cell Res 22(3): 457–472

85. Loeffler M, Krüger JA, Niethammer AG, Reisfeld RA (2006) Targeting tumor-associated fibroblasts improves cancer chemotherapy by increasing intratumoral drug uptake. J Clin Invest 116(7):1955–1962

86. Rafii A, Mirshahi P, Poupot M, Faussat AM, Simon A, Ducros E et al (2008) Oncologic trogocytosis of an original stromal cells induces chemoresistance of ovarian tumours. PLoS One 3(12):e3894

87. Shibue T, Weinberg RA (2017) EMT, CSCs, and drug resistance: the mechanistic link and clinical implications. Nat Rev Clin Oncol 14(10):611–629

88. Lewis CE, Pollard JW (2006) Distinct role of macrophages in different tumor microenvironments. Cancer Res 66(2):605–612

89. Condeelis J, Pollard JW (2006) Macrophages: obligate partners for tumor cell migration, invasion, and metastasis. Cell 124(2):263–266
90. Bonde AK, Tischler V, Kumar S, Soltermann A, Schwendener RA (2012) Intratumoral macrophages contribute to epithelial-mesenchymal transition in solid tumors. BMC Cancer 12:35
91. Korkaya H, Kim GI, Davis A, Malik F, Henry NL, Ithimakin S et al (2012) Activation of an IL6 inflammatory loop mediates trastuzumab resistance in HER2+ breast cancer by expanding the cancer stem cell population. Mol Cell 47(4):570–584
92. Calabrese C, Poppleton H, Kocak M, Hogg TL, Fuller C, Hamner B et al (2007) A perivascular niche for brain tumor stem cells. Cancer Cell 11(1):69–82
93. Krishnamurthy S, Dong Z, Vodopyanov D, Imai A, Helman JI, Prince ME et al (2010) Endothelial cell-initiated signaling promotes the survival and self-renewal of cancer stem cells. Cancer Res 70(23):9969–9978
94. Frank NY, Schatton T, Frank MH (2010) The therapeutic promise of the cancer stem cell concept. J Clin Invest 120(1):41–50
95. Zhang Z, Dong Z, Lauxen IS, Filho MS, Nör JE (2014) Endothelial cell-secreted EGF induces epithelial to mesenchymal transition and endows head and neck cancer cells with stem-like phenotype. Cancer Res 74(10):2869–2881
96. Fukumura D, Jain RK (2007) Tumor microenvironment abnormalities: causes, consequences, and strategies to normalize. J Cell Biochem 101(4):937–949
97. Wong GS, Rustgi AK (2013) Matricellular proteins: priming the tumour microenvironment for cancer development and metastasis. Br J Cancer 108(4):755–761
98. Murai T (2015) Lipid raft-mediated regulation of hyaluronan-CD44 interactions in inflammation and cancer. Front Immunol 6:420
99. Oskarsson T, Acharyya S, Zhang XH, Vanharanta S, Tavazoie SF, Morris PG et al (2011) Breast cancer cells produce tenascin C as a metastatic niche component to colonize the lungs. Nat Med 17(7):867–874

Part III
Systemic *Onco-Sphere*

Chapter 18
Systemic *Onco-sphere*: An Overview from the Host's Perspective

Phei Er Saw and Erwei Song

Abstract Cancer is a systemic disease. Although many researchers are trying to eradicate cancer, their efforts are incomplete if the treatment modality does not take into account the host factor. Recently, researches were done to focus on the impact of host multiple characteristics, including age, comorbidity, and gender, to their treatment efficacy. There are complex physiological changes that are associated with aging, and common phenomena include the following: (1) decrease in metabolic function, (2) decrease in bone marrow reserve and self-renewal process, (3) alteration in hepatic and renal function, and many others. These physiological changes may lead to significant changes in drug pharmacokinetics (absorption, distribution, metabolism, and elimination) and drug toxicity, which renders anticancer drugs only pertain sub-optimal result in aging patients. Importantly, aging is parallel with comorbidity, and comorbidity has a strong link with cancer growth and progression. Therefore, in this chapter, we will highlight the importance of host physiological factors in cancer.

P. E. Saw
Guangdong Provincial Key Laboratory of Malignant Tumor Epigenetics and Gene Regulation, Guangdong-Hong Kong Joint Laboratory for RNA Medicine, Medical Research Center, Sun Yat-sen Memorial Hospital, Sun Yat-sen University, Guangzhou, China

Nanhai Translational Innovation Center of Precision Immunology, Sun Yat-sen Memorial Hospital, Sun Yat-sen University, Foshan, China

E. Song (✉)
Guangdong Provincial Key Laboratory of Malignant Tumor Epigenetics and Gene Regulation, Guangdong-Hong Kong Joint Laboratory for RNA Medicine, Medical Research Center, Sun Yat-sen Memorial Hospital, Sun Yat-sen University, Guangzhou, China

Nanhai Translational Innovation Center of Precision Immunology, Sun Yat-sen Memorial Hospital, Sun Yat-sen University, Foshan, China

Breast Tumor Center, Sun Yat-sen Memorial Hospital, Sun Yat-sen University, Guangzhou, China
e-mail: songew@mail.sysu.edu.cn

Introduction

Recently, researches were done to focus on the impact of host multiple characteristics, including age, comorbidity, and gender, to their treatment efficacy [1]. There are complex physiological changes that are associated with aging, and common phenomena include the following: (1) decrease in metabolic function, (2) decrease in bone marrow reserve and self-renewal process, (3) alteration in hepatic and renal function, and many others. These physiological changes may lead to significant changes in drug pharmacokinetics (absorption, distribution, metabolism, and elimination) and drug toxicity, which renders anticancer drugs only pertaining sub-optimal result in aging patients. Importantly, aging is parallel with comorbidity, and comorbidity has a strong link with cancer growth and progression. For example, in colon cancer patients, being diabetic increases the risk of cancer recurrence and mortality. In gender difference, biological features can vary significantly. For example, EGFR mutation, dihydropyrimidine dehydrogenase polymorphism, and hormone levels) may influence therapeutic toxicity and leads to therapeutic efficacy difference in female and male patients. So far, we have discussed the importance of viewing cancer as an ecosystem, from the disease point of view. Herein, we will look at the overview of the systemic *onco-sphere* from the host's point of view and how host (the systemic *onco-sphere*) could determine the outcome of cancer and their progression.

Host Physiological Factor in Cancer

Age

The majority of cancer diagnoses and deaths occur in patients over the age of 65, and in the US alone, population is aging at an alarming rate, with the number of persons over the age of 65 is expected to get double between the years 2000 and 2030. A sharp rise in the number of new cancer diagnoses is anticipated over the next 20 years due to the aging of the US population and the proven link between aging and cancer. By 2030, it is expected that cancer diagnoses will affect 70% of individuals over the age of 65. There are various explanations regarding this biological link between aging and cancer, including (1) increased DNA stability leading to potentially higher mutation, (2) telomere shortening leading to shorter life-span, (3) immune dysregulation, and (4) increased oxidative stress and other biochemical changes. Note that these links are usually bi-directional [2–5]. Although these theories are logically connected between aging and cancer, these theories did not clearly identify why some aged persons are more prone to one cancer when compared to another. Although little research has looked at cancer frequency and death at the extremes of age, suggestive data point to a possible decline in cancer prevalence around 85 years of age. Large cohort-based studies show a consistent increase in the likelihood of acquiring cancer over the age spectrum [6, 7].

Understanding the relationship between the biology of certain tumors and aging might assist direct therapeutic therapy. Cancer biology may also change depending on the age of presentation. For instance, in cases of acute myeloid leukemia, older persons had higher rates of unfavorable cytogenetics and more antecedent myelodysplasia [8]. Similar to this, the features of tumors in breast cancer change with age. HER2 overexpression decreases with age, although the prevalence of cancers that express hormone receptors rises [9]. The loss of physiologic reserve is correlated with aging. Due to physiologic changes that take place in several organ systems, this diminished reserve may alter how well patients tolerate anticancer treatment. Cytotoxic drugs excreted by the kidneys, such as cisplatin, carboplatin, etoposide, and methotrexate, may no longer be cleared as effectively as they once were as a result of age-related decreases in renal blood flow and glomerular filtration [10–13].

Due to aging-related muscle loss, serum creatinine may not correctly represent the renal function in older persons. To offer a more precise estimation of renal function with advancing age, a measure of glomerular filtration rate is necessary. Aging is also linked to reduced splanchnic blood flow and stomach enzyme production, which might affect the gastrointestinal absorption of oral medications like capecitabine [14, 15]. Although the clinical significance of these alterations is debatable, it is certain that as people age, their liver mass and cytochrome p450 content decrease [16, 17]. In older persons, decreased bone marrow reserve may lead to higher toxicity from myelosuppressive medications [13]. As a result, 65 years of age is included as a clinical determinant in the National Comprehensive Cancer Network and American Society of Clinical Oncology recommendations for primary prophylaxis with WBC growth factors [18, 19]. Numerous studies have sought to identify changes in pharmacokinetic parameters and resulting toxicities in older persons because of the complicated physiologic changes that come with age [20–31].

Comorbidity

The prevalence of comorbid diseases rises with age. In a study of 7,600 cancer patients over the age of 55, individuals between the ages of 55 and 64 had an average of 2.9 comorbid diseases, compared to those over the age of 75, who had an average of 4.2 comorbid disorders. The prevalence of comorbid diseases rises with age. In a study of 7600 cancer patients over the age of 55, individuals between the ages of 55 and 64 had an average of 2.9 comorbid diseases, compared to those over the age of 75, wh   average of 4.2 comorbid disorders [32]. A large cohort observa-
712) multiple cancer type cancers revealed that as comorbidities
s affected, in a dose-dependent fashion. Oncologists compare
y to that of a concomitant disease on life expectancy when
nt strategy. Although there are no clear rules, it seems that
onsidered in practice. Interestingly, patients with comorbid-
ld also affect the surgical outcome. For breast, prostate, and
ices such as axillary dissection, radical prostatectomy, and
enced by the existence and severity of comorbidity [33–

35]. Similarly, comorbidity seems to influence how chemotherapy is used across many cancers [36–38]. Although there is mixed evidence, it is probable that the latter trend reflects research that shows patients with comorbidity have increased chemotherapy-related toxicity [39–41].

Certain comorbidities may uniquely impact the prognosis and treatment result. Hormone treatment usage was linked to a greater risk of all-cause death including radiation and neoadjuvant hormone therapy for localized prostate cancer 5077 patients, who also had coronary artery disease, congestive heart failure, or a previous myocardial infarction [42]. In contrast, neither men with comorbid conditions nor those with just one risk factor for coronary artery disease saw an elevated mortality risk. Other research has looked at how diabetes affects the development of cancer. Several other studies found a higher risk of overall death incidence in colon cancer patients with diabetes (INT-0089) [43–45]. Elevated blood insulin levels, which accelerate colorectal cell line growth, may be the molecular cause of this condition [46]. Comorbidities may also affect a patient's tolerance to a particular therapy. For instance, early research on paclitaxel treatment revealed that individuals with a concurrent diagnosis of diabetes had a higher chance of developing severe neuropathy [47]. Similarly, individuals with pre-existing hypertension are more susceptible to cardiac toxicity when treated with trastuzuman (HER2-directed monoclonal antibody) [48, 49]. It is important to stress that it is important to differentiate between comorbidity and treatment-related toxicity since they may have distinct prognostic consequences. For instance, in clinical trials for various cancers, the vascular endothelial growth factor-targeting antibody bevacizumab has been shown to increase blood pressure [50–52].

Comorbidity: Host Obesity and Cancer

Obesity is a recognized epidemiologic risk factor for various malignancies, and it also has a detrimental impact on the prognosis for many but not all cancers [53–56]. Although obesity has steadily increased in prevalence over the past few [57, 58], the causes of the worse outcomes in many obese cancer patients and cancer survivors are complex. Not only does obesity itself is directly affecting patients OS, but also obesity-related biochemical changes in host. Numerous energy balance-related host variables have been shown to impact tumor growth and/or therapy response when cancer develops, even though they may also affect survival. As a consequence of metabolic and inflammatory alterations, obesity is often linked to increased oxidative stress, which is defined by an increased abundance of ROS [59, 60]. Singlet oxygen and superoxide molecules are produced as a consequence of the extremely reactive free radicals left behind after the incomplete reduction of oxygen. These free radicals may harm lipids, proteins, and nucleic acids if antioxidant defense systems in the cell are not able to neutralize them. In addition, various obesity-related cytokines and growth factors have been demonstrated to activate the P13K pathway by producing ROS, which has been linked to mutagenesis al tumor development, and metastasis [61, 62].

Comorbidity: Host Insulin Resistance and Cancer

Numerous malignancies, including colorectal, pancreatic, post-menopausal breast, and endometrial cancers, are more likely to develop and spread due to insulin resistance or hyperinsulinemia [63–66]. Insulin either directly affects preneoplastic and neoplastic cells through the insulin receptor (IR) or hybrid IR/IGF-1 receptors (IGF-1Rs) or indirectly affects them via IGF-1, estrogens, or other hormones. Insulin or IGF-1 can bind to surface receptors that are overexpressed on tumors (or pre-cancerous cells), to activate PI3K/AKT pathways, which in turn activates mTOR complex. mTOR is a key regulator in cell growth [67]. Furthermore, high insulin levels stimulate hepatic IGF-1 synthesis while suppressing the formation of IGF binding protein (BP)-1, increasing the biologic activity of IGF-1 [67, 68]. Therefore, insulin and IGF-1 are considered mitogens that are capable of stimulating cancer growth, while inhibiting apoptosis [68]. In fast-growing countries, intra-abdominal obesity is increasing at an alarming rate. Intra-abdominal obesity is defined as "uneven body fat distribution, especially intra-abdominal adipose tissue accumulation" in the waist area, a common phenomenon in middle-aged men. Intra-abdomninal obesity encourages insulin resistance, which is a condition in which tissues are less receptive to the physiological effects of insulin [69]. In type 2 diabetes, patients are often characterized by persistent hyperinsulinemia and insulin resistance, and both physiological conditions are now linked to a poor prognosis in many different cancers [53–56, 67–69] (Fig. 18.1).

Comorbidity: Host Metabolic Syndrome and Cancer

It has become widely accepted that metabolic syndrome is linked to an increased risk of cardiovascular disease [70]. Metabolic syndrome includes central obesity, high

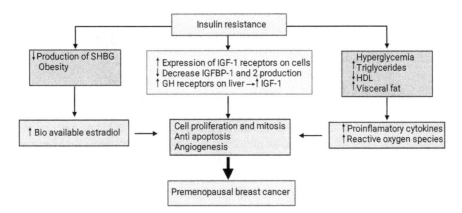

Fig. 18.1 Detailed mechanism of insulin resistance, obesity, and cellular biochemical changes that leads to an increment in pre-menopausal breast cancer

blood pressure, high fasting blood sugar, and dyslipidemia, the latter of which includes high triglyceridemia and low levels of HDL [71]. Increases in various pro-cancerous factors, such as inflammatory cytokines and chemokines, insulin and IGF-1, adipokines, etc., are often seen in patients with metabolic syndrome [71, 72]. Therefore, obese individuals with cancer who also have metabolic syndrome may be vulnerable to various variables operating synergistically to accelerate tumor development. Furthermore, any one of these associated factors might have an impact on tumor growth and progression [73, 74]. Metabolic syndrome has been linked to post-menopausal breast, colon, and other cancers [72–74]. These findings highlight the significance of preventing metabolic syndrome as a whole and/or developing methods to block crucial downstream sites of convergence, such as mTOR, which is a key player in mediating the proliferative and cell-growth impacts of several of these variables.

Comorbidity: Host Inflammation and Cancer

The relationship between inflammation (mostly chronic inflammation) and cancer are well-documented [75]. In short, inflammation influences all stages of tumorigenesis to promote the development of cancer. A series of changes could be seen in both innate and immune system, in response to inflammatory environment of the host. The cytokines (i.e., TNFα, soluble TNFR, IL-1, and IL-6) all show significant increases in circulation levels when there is chronic, low-grade systemic inflammation that often goes along with obesity [76]. The inflammatory environment is mostly mediated by macrophages or stromal adipocytes, where they could secrete cytokines to increase inflammation [76]. Depending on the cytokine and chemokine environments, macrophages could be activated to display either a traditional proinflammatory M1-like phenotype or an immunosuppressive M2-like phenotype [77, 78]. These details will be discussed in Chap. 21.

Inter-*onco Spherical* Communication: Host Physiological Factors Stress Response

Stress Effects on Angiogenesis

The creation of a blood supply is essential for the development and spread of tumors. VEGF, IL-6, TGF-β, and TNF-α are some factors that encourage angiogenesis [79, 80]. In both serum and tumor tissue, it has been shown that ovarian cancer patients had lower levels of VEGF if given perisurgical social support [81, 82]. Additionally, prolonged constraint stress enhanced tumor burden and invasiveness in orthotopic animal models of ovarian cancer, which was mediated by norepinephrine (NE)-driven elevations in VEGF and angiogenesis [83]. The fact that applying an α-blocker reversed the effects of the agonist isoproterenol confirmed the critical role played by adrenergic receptor signaling in mediating these effects. A shift in pro- to anti-angiogenic factors ratio may also promote angiogenesis. This balance is upset by the significant angiogenic factor IL-6, which is generated by tumor cells [84, 85]. Clinically, IL-6 levels in plasma and ascites were greater in ovarian cancer patients who had less social support [86]. Furthermore, NE could activate IL6/Src axis in the tumor cells, to trigger stress pathways that are essential for their expansion [83]. STAT3 is known to have a role in stress-induced tumor-associated angiogenesis. Through the activation of downstream targets to encourage proliferation and hinder apoptosis, STAT3 participates in various protumorigenic pathways. Usually, STAT3 activation requires cytokines and GFs such as VEGF and IL6, stress hormones (epinephrine and norepinephrine) can activate STAT3 in an IL-6-independent manner. Although STAT3 is activated in a non-cannonical manner, this still induces the nucleus translocation of STAT3, leading to increased gen transcription to induce cell survival, prolieferation, and angiogenesis [87].

Stress Effects on Tumor Growth and Invasion

Stress hormones may impact the growth and invasion of primary tumor cells by encouraging these cells to produce more MMPs and acting as chemoattractants to encourage cell migration. The antagonist propranolol fully prevented stress levels of NE from increasing the *in vitro* invasive potential of ovarian cancer cells by 89–198% [88]. Additional investigations showed that NE and E greatly boosted ovarian cancer cells' synthesis of MMP-2 and MMP-9 by triggering the adrenergic system [88]. Similar results have been observed in several other tumor types, including colon and head and neck malignancies [89–92]. In ovarian cancer patients, MMP-9 released by TAMs has been clinically linked to both depression and stress. Social support is believed to reduce both the effects of stress and have direct implications for health outcomes [93]. For instance, it was shown that those with little social support had reduced glucocorticoid response gene transcription and increased activity in proinflammatory transcription regulatory pathways [94]. Social isolation has been linked to enhanced tumor development in a mouse breast cancer model and raised mammary gland expression of many important metabolic genes involved in human carcinogenesis [95]. In a large cohort study, gene transcripts were obtained from ovarian cancer patients with serious depression and low levels of social supports. In these patients, a total of 200 gene transcripts were found to be upregulated as compared to their counterpartism and these transcripts (such as

CREB, NFKB, STAT, and ELK1) are important in the activation of signaling pathway in tumor growth [96].

Stress and Immune Response

The host immune response is downregulated by psychological conditions such as long-term stress, loneliness, and depression [97–99], mostly via adrenergic and glucocorticoid signaling pathways. Animal models used in experimental studies have shown that chronic stress, including surgical stress, can worsen tumor incidence and progression by inhibiting the cytotoxic activities of T cells (mainly Th1 cytokines) and NK cells, degrading antigen presentation, and boosting the activities of Treg cells [100–103]. After surgery, stress has been linked to declines in various cellular immunity indicators in breast cancer patients, including reduced Th1 vs Th2 cytokine production by T cells [104], decreased T-cell responsiveness to mitogen stimulation, and reduced NK cell cytotoxicity. Depression has been linked to a decreased cellular immune response to a range of particular antigens in individuals with metastatic breast cancer [105–107]. Interestingly, social support has been linked to higher NK activity in both peripheral blood and TIL [108, 109]. A detailed review on the link between inflammatory cytokines and depression and weariness could be found in [110–113].

Stress and Neuroendocrine Circadian Dysregulation

Clinical research has shown that stress may interfere with the daytime production of neuroendocrine hormones like cortisol. Cortisol dysregulation has been linked to a worse quality of life and worse outcomes in certain cancer patients. Diurnal serum cortisol rhythms have been documented to undergo significant modifications in tumor-affected animals and various cancer patients [114, 115]. It is unclear if these diurnal cortisol dysregulations result from tumor-produced inflammatory chemicals, stress and depression, or both [111, 116, 117]. Furthermore, dysregulations of diurnal cortisol have been closely linked to functional disability [118], fatigue [119], and poorer survival breast cancer patients [120]. There is evidence of a direct connection between glucocorticoids and cancer development. For instance, a breast tumor cell line's glucocorticoids directly boost a survival pathway and blocks apoptosis [121], downregulates BRCA1 and other DNA repair genes' expression [122]. Higher mean diurnal cortisol levels were seen in patients with advanced breast cancer who also had reduced cellular immunity to many antigens [107]. Indeed, glucocorticoids may impact aspects of quality of life, immunosurveillance, and tumor growth and progression; therefore, it should be investigated in deeper length.

Box 18.1 Stress, Cancer-Induced Depression (CID), Gut Microbiome, and Cancer

Chronic and acute stress can both lead to emotional disorder in individuals. Cancer induced depression (CID) is the most common emotional disorder in cancer patients, which has also been shown to be an important predictor of disease progression and elevated mortality [123, 124]. For example, it was reported that over 25% of women with breast cancer had elevated levels of depressive symptoms before their cancer diagnosis [125]. The pathological mechanism of the relationship between CID and cancer prognosis is very complex, CID may affect cancer progression by affecting the hypothalamic-pituitary-adrenocortical-immune   axis   (HPA   axis)   network [126, 127]. Recently, more evidences are pointing towards the microbiome-gut-brain (MGB) axis as a potent regulator of cancer [128]. Within this axis, the microbiota in the gut affect brain function, behaviors, and emotion through the immunoregulatory, neuroendocrine, and vagus pathways [129], and this axis is bi-directional. At the same time, emotional and mental states can also influence an individual's commensal microbes. On the one hand, depressive symptoms can affect the normal metabolism and growth and reproduction of gut microbiota, leading to the intestinal dysbiosis [130], which in turn leads to the microbiota's dysfunction of synthesizing or regulation of certain neuro-transmitters (such as γ-aminobutyric acid, 5-Serotonin, norepinephrine, etc.) [131], and induce abnormal immune response [132] and irregular inflamma-tion [133], causing dysfunction of HPA axis, which leads to the further development of depressive symptoms. For example, probiotic intervention can reduce individual cortisol levels and show antidepressant-like effects [134]. On the other hand, microbiome can affect the occurrence and develop-ment of malignant tumors by regulating host inflammation and immunity via participating in material metabolism, and destroying gene stability [135–137]. For example, researchers have found that gut microbes can not only significantly affect host immune abnormalities caused by antitumor drugs [135, 136], but also affect the antitumor treatment response of extraintestinal organs by affecting drug activity [137, 138]. In mouse models, supplementa-tion with Lactobacillus acidophilus and Bifidobacterium showed an anti-tumor effect by enhancing the immune response [139, 140]. It is interesting to note that stress, depression, and gut microbiome had been closely linked to the occurrence of cancer, revealing the intertwined relationship between host systemic onco-sphere and cancer, as we will discuss in detail in the following chapters (Fig. 18.2).

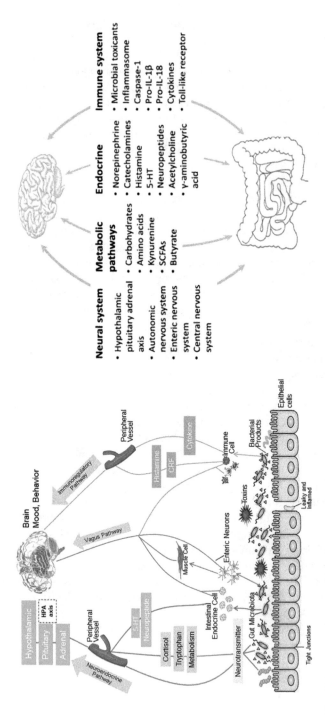

Fig. 18.2 The mechanism of intestinal microbiota in regulating brain function through the microbiome-gut-brain axis (left). Communication pathways gut microbes and brain are bi-diectional (right). In this axis, all host systemic *onco-sphere* are closely involved including host nervous system, host metabolic system, host endocrine system, and host immune system

stemic *Onco-sphere*: Sex Hormones on Cancer
ssion

Some of the most often diagnosed malignancies in industrialized nations are those that affect hormone-sensitive organs, including the breast, prostate, and, less frequently, the colon [141, 142]. The development of hormone-sensitive malignancies is etiologically related to host characteristics such as lifestyle, body composition, and endogenous hormone levels. Additionally, the three classes of steroids that make up sex hormones—estrogens, androgens, and progestogens—influence the development of several malignancies, and treatment approaches intended to alter hormone levels have significant clinical advantages. Growth of the initial lesion, lymph node status, and/or the emergence of a secondary metastasis are indicators of the impact of elements such as sex hormones on the development of the illness. The effectiveness of hormone withdrawal therapy utilizing certain inhibitors, which in this regard operate as pharmacologic probes, may be able to demonstrate this role in particular. Evidence of a tight connection with illness development may be obtained by correlating clinical effectiveness with the degree of hormone withdrawal [143, 144]. Additional proof may be found in relationships between prognosis and baseline tissue levels or circulating sex hormone levels. Last but not least, new analyses of gene expression patterns in conjunction with hormone production and disposition [145, 146] have shed light on the functional relationships between hormones and the clinical behavior of malignancies.

Host Endogenous Steroids

The main androgens are testosterone and androstenedione, which are transformed into estradiol and estrone, respectively, in a process (aromatization) mediated by aromatase, so named because it creates the aromatic A ring, which is the key characteristic of estrogens. Follicle-stimulating hormone levels serve as a feedback control mechanism for its action in gonadal tissues. Aromatase is also present in various organs such as breast, adipose tissue, brain, including the musciles, where its activity is controlled by mainly prostaglandin E2, c-AMP, and glucocorticoids [147]. Female peripheral tissues convert circulating adrenal androgens to estrogens after menopause when ovarian estrogen synthesis stops. Depending on the particular hormone, this seems to be tied to varying degrees of heredity and shared environmental factors [148–150]. A few genetic polymorphisms have been discovered that help to partially explain the genetic component [151, 152]. Two distinct genes in which each encode one of the two isoforms of the estrogen receptor (ER) [153, 154]. Estradiol is a high-affinity ligand for both receptors despite the fact that the two have significantly differing affinities for certain ligands. The binding of testosterone or 5-dihydrotestosterone activates the androgen receptor (AR). While the receptors are more receptive to these high-affinity ligands, binding of alternative lower affinity hormones may activate transcription when the most beneficial hormone is depleted, leading to the development of illness [155, 156]. In response to ligand binding to receptors, there are conformational changes, heat shock protein dissociation, phosphorylation, and dimerization [157, 158]. The target genes' promotor regions include response elements that the dimers bind to, which triggers the transcription of the target genes [159]. A tumor's response to steroidal stimulation seems to be significantly influenced by the expression of these coregulators.

In summary, we have seen interconnected links between systemic onco-spheres in the host that could cross-communicate with each other to protect the host from pathogenic invasion, especially cancer. However, upon losing this homeostasis, the cancer cell could hijack any part of the host ecosystem to favor their growth. Some of the current findings in host systemic onco-sphere-cancer relationship are summarized in Table 18.1.

Clinical Focus: Case Studies in Various Cancers

Case Study 1: Breast Cancer

Age has such an effect on breast cancer risk that risk increases by around 8.5% a year from menarche to menopause but by just 2.5% annually after menopause [176]. This implies that risk factors may have different effects on pre- and post-menopausal women. As a result, the frequency of breast cancer may provide several insights into the time of exposure and risk. The strongest evidence on radiation and risk, for instance, comes from the follow-up of women who were exposed to the atomic bomb, and it demonstrates that the dose and age at exposure have a significant impact on the risk of breast cancer [177]. Additionally, the influence of obesity on risk varies noticeably during life. Premenopausal incidence is negatively correlated with childhood and teenage obesity [178], as does obesity in early adulthood [179], but obesity after menopause causes breast cancer [180] and lowers survival rates after diagnosis.

Exercise is the other element of energy balance. Unlike obesity, it shows very consistent relationships with incidence and survival, with greater levels of physical activity being associated with a decreased risk of breast cancer incidence throughout premenopausal years [181] and among post-menopausal women [182]. Higher levels of physical activity are linked to a lower chance of breast cancer recurrence after diagnosis [183]. Alcohol use has been linked to a precursor or premalignant breast lesions, such as proliferative benign breast disease, and significantly impacts the likelihood of developing breast cancer [184]. According to feeding studies, hormone alterations may be a route through which alcohol causes breast cancer [185]. Data from many meta-analyses, prospective cohort studies, the more recent MillionWomenStudy, and prospective cohort studies together demonstrate a continuous monotonic rise in risk with increased alcohol consumption, with risk increasing by around 7% for every 10 g of alcohol consumed per day [186–188]. Although not

Table 18.1 Effect of host systemic onco-sphere on cancer

Effect of host systemic effect on cancer				
		Effect to local onco-sphere	Major findings	References
Metabolic regulation	Obesity	Immunosuppressive	• High-fat diet (HFD)-induced obesity increased CXCL1 concentration in the TME, driving CXCR2-mediated chemotaxis and accumulation of MDSCs in tumors • Moreover, in an HFD MMTV-PyMT breast cancer mouse model, leptin induced STAT3 activation in CD8$^+$ T effector cells to promote fatty acid oxidation and inhibited glycolysis and IFN-γ production of CD8$^+$ T cells, leading to CD8$^+$ T cell exhaustion	[160, 161]
	Obesity	Immunostimulatory	• In NSCLC and melanoma patients, higher body mass index correlated with better immunotherapy outcomes • Diet-induced metabolism alterations such as fasting-mimicking diet (FMD) could boost antitumor immunity • Reduced immunosuppressive MDSC numbers and increased numbers of activated CD8$^+$ T and NK cells in both peripheral blood and tumors	[162–164]
Hormone dysregulation	Exogenous corticosteroid administration	Immunosuppressive	• May impair ICB efficacy in melanoma patients and mouse models	[165, 166]
	Endogenous glucocorticoids (by tumor-	Immunosuppressive	• Activated the expression of multiple checkpoint receptors,	[166]

(continued)

Table 18.1 (continued)

Effect of host systemic effect on cancer				
		Effect to local onco-sphere	Major findings	References
	associated mye-loid cells)		such as PD-1, TIM3, and LAG3, in CD8$^+$ TILs, leading to T cell dysfunction	
The nervous system	Increased sympa-thetic nerve density	Immunosuppressive	• Sympathetic β-adrenergic norepi-nephrine derived from nontumor host cells impairs CTL infiltra-tion, facilitates MDSC infiltration, and improves their survival	[167, 168]
	Abrogating β-adrenergic signaling	Immunostimulatory	• Increased CD8$^+$ T cell infiltration, ele-vated CD8/Treg ratios, and decreased PD-1 expression, turning the TME into an immune-hot phenotype	[169]
	Tumor cell-derived GABA	Immunosuppressive	• Inhibited the infiltra-tion and function of CD8$^+$ T cells through β-catenin-induced CCL4/CCL5 downregulation • GABA signaling inhibition demon-strated higher CD4$^+$ and CD8$^+$ T cell and CD103$^+$ DC infiltra-tion, as well as better tumor control	[170]
	B cell-derived GABA	Immunosuppressive	• Promoted macro-phage anti-inflammatory polari-zation in mice and decreased cytotoxic CD8$^+$ T cell infiltra-tion in the TME	[171]
The microbiome	The gut microbiome	Immunostimulatory	• Modulate ICB responsiveness in non-gastrointestinal cancers • Transplanting fecal bacteria from ICB-responsive	[172]

(continued)

Table 18.1 (continued)

Effect of host systemic effect on cancer				
		Effect to local onco-sphere	Major findings	References
			melanoma patients into germ-free recipient mice have significantly boosted their immunity, as evidenced by higher CD8$^+$ T cell infiltration, which restored ICB sensitivity	
	Microbiota-derived products (cyclic di-adenosine monophosphate (c-di-AMP)	Immunostimulatory	Act as STING agonists and facilitate monocyte IFN-α/β production in the CRC mouse model	[173]
	Microbial metabolites (i.e., butyrate, inosine)	Immunostimulatory	Boost Th$_1$ and CTL responses	[174, 175]

all studies support this possible protection, greater folate consumption may counteract the negative impact of alcohol on incidence [189–191]. Alcohol use before diagnosis has been linked in certain studies to lower mortality, however alcohol consumption after diagnosis had no relation to survival outcomes [192–194].

Case Study 2: Colon Cancer

Through the study of colon polyps, an intermediate marker of colon cancer that likely takes 10–20 years of development before becoming invasive, we may more precisely comprehend the actions of causative and protective variables. As a result, we can assess the risk factors for mortality, invasive cancer, and polyps. Folate, for instance, may affect colorectal cancer risk differently depending on when it is exposed to the body, according to compelling research that is emerging in this area. The link between folic acid supplementation and the return of anemia has been shown to be null or positive in more recent animal [195] and epidemiologic investigations [196, 197]. The Aspirin/Folate Polyp Prevention Trial found that the folic acid supplementation group had a 67% higher chance of advanced lesions with high malignant potential and a less than twice higher probability of having at least three adenomas. Additional analyses of this research corroborate the idea that getting enough folate has advantages, but only up to a point beyond which there are no more advantages [198]. The dual function of folate in DNA pathways helps to explain these seeming discrepancies. Lack of folate may cause DNA instability and uracil misincorporation in the context of healthy mucosa [199], therefore, having enough folate in daily diet will lower the chance of developing colorectal cancer in its early, transformational phases. However, folate deficiency may work similarly to chemotherapy in the context of a preneoplasic lesion, which is going through faster cell divisions by impairing DNA synthesis and preventing the progression of a small adenoma toward cancer [200]. Folate deficiency or supplementation increases the risk that a minor lesion may advance by supplying the substrates for tumor replication and growth in preneoplastic or neoplastic tissue. Once a colon tumor has grown, chemotherapy drugs like fluorouracil depend on antifolate action to slow its development. Although the impact of folate status on colorectal cancer prognosis has received less research, prediagnostic plasma folate levels did increase or predict subsequent death [201]. A recent meta-analysis demonstrating that current smokers had a greater risk of colorectal cancer than non-smokers, which raises the possibility that smoking may induce permanent early-stage damage to healthy, normal colorectal mucosa [202]. Other dietary variables serve as excellent examples of the significance of determining how a risk factor may affect a disease's progress over time. For instance, studies on the effects of calcium supplementation show a negative correlation between calcium intake (1200–2000 mg/day) and the recurrence of colorectal adenoma [203] that persists for years after the supplement has been stopped [204].

Case Study 3: Lung Cancer

The relationship between smoking and lung cancer has been modeled to have high effects on smoking duration and age at onset, suggesting both an initiating and an extra later promoter impact [205]. It is widely known that genetic processes underpin the development of invasive lung carcinoma, squamous metaplasia, dysplasia, hyperplasia, and dysplasia from the normal epithelium [206]. The quick decline in incidence that follows smoking cessation provides further proof of the significance of the present smoking among middle-aged and older persons as a late promoter [207]. Smoking after diagnosis has additional negative consequences on lung cancer patients, increasing the probability of developing secondary malignancies and decreasing survival [208]. Both the etiologic effects of smoking and the effects of smoking after diagnosis are abundantly seen in head and neck cancer. Smoking is linked to an increased risk of lung, esophageal, oral cavity, and pharyngeal cancers after an oral cancer diagnosis. The risk of a second cancer is much lower five or more years after quitting [209], and those who stop are more likely to live for at least 18 months. These findings emphasize the need for cessation treatments for all smokers receiving cancer treatment [210].

Case Study 4: Prostate Cancer

The evidence supporting a link between obesity and prostate cancer is generally ambiguous. Recent investigations, however, have revealed that this could be the outcome of a failure to distinguish between low-grade and aggressive and metastatic malignancies [211]. Low testosterone levels in obese men may reduce their chance of lower-grade tumor development. However, cancers may become more aggressive in this low testosterone environment [212]. According to a meta-analysis, obesity was only linked to a higher chance of developing advanced illness when the tumors were looked at independently [213]. Subsequent investigations that also discovered an adverse relationship between obesity and low-grade cancers backed up this conclusion [214, 215]. In contrast, evidence points to lycopene's potential to help prevent prostate cancer and its recurrence. The evidence is somewhat scant, however. Similar to obesity, data points to various relationships depending on tumor grade. According to a recent qualitative study, lycopene is not linked to low-grade cancers, most of which are found via PSA screening, but it is protective against advanced and metastatic illnesses [216].

Conclusion

In this chapter, we looked at cancer ecosystem from the host point of view. We now understood that cancer is indeed a systemic disease, with complex interconnected communication from all angles, in the local, distal, and systemic *onco-spheres*. These information could be inter-communicated among these *onco-spheres* to ensure cancer growth and progression. Part 3 of this book will entail the role of each host systemic *onco-spheres* and how they were hijacked for cancer growth and metastasis.

References

1. Schilsky RL (2009) Personalizing cancer care: American Society of Clinical Oncology presidential address 2009. J Clin Oncol 27(23):3725–3730
2. Lustgarten J (2009) Cancer, aging and immunotherapy: lessons learned from animal models. Cancer Immunol Immunother 58(12):1979–1989
3. Slebos RJ, Li M, Vadivelu S, Burkey BB, Netterville JL, Sinard R et al (2008) Microsatellite mutations in buccal cells are associated with aging and head and neck carcinoma. Br J Cancer 98(3):619–626
4. Campisi J, Kim SH, Lim CS, Rubio M (2001) Cellular senescence, cancer and aging: the telomere connection. Exp Gerontol 36(10):1619–1637
5. Song YS, Lee BY, Hwang ES (2005) Dinstinct ROS and biochemical profiles in cells undergoing DNA damage-induced senescence and apoptosis. Mech Ageing Dev 126(5): 580–590

6. Stanta G, Campagner L, Cavallieri F, Giarelli L (1997) Cancer of the oldest old. What we have learned from autopsy studies. Clin Geriatr Med 13(1):55–68
7. Kanapuru B, Posani K, Muller D, Ershler WB (2008) Decreased cancer prevalence in the nursing home. J Am Geriatr Soc 56(11):2165–2166
8. Appelbaum FR, Gundacker H, Head DR, Slovak ML, Willman CL, Godwin JE et al (2006) Age and acute myeloid leukemia. Blood 107(9):3481–3485
9. Diab SG, Elledge RM, Clark GM (2000) Tumor characteristics and clinical outcome of elderly women with breast cancer. J Natl Cancer Inst 92(7):550–556
10. Bressolle F, Bologna C, Kinowski JM, Sany J, Combe B (1998) Effects of moderate renal insufficiency on pharmacokinetics of methotrexate in rheumatoid arthritis patients. Ann Rheum Dis 57(2):110–113
11. Toffoli G, Corona G, Sorio R, Robieux I, Basso B, Colussi AM et al (2001) Population pharmacokinetics and pharmacodynamics of oral etoposide. Br J Clin Pharmacol 52(5): 511–519
12. Go RS, Adjei AA (1999) Review of the comparative pharmacology and clinical activity of cisplatin and carboplatin. J Clin Oncol 17(1):409–422
13. Vestal RE (1997) Aging and pharmacology. Cancer 80(7):1302–1310
14. Yuen GJ (1990) Altered pharmacokinetics in the elderly. Clin Geriatr Med 6(2):257–267
15. Baker SD, Grochow LB (1997) Pharmacology of cancer chemotherapy in the older person. Clin Geriatr Med 13(1):169–183
16. Sawhney R, Sehl M, Naeim A (2005) Physiologic aspects of aging: impact on cancer management and decision making, part I. Cancer J 11(6):449–460
17. Sotaniemi EA, Arranto AJ, Pelkonen O, Pasanen M (1997) Age and cytochrome P450-linked drug metabolism in humans: an analysis of 226 subjects with equal histopathologic conditions. Clin Pharmacol Ther 61(3):331–339
18. Smith TJ, Khatcheressian J, Lyman GH, Ozer H, Armitage JO, Balducci L et al (2006) 2006 update of recommendations for the use of white blood cell growth factors: an evidence-based clinical practice guideline. J Clin Oncol 24(19):3187–3205
19. Crawford J, Armitage J, Balducci L, Bennett C, Blayney DW, Cataland SR et al (2009) Myeloid growth factors. J Natl Compr Cancer Netw 7(1):64–83
20. Sorio R, Robieux I, Galligioni E, Freschi A, Colussi AM, Crivellari D et al (1997) Pharmacokinetics and tolerance of vinorelbine in elderly patients with metastatic breast cancer. Eur J Cancer 33(2):301–303
21. Gauvin A, Pinguet F, Culine S, Astre C, Gomeni R, Bressolle F (2000) Bayesian estimate of vinorelbine pharmacokinetic parameters in elderly patients with advanced metastatic cancer. Clin Cancer Res 6(7):2690–2695
22. Jen JF, Cutler DL, Pai SM, Batra VK, Affrime MB, Zambas DN et al (2000) Population pharmacokinetics of temozolomide in cancer patients. Pharm Res 17(10):1284–1289
23. Fidias P, Supko JG, Martins R, Boral A, Carey R, Grossbard M et al (2001) A phase II study of weekly paclitaxel in elderly patients with advanced non-small cell lung cancer. Clin Cancer Res 7(12):3942–3949
24. Lichtman SM, Hollis D, Miller AA, Rosner GL, Rhoades CA, Lester EP et al (2006) Prospective evaluation of the relationship of patient age and paclitaxel clinical pharmacology: Cancer and Leukemia Group B (CALGB 9762). J Clin Oncol 24(12):1846–1851
25. Graham MA, Lockwood GF, Greenslade D, Brienza S, Bayssas M, Gamelin E (2000) Clinical pharmacokinetics of oxaliplatin: a critical review. Clin Cancer Res 6(4):1205–1218
26. Ando M, Minami H, Ando Y, Sakai S, Shimono Y, Sugiura S et al (1999) Pharmacological analysis of etoposide in elderly patients with lung cancer. Clin Cancer Res 5(7):1690–1695
27. Li J, Gwilt PR (2003) The effect of age on the early disposition of doxorubicin. Cancer Chemother Pharmacol 51(5):395–402
28. ten Tije AJ, Verweij J, Carducci MA, Graveland W, Rogers T, Pronk T et al (2005) Prospective evaluation of the pharmacokinetics and toxicity profile of docetaxel in the elderly. J Clin Oncol 23(6):1070–1077

29. Slaviero KA, Clarke SJ, McLachlan AJ, Blair EY, Rivory LP (2004) Population pharmaco-kinetics of weekly docetaxel in patients with advanced cancer. Br J Clin Pharmacol 57(1): 44–53

30. Cassidy J, Twelves C, Cameron D, Steward W, O'Byrne K, Jodrell D et al (1999) Bioequiv-alence of two tablet formulations of capecitabine and exploration of age, gender, body surface area, and creatinine clearance as factors influencing systemic exposure in cancer patients. Cancer Chemother Pharmacol 44(6):453–460

31. Milano G, Etienne MC, Cassuto-Viguier E, Thyss A, Santini J, Frenay M et al (1992) Influence of sex and age on fluorouracil clearance. J Clin Oncol 10(7):1171–1175

32. Yancik R (1997) Cancer burden in the aged: an epidemiologic and demographic overview. Cancer 80(7):1273–1283

33. Yancik R, Wesley MN, Ries LA, Havlik RJ, Edwards BK, Yates JW (2001) Effect of age and comorbidity in postmenopausal breast cancer patients aged 55 years and older. JAMA 285(7): 885–892

34. Smith TJ, Penberthy L, Desch CE, Whittemore M, Newschaffer C, Hillner BE et al (1995) Differences in initial treatment patterns and outcomes of lung cancer in the elderly. Lung Cancer 13(3):235–252

35. Konety BR, Cowan JE, Carroll PR (2008) Patterns of primary and secondary therapy for prostate cancer in elderly men: analysis of data from CaPSURE. J Urol 179(5):1797–1803. discussion 803.

36. Blanco JA, Toste IS, Alvarez RF, Cuadrado GR, Gonzalvez AM, Martín IJ (2008) Age, comorbidity, treatment decision and prognosis in lung cancer. Age Ageing 37(6):715 718

37. Hurria A, Wong FL, Villaluna D, Bhatia S, Chung CT, Mortimer J et al (2008) Role of age and health in treatment recommendations for older adults with breast cancer: the perspective of oncologists and primary care providers. J Clin Oncol 26(33):5386–5392

38. Keating NL, Landrum MB, Klabunde CN, Fletcher RH, Rogers SO, Doucette WR et al (2008) Adjuvant chemotherapy for stage III colon cancer: do physicians agree about the importance of patient age and comorbidity? J Clin Oncol 26(15):2532–2537

39. Moscetti L, Nelli F, Padalino D, Sperduti I, Giannarelli D, Pollera CF (2005) Gemcitabine and cisplatin in the treatment of elderly patients with advanced non-small cell lung cancer: impact of comorbidities on safety and efficacy outcome. J Chemother 17(6):685–692

40. Asmis TR, Ding K, Seymour L, Shepherd FA, Leighl NB, Winton TL et al (2008) Age and comorbidity as independent prognostic factors in the treatment of non small-cell lung cancer: a review of National Cancer Institute of Canada Clinical Trials Group trials. J Clin Oncol 26(1): 54–59

41. Aparicio T, Desramé J, Lecomte T, Mitry E, Belloc J, Etienney I et al (2003) Oxaliplatin- or irinotecan-based chemotherapy for metastatic colorectal cancer in the elderly. Br J Cancer 89(8):1439–1444

42. Nanda A, Chen MH, Braccioforte MH, Moran BJ, D'Amico AV (2009) Hormonal therapy use for prostate cancer and mortality in men with coronary artery disease-induced congestive heart failure or myocardial infarction. JAMA 302(8):866–873

43. Yancik R, Wesley MN, Ries LA, Havlik RJ, Long S, Edwards BK et al (1998) Comorbidity and age as predictors of risk for early mortality of male and female colon carcinoma patients: a population-based study. Cancer 82(11):2123–2134

44. Payne JE, Meyer HJ (1995) The influence of other diseases upon the outcome of colorectal cancer patients. Aust N Z J Surg 65(6):398–402

45. Meyerhardt JA, Catalano PJ, Haller DG, Mayer RJ, Macdonald JS, Benson AB 3rd et al (2003) Impact of diabetes mellitus on outcomes in patients with colon cancer. J Clin Oncol 21(3): 433–440

46. Tran TT, Medline A, Bruce WR (1996) Insulin promotion of colon tumors in rats. Cancer Epidemiol Biomark Prev 5(12):1013–1015

47. Rowinsky EK, Eisenhauer EA, Chaudhry V, Arbuck SG, Donehower RC (1993) Clinical toxicities encountered with paclitaxel (Taxol). Semin Oncol 20(4 Suppl 3):1–15

48. Suter TM, Procter M, van Veldhuisen DJ, Muscholl M, Bergh J, Carlomagno C et al (2007) Trastuzumab-associated cardiac adverse effects in the herceptin adjuvant trial. J Clin Oncol 25(25):3859–3865
49. Perez EA, Suman VJ, Davidson NE, Sledge GW, Kaufman PA, Hudis CA et al (2008) Cardiac safety analysis of doxorubicin and cyclophosphamide followed by paclitaxel with or without trastuzumab in the North Central Cancer Treatment Group N9831 adjuvant breast cancer trial. J Clin Oncol 26(8):1231–1238
50. Sandler A, Gray R, Perry MC, Brahmer J, Schiller JH, Dowlati A et al (2006) Paclitaxel-carboplatin alone or with bevacizumab for non-small-cell lung cancer. N Engl J Med 355(24):2542–2550
51. Miller K, Wang M, Gralow J, Dickler M, Cobleigh M, Perez EA et al (2007) Paclitaxel plus bevacizumab versus paclitaxel alone for metastatic breast cancer. N Engl J Med 357(26):2666–2676
52. Hurwitz H, Fehrenbacher L, Novotny W, Cartwright T, Hainsworth J, Heim W et al (2004) Bevacizumab plus irinotecan, fluorouracil, and leucovorin for metastatic colorectal cancer. N Engl J Med 350(23):2335–2342
53. LeRoith D, Novosyadlyy R, Gallagher EJ, Lann D, Vijayakumar A, Yakar S (2008) Obesity and type 2 diabetes are associated with an increased risk of developing cancer and a worse prognosis; epidemiological and mechanistic evidence. Exp Clin Endocrinol Diabetes 116 (Suppl 1):4–6
54. Parekh N, Okada T, Lu-Yao GL (2009) Obesity, insulin resistance, and cancer prognosis: implications for practice for providing care among cancer survivors. J Am Diet Assoc 109(8):1346–1353
55. Wiseman M (2008) The second World Cancer Research Fund/American Institute for Cancer Research expert report. Food, nutrition, physical activity, and the prevention of cancer: a global perspective. Proc Nutr Soc 67(3):253–256
56. Calle EE, Rodriguez C, Walker-Thurmond K, Thun MJ (2003) Overweight, obesity, and mortality from cancer in a prospectively studied cohort of U.S. adults. N Engl J Med 348(17):1625–1638
57. James PT, Leach R, Kalamara E, Shayeghi M (2001) The worldwide obesity epidemic. Obes Res 9(Suppl 4):228s–233s
58. Hedley AA, Ogden CL, Johnson CL, Carroll MD, Curtin LR, Flegal KM (2004) Prevalence of overweight and obesity among US children, adolescents, and adults, 1999-2002. JAMA 291(23):2847–2850
59. Valko M, Izakovic M, Mazur M, Rhodes CJ, Telser J (2004) Role of oxygen radicals in DNA damage and cancer incidence. Mol Cell Biochem 266(1-2):37–56
60. Furukawa S, Fujita T, Shimabukuro M, Iwaki M, Yamada Y, Nakajima Y et al (2004) Increased oxidative stress in obesity and its impact on metabolic syndrome. J Clin Invest 114(12):1752–1761
61. Cooke MS, Evans MD, Dizdaroglu M, Lunec J (2003) Oxidative DNA damage: mechanisms, mutation, and disease. FASEB J 17(10):1195–1214
62. Loft S, Poulsen HE (1996) Cancer risk and oxidative DNA damage in man. J Mol Med 74(6):297–312
63. Lukanova A, Zeleniuch-Jacquotte A, Lundin E, Micheli A, Arslan AA, Rinaldi S et al (2004) Prediagnostic levels of C-peptide, IGF-I, IGFBP -1, -2 and -3 and risk of endometrial cancer. Int J Cancer 108(2):262–268
64. Schairer C, Hill D, Sturgeon SR, Fears T, Pollak M, Mies C et al (2004) Serum concentrations of IGF-I, IGFBP-3 and c-peptide and risk of hyperplasia and cancer of the breast in postmenopausal women. Int J Cancer 108(5):773–779
65. Michaud DS, Wolpin B, Giovannucci E, Liu S, Cochrane B, Manson JE et al (2007) Prediagnostic plasma C-peptide and pancreatic cancer risk in men and women. Cancer Epidemiol Biomark Prev 16(10):2101–2109

66. Ma J, Giovannucci E, Pollak M, Leavitt A, Tao Y, Gaziano JM et al (2004) A prospective study of plasma C-peptide and colorectal cancer risk in men. J Natl Cancer Inst 96(7):546–553
67. Pollak M (2008) Insulin and insulin-like growth factor signalling in neoplasia. Nat Rev Cancer 8(12):915–928
68. Renehan AG, Frystyk J, Flyvbjerg A (2006) Obesity and cancer risk: the role of the insulin-IGF axis. Trends Endocrinol Metab 17(8):328–336
69. Calle EE, Kaaks R (2004) Overweight, obesity and cancer: epidemiological evidence and proposed mechanisms. Nat Rev Cancer 4(8):579–591
70. Alberti KG, Eckel RH, Grundy SM, Zimmet PZ, Cleeman JI, Donato KA et al (2009) Harmonizing the metabolic syndrome: a joint interim statement of the International Diabetes Federation Task Force on Epidemiology and Prevention; National Heart, Lung, and Blood Institute; American Heart Association; World Heart Federation; International Atherosclerosis Society; and International Association for the Study of Obesity. Circulation 120(16): 1640–1645
71. Cowey S, Hardy RW (2006) The metabolic syndrome: a high-risk state for cancer? Am J Pathol 169(5):1505–1522
72. Giovannucci E (2007) Metabolic syndrome, hyperinsulinemia, and colon cancer: a review. Am J Clin Nutr 86(3):s836–s842
73. Pothiwala P, Jain SK, Yaturu S (2009) Metabolic syndrome and cancer. Metab Syndr Relat Disord 7(4):279–288
74. Xue F, Michels KB (2007) Diabetes, metabolic syndrome, and breast cancer: a review of the current evidence. Am J Clin Nutr 86(3):s823–s835
75. Coussens LM, Werb Z (2002) Inflammation and cancer. Nature 420(6917):860–867
76. Ceciliani F, Giordano A, Spagnolo V (2002) The systemic reaction during inflammation: the acute-phase proteins. Protein Pept Lett 9(3):211–223
77. Sica A, Larghi P, Mancino A, Rubino L, Porta C, Totaro MG et al (2008) Macrophage polarization in tumour progression. Semin Cancer Biol 18(5):349–355
78. Mantovani A, Sozzani S, Locati M, Allavena P, Sica A (2002) Macrophage polarization: tumor-associated macrophages as a paradigm for polarized M2 mononuclear phagocytes. Trends Immunol 23(11):549–555
79. Spannuth WA, Sood AK, Coleman RL (2008) Angiogenesis as a strategic target for ovarian cancer therapy. Nat Clin Pract Oncol 5(4):194–204
80. Senger DR, Galli SJ, Dvorak AM, Perruzzi CA, Harvey VS, Dvorak HF (1983) Tumor cells secrete a vascular permeability factor that promotes accumulation of ascites fluid. Science 219(4587):983–985
81. Lutgendorf SK, Johnsen EL, Cooper B, Anderson B, Sorosky JI, Buller RE et al (2002) Vascular endothelial growth factor and social support in patients with ovarian carcinoma. Cancer 95(4):808–815
82. Lutgendorf SK, Lamkin DM, Jennings NB, Arevalo JM, Penedo F, DeGeest K et al (2008) Biobehavioral influences on matrix metalloproteinase expression in ovarian carcinoma. Clin Cancer Res 14(21):6839–6846
83. Nilsson MB, Armaiz-Pena G, Takahashi R, Lin YG, Trevino J, Li Y et al (2007) Stress hormones regulate interleukin-6 expression by human ovarian carcinoma cells through a Src-dependent mechanism. J Biol Chem 282(41):29919–29926
84. Cohen T, Nahari D, Cerem LW, Neufeld G, Levi BZ (1996) Interleukin 6 induces the expression of vascular endothelial growth factor. J Biol Chem 271(2):736–741
85. Nilsson MB, Langley RR, Fidler IJ (2005) Interleukin-6, secreted by human ovarian carcinoma cells, is a potent proangiogenic cytokine. Cancer Res 65(23):10794–10800
86. Costanzo ES, Lutgendorf SK, Sood AK, Anderson B, Sorosky J, Lubaroff DM (2005) Psychosocial factors and interleukin-6 among women with advanced ovarian cancer. Cancer 104(2):305–313

87. Landen CN Jr, Lin YG, Armaiz Pena GN, Das PD, Arevalo JM, Kamat AA et al (2007) Neuroendocrine modulation of signal transducer and activator of transcription-3 in ovarian cancer. Cancer Res 67(21):10389–10396

88. Sood AK, Bhatty R, Kamat AA, Landen CN, Han L, Thaker PH et al (2006) Stress hormone-mediated invasion of ovarian cancer cells. Clin Cancer Res 12(2):369–375

89. Yang EV, Sood AK, Chen M, Li Y, Eubank TD, Marsh CB et al (2006) Norepinephrine up-regulates the expression of vascular endothelial growth factor, matrix metalloproteinase (MMP)-2, and MMP-9 in nasopharyngeal carcinoma tumor cells. Cancer Res 66(21): 10357–10364

90. Yang EV, Bane CM, MacCallum RC, Kiecolt-Glaser JK, Malarkey WB, Glaser R (2002) Stress-related modulation of matrix metalloproteinase expression. J Neuroimmunol 133(1-2): 144–150

91. Drell TL, Joseph J, Lang K, Niggemann B, Zaenker KS, Entschladen F (2003) Effects of neurotransmitters on the chemokinesis and chemotaxis of MDA-MB-468 human breast carcinoma cells. Breast Cancer Res Treat 80(1):63–70

92. Masur K, Niggemann B, Zanker KS, Entschladen F (2001) Norepinephrine-induced migration of SW 480 colon carcinoma cells is inhibited by beta-blockers. Cancer Res 61(7):2866–2869

93. Cohen S (2004) Social relationships and health. Am Psychol 59(8):676–684

94. Cole SW, Hawkley LC, Arevalo JM, Sung CY, Rose RM, Cacioppo JT (2007) Social regulation of gene expression in human leukocytes. Genome Biol 8(9):R189

95. Williams JB, Pang D, Delgado B, Kocherginsky M, Tretiakova M, Krausz T et al (2009) A model of gene-environment interaction reveals altered mammary gland gene expression and increased tumor growth following social isolation. Cancer Prev Res 2(10):850–861

96. Lutgendorf SK, DeGeest K, Sung CY, Arevalo JM, Penedo F, Lucci J et al (2009) Depression, social support, and beta-adrenergic transcription control in human ovarian cancer. Brain Behav Immun 23(2):176–183

97. Irwin M (2002) Psychoneuroimmunology of depression: clinical implications. Brain Behav Immun 16(1):1–16

98. Zorrilla EP, Luborsky L, McKay JR, Rosenthal R, Houldin A, Tax A et al (2001) The relationship of depression and stressors to immunological assays: a meta-analytic review. Brain Behav Immun 15(3):199–226

99. Kiecolt-Glaser JK, Fisher LD, Ogrocki P, Stout JC, Speicher CE, Glaser R (1987) Marital quality, marital disruption, and immune function. Psychosom Med 49(1):13–34

100. Greenfeld K, Avraham R, Benish M, Goldfarb Y, Rosenne E, Shapira Y et al (2007) Immune suppression while awaiting surgery and following it: dissociations between plasma cytokine levels, their induced production, and NK cell cytotoxicity. Brain Behav Immun 21(4):503–513

101. Ben-Eliyahu S, Yirmiya R, Liebeskind JC, Taylor AN, Gale RP (1991) Stress increases metastatic spread of a mammary tumor in rats: evidence for mediation by the immune system. Brain Behav Immun 5(2):193–205

102. Ben-Eliyahu S, Page GG, Yirmiya R, Shakhar G (1999) Evidence that stress and surgical interventions promote tumor development by suppressing natural killer cell activity. Int J Cancer 80(6):880–888

103. Saul AN, Oberyszyn TM, Daugherty C, Kusewitt D, Jones S, Jewell S et al (2005) Chronic stress and susceptibility to skin cancer. J Natl Cancer Inst 97(23):1760–1767

104. Blomberg BB, Alvarez JP, Diaz A, Romero MG, Lechner SC, Carver CS et al (2009) Psychosocial adaptation and cellular immunity in breast cancer patients in the weeks after surgery: an exploratory study. J Psychosom Res 67(5):369–376

105. Thornton LM, Andersen BL, Crespin TR, Carson WE (2007) Individual trajectories in stress covary with immunity during recovery from cancer diagnosis and treatments. Brain Behav Immun 21(2):185–194

106. Andersen BL, Farrar WB, Golden-Kreutz D, Kutz LA, MacCallum R, Courtney ME et al (1998) Stress and immune responses after surgical treatment for regional breast cancer. J Natl Cancer Inst 90(1):30–36

107. Sephton SE, Dhabhar FS, Keuroghlian AS, Giese-Davis J, McEwen BS, Ionan AC et al (2009) Depression, cortisol, and suppressed cell-mediated immunity in metastatic breast cancer. Brain Behav Immun 23(8):1148–1155
108. Lutgendorf SK, Lamkin DM, DeGeest K, Anderson B, Dao M, McGinn S et al (2008) Depressed and anxious mood and T-cell cytokine expressing populations in ovarian cancer patients. Brain Behav Immun 22(6):890–900
109. Lutgendorf SK, Sood AK, Anderson B, McGinn S, Maiseri H, Dao M et al (2005) Social support, psychological distress, and natural killer cell activity in ovarian cancer. J Clin Oncol 23(28):7105–7113
110. Maier SF, Watkins LR (1998) Cytokines for psychologists: implications of bidirectional immune-to-brain communication for understanding behavior, mood, and cognition. Psychol Rev 105(1):83–107
111. Lutgendorf SK, Weinrib AZ, Penedo F, Russell D, DeGeest K, Costanzo ES et al (2008) Interleukin-6, cortisol, and depressive symptoms in ovarian cancer patients. J Clin Oncol 26(29):4820–4827
112. Bower JE (2007) Cancer-related fatigue: links with inflammation in cancer patients and survivors. Brain Behav Immun 21(7):863–871
113. Collado-Hidalgo A, Bower JE, Ganz PA, Cole SW, Irwin MR (2006) Inflammatory biomarkers for persistent fatigue in breast cancer survivors. Clin Cancer Res 12(9):2759–2766
114. Touitou Y, Bogdan A, Lévi F, Benavides M, Auzéby A (1996) Disruption of the circadian patterns of serum cortisol in breast and ovarian cancer patients: relationships with tumour marker antigens. Br J Cancer 74(8):1248–1252
115. Sephton S, Spiegel D (2003) Circadian disruption in cancer: a neuroendocrine-immune pathway from stress to disease? Brain Behav Immun 17(5):321–328
116. Jehn CF, Kuehnhardt D, Bartholomae A, Pfeiffer S, Krebs M, Regierer AC et al (2006) Biomarkers of depression in cancer patients. Cancer 107(11):2723–2729
117. Musselman DL, Miller AH, Porter MR, Manatunga A, Gao F, Penna S et al (2001) Higher than normal plasma interleukin-6 concentrations in cancer patients with depression: preliminary findings. Am J Psychiatry 158(8):1252–1257
118. Touitou Y, Lévi F, Bogdan A, Benavides M, Bailleul F, Misset JL (1995) Rhythm alteration in patients with metastatic breast cancer and poor prognostic factors. J Cancer Res Clin Oncol 121(3):181–188
119. Bower JE, Ganz PA, Dickerson SS, Petersen L, Aziz N, Fahey JL (2005) Diurnal cortisol rhythm and fatigue in breast cancer survivors. Psychoneuroendocrinology 30(1):92–100
120. Sephton SE, Sapolsky RM, Kraemer HC, Spiegel D (2000) Diurnal cortisol rhythm as a predictor of breast cancer survival. J Natl Cancer Inst 92(12):994–1000
121. Moran TJ, Gray S, Mikosz CA, Conzen SD (2000) The glucocorticoid receptor mediates a survival signal in human mammary epithelial cells. Cancer Res 60(4):867–872
122. Antonova L, Mueller CR (2008) Hydrocortisone down-regulates the tumor suppressor gene BRCA1 in mammary cells: a possible molecular link between stress and breast cancer. Genes Chromosomes Cancer 47(4):341–352
123. Pinquart M, Duberstein PR (2010) Depression and cancer mortality: a meta-analysis. Psychol Med 40(11):1797–1810
124. Schneider S, Moyer A (2010) Depression as a predictor of disease progression and mortality in cancer patients: a meta-analysis. Cancer 116(13):3304; author reply 5.
125. Van Esch L, Roukema JA, Ernst MF, Nieuwenhuijzen GA, De Vries J (2012) Combined anxiety and depressive symptoms before diagnosis of breast cancer. J Affect Disord 136(3): 895–901
126. Bortolato B, Hyphantis TN, Valpione S, Perini G, Maes M, Morris G et al (2017) Depression in cancer: the many biobehavioral pathways driving tumor progression. Cancer Treat Rev 52: 58–70

127. Ahmad MH, Rizvi MA, Fatima M, Mondal AC (2021) Pathophysiological implications of neuroinflammation mediated HPA axis dysregulation in the prognosis of cancer and depression. Mol Cell Endocrinol 520:111093
128. Margolis KG, Cryan JF, Mayer EA (2021) The microbiota-gut-brain axis: from motility to mood. Gastroenterology 160(5):1486–1501
129. Li Y, Hao Y, Fan F, Zhang B (2018) The role of microbiome in insomnia, circadian disturbance and depression. Front Psych 9:669
130. Sun Y, Zhang M, Chen CC, Gillilland M, Sun X, El-Zaatari M et al (2013) Stress-induced corticotropin-releasing hormone-mediated NLRP6 inflammasome inhibition and transmissible enteritis in mice. Gastroenterology 144(7):1478–1487, 87e1-8.
131. Rieder R, Wisniewski PJ, Alderman BL, Campbell SC (2017) Microbes and mental health: a review. Brain Behav Immun 66:9–17
132. Beurel E, Toups M, Nemeroff CB (2020) The bidirectional relationship of depression and inflammation: double trouble. Neuron 107(2):234–256
133. Sha Q, Madaj Z, Keaton S, Escobar Galvis ML, Smart L, Krzyzanowski S et al (2022) Cytokines and tryptophan metabolites can predict depressive symptoms in pregnancy. Transl Psychiatry 12(1):35
134. Burokas A, Arboleya S, Moloney RD, Peterson VL, Murphy K, Clarke G et al (2017) Targeting the microbiota-gut-brain axis: prebiotics have anxiolytic and antidepressant-like effects and reverse the impact of chronic stress in mice. Biol Psychiatry 82(7):472–487
135. McQuade JL, Daniel CR, Helmink BA, Wargo JA (2019) Modulating the microbiome to improve therapeutic response in cancer. Lancet Oncol 20(2):e77–e91
136. Routy B, Le Chatelier E, Derosa L, Duong CPM, Alou MT, Daillere R et al (2018) Gut microbiome influences efficacy of PD-1-based immunotherapy against epithelial tumors. Science 359(6371):91–97
137. Oliva M, Mulet-Margalef N, Ochoa-De-Olza M, Napoli S, Mas J, Laquente B et al (2021) Tumor-associated microbiome: where do we stand? Int J Mol Sci 22:3
138. Pennisi E (2013) Biomedicine. Cancer therapies use a little help from microbial friends. Science 342(6161):921
139. Imani Fooladi AA, Yazdi MH, Pourmand MR, Mirshafiey A, Hassan ZM, Azizi T et al (2015) Th1 cytokine production induced by Lactobacillus acidophilus in BALB/c mice bearing transplanted breast tumor. Jundishapur J Microbiol 8(4):e17354
140. Sivan A, Corrales L, Hubert N, Williams JB, Aquino-Michaels K, Earley ZM et al (2015) Commensal Bifidobacterium promotes antitumor immunity and facilitates anti-PD-L1 efficacy. Science 350(6264):1084–1089
141. Folkerd EJ, Dowsett M (2010) Influence of sex hormones on cancer progression. J Clin Oncol 28(26):4038–4044
142. Greenlee RT, Hill-Harmon MB, Murray T, Thun M (2001) Cancer statistics, 2001. CA Cancer J Clin 51(1):15–36
143. MacNeill FA, Jones AL, Jacobs S, Lønning PE, Powles TJ, Dowsett M (1992) The influence of aminoglutethimide and its analogue rogletimide on peripheral aromatisation in breast cancer. Br J Cancer 66(4):692–697
144. Gershanovich M, Chaudri HA, Campos D, Lurie H, Bonaventura A, Jeffrey M et al (1998) Letrozole, a new oral aromatase inhibitor: randomised trial comparing 2.5 mg daily, 0.5 mg daily and aminoglutethimide in postmenopausal women with advanced breast cancer. Letrozole International Trial Group (AR/BC3). Ann Oncol 9(6):639–645
145. Kristensen VN, Sørlie T, Geisler J, Langerød A, Yoshimura N, Kåresen R et al (2005) Gene expression profiling of breast cancer in relation to estrogen receptor status and estrogen-metabolizing enzymes: clinical implications. Clin Cancer Res 11(2 Pt 2):878s–883s
146. Dutertre M, Gratadou L, Dardenne E, Germann S, Samaan S, Lidereau R et al (2010) Estrogen regulation and physiopathologic significance of alternative promoters in breast cancer. Cancer Res 70(9):3760–3770

147. Simpson ER, Mahendroo MS, Means GD, Kilgore MW, Corbin CJ, Mendelson CR (1993) Tissue-specific promoters regulate aromatase cytochrome P450 expression. J Steroid Biochem Mol Biol 44(4-6):321–330

148. Stone J, Folkerd E, Doody D, Schroen C, Treloar SA, Giles GG et al (2009) Familial correlations in postmenopausal serum concentrations of sex steroid hormones and other mitogens: a twins and sisters study. J Clin Endocrinol Metab 94(12):4793–4800

149. Kuijper EA, Lambalk CB, Boomsma DI, van der Sluis S, Blankenstein MA, de Geus EJ et al (2007) Heritability of reproductive hormones in adult male twins. Hum Reprod 22(8): 2153–2159

150. Ring HZ, Lessov CN, Reed T, Marcus R, Holloway L, Swan GE et al (2005) Heritability of plasma sex hormones and hormone binding globulin in adult male twins. J Clin Endocrinol Metab 90(6):3653–3658

151. Eriksson AL, Lorentzon M, Vandenput L, Labrie F, Lindersson M, Syvänen AC et al (2009) Genetic variations in sex steroid-related genes as predictors of serum estrogen levels in men. J Clin Endocrinol Metab 94(3):1033–1041

152. Dunning AM, Dowsett M, Healey CS, Tee L, Luben RN, Folkerd E et al (2004) Polymorphisms associated with circulating sex hormone levels in postmenopausal women. J Natl Cancer Inst 96(12):936–945

153. Fox EM, Davis RJ, Shupnik MA (2008) ERbeta in breast cancer–onlooker, passive player, or active protector? Steroids 73(11):1039–1051

154. Nilsson S, Mäkelä S, Treuter E, Tujague M, Thomsen J, Andersson G et al (2001) Mechanisms of estrogen action. Physiol Rev 81(4):1535–1565

155. Dorgan JF, Stanczyk FZ, Longcope C, Stephenson HE Jr, Chang L, Miller R et al (1997) Relationship of serum dehydroepiandrosterone (DHEA), DHEA sulfate, and 5-androstene-3 beta, 17 beta-diol to risk of breast cancer in postmenopausal women. Cancer Epidemiol Biomark Prev 6(3):177–181

156. Sikora MJ, Cordero KE, Larios JM, Johnson MD, Lippman ME, Rae JM (2009) The androgen metabolite 5alpha-androstane-3beta,17beta-diol (3betaAdiol) induces breast cancer growth via estrogen receptor: implications for aromatase inhibitor resistance. Breast Cancer Res Treat 115(2):289–296

157. Kumar V, Chambon P (1988) The estrogen receptor binds tightly to its responsive element as a ligand-induced homodimer. Cell 55(1):145–156

158. Le Goff P, Montano MM, Schodin DJ, Katzenellenbogen BS (1994) Phosphorylation of the human estrogen receptor. Identification of hormone-regulated sites and examination of their influence on transcriptional activity. J Biol Chem 269(6):4458–4466

159. McKenna NJ, Lanz RB, O'Malley BW (1999) Nuclear receptor coregulators: cellular and molecular biology. Endocr Rev 20(3):321–344

160. Gibson JT, Orlandella RM, Turbitt WJ, Behring M, Manne U, Sorge RE et al (2020) Obesity-associated myeloid-derived suppressor cells promote apoptosis of tumor-infiltrating CD8 T cells and immunotherapy resistance in breast cancer. Front Immunol 11:590794

161. Zhang C, Yue C, Herrmann A, Song J, Egelston C, Wang T et al (2020) STAT3 activation-induced fatty acid oxidation in CD8(+) T effector cells is critical for obesity-promoted breast tumor growth. Cell Metab 31(1):148–161

162. Kichenadasse G, Miners JO, Mangoni AA, Rowland A, Hopkins AM, Sorich MJ (2020) Association between body mass index and overall survival with immune checkpoint inhibitor therapy for advanced non-small cell lung cancer. JAMA Oncol 6(4):512–518

163. McQuade JL, Daniel CR, Hess KR, Mak C, Wang DY, Rai RR et al (2018) Association of body-mass index and outcomes in patients with metastatic melanoma treated with targeted therapy, immunotherapy, or chemotherapy: a retrospective, multicohort analysis. Lancet Oncol 19(3):310–322

164. Vernieri C, Fuca G, Ligorio F, Huber V, Vingiani A, Iannelli F et al (2022) Fasting-mimicking diet is safe and reshapes metabolism and antitumor immunity in patients with cancer. Cancer Discov 12(1):90–107

165. Bai X, Hu J, Betof Warner A, Quach HT, Cann CG, Zhang MZ et al (2021) Early use of high-dose glucocorticoid for the management of irAE is associated with poorer survival in patients with advanced melanoma treated with anti-PD-1 monotherapy. Clin Cancer Res 27(21): 5993–6000

166. Acharya N, Madi A, Zhang H, Klapholz M, Escobar G, Dulberg S et al (2020) Endogenous glucocorticoid signaling regulates CD8(+) T cell differentiation and development of dysfunction in the tumor microenvironment. Immunity 53(3):658–71 e6

167. Mohammadpour H, MacDonald CR, Qiao G, Chen M, Dong B, Hylander BL et al (2019) Beta2 adrenergic receptor-mediated signaling regulates the immunosuppressive potential of myeloid-derived suppressor cells. J Clin Invest 129(12):5537–5552

168. Bucsek MJ, Qiao G, MacDonald CR, Giridharan T, Evans L, Niedzwecki B et al (2017) Beta-adrenergic signaling in mice housed at standard temperatures suppresses an effector phenotype in CD8(+) T cells and undermines checkpoint inhibitor therapy. Cancer Res 77(20): 5639–5651

169. Qiao G, Bucsek MJ, Winder NM, Chen M, Giridharan T, Olejniczak SH, Hylander BL, Repasky EA (2019) β-Adrenergic signaling blocks murine CD8+ T-cell metabolic reprogramming during activation: a mechanism for immunosuppression by adrenergic stress. Cancer Immunol Immunother 68(1):11–22. https://doi.org/10.1007/s00262-018-2243-8

170. Huang WY, Thompson JW, Yin T, Alexander PB, Qin D et al (2022) Cancer-cell-derived GABA promotes beta-catenin-mediated tumour growth and immunosuppression. Nat Cell Biol 24(2):230–241

171. Zhang B, Vogelzang A, Miyajima M, Sugiura Y, Wu Y, Chamoto K et al (2021) B cell-derived GABA elicits IL-10(+) macrophages to limit anti-tumour immunity. Nature 599(7885):471–476

172. Helmink BA, Khan MAW, Hermann A, Gopalakrishnan V, Wargo JA (2019) The microbiome, cancer, and cancer therapy. Nat Med 25(3):377–388

173. Lam KC, Araya RE, Huang A, Chen Q, Di Modica M, Rodrigues RR et al (2021) Microbiota triggers STING-type I IFN-dependent monocyte reprogramming of the tumor microenvironment. Cell 184(21):5338–5356

174. He Y, Fu L, Li Y, Wang W, Gong M, Zhang J et al (2021) Gut microbial metabolites facilitate anticancer therapy efficacy by modulating cytotoxic CD8(+) T cell immunity. Cell Metab 33(5):988–1000

175. Mager LF, Burkhard R, Pett N, Cooke NCA, Brown K, Ramay H et al (2020) Microbiome-derived inosine modulates response to checkpoint inhibitor immunotherapy. Science 369(6510):1481–1489

176. Colditz GA, Rosner B (2000) Cumulative risk of breast cancer to age 70 years according to risk factor status: data from the Nurses' Health Study. Am J Epidemiol 152(10):950–964

177. Land CE, Tokunaga M, Koyama K, Soda M, Preston DL, Nishimori I et al (2003) Incidence of female breast cancer among atomic bomb survivors, Hiroshima and Nagasaki, 1950-1990. Radiat Res 160(6):707–717

178. Baer HJ, Colditz GA, Rosner B, Michels KB, Rich-Edwards JW, Hunter DJ et al (2005) Body fatness during childhood and adolescence and incidence of breast cancer in premenopausal women: a prospective cohort study. Breast Cancer Res 7(3):R314–R325

179. Willett WC, Browne ML, Bain C, Lipnick RJ, Stampfer MJ, Rosner B et al (1985) Relative weight and risk of breast cancer among premenopausal women. Am J Epidemiol 122(5): 731–740

180. Bianchini F, Kaaks R, Vainio H (2002) Weight control and physical activity in cancer prevention. Obes Rev 3(1):5–8

181. Maruti SS, Willett WC, Feskanich D, Rosner B, Colditz GA (2008) A prospective study of age-specific physical activity and premenopausal breast cancer. J Natl Cancer Inst 100(10): 728–737

182. Rockhill B, Willett WC, Hunter DJ, Manson JE, Hankinson SE, Colditz GA (1999) A prospective study of recreational physical activity and breast cancer risk. Arch Intern Med 159(19):2290–2296

183. Holmes MD, Chen WY, Feskanich D, Kroenke CH, Colditz GA (2005) Physical activity and survival after breast cancer diagnosis. JAMA 293(20):2479–2486

184. Willett WC, Stampfer MJ, Colditz GA, Rosner BA, Hennekens CH, Speizer FE (1987) Moderate alcohol consumption and the risk of breast cancer. N Engl J Med 316(19): 1174–1180

185. Reichman ME, Judd JT, Longcope C, Schatzkin A, Clevidence BA, Nair PP et al (1993) Effects of alcohol consumption on plasma and urinary hormone concentrations in premenopausal women. J Natl Cancer Inst 85(9):722–727

186. Smith-Warner SA, Spiegelman D, Yaun SS, van den Brandt PA, Folsom AR, Goldbohm RA et al (1998) Alcohol and breast cancer in women: a pooled analysis of cohort studies. JAMA 279(7):535–540

187. Allen NE, Beral V, Casabonne D, Kan SW, Reeves GK, Brown A et al (2009) Moderate alcohol intake and cancer incidence in women. J Natl Cancer Inst 101(5):296–305

188. Hamajima N, Hirose K, Tajima K, Rohan T, Calle EE, Heath CW Jr et al (2002) Alcohol, tobacco and breast cancer–collaborative reanalysis of individual data from 53 epidemiological studies, including 58,515 women with breast cancer and 95,067 women without the disease. Br J Cancer 87(11):1234–1245

189. Sellers TA, Kushi LH, Cerhan JR, Vierkant RA, Gapstur SM, Vachon CM et al (2001) Dietary folate intake, alcohol, and risk of breast cancer in a prospective study of postmenopausal women. Epidemiology 12(4):420–428

190. Zhang SM, Willett WC, Selhub J, Hunter DJ, Giovannucci EL, Holmes MD et al (2003) Plasma folate, vitamin B6, vitamin B12, homocysteine, and risk of breast cancer. J Natl Cancer Inst 95(5):373–380

191. Lin J, Lee IM, Cook NR, Selhub J, Manson JE, Buring JE et al (2008) Plasma folate, vitamin B-6, vitamin B-12, and risk of breast cancer in women. Am J Clin Nutr 87(3):734–743

192. Holmes MD, Stampfer MJ, Colditz GA, Rosner B, Hunter DJ, Willett WC (1999) Dietary factors and the survival of women with breast carcinoma. Cancer 86(5):826–835

193. Reding KW, Daling JR, Doody DR, O'Brien CA, Porter PL, Malone KE (2008) Effect of prediagnostic alcohol consumption on survival after breast cancer in young women. Cancer Epidemiol Biomark Prev 17(8):1988–1996

194. Barnett GC, Shah M, Redman K, Easton DF, Ponder BA, Pharoah PD (2008) Risk factors for the incidence of breast cancer: do they affect survival from the disease? J Clin Oncol 26(20): 3310–3316

195. Song J, Sohn KJ, Medline A, Ash C, Gallinger S, Kim YI (2000) Chemopreventive effects of dietary folate on intestinal polyps in Apc+/-Msh2-/- mice. Cancer Res 60(12):3191–3199

196. Logan RF, Grainge MJ, Shepherd VC, Armitage NC, Muir KR (2008) Aspirin and folic acid for the prevention of recurrent colorectal adenomas. Gastroenterology 134(1):29–38

197. Cole BF, Baron JA, Sandler RS, Haile RW, Ahnen DJ, Bresalier RS et al (2007) Folic acid for the prevention of colorectal adenomas: a randomized clinical trial. JAMA 297(21):2351–2359

198. Figueiredo JC, Levine AJ, Grau MV, Barry EL, Ueland PM, Ahnen DJ et al (2008) Colorectal adenomas in a randomized folate trial: the role of baseline dietary and circulating folate levels. Cancer Epidemiol Biomark Prev 17(10):2625–2631

199. Wickramasinghe SN, Fida S (1993) Misincorporation of uracil into the DNA of folate- and B12-deficient HL60 cells. Eur J Haematol 50(3):127–132

200. Kim YI (2007) Folate and colorectal cancer: an evidence-based critical review. Mol Nutr Food Res 51(3):267–292

201. Wolpin BM, Wei EK, Ng K, Meyerhardt JA, Chan JA, Selhub J et al (2008) Prediagnostic plasma folate and the risk of death in patients with colorectal cancer. J Clin Oncol 26(19): 3222–3228

202. Liang PS, Chen TY, Giovannucci E (2009) Cigarette smoking and colorectal cancer incidence and mortality: systematic review and meta-analysis. Int J Cancer 124(10):2406–2415

203. Baron JA, Beach M, Mandel JS, van Stolk RU, Haile RW, Sandler RS et al (1999) Calcium supplements for the prevention of colorectal adenomas. Calcium Polyp Prevention Study Group. N Engl J Med 340(2):101–107

204. Grau MV, Baron JA, Sandler RS, Wallace K, Haile RW, Church TR et al (2007) Prolonged effect of calcium supplementation on risk of colorectal adenomas in a randomized trial. J Natl Cancer Inst 99(2):129–136

205. Brown CC, Chu KC (1987) Use of multistage models to infer stage affected by carcinogenic exposure: example of lung cancer and cigarette smoking. J Chronic Dis 40(Suppl 2):171s–179s

206. Minna JD, Roth JA, Gazdar AF (2002) Focus on lung cancer. Cancer Cell 1(1):49–52

207. Kenfield SA, Stampfer MJ, Rosner BA, Colditz GA (2008) Smoking and smoking cessation in relation to mortality in women. JAMA 299(17):2037–2047

208. Johnson BE (1998) Second lung cancers in patients after treatment for an initial lung cancer. J Natl Cancer Inst 90(18):1335–1345

209. Day GL, Blot WJ, Shore RE, McLaughlin JK, Austin DF, Greenberg RS et al (1994) Second cancers following oral and pharyngeal cancers: role of tobacco and alcohol. J Natl Cancer Inst 86(2):131–137

210. Browman GP, Wong G, Hodson I, Sathya J, Russell R, McAlpine L et al (1993) Influence of cigarette smoking on the efficacy of radiation therapy in head and neck cancer. N Engl J Med 328(3):159–163

211. Freedland SJ, Platz EA (2007) Obesity and prostate cancer: making sense out of apparently conflicting data. Epidemiol Rev 29:88–97

212. Skolarus TA, Wolin KY, Grubb RL (2007) The effect of body mass index on PSA levels and the development, screening and treatment of prostate cancer. Nat Clin Pract Urol 4(11):605–614

213. MacInnis RJ, English DR (2006) Body size and composition and prostate cancer risk: systematic review and meta-regression analysis. Cancer Causes Control 17(8):989–1003

214. Rodriguez C, Freedland SJ, Deka A, Jacobs EJ, McCullough ML, Patel AV et al (2007) Body mass index, weight change, and risk of prostate cancer in the Cancer Prevention Study II Nutrition Cohort. Cancer Epidemiol Biomark Prev 16(1):63–69

215. Wright ME, Chang SC, Schatzkin A, Albanes D, Kipnis V, Mouw T et al (2007) Prospective study of adiposity and weight change in relation to prostate cancer incidence and mortality. Cancer 109(4):675–684

216. Giovannucci E (2007) Does prostate-specific antigen screening influence the results of studies of tomatoes, lycopene, and prostate cancer risk? J Natl Cancer Inst 99(14):1060–1062

Chapter 19
Systemic *Oncosphere:* Host Innate Immune System

Phei Er Saw and Erwei Song

Abstract Immune system has been known as the "predator" of cancer cells. Their original function is the prey upon non-self-cells, including during infections and malignancy. Host homeostasis is regulated by a normal "predator-prey" relationship, and malignancy occurs when this balance is disrupted. In this disruption, predatory immune cells are now seeing cancer cells as friends, and the relationship between them became a symbiotic relationship, which cancer cells could also secrete factors that produce more immunoregulatory phenotypes, rather than the cancer cell killing phenotype. In this chapter, we will highlight the importance of the host innate immune system and the role of their key components (i.e. NK cells, macrophages, dendritic cells, mast cells and other leukocytes) to activate host innate immune systems in cancer eradication.

P. E. Saw
Guangdong Provincial Key Laboratory of Malignant Tumor Epigenetics and Gene Regulation, Guangdong-Hong Kong Joint Laboratory for RNA Medicine, Medical Research Center, Sun Yat-sen Memorial Hospital, Sun Yat-sen University, Guangzhou, China

Nanhai Translational Innovation Center of Precision Immunology, Sun Yat-sen Memorial Hospital, Sun Yat-sen University, Foshan, China

E. Song (✉)
Guangdong Provincial Key Laboratory of Malignant Tumor Epigenetics and Gene Regulation, Guangdong-Hong Kong Joint Laboratory for RNA Medicine, Medical Research Center, Sun Yat-sen Memorial Hospital, Sun Yat-sen University, Guangzhou, China

Nanhai Translational Innovation Center of Precision Immunology, Sun Yat-sen Memorial Hospital, Sun Yat-sen University, Foshan, China

Breast Tumor Center, Sun Yat-sen Memorial Hospital, Sun Yat-sen University, Guangzhou, China
e-mail: songew@mail.sysu.edu.cn

Introduction

Immune system has been known as the "predator" of cancer cells. Their original function is the prey upon nonself-cells, including during infections and malignancy. Host homeostasis is regulated by a normal "predator-prey" relationship, and malignancy occurs when this balance is disrupted. In this disruption, predatory immune cells are now seeing cancer cells as friends, and the relationship between them became a symbiotic relationship, which cancer cells could also secrete factors that produce more immunoregulatory phenotypes, rather than the cancer cell killing phenotype. Current immunotherapies are focusing to reconstitute this balance by reeducating immune cells to act upon the cancerous cells, usually by means of immune-checkpoint inhibitors (ICIs). However, most, if not all ICIs are focused in adaptive immunity (i.e., PD-L1, CTLA-4 therapies). Although the major cancer immunotherapy focuses on the activation of adaptive immune responses against tumor, not all patients benefit. These treatments are limited to a fraction of patients (i.e., PD-L1[+], CTLA[+] patient subset), which only accounts for about 20% across malignancies. More importantly, the success of these ICIs is limited to the high T cell-infiltrated "hot" tumors. "Cold" tumors, which are gaining more importance, prevent T cell invasion by orchestrating an immunosuppressive TME composed of cell lines such as TAMs and MDSCs [1–3]. As a result, there is a serious unfulfilled requirement of treatment methods that trigger an intrinsic immune reaction and boost T cell invasion in immunologically "cold" malignancies.

As we recently mentioned in our publication, we should use the concept of EICD "Effector Immune Cell Deployment" which takes into account all possible mechanisms in innate and adaptive immunity to stratify patients immunologically [4]. A considerable proportion of commonly prevalent tumors, particularly prostate, breast, and pancreatic cancers, have "cold" TMEs and have previously not been profited by ICI. The innate immune system comprising of natural killer (NK) cells, DCs, and macrophages, among others assists in tumor eradication by killing tumor cells explicitly via phagocytosis and cytotoxic processes, respectively. Recently, more strategies are emerging to include therapeutics which enhances the activation of innate immune systems, such as Toll-like Receptors (TLRs), Pattern Recognition Receptors (PPRs), nucleotide-binding oligomerization domain-like receptors (NLRs), RIG-I-like receptors (RLRs), and DNA sensing cGAS/STING pathway; just to name a few. In a complete cancer-immunity cycle, both host immunity (innate and adaptive) should work together closely to fully eradicate tumor (Fig. 19.2). In this chapter, we will focus on the innate immunity, and the advancement of harnessing innate immunity of the host for anticancer therapy. In the next chapter (Chap. 19), we will focus on host systemic adaptive immunity.

Key Component of Innate Immunity

Natural Killer (NK) Cells

NK cells are the major intrinsic immunity cell types accountable for eliminating non-MHC-producing cancer cells by secreting tiny cytotoxic protein molecules like perforin and granzyme that trigger death in target cells. The surface of NK cells possesses two types of receptors, namely stimulatory receptors and inhibitory receptors. The most significant stimulatory receptor includes the natural killer group 2D (NKG2D) molecules [1], which binds to MHC class-I-chain-linked protein A (MICA) [2], MICB [3, 5], and UL16 adhesive protein [6] on tumor cells, activating NK cells (with the help of cytokine secretion) to induce the secretion of IFN-γ and perforin, to induce tumor cell apoptosis (Fig. 19.1). Apart from NKG2D, other NK cell-activating receptors (NKp30 [7], NKp44 [8], and NKp46 [9]) had also been identified in human. Reciprocally, NK-inhibiting receptors were also identified, such as killer-cell immunoglobulin-like receptors (KIR) [10, 11] and NKG2A-CD94 lectin-like receptors [12]. HLA-G, a noncustomary MHC-I is found to be overexpressed in cancer cells, which can act to bind to KIR to suppress NK cells' toxicity. Another subset of MHC I is HLA-E, which binds to NKG2A/CD94 heterodimer receptor sites, also inhibiting NK cells toxicity [13]. Apart from the above ligands, NK cell surface membrane is characterized by upregulated expression of TNF group ligands, such as TNFα, TRAIL, FasL, lymphotoxin, Fas ligand (FasL), OX40, CD40, CD30, and CD27. Reciprocally, cancer cells overexpressed these receptors that correspond to the above ligands [14–18]. Once ligand-receptors are bound, they can trigger tumor cell

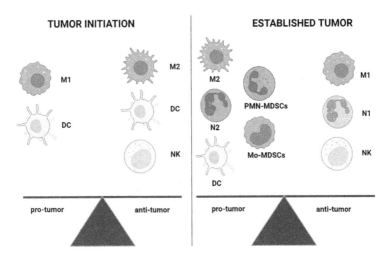

Fig. 19.1 Balancing of the intrinsic immune system. A diverse range of intrinsic immune cells' protumor versus antitumor functions might change on the basis of tumor setting, i.e., "tumor initiation" or "established tumor," rendering it hard to distinguish friendly cells from opponents. Cancer progression will ultimately be determined by the balance between intrinsic immunity cells

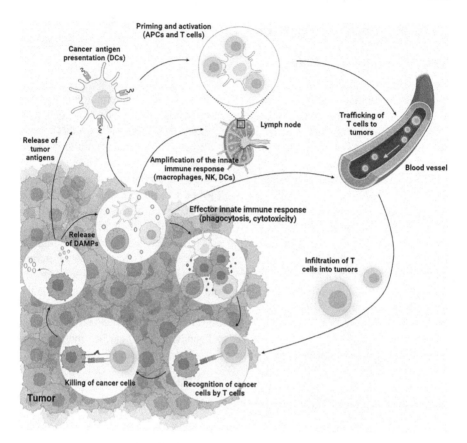

Fig. 19.2 The cancer immunity cycle (CIC). A full CIC comprises of a connection between innate and adaptive immunity. When tumor antigens are released by cancer cells, these antigens (or sometimes DAMPs) could be up taken by innate immune cells, while DCs will take up the tumor antigens and process them into small peptides, while moving into the lymph node. For innate immune cells, upon DAMP signal activation, they could (1) amplify their immune response and exert killing mechanism, or (2) induce phagocytosis of the tumor cells. The antigen presentation of antigen to T cells happens in the lymph node, then these activated T cells are transported back into the tumor to exert T cell-specific antitumor effect. Generally, both pathways could be activated, although not necessary at the exact same time

apoptosis; making TNF family ligands a promising target for immunotherapy [19–21]. Antibody-coated tumors can be identified directly by numerous intrinsic immune cells via Fc receptors (FcR). FcR for IgG (FcR) receptors are divided into two types: stimulating and inhibiting receptors. When these antibodies are bound to tumor cells, FcγR-expressing NK cells or macrophage could then induce ADCC to destroy antibody-coated tumor cells [22, 23].

Macrophages

To prevent autoimmunity, apoptotic tumor cells produce "eat me" proteins on their cell surfaces, which allow macrophages to recognize them for phagocytosis (Fig. 19.2); a classic predator-prey relationship. These "eat me" signals commonly known are phosphatidylserine (PS) or its oxidized form, the oxidized subset of low-density lipoprotein (oxLDL), and calreticulin (CRT) [24–26]. CD91 receptor on macrophage acts upon CRT overexpression, and along with protein C1q and its ligand PS, works to ingest apoptotic cells. Predating receptors like SR-A, CLA-1, CD36, CD68, LOX-1, and stabilin-2 are highly expressed on macrophage, and they have the potential to bind apoptotic tumor cells with ox-PS and oxLDL motifs. Another family of T cell Immunoglobulin Mucin (TIM) proteins, comprising of TIM-1, TIM-3, and TIM-4, are main receptors that react to PS [27–29]. Interestingly, macrophages are capable of simultaneous production of both stimulating and suppressive FcγR. Activating FcγR causes tumor cells to become cytotoxic while inhibiting FcγR diminishes the tumor killing activity. In this family, only one receptor is inhibitory, FcγRIIB. When expressed on mice macrophages, it is accountable for suppressive phagocytic functions of macrophages, reduction of cytokine synthesis, superoxide formation, and inhibition of the TLR4 signaling pathway [30]. Taken together, macrophages are perceived as key partakers of the persistent inflammation that creates an immunosuppressant environment that promotes tumor development [31].

Dendritic Cells

As the most important class of antigen-presenting cells (APCs), DCs stand as a connective bridge, the most potent cell that allows direct innate-adaptive cell communication. Not only DCs are efficient, DCs are also very specific in their communicative directions. DCs are divided into myeloid DC (mDCs) and plasmacytoid DC (pDCs). DCs are also subclassified with various terms depending on their location in the host. Even in a thin layer of skin, there are differences in DC subtypes seen in them. For example, epidermal Langerhans cells only reside on the epidermal layer, and dermal interstitial DCs are found in large quantity on the dermis layer. Although they are only micrometers apart, all DC subsets have unique immunity-inducing capabilities. For example, activated epidermal Langerhans cells release IL-15, and IL-15 is important for the priming of CD4$^+$ and CD8$^+$ T cell, while dermal interstitial DCs promote B cell priming, which are able to generate humoral immunity to produce plasma cells or antibody, also inducing innate immunity [32, 33].

One of the most unique features of DC is that immature DC can have a phagocytic response to cancer cell, while mature DC do not. When DC is in an immature state, they express CD36 and αvβ5 integrin, and these receptors are downregulated upon DC maturation. Interestingly, these DCs are able to cross-present the antigens (after phagocytosis of tumor cells) on MHC-I complex to induce T cell activation, which is unique and specialized to immature DCs [34]. Due to the presence of endocytic receptors, predator receptors, and TIM receptors on DCs, like macrophages, DCs may sense "eat me" cues that are presented on apoptotic cells. Furthermore, TAMs also overexpress similar receptors that are found on DCs (tyrosine kinase receptors; TYRO3, AXL, and MER). Therefore, TAMs could assist DCs in capturing the apoptotic cell marker PS with the aid of molecular dimers Gas6/protein S and via αvβ3 integrin via linking protein MFG-E8 [35–37]. The integrin αvβ3 complex can drive the uptake of apoptotic tumor cells [38, 39]. In the dearth of warning signals, DCs ingest apoptotic tumor cells, leading to immunological resistance. DCs are characterized by the presence of both stimulating and inhibiting FcγR. When tumor cells are bound by targeted antibodies, the Fc region of the antibodies could be captured by macrophages, DCs, or NK cells to induce ADCC. In this case, FcγR on DC will be able to effectively bind to these tumor cells, activate the expression of MHC-I and II-restricted antigen, and production of tumor-specific effector and memory T cells [40].

Mast Cells and Polymorphonuclear (PMN) Leukocytes

Mast cells and PMNs have been associated with carcinogenesis and metastasis [41], although their mechanism is yet to be fully understood. One of the most important phenomena is the expression of both stimulating and suppressing FcγR on PMN and mast cells, which best exemplify their engagement with antibody-coated Fc on tumor cells. If FcγR on PMN and mast cells are activated, this could lead to production of various proinflammatory chemokines and cytokines by neutrophils, which further induce DCs and macrophage recruitment into the tumor milieu [42, 43]. Similar to neutrophil, activating inhibitory FcγRIIB reduces the production of ROS, which could be lethal to malignant cells. Stimulation of FcγRIIB in mast cells tends to reduce Ig-E-controlled production of granules, histamine, or IL-4, all of which cause an inflammatory reaction in the tumor milieu [30]. According to a study in mouse model, direct interaction between PMNs and tumor cells causes resistance to therapeutics, which originally fatal to cancer cells [44, 45], indicating a possible immunoinhibitory effect of mast cells (summarized in Fig. 19.3).

Activating the Host Innate Immune System

As we mentioned above, the tumor milieu is composed of various innate immune cells. The intrinsic and effective pathways that these immune cells can trigger host innate immunity should be discussed in detail in order to bring upon novel

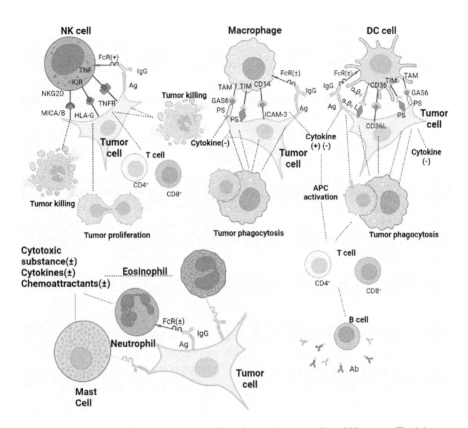

Fig. 19.3 Direct and indirect mechanisms of host innate immune cells to kill cancer. The inherent immune system consists of NK cells, macrophages, DC, neutrophils, eosinophils, and mast cells. NKG2D, an NK cell-based stimulating receptor, particularly detects MICA/B on cancer cells for initiating cell death. NK cell cytotoxicity can be restricted HLA-G on tumors by inhibitory receptors like KIR. TNF group ligands on NK cells bind to TNFRs on tumor cells, causing cancer cells' death and the generation of successive CD4+ and CD8+ T lymphocytes. The role of NK cells is likewise controlled by FcR/CD16 activation via ADCC. CD14, TIM, TAM, and FcR receptors assist macrophages in conducting phagocytosis of dead cancer cells by interacting with ICAM-3, PS, PS/Gas6. Macrophages have two Fc receptors (FcR+, activating; FcR, inhibitory). Apoptotic tumor cells may be taken up by DC via various receptors. Cytokines released by DC and macrophages result in a cellular and humoral adaptable immune reaction. FcR activation on DC aids in tumor cell antigen expression. Stimulating and inhibiting FcR are also present on neutrophils, eosinophils, and mast cells

techniques that can harness the innate immune system for cancer therapeutics. Herein, we will discuss more on the major pathways in innate immune systems, including: TLRs, NLRP3, cGAS/STING pathway, RIG-I-like receptors (RLRs) among others. Every section evaluates reasonable immune-oncology fusion methods that engage the intrinsic immune system, hence improving the effectiveness of existing immunotherapies.

Toll-Like Receptors (TLRs)

Toll-like receptors (TLRs) are a family of transmembrane receptors with a wide spectrum of microbial recognition by their ten major family members. Activation of TLRs is usually closely related to microbe infection, and TLR activation can trigger many signaling pathways that are involved in the defensive mechanism [46]. In humans, ten TLRs have been identified. TLRs could be divided into two categories, plasma membrane-bound TLRs (TLRs 1, 2, 5, and 6) and endosome-bound TLRs (TLRs 3, 4, 7, 8, and 9). Only TLR4 is found on both [47]. Membrane-bound TLRs mainly recognize lipid and protein/peptide antigen, while endosome-bound TLRs are proficient in nucleic acid recognition. TLR signaling is triggered by the stimulation of adaptor proteins, such as MyD88, interferon regulatory factor 3 (IRF-3), NF-kB, and activating protein-1 (AP-1), which could enhance the production of proinflammatory cascades upon activation [48]. TLRs exert a pleiotropic impact on tumor immunoregulation. TLRs, when triggered on immune cells, regulate a wide spectrum of immunostimulatory activities that increase anticancer T cell responses [49]. For example, chemotherapy initiates DMAP, which stimulates TLR4 and resulting in DC maturity [50]. TLR9 signaling has been demonstrated to stimulate pDCs and cause significant amounts of IFN-I release [51]. Activating TLR7 and TLR8 resulted in the transformation of the tumor-favoring M2 TAM phenotype into the antitumoral M1 phenotype [52, 53]. Furthermore, constitutive TLR stimulation can result in permanent inflammatory conditions as the tumor recruits immunosuppressive MDSCs [54–56]. Preclinical and clinical studies of TLR-based therapeutics are summarized in Table 19.1.

NLRP3 Inflammasome

Inflammasomes are huge aggregates made of multiple proteins and are found in the cytosol; these regulate essential inflammatory intrinsic immune reactions in the host's defense system against microbiological invaders. NOD-like receptors, also known as nucleotide-attaching oligomerization domain-like receptors (NLRs), form a large family of intracellular PRRs. Among the members, NLRP3 is the widely studied. NLRP3 is mainly produced by innate immune cells (macrophages, DCs, and lymphocytes), though it has been also found in nonimmune epithelial cells [70]. Cellular stress-induced PAMPs or DAMPs (i.e., ATP, extracellular glucose, and ROS) can drive NLRP3 inflammasome excitation [71–75]. Oligomerization of NLRP3 results in the breakdown of procaspase-1 to caspase-1, resulting in secretion of IL-18 and IL-1β, causing proteolysis of these cytokines, leading to tumor death. Among the members of inflammasome, Gasdermin-D is a key element that can permeate the cell membrane and favors the pyroptosis pathway rather than apoptosis [76–78]. Inflammasome-induced pyroptosis is uniquely activated by caspase-1, an

Table 19.1 Concept of ECID: innate immune cells that are activated during cancer progression

Innate immune cell components				
Immune cell type	Subset/secreted factor	Effect to local *oncosphere*	Major findings	Ref
Dendritic cells (DCs)	PD-L1$^+$	Immunosuppressive	Sequesters CD80 and dampens its binding to CD28 on T cells	[57, 58]
	PD-L1$^+$ (in tumor-draining lymph nodes (TDLNs)	Immunosuppressive	Low-dose intrapleural PD-L1 antibody treatment selectively blocked PD-L1/PD-1 in TDLNs but not in the local oncosphere	[57]
Mature DCs	T cells	Immunostimulatory	Upregulate costimulators such as CD80, CD86, and CD40; stimulating T cell priming, subsequently reflecting a secondary signal for activation and subsequent clonal expansion	[57, 58]
Immature DCs		Immunosuppressive	Coinhibitor receptors that block T cell activation	[58]
NK cells	PD-1$^+$, PD-LI$^+$ NK	Immunostimulatory	Indispensable for the therapeutic effect of PD-1/PD-L1 blockade in various mouse models	[59, 60]
	Expresses KLRB1, NKG2A, TIGIT, and IL18BP	Immunosuppressive	Shared inhibitory receptors with T cells	[61–64]
	Inducing DC maturation	Immunostimulatory	Secreting IFN-γ to orchestrate adaptive immune responses	
	NK-derived CCL5 and XCL-1	Immunostimulatory	Recruit type I conventional DCs (cDC1s), the main DC subset that cross-presents tumor antigens and primes CD8$^+$ T cells	[65]
	NK cell-derived FLT3L	Immunostimulatory	Prolongs cDC1 survival enhancement of T cell-mediated antitumor immune responses	[66]
TAMs	Secrete CCL18	Immunosuppressive	Recruit naive CD4$^+$ T cells which can further differentiate into T$_{reg}$ cells	[67]
	Restrict CD8$^+$ T cell motility	Immunosuppressive	Restrict CD8$^+$ T cell motility from infiltrating into tumor islets through long-lasting contact	[68]
	IDO1 expression, PI3Kγ activation	Immunosuppressive	Did not respond well to ICB, as evidenced by a shorter nonprogression rate relative to controls	[69]

activated form of PCD wherein the cytoplasmic contents of target cells are liberated to cause inflammation [79].

Preclinical studies have shown that, during innate immune system activation, NLRP3 could induce the upregulation of two cytokines, namely IL-1β and IL-18, which then induces IFN-γ expression in the tumor secretome. High IFN-γ concentration will then induce CD8+ T activation, which ultimately leads to tumor cell death [80, 81]. In hepatocellular carcinoma, when NLRP3 inflammasome is induced via estrogen receptor signaling, caspase-1 is activated, leading to cancer cell pyroptosis, along with autophagy, a self-induced death mechanism [82]. Mice lacking the NLRP3 inflammasome showed higher metastatic development as these cells are presented with defective IL-18 signaling, which in turn affect the normal maturation of NK cells [83]. In several solid tumor mouse models, downregulated NLRP3 inflammasome stimulation has also been shown to enhance carcinogenesis. MCA-induced sarcomas in mice lacking NLRP3 had a lower tumor volume than wild-type, which was linked to NLRP3-driven reduction of NK cell infiltration [84]. In OSCC, NLRP3 inflammasome stimulation and IL-1β release were linked to tumor development, metastasis, and invasion of immunosuppressant myeloid cells, like TAMs and MDSCs [85–87]. Furthermore, the latest research has revealed that activation of intratumoral NLRP3 inflammasome might confer resistance to anti-PD-1 therapy [88].

cGAS/STING Pathway

cGAS-STING pathway detects viral DNA contamination in the cytosolic DNA. cGAS detects cytosolic DNA and triggers the stimulation of IFN genes (STING) via cyclic dinucleotide GMP-AMP production (cGAMP) [89, 90]. STING is first activated in the ER, which is then transported into the Golgi, stimulating IRF-3 and NF-kB, to cause the production and release of IFN-I [91, 92]. STING is also produced by a variety of immune and nonimmune cells, and therefore could be utilized to detect tumor-generated DNA can be used therapeutically to treat cancer. STING-based cytosolic DNA detection by tumor-located DCs was discovered to trigger IFN-1 expression and was essential for CD8+ T cell infiltration and results in enhanced tumor inhibition [93]. In preclinical studies, intratumoral administration of STING activators mimicked similar proinflammatory responses and resulted in significant tumor regression [94], summarized in Table 19.1. It is important to note, however, that although cGAS/STING pathway is promising, certain complexities regarding the context and dose-dependent consequences are surfacing. Recent studies have shown that in tumors with chromosomal instability (CIN), the tumor's inherent high level of cytosolic DNA is sufficient to trigger activation of endogenous cGAS/STING pathway. An intrinsic activation leads to the promotion of carcinogenesis, immune escape, enhanced metastasis, and prolonged survival [90]. Therefore, patient stratification is crucial, and patients with this phenotype should not be considered for continuous therapeutics.

Retinoic Acid-Inducible Gene-I-like Receptors (RLRs) and RIG-I

RLRs refer to PRRs that recognize cytosolic RNA in the physiological setting of viral diseases [95]. RIG-I, MDA5, and LGP2 are the most extensively investigated RLRs. RIG-I preferentially attaches shorter dsRNA fragments, while MDA-5 binds longer components [96]. Like the cGAS/STING pathway, RLRs activation leads to a conformational shift that reveals a CARD domain, which triggers downstream targets that boost the transcription agents IRF-1. CARD domain is vital for inflammasome stimulation [97]. RIG-I regulates a multitude of immunostimulatory processes, such as DC maturation, T cell priming, and increased NK cell degranulation and cytolytic function [98, 99]. RIG-I is also able to induce pyroptosis via intrinsic and extrinsic apoptotic mechanisms [98]. Moreover, recent research suggests the significance of RIG-I for an appropriate reaction to anti-CTLA-4 therapies by triggering caspase-3-driven apoptosis, which leads to presentation of tumor-associated antigens to T cells, activating these T cells into functional CD8+ T cell to mediate tumor cell death [100].

CD40

CD40 is a well-studied costimulatory protein that belongs to the TNFR superfamily. CD40 is abundantly expressed on antigen-presenting cells such as DCs, and other innate immune cells such as macrophages, and B cells [101]. Its corresponding ligand CD40L could be found on T cells. Therefore, when CD40 binds to CD40L, MHC and other costimulatory molecules are overexpressed, leading to the release of IFN-γ and IL-12a [102–105]. It was found that CD40-regulated CD8+ T cell stimulation is not related and independent of CD4+ T cells or other innate immune cells [106, 107]. Additionally, CD40 also converts TAMs to antitumoral M1-like phenotype, which could enhance ECM remodeling, leading to enhancement of chemotherapeutic effects [108, 109].

Colony-Stimulating Factor 1 (CSF-1)

In mouse model, when macrophage CSF-1/CSF-1R is blocked, macrophage is skewed toward M1-like antitumoral phenotype, leading to tumor inhibition [110]. This, combined with anti-PD-1 and anti-CTLA-4 ICI treatment, synergistic effect was observed [111]. Currently, antibodies/small molecule inhibitors of CSF-1R are being tested in clinical studies as monotherapeutic, or in combination therapy (ADC + chemotherapy or ADC + ICI) [112, 113] (Table 19.1).

PI3K-γ Inhibition

Activating PI3K by p110 isoform promotes polarization to a protumorigenic M2 phenotype in macrophages [114]. In various solid tumor models, suppression of the PI3K-γ has shown to enhance polarization of TAMs into antitumoral M1-like phenotype, elevating proinflammatory cytokines, leading to stimulated antitumor responsiveness and reduced tumor growth [115, 116].

CD47-SIRPα

CD47 is a membrane glycoprotein on immune cells, and is a "don't eat me" marker generated on both tumor and immune cells. CD47 binds to SIRPα on macrophages for prevention of phagocytosis. In vitro inhibition of CD47-SIRPα via CD47 antibodies was demonstrated to reactive tumor cell phagocytosis by TAMs, boost antigen-specific T lymphocytes, and restrict tumor development in animal models [117].

DC-SIGN

DC-SIGN (or CD209), is an immunosuppressive TAM marker. In clinical samples, DC-SIGN+ TAM invasion corresponds to an increase in the number of exhausted CD8+ T cells and Tregs. In vitro, treatment of bladder cancer cells with a monoclonal antibody addressing acting upon DC-SIGN in conjunction with PD-1 inhibition revealed higher anticancer efficacy than monotherapy, thus presenting a justification for clinical formulation [118].

Natural-Killer Group 2-Member (NKG2A and D) Ligands

The most widely investigated NK cell-stimulating receptors are NKG2D and its ligands, MICA and MICB. In their attempt to increase survival, many cancer cells (especially malignant cancers) lose MICA and MICB via proteolytic processing by MMP families (i.e., ADAM10, ADAM17, and MMP14 [119]). Small molecule inhibitors of MMPs have lately been produced to counteract MICA and MICB proteolytic breakdown [120]. Other techniques such as producing an antibody specifically targeting MICA/B-α3 section can also be employed for reducing MICA and MICB shedding. In mice, MICA/B-α3 antibodies were demonstrated to generate a substantial NK-regulated antitumoral reaction [121]. Likewise, proteasome blockers like bortezomib may block MICA/B breakdown and improve

NK cells' invasion of tumor cells [122]. Also, cancer cells can develop resistance to NKG2D, which results in modification of NKG2D ligand [123, 124]. Hence, histone deacetylase blockers have been studied as therapies to increase NKG2D ligand transcription [125, 126]. NKG2A, on the other hand, is a suppressive immunological barrier protein produced on NK cells and a subgroup of α/β T cells [61, 127, 128]. In a current Phase III clinical trials for HNSCC, Monalizumab, a first-in-class ICI targeting the NKG2A receptor cells was given to the patient, hoping to concurrently activating NK cells and CD8$^+$ T cells [129].

NK Cell Engagers (NKCEs)

Apart from mono-antibody, bi-targeting or tri-targeting antibody complexes could be a great alternative. These antibodies could attach several antigens and drive NK cells toward the tumor in order to trigger an immune reaction to induce tumor inhibition [130]. Multitargeting NKCEs having a tri-specific engager as they are equipped with two NK cell activation receptors, namely NKp46 and CD16, and another receptor bound to TAAs of cancer cells. Treatment using NKCEs was shown to cause considerable tumor suppression in solid tumor mouse models with no major damage [131]. These investigations lay the groundwork for the therapeutic development of these compounds.

> **Box 19.1 EICD Concept to Include Activated Innate Immune Cells as "Hot Tumor" Classification**
> Current evaluation of ICB effectiveness is based on CD8$^+$ T cell infiltration and to reinvigorate CD8$^+$ T cells in tumors [132]. In ICB therapy, responders exhibit a "hot" ("immune-inflamed") phenotype, characterized by T lymphocyte infiltration, whereas nonresponders may exhibit a "cold" ("immune-desert"/"immune-excluded") phenotype, characterized by the absence or exclusion of T cells in the tumor parenchyma [133]. Although ICB therapies have revolutionized cancer treatment, only a subset of patients elicit favorable responses [57]. Through the years, fluctuations were seen in treatment responses in clinical trials. Increasing evidence suggests that tumors with poor T cell infiltration might demonstrate a considerable response to ICB, whereas poor response to ICB might be observed in tumors even with high T cell infiltration [57, 59]. Moreover, other immune-related factors, such as tumor mutational burden (TMB), can help predict therapeutic efficacy independent of T cell infiltration [134, 135]. These findings suggest that T cell infiltration may be necessary but insufficient for ICB responsiveness, raising questions on how to identify ICB responders precisely. Taken together, the notion of evaluating ICB therapeutic efficacy based on CD8+ T cell infiltration

(continued)

Box 19.1 (continued)

is insufficient, and should not be the sole factor being considered in the design of ICB therapeutics.

We recognized that the current "hot" tumor classification is inadequate, and should be revamped in order to achieve a precise and comprehensive classification of "hot" tumors. In this *featured review*, we propose the concept of effector immune cell deployment (EICD), which quantifies every aspect of tumor characteristics, including (1) the priming, circulation, activity, trafficking, and fate of *all* antitumor effector immune cells (i.e., T cells, NK cells), (2) the effect of stromal cells in the TME (i.e., CAFs, MDSCs, TAMs), (3) the effect of local TME environment (i.e., cytokines, chemokines), and (iv) host systemic effect on the TME (i.e., host metabolic activity) as summarized in Table 19.1. In this table, EICD concepts on innate immune cells are specially highlighted. Herein, we emphasize on the importance of analyzing cancer as a whole ecosystem, to scrutinize changes that occur not only in the cancer cells or its surrounding (local oncosphere), but also take into consideration the host systemic oncosphere (i.e., host innate and adaptive immune systems, host neuroendocrine system, host metabolic system) to demonstrate a fully comprehensive analysis of a cancer.

Examples of Innate Effector Immune Cells in Immunotherapy

Adoptive DC Strategies

Adoptive therapies using DC are defined as the DC immunization with TAAs or specifically tailored TSAs. Under this technique, autologous DC subsets are extracted from the patient's own blood. These DCs are then electroporated with the TSAs from the patients, known as the ex vivo activation step. Then, these DCs are reintroduced into the patient's body through in vivo transfusion. Such types of DC immunization techniques have drawn interest for a long time, wherein over 200 clinical studies have investigated their effectiveness. One of the famous examples is Sipuleucel-T, an autologous DC vaccine which was approved by the FDA. Sipuleucel-T is an ex vivo culture DCs loaded with a recombinant protein GM-CSF/PSA to cure CRPCs [136]. CM-CSF/PSA are common cancer antigens (TAAs) which could be used in majority of patients in similar cancer subtypes. However, to go one step further, one should consider using each patient's tumor-specific antigen (TSAs) to be introduced into the DCs, creating the real personalized adoptive DC [137].

Adoptive NK Cell Strategies

Adoptive NK treatment (ACT) techniques have been a focus of recent research due to the significant physiological involvement of NK cells in tumor immunity. In ACT, allogeneic NK cells are obtained from peripheral circulation from patient. Since patient's NK cells normally are inhibited (or mutated), these NK cells are reintroduced with NK-stimulating receptors (such as NKG2DR) and further grown ex vivo for its reinfusion [138]. In comparison to adoptive T cell approaches, NK cell ACT has exhibited substantial suppression of initial metastasis, tumor selectivity, and toxicity characteristics of higher conduciveness. However, there are few doubts regarding the effectiveness of NK cell ACT in solid tumors, such as low proliferation capability, tumor penetrability, and the existence of intrinsic immunosuppressive systems inside the local *oncosphere* [139, 140]. Techniques like HLA reduction are being explored to increase the lifespan of NK cells after infusion, and to reduce the probability of recipient's host rejection [141]. Furthermore, NK cell activity is very much influenced by the cancer secretome, which can easily deactivate NK cell activity. For example, tumors can secrete immunosuppressive TGF-β and adenosine, tryptophan or other metabolites to increase the expression of IDO, releasing MICA and MICB proteins, which ultimately attracts immunosuppressive immune cells [142–144]. Therefore, concurrent or combination therapy focusing on these processes could be synergistic to reactivate a dormant NK cell. Some major clinical developments of innate immune cell-based therapy are shown in Table 19.2.

Conclusion

Substantial progress has been achieved in our comprehension of the innate immune system and their involvement and responsiveness to carcinogenesis. Excitement for emerging intrinsic immune approaches must be balanced with a realistic assessment of the danger of immunological-linked negative impacts (irAEs). The danger of off-target cytotoxicity cannot be regarded as negligible due to the targeted antigen-free on-target actions of stimulating highly powerful and conserved proinflammatory pathways. Given extensive clinical usage, it will be critical to separate irAEs unique to intrinsic immune exploratory drugs from ICI-caused induction of irAEs, due to the involvement of ICI pairing in multiple experimental techniques. There is an unfulfilled therapeutic requirement for establishing innovative, evidence-based toxicity management procedures that recognize the rising importance of combined methods. Therefore, it is crucial to further identify the situational functions of intrinsic immune mechanisms in various tumor and genetic subgroups.

Table 19.2 Clinical development of major PRRs

Route of administration	PRR	Active compound	Cancer type	Phase
Intratumoral	TLR 8	Motilomod (VTX-2337)	Ovarian cancer, HSNCC	Phase I, II
	TLR 7/8	NKTR-262	Not defined (solid tumors)	Phase I, II
	TLR 9	SD-101	Not defined (solid tumors)	Phase I, II
		Tilsotolimod (IMO-2125)	Not defined (solid tumors)	Phase I, II
		CMP-001	Not defined (solid tumors)	Phase I, II
	RIG-1	SLR-14	Not defined (solid tumors)	Preclinical
		RGT-100 (MK-4621)	Not defined (solid tumors)	Preclinical
	MDA-5	BO-112	Not defined (solid tumors)	Phase I
	STING	MK1454	Not defined (solid tumors)	Phase I, II
		BMS-986301	Not defined (solid tumors)	Phase I
Subcutaneous injections	TLR 9	EMD 1201081	HSNCC	Phase I, II
		CPG 7909	Lymphomas	Phase I, II
Intravenous injections	STING	E7766	Not defined (solid tumors)	Phase I
		GSK3745417	Not defined (solid tumors)	Phase I
	CSF-1R	Cabiralizumab	Not defined (solid tumors)	Phase I, II
		JNJ-40346527	Advanced prostate cancers	Phase I, II
		IMC-CS4	Not defined (solid tumors)	Phase I
	CD40	APX005M	Not defined (solid tumors)	Phase I, II
		CP780, CP-893	Not defined (solid tumors)	Phase I
		Selicrelumab	Not defined (solid tumors)	Phase I, II
	STAT3 inhibitors	Siltuzumab	Not defined (solid tumor)	Phase I, II
Oral administration	CSF-1R	PLX3397, MCS 110	Not defined (solid tumors)	Phase I, II
	PI3K inhibitors	IPI-549	Not defined (solid tumors)	Phase I, II
		TMP-195		Preclinical

(continued)

Table 19.2 (continued)

Route of administration	PRR	Active compound	Cancer type	Phase
	Histone deacetylase inhibitor		Not defined (solid tumor)	
	IDO inhibitor	Indoximod	Not defined (solid tumor)	Phase I, II

References

1. Yokoyama WM, Plougastel BF (2003) Immune functions encoded by the natural killer gene complex. Nat Rev Immunol 3(4):304–316
2. Bauer S, Groh V, Wu J, Steinle A, Phillips JH, Lanier LL et al (1999) Pillars Article: Activation of NK cells and T cells by NKG2D, a receptor for stress-inducible MICA. Science 285:727–729
3. Salih HR, Antropius H, Gieseke F, Lutz SZ, Kanz L, Rammensee HG et al (2003) Functional expression and release of ligands for the activating immunoreceptor NKG2D in leukemia. Blood 102(4):1389–1396
4. Zhang J, Huang D, Saw PE, Song E (2022) Turning cold tumors hot: from molecular mechanisms to clinical applications. Trends Immunol 43(7):523–545
5. Vetter CS, Groh V, Thor Straten P, Spies T, Bröcker EB, Becker JC (2002) Expression of stress-induced MHC class I-related chain molecules on human melanoma. J Invest Dermatol 118(4):600–605
6. Champsaur M, Lanier LL (2010) Effect of NKG2D ligand expression on host immune responses. Immunol Rev 235(1):267–285
7. Pende D, Parolini S, Pessino A, Sivori S, Augugliaro R, Morelli L et al (1999) Identification and molecular characterization of NKp30, a novel triggering receptor involved in natural cytotoxicity mediated by human natural killer cells. J Exp Med 190(10):1505–1516
8. Vitale M, Bottino C, Sivori S, Sanseverino L, Castriconi R, Marcenaro E et al (1998) NKp44, a novel triggering surface molecule specifically expressed by activated natural killer cells, is involved in non-major histocompatibility complex-restricted tumor cell lysis. J Exp Med 187(12):2065–2072
9. Sivori S, Pende D, Bottino C, Marcenaro E, Pessino A, Biassoni R et al (1999) NKp46 is the major triggering receptor involved in the natural cytotoxicity of fresh or cultured human NK cells. Correlation between surface density of NKp46 and natural cytotoxicity against autologous, allogeneic or xenogeneic target cells. Eur J Immunol 29(5):1656–1666
10. Long EO (1999) Regulation of immune responses through inhibitory receptors. Annu Rev Immunol 17:875–904
11. Moretta L, Biassoni R, Bottino C, Mingari MC, Moretta A (2000) Human NK-cell receptors. Immunol Today 21(9):420–422
12. Plougastel B, Jones T, Trowsdale J (1996) Genomic structure, chromosome location, and alternative splicing of the human NKG2A gene. Immunogenetics 44(4):286–291
13. Braud VM, Allan DS, O'Callaghan CA, Söderström K, D'Andrea A, Ogg GS et al (1998) HLA-E binds to natural killer cell receptors CD94/NKG2A. Nature 391(6669):795–799
14. Beutler B, van Huffel C (1994) Unraveling function in the TNF ligand and receptor families. Science 264(5159):667–668
15. Gruss HJ (1996) Molecular, structural, and biological characteristics of the tumor necrosis factor ligand superfamily. Int J Clin Lab Res 26(3):143–159
16. Nagata S (1997) Apoptosis by death factor. Cell 88(3):355–365

17. Anderson DM, Maraskovsky E, Billingsley WL, Dougall WC, Tometsko ME, Roux ER et al (1997) A homologue of the TNF receptor and its ligand enhance T-cell growth and dendritic-cell function. Nature 390(6656):175–179
18. Smith CA, Farrah T, Goodwin RG (1994) The TNF receptor superfamily of cellular and viral proteins: activation, costimulation, and death. Cell 76(6):959–962
19. Wang YG, Kim KD, Wang J, Yu P, Fu YX (2005) Stimulating lymphotoxin beta receptor on the dendritic cells is critical for their homeostasis and expansion. J Immunol 175(10): 6997–7002
20. Yu P, Fu YX (2008) Targeting tumors with LIGHT to generate metastasis-clearing immunity. Cytokine Growth Factor Rev 19(3-4):285–294
21. Fan Z, Yu P, Wang Y, Wang Y, Fu ML, Liu W et al (2006) NK-cell activation by LIGHT triggers tumor-specific CD8+ T-cell immunity to reject established tumors. Blood 107(4): 1342–1351
22. Nakamura A, Kubo T, Takai T (2008) Fc receptor targeting in the treatment of allergy, autoimmune diseases and cancer. Adv Exp Med Biol 640:220–233
23. Nimmerjahn F, Ravetch JV (2008) Fcgamma receptors as regulators of immune responses. Nat Rev Immunol 8(1):34–47
24. Jeannin P, Jaillon S, Delneste Y (2008) Pattern recognition receptors in the immune response against dying cells. Curr Opin Immunol 20(5):530–537
25. Gardai SJ, Bratton DL, Ogden CA, Henson PM (2006) Recognition ligands on apoptotic cells: a perspective. J Leukoc Biol 79(5):896–903
26. Gardai SJ, McPhillips KA, Frasch SC, Janssen WJ, Starefeldt A, Murphy-Ullrich JE et al (2005) Cell-surface calreticulin initiates clearance of viable or apoptotic cells through trans-activation of LRP on the phagocyte. Cell 123(2):321–334
27. Kobayashi N, Karisola P, Peña-Cruz V, Dorfman DM, Jinushi M, Umetsu SE et al (2007) TIM-1 and TIM-4 glycoproteins bind phosphatidylserine and mediate uptake of apoptotic cells. Immunity 27(6):927–940
28. Miyanishi M, Tada K, Koike M, Uchiyama Y, Kitamura T, Nagata S (2007) Identification of Tim4 as a phosphatidylserine receptor. Nature 450(7168):435–439
29. Nakayama M, Akiba H, Takeda K, Kojima Y, Hashiguchi M, Azuma M et al (2009) Tim-3 mediates phagocytosis of apoptotic cells and cross-presentation. Blood 113(16):3821–3830
30. Smith KG, Clatworthy MR (2010) FcgammaRIIB in autoimmunity and infection: evolutionary and therapeutic implications. Nat Rev Immunol 10(5):328–343
31. Ostrand-Rosenberg S (2008) Immune surveillance: a balance between protumor and antitumor immunity. Curr Opin Genet Dev 18(1):11–18
32. Klechevsky E, Morita R, Liu M, Cao Y, Coquery S, Thompson-Snipes L et al (2008) Functional specializations of human epidermal Langerhans cells and CD14+ dermal dendritic cells. Immunity 29(3):497–510
33. Palucka K, Ueno H, Zurawski G, Fay J, Banchereau J (2010) Building on dendritic cell subsets to improve cancer vaccines. Curr Opin Immunol 22(2):258–263
34. Albert ML, Pearce SF, Francisco LM, Sauter B, Roy P, Silverstein RL et al (1998) Immature dendritic cells phagocytose apoptotic cells via alphavbeta5 and CD36, and cross-present antigens to cytotoxic T lymphocytes. J Exp Med 188(7):1359–1368
35. Lai C, Lemke G (1991) An extended family of protein-tyrosine kinase genes differentially expressed in the vertebrate nervous system. Neuron 6(5):691–704
36. Stitt TN, Conn G, Gore M, Lai C, Bruno J, Radziejewski C et al (1995) The anticoagulation factor protein S and its relative, Gas6, are ligands for the Tyro 3/Axl family of receptor tyrosine kinases. Cell 80(4):661–670
37. Lemke G, Rothlin CV (2008) Immunobiology of the TAM receptors. Nat Rev Immunol 8(5): 327–336
38. Hanayama R, Tanaka M, Miwa K, Shinohara A, Iwamatsu A, Nagata S (2002) Identification of a factor that links apoptotic cells to phagocytes. Nature 417(6885):182–187

39. Wu Y, Tibrewal N, Birge RB (2006) Phosphatidylserine recognition by phagocytes: a view to a kill. Trends Cell Biol 16(4):189–197
40. Regnault A, Lankar D, Lacabanne V, Rodriguez A, Théry C, Rescigno M et al (1999) Fcgamma receptor-mediated induction of dendritic cell maturation and major histocompatibility complex class I-restricted antigen presentation after immune complex internalization. J Exp Med 189(2):371–380
41. Gregory AD, Houghton AM (2011) Tumor-associated neutrophils: new targets for cancer therapy. Cancer Res 71(7):2411–2416
42. Amulic B, Cazalet C, Hayes GL, Metzler KD, Zychlinsky A (2012) Neutrophil function: from mechanisms to disease. Annu Rev Immunol 30:459–489
43. Scapini P, Laudanna C, Pinardi C, Allavena P, Mantovani A, Sozzani S et al (2001) Neutrophils produce biologically active macrophage inflammatory protein-3alpha (MIP-3alpha)/CCL20 and MIP-3beta/CCL19. Eur J Immunol 31(7):1981–1988
44. Hicks AM, Riedlinger G, Willingham MC, Alexander-Miller MA, Von Kap-Herr C, Pettenati MJ et al (2006) Transferable anticancer innate immunity in spontaneous regression/complete resistance mice. Proc Natl Acad Sci U S A 103(20):7753–7758
45. Riedlinger G, Adams J, Stehle JR Jr, Blanks MJ, Sanders AM, Hicks AM et al (2010) The spectrum of resistance in SR/CR mice: the critical role of chemoattraction in the cancer/leukocyte interaction. BMC Cancer 10:179
46. Montero Vega MT, de Andres MA (2009) The significance of toll-like receptors in human diseases. Allergol Immunopathol 37(5):252–263
47. Gangloff M (2012) Different dimerisation mode for TLR4 upon endosomal acidification? Trends Biochem Sci 37(3):92–98
48. Satoh T, Akira S (2016) Toll-like receptor signaling and its inducible proteins. Microbiology 4:6
49. Adams S (2009) Toll-like receptor agonists in cancer therapy. Immunotherapy 1(6):949–964
50. Apetoh L, Ghiringhelli F, Tesniere A, Obeid M, Ortiz C, Criollo A et al (2007) Toll-like receptor 4-dependent contribution of the immune system to anticancer chemotherapy and radiotherapy. Nat Med 13(9):1050–1059
51. Liu YJ (2005) IPC: professional type 1 interferon-producing cells and plasmacytoid dendritic cell precursors. Annu Rev Immunol 23:275–306
52. Rodell CB, Arlauckas SP, Cuccarese MF, Garris CS, Li R, Ahmed MS et al (2018) TLR7/8-agonist-loaded nanoparticles promote the polarization of tumour-associated macrophages to enhance cancer immunotherapy. Nat Biomed Eng 2(8):578–588
53. Vidyarthi A, Khan N, Agnihotri T, Negi S, Das DK, Aqdas M et al (2018) TLR-3 stimulation skews M2 macrophages to M1 through IFN-$\alpha\beta$ signaling and restricts tumor progression. Front Immunol 9:1650
54. Dajon M, Iribarren K, Petitprez F, Marmier S, Lupo A, Gillard M et al (2019) Toll-like receptor 7 expressed by malignant cells promotes tumor progression and metastasis through the recruitment of myeloid-derived suppressor cells. Onco Targets Ther 8(1):e1505174
55. Jouhi L, Renkonen S, Atula T, Mäkitie A, Haglund C, Hagström J (2014) Different toll-like receptor expression patterns in progression toward cancer. Front Immunol 5:638
56. Hao B, Chen Z, Bi B, Yu M, Yao S, Feng Y et al (2018) Role of TLR4 as a prognostic factor for survival in various cancers: a meta-analysis. Oncotarget 9(16):13088–13099
57. Dammeijer F, van Gulijk M, Mulder EE, Lukkes M, Klaase L, van den Bosch T et al (2020) The PD-1/PD-L1-checkpoint restrains T cell immunity in tumor-draining lymph nodes. Cancer Cell 38(5):685–700
58. Mayoux M, Roller A, Pulko V, Sammicheli S, Chen S, Sum E et al (2020) Dendritic cells dictate responses to PD-L1 blockade cancer immunotherapy. Sci Transl Med 12:534
59. Hsu J, Hodgins JJ, Marathe M, Nicolai CJ, Bourgeois-Daigneault MC, Trevino TN et al (2018) Contribution of NK cells to immunotherapy mediated by PD-1/PD-L1 blockade. J Clin Invest 128(10):4654–4668

60. Dong W, Wu X, Ma S, Wang Y, Nalin AP, Zhu Z et al (2019) The Mechanism of anti-PD-L1 antibody efficacy against PD-L1-negative tumors identifies NK cells expressing PD-L1 as a cytolytic effector. Cancer Discov 9(10):1422–1437
61. Andre P, Denis C, Soulas C, Bourbon-Caillet C, Lopez J, Arnoux T et al (2018) Anti-NKG2A mAb is a checkpoint inhibitor that promotes anti-tumor immunity by unleashing both T and NK cells. Cell 175(7):1731–1743
62. Mathewson ND, Ashenberg O, Tirosh I, Gritsch S, Perez EM, Marx S et al (2021) Inhibitory CD161 receptor identified in glioma-infiltrating T cells by single-cell analysis. Cell 184(5): 1281–1298
63. Zhang Q, Bi J, Zheng X, Chen Y, Wang H, Wu W et al (2018) Blockade of the checkpoint receptor TIGIT prevents NK cell exhaustion and elicits potent anti-tumor immunity. Nat Immunol 19(7):723–732
64. Zhou T, Damsky W, Weizman OE, McGeary MK, Hartmann KP, Rosen CE et al (2020) IL-18BP is a secreted immune checkpoint and barrier to IL-18 immunotherapy. Nature 583(7817):609–614
65. Bottcher JP, Bonavita E, Chakravarty P, Blees H, Cabeza-Cabrerizo M, Sammicheli S et al (2018) NK cells stimulate recruitment of cDC1 into the tumor microenvironment promoting cancer immune control. Cell 172(5):1022–1037
66. Barry KC, Hsu J, Broz ML, Cueto FJ, Binnewies M, Combes AJ et al (2018) A natural killer-dendritic cell axis defines checkpoint therapy-responsive tumor microenvironments. Nat Med 24(8):1178–1191
67. Su S, Liao J, Liu J, Huang D, He C, Chen F et al (2017) Blocking the recruitment of naive CD4 (+) T cells reverses immunosuppression in breast cancer. Cell Res 27(4):461–482
68. Peranzoni E, Lemoine J, Vimeux L, Feuillet V, Barrin S, Kantari-Mimoun C et al (2018) Macrophages impede CD8 T cells from reaching tumor cells and limit the efficacy of anti-PD-1 treatment. Proc Natl Acad Sci U S A 115(17):4041–4050
69. Toulmonde M, Penel N, Adam J, Chevreau C, Blay JY, Le Cesne A et al (2018) Use of PD-1 targeting, macrophage infiltration, and IDO pathway activation in sarcomas: a phase 2 clinical trial. JAMA Oncol 4(1):93–97
70. Franchi L, Warner N, Viani K, Nuñez G (2009) Function of Nod-like receptors in microbial recognition and host defense. Immunol Rev 227(1):106–128
71. Swanson KV, Deng M, Ting JP (2019) The NLRP3 inflammasome: molecular activation and regulation to therapeutics. Nat Rev Immunol 19(8):477–489
72. Gong T, Yang Y, Jin T, Jiang W, Zhou R (2018) Orchestration of NLRP3 inflammasome activation by ion fluxes. Trends Immunol 39(5):393–406
73. Hughes MM, O'Neill LAJ (2018) Metabolic regulation of NLRP3. Immunol Rev 281(1): 88–98
74. Martínez-García JJ, Martínez-Banaclocha H, Angosto-Bazarra D, de Torre-Minguela C, Baroja-Mazo A, Alarcón-Vila C et al (2019) P2X7 receptor induces mitochondrial failure in monocytes and compromises NLRP3 inflammasome activation during sepsis. Nat Commun 10(1):2711
75. Karki R, Man SM, Kanneganti TD (2017) Inflammasomes and cancer. Cancer Immunol Res 5(2):94–99
76. Martinon F, Burns K, Tschopp J (2002) The inflammasome: a molecular platform triggering activation of inflammatory caspases and processing of proIL-beta. Mol Cell 10(2):417–426
77. He WT, Wan H, Hu L, Chen P, Wang X, Huang Z et al (2015) Gasdermin D is an executor of pyroptosis and required for interleukin-1β secretion. Cell Res 25(12):1285–1298
78. Salcedo R, Worschech A, Cardone M, Jones Y, Gyulai Z, Dai RM et al (2010) MyD88-mediated signaling prevents development of adenocarcinomas of the colon: role of interleukin 18. J Exp Med 207(8):1625–1636
79. Broz P, Dixit VM (2016) Inflammasomes: mechanism of assembly, regulation and signalling. Nat Rev Immunol 16(7):407–420

80. Allen IC, TeKippe EM, Woodford RM, Uronis JM, Holl EK, Rogers AB et al (2010) The NLRP3 inflammasome functions as a negative regulator of tumorigenesis during colitis-associated cancer. J Exp Med 207(5):1045–1056
81. Ghiringhelli F, Apetoh L, Tesniere A, Aymeric L, Ma Y, Ortiz C et al (2009) Activation of the NLRP3 inflammasome in dendritic cells induces IL-1beta-dependent adaptive immunity against tumors. Nat Med 15(10):1170–1178
82. Wei Q, Zhu R, Zhu J, Zhao R, Li M (2019) E2-induced activation of the NLRP3 inflammasome triggers pyroptosis and inhibits autophagy in HCC cells. Oncol Res 27(7): 827–834
83. Dupaul-Chicoine J, Arabzadeh A, Dagenais M, Douglas T, Champagne C, Morizot A et al (2015) The Nlrp3 inflammasome suppresses colorectal cancer metastatic growth in the liver by promoting natural killer cell tumoricidal activity. Immunity 43(4):751–763
84. Chow MT, Sceneay J, Paget C, Wong CS, Duret H, Tschopp J et al (2012) NLRP3 suppresses NK cell-mediated responses to carcinogen-induced tumors and metastases. Cancer Res 72(22): 5721–5732
85. Wang H, Luo Q, Feng X, Zhang R, Li J, Chen F (2018) NLRP3 promotes tumor growth and metastasis in human oral squamous cell carcinoma. BMC Cancer 18(1):500
86. Daley D, Mani VR, Mohan N, Akkad N, Pandian G, Savadkar S et al (2017) NLRP3 signaling drives macrophage-induced adaptive immune suppression in pancreatic carcinoma. J Exp Med 214(6):1711–1724
87. Guo B, Fu S, Zhang J, Liu B, Li Z (2016) Targeting inflammasome/IL-1 pathways for cancer immunotherapy. Sci Rep 6:36107
88. Theivanthiran B, Evans KS, DeVito NC, Plebanek M, Sturdivant M, Wachsmuth LP et al (2020) A tumor-intrinsic PD-L1/NLRP3 inflammasome signaling pathway drives resistance to anti-PD-1 immunotherapy. J Clin Invest 130(5):2570–2586
89. Wu J, Sun L, Chen X, Du F, Shi H, Chen C et al (2013) Cyclic GMP-AMP is an endogenous second messenger in innate immune signaling by cytosolic DNA. Science 339(6121):826–830
90. Wu JJ, Zhao L, Hu HG, Li WH, Li YM (2020) Agonists and inhibitors of the STING pathway: potential agents for immunotherapy. Med Res Rev 40(3):1117–1141
91. Liu S, Cai X, Wu J, Cong Q, Chen X, Li T et al (2015) Phosphorylation of innate immune adaptor proteins MAVS, STING, and TRIF induces IRF3 activation. Science 347(6227):2630
92. Ishikawa H, Barber GN (2008) STING is an endoplasmic reticulum adaptor that facilitates innate immune signalling. Nature 455(7213):674–678
93. Woo SR, Fuertes MB, Corrales L, Spranger S, Furdyna MJ, Leung MY et al (2014) STING-dependent cytosolic DNA sensing mediates innate immune recognition of immunogenic tumors. Immunity 41(5):830–842
94. Corrales L, Glickman LH, McWhirter SM, Kanne DB, Sivick KE, Katibah GE et al (2015) Direct activation of STING in the tumor microenvironment leads to potent and systemic tumor regression and immunity. Cell Rep 11(7):1018–1030
95. Loo YM, Gale M Jr (2011) Immune signaling by RIG-I-like receptors. Immunity 34(5): 680–692
96. Kato H, Takeuchi O, Sato S, Yoneyama M, Yamamoto M, Matsui K et al (2006) Differential roles of MDA5 and RIG-I helicases in the recognition of RNA viruses. Nature 441(7089): 101–105
97. Poeck H, Bscheider M, Gross O, Finger K, Roth S, Rebsamen M et al (2010) Recognition of RNA virus by RIG-I results in activation of CARD9 and inflammasome signaling for interleukin 1 beta production. Nat Immunol 11(1):63–69
98. Elion DL, Cook RS (2018) Harnessing RIG-I and intrinsic immunity in the tumor microenvironment for therapeutic cancer treatment. Oncotarget 9(48):29007–29017
99. Jiang X, Kinch LN, Brautigam CA, Chen X, Du F, Grishin NV et al (2012) Ubiquitin-induced oligomerization of the RNA sensors RIG-I and MDA5 activates antiviral innate immune response. Immunity 36(6):959–973

100. Heidegger S, Wintges A, Stritzke F, Bek S, Steiger K, Koenig PA et al (2019) RIG-I activation is critical for responsiveness to checkpoint blockade. Sci Immunol 4:39
101. van Kooten C, Banchereau J (2000) CD40-CD40 ligand. J Leukoc Biol 67(1):2–17
102. Todryk SM, Tutt AL, Green MH, Smallwood JA, Halanek N, Dalgleish AG et al (2001) CD40 ligation for immunotherapy of solid tumours. J Immunol Methods 248(1-2):139–147
103. van Mierlo GJ, den Boer AT, Medema JP, van der Voort EI, Fransen MF, Offringa R et al (2002) CD40 stimulation leads to effective therapy of CD40(-) tumors through induction of strong systemic cytotoxic T lymphocyte immunity. Proc Natl Acad Sci U S A 99(8): 5561–5566
104. Buhtoiarov IN, Lum H, Berke G, Paulnock DM, Sondel PM, Rakhmilevich AL (2005) CD40 ligation activates murine macrophages via an IFN-gamma-dependent mechanism resulting in tumor cell destruction in vitro. J Immunol 174(10):6013–6022
105. Elgueta R, Benson MJ, de Vries VC, Wasiuk A, Guo Y, Noelle RJ (2009) Molecular mechanism and function of CD40/CD40L engagement in the immune system. Immunol Rev 229(1):152–172
106. Bennett SR, Carbone FR, Karamalis F, Flavell RA, Miller JF, Heath WR (1998) Help for cytotoxic-T-cell responses is mediated by CD40 signalling. Nature 393(6684):478–480
107. Byrne KT, Vonderheide RH (2016) CD40 stimulation obviates innate sensors and drives T cell immunity in cancer. Cell Rep 15(12):2719–2732
108. Beatty GL, Chiorean EG, Fishman MP, Saboury B, Teitelbaum UR, Sun W et al (2011) CD40 agonists alter tumor stroma and show efficacy against pancreatic carcinoma in mice and humans. Science 331(6024):1612–1616
109. Long KB, Gladney WL, Tooker GM, Graham K, Fraietta JA, Beatty GL (2016) IFNγ and CCL2 cooperate to redirect tumor-infiltrating monocytes to degrade fibrosis and enhance chemotherapy efficacy in pancreatic carcinoma. Cancer Discov 6(4):400–413
110. Jeannin P, Paolini L, Adam C, Delneste Y (2018) The roles of CSFs on the functional polarization of tumor-associated macrophages. FEBS J 285(4):680–699
111. Zhu Y, Knolhoff BL, Meyer MA, Nywening TM, West BL, Luo J et al (2014) CSF1/CSF1R blockade reprograms tumor-infiltrating macrophages and improves response to T-cell checkpoint immunotherapy in pancreatic cancer models. Cancer Res 74(18):5057–5069
112. Papadopoulos KP, Gluck L, Martin LP, Olszanski AJ, Tolcher AW, Ngarmchamnanrith G et al (2017) First-in-human study of AMG 820, a monoclonal anti-colony-stimulating factor 1 receptor antibody, in patients with advanced solid tumors. Clin Cancer Res 23(19): 5703–5710
113. Dowlati A, Harvey RD, Carvajal RD, Hamid O, Klempner SJ, Kauh JSW et al (2021) LY3022855, an anti-colony-stimulating factor-1 receptor (CSF-1R) monoclonal antibody, in patients with advanced solid tumors refractory to standard therapy: phase 1 dose-escalation trial. Investig New Drugs 39(4):1057–1071
114. Vergadi E, Ieronymaki E, Lyroni K, Vaporidi K, Tsatsanis C (2017) Akt signaling pathway in macrophage activation and M1/M2 polarization. J Immunol 198(3):1006–1014
115. Kaneda MM, Messer KS, Ralainirina N, Li H, Leem CJ, Gorjestani S et al (2016) PI3Kgamma is a molecular switch that controls immune suppression. Nature 539(7629):437–442
116. Kaneda MM, Cappello P, Nguyen AV, Ralainirina N, Hardamon CR, Foubert P et al (2016) Macrophage PI3Kgamma drives pancreatic ductal adenocarcinoma progression. Cancer Discov 6(8):870–885
117. Tseng D, Volkmer JP, Willingham SB, Contreras-Trujillo H, Fathman JW, Fernhoff NB et al (2013) Anti-CD47 antibody-mediated phagocytosis of cancer by macrophages primes an effective antitumor T-cell response. Proc Natl Acad Sci U S A 110(27):11103–11108
118. Hu B, Wang Z, Zeng H, Qi Y, Chen Y, Wang T et al (2020) Blockade of DC-SIGN(+) tumor-associated macrophages reactivates antitumor immunity and improves immunotherapy in muscle-invasive bladder cancer. Cancer Res 80(8):1707–1719
119. Chitadze G, Lettau M, Bhat J, Wesch D, Steinle A, Furst D et al (2013) Shedding of endogenous MHC class I-related chain molecules A and B from different human tumor

entities: heterogeneous involvement of the "a disintegrin and metalloproteases" 10 and 17. Int J Cancer 133(7):1557–1566

120. Cathcart J, Pulkoski-Gross A, Cao J (2015) Targeting matrix metalloproteinases in cancer: bringing new life to old ideas. Genes Dis 2(1):26–34

121. Ferrari de Andrade L, Tay RE, Pan D, Luoma AM, Ito Y, Badrinath S et al (2018) Antibody-mediated inhibition of MICA and MICB shedding promotes NK cell-driven tumor immunity. Science 359(6383):1537–1542

122. Bekaert S, Rocks N, Vanwinge C, Noel A, Cataldo D (2021) Asthma-related inflammation promotes lung metastasis of breast cancer cells through CCL11-CCR3 pathway. Respir Res 22(1):61

123. Lopez-Soto A, Folgueras AR, Seto E, Gonzalez S (2009) HDAC3 represses the expression of NKG2D ligands ULBPs in epithelial tumour cells: potential implications for the immunosurveillance of cancer. Oncogene 28(25):2370–2382

124. O'Sullivan T, Dunn GP, Lacoursiere DY, Schreiber RD, Bui JD (2011) Cancer immunoediting of the NK group 2D ligand H60a. J Immunol 187(7):3538–3545

125. Armeanu S, Bitzer M, Lauer UM, Venturelli S, Pathil A, Krusch M et al (2005) Natural killer cell-mediated lysis of hepatoma cells via specific induction of NKG2D ligands by the histone deacetylase inhibitor sodium valproate. Cancer Res 65(14):6321–6329

126. Hervieu A, Rebe C, Vegran F, Chalmin F, Bruchard M, Vabres P et al (2013) Dacarbazine-mediated upregulation of NKG2D ligands on tumor cells activates NK and CD8 T cells and restrains melanoma growth. J Invest Dermatol 133(2):499–508

127. van Montfoort N, Borst L, Korrer MJ, Sluijter M, Marijt KA, Santegoets SJ et al (2018) NKG2A blockade potentiates CD8 T cell immunity induced by cancer vaccines. Cell 175(7):1744–1755

128. Creelan BC, Antonia SJ (2019) The NKG2A immune checkpoint - a new direction in cancer immunotherapy. Nat Rev Clin Oncol 16(5):277–278

129. van Hall T, Andre P, Horowitz A, Ruan DF, Borst L, Zerbib R et al (2019) Monalizumab: inhibiting the novel immune checkpoint NKG2A. J Immunother Cancer 7(1):263

130. Anagnostou E, Kosmopoulou MN, Chrysina ED, Leonidas DD, Hadjiloi T, Tiraidis C et al (2006) Crystallographic studies on two bioisosteric analogues, N-acetyl-beta-D-glucopyranosylamine and N-trifluoroacetyl-beta-D-glucopyranosylamine, potent inhibitors of muscle glycogen phosphorylase. Bioorg Med Chem 14(1):181–189

131. Gauthier L, Morel A, Anceriz N, Rossi B, Blanchard-Alvarez A, Grondin G et al (2019) Multifunctional natural killer cell engagers targeting NKp46 trigger protective tumor immunity. Cell 177(7):1701–1713

132. Sharma P, Allison JP (2015) The future of immune checkpoint therapy. Science 348(6230):56–61

133. Chen DS, Mellman I (2017) Elements of cancer immunity and the cancer-immune set point. Nature 541(7637):321–330

134. Cristescu R, Mogg R, Ayers M, Albright A, Murphy E, Yearley J, Sher X, Liu XQ, Lu H, Nebozhyn M, Zhang C, Lunceford JK, Joe A, Cheng J, Webber AL, Ibrahim N, Plimack ER, Ott PA, Seiwert TY, Ribas A, McClanahan TK, Tomassini JE, Loboda A, Kaufman D (2019) Erratum: Pan-tumor genomic biomarkers for PD-1 checkpoint blockade-based immunotherapy. Science 363:6430

135. Cristescu R, Mogg R, Ayers M, Albright A, Murphy E, Yearley J et al (2018) Pan-tumor genomic biomarkers for PD-1 checkpoint blockade-based immunotherapy. Science 362:6411

136. Cheever MA, Higano CS (2011) PROVENGE (Sipuleucel-T) in prostate cancer: the first FDA-approved therapeutic cancer vaccine. Clin Cancer Res 17(11):3520–3526

137. Carreno BM, Magrini V, Becker-Hapak M, Kaabinejadian S, Hundal J, Petti AA et al (2015) Cancer immunotherapy. A dendritic cell vaccine increases the breadth and diversity of melanoma neoantigen-specific T cells. Science 348(6236):803–808

138. Miller JS, Soignier Y, Panoskaltsis-Mortari A, McNearney SA, Yun GH, Fautsch SK et al (2005) Successful adoptive transfer and in vivo expansion of human haploidentical NK cells in patients with cancer. Blood 105(8):3051–3057

139. Miller JS, Lanier LL (2019) Natural Killer Cells in Cancer Immunotherapy. Annu Rev Cancer Biol 3(1):77–103

140. Bald T, Krummel MF, Smyth MJ, Barry KC (2020) The NK cell-cancer cycle: advances and new challenges in NK cell-based immunotherapies. Nat Immunol 21(8):835–847

141. Torikai H, Reik A, Soldner F, Warren EH, Yuen C, Zhou Y et al (2013) Toward eliminating HLA class I expression to generate universal cells from allogeneic donors. Blood 122(8): 1341–1349

142. Trzonkowski P, Szmit E, Mysliwska J, Dobyszuk A, Mysliwski A (2004) CD4+CD25+ T regulatory cells inhibit cytotoxic activity of T CD8+ and NK lymphocytes in the direct cell-to-cell interaction. Clin Immunol 112(3):258–267

143. Li H, Han Y, Guo Q, Zhang M, Cao X (2009) Cancer-expanded myeloid-derived suppressor cells induce energy of NK cells through membrane-bound TGF-beta 1. J Immunol 182(1): 240–249

144. Labadie BW, Bao R, Luke JJ (2019) Reimagining IDO pathway inhibition in cancer immunotherapy via downstream focus on the tryptophan-kynurenine-aryl hydrocarbon axis. Clin Cancer Res 25(5):1462–1471

Chapter 20
Systemic Onco-sphere: Host Adaptive Immune System

Phei Er Saw and Erwei Song

Abstract When antigenic tumor cells contact the immune system, they set off both innate and adaptive immune system. In the previous chapter, we have described the host innate immune system and how it influences cancer growth and progression. For T cells, adaptive immune system must be activated by innate immune system, especially by the presentation of antigens from APCs to T cells in order to be activated. For B cells, the system can activate two pathways (1) secretion of plasma cells, producing tumor-specific antibody, or (2) releasing cytokines that have tumor inhibition effect. In this chapter, we will summarize the pivotal role of host adaptive immune cells in tumor growth.

Introduction

When antigenic tumor cells contact the immune system, they set off both innate and adaptive immune system. In the previous chapter, we have described the host innate immune system and how it influences cancer growth and progression. For T cells,

P. E. Saw
Guangdong Provincial Key Laboratory of Malignant Tumor Epigenetics and Gene Regulation, Guangdong-Hong Kong Joint Laboratory for RNA Medicine, Medical Research Center, Sun Yat-sen Memorial Hospital, Sun Yat-sen University, Guangzhou, China

Nanhai Translational Innovation Center of Precision Immunology, Sun Yat-sen Memorial Hospital, Sun Yat-sen University, Foshan, China

E. Song (✉)
Guangdong Provincial Key Laboratory of Malignant Tumor Epigenetics and Gene Regulation, Guangdong-Hong Kong Joint Laboratory for RNA Medicine, Medical Research Center, Sun Yat-sen Memorial Hospital, Sun Yat-sen University, Guangzhou, China

Nanhai Translational Innovation Center of Precision Immunology, Sun Yat-sen Memorial Hospital, Sun Yat-sen University, Foshan, China

Breast Tumor Center, Sun Yat-sen Memorial Hospital, Sun Yat-sen University, Guangzhou, China
e-mail: songew@mail.sysu.edu.cn

adaptive immune system must be activated by innate immune system, especially by the presentation of antigens from APCs to T cells in order to be activated. For B cells, the system can activate two pathways (1) secretion of plasma cells, producing tumor-specific antibody, or (2) releasing cytokines that have tumor inhibition effect [1]. Mounting evidences are pointing toward the feasibility of harnessing the antitumor activity of T and B cells, as they have proven to be effective in multiple solid tumors [2, 3]. Over the past decade, immune checkpoint inhibitors (ICIs), especially antibodies targeting CLTA-4 and PD-1/PD-L1 axis, have shown impressive results, with proofs of long-term survival of cancer patients [4, 5]. However, the rule of thumb in this therapy is the prerequisite of effector immune cell activation, this could include NK cells as well (discussed in detail in [6]). In adaptive immunity, this assumption is mainly targeted toward T cells, as their activation is a must for ICI to work [7]. However, as we seen throughout this book, cancer cells are smart enough to modulate their ecosystem toward one that favors their own survival, and that includes overexpression of ligands that can counteract the ICI receptors on effector cells, causing exhaustive phenotype of immunoregulatory phenotype, rendering immunotherapy ineffective [8, 9]. Herein, we discuss the host adaptive immune system should be normally working, and how it changes as the tumor cells in the local *oncosphere* create their own niche to transform host immune system.

Host Adaptive Immunity and Tumor Growth

Tumor-associated antigens, or TAAs, are crucial components to trigger immune response. These TAAs and even tumor-specific antigens (TSAs) are crucial to the activation of T cell response. This T cell response is mediated through the major histocompatibility complex (MHC), a key defense line against tumor growth. Even though TAAs are made in different ways, APCs presented these antigens to the T cells in a standardized manner: as a small peptides bound on their MHC class I or class II molecules. This causes chemokines and cytokines to be released and costimulatory molecules on T cells are also induced to be expressed. Together, they lead to the clonal expansion of T cells, while encouraging other immune cells to infiltrate the tumor. CD4 T cells, also called T helper cells, release chemicals called cytokines that could modulate different response of the immune environment. The two major types of CD4 are Th1 and Th2 subsets. Th1 cells' major activity is to enhance antitumor efficacy by activating CD8 T cells, while Th2 cells work closely with B cells to aid in humoral immunity [10]. The prerequisite of a potent effector immune cell activation lies in how these antigens are presented to the T cells, and therefore, the APCs play a major role in T cell priming (Fig. 20.1).

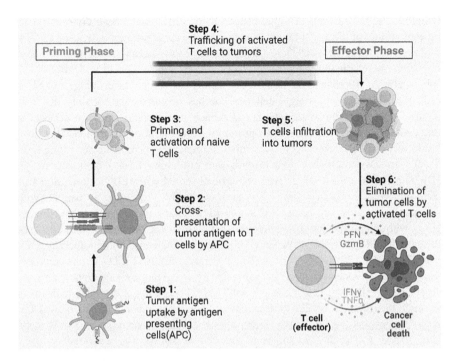

Fig. 20.1 The importance of APCs as the bridge that connects the innate immune system and the adaptive immune systems. DCs are the major APCs in immune system, activating effector T cells in both the tumor microenvironment (local oncosphere, right) and the tumor-draining lymph nodes (regional oncosphere, left)

DCs: A Potent APCs for Priming T Cells

DC Major Subsets

Although DCs are categorized as innate immune cells, they are the bridge and the key players of adaptive antitumor immunity, by cross-presentation of antigens to naïve T cells, thereby activating these T cell to exert their tumor killing ability [11]. Conventional DCs (cDCs) could be divided into (1) CD103$^+$ cDC1 lineage (priming CD8$^+$ T cells); and (2) CD11b$^+$ cDC2 lineage (priming of helper CD4$^+$ T cells) [12]. Interestingly, although cDC1s are found in lesser amount in tumors, this subset is critical for T cell infiltration. Only a small amount of cDC1 is required to process antigens which they took up from phagocytosed tumor cells [13, 14]. In a murine melanoma model, in order to successfully recruit CTL to the tumor site, Batf3$^+$ CD103$^+$ cDC1s' subset is required. Mechanistically, Batf3$^+$ CD103$^+$ cDC1s secrete CXCL9 and CXCL10 to attract T cells to the local *oncosphere* [15]. Furthermore, CD103$^+$ cDC1 could migrate from the local *oncosphere* to the regional *oncosphere* (lymph node) to cross-present these antigens to naïve T cells in the lymph nodes [16]. Given its significance, many studies have been done to derive strategic usage of cDC1s at tumor sites to improve cancer immunotherapy [13, 17].

Another DC subset, cDC2 has been getting more attention recently, as more researches are elucidating their role in immunosurveillance regulation. Unlike cDC1 subset, cDC2 is more heterogenous. They mostly coordinate the priming of CD4$^+$ T cells [18]. Interestingly, single cell analysis has revealed that not only cDC2 is composed of a variety of subsets, but also each subset could have distinct role in the regulation of CD4 T cells. Both protumoral and antitumoral features have been found within cDC2 subsets [19]. Nevertheless, generally, cDC2s are activating CD4 T cells, thereby improving their priming and promoting CD4 T cells activity. In HNCC patients, a decrease in Treg could be observed when cDC2 expression was increased, which was indicative of an increase in PFS [18]. Also, in patients with melanoma, patients who responded to anti-PD1 therapy were found to have higher cDC2 within their tumors [18]. Therefore, the relationship between cDC2s and Treg balance should be carefully considered in designing DC-based immunotherapy. DCs could be loaded with antigen, but without the right conditions, CD4 T cells could not be activated. This step is called "licensing," in a way, giving DCs the right to activate T cells for T cells to have a "license to kill" [20, 21]. The major licensing pathway is through the binding of CD40 (expressed abundantly on APCs, such as DCs, macrophages, and even on B cells) with CD40L on activated CD4 T cells [22]. Upon CD40/CD40L binding, the CD40 pathway is activated in DCs [23, 24], increasing their expression of MHC-II, CD80, and CD86 (all supportive of T cell priming) [25, 26]. A study reveals that during CD4$^+$ T cell-mediated DCs licensing, CCL5 is secreted by the DCs that could recruit CCR5 naïve CD8$^+$ T cells, which could lead to the activation of CD8$^+$ T cells as well [27]. Therefore, regardless of DCs subset, they can both be useful in activating adaptive immune response.

Adaptive Immunity: Immune Editing and Evasion

Tumor cells can be educated to avoid being recognized as "foreign entity" by the immune system through various pathways. Some tumors have been shown to stop making MHC molecules, preventing them from presenting tumor antigens and letting T cells recognize them. Some tumors secrete immunosuppressive cytokines, i.e., IL-10. Some tumors grow in places where the immune system does not attack. They make physical barriers, like collagen and fibrin, that hide them from the immune system [28]. Immune tolerance is achieved by certain regulatory cells and inhibitory receptors. Immunosuppressive Tregs release IL-10 and TGF-β, which cause effector B and T cells to be inactive [29]. Costimulatory signals (i.e., CTLA-4, PD-1) educate T cells to not respond to stimuli. Therefore, downregulating immune checkpoint proteins are being looked at to boost the immune system's ability to fight cancer.

Pivotal Role of CTLs in Cancer Immunity

CTLs are a key part of cytotoxic activity against autologous tumor cells restricted by HLA class I. CTLs can recognize different neoantigens that are only found in tumors and cause antitumor immunity. Activated CTLs bound to target cells, in this case, tumor self, causing T cell to secrete and release cytotoxic granules, such as perforin, granulysin, and granzymes (Fig. 20.2), which kill the target cells [30]. Activated T cells also secrete cytokines that can act in a paracrine manner to induce cell death in cancer. CD8$^+$ CTL infiltration is directly linked to a favorable outcome in various cancers [31–33]. Interestingly, when CTLs recognize tumor-specific antigens (TSAs), these T cells are able to kill tumor cells without the inclusion or infiltration of CD4$^+$ T cells or the expression of costimulatory molecules, just like it has been shown that viral antigen recognition [34]. In another study, the CD3 molecule was used to stimulate T cells taken from the lymph nodes of people with head and neck cancers that had already spread. It was found that patients who did not respond well to CD3 stimulation had a higher rate of recurrent cancer [35]. Bladder cancer patients with higher CD8$^+$ CTLs were also more likely to have longer OS [36]. Interestingly, the ratio of CD8$^+$ CTL to Treg is important in NAC therapy, as higher CTL/Treg ratio can lead to good clinical response [36, 37]. This observation shows that immunotherapy should be stratified to certain population of patients. In ovarian cancer patients, not only those with higher intraepithelial CTLs have longer OS, higher CTL/Treg ratio, they also have an increment of CD8$^+$ effector memory T cells and an increased level of CXCL9. This is interesting as CXCL9 is an antitumoral chemokine that could attract the infiltration of CD8 T cells [38, 39]. In breast cancer, it has been shown that TILs in the stroma are linked to better outcomes in some subgroups of patients [40].

However, research also found that CD8$^+$ T cells play a double role in RCC patients, where higher CD8$^+$ T cells were linked to a shorter OS [41]. When CTLs were added to cytarabine treatment in AML patients, it made it easier to inhibit the expression of BCL-2 [42]. Also, when chemotherapy is combined with CTLs, a strong immune response against the tumor can be triggered. The latter seems to improve the effectiveness of immunotherapy by getting rid of Treg cells and improved CTLs efficacy [43]. Lastly, CD8$^+$ memory stem T cells (TSCM) have been described. These cells can self-renew and can change into powerful effector cells [44, 45]. These cells could have much clinical potential because they could be used in adoptive T cell therapy to create long-lasting and effective immunity against tumors [46].

Th1 Cells in Antitumor Immunity

Th1 cells can be seen as generally good for triggering an effective immune response against many tumors as Th1 is an antitumoral phenotype. High infiltration of Th1 cells is indicative of favorable prognosis in many cancers [31, 47–49]. In brain

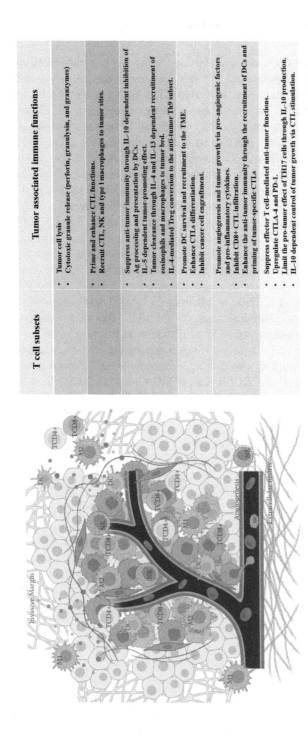

T cell subsets	Tumor associated immune functions
	• Tumor cell lysis • Cytotoxic granule release (perforin, granulysin, and granzymes)
	• Prime and enhance CTL functions. • Recruit CTL, NK and type I macrophages to tumor sites.
	• Suppress anti-tumor immunity through IL–10 dependent inhibition of Ag processing and presentation by DCs. • IL–5 dependent tumor-promoting effect. • Tumor clearance through IL–4 and IL–13 dependent recruitment of eosinophils and macrophages to tumor bed. • IL–4-mediated Treg conversion to the anti-tumor Th9 subset.
	• Promote DC survival and recruitment to the TME. • Enhance CTLs differentiation. • Inhibit cancer cell engraftment.
	• Promote angiogenesis and tumor growth via pro-angiogenic factors and pro-inflammatory cytokines. • Inhibit CD8+ CTL infiltration. • Enhance the anti-tumor immunity through the recruitment of DCs and priming of tumor-specific CTLs
	• Suppress effector T cell-mediated anti-tumor functions. • Upregulate CTLA-4 and PD-1. • Limit the pro-tumor effect of TH17 cells through IL–10 production. • IL–10 dependent control of tumor growth via CTL stimulation.

Fig. 20.2 The presence and function of the main types of T cells in the microenvironment of a tumor. (Left) There are different subset of T cells that are concurrently existing in a tumor *oncosphere*. (Right) The table shows the functions of each T cell subsets

cancer, tumor-specific Th1 cells were responsible for CD8 T cell infiltration. Also, mice with brain tumors would have a stronger immune response against the tumor if CD4 Th1 cells and CD8 T cells were simultaneously given. High levels of IFN-γ were linked to a good prognosis of colorectal cancer [50]. Therefore, Th1 cell responses are mostly helpful when mounting an effective immune response against a tumor. However, Th1 cells could cause chronic inflammation through IL-1β, IL-2, IFN-γ, and TNF-α production, which is protumoral [51, 52]. Th1 phenotype is very important for developing an effective immune response against tumors, especially when it comes to boosting CTL activity [53]. The outcome of the immune response could be changed by cytokines that could affect this phenotype. It has been suggested that the cytokine-induced STAT3 promotes Th1 conversion [54], while the same STAT3 stimulated by IFN-α or IFN-γ receptor works to stabilize Th1 phenotype [54].

Th2 Cells in Tumor Immunity

In its antitumoral activity, Th2 T cells do not kill tumor cells directly, rather they secrete cytokines to activate other types of immune cells [55, 56]. Cytokines released by Th2 cells are linked to lowering the immune response against tumors [57, 58]. This effect could be caused by IL-10 through the blockade of DC antigen processing, presentation, and/or activating immunosuppressing Treg cells [59]. Th2-secreted factors and components have been implicated and also play a role in the death of tumor cells [60, 61]. It was shown that the Th2 cytokine IL-4 was associated to tumor eradication by attracting eosinophils and macrophages to attack the tumor [62]. CLL patients with good prognosis have more Th2 cells, compared to progressive patients [63]. Also, cytokine secretion analyses from previous studies have shown that during the progression of CLL, perforin-expressing CD4$^+$ T cells release abundant IL-4 [64].

Th17 Cells in Cancer Immunity: Dual Properties

Depending on the type of cancer, Th17 cells can either be pro- or antitumorigenic [65, 66]. For example, the high level of IL-17 is indicative of worse prognosis in breast cancer [67]. However, in multiple myeloma patients, DCs can activate Th17 cells to produce high levels of IL-17 through CCL20 axis [68, 69]. Blood level of IL-17 has been linked to the formation of angiogenesis [69, 70]. CD45RO$^+$CD45RA Th17 cells express surface receptors CD49 and CCR2, CCR5, and CCR7 that attract them to the tumor sites [71, 72]. Interestingly, Th17 cells may have different effects on tumor growth, depending on their phenotype and cytokine profile. In the presence of CXCL2 and CXCL9 (antiangiogenic chemokines), the proinflammatory effect of IL-17 is reduced, leading to an antiangiogenic effect from Th17 [73, 74]. It has been recently found that Th17 cells directly work CD8$^+$ CTLs to kill tumor cells [75]. However, in melanoma, Th17 cells have been identified to produce the protumoral CCD20 chemokine [76, 77]. Using a human gastric adenocarcinoma cell line, IL-17 is involved in higher levels of MAPK and the recruitment of neutrophils to cause chronic proinflammatory process leading to worse outcome [78]. In glioma mouse models, IL-10 and Treg cells were higher compared to control. These results showed that the antitumor effect of Th17 cells could be affected by the cytokines released by Treg cells [79]. This could be an example of the "environmental conditioning," which occurs in a tumor niche in order to elevate their own survival.

Emerging Role of Th9 Cells in Cancer Immunity

Contradicting data were found on the effect of Th9 subsets and their role in cancer immunity. Some studies presented a protumoral activity of Th9, while others support an antitumoral role of Th9 in cancers [80]. For example, in a melanoma murine model, Th9 cells showed strong antitumor effect. When Th9-secreted IL9 is depleted, the mouse lost its ability to fight against cancer. Similarly, when the DCs are activated by dentin-1, this activation leads to the induction of a Th9-mediated antitumor immunity, therefore indicating a strong antitumoral functions of Th9 cell [81, 82]. CD8$^+$ T cytotoxic 9 (Tc9) cells were more effective at killing tumors than regular CD8$^+$ Tc1 cells when they mature in a Th9-polarized environment. In IL-9-rich environment, the transferred Tc9 cells are long-lived and have self-renewing ability [83]. Vaccinating mice with the carcinoembryonic antigen (CEA) led to the production of CEA-specific Th9 cells. Together with activated mast cells, these cells were able to cause long-term immune surveillance and stop CTCs from creating a new distal *oncosphere* [84]. IL-9 is overexpressed in CLL and that IL-9 directly contributes to CLL development. IL-9 is a cytokine that is only made by Th9 when the STAT6 is present, as silencing STAT6 reduces IL-9 production. Contrastingly, overexpression of IL-4 could lead STAT-6 phosphorylation, which leads to an overexpression of IL-9, providing a new avenue for CLL therapy [85].

Treg Cells in Cancer Immunity

Many cancers have clear indication of excessive Tregs in the tumor [86, 87]. The presence or abundance of Tregs have been shown to inhibit the antitumoral functions to effector T cells [60]. In colorectal and pancreatic cancers, studies have shown that IL-10 and IL-17-producing RORγt$^+$ FOXP3$^+$ Treg cells are more abundant in cancer tissues compared to controls. Patients with higher subset of RORγt$^+$ FOXP3$^+$ Treg cells have shown to have worse diagnosis [88, 89]. There is much information about how the exhaustion process works for effector T cells, but not for Tregs. It was found that PD-1^{high} Treg cells had lesser suppressive activity, with high IFN-γ expression, with hints of molecules linked to the exhaustion phenotype [90]. There are ligands that are expressed on Tregs, namely, ICOS, LAG-3, and TIM-3 that are regularly coexpressed on the surface of Tregs. These ligands have been found to bind to PD-1 in tumors [90]. The presence of both tumor-specific Tregs and effector T cells leads to suppressive functions of Tregs and suppresses immune response against CRC. It has been found that FoxP3$^+$ Helios$^+$ Treg subsets could halt their activities by expressing both PD-1 and CD39 simultaneously [91]. These Treg subsets of cells could also express both PD-1 and CTLA-4, slow down T cell activation, and stop them from making an effective immune response against cancer [91]. Interestingly, in melanoma patients treated with ipilimumab, the intratumoral Treg cells seemed to be changed as they stop affecting the effector T cells, resulting in better clinical outcome [92], a phenomenon seen in many types of cancer, like head and neck, colorectal, ovarian, and bladder [93]. Treg cells release a powerful anti-inflammatory cytokine, IL-10, which was thought to slow down the immune response against tumors. However, there are proofs that IL-10 may activate tumor-specific CD8$^+$ T cells. When PEGylated IL-10 was injected into mice, it activated IFN-γ$^+$ tumor-specific CD8$^+$ T cells which then inhibit tumor growth [94, 95]. Untreated CLL patients had more Treg cells compared to treated patients [63] while in AML patients undergoing immunotherapy, Treg cells might affect the risk of relapse [96].

B Cells in Antitumor Response: Antibody-Mediated Tumor Immunity

Protumoral Effect of Antibody in Cancer Immunology

Why do some antitumor antibodies speed up the growth of tumors? There may be a link between the ability of antitumor antibodies to make circulating immune complexes (CICs) and the progression of the disease [97]. In cancer, CICs in the blood or tumor tissue indicate that the patient's condition is getting worse [98, 99]. In a murine SCC model, CICs, when they are produced, are then absorbed by cancerous and precancerous tissues. This in turn activates Fcγ receptors on infiltrating myeloid cells, including mast cells and macrophages to be skewed toward a protumoral phenotype [100]. Simultaneously, this also activates the complement pathways, where the proangiogenic programming of tissue is activated. In a study using melanoma cell lines, the EVs that are secreted by the tumors could carry antibodies that are protumoral [101], indicating that EVs from tumors could encapsulate proteins or other biomolecules in their compartments that can trigger adaptive immune responses [102]. Another camouflage method used by the tumor cells is to produce tumor antigens that are not actually antigenic, but still incur B cells to produce antibodies specific to these antigens. When this happens, not only these antibodies do not possess any tumor cell killing activity, but also they are still able to bind with infiltrated myeloid cells, binding Fcγ receptors on these cells, and causing a suppression in myeloid cell activity, which ultimately leads to tumor growth (Fig. 20.2).

B Cells-Secreted Protumorigenic Factors

Lymphangiogenesis is one of the main pathways for tumor metastasis [103]. Inflammation can help lymphangiogenesis, making it easier for immune cells to move toward the lymphatic system. As we emphasized in this book, the intercellular communications between cells are crucial in every step of carcinogenesis, and this is true also for lymphangiogenesis as lymphotoxin is mainly produced by B, and it is a crucial factor in activating the angiogenesis and lymphangiogenesis of tumor cells. Furthermore, chemokine secretion is also crucial for B cells. In a model of prostate cancer in mouse, when the androgen is cut off by castration, the cancer cell could not survive, leading to apoptosis of the cancer cell, damaging the stromal cells and making it easier for white blood cells to fenestrate into the tumor. After the deprivation of androgen CXCL13 production is increased, increment of CXCL13 attracts B cells into the tumor parenchyma [104, 105]. These B cells (infiltrated B cells) then release lymphotoxin, which turns on NF-κB and STAT3 signaling, causing them to grow without the help of androgens and the tumor to spread [106, 107]. Also, in bladder cancer, B cells activate IL-8 to modulate androgen receptor and MMPs remodeling toward a protumoral phenotype [108].

Bregs are cells that release IL-10, but some Bregs can also release TGFβ, and others can make IL-35 [109, 110]. Also, it seems that many of these Bregs are different in how they look and how they work. Some Bregs make IL-10, make inflammation worse, and help cancer grow [30, 37] while some prevent CD4$^+$ T cell responses [111]. In autoimmune disease, B cell-suppressing Th1 responses are helpful; however, this mechanism in tumor is not favorable toward the host. The abundance of Bregs increases the tumor cell ability to survive in a chronically inflamed environment. This is exemplified by the tumor's high expression of 5-lipoxygenase metabolites (like leukotriene B4), where these metabolites could activate PPARα pathway in B cells, transforming them into Bregs [112]. Bregs also secrete high levels of TGFβ, and this can trigger phenotype changes of a CD4$^+$ T cells into Foxp3$^+$ Tregs. When Tregs ratio increases, these cells in turn block the TILs in tumor, especially NK cells and effector CD8$^+$ CTLs, reducing their antitumor efficacy [109, 113]. As these tumor-induced Bregs set off a chain of events that end up suppressing the immune system, they will likely continue to be made as long as the cancer cells are still there [114]. This shows how important it is to find ways to control and get rid of these cells as part of a treatment plan.

Breg phenotypes can also be caused by immune cells at the tumor site or in a lymph node that drains the tumor. It has also been shown that when Tregs make IL-21, this encourages B cells to secrete more IL-10, IDO, and granzyme B [115]. Normally, granzyme B is important for effector cells such as cytotoxic NK cells, CD8$^+$ CTLs, and CD4$^+$ CTLs. However, recently, granzyme B has been associated with an immunomodulatory role. When Bregs secrete granzyme B, this paracrine mode of T cell uptake of granzyme can lead to a breakdown of their receptor (in zeta chain), which renders the T cell to be inefficient [115]. In one B16F10 melanoma mouse model, B cells tend to collect in the lymph nodes that the tumor drained into. The specific subset of B cells that caused remodeling of the lymph nodes that the tumor drained into and helped the cancer spread was found using phenotypic analysis. These cells were T2-MZP "marginal zone precursors; $IgM^{hi}IgD^{hi}CD1d^{hi}CD21^{hi}$" B cells, which, unlike their Breg counterparts in the spleen [116], did not make more IL-10 or help make more Tregs. These T2-MZP Bregs seemed to be put into the lymph node as "seeds" that could modulate an immunosuppressive environments in lymph nodes and during metastasis [117, 118].

B cells are also needed to fully activate MDSCs to help B cells with halting $CD4^+$ and $CD8^+$ T cells from activation. As mentioned above, Bregs in the tumor niche secrete TGFβ, which then encourages MDSC subsets of monocytes and granulocytes to increase the production of ROS and NO, which have serious repercussion on antitumor $CD4^+$ and $CD8^+$ T cells activity [109]. As seen in one study on prostate cancer murine model, tumors do not respond to oxaliplatin treatment, unless B cells were fully removed from the system [119]. As one of the effect of oxaliplatin is to induce tumoral secretion of TGFβ, this environment became favorable to infiltrating B cells to be transformed into IgA-secreting plasmacytes, which also secrete IL-10 and overexpress death-receptor-mediated ligands such as PD-L1 and Fas-L, again, leaning toward an immunosuppressive environment [113, 120, 121] (Fig. 20.3). More and more evidence shows that Bregs are present in some human tumors. However, while anti-CD20 and other reagents can be used to get rid of more B cells overall, there are currently no ways to remove only Bregs. Also, B cell depletion has had mixed results in antitumor efficacy in mouse models. For example, one study revealed that when B cell is depleted with an anti-CD20 antibody, tumor growth was halted [122].

B Cell-Production of Antibodies That Promote Tumor Inhibition

Tumor antigen-specific antibodies are often found in the serum and blood of cancer patients, indicating that the host immune system has been identifying these tumors as foreign in these patients [123]. For example, antibodies that target an abnormally expressed β-actin (abnormally expressed on apoptotic tumor cells) could be detected in breast cancer patients [124, 125]. Many subsequent studies also affirm the importance of the antibody, as they suggested a good clinical outcome with increment of lymphoplasmacytic infiltrates in the tumor [126, 127]. Even though the research is not always in agreement, some identified anti-p53 antibodies as a factor that could lead to better prognosis in lung cancer [99]. In an orthotopic model, when human lung cancer tissue was transplanted into SCID mice, tumor growth was

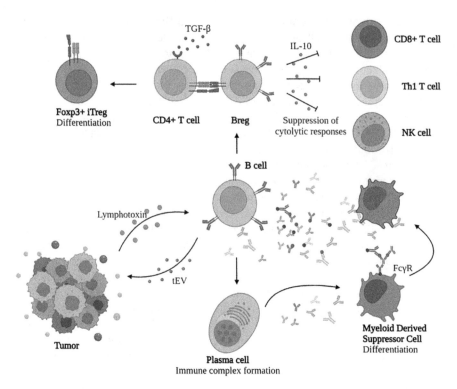

Fig. 20.3 A summary of how B cells can be protumorigenic. Lymphotoxins secreted from B cells can cause tumor angiogenesis. EVs that are derived from a tumor can stimulate B cells to make antibodies, which can bind antigens and form circulating immune complexes (CICs). CICs in the blood can turn on Fcγ receptors on myeloid cells, causing them to change into MDSCs, which then secrete various cytokines and chemokines that are protumoral, which in turn inhibit the activity of CD4$^+$ and CD8$^+$ T cells. Bregs can also release TGF-β, which makes CD4$^+$ T cells into Foxp3$^+$ CD4$^+$ Tregs, and IL-10, which inhibits CD4$^+$ Th1 cells, NK cells, CD8$^+$ cytotoxic T cells from exerting their antitumoral effect

inhibited. Results indicated that the mice B cells had produced tumor-specific IgG, that leads to tumor growth inhibition [128]. Using TCGA data and single-cell profiling of the transcriptome, data revealed that there is a direct correlation between the between the expression of complement genes and the "inferred" number of T cells in many tumors [129]. Even though there is not much experimental evidence in the case of cancer, it is possible that immune complexes with antigen, antibody, and complement help cause inflammation that makes it easier for T cells to infiltrate into tumors. In an interesting approach, mice were vaccinated with immunogenic epitopes, which were derived by tumor-derived cRNA libraries, lead to the generation of antibodies that enhance CD8$^+$ T cells activity in killing tumor cells [130]. By coinjecting tumor-binding allogeneic natural IgG antibodies and DCs, the antibodies

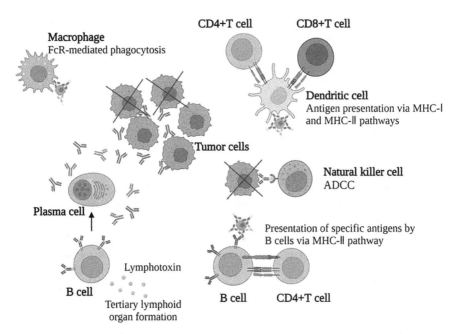

Fig. 20.4 B cells as positive mediators of the antitumor response. B cells can make lymphotoxin, which helps form tertiary lymphoid organs, which is a good sign for how the disease will turn out and how long the patient will live. Plasma cells produces antibodies, which help the immune system fight tumors in many ways. Fc receptor on antibodies can activate (1) Fc-mediated phagocytosis by macrophages, (2) ADCC through NK cells, (3) bind to Fcγ on DCs, bringing DCs closer to the tumor cells. Then, the DCs can easily engulf the tumor cells, process their tumor antigen, and cross-present them to CD8+ T cells. Specific subsets of B cells are also capable of processing tumor antigens, and these are presented to CD4 T cells

enhance the ability of DC to bind to tumor cells through the Fcγ receptors, as the Fc region of antibodies is now attached on tumor surface. Then, these DCs, after uptaking the tumor antigen, then present them to tumor-specific CD8+ T cells, leading to an enhanced and strong antitumoral (Fig. 20.4).

B cells are good APCs, although not as common as DCs. In fact, B cells could present small fractions of tumor antigens on their B cell receptors (BCRs) and even presenting them successfully to CD4 T cells. Once DCs undergo apoptosis after acute immunoactivation, B cells at this time would present antigens to T cells, but in order for them to grow into memory T cells [131, 132], a phenomenon that recognizes the importance of B cell-T cell interactions. In another murine melanoma model, depletion of B cells using anti-CD20 antibody leads to a significant decrease of CD4+ and CD8+ T cell responses, and the tumor grew to twice the size, while having incidences of lung metastasis, indicating the importance of B cells in the adaptive immune activation [133]. Even though lymphotoxin can help tumors grow [106, 134], this cytokine made by B cells can also help tertiary lymphoid organs

(TLOs) grow in favor of antitumor response [110, 135]. In both human and mouse models, the number of TLOs are directly linked to positive outcomes [33, 136]. In fact, in lung cancer patients, having increased amount of B cells in TLOs is directly correlated with longer survival [137]. In addition to making cytokines, B cells also secrete some chemokines that could attract other immune cells to secondary lymphoid organs, TLOs, and effector sites [132, 138, 139]. Through interactions between CD27 and CD70, antitumor B cells can help cytolytic T cells kill tumor cells even when they do not recognize the tumor [140] (Boxes 20.1 and 20.2).

Box 20.1 Macrophages and T Cell Activation
Macrophages are one of the main innate immune cells, as described in the previous chapters. Although in tumors, they are mostly presented as protumoral M2-like phenotype, certain macrophages can promote T-cell mediated immune response by behaving as an APCs if they are in M1-like phenotypes [141]. Even inherent macrophages (tissue-resident) could also enhance DCs ability to activate T cells. In the spleen, marginal zone macrophages have shown to be able to phagocytose tumor cells, and present these antigens to DCs [27, 142, 143]. However, due to the influence of the tumor, macrophages are usually skewed toward M2-like phenotypes that could support tumoral growth by suppressing their ability in activating T cells. For example, M2-like macrophages are known to express high levels of IL-10 that could in turn enhance the expression of N-glycan on effector T cells, which could disrupt the normal binding of TCR to CD8 [144]. After infiltrating the tumor, macrophages can be induced to express PD-L1 and B7-H4, receptors that could bind to respective ligands on T cell to inhibit their activation [145, 146].

Specific subsets of macrophages are also seen in various tissues that can be accomplices. For example, CD169$^+$ subcapsular sinus (SCS) macrophages have been identified to be localized in tumor-draining lymph nodes [147, 148]. Apparently, due to their homing location, SCS macrophages are among the first to have contact with TAAs or cell debris from apoptotic cells, making them a potential candidate to uptake these antigens and to present them as APCs to effector CD8$^+$ T cells [149, 150]. However, there are contradicting results regarding CD169$^+$ macrophages. Some studies had indicated that these macrophages can also be immunosuppressive [151, 152]. One possibility could be due to the inherent property of CD169$^+$ macrophages to capture antigens, and in cancer environment, this may be seen as "hoarding" the TAAs, preventing their cross-presentation to CD8$^+$ T cells (Table 20.1).

Table 20.1 Examples of innate immune cells' subsets and their regulation of adaptive immune cells

Components	Subsets	Functions	References
APCs	CXCL9 secretion	IFNγ stimulation, promotes the recruitment of CXCR3-expressing T cells into tumors	[153]
CD8α⁺ DCs	CXCL10 secretion	Promotes the infiltration of CXCR3⁺ activated T cells into the tumor, in a Batf3-dependent pathway	[153]
CD163⁺ macrophages and CD66b⁺ granulocytes	Multiple cytokines and chemokines	Predictive of reduced overall survival and poor response to neoadjuvant immunotherapy	[154]
Myeloid cell infiltration		Inversely correlates with CD8⁺ T cell infiltrates in breast cancer	[155]
Colony-stimulating factor-1 receptor (CSF-1R)+ TAMs		Decrease tumor-infiltrating CD8⁺ T cells	[155]
Ly6C^{lo}F4/80⁺ extratumoral macrophages	Secretion of reactive nitrogen species (RNS)	Decrease tumor-infiltrating CD8⁺ T cells	[156]
Myeloid cells	CCL2 (due to RNS)	Restricts T cells to the peritumoral stroma and impedes their direct entry into the tumor	[157]
Stromal leukocytes + CAFs	Initiating the activation of TGF-β	May inhibit T cell entry	[158, 159]

Box 20.2 Cancer Cell-Intrinsic Mechanisms Suppress Adaptive Immunity

To inhibit adaptive immunity, cancer cells can have intrinsic mechanism to ensure their survival, and their mechanisms covered all the stages: from antigen-presentation, to inhibiting immune cell infiltration, or hindering immune cell activation.

Level 1: Disruption of Antigen-Presenting Mechanism

For one, cancer cells can inhibit the movement of CD103⁺ DCs. Mechanistically, it was found that in a murine model of melanoma, PTEN loss could induce continuous activation of Wnt/β-catenin signaling, which suppresses CCL4 expression, and finally halts the migration of CD103⁺ DCs [160, 161]. In another study, liver X receptor-α, a metabolite of cholesterol derived by tumor cells, could suppress CCR7 expression on DCs, which in turn inhibit the migration of the antigen-loaded DCs from the local *oncosphere* to the regional *oncosphere* (in this case, tumor-draining lymph nodes) [162]. Tumor-derived cytokines (i.e., IL-6 and IL-10) can also promote the formation of regulatory/tolerogenic DCs that are unable to elicit adaptive

(continued)

Box 20.2 (continued)

immune response [163]. Tumor-derived VEGFs can also inhibit the maturation of DCs from their progenitor cells [164].

Level 2: Inhibition of Effector Cell Infiltration and Activation

One of the most direct observations is the upregulation of PD-L1 on tumor that could bind to PD-1 on T cells, resulting in T cell exhaustion [165]. In line with this, current studies also observed that tumor-derived exosomes are also expressing PD-L1 on the exosome membrane which suggests a long-distance communication of these tumor cells to inhibit adaptive immunity in the regional or distal *oncosphere* [166]. Besides that, biochemical changes in the local *oncosphere* (mainly resulted from tumor cell metabolism), can also lead to T cell dysfunction, exhaustion or anergy. For example, the elevated level of IDO by tumor cells leads to the breakdown of tryptophan to kynurenine [167]. As T cell proliferation requires tryptophan, this change in the metabolic environment greatly disrupts the T cell growth, which later leads to minimal T cell infiltration [168]. As mentioned above, tumor cells actively secrete TGF-β. An elevated level of TGF-β can suppress the expression of granzyme-B and perforin, at the transcriptional level, which renders the effector T cells inactive [169]. Tumor cells are also known to secrete a plethora of chemokines that could engage various innate immune cells to create a positive feedback mechanism that enhances tumor growth, mostly in a commensal or symbiotic relationship. For example, tumor-derived chemokines can attract CCR2+ and CSF1R+ macrophages, or CXCR2+ granulocytes to start the cycle mentioned above.

Level 3: Recruitment of Protumoral Comrades

To survive and thrive, tumors can exploit the neighboring cells in the local *oncosphere*, giving the tumors the "immune privilege," to be seen as self by these immune cells, rather than a foe that needs to be eradicated [170, 171]. Through changing the plasticity, tumors can establish an immunotolerant environment through various mechanisms, which are done through the recruitment of their immunosuppressive cells. As tumor cells secrete many ctyokines and chemokines (i.e., IL-4, IL-13, IL-1β, CXCL1, GM-CSF), these are the chemoattractants that could attract immune cells to the local *oncosphere* [172, 173]. For example, CD11b+Gr1+ myeloid cells have been observed to be attracted to the tumor in a model of pancreatic cancer via GM-CSF [174]. Myeloid cells that possess CD11b+Gr1+ subsets include monocytes and neutrophils. These CD11b+Gr1+ subsets are affecting adaptive immune cell activation in a few ways: (1) CD11b+Gr1+ neutrophils could release soluble arginase-1 to degrade arginine. The depletion of arginine leads to the downregulation of CD3ζ (a critical component of the TCR to induce T cell activation), which ultimately inhibits proliferative capacity of T cells [175, 176]. (2) CD11b+Gr1+ myeloid cells have shown to be activating

(continued)

Box 20.2 (continued)

NF-kB signaling due to IL-1β secretion by tumor cells [177]. In a recent study, epithelial cells have been implicated with TLR4 activation, which drives NLRP3 inflammasome activation, releasing IL-1β. High levels of IL-1β are indicative of an environment that is immunosuppressive [178]. Even during tumor cell apoptosis, they are still sending out signals that are protumoral. For example, during apoptosis, tumor cells release high amount of extracellular ATP (eATP). eATP is a common DAMP that could act as a chemoattractant for neutrophils, which could elicit inflammation when recruited to the tumor site [179–181]. eATP is also processed by ectonucleotidases to generate adenosine, which promotes immunosuppression. As mentioned above, adenosine can bind to the A2 receptors on T cell to impair T cell function [182].

Conclusion

Given the complexity of the host immune system, it is insufficient to predict cancer prognosis by only looking at one specific point. In cancer immunology, the complex interaction between host innate and adaptive immune system in predicting the outcome is seen as the "tip of the iceberg." As we mentioned as the core concept of this book, is to be able to view cancer as a self-sustainable ecosystem, and how each component can work together in realizing cancer ecosystem-directed therapeutics, which will be discussed in the final chapter of this book. As host immune system is one major component in the systemic *oncosphere*, we should consider each cancer patient as a separate entity with unique immune-environment. Understanding how immune system works in each patient might allow a better therapeutic regimen for cancer patients.

References

1. Woo SR, Corrales L, Gajewski TF (2015) Innate immune recognition of cancer. Annu Rev Immunol 33:445–474
2. Wouters MCA, Nelson BH (2018) Prognostic significance of tumor-infiltrating B cells and plasma cells in human cancer. Clin Cancer Res 24(24):6125–6135
3. Denkert C, von Minckwitz G, Darb-Esfahani S, Lederer B, Heppner BI, Weber KE et al (2018) Tumour-infiltrating lymphocytes and prognosis in different subtypes of breast cancer: a pooled analysis of 3771 patients treated with neoadjuvant therapy. Lancet Oncol 19(1):40–50
4. Ribas A, Wolchok JD (2018) Cancer immunotherapy using checkpoint blockade. Science 359(6382):1350–1355
5. Sharma P, Allison JP (2015) The future of immune checkpoint therapy. Science 348(6230): 56–61
6. Zhang J, Huang D, Saw PE, Song E (2022) Turning cold tumors hot: from molecular mechanisms to clinical applications. Trends Immunol 43:523

7. Wei SC, Levine JH, Cogdill AP, Zhao Y, Anang NAS, Andrews MC et al (2017) Distinct cellular mechanisms underlie anti-CTLA-4 and anti-PD-1 checkpoint blockade. Cell 170(6): 1120–33.e17

8. Schreiber RD, Old LJ, Smyth MJ (2011) Cancer immunoediting: integrating immunity's roles in cancer suppression and promotion. Science 331(6024):1565–1570

9. de Visser KE, Eichten A, Coussens LM (2006) Paradoxical roles of the immune system during cancer development. Nat Rev Cancer 6(1):24–37

10. Janeway CA et al (2005) Immunobiology: the immune system in health and disease, 6th edn. Churchill Livingstone, London

11. Mildner A, Jung S (2014) Development and function of dendritic cell subsets. Immunity 40(5): 642–656

12. Gardner A, Ruffell B (2016) Dendritic cells and cancer immunity. Trends Immunol 37(12): 855–865

13. Broz ML, Binnewies M, Boldajipour B, Nelson AE, Pollack JL, Erle DJ et al (2014) Dissecting the tumor myeloid compartment reveals rare activating antigen-presenting cells critical for T cell immunity. Cancer Cell 26(5):638–652

14. Kotera Y, Shimizu K, Mulé JJ (2001) Comparative analysis of necrotic and apoptotic tumor cells as a source of antigen(s) in dendritic cell-based immunization. Cancer Res 61(22): 8105–8109

15. Spranger S, Dai D, Horton B, Gajewski TF (2017) Tumor-residing Batf3 dendritic cells are required for effector T cell trafficking and adoptive T cell therapy. Cancer Cell 31(5): 711–23.e4

16. Roberts EW, Broz ML, Binnewies M, Headley MB, Nelson AE, Wolf DM et al (2016) Critical role for CD103(+)/CD141(+) dendritic cells bearing CCR7 for tumor antigen trafficking and priming of T cell immunity in melanoma. Cancer Cell 30(2):324–336

17. Salmon H, Idoyaga J, Rahman A, Leboeuf M, Remark R, Jordan S et al (2016) Expansion and activation of CD103(+) dendritic cell progenitors at the tumor site enhances tumor responses to therapeutic PD-L1 and BRAF inhibition. Immunity 44(4):924–938

18. Binnewies M, Mujal AM, Pollack JL, Combes AJ, Hardison EA, Barry KC et al (2019) Unleashing type-2 dendritic cells to drive protective antitumor CD4(+) T cell immunity. Cell 177(3):556–71.e16

19. Brown CC, Gudjonson H, Pritykin Y, Deep D, Lavallée VP, Mendoza A et al (2019) Transcriptional basis of mouse and human dendritic cell heterogeneity. Cell 179(4): 846–63.e24

20. Reis e Sousa C (2006) Dendritic cells in a mature age. Nat Rev Immunol 6(6):476–483

21. Lanzavecchia A (1998) Immunology. Licence to kill. Nature 393(6684):413–414

22. Elgueta R, Benson MJ, de Vries VC, Wasiuk A, Guo Y, Noelle RJ (2009) Molecular mechanism and function of CD40/CD40L engagement in the immune system. Immunol Rev 229(1):152–172

23. Hernandez MG, Shen L, Rock KL (2007) CD40-CD40 ligand interaction between dendritic cells and CD8+ T cells is needed to stimulate maximal T cell responses in the absence of CD4+ T cell help. J Immunol 178(5):2844–2852

24. Flinsenberg TW, Spel L, Jansen M, Koning D, de Haar C, Plantinga M et al (2015) Cognate CD4 T-cell licensing of dendritic cells heralds anti-cytomegalovirus CD8 T-cell immunity after human allogeneic umbilical cord blood transplantation. J Virol 89(2):1058–1069

25. Vonderheide RH, Bajor DL, Winograd R, Evans RA, Bayne LJ, Beatty GL (2013) CD40 immunotherapy for pancreatic cancer. Cancer Immunol Immunother 62(5):949–954

26. Beyranvand Nejad E, van der Sluis TC, van Duikeren S, Yagita H, Janssen GM, van Veelen PA et al (2016) Tumor eradication by cisplatin is sustained by CD80/86-mediated costimulation of CD8+ T cells. Cancer Res 76(20):6017–6029

27. Kurts C, Robinson BW, Knolle PA (2010) Cross-priming in health and disease. Nat Rev Immunol 10(6):403–414

28. Zou W, Chen L (2008) Inhibitory B7-family molecules in the tumour microenvironment. Nat Rev Immunol 8(6):467–477

29. Vignali DA, Collison LW, Workman CJ (2008) How regulatory T cells work. Nat Rev Immunol 8(7):523–532

30. Lieberman J (2003) The ABCs of granule-mediated cytotoxicity: new weapons in the arsenal. Nat Rev Immunol 3(5):361–370

31. Fridman WH, Pages F, Sautes-Fridman C, Galon J (2012) The immune contexture in human tumours: impact on clinical outcome. Nat Rev Cancer 12(4):298–306

32. Al-Shibli KI, Donnem T, Al-Saad S, Persson M, Bremnes RM, Busund LT (2008) Prognostic effect of epithelial and stromal lymphocyte infiltration in non-small cell lung cancer. Clin Cancer Res 14(16):5220–5227

33. Dieu-Nosjean MC, Antoine M, Danel C, Heudes D, Wislez M, Poulot V et al (2008) Long-term survival for patients with non-small-cell lung cancer with intratumoral lymphoid structures. J Clin Oncol 26(27):4410–4417

34. Zhang N, Bevan MJ (2011) CD8(+) T cells: foot soldiers of the immune system. Immunity 35(2):161–168

35. Shibuya TY, Nugyen N, McLaren CE, Li KT, Wei WZ, Kim S et al (2002) Clinical significance of poor CD3 response in head and neck cancer. Clin Cancer Res 8(3):745–751

36. Fluxá P, Rojas-Sepúlveda D, Gleisner MA, Tittarelli A, Villegas P, Tapia L et al (2018) High CD8(+) and absence of Foxp3(+) T lymphocytes infiltration in gallbladder tumors correlate with prolonged patients survival. BMC Cancer 18(1):243

37. Baras AS, Drake C, Liu JJ, Gandhi N, Kates M, Hoque MO et al (2016) The ratio of CD8 to Treg tumor-infiltrating lymphocytes is associated with response to cisplatin-based neoadjuvant chemotherapy in patients with muscle invasive urothelial carcinoma of the bladder. Oncoimmunology 5(5):e1134412

38. Sato E, Olson SH, Ahn J, Bundy B, Nishikawa H, Qian F et al (2005) Intraepithelial CD8+ tumor-infiltrating lymphocytes and a high CD8+/regulatory T cell ratio are associated with favorable prognosis in ovarian cancer. Proc Natl Acad Sci U S A 102(51):18538–18543

39. Lieber S, Reinartz S, Raifer H, Finkernagel F, Dreyer T, Bronger H et al (2018) Prognosis of ovarian cancer is associated with effector memory CD8(+) T cell accumulation in ascites, CXCL9 levels and activation-triggered signal transduction in T cells. Oncoimmunology 7(5): e1424672

40. de Melo Gagliato D, Cortes J, Curigliano G, Loi S, Denkert C, Perez-Garcia J et al (2017) Tumor-infiltrating lymphocytes in Breast Cancer and implications for clinical practice. Biochim Biophys Acta Rev Cancer 1868(2):527–537

41. Nakano O, Sato M, Naito Y, Suzuki K, Orikasa S, Aizawa M et al (2001) Proliferative activity of intratumoral CD8(+) T-lymphocytes as a prognostic factor in human renal cell carcinoma: clinicopathologic demonstration of antitumor immunity. Cancer Res 61(13):5132–5136

42. Deng R, Fan FY, Yi H, Fu L, Zeng Y, Wang Y et al (2017) Cytotoxic T lymphocytes promote cytarabine-induced acute myeloid leukemia cell apoptosis via inhibiting Bcl-2 expression. Exp Therapeut Med 14(2):1081–1085

43. Ramakrishnan R, Assudani D, Nagaraj S, Hunter T, Cho HI, Antonia S et al (2010) Chemotherapy enhances tumor cell susceptibility to CTL-mediated killing during cancer immunotherapy in mice. J Clin Invest 120(4):1111–1124

44. Gattinoni L, Zhong XS, Palmer DC, Ji Y, Hinrichs CS, Yu Z et al (2009) Wnt signaling arrests effector T cell differentiation and generates CD8+ memory stem cells. Nat Med 15(7):808–813

45. Gattinoni L, Lugli E, Ji Y, Pos Z, Paulos CM, Quigley MF et al (2011) A human memory T cell subset with stem cell-like properties. Nat Med 17(10):1290–1297

46. Cieri N, Camisa B, Cocchiarella F, Forcato M, Oliveira G, Provasi E et al (2013) IL-7 and IL-15 instruct the generation of human memory stem T cells from naive precursors. Blood 121(4):573–584

47. Sasaki K, Pardee AD, Qu Y, Zhao X, Ueda R, Kohanbash G et al (2009) IL-4 suppresses very late antigen-4 expression which is required for therapeutic Th1 T-cell trafficking into tumors. J Immunother 32(8):793–802

48. Xu X, Wang R, Su Q, Huang H, Zhou P, Luan J et al (2016) Expression of Th1- Th2- and Th17-associated cytokines in laryngeal carcinoma. Oncol Lett 12(3):1941–1948

49. Hoepner S, Loh JM, Riccadonna C, Derouazi M, Maroun CY, Dietrich PY et al (2013) Synergy between CD8 T cells and Th1 or Th2 polarised CD4 T cells for adoptive immunotherapy of brain tumours. PLoS One 8(5):e63933

50. Slattery ML, Lundgreen A, Bondurant KL, Wolff RK (2011) Interferon-signaling pathway: associations with colon and rectal cancer risk and subsequent survival. Carcinogenesis 32(11): 1660–1667

51. Konishi N, Miki C, Yoshida T, Tanaka K, Toiyama Y, Kusunoki M (2005) Interleukin-1 receptor antagonist inhibits the expression of vascular endothelial growth factor in colorectal carcinoma. Oncology 68(2–3):138–145

52. Wetzler M, Kurzrock R, Estrov Z, Kantarjian H, Gisslinger H, Underbrink MP et al (1994) Altered levels of interleukin-1 beta and interleukin-1 receptor antagonist in chronic myelogenous leukemia: clinical and prognostic correlates. Blood 84(9):3142–3147

53. Knutson KL, Disis ML (2005) Tumor antigen-specific T helper cells in cancer immunity and immunotherapy. Cancer Immunol Immunother 54(8):721–728

54. Mullen AC, High FA, Hutchins AS, Lee HW, Villarino AV, Livingston DM et al (2001) Role of T-bet in commitment of TH1 cells before IL-12-dependent selection. Science 292(5523): 1907–1910

55. Anthony RM, Urban JF Jr, Alem F, Hamed HA, Rozo CT, Boucher JL et al (2006) Memory T (H)2 cells induce alternatively activated macrophages to mediate protection against nematode parasites. Nat Med 12(8):955–960

56. Lorvik KB, Hammarström C, Fauskanger M, Haabeth OA, Zangani M, Haraldsen G et al (2016) Adoptive transfer of tumor-specific Th2 cells eradicates tumors by triggering an in situ inflammatory immune response. Cancer Res 76(23):6864–6876

57. Kusuda T, Shigemasa K, Arihiro K, Fujii T, Nagai N, Ohama K (2005) Relative expression levels of Th1 and Th2 cytokine mRNA are independent prognostic factors in patients with ovarian cancer. Oncol Rep 13(6):1153–1158

58. Ubukata H, Motohashi G, Tabuchi T, Nagata H, Konishi S, Tabuchi T (2010) Evaluations of interferon-γ/interleukin-4 ratio and neutrophil/lymphocyte ratio as prognostic indicators in gastric cancer patients. J Surg Oncol 102(7):742–747

59. Ellyard JI, Simson L, Parish CR (2007) Th2-mediated anti-tumour immunity: friend or foe? Tissue Antigens 70(1):1–11

60. Schreck S, Friebel D, Buettner M, Distel L, Grabenbauer G, Young LS et al (2009) Prognostic impact of tumour-infiltrating Th2 and regulatory T cells in classical Hodgkin lymphoma. Hematol Oncol 27(1):31–39

61. Tosolini M, Kirilovsky A, Mlecnik B, Fredriksen T, Mauger S, Bindea G et al (2011) Clinical impact of different classes of infiltrating T cytotoxic and helper cells (Th1, th2, treg, th17) in patients with colorectal cancer. Cancer Res 71(4):1263–1271

62. Tepper RI, Coffman RL, Leder P (1992) An eosinophil-dependent mechanism for the antitumor effect of interleukin-4. Science 257(5069):548–551

63. Palma M, Gentilcore G, Heimersson K, Mozaffari F, Näsman-Glaser B, Young E et al (2017) T cells in chronic lymphocytic leukemia display dysregulated expression of immune checkpoints and activation markers. Haematologica 102(3):562–572

64. Porakishvili N, Roschupkina T, Kalber T, Jewell AP, Patterson K, Yong K et al (2001) Expansion of CD4+ T cells with a cytotoxic phenotype in patients with B-chronic lymphocytic leukaemia (B-CLL). Clin Exp Immunol 126(1):29–36

65. Chen X, Wan J, Liu J, Xie W, Diao X, Xu J et al (2010) Increased IL-17-producing cells correlate with poor survival and lymphangiogenesis in NSCLC patients. Lung Cancer 69(3): 348–354

66. Liu J, Duan Y, Cheng X, Chen X, Xie W, Long H et al (2011) IL-17 is associated with poor prognosis and promotes angiogenesis via stimulating VEGF production of cancer cells in colorectal carcinoma. Biochem Biophys Res Commun 407(2):348–354
67. Chen WC, Lai YH, Chen HY, Guo HR, Su IJ, Chen HH (2013) Interleukin-17-producing cell infiltration in the breast cancer tumour microenvironment is a poor prognostic factor. Histopathology 63(2):225–233
68. Ouyang W, Kolls JK, Zheng Y (2008) The biological functions of T helper 17 cell effector cytokines in inflammation. Immunity 28(4):454–467
69. Dhodapkar KM, Barbuto S, Matthews P, Kukreja A, Mazumder A, Vesole D et al (2008) Dendritic cells mediate the induction of polyfunctional human IL17-producing cells (Th17-1 cells) enriched in the bone marrow of patients with myeloma. Blood 112(7):2878–2885
70. Niemöller K, Jakob C, Heider U, Zavrski I, Eucker J, Kaufmann O et al (2003) Bone marrow angiogenesis and its correlation with other disease characteristics in multiple myeloma in stage I versus stage II-III. J Cancer Res Clin Oncol 129(4):234–238
71. Kryczek I, Banerjee M, Cheng P, Vatan L, Szeliga W, Wei S et al (2009) Phenotype, distribution, generation, and functional and clinical relevance of Th17 cells in the human tumor environments. Blood 114(6):1141–1149
72. Martin-Orozco N, Muranski P, Chung Y, Yang XO, Yamazaki T, Lu S et al (2009) T helper 17 cells promote cytotoxic T cell activation in tumor immunity. Immunity 31(5):787–798
73. Kryczek I, Wei S, Gong W, Shu X, Szeliga W, Vatan L et al (2008) Cutting edge: IFN-gamma enables APC to promote memory Th17 and abate Th1 cell development. J Immunol 181(9):5842–5846
74. Carmeliet P, Jain RK (2000) Angiogenesis in cancer and other diseases. Nature 407(6801):249–257
75. Bowers JS, Nelson MH, Majchrzak K, Bailey SR, Rohrer B, Kaiser AD et al (2017) Th17 cells are refractory to senescence and retain robust antitumor activity after long-term ex vivo expansion. JCI Insight 2(5):e90772
76. Fabre J, Giustiniani J, Garbar C, Antonicelli F, Merrouche Y, Bensussan A et al (2016) Targeting the tumor microenvironment: the protumor effects of IL-17 related to cancer type. Int J Mol Sci 17(9):1433
77. Ghadjar P, Rubie C, Aebersold DM, Keilholz U (2009) The chemokine CCL20 and its receptor CCR6 in human malignancy with focus on colorectal cancer. Int J Cancer 125(4):741–745
78. Zhou Y, Toh ML, Zrioual S, Miossec P (2007) IL-17A versus IL-17F induced intracellular signal transduction pathways and modulation by IL-17RA and IL-17RC RNA interference in AGS gastric adenocarcinoma cells. Cytokine 38(3):157–164
79. Cantini G, Pisati F, Mastropietro A, Frattini V, Iwakura Y, Finocchiaro G et al (2011) A critical role for regulatory T cells in driving cytokine profiles of Th17 cells and their modulation of glioma microenvironment. Cancer Immunol Immunother 60(12):1739–1750
80. Li H, Rostami A (2010) IL-9: basic biology, signaling pathways in CD4+ T cells and implications for autoimmunity. J NeuroImmune Pharmacol 5(2):198–209
81. Chen J, Zhao Y, Chu X, Lu Y, Wang S, Yi Q (2016) Dectin-1-activated dendritic cells: a potent Th9 cell inducer for tumor immunotherapy. Oncoimmunology 5(11):e1238558
82. Zhao Y, Chu X, Chen J, Wang Y, Gao S, Jiang Y et al (2016) Dectin-1-activated dendritic cells trigger potent antitumour immunity through the induction of Th9 cells. Nat Commun 7:12368
83. Lu Y, Hong B, Li H, Zheng Y, Zhang M, Wang S et al (2014) Tumor-specific IL-9-producing CD8+ Tc9 cells are superior effector than type-I cytotoxic Tc1 cells for adoptive immunotherapy of cancers. Proc Natl Acad Sci U S A 111(6):2265–2270
84. Abdul-Wahid A, Cydzik M, Prodeus A, Alwash M, Stanojcic M, Thompson M et al (2016) Induction of antigen-specific TH 9 immunity accompanied by mast cell activation blocks tumor cell engraftment. Int J Cancer 139(4):841–853
85. Chen N, Lv X, Li P, Lu K, Wang X (2014) Role of high expression of IL-9 in prognosis of CLL. Int J Clin Exp Pathol 7(2):716–721

86. Ward ST, Li KK, Hepburn E, Weston CJ, Curbishley SM, Reynolds GM et al (2015) The effects of CCR5 inhibition on regulatory T-cell recruitment to colorectal cancer. Br J Cancer 112(2):319–328

87. Ladányi A, Mohos A, Somlai B, Liszkay G, Gilde K, Fejos Z et al (2010) FOXP3+ cell density in primary tumor has no prognostic impact in patients with cutaneous malignant melanoma. Pathol Oncol Res 16(3):303–309

88. Chellappa S, Hugenschmidt H, Hagness M, Line PD, Labori KJ, Wiedswang G et al (2016) Regulatory T cells that co-express RORγt and FOXP3 are pro-inflammatory and immunosuppressive and expand in human pancreatic cancer. Oncoimmunology 5(4):e1102828

89. Blatner NR, Mulcahy MF, Dennis KL, Scholtens D, Bentrem DJ, Phillips JD et al (2012) Expression of RORγt marks a pathogenic regulatory T cell subset in human colon cancer. Sci Transl Med 4(164):164ra59

90. Lowther DE, Goods BA, Lucca LE, Lerner BA, Raddassi K, van Dijk D et al (2016) PD-1 marks dysfunctional regulatory T cells in malignant gliomas. JCI Insight 1(5):e85935

91. Syed Khaja AS, Toor SM, El Salhat H, Ali BR, Elkord E (2017) Intratumoral FoxP3(+)Helios (+) regulatory T cells upregulating immunosuppressive molecules are expanded in human colorectal cancer. Front Immunol 8:619

92. Tarhini AA, Edington H, Butterfield LH, Lin Y, Shuai Y, Tawbi H et al (2014) Immune monitoring of the circulation and the tumor microenvironment in patients with regionally advanced melanoma receiving neoadjuvant ipilimumab. PLoS One 9(2):e87705

93. Winerdal ME, Marits P, Winerdal M, Hasan M, Rosenblatt R, Tolf A et al (2011) FOXP3 and survival in urinary bladder cancer. BJU Int 108(10):1672–1678

94. Mumm JB, Emmerich J, Zhang X, Chan I, Wu L, Mauze S et al (2011) IL-10 elicits IFNγ-dependent tumor immune surveillance. Cancer Cell 20(6):781–796

95. Mumm JB, Oft M (2013) Pegylated IL-10 induces cancer immunity: the surprising role of IL-10 as a potent inducer of IFN-γ-mediated CD8(+) T cell cytotoxicity. BioEssays 35(7): 623–631

96. Sander FE, Nilsson M, Rydström A, Aurelius J, Riise RE, Movitz C et al (2017) Role of regulatory T cells in acute myeloid leukemia patients undergoing relapse-preventive immunotherapy. Cancer Immunol Immunother 66(11):1473–1484

97. Gunderson AJ, Coussens LM (2013) B cells and their mediators as targets for therapy in solid tumors. Exp Cell Res 319(11):1644–1649

98. Tan TT, Coussens LM (2007) Humoral immunity, inflammation and cancer. Curr Opin Immunol 19(2):209–216

99. Kumar S, Mohan A, Guleria R (2009) Prognostic implications of circulating anti-p53 antibodies in lung cancer--a review. Eur J Cancer Care 18(3):248–254

100. Andreu P, Johansson M, Affara NI, Pucci F, Tan T, Junankar S et al (2010) FcRgamma activation regulates inflammation-associated squamous carcinogenesis. Cancer Cell 17(2): 121–134

101. Pucci F, Garris C, Lai CP, Newton A, Pfirschke C, Engblom C et al (2016) SCS macrophages suppress melanoma by restricting tumor-derived vesicle-B cell interactions. Science 352(6282):242–246

102. Raposo G, Nijman HW, Stoorvogel W, Liejendekker R, Harding CV, Melief CJ et al (1996) B lymphocytes secrete antigen-presenting vesicles. J Exp Med 183(3):1161–1172

103. Folkman J (1971) Tumor angiogenesis: therapeutic implications. N Engl J Med 285(21): 1182–1186

104. Bindea G, Mlecnik B, Angell HK, Galon J (2014) The immune landscape of human tumors: implications for cancer immunotherapy. Oncoimmunology 3(1):e27456

105. Teng MW, Galon J, Fridman WH, Smyth MJ (2015) From mice to humans: developments in cancer immunoediting. J Clin Invest 125(9):3338–3346

106. Ammirante M, Luo JL, Grivennikov S, Nedospasov S, Karin M (2010) B-cell-derived lymphotoxin promotes castration-resistant prostate cancer. Nature 464(7286):302–305

107. Woo JR, Liss MA, Muldong MT, Palazzi K, Strasner A, Ammirante M et al (2014) Tumor infiltrating B-cells are increased in prostate cancer tissue. J Transl Med 12:30
108. Ou Z, Wang Y, Liu L, Li L, Yeh S, Qi L et al (2015) Tumor microenvironment B cells increase bladder cancer metastasis via modulation of the IL-8/androgen receptor (AR)/MMPs signals. Oncotarget 6(28):26065–26078
109. Bodogai M, Moritoh K, Lee-Chang C, Hollander CM, Sherman-Baust CA, Wersto RP et al (2015) Immunosuppressive and prometastatic functions of myeloid-derived suppressive cells rely upon education from tumor-associated B cells. Cancer Res 75(17):3456–3465
110. Shen P, Fillatreau S (2015) Antibody-independent functions of B cells: a focus on cytokines. Nat Rev Immunol 15(7):441–451
111. Qin Z, Richter G, Schüler T, Ibe S, Cao X, Blankenstein T (1998) B cells inhibit induction of T cell-dependent tumor immunity. Nat Med 4(5):627–630
112. Wejksza K, Lee-Chang C, Bodogai M, Bonzo J, Gonzalez FJ, Lehrmann E et al (2013) Cancer-produced metabolites of 5-lipoxygenase induce tumor-evoked regulatory B cells via peroxisome proliferator-activated receptor α. J Immunol 190(6):2575–2584
113. Olkhanud PB, Damdinsuren B, Bodogai M, Gress RE, Sen R, Wejksza K et al (2011) Tumor-evoked regulatory B cells promote breast cancer metastasis by converting resting CD4$^+$ T cells to T-regulatory cells. Cancer Res 71(10):3505–3515
114. Lee-Chang C, Bodogai M, Martin-Montalvo A, Wejksza K, Sanghvi M, Moaddel R et al (2013) Inhibition of breast cancer metastasis by resveratrol-mediated inactivation of tumor-evoked regulatory B cells. J Immunol 191(8):4141–4151
115. Lindner S, Dahlke K, Sontheimer K, Hagn M, Kaltenmeier C, Barth TF et al (2013) Interleukin 21-induced granzyme B-expressing B cells infiltrate tumors and regulate T cells. Cancer Res 73(8):2468–2479
116. Ganti SN, Albershardt TC, Iritani BM, Ruddell A (2015) Regulatory B cells preferentially accumulate in tumor-draining lymph nodes and promote tumor growth. Sci Rep 5:12255
117. Cariappa A, Pillai S (2002) Antigen-dependent B-cell development. Curr Opin Immunol 14(2):241–249
118. Pillai S, Cariappa A, Moran ST (2004) Positive selection and lineage commitment during peripheral B-lymphocyte development. Immunol Rev 197:206–218
119. Shalapour S, Font-Burgada J, Di Caro G, Zhong Z, Sanchez-Lopez E, Dhar D et al (2015) Immunosuppressive plasma cells impede T-cell-dependent immunogenic chemotherapy. Nature 521(7550):94–98
120. Schioppa T, Moore R, Thompson RG, Rosser EC, Kulbe H, Nedospasov S et al (2011) B regulatory cells and the tumor-promoting actions of TNF-α during squamous carcinogenesis. Proc Natl Acad Sci U S A 108(26):10662–10667
121. Tadmor T, Zhang Y, Cho HM, Podack ER, Rosenblatt JD (2011) The absence of B lymphocytes reduces the number and function of T-regulatory cells and enhances the anti-tumor response in a murine tumor model. Cancer Immunol Immunother 60(5):609–619
122. Kim S, Fridlender ZG, Dunn R, Kehry MR, Kapoor V, Blouin A et al (2008) B-cell depletion using an anti-CD20 antibody augments antitumor immune responses and immunotherapy in nonhematopoietic murine tumor models. J Immunother 31(5):446–457
123. Reuschenbach M, von Knebel Doeberitz M, Wentzensen N (2009) A systematic review of humoral immune responses against tumor antigens. Cancer Immunol Immunother 58(10): 1535–1544
124. Hansen MH, Nielsen HV, Ditzel HJ (2002) Translocation of an intracellular antigen to the surface of medullary breast cancer cells early in apoptosis allows for an antigen-driven antibody response elicited by tumor-infiltrating B cells. J Immunol 169(5):2701–2711
125. Hansen MH, Nielsen H, Ditzel HJ (2001) The tumor-infiltrating B cell response in medullary breast cancer is oligoclonal and directed against the autoantigen actin exposed on the surface of apoptotic cancer cells. Proc Natl Acad Sci U S A 98(22):12659–12664

126. Bacus SS, Zelnick CR, Chin DM, Yarden Y, Kaminsky DB, Bennington J et al (1994) Medullary carcinoma is associated with expression of intercellular adhesion molecule-1. Implication to its morphology and its clinical behavior. Am J Pathol 145(6):1337–1348
127. Gaffey MJ, Frierson HF Jr, Mills SE, Boyd JC, Zarbo RJ, Simpson JF et al (1993) Medullary carcinoma of the breast. Identification of lymphocyte subpopulations and their significance. Mod Pathol 6(6):721–728
128. Mizukami M, Hanagiri T, Shigematsu Y, Baba T, Fukuyama T, Nagata Y et al (2006) Effect of IgG produced by tumor-infiltrating B lymphocytes on lung tumor growth. Anticancer Res 26(3a):1827–1831
129. Tirosh I, Izar B, Prakadan SM, Wadsworth MH II, Treacy D, Trombetta JJ et al (2016) Dissecting the multicellular ecosystem of metastatic melanoma by single-cell RNA-seq. Science 352(6282):189–196
130. Nishikawa H, Tanida K, Ikeda H, Sakakura M, Miyahara Y, Aota T et al (2001) Role of SEREX-defined immunogenic wild-type cellular molecules in the development of tumor-specific immunity. Proc Natl Acad Sci U S A 98(25):14571–14576
131. Rodríguez-Pinto D (2005) B cells as antigen-presenting cells. Cell Immunol 238(2):67–75
132. Yanaba K, Bouaziz JD, Matsushita T, Magro CM, St Clair EW, Tedder TF (2008) B-lymphocyte contributions to human autoimmune disease. Immunol Rev 223:284–299
133. DiLillo DJ, Yanaba K, Tedder TF (2010) B cells are required for optimal CD4+ and CD8+ T cell tumor immunity: therapeutic B cell depletion enhances B16 melanoma growth in mice. J Immunol 184(7):4006–4016
134. Schrama D, Thor Straten P, Fischer WH, McLellan AD, Bröcker EB, Reisfeld RA et al (2001) Targeting of lymphotoxin-alpha to the tumor elicits an efficient immune response associated with induction of peripheral lymphoid-like tissue. Immunity 14(2):111–121
135. Luther SA, Lopez T, Bai W, Hanahan D, Cyster JG (2000) BLC expression in pancreatic islets causes B cell recruitment and lymphotoxin-dependent lymphoid neogenesis. Immunity 12(5):471–481
136. Pimenta EM, Barnes BJ (2014) Role of tertiary lymphoid structures (TLS) in anti-tumor immunity: potential tumor-induced cytokines/chemokines that regulate TLS formation in epithelial-derived cancers. Cancers 6(2):969–997
137. Germain C, Gnjatic S, Tamzalit F, Knockaert S, Remark R, Goc J et al (2014) Presence of B cells in tertiary lymphoid structures is associated with a protective immunity in patients with lung cancer. Am J Respir Crit Care Med 189(7):832–844
138. Hoff ST, Salman AM, Ruhwald M, Ravn P, Brock I, Elsheikh N et al (2015) Human B cells produce chemokine CXCL10 in the presence of Mycobacterium tuberculosis specific T cells. Tuberculosis 95(1):40–47
139. Menard LC, Minns LA, Darche S, Mielcarz DW, Foureau DM, Roos D et al (2007) B cells amplify IFN-gamma production by T cells via a TNF-alpha-mediated mechanism. J Immunol 179(7):4857–4866
140. Deola S, Panelli MC, Maric D, Selleri S, Dmitrieva NI, Voss CY et al (2008) Helper B cells promote cytotoxic T cell survival and proliferation independently of antigen presentation through CD27/CD70 interactions. J Immunol 180(3):1362–1372
141. Tseng D, Volkmer JP, Willingham SB, Contreras-Trujillo H, Fathman JW, Fernhoff NB et al (2013) Anti-CD47 antibody-mediated phagocytosis of cancer by macrophages primes an effective antitumor T-cell response. Proc Natl Acad Sci U S A 110(27):11103–11108
142. Backer R, Schwandt T, Greuter M, Oosting M, Jüngerkes F, Tüting T et al (2010) Effective collaboration between marginal metallophilic macrophages and CD8+ dendritic cells in the generation of cytotoxic T cells. Proc Natl Acad Sci U S A 107(1):216–221
143. van Dinther D, Veninga H, Iborra S, Borg EGF, Hoogterp L, Olesek K et al (2018) Functional CD169 on macrophages mediates interaction with dendritic cells for CD8(+) T cell cross-priming. Cell Rep 22(6):1484–1495

144. Smith LK, Boukhaled GM, Condotta SA, Mazouz S, Guthmiller JJ, Vijay R et al (2018) Interleukin-10 directly inhibits CD8(+) T cell function by enhancing N-glycan branching to decrease antigen sensitivity. Immunity 48(2):299–312.e5

145. Kuang DM, Zhao Q, Peng C, Xu J, Zhang JP, Wu C et al (2009) Activated monocytes in peritumoral stroma of hepatocellular carcinoma foster immune privilege and disease progression through PD-L1. J Exp Med 206(6):1327–1337

146. DeNardo DG, Ruffell B (2019) Macrophages as regulators of tumour immunity and immunotherapy. Nat Rev Immunol 19(6):369–382

147. Asano K, Kikuchi K, Tanaka M (2018) CD169 macrophages regulate immune responses toward particulate materials in the circulating fluid. J Biochem 164(2):77–85

148. Moran I, Grootveld AK, Nguyen A, Phan TG (2019) Subcapsular sinus macrophages: the seat of innate and adaptive memory in murine lymph nodes. Trends Immunol 40(1):35–48

149. Louie DAP, Liao S (2019) Lymph node subcapsular sinus macrophages as the frontline of lymphatic immune defense. Front Immunol 10:347

150. Asano K, Nabeyama A, Miyake Y, Qiu CH, Kurita A, Tomura M et al (2011) CD169-positive macrophages dominate antitumor immunity by cross presenting dead cell-associated antigens. Immunity 34(1):85–95

151. McGaha TL, Chen Y, Ravishankar B, van Rooijen N, Karlsson MC (2011) Marginal zone macrophages suppress innate and adaptive immunity to apoptotic cells in the spleen. Blood 117(20):5403–5412

152. Qiu CH, Miyake Y, Kaise H, Kitamura H, Ohara O, Tanaka M (2009) Novel subset of CD8 {alpha}+ dendritic cells localized in the marginal zone is responsible for tolerance to cell-associated antigens. J Immunol 182(7):4127–4136

153. Dangaj D, Bruand M, Grimm AJ, Ronet C, Barras D, Duttagupta PA et al (2019) Cooperation between constitutive and inducible chemokines enables T cell engraftment and immune attack in solid tumors. Cancer Cell 35(6):885–900.e10

154. Tsujikawa T, Kumar S, Borkar RN, Azimi V, Thibault G, Chang YH et al (2017) Quantitative multiplex immunohistochemistry reveals myeloid-inflamed tumor-immune complexity associated with poor prognosis. Cell Rep 19(1):203–217

155. DeNardo DG, Brennan DJ, Rexhepaj E, Ruffell B, Shiao SL, Madden SF et al (2011) Leukocyte complexity predicts breast cancer survival and functionally regulates response to chemotherapy. Cancer Discov 1(1):54–67

156. Beatty GL, Winograd R, Evans RA, Long KB, Luque SL, Lee JW et al (2015) Exclusion of T cells from pancreatic carcinomas in mice is regulated by Ly6C(low) F4/80(+) extratumoral macrophages. Gastroenterology 149(1):201–210

157. Molon B, Ugel S, Del Pozzo F, Soldani C, Zilio S, Avella D et al (2011) Chemokine nitration prevents intratumoral infiltration of antigen-specific T cells. J Exp Med 208(10):1949–1962

158. Mariathasan S, Turley SJ, Nickles D, Castiglioni A, Yuen K, Wang Y et al (2018) TGFβ attenuates tumour response to PD-L1 blockade by contributing to exclusion of T cells. Nature 554(7693):544–548

159. Tauriello DVF, Palomo-Ponce S, Stork D, Berenguer-Llergo A, Badia-Ramentol J, Iglesias M et al (2018) TGFβ drives immune evasion in genetically reconstituted colon cancer metastasis. Nature 554(7693):538–543

160. Spranger S, Bao R, Gajewski TF (2015) Melanoma-intrinsic β-catenin signalling prevents anti-tumour immunity. Nature 523(7559):231–235

161. Spranger S, Gajewski TF (2015) A new paradigm for tumor immune escape: β-catenin-driven immune exclusion. J Immunother Cancer 3:43

162. Villablanca EJ, Raccosta L, Zhou D, Fontana R, Maggioni D, Negro A et al (2010) Tumor-mediated liver X receptor-alpha activation inhibits CC chemokine receptor-7 expression on dendritic cells and dampens antitumor responses. Nat Med 16(1):98–105

163. Binnewies M, Roberts EW, Kersten K, Chan V, Fearon DF, Merad M et al (2018) Understanding the tumor immune microenvironment (TIME) for effective therapy. Nat Med 24(5): 541–550

164. Oyama T, Ran S, Ishida T, Nadaf S, Kerr L, Carbone DP et al (1998) Vascular endothelial growth factor affects dendritic cell maturation through the inhibition of nuclear factor-kappa B activation in hemopoietic progenitor cells. J Immunol 160(3):1224–1232
165. Dong H, Strome SE, Salomao DR, Tamura H, Hirano F, Flies DB et al (2002) Tumor-associated B7-H1 promotes T-cell apoptosis: a potential mechanism of immune evasion. Nat Med 8(8):793–800
166. Chen G, Huang AC, Zhang W, Zhang G, Wu M, Xu W et al (2018) Exosomal PD-L1 contributes to immunosuppression and is associated with anti-PD-1 response. Nature 560(7718):382–386
167. Munn DH, Mellor AL (2016) IDO in the tumor microenvironment: inflammation, counter-regulation, and tolerance. Trends Immunol 37(3):193–207
168. Uyttenhove C, Pilotte L, Théate I, Stroobant V, Colau D, Parmentier N et al (2003) Evidence for a tumoral immune resistance mechanism based on tryptophan degradation by indoleamine 2,3-dioxygenase. Nat Med 9(10):1269–1274
169. Yang L, Pang Y, Moses HL (2010) TGF-beta and immune cells: an important regulatory axis in the tumor microenvironment and progression. Trends Immunol 31(6):220–227
170. Beatty GL, Gladney WL (2015) Immune escape mechanisms as a guide for cancer immuno-therapy. Clin Cancer Res 21(4):687–692
171. Stone ML, Beatty GL (2019) Cellular determinants and therapeutic implications of inflamma-tion in pancreatic cancer. Pharmacol Ther 201:202–213
172. Vesely MD, Kershaw MH, Schreiber RD, Smyth MJ (2011) Natural innate and adaptive immunity to cancer. Annu Rev Immunol 29:235–271
173. Li J, Byrne KT, Yan F, Yamazoe T, Chen Z, Baslan T et al (2018) Tumor cell-intrinsic factors underlie heterogeneity of immune cell infiltration and response to immunotherapy. Immunity 49(1):178–93.e7
174. Bayne LJ, Beatty GL, Jhala N, Clark CE, Rhim AD, Stanger BZ et al (2012) Tumor-derived granulocyte-macrophage colony-stimulating factor regulates myeloid inflammation and T cell immunity in pancreatic cancer. Cancer Cell 21(6):822–835
175. Mollinedo F (2019) Neutrophil degranulation, plasticity, and cancer metastasis. Trends Immunol 40(3):228–242
176. Geiger R, Rieckmann JC, Wolf T, Basso C, Feng Y, Fuhrer T et al (2016) L-arginine modulates T cell metabolism and enhances survival and anti-tumor activity. Cell 167(3): 829–42.e13
177. Tu S, Bhagat G, Cui G, Takaishi S, Kurt-Jones EA, Rickman B et al (2008) Overexpression of interleukin-1beta induces gastric inflammation and cancer and mobilizes myeloid-derived suppressor cells in mice. Cancer Cell 14(5):408–419
178. Das S, Shapiro B, Vucic EA, Vogt S, Bar-Sagi D (2020) Tumor cell-derived IL1β promotes desmoplasia and immune suppression in pancreatic cancer. Cancer Res 80(5):1088–1101
179. Di Virgilio F, Dal Ben D, Sarti AC, Giuliani AL, Falzoni S (2017) The P2X7 Receptor in Infection and Inflammation. Immunity 47(1):15–31
180. Idzko M, Ferrari D, Eltzschig HK (2014) Nucleotide signalling during inflammation. Nature 509(7500):310–317
181. Cauwels A, Rogge E, Vandendriessche B, Shiva S, Brouckaert P (2014) Extracellular ATP drives systemic inflammation, tissue damage and mortality. Cell Death Dis 5(3):e1102
182. Vijayan D, Young A, Teng MWL, Smyth MJ (2017) Targeting immunosuppressive adenosine in cancer. Nat Rev Cancer 17(12):709–724

Chapter 21
Systemic *Oncospheres:* Host Inflammation and Cancer

Phei Er Saw and Erwei Song

Abstract Inflammation is a double-edged sword in a sense that it can eradicate pathogens and encourages tissue repair under homeostatic condition. However, dysregulated inflammation, especially in the immune system, can lead to uncontrolled and chronic inflammation, which ultimately leads to cancer lesions. Therefore, uncovering biological molecular pathways underlying inflammation is crucial, as well as understanding how host inflammatory system works in relation to chronic inflammation caused by cancer. In this chapter, we look at how host inflammatory system communicate with the local onco-sphere; and the importance of balancing host inflammation to eradicate cancer.

Introduction

Virchow first proposed in 1863 that cancer occurred in areas of persistent inflammation, establishing a link between inflammation and cancer. In support of this notion, he stated that when a tissue is given certain kinds of irritant, this leads to

P. E. Saw
Guangdong Provincial Key Laboratory of Malignant Tumor Epigenetics and Gene Regulation, Guangdong-Hong Kong Joint Laboratory for RNA Medicine, Medical Research Center, Sun Yat-sen Memorial Hospital, Sun Yat-sen University, Guangzhou, China

Nanhai Translational Innovation Center of Precision Immunology, Sun Yat-sen Memorial Hospital, Sun Yat-sen University, Foshan, China

E. Song (✉)
Guangdong Provincial Key Laboratory of Malignant Tumor Epigenetics and Gene Regulation, Guangdong-Hong Kong Joint Laboratory for RNA Medicine, Medical Research Center, Sun Yat-sen Memorial Hospital, Sun Yat-sen University, Guangzhou, China

Nanhai Translational Innovation Center of Precision Immunology, Sun Yat-sen Memorial Hospital, Sun Yat-sen University, Foshan, China

Breast Tumor Center, Sun Yat-sen Memorial Hospital, Sun Yat-sen University, Guangzhou, China
e-mail: songew@mail.sysu.edu.cn

tissue damage, promoting subsequent inflammation, and ultimately leads to cellular proliferation [1]. Although it is now known that cell division alone cannot cause cancer, continuous cell division in a certain milieu containing inflammatory cells, growth hormones, active stroma, and DNA damage-promoting chemicals increases and/or promotes the chance of developing cancer. Tumors resemble wounds that do not mend in a certain sense [2]. Inflammation and cancer are regarded as having a causal link; nevertheless, many of the cellular and molecular processes regulating this relationship are still unclear. Furthermore, to promote their colonization of the host systemic oncosphere, tumor cells may commandeer crucial processes through which inflammation and cancer interact (Fig. 21.1).

The relationship between inflammation, immune system, and tumor progression is indispensable [3]. Therefore, to harness inflammation as an efficient anticancer therapy seems like a logical approach. One of the famous examples is aspirin, a non-steroidal anti-inflammatory drug (NSAIDs) that has been shown to have significant chemopreventive effect [4, 5]. Also in many studies, the statin families have been reported to be closely related with cancer risks in multiple cancers [6, 7]. In using immunotherapies such as CAR T indeed has shown plausible anticancer effect in patients [8]. Although many patients benefit, the side effects of these immune-based therapy such as cytokine storm should not be neglected [9]. This fact also reminded us that immunotherapy influences the host to activate inflammation events, which are harmful to these patients. Therefore, prior to implementing these treatments, we should think of ways to reduce systemic inflammations that would be detrimental to cancer patients. In fact, numerous studies have shown that cancer-related chronic inflammation (not acute inflammation in wound healing process) is one of the main causes of immunosuppression in the local *oncosphere*. Understanding the complex relationship between host inflammation and cancer is crucial to comprehending the systemic oncosphere.

Inflammatory Condition: A Background

The inflammatory response is usually started with a wound and therefore a breach in the blood vessels. The most initial step of the response is to marginalize leukocytes. Usually, inflammatory cells do not migrate to the side of the walls. Blood flow and interstitial pressure will keep these leukocytes flowing under normal circumstances. Major changes of leukocytes during the inflammatory process are outlined below in a timeline.

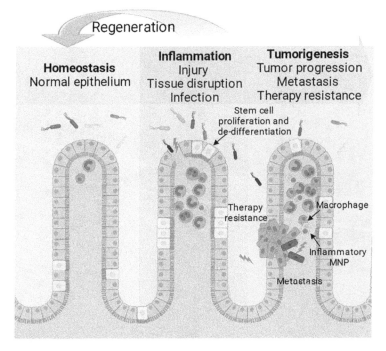

Fig. 21.1 Healing of a wound vs. invasive tumor growth. Normal structure: having an isolated, well-organized structure, and normal tissues. The vascularized stromal (dermis) compartment's removed basement membrane is positioned on top of epithelial cells. As a result of being injured, the first responder is the platelets. Upon activation, platelets then aggregated at the wound site and a hemostatic plug. Within this plug, platelets release vasoactive mediators that reduce vascular permeability, allowing more fibrinogen to penetrate through the blood vessel to form the fibrin clot. TGF-β and other GFs as well proteolytic enzymes are secreted from the platelets to begin the creation of the granulation tissue. In tumorigenesis, less organization can be seen in invasive carcinomas. In order to facilitate communication between neoplastic cells and many other types of cells (mesenchymal, hematopoietic, and lymphoid cells) as well as a modified extracellular matrix, neoplasia-associated angiogenesis, and lymphangiogenesis organize the lymphatic system and blood vessels in a complex way. While there are not as many reciprocal contacts going on at once as there are while a wound is being healed, the vascular pathway is nevertheless disrupted in a similar way during the evolution of a tumor. Neoplastic cells release cytokines and chemokines that are chemo-attractants for mast cells, fibroblasts, granulocytes, monocytes/macrophages, and endothelial cells as well as mitogens for these cells. In addition, CAFs and invasive inflammatory cells activate endothelial cells, which secretes various lymphangiogenic and angiogenic factors. Via their interactions with the lymphatic or venous networks, all of this supports angiogenesis, encourages fibroblast migration and proliferation, and contributes to the growth of the tumor

Heparin sulfate glycosaminoglycans on endothelial surface activated by chemokies binds with specific leukocyte receptors to activate integrins on inflammatory cells

Main ligand of β1-integrins are icam-1 and ICAM-2, present on endothelium. Others include VLA-4, cd49d/CD29, α4β1; which binds to VCAM.

Integrin binds leukocytes tightly, leading to complete arrest. Leukocytes "crawl" to the contact point of endothelial cells, preparing for extravasation.

A few hours after the onset of inflammation, e-selectin appears on endothelial surface, mediate slow shear stress (leukocyte rolling), along with partial leukocyte integrin activation

A dynamic process of constant binding and rapid dissociation between leukocyte and endothelium

PSGL-1, are capable of modifying glycoproteins, such as CD34 on the endothelial cell surface to become l-selectin receptors

Inflammation triggers upregulation of TNF-α and histamine, activating p-selectin

P-selectin translocation from weibel-palada corspuscles to the endothelial cell membrane

Selectin could interact with sialyl-lewis antigens, which are heavily sialyted or fucosylated. These antigens act as the ligand for p-selectin to help with their binding to ecs to facilitate their translocation.

Inflammation: A Double-Edged Sword

The fundamental role of inflammation is to protect host from infection and tissue damage, similar to the role of blood-brain barrier in the brain, to protect the nervous system from being invaded by lethal viruses and bacteria. The process of inflammation not only prevents the spread of pathogens, but inflammation also triggers appropriate mechanism to promote tissue repair. The normal highly programmed inflammatory cascade is summarized below: (1) when PAMPs are recognized by innate immune cells (i.e., macrophages/mast cells), they secrete pro-inflammatory soluble factors, such as cytokines, chemokines, vasoactive modulators to trigger early inflammation stage and (2) the secretion of the above pro-inflammatory mediators then works together to increase the permeability of vasculature, leading to the penetration and influx of plasma into the inflammation area. This plasma contains antibodies and soluble factors. Not only that, injury site can also trigger their own response to increase inflammation, including the recruitment of monocytes and neutrophils. (3) As the inflammation progresses, the host would initiate a neutralization process to stop the inflammation. At this time, macrophages are activated to clear apoptotic inflammatory cells (after being activated). (4) Finally, during the resolving period of inflammation, the host activates a tissue repair process, suppresses the inflammatory response, and thereby re-creating a homeostatic environment [10–13].

The Two Categories of Inflammation: Acute and Chronic Inflammation

In short, acute inflammation is not always bad. It is the initial response to pathogens, and usually its activated within a couple of days (max weeks), and will be resolved by the mechanisms mentioned above. In acute inflammation site, most of the infiltrated cells are granulocytes [14]. In contrast, chronic inflammation occurs when the process of tissue destruction and healing process occurs concurrently. The main immune cells infiltrating into the chronic inflamed site are lymphocytes and macrophages [15]. If not resolved, these pro-inflammatory stimuli will cause autoimmunity, tissue fibrosis, and finally, necrosis of the tissue. The most dangerous inflammation is "sustained acute inflammation without observable symptoms." Some examples of diseases in this category are chronic cholecystitis and chronic pyelonephritis [16]. Another cause of chronic inflammation includes viral infections. *Mycobacterium tuberculosis* infection does not show any symptom, but could trigger chronic inflammation without going through acute inflammation process, most probably through IFN-I pathway [17]. Chemical carcinogens are also a major source of toxicity. For example, long-term exposure to silicon or asbestos is linked to an increase in rheumatoid arthritis [18]. Not only that, major diseases such as atherosclerosis, myocardial infarction, chronic heart failure, Parkinson's disease, and Alzheimer's disease have been associated with chronic inflammation [19]. Interestingly, almost 20% of all human cancers are linked to chronic inflammation [20], which includes *H. pylori* infection, HBV, HCV, or HPV infections, which we will discuss further in Chaps. 26 and 27, respectively.

Inflammation and Cancer Progression

Peyton Rous was the first to observe that when cells are challenged with external stress, such as chemical or biological carcinogens (i.e., bacterial/virus); these cell cancers are transformed into "subthreshold neoplastic states," triggering somatic changes that are mostly irreversible [21, 22]. These states entail DNA modifications, are irreversible, and last an unlimited amount of time in otherwise normal tissues. This stage is called the "initiation stage." The cells will stay in this stage until the second phase of stimulation. In this "promotion" stage, cells are now having tumor-initiating properties, and as they are exposed to yet another carcinogen, these cells are now triggered into a second stage of inflammatory-like process. At this point, cellular biologic behavior changes and many pathways are being triggered, including promoters of pathways favoring cellular proliferation, which can also indirectly attract many immune cells into the niche, leading to an ongoing loop of inflammatory environment. In tissues that are chronically inflamed, cell death and/or restoration systems are reversed, which causes the replication of DNA and the proliferation of cells that are no longer in control of their own growth. As anti-inflammatory cytokines replace pro-inflammatory cytokines in the production process, normal inflammation is self-regulatory. But starting events or a breakdown of compensatory mechanisms that control the inflammatory response could cause chronic inflammation to become active. The summary of inflammation and cancer is summarized in Fig. 21.2.

Cancer-Promoting Inflammation

The body's vulnerability to various cancer forms has been linked to a change in biochemical pathways due to immune cell over-activation triggering chronic inflammation [23]. Although the specific mechanism by which this association is developed is still not fully known, evidence suggests that up to 25% of malignancies are linked to chronic inflammatory illnesses [24]. Clinical research has identified some chronic inflammatory malignancies as precancerous tumor lesions. For instance, it is well known that inflammatory bowel disease (IBD) is a precancerous lesion of colorectal cancer (CRC). Depending on each patient, IBD is indeed a risk factor that could develop into malignant CRCs. In addition, the chemical stimulation of IBD is thought to be a traditional technique for causing CRC in mouse models [25, 26]. IBD-related colon cancer reveals different patterns of DNA methylation

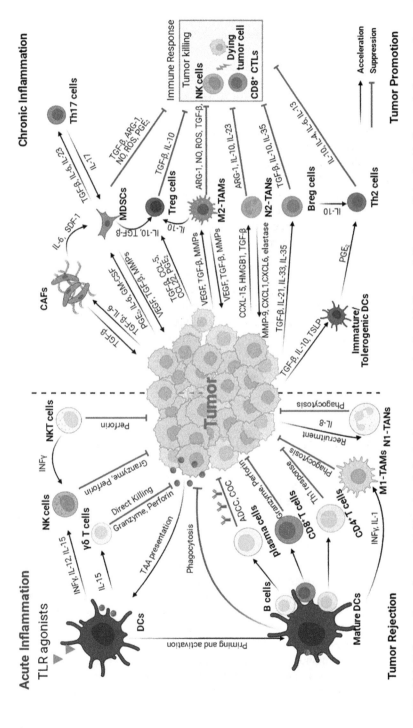

Fig. 21.2 Inflammation and cancer. (**a**) There is a distinction between a tumorigenic epithelium, an inflammatory/injured epithelium, and a homeostatic normal epithelium. (**b**) The production of auxiliary cells, the regulation of mechanical and metabolic processes, or the indirect stimulation of cytokines to stimulate tumor growth are all examples of how inflammation is implicated in the regulation of TME

levels, as compared to non-IBD colon cancer patients [27]. In addition, studies using single-cell multi-omics analysis of human CRC have demonstrated that inherent epigenetic changes are a key risk factor in both the formation and incidence of CRC [28]. The development of cancer has also been linked to some chronic inflammatory conditions brought on by viruses and bacteria. For instance, it has been demonstrated that *Helicobacter pylori* (*H. pylori*) infection causes stomach cancer and gastritis [29, 30]. In the case of mice lacking of intestinal microbiota or other microbial products, IBD alone was not sufficient to cause CRC [31], indicating the importance of *H. pylori*-dependent inflammatory response in host that in turn leads to CRC malignancy. HBV infection is known to cause hepatitis, which, in turn, is a risk factor for transformation into primary hepatocellular carcinoma [32, 33], while HPV infection is thought to be a cause of cervical cancer [34].

In all these bacterial/virus-related inflammation, the underlying mechanism is similar. First, the bacteria/virus invaded the host, and they produce metabolites to activate host immune system, causing the host to over-activate their immune system to favor inflammatory phenotype, such as M2-like macrophages, Treg cells that in turn leads to an immunosuppressive environment, favoring tumor growth [25–32, 34–42]. Immunotherapy effectiveness was markedly improved by treatments that target the gut microbiome [43], and this will be discussed further in Chap. 26, Host microbiome in systemic *oncosphere*. Additionally, the development of tumors has also been linked to a few chronic autoimmune illnesses [44]. A significant number of immunosuppressive cells prevent T cells from killing and aid immune escape in the severe inflammatory milieu, which encourages the growth of tumor cells. Additionally, research has shown that persistent inflammatory stimuli raise the likelihood of developing cancer, help it advance, and aid in the spread of metastatic disease [23].

Inter-*Oncospherical* Crosstalk: Cancer Cells Facilitate Systemic Inflammation

One of the main characteristics of malignancy is systemic inflammation, and it is known that individuals who have systemic inflammation always experience worse results [45]. It has been demonstrated how poor systemic inflammation is linked to obesity or depression, which in turn causing changes in the immune cell composition and accelerates the development of cancer [46, 47]. The risk of several cancers is increased by obesity, which is characterized by persistent inflammation. Obesity is also associated with poor outcomes [48]. Excessive nutrient intake is always a factor in the promotion of obesity-related inflammation [49]. A few examples of inflammatory chemicals are TNF-α, IL-6, IL-1β, and CCL2 that white adipose cells secreted, which has pro-tumoral properties [50, 51]. These cytokines also activated macrophages and lymphocytes to secrete more of these cytokines, creating a long-lasting inflammatory milieu. Cancer-associated adipocytes, for instance, can increase radioresistance by releasing IL-6 [52]. Since white adipocytes are pro-tumoral, one of the cancer treatment modalities is to change the white adipose tissues to brown one. The brown adipose metabolism activities include promoting insulin resistance, reducing inflammation, and increasing the release of anti-inflammatory chemicals, could be activated, which will result in a milieu that is antitumorigenic [53]. However, in breast cancer, forcing while adipocytes into pink adipocytes lead to a loss of PPARγ expression ability of mammary epithelial secretory cells, which in turn leads to a pro-tumorigenic phenotype [54]. Therefore, phenotype switching should not be generalized.

Chronic stress, depression, or social withdrawal alters immune system functioning and the inflammatory response, which gives it a pro-tumoral role in the development of cancers [55, 56]. First of all, long-term stress activates the conventional neuroendocrine system, which comprises the sympathetic nervous system (SNS) and the hypothalamic–pituitary–adrenal (HPA) axis. This, in turn, causes the hippocampus and the prefrontal cortex to become dysfunctional. Stress hormones released as a result of the HPA axis and SNS activation can then promote carcinogenesis and cancer growth through a variety of mechanisms, including those that cause DNA damage, quicken p53 degradation, and control local oncospheric TME regulation [57, 58]. Chronic stress has the power to activate the inflammatory response and the exchange of information between inflammatory and malignant cells, resulting in the development of the inflammatory TME and an increase in carcinogenesis [59, 60] (Box 21.1).

Box 21.1 Adipocytes: An Emerging Player in the Host Inflammatory System

A vital regulator of body homeostasis and systemic metabolism, adipose tissue has both paracrine and endocrine roles. It consists of adult adipocytes and the stromal vascular fraction (SVF), which is made up of endothelial cells, various immune cell subsets, and adipocyte progenitors (adipose-derived stem cells). To study adipocyte functions in cellular models, adipocytes from various adipose depots must be isolated, cultured, and differentiated. Centrifugation and collagenase digestion can be used to separate mature adipocytes and SVF from adipose tissue. Nearly 90% of the adipose tissue is made up of mature adipocytes, which float in liquid because of the high triacylglycerol content. Additionally, mature adipocytes cannot be multiplied in vitro since they are extremely fragile and have a short lifespan. They must be employed right away for a week following isolation because they are simple to rupture and consequently leak lipids during the process. As a result, many attempts have been undertaken to establish methods to increase the longevity of mature adipocytes, as well as culturing adipose tissue explants and embedding mature adipocytes in semi-solid matrixes [59, 60].

Adipocyte progenitors can also be chosen from other cell subsets in SVF via adherent cell culture. Using flow cytometry, it is possible to determine the

(continued)

Box 21.1 (continued)
phenotype of the adipocyte progenitors and their functional characteristics based on their capacity to differentiate into adipocytes. Although the precise underlying mechanisms of adipogenesis are still unknown, the diversification of adipocyte progenitors has been demonstrated in vitro. A confluent population of adipocyte progenitors can be developed into immature adipocytes that contain multilocular lipid droplets in a defined media that also contains a variety of pro-adipogenic substances like insulin, T3, glucocorticoids, IBMX, and PPAR agonists [61]. Notably, in 2D culture, the fully differentiated state, which is the acquisition of a unilocular lipid droplet in white adipocyte, is not yet attained. According to several studies, the production of unilocular lipid droplets shows that 3D-cultured cells have higher levels of differentiation. In a very recent publication in Nature Immunology, Nicholas Bernard summarized that adipocytes interact very closely indeed with the host immune cells to create a pro-tumorigenic environment, while regulating host metabolic system [62]. This further strengthen our ideology of the importance of each component of the local onco-sphere in the host inflammation-cancer axis.

Crosstalk with Host Innate and Adaptive Immune Systems

Host Innate Immunity

Cancer-Promoting Inflammation

Numerous innate immune cells have been linked to the promotion of cancer progression. The TME, which is found to be the site promoting tumor cell proliferation and angiogenesis, is where collagen is deposited and various ECM components are present [63, 64]. Additionally, because CAFs release several cytokines and chemokines, including osteopontin, IL-6, IL-1, CXCL1, CXCL2, CXCL12, CXCL13, and CCL-5, they play a critical role in the immune system [65]. Additionally, therapy-induced hypoxia can activate CAFs, which trigger the release of TGF-β and a variety of chemokines, including CXCL1 [65]. Once TGF-β is released by CAFs, TGF-β prevents the activation of both CTLs and NK cells, while favoring the changes of T cells into Treg phenotype and encouraging infiltration of immunosuppressive plasmocytes [66, 67]. Furthermore, CAF-produced CXCL13 drives B-cell recruitment to prostate cancer, resulting in resistance [68, 69].

When innate immune cells respond to infections, irritants, and pro-inflammatory or toxic substances, mast cells are the first responders [70]. In addition to rapidly releasing several biologically active mediators from their cytoplasmic granules, such as histamine, TNF-α, proteoglycans, and serotonin, among several other proteases, mast cells also released newly synthesized lipid mediators, including prostaglandins and leukotrienes, along with cytokines, leukotrienes, chemokines, and GFs after activation [71]. In addition, several mediators released by mast cells, including

IL-1β, IL-6, PGE2, TNF-α, LTB4, and leukotriene D4 (LTD4), can stimulate immunological, epithelial, endothelial, stromal cells. Numerous inflammatory conditions and various cancers have been linked to an abundance of DCs [72–74]. In addition, pancreatic cancer, CRC, and lung cancer were all found to have poorer clinical outcomes when mast cells were present in high numbers [75–77]. Interestingly, murine mast cells have also been shown to express high levels of checkpoint inhibitors' ligand, namely, PD-L1 and PD-L2. This finding indicates that mast cell could be involved in a mast cell-driven pathway of the PD-1/PD-L1 axis. Mast cells have been indicated to be involved in cancer progression by creating a pro-inflammatory local *oncosphere* for immune evasion. Additionally, mast cells promote tumor growth and metastasis by secreting lysozyme or heparin to dissolve nearby stromal tissue, which in turn promotes the formation of endothelial cells and angiogenesis [70, 71].

TAMs are a model for tumor-promoting inflammation by preventing T cells from killing and producing cytokines to stabilize the immunosuppressive condition in the local *oncosphere* [78, 79]. M2-like TAMs have also been shown to control the alteration of adaptive mechanisms, cell growth, angiogenesis deposition, and stromal cell reorganization in the TME [80]. The signals and impulses from tumor cells, T cells, and B cells were shown to be regulated by the functional reconditioning of TAMs. Even though different tumors have diverse phenotypes and communication pathways, TAMs often have M2-like traits that are comparable to immune-tolerant macrophages [80]. As the first line of defense mechanism, neutrophils' persistent infiltration is an indication of chronic inflammation, which causes tissue damage [72, 81]. They are referred to as "kamikaze" cells, which kill themselves by phagocytosis, hypochlorous acid, the release of ROS, the secretion of antimicrobial proteins, or the protuberance of DNA to produce NETs. Tumor-associated neutrophils (TANs) have also been shown to promote tumor progression by impairing the adaptive immune response [73, 74, 82]. In cancer patients, an elevation in TANs is inversely connected with the emergence of severe illness and subpar results [83]. As was noted in the previous chapters, neutrophil polarization influences the actions of TANs in the TME, which are further divided into N1 antitumor and N2 pro-tumor groups [83]. N2 are similar in M2-like macrophage, behave as a pro-tumoral neutrophil phenotype, modulating the local *oncosphere* to trigger the switching of tumor angiogenesis during the early progression of the tumor, reshape the ECM to boost the growth of tumor cells, and boost metastasis [84].

By exposing antigens to T cells and releasing immunomodulatory chemicals, eosinophils, which have vast secretory granules in their cytoplasm, control the immunological response [85]. In response to these cues, they move toward the sites of inflammation and synthesize a variety of immunomodulatory chemicals, including granule proteins that can eradicate tumor cells [86]. In addition, eosinophils can create soluble mediators that alter the matrix and promote angiogenesis, which both speed up the development of tumors. Additionally, tumor-associated tissue eosinophilia (TATE), which has a significant predictive value [87], has been discovered in several hematological and solid malignancies, confirming eosinophils' function in the antitumor response. Eosinophils have been observed to exhibit cytotoxicity via granule protein production, which contains granzyme B, and TNF-α, a similar model of effector T-cell toxicity [88]. Not only that, proteins in the granule can also direct the phenotype change of TAMs into an inflammatory (M1) phenotype [89]. When eosinophil is activated by IL-10 and IL-12, eosinophil can increase the production of adhesion molecules (such as E-cadherin) so that the dissemination of cells was reduced [90]. However, not all cancer showed benefit of TATE. In Hodgkin lymphoma and OSCCs, TATE is linked to a poor prognosis [91, 92]. Furthermore, in cervical cancer, tumor-derived thymic stromal lymphopoietin (TSLP) can promote cancer cells to secrete anti-inflammatory cytokines (i.e., IL-4, IL-5, IL-10, IL-13) which can result in decreasing CD80 and CD86 on eosinophils. Furthermore, some studies have also shown that eosinophil is pro-tumoral by secreting MMP9, FGFs, VEGFs, and PDGFs, which promote angiogenesis and tumor metastasis. By secretion of IL-4 and IL-13, they can also polarize TAM into M2-like phenotype, which is the opposite of TATE mentioned above [93]. Therefore, the environment is important to determine the function of eosinophil and whether these cells are skewed toward a pro-tumoral or antitumoral phenotype. It is generally established that MDSCs play a tumor-promoting role in cancer and store themselves in peripheral tissues. More specifically, MDSCs produce Arg-1, IL-10, iNOS, TGF-β, and COX-2 to prevent T cells from developing and functioning normally [94]. Additionally, DSCs can promote tumor angiogenesis by producing cytokines like VEGF and FGF and can speed up tumor growth by altering the TME [95]. Additionally, it was discovered that MDSCs contributed to the growth of premetastatic lesions and also metastasis via invasive primary tumors. In the case of spontaneous prostate cancer, they prevented cellular senescence by blocking the IL-1 signaling pathway. Additionally, using g-MDSCs increased IBD and had an impact on CRC formation [96].

Host Adaptive Immunity

The adaptive immune response is often a distinct reaction to lymphocyte-stimulated antigens, followed by the immunological memory effect [97]. The T-cell receptor (TCR), which recognizes antigens, is presented by antigen-presenting cells (APCs). When antigen is presented to T cells, this will activate T cells to secrete soluble factors such as IFN-γ and granzymes, through the actions of co-stimulatory molecules. One of the T-cell subset, T helper cells (Th family; Th1, Th2, Th17), also releases cytokines that activate B cells, which then secrete antibodies that trigger ADCC [98, 99]. It is well accepted that adaptive immune responses obstruct carcinogenesis and tumor growth. However, some T-cell subsets primarily engage in response to acquired immunity, which promotes tumor progression. Additionally, Treg cells, Th2 cells, and Th17 cells have frequently been linked to the development of tumors and a poor prognosis [99]. For example, Th2 is essential for orchestrating tumor progression as well as metastasis [100]. In breast cancer, Th2 and its secretion of related cytokines can stimulate the TAMs to promote M2-like phenotype, further promoting tumor metastasis [101]. These Th2-secreted cytokines (especially IL-4) are positively related with the number of $CD4^+$ T cell infiltration [102, 103]. Another subset of CD4 T cell is the Th17 subset of T helper cells. As the name implies, Th17 cells are named as they mainly secrete IL-17. Th17 is immunosuppressive as high amount of this subset have shown to be correlated to tumor growth and angiogenesis. Additionally, certain $IL\text{-}17^+$ $\gamma\delta$T cell subsets were discovered to be highly influential in encouraging tumor development and progression. By secreting various cytokines as regulatory Th17/Treg/Th2 cells, they produce an immunosuppressive milieu and promote angiogenesis [104]. These pro-tumor $IL\text{-}17^+$ $\gamma\delta$T-cells can limit DC growth and activity, which suppresses antitumor immunity via activating the PD-1/PD-L1 pathway [105–107]. According to various studies, Tregs can prevent DCs from maturing, impeding their function to phagocytose tumor cells, and restrict CTL activation, in which all of these functions lead to tumor progression [108]. Generally, Treg cells encourage the growth of tumors by impairing the antitumor immune response in the local *oncosphere*, as a whole. Specifically, Treg cells assist in immune suppression by preventing CTLA-4-mediated immunosuppression, which requires co-stimulatory signals from CD80 and CD86. Also, Tregs can produce inhibitory cytokines to diminish the antitumoral effect of TILs [109]. Tregs can also be guided toward the tumor by chemokines. For example, CCR4-CCL17/22 axis and CXCR3-CCL9/10/11 axis can attract and active Treg cells [110]. High Treg cell counts in patients are correlated with lower survival [111].

B cells also represent a major subtype of adaptive immune cells. In B-cell subtypes, there are also pro-tumoral regulatory phenotypes, known as Breg cells, which can also inhibit the immune system [112]. Breg cells also exhibit specific immunosuppressive effects in studies using both human and murine models. They do this by producing cytokines like IL-10 and TGF-β or by activating immunomodulatory ligands such as PD-L1 and CTLA-4, which reduce the response of T and NK cells and increase the cancerous effects of Treg cells, TAMs, and MDSCs [113].

Cancer-Suppressing Inflammation

Although persistent inflammation can cause cancer, the majority of inflammatory cells have antipathogenic, tissue repair, and tumor-suppressive functions. Non-specific and specific immune responses block the growth and development of tumors [114]. Cancer immune surveillance, a method through which the immune system can detect and remove emerging tumor cells, plays a crucial role in the prevention of cancer. Some strong evidence recently emerged from a huge body of research on cancer patients and mouse models, demonstrating that specific immune cell types such as innate and adaptive, as well as effector chemicals and pathways, can occasionally function as endogenous tumor suppression factors [109]. However, it is worthy to note that in an adaptive immune response to tumors, the activation is almost always initiated by innate immune cells, which triggers the adaptive immune system, mostly through DC presentation of tumor-specific antigen to T cells or through B-cell humoral immunity.

Host Innate Immunity

As the mediator of innate-adaptive immune system, DCs can regulate immune responses by various mechanisms, including activating adaptive immunity by triggering T-cell activation [115]. Additionally, by secreting IL-22BP, which can counteract the effects of IL-22 [116], DCs can prevent the malignant growth of colitis-associated colorectal cancer (CAC), whereas IL-15-cultured DCs can encourage T cells' antitumor responses by γδT cells [117]. However, it has been suggested that tumor cells may use DCs as a pawn to increase chronic inflammation and decrease TAA presentation, speeding tumor growth. For example, the IL-6 and M-CSF, together with other intrinsic signaling proteins of DCs, particularly STAT3, can redirect the development of monocytes to macrophages instead of to DCs, preventing the stimulating of tumor-related T cells [118, 119]. Furthermore, inflammatory DCs (infDCs), a subset of DCs that is linked directly to inflammatory responses, are essential for the antitumor immune response [120]. For example, depending on the inflammatory environment, fDCs might travel to lymphoid nodes and deliver antigens to immature CD4$^+$ T cells. This causes the cells to differentiate into Th1, Th2, or Th17 cells [121–123]. As a result, inflammatory DCs manifest in vitro experiments of inflammatory disorders, such as those affecting people with cancer or rheumatoid arthritis, as well as during pathogenic inflammation [124]. In conclusion, by using and activating a variety of immune cells, DCs can provide effective antitumor immunity. However, TME is abundant in immunosuppressive substances (such as VEGF, IL-6, PGE2, and IL-10) that prevent DCs from acting as immunostimulatory agents and move them toward an anti-inflammatory phenotype [125].

TAMs have a crucial role in orchestrating the inflammatory response to malignancy. In fact, TAMs display a pro-inflammatory M1-like phenotype in early cancers, in contrast to the M2-like phenotype during tumor growth. M1-like phenotype is antitumoral; therefore, they can eradicate immunogenic tumor cells through activation of Th1 response [126]. Additionally, M1-like polarized macrophages are recognized for their effective antigen presentation, increased expression of key MHC-II and co-stimulatory substances, an increased supply of pro-inflammatory cytokines (including TNF-α, IL-1β, CXCL9, IL-6, IL-12, and CXCL10), NOS, and ROS intermediates, but reduced expression of IL-10 and arginase [127, 128]. Furthermore, this phenotype of macrophage (M1-like) secretes IL-12, CXCL9, and CXCL10, which can work together to polarize and recruit Th1 cells, leading to an enhanced phagocytic activity of the macrophage toward these tumor cells [129]. LPS and IFN-γ are two important soluble factors that can stimulate macrophage polarization to M1-like. Apart from that, CpG-mediated TLR9 activation, overexpression of IL-10R is several important stimuli that can skew macrophage from M2 to M1-like phenotype. These macrophages possess high expression of HLA-DR (MHC-II) [129].

Tumor-inhibitory N1-TANs secrete CCL2, CCL3, IL-6, CXCL8, IFN-γ, and TNF-α. These soluble factors can help N1-TAN to stimulate other immune cells, such as DCs and CD8$^+$ T cells [130]. Furthermore, specific expression of co-stimulatory molecules on N1-TANs could activate CD4$^+$ and CD8$^+$ T cells, which further affects immune responses against tumors [131]. Various studies have also shown a link between the powerful antitumor effects of N1-TANs and ADCC, ROS generation, NET formation, among others [132, 133]. Other lymphoid cell subgroups, such as ILC1, ILC2, and ILC3, also performed many antitumoral activity by promoting inflammatory condition [134]. ILCs were formally recognized, which improved our understanding of their anatomical structure and outlined their crucial roles in many physiological mechanisms. Pathogen resistance, autoimmune inflammation control, tissue remodeling, cancer prevention, and metabolic balance were a few of them [31]. In cases of tissue damage, ILCs are the primary cytokine producers and important inflammatory response controllers. However, nothing is known about their specific functions in cellular change or the onset of cancer. The distinctive cytokine production patterns of the ILC family subgroups are essentially what distinguishes them. ILC1 produces IFN-γ, whereas ILC2 and ILC3 produce IL-5 and IL-13, and ILC3 produces IL-17 and IL-22 [135].

NK cells are a vital component of the immune response because of their function in inhibiting tumor progression [120]. NK cells can trigger cell apoptosis after they are activated by either secreting perforin and granzymes or by expressing FAS-L and TRAIL on their surface [136, 137]. NK cells can produce a variety of cytokines, chemokines, and growth factors in addition to their capability for cytotoxicity, including IFN-γ, TNF, IL-13, FLT3L, CCL5, CCL4, CCL3, lymphotactin (XCL1), and GM-CSF [138]. Additionally, by generating IFN-γ, which increases the expression of MHC-I on cancer cells as well as MHC-II on APCs including monocytes, macrophages, and DCs, NK cells act as a bridge that links both innate and adaptive immune system. A higher incidence of several cancers has been linked to NK cell depletion or defective NK cells [134, 139].

Notably, innate immunity depends heavily on NK-T cells because they can recognize lipid antigens presented by CD1d by expressing both the TCR of T cells and the natural killer cell receptor (NKR)-P1 receptor of NK cells [140]. Additionally, NK-T is found to release more cytokines than those associated with Th1 and Th2 even while having similar CD8$^+$ T-cell targets for killing [140]. The immune response is significantly impacted following the activation of the NK-T cells since they are frequently linked to the T-cell activation, B cells, and NK cells [134, 141]. Even though IL-17-secreting γδ-T cells have been shown to promote the growth of tumors in some circumstances, they are typically thought of as antitumor as they could provide IFN-γ mediated protective responses when necessary, indicating pn the possible plasticity of γδ-T cells in tumor immunity. Natural killer cell receptors (NKR) and TCR enable γδ-T cells to directly recognize tumor cells and eradicate tumor cells immediately, mostly through the activation of TRAIL pathway [142].

Additionally, immune cells' anti-inflammatory metabolites are crucial for the reduction of inflammation. A class of endogenous lipid mediators known as proresolving mediators (SPM), which includes resolvins, protectins, lipoxins, and maresins, exhibit proresolving and anti-inflammatory properties without impairing the immune response [142]. When inflammation first begins, macrophages release SPM, which aids in its resolution and increases vascular permeability, allowing PMN to infiltrate the inflamed tissues. SPM has also been discovered to encourage self-limited non-specific responses and increase innate microbial clearance, eliminating chronic inflammation by stopping the spread of malignancy [143]. Resolvin (RvD1 and RvD2) also can prevent A549 metastasis by minimizing EMT brought on by TGF-β1 [144]. Similarly, RvD1 activates caspase-3, increasing pancreatic ductal adenocarcinoma cells in vitro apoptosis [145]. Additionally, SPM's target immune cells can have antitumor capabilities. For instance, an LXA4 isomer may inhibit neutrophil infiltration and reduce the generation of pro-inflammatory cytokines, inhibiting the crucial aspects of colitis in animal models [146]. By targeting Breg cells that secrete IL-10 and preferentially converting M2-TAMs to the M1 phenotype, LXA4 significantly slowed the growth of tumors in tumor-bearing mice [147]. This action triggered tumor cell death, which slowed the tumor's progression [147, 148]. RvD1 was also found to enhance NK cells' capacity to kill in PDACs [149]. SPM has also been shown to stop tumor growth by concentrating on precancerous areas. RvE1, for instance, could improve colitis regression and increase survival rates [146]. Similar to this, it was also discovered that Maresin receptor 1 (MaR1) has an inhibitory effect on animals with colitis [150]. To sum up, SPM has a crucial role in reducing inflammation that supports tumors, halting the growth and spread of tumors, and boosting antitumor immunity.

Cancer-Suppressing Inflammation in Host Adaptive Immunity

The antitumor immune response heavily relies on adaptive immunity, as they are very potent in tumor cell killing mechanisms [98, 99, 151]. It has been noted that immune responses frequently include CD4+ Th1 cells, activated CD8+ T cells, and $\gamma\delta$T T cells [152]. CTLs, particularly CD8+ T cells, can recognize the tumor-specific antigens (TSAs) present in tumor cells. When a tumor cell is recognized, CTLs are activated to secrete large amount of granzyme and perforin to cause direct tumor death. CTLs will also over-express Fas-L, to enable them to directly interact on the Fas receptor on tumor cells to activate Fas-mediated cell death signaling pathways.

Th1 cells, a subset of CD4+ effector T cells known for secreting IL-2, lymphotoxin, IFN-γ, and TNF, are mainly in charge of stimulating and controlling CTL proliferation and persistence. For instance, Th1 cells can generate IFN-γ, which encourages the upregulation of LMP2, MECL, LMP7, PA28, and MHC class I molecules on APCs, all of which boost the antigen presentation to CTLs [153]. Additionally, Th1 cells are also able to orchestrate the infiltration of many other inflammatory cells within the tumor, to induce their activation and enhancing their capacity in antigen presentation to CD8+ CTLs [154]. Furthermore, Th1 cells can secrete antitumoral cytokines and lymphotoxins that could directly kill tumor cells, or by triggering the activation of death receptors on the surface of cancer cells [155].

B cells and humoral immunity can exert antitumor immunity through B cell or plasma cell specific mechanisms, such as the expression of cytokines like IL-10 or IL-35, the activation of C5a or C3a complement system components, or antibody-mediated cytotoxicity via NK cells [156]. It is important to note that B cells are also play a dual role in immunity. Some studies revealed that immunosuppressive subtypes of B cells may encourage tumor growth. For instance, tumor-infiltrating B lymphocytes (B-TILs) were seen in lung cancer at all stages [157]. It has been demonstrated that the presence of TIBs varies in different phases and histological subtypes, pointing to a critical function for B cells during the development of lung cancer [158]. It is interesting to note that activated B cells can also lyse cancer cells directly. Furthermore, TIBs can produce granzyme B and TRAIL, which can have lethal effects on hepatoma cells. In one of these studies, B cells activated by IFN-α- and TLR agonists produced functional TRAIL that was cytotoxic to melanoma cell types [159]. Numerous studies have used immunohistochemistry CD20 to examine the role of TIL-B [160]. From all these researches, 50.0% indicated a predictive effect for $CD20^+$TIBs that was positive, whereas the remaining studies revealed neutral as well as adverse effects. The antitumor activity of T cells was generally more powerful when B-TILs were present, and the prognostic importance of TIBs was primarily observed to be coherent with $CD3^+$ and $CD8^+$ T cells [160]. Finally, mounting evidence has demonstrated that B-TILs have a beneficial role in antitumor immunity, suggesting that future cancer immunotherapies should consider ways to improve these responses [161] (Box 21.2).

Box 21.2 The Host Connection: Therapy-Elicited Inflammation
Inflammation brought on by anticancer treatment has recently been discovered to be a powerful TME modulator. Different traditional chemoradiotherapy can cause immunogenic cell death (ICD) of tumor cells and cause these dying tumor cells to produce DAMPs [162–164]. As a result, CTL response is activated, in response to the ICD-induced DAMPs. The immunological response of the host affects the therapeutic effectiveness of several of these medications [162]. Chemotherapeutic medications are cytotoxic. They usually kill off cancer by obstructing cellular processes that are not only necessary for the growth and survival of tumor cells, but also important for normal cells, leading to unwanted side effects during and post-chemoradiotherapy. On the good side, chemotherapy can stimulate immunological responses and increase the stimulation of effector T cells or CTLs, thereby severing the tumor immunosuppressive environment [149, 165]. However, one of the main variables limiting the clinical outcome and therapeutic efficacy is drug resistance [2, 166]. Some chemotherapy medications cause inflammation, which is extremely important for tumor angiogenesis, metastasis, and therapy failure [167]. For instance, one of the best treatments for a solid tumor is a platinum-based drug cisplatin [168]. The stimulation of NF-κB, COX-2, and TNF-α is

(continued)

Box 21.2 (continued)

just a few of the mechanisms through which cisplatin induces inflammation [168, 169]. COX2 inhibitor celecoxib increases the antitumor effects of cisplatin in multiple cancers [170–172]. Paclitaxel causes cell arrest by stabilizing microtubules, which cause cancer cell apoptosis [170, 173]. However, numerous inflammatory factors and signaling pathways, including IL-1β, IL-6, IL-8, and NF-κB can be activated in response to the administration of paclitaxel [174–177].

Radiotherapy is currently one of the major choices for cancer treatment, totaling almost 50% of all cancer treatments [178]. Radiation activates multiple cytokines, ROS/RNS, adhesion molecules, and DAMPs, a self-amplifying cascade that could result in either triggering pro-inflammatory or anti-inflammatory environment, that could determine the fate of tumor cell death [158, 178]. On the one hand, radiation-induced inflammation induces adaptive immune responses that cross-communicate with the host during radiotherapy, potentially curing the malignancy [99, 179]. On the other hand, persistent inflammatory responses brought on by radiation may result in a rise in immunosuppressive populations, such as M2 macrophages, Tregs, and MDSCs [180]. For example, radiation can activate the IL-6/STAT3 signaling system, which promotes tumor invasion and increases tumor cells' capacity to survive after treatment, so presenting a therapeutic resistance [181, 182]. Additionally, suppressing IL-6 via siRNA prevents prostate cancer patients' tumors from recur after radiotherapy while making tumor cells more sensitive to radiation [183]. Chronic inflammation significantly contributes to tumor cell proliferation, immunosuppression, and angiogenesis [184, 185]. In ICB and CAR T treatment, the possibility of patients having a "cytokine storm" has limited their application, suggesting that the amelioration of this detrimental immunotherapy-related inflammation would be helpful for a successful outcome for cancer patients [9, 186, 187]. The potency of immunotherapy can, however, be enhanced by acute inflammation brought on by other treatments. For example, stimulation of the type 1 IFN response could enhance the efficiency of anticancer medicines by working in concert with them [188]. Radiation therapy can also cause an immediate local inflammatory response that makes tumor cells more susceptible to ICB therapy [189]. Nevertheless, it is possible to combine radiotherapy or chemotherapy with medicines that trigger acute inflammation, but not chronic inflammation. Since acute inflammation is beneficial to the host, this pathway should be considered in the future.

Conclusion

In antitumor therapy, one of the most crucial issues is figuring out how the immune system affects the formation and progression of cancer. The host immune system and chronic inflammation that make up the local *oncosphere* are intricately linked and can either promote or inhibit tumor growth and progression. Identifying the link between inflammation and malignant growth will provide new opportunities for long-lasting and effective tumor management due to its critical role in the development of cancer and its antitumor therapeutic effects.

References

1. Balkwill F, Mantovani A (2001) Inflammation and cancer: back to Virchow? Lancet 357(9255):539–545
2. Dvorak HF (1986) Tumors: wounds that do not heal. Similarities between tumor stroma generation and wound healing. N Engl J Med 315(26):1650–1659
3. Ma Y, Adjemian S, Mattarollo SR, Yamazaki T, Aymeric L, Yang H et al (2013) Anticancer chemotherapy-induced intratumoral recruitment and differentiation of antigen-presenting cells. Immunity 38(4):729–741
4. Cuzick J, Otto F, Baron JA, Brown PH, Burn J, Greenwald P et al (2009) Aspirin and non-steroidal anti-inflammatory drugs for cancer prevention: an international consensus statement. Lancet Oncol 10(5):501–507
5. Rothwell PM, Fowkes FG, Belch JF, Ogawa H, Warlow CP, Meade TW (2011) Effect of daily aspirin on long-term risk of death due to cancer: analysis of individual patient data from randomised trials. Lancet 377(9759):31–41
6. Undela K, Srikanth V, Bansal D (2012) Statin use and risk of breast cancer: a meta-analysis of observational studies. Breast Cancer Res Treat 135(1):261–269
7. Bonovas S, Nikolopoulos G, Sitaras NM (2013) Statins and reduced risk of hepatocellular carcinoma in patients with hepatitis C virus infection: further evidence is warranted. J Clin Oncol 31(32):4160
8. Rameshbabu S, Labadie BW, Argulian A, Patnaik A (2021) Targeting innate immunity in cancer therapy. Vaccines 9(2):138
9. Bonifant CL, Jackson HJ, Brentjens RJ, Curran KJ (2016) Toxicity and management in CAR T-cell therapy. Mol Ther Oncolyt 3:16011
10. Medzhitov R (2008) Origin and physiological roles of inflammation. Nature 454(7203): 428–435
11. Kono H, Rock KL (2008) How dying cells alert the immune system to danger. Nat Rev Immunol 8(4):279–289
12. Nathan C (2002) Points of control in inflammation. Nature 420(6917):846–852
13. Headland SE, Norling LV (2015) The resolution of inflammation: principles and challenges. Semin Immunol 27(3):149–160
14. Kumar R, Clermont G, Vodovotz Y, Chow CC (2004) The dynamics of acute inflammation. J Theor Biol 230(2):145–155
15. Serhan CN (2008) Controlling the resolution of acute inflammation: a new genus of dual anti-inflammatory and proresolving mediators. J Periodontol 79(8 Suppl):1520–1526
16. Nasef NA, Mehta S, Ferguson LR (2017) Susceptibility to chronic inflammation: an update. Arch Toxicol 91(3):1131–1141

17. Snell LM, McGaha TL, Brooks DG (2017) Type I interferon in chronic virus infection and cancer. Trends Immunol 38(8):542–557
18. Monteiro R, Azevedo I (2010) Chronic inflammation in obesity and the metabolic syndrome. Mediat Inflamm 2010:289645
19. Glass CK, Saijo K, Winner B, Marchetto MC, Gage FH (2010) Mechanisms underlying inflammation in neurodegeneration. Cell 140(6):918–934
20. Coussens LM, Werb Z (2002) Inflammation and cancer. Nature 420(6917):860–867
21. Mackenzie I, Rous P (1941) The experimental disclosure of latent neoplastic changes in tarred skin. J Exp Med 73(3):391–416
22. Rous P, Kidd JG (1941) Conditional neoplasms and subthreshold neoplastic states: a study of the tar tumors of rabbits. J Exp Med 73(3):365–390
23. Hanahan D, Weinberg RA (2011) Hallmarks of cancer: the next generation. Cell 144(5): 646–674
24. Murata M (2018) Inflammation and cancer. Environ Health Prev Med 23(1):50
25. Keller DS, Windsor A, Cohen R, Chand M (2019) Colorectal cancer in inflammatory bowel disease: review of the evidence. Tech Coloproctol 23(1):3–13
26. Jess T, Simonsen J, Jørgensen KT, Pedersen BV, Nielsen NM, Frisch M (2012) Decreasing risk of colorectal cancer in patients with inflammatory bowel disease over 30 years. Gastroenterology 143(2):375–81.e1; quiz e13–4.
27. Pekow J, Hernandez K, Meckel K, Deng Z, Haider HI, Khalil A et al (2019) IBD-associated colon cancers differ in DNA methylation and gene expression profiles compared with sporadic colon cancers. J Crohns Colit 13(7):884–893
28. Bian S, Hou Y, Zhou X, Li X, Yong J, Wang Y et al (2018) Single-cell multiomics sequencing and analyses of human colorectal cancer. Science 362(6418):1060–1063
29. Loor A, Dumitraşcu DL (2016) Helicobacter pylori infection, gastric cancer and gastropanel. Rom J Intern Med 54(3):151–156
30. Gottlieb M, Nakitende D (2017) Comparison of tamsulosin, nifedipine, and placebo for ureteric colic. CJEM 19(2):156–158
31. Bain CC, Mowat AM (2014) Macrophages in intestinal homeostasis and inflammation. Immunol Rev 260(1):102–117
32. Chen Y, Tian Z (2019) HBV-induced immune imbalance in the development of HCC. Front Immunol 10:2048
33. Grivennikov SI, Greten FR, Karin M (2010) Immunity, inflammation, and cancer. Cell 140(6): 883–899
34. Schiffman M, Castle PE, Jeronimo J, Rodriguez AC, Wacholder S (2007) Human papillomavirus and cervical cancer. Lancet 370(9590):890–907
35. Ma C, Han M, Heinrich B, Fu Q, Zhang Q, Sandhu M et al (2018) Gut microbiome-mediated bile acid metabolism regulates liver cancer via NKT cells. Science 360(6391):eaan5931
36. Routy B, Le Chatelier E, Derosa L, Duong CPM, Alou MT, Daillère R et al (2018) Gut microbiome influences efficacy of PD-1-based immunotherapy against epithelial tumors. Science 359(6371):91–97
37. Arpaia N, Campbell C, Fan X, Dikiy S, van der Veeken J, deRoos P et al (2013) Metabolites produced by commensal bacteria promote peripheral regulatory T-cell generation. Nature 504(7480):451–455
38. Furusawa Y, Obata Y, Fukuda S, Endo TA, Nakato G, Takahashi D et al (2013) Commensal microbe-derived butyrate induces the differentiation of colonic regulatory T cells. Nature 504(7480):446–450
39. Smith PM, Howitt MR, Panikov N, Michaud M, Gallini CA, Bohlooly YM et al (2013) The microbial metabolites, short-chain fatty acids, regulate colonic Treg cell homeostasis. Science 341(6145):569–573
40. Kalafati L, Kourtzelis I, Schulte-Schrepping J, Li X, Hatzioannou A, Grinenko T et al (2020) Innate immune training of granulopoiesis promotes anti-tumor activity. Cell 183(3): 771–85.e12

41. Li R, Zhou R, Wang H, Li W, Pan M, Yao X et al (2019) Gut microbiota-stimulated cathepsin K secretion mediates TLR4-dependent M2 macrophage polarization and promotes tumor metastasis in colorectal cancer. Cell Death Differ 26(11):2447–2463

42. Yang H, Wang W, Romano KA, Gu M, Sanidad KZ, Kim D et al (2018) A common antimicrobial additive increases colonic inflammation and colitis-associated colon tumorigenesis in mice. Sci Transl Med 10(443):eaan4116

43. Elkrief A, Derosa L, Zitvogel L, Kroemer G, Routy B (2019) The intimate relationship between gut microbiota and cancer immunotherapy. Gut Microbes 10(3):424–428

44. Jin S, Chen H, Li Y, Zhong H, Sun W, Wang J et al (2018) Maresin 1 improves the Treg/Th17 imbalance in rheumatoid arthritis through miR-21. Ann Rheum Dis 77(11):1644–1652

45. Laird BJ, McMillan DC, Fayers P, Fearon K, Kaasa S, Fallon MT et al (2013) The systemic inflammatory response and its relationship to pain and other symptoms in advanced cancer. Oncologist 18(9):1050–1055

46. Reiche EM, Nunes SO, Morimoto HK (2004) Stress, depression, the immune system, and cancer. Lancet Oncol 5(10):617–625

47. Avgerinos KI, Spyrou N, Mantzoros CS, Dalamaga M (2019) Obesity and cancer risk: emerging biological mechanisms and perspectives. Metabolism 92:121–135

48. Calle EE, Rodriguez C, Walker-Thurmond K, Thun MJ (2003) Overweight, obesity, and mortality from cancer in a prospectively studied cohort of U.S. adults. N Engl J Med 348(17): 1625–1638

49. Saltiel AR, Olefsky JM (2017) Inflammatory mechanisms linking obesity and metabolic disease. J Clin Invest 127(1):1–4

50. Howe LR, Subbaramaiah K, Hudis CA, Dannenberg AJ (2013) Molecular pathways: adipose inflammation as a mediator of obesity-associated cancer. Clin Cancer Res 19(22):6074–6083

51. Rogers NH, Perfield JW II, Strissel KJ, Obin MS, Greenberg AS (2009) Reduced energy expenditure and increased inflammation are early events in the development of ovariectomy-induced obesity. Endocrinology 150(5):2161–2168

52. Bochet L, Meulle A, Imbert S, Salles B, Valet P, Muller C (2011) Cancer-associated adipocytes promotes breast tumor radioresistance. Biochem Biophys Res Commun 411(1):102–106

53. Lee YH, Jung YS, Choi D (2014) Recent advance in brown adipose physiology and its therapeutic potential. Exp Mol Med 46(2):e78

54. Apostoli AJ, Skelhorne-Gross GE, Rubino RE, Peterson NT, Di Lena MA, Schneider MM et al (2014) Loss of PPARγ expression in mammary secretory epithelial cells creates a pro-breast tumorigenic environment. Int J Cancer 134(5):1055–1066

55. Chrousos GP (1995) The hypothalamic-pituitary-adrenal axis and immune-mediated inflammation. N Engl J Med 332(20):1351–1362

56. Stein M (1989) Stress, depression, and the immune system. J Clin Psychiatry 50 (Suppl):35–40; discussion 1–2.

57. Gao X, Cao Q, Cheng Y, Zhao D, Wang Z, Yang H et al (2018) Chronic stress promotes colitis by disturbing the gut microbiota and triggering immune system response. Proc Natl Acad Sci U S A 115(13):E2960–E29e9

58. Miller ES, Apple CG, Kannan KB, Funk ZM, Plazas JM, Efron PA et al (2019) Chronic stress induces persistent low-grade inflammation. Am J Surg 218(4):677–683

59. Yang H, Xia L, Chen J, Zhang S, Martin V, Li Q et al (2019) Stress-glucocorticoid-TSC22D3 axis compromises therapy-induced antitumor immunity. Nat Med 25(9):1428–1441

60. Curtin NM, Boyle NT, Mills KH, Connor TJ (2009) Psychological stress suppresses innate IFN-gamma production via glucocorticoid receptor activation: reversal by the anxiolytic chlordiazepoxide. Brain Behav Immun 23(4):535–547

61. Dufau J, Shen JX, Couchet M, De Castro T, Barbosa NM, Massier L, Griseti E, Mouisel E, Amri E-Z, Lauschke VM, Rydén M, Langin D (2021) In vitro and ex vivo models of adipocytes. Am J Physiol Cell Physiol 320(5):C822–C841. https://doi.org/10.1152/ajpcell. 00519.2020

62. Bernard NJ (2022) Adipocytes behaving like immune cells. Nat Immunol 23(6):817. https://doi.org/10.1038/s41590-022-01236-9
63. Bhowmick NA, Neilson EG, Moses HL (2004) Stromal fibroblasts in cancer initiation and progression. Nature 432(7015):332–337
64. Orimo A, Gupta PB, Sgroi DC, Arenzana-Seisdedos F, Delaunay T, Naeem R et al (2005) Stromal fibroblasts present in invasive human breast carcinomas promote tumor growth and angiogenesis through elevated SDF-1/CXCL12 secretion. Cell 121(3):335–348
65. Wong VW, Rustad KC, Akaishi S, Sorkin M, Glotzbach JP, Januszyk M et al (2011) Focal adhesion kinase links mechanical force to skin fibrosis via inflammatory signaling. Nat Med 18(1):148–152
66. Yang L, Pang Y, Moses HL (2010) TGF-beta and immune cells: an important regulatory axis in the tumor microenvironment and progression. Trends Immunol 31(6):220–227
67. Shalapour S, Font-Burgada J, Di Caro G, Zhong Z, Sanchez-Lopez E, Dhar D et al (2015) Immunosuppressive plasma cells impede T-cell-dependent immunogenic chemotherapy. Nature 521(7550):94–98
68. Ammirante M, Luo JL, Grivennikov S, Nedospasov S, Karin M (2010) B-cell-derived lymphotoxin promotes castration-resistant prostate cancer. Nature 464(7286):302–305
69. Ammirante M, Shalapour S, Kang Y, Jamieson CA, Karin M (2014) Tissue injury and hypoxia promote malignant progression of prostate cancer by inducing CXCL13 expression in tumor myofibroblasts. Proc Natl Acad Sci U S A 111(41):14776–14781
70. Galli SJ, Kalesnikoff J, Grimbaldeston MA, Piliponsky AM, Williams CM, Tsai M (2005) Mast cells as "tunable" effector and immunoregulatory cells: recent advances. Annu Rev Immunol 23:749–786
71. Bulfone-Paus S, Nilsson G, Draber P, Blank U, Levi-Schaffer F (2017) Positive and negative signals in mast cell activation. Trends Immunol 38(9):657–667
72. Giese MA, Hind LE, Huttenlocher A (2019) Neutrophil plasticity in the tumor microenvironment. Blood 133(20):2159–2167
73. Castanheira FVS, Kubes P (2019) Neutrophils and NETs in modulating acute and chronic inflammation. Blood 133(20):2178–2185
74. Nicolás-Ávila J, Adrover JM, Hidalgo A (2017) Neutrophils in Homeostasis, Immunity, and Cancer. Immunity 46(1):15–28
75. Kischer CW, Bunce H III, Shetlah MR (1978) Mast cell analyses in hypertrophic scars, hypertrophic scars treated with pressure and mature scars. J Invest Dermatol 70(6):355–357
76. Khazaie K, Blatner NR, Khan MW, Gounari F, Gounaris E, Dennis K et al (2011) The significant role of mast cells in cancer. Cancer Metastasis Rev 30(1):45–60
77. Aller MA, Arias JI, Arias J (2010) Pathological axes of wound repair: gastrulation revisited. Theor Biol Med Model 7:37
78. Noy R, Pollard JW (2014) Tumor-associated macrophages: from mechanisms to therapy. Immunity 41(1):49–61
79. Salmaninejad A, Valilou SF, Soltani A, Ahmadi S, Abarghan YJ, Rosengren RJ et al (2019) Tumor-associated macrophages: role in cancer development and therapeutic implications. Cell Oncol 42(5):591–608
80. Kim J, Bae JS (2016) Tumor-associated macrophages and neutrophils in tumor microenvironment. Mediat Inflamm 2016:6058147
81. Hidalgo A, Chilvers ER, Summers C, Koenderman L (2019) The neutrophil life cycle. Trends Immunol 40(7):584–597
82. Fridlender ZG, Sun J, Kim S, Kapoor V, Cheng G, Ling L et al (2009) Polarization of tumor-associated neutrophil phenotype by TGF-beta: "N1" versus "N2" TAN. Cancer Cell 16(3):183–194
83. Shaul ME, Fridlender ZG (2018) Cancer-related circulating and tumor-associated neutrophils - subtypes, sources and function. FEBS J 285(23):4316–4342
84. Ocana A, Nieto-Jiménez C, Pandiella A, Templeton AJ (2017) Neutrophils in cancer: prognostic role and therapeutic strategies. Mol Cancer 16(1):137

85. Sastre B, Rodrigo-Muñoz JM, Garcia-Sanchez DA, Cañas JA, Del Pozo V (2018) Eosinophils: old players in a new game. J Investig Allergol Clin Immunol 28(5):289–304
86. Gleich GJ, Adolphson CR, Leiferman KM (1993) The biology of the eosinophilic leukocyte. Annu Rev Med 44:85–101
87. Gatault S, Legrand F, Delbeke M, Loiseau S, Capron M (2012) Involvement of eosinophils in the anti-tumor response. Cancer Immunol Immunother 61(9):1527–1534
88. Legrand F, Driss V, Delbeke M, Loiseau S, Hermann E, Dombrowicz D et al (2010) Human eosinophils exert TNF-α and granzyme A-mediated tumoricidal activity toward colon carcinoma cells. J Immunol 185(12):7443–7451
89. Carretero R, Sektioglu IM, Garbi N, Salgado OC, Beckhove P, Hämmerling GJ (2015) Eosinophils orchestrate cancer rejection by normalizing tumor vessels and enhancing infiltration of CD8(+) T cells. Nat Immunol 16(6):609–617
90. Furbert-Harris PM, Parish-Gause D, Hunter KA, Vaughn TR, Howland C, Okomo-Awich J et al (2003) Activated eosinophils upregulate the metastasis suppressor molecule E-cadherin on prostate tumor cells. Cell Mol Biol 49(7):1009–1016
91. von Wasielewski R, Seth S, Franklin J, Fischer R, Hübner K, Hansmann ML et al (2000) Tissue eosinophilia correlates strongly with poor prognosis in nodular sclerosing Hodgkin's disease, allowing for known prognostic factors. Blood 95(4):1207–1213
92. Alaarg A, Pérez-Medina C, Metselaar JM, Nahrendorf M, Fayad ZA, Storm G et al (2017) Applying nanomedicine in maladaptive inflammation and angiogenesis. Adv Drug Deliv Rev 119:143–158
93. Reichman H, Karo-Atar D, Munitz A (2016) Emerging roles for eosinophils in the tumor microenvironment. Trends Cancer 2(11):664–675
94. Gabrilovich DI, Nagaraj S (2009) Myeloid-derived suppressor cells as regulators of the immune system. Nat Rev Immunol 9(3):162–174
95. Kumar V, Patel S, Tcyganov E, Gabrilovich DI (2016) The nature of myeloid-derived suppressor cells in the tumor microenvironment. Trends Immunol 37(3):208–220
96. Wang C, Xiao M, Liu X, Ni C, Liu J, Erben U et al (2013) IFN-γ-mediated downregulation of LXA4 is necessary for the maintenance of nonresolving inflammation and papilloma persistence. Cancer Res 73(6):1742–1751
97. Iwasaki A, Medzhitov R (2015) Control of adaptive immunity by the innate immune system. Nat Immunol 16(4):343–353
98. Vesely MD, Kershaw MH, Schreiber RD, Smyth MJ (2011) Natural innate and adaptive immunity to cancer. Annu Rev Immunol 29:235–271
99. Gajewski TF, Schreiber H, Fu YX (2013) Innate and adaptive immune cells in the tumor microenvironment. Nat Immunol 14(10):1014–1022
100. Coussens LM, Zitvogel L, Palucka AK (2013) Neutralizing tumor-promoting chronic inflammation: a magic bullet? Science 339(6117):286–291
101. Dong C (2017) Helper T cells and cancer-associated inflammation: a new direction for immunotherapy? J Interf Cytokine Res 37(9):383–385
102. Kohrt HE, Nouri N, Nowels K, Johnson D, Holmes S, Lee PP (2005) Profile of immune cells in axillary lymph nodes predicts disease-free survival in breast cancer. PLoS Med 2(9):e284
103. Pedroza-Gonzalez A, Xu K, Wu TC, Aspord C, Tindle S, Marches F et al (2011) Thymic stromal lymphopoietin fosters human breast tumor growth by promoting type 2 inflammation. J Exp Med 208(3):479–490
104. Guéry L, Hugues S (2015) Th17 cell plasticity and functions in cancer immunity. Biomed Res Int 2015:314620
105. Fleming C, Cai Y, Sun X, Jala VR, Xue F, Morrissey S et al (2017) Microbiota-activated CD103(+) DCs stemming from microbiota adaptation specifically drive γδT17 proliferation and activation. Microbiome 5(1):46
106. Ye J, Ma C, Hsueh EC, Eickhoff CS, Zhang Y, Varvares MA et al (2013) Tumor-derived γδ regulatory T cells suppress innate and adaptive immunity through the induction of immunosenescence. J Immunol 190(5):2403–2414

107. Fleming C, Morrissey S, Cai Y, Yan J (2017) γδ T Cells: unexpected regulators of cancer development and progression. Trends Cancer 3(8):561–570

108. Knochelmann HM, Dwyer CJ, Bailey SR, Amaya SM, Elston DM, Mazza-McCrann JM et al (2018) When worlds collide: Th17 and Treg cells in cancer and autoimmunity. Cell Mol Immunol 15(5):458–469

109. Ohue Y, Nishikawa H (2019) Regulatory T (Treg) cells in cancer: can Treg cells be a new therapeutic target? Cancer Sci 110(7):2080–2089

110. Bromley SK, Mempel TR, Luster AD (2008) Orchestrating the orchestrators: chemokines in control of T cell traffic. Nat Immunol 9(9):970–980

111. van Herk EH, Te Velde AA (2016) Treg subsets in inflammatory bowel disease and colorectal carcinoma: characteristics, role, and therapeutic targets. J Gastroenterol Hepatol 31(8): 1393–1404

112. Alhabbab RY, Nova-Lamperti E, Aravena O, Burton HM, Lechler RI, Dorling A et al (2019) Regulatory B cells: development, phenotypes, functions, and role in transplantation. Immunol Rev 292(1):164–179

113. Zhang Y, Gallastegui N, Rosenblatt JD (2015) Regulatory B cells in anti-tumor immunity. Int Immunol 27(10):521–530

114. Schreiber RD, Old LJ, Smyth MJ (2011) Cancer immunoediting: integrating immunity's roles in cancer suppression and promotion. Science 331(6024):1565–1570

115. Schraml BU, Reis e Sousa C (2015) Defining dendritic cells. Curr Opin Immunol 32:13–20

116. Martin JC, Bériou G, Heslan M, Chauvin C, Utriainen L, Aumeunier A et al (2014) Interleukin-22 binding protein (IL-22BP) is constitutively expressed by a subset of conventional dendritic cells and is strongly induced by retinoic acid. Mucosal Immunol 7(1):101–113

117. Van Acker HH, Anguille S, De Reu H, Berneman ZN, Smits EL, Van Tendeloo VF (2018) Interleukin-15-cultured dendritic cells enhance anti-tumor gamma delta T cell functions through IL-15 secretion. Front Immunol 9:658

118. Chomarat P, Dantin C, Bennett L, Banchereau J, Palucka AK (2003) TNF skews monocyte differentiation from macrophages to dendritic cells. J Immunol 171(5):2262–2269

119. Chomarat P, Banchereau J, Davoust J, Palucka AK (2000) IL-6 switches the differentiation of monocytes from dendritic cells to macrophages. Nat Immunol 1(6):510–514

120. Morvan MG, Lanier LL (2016) NK cells and cancer: you can teach innate cells new tricks. Nat Rev Cancer 16(1):7–19

121. Hammad H, Plantinga M, Deswarte K, Pouliot P, Willart MA, Kool M et al (2010) Inflammatory dendritic cells--not basophils--are necessary and sufficient for induction of Th2 immunity to inhaled house dust mite allergen. J Exp Med 207(10):2097–2111

122. Fei M, Bhatia S, Oriss TB, Yarlagadda M, Khare A, Akira S et al (2011) TNF-alpha from inflammatory dendritic cells (DCs) regulates lung IL-17A/IL-5 levels and neutrophilia versus eosinophilia during persistent fungal infection. Proc Natl Acad Sci U S A 108(13):5360–5365

123. León B, López-Bravo M, Ardavín C (2007) Monocyte-derived dendritic cells formed at the infection site control the induction of protective T helper 1 responses against Leishmania. Immunity 26(4):519–531

124. Qian C, Cao X (2018) Dendritic cells in the regulation of immunity and inflammation. Semin Immunol 35:3–11

125. Wculek SK, Cueto FJ, Mujal AM, Melero I, Krummel MF, Sancho D (2020) Dendritic cells in cancer immunology and immunotherapy. Nat Rev Immunol 20(1):7–24

126. Lewis CE, Pollard JW (2006) Distinct role of macrophages in different tumor microenvironments. Cancer Res 66(2):605–612

127. Germano G, Frapolli R, Belgiovine C, Anselmo A, Pesce S, Liguori M et al (2013) Role of macrophage targeting in the antitumor activity of trabectedin. Cancer Cell 23(2):249–262

128. Cook J, Hagemann T (2013) Tumour-associated macrophages and cancer. Curr Opin Pharmacol 13(4):595–601

129. Mantovani A, Marchesi F, Malesci A, Laghi L, Allavena P (2017) Tumour-associated macrophages as treatment targets in oncology. Nat Rev Clin Oncol 14(7):399–416

130. Scapini P, Laudanna C, Pinardi C, Allavena P, Mantovani A, Sozzani S et al (2001) Neutrophils produce biologically active macrophage inflammatory protein-3alpha (MIP-3alpha)/CCL20 and MIP-3beta/CCL19. Eur J Immunol 31(7):1981–1988
131. Eruslanov EB, Bhojnagarwala PS, Quatromoni JG, Stephen TL, Ranganathan A, Deshpande C et al (2014) Tumor-associated neutrophils stimulate T cell responses in early-stage human lung cancer. J Clin Invest 124(12):5466–5480
132. Amulic B, Cazalet C, Hayes GL, Metzler KD, Zychlinsky A (2012) Neutrophil function: from mechanisms to disease. Annu Rev Immunol 30:459–489
133. Wu L, Saxena S, Awaji M, Singh RK (2019) Tumor-associated neutrophils in cancer: going pro. Cancers 11(4):564
134. Chiossone L, Dumas PY, Vienne M, Vivier E (2018) Natural killer cells and other innate lymphoid cells in cancer. Nat Rev Immunol 18(11):671–688
135. Vacca P, Munari E, Tumino N, Moretta F, Pietra G, Vitale M et al (2018) Human natural killer cells and other innate lymphoid cells in cancer: friends or foes? Immunol Lett 201:14–19
136. Smyth MJ, Cretney E, Kelly JM, Westwood JA, Street SE, Yagita H et al (2005) Activation of NK cell cytotoxicity. Mol Immunol 42(4):501–510
137. Smyth MJ, Swann J, Cretney E, Zerafa N, Yokoyama WM, Hayakawa Y (2005) NKG2D function protects the host from tumor initiation. J Exp Med 202(5):583–588
138. Vivier E, Tomasello E, Baratin M, Walzer T, Ugolini S (2008) Functions of natural killer cells. Nat Immunol 9(5):503–510
139. Artis D, Spits H (2015) The biology of innate lymphoid cells. Nature 517(7534):293–301
140. Krijgsman D, Hokland M, Kuppen PJK (2018) The role of natural killer T cells in cancer-a phenotypical and functional approach. Front Immunol 9:367
141. Bae EA, Seo H, Kim IK, Jeon I, Kang CY (2019) Roles of NKT cells in cancer immunotherapy. Arch Pharm Res 42(7):543–548
142. Gertner-Dardenne J, Bonnafous C, Bezombes C, Capietto AH, Scaglione V, Ingoure S et al (2009) Bromohydrin pyrophosphate enhances antibody-dependent cell-mediated cytotoxicity induced by therapeutic antibodies. Blood 113(20):4875–4884
143. Buckley CD, Gilroy DW, Serhan CN (2014) Proresolving lipid mediators and mechanisms in the resolution of acute inflammation. Immunity 40(3):315–327
144. Lee HJ, Park MK, Lee EJ, Lee CH (2013) Resolvin D1 inhibits TGF-β1-induced epithelial mesenchymal transition of A549 lung cancer cells via lipoxin A4 receptor/formyl peptide receptor 2 and GPR32. Int J Biochem Cell Biol 45(12):2801–2807
145. Halder RC, Almasi A, Sagong B, Leung J, Jewett A, Fiala M (2015) Curcuminoids and ω-3 fatty acids with anti-oxidants potentiate cytotoxicity of natural killer cells against pancreatic ductal adenocarcinoma cells and inhibit interferon γ production. Front Physiol 6:129
146. Arita M, Bianchini F, Aliberti J, Sher A, Chiang N, Hong S et al (2005) Stereochemical assignment, antiinflammatory properties, and receptor for the omega-3 lipid mediator resolvin E1. J Exp Med 201(5):713–722
147. Gewirtz AT, Collier-Hyams LS, Young AN, Kucharzik T, Guilford WJ, Parkinson JF et al (2002) Lipoxin a4 analogs attenuate induction of intestinal epithelial proinflammatory gene expression and reduce the severity of dextran sodium sulfate-induced colitis. J Immunol 168(10):5260–5267
148. Wang Z, Cheng Q, Tang K, Sun Y, Zhang K, Zhang Y et al (2015) Lipid mediator lipoxin A4 inhibits tumor growth by targeting IL-10-producing regulatory B (Breg) cells. Cancer Lett 364(2):118–124
149. Hirata E, Sahai E (2017) Tumor microenvironment and differential responses to therapy. Cold Spring Harb Perspect Med 7(7):a026781
150. Marcon R, Bento AF, Dutra RC, Bicca MA, Leite DF, Calixto JB (2013) Maresin 1, a proresolving lipid mediator derived from omega-3 polyunsaturated fatty acids, exerts protective actions in murine models of colitis. J Immunol 191(8):4288–4298
151. Cronkite DA, Strutt TM (2018) The regulation of inflammation by innate and adaptive lymphocytes. J Immunol Res 2018:1467538

152. Cheng M, Hu S (2017) Lung-resident γδ T cells and their roles in lung diseases. Immunology 151(4):375–384
153. Thommen DS, Schumacher TN (2018) T cell dysfunction in cancer. Cancer Cell 33(4): 547–562
154. Crespo J, Sun H, Welling TH, Tian Z, Zou W (2013) T cell anergy, exhaustion, senescence, and stemness in the tumor microenvironment. Curr Opin Immunol 25(2):214–221
155. Früh K, Yang Y (1999) Antigen presentation by MHC class I and its regulation by interferon gamma. Curr Opin Immunol 11(1):76–81
156. Sarvaria A, Madrigal JA, Saudemont A (2017) B cell regulation in cancer and anti-tumor immunity. Cell Mol Immunol 14(8):662–674
157. Dieu-Nosjean MC, Goc J, Giraldo NA, Sautès-Fridman C, Fridman WH (2014) Tertiary lymphoid structures in cancer and beyond. Trends Immunol 35(11):571–580
158. Schaue D, Micewicz ED, Ratikan JA, Xie MW, Cheng G, McBride WH (2015) Radiation and inflammation. Semin Radiat Oncol 25(1):4–10
159. Schwartz M, Zhang Y, Rosenblatt JD (2016) B cell regulation of the anti-tumor response and role in carcinogenesis. J Immunother Cancer 4:40
160. Wouters MCA, Nelson BH (2018) Prognostic significance of tumor-infiltrating B cells and plasma cells in human cancer. Clin Cancer Res 24(24):6125–6135
161. Wang SS, Liu W, Ly D, Xu H, Qu L, Zhang L (2019) Tumor-infiltrating B cells: their role and application in anti-tumor immunity in lung cancer. Cell Mol Immunol 16(1):6–18
162. Kroemer G, Galluzzi L, Kepp O, Zitvogel L (2013) Immunogenic cell death in cancer therapy. Annu Rev Immunol 31:51–72
163. Krysko DV, Garg AD, Kaczmarek A, Krysko O, Agostinis P, Vandenabeele P (2012) Immunogenic cell death and DAMPs in cancer therapy. Nat Rev Cancer 12(12):860–875
164. Barker HE, Paget JT, Khan AA, Harrington KJ (2015) The tumour microenvironment after radiotherapy: mechanisms of resistance and recurrence. Nat Rev Cancer 15(7):409–425
165. Li H, Zhou L, Zhou J, Li Q, Ji Q (2021) Underlying mechanisms and drug intervention strategies for the tumour microenvironment. J Exp Clin Cancer Res 40(1):97
166. Rivera G, Wakelee HA (2016) Resistance to therapy. Cancer Treat Res 170:183–202
167. Karagiannis GS, Condeelis JS, Oktay MH (2019) Chemotherapy-induced metastasis: molecular mechanisms, clinical manifestations, therapeutic interventions. Cancer Res 79(18): 4567–4576
168. Yao X, Panichpisal K, Kurtzman N, Nugent K (2007) Cisplatin nephrotoxicity: a review. Am J Med Sci 334(2):115–124
169. Grabosch S, Bulatovic M, Zeng F, Ma T, Zhang L, Ross M et al (2019) Cisplatin-induced immune modulation in ovarian cancer mouse models with distinct inflammation profiles. Oncogene 38(13):2380–2393
170. Robledo-Cadena DX, Gallardo-Pérez JC, Dávila-Borja V, Pacheco-Velázquez SC, Belmont-Díaz JA, Ralph SJ et al (2020) Non-steroidal anti-inflammatory drugs increase cisplatin, paclitaxel, and doxorubicin efficacy against human cervix cancer cells. Pharmaceuticals (Basel) 13(12):463
171. Xu HB, Shen FM, Lv QZ (2016) Celecoxib enhanced the cytotoxic effect of cisplatin in chemo-resistant gastric cancer xenograft mouse models through a cyclooxygenase-2-dependent manner. Eur J Pharmacol 776:1–8
172. Kashiwagi E, Inoue S, Mizushima T, Chen J, Ide H, Kawahara T et al (2018) Prostaglandin receptors induce urothelial tumourigenesis as well as bladder cancer progression and cisplatin resistance presumably via modulating PTEN expression. Br J Cancer 118(2):213–223
173. Rowinsky EK (1997) The development and clinical utility of the taxane class of antimicrotubule chemotherapy agents. Annu Rev Med 48:353–374
174. White CM, Martin BK, Lee LF, Haskill JS, Ting JP (1998) Effects of paclitaxel on cytokine synthesis by unprimed human monocytes, T lymphocytes, and breast cancer cells. Cancer Immunol Immunother 46(2):104–112

175. Lee LF, Haskill JS, Mukaida N, Matsushima K, Ting JP (1997) Identification of tumor-specific paclitaxel (Taxol)-responsive regulatory elements in the interleukin-8 promoter. Mol Cell Biol 17(9):5097–5105

176. Pusztai L, Mendoza TR, Reuben JM, Martinez MM, Willey JS, Lara J et al (2004) Changes in plasma levels of inflammatory cytokines in response to paclitaxel chemotherapy. Cytokine 25(3):94–102

177. Volk LD, Flister MJ, Bivens CM, Stutzman A, Desai N, Trieu V et al (2008) Nab-paclitaxel efficacy in the orthotopic model of human breast cancer is significantly enhanced by concurrent anti-vascular endothelial growth factor A therapy. Neoplasia 10(6):613–623

178. Jaffray DA (2012) Image-guided radiotherapy: from current concept to future perspectives. Nat Rev Clin Oncol 9(12):688–699

179. Yang X, Zhang X, Fu ML, Weichselbaum RR, Gajewski TF, Guo Y et al (2014) Targeting the tumor microenvironment with interferon-β bridges innate and adaptive immune responses. Cancer Cell 25(1):37–48

180. McLaughlin M, Patin EC, Pedersen M, Wilkins A, Dillon MT, Melcher AA et al (2020) Inflammatory microenvironment remodelling by tumour cells after radiotherapy. Nat Rev Cancer 20(4):203–217

181. Chen MF, Chen PT, Lu MS, Lin PY, Chen WC, Lee KD (2013) IL-6 expression predicts treatment response and outcome in squamous cell carcinoma of the esophagus. Mol Cancer 12: 26

182. Wu CT, Chen MF, Chen WC, Hsieh CC (2013) The role of IL-6 in the radiation response of prostate cancer. Radiat Oncol 8:159

183. Culig Z, Puhr M (2012) Interleukin-6: a multifunctional targetable cytokine in human prostate cancer. Mol Cell Endocrinol 360(1–2):52–58

184. Hou J, Karin M, Sun B (2021) Targeting cancer-promoting inflammation - have anti-inflammatory therapies come of age? Nat Rev Clin Oncol 18(5):261–279

185. Crusz SM, Balkwill FR (2015) Inflammation and cancer: advances and new agents. Nat Rev Clin Oncol 12(10):584–596

186. Braaten TJ, Brahmer JR, Forde PM, Le D, Lipson EJ, Naidoo J et al (2020) Immune checkpoint inhibitor-induced inflammatory arthritis persists after immunotherapy cessation. Ann Rheum Dis 79(3):332–338

187. Davila ML, Riviere I, Wang X, Bartido S, Park J, Curran K et al (2014) Efficacy and toxicity management of 19-28z CAR T cell therapy in B cell acute lymphoblastic leukemia. Sci Transl Med 6(224):224ra25

188. Zitvogel L, Galluzzi L, Kepp O, Smyth MJ, Kroemer G (2015) Type I interferons in anticancer immunity. Nat Rev Immunol 15(7):405–414

189. Spiotto M, Fu YX, Weichselbaum RR (2016) The intersection of radiotherapy and immunotherapy: mechanisms and clinical implications. Sci Immunol 1(3):EAAG1266

Chapter 22
Systemic *Oncosphere*: Host Endocrine System

Phei Er Saw and Erwei Song

Abstract Host endocrine system is a complicated network of glands, that precisely secrete hormones, chemicals or peptides to regulate most, if not all host systemic activity. Although there has been hint on the effect of endocrine system in tumor growth, the in-depth mechanism remains ambiguous. In this chapter, not only we are looking at endocrine cancers and how these tumors can reciprocally dysregulate hormone production, more importantly, we are deciphering the effect of host endocrine system (i.e. age, metabolism, gender, etc.) towards solid tumor progression, solidifying our tumor ecosystem concept of host systemic influence on the local onco-sphere.

Introduction

It has been known for a long time that exposures and factors in the host play important roles in the cause of cancer. However, except for cancers sensitive to sex hormones (i.e., certain subsets in breast cancer and prostate cancers), these

P. E. Saw
Guangdong Provincial Key Laboratory of Malignant Tumor Epigenetics and Gene Regulation, Guangdong-Hong Kong Joint Laboratory for RNA Medicine, Medical Research Center, Sun Yat-sen Memorial Hospital, Sun Yat-sen University, Guangzhou, China

Nanhai Translational Innovation Center of Precision Immunology, Sun Yat-sen Memorial Hospital, Sun Yat-sen University, Foshan, China

E. Song (✉)
Guangdong Provincial Key Laboratory of Malignant Tumor Epigenetics and Gene Regulation, Guangdong-Hong Kong Joint Laboratory for RNA Medicine, Medical Research Center, Sun Yat-sen Memorial Hospital, Sun Yat-sen University, Guangzhou, China

Nanhai Translational Innovation Center of Precision Immunology, Sun Yat-sen Memorial Hospital, Sun Yat-sen University, Foshan, China

Breast Tumor Center, Sun Yat-sen Memorial Hospital, Sun Yat-sen University, Guangzhou, China
e-mail: songew@mail.sysu.edu.cn

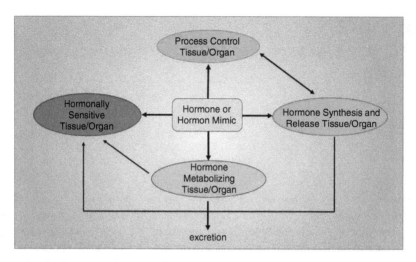

Fig. 22.1 Five main parts of an endocrine system: a tissue or organ that makes and releases hormones, a tissue or organ that breaks down hormones, tissue or organ that responds to signals from hormones, tissue or organ that controls feedback signals that control how hormones are made and released, and blood or lymphatic tissue that transfers hormones between organs

factors have not been thought to affect the clinical course of cancer as much as they could. Ongoing research in both basic and clinical areas has found more and more evidence that these host-related factors may be very important in determining a cancer patient's prognosis and how well their treatment works. To understand how the environment can affect the endocrine system(s), we must first look at what an endocrine signaling system looks like at its most basic level [1]. Figure 22.1 shows the five main parts of an endocrine system: a tissue or organ that makes and releases hormones, a tissue or organ that breaks down hormones, tissue or organ that responds to signals from hormones, tissue or organ that controls feedback signals that control how hormones are made and released, and blood or lymphatic tissue that moves hormones between organs. These organs do not have to be different or independent, and each system could have more than one organ that does the same thing. This simplified figure only shows the major feedback between synthesis and control, for readability purposes. Nevertheless, this figure can be very helpful for showing how things outside of the body can change the endocrine system [2].

Disruptions in Hormone Synthesis and Release

When making hormones, the precursor peptides follow the classic model of transcription, modification after transcription, translation, and modification after translation. The main thing that could go wrong in this part of an endocrine system would be mutations in the genes that control how the message is made, mutations in the genes that control how the precursor peptide is changed after it is made, or environmental agents that bind to the promoter regions of these genes and make them

agonists block the natural ligand as antagonists. There are examples of germline mutations in genes that control the production of hormones that cause health problems (for example, a mutation in the gene for the antimullerian hormone can lead to bilateral cryptorchidism) [2], but it is unlikely that a somatic mutation in any of these genes will have a similar effect without clonal expansion of the cells carrying the mutation; no such examples exist in the literature. However, there are cases where xenobiotic agents can change the expression of either the gene that makes the hormone or the enzymes that change the hormone after it has been made.

Disruptions in Hormone Metabolism

Like most biochemicals in the body, hormones are made and then taken out of the body through their primary activity (like binding to receptors) and/or by being broken down. Mutations can cause changes in the metabolism of hormones in the key enzymes involved in this metabolism or by direct and indirect changes in the levels of the key enzymes in tissues and organs that are involved in this metabolism (e.g., the liver). As with hormone synthesis, it is unlikely that somatic mutations in genes that control the enzymes for hormone metabolism will have a big effect on hormone levels unless the mutated cells clonally grow and replace normal cells. Nevertheless, most of the work that has been done on how genes interact with the environment has shown how important germline mutations are in metabolizing genes. For example, the high-activity Val_{432} allele of the CYP1B1 gene [3], which may be linked to oxidative stress through high levels of 4-hydroxylated catechol estrogen formation, was linked to a higher risk of ovarian cancer [3]. Changes in the expression of the CYP1B1 gene will change the amount of estrogen in the blood. It has been shown that xenobiotics can both upregulate the gene (for example, dioxin) and downregulate the gene (12-*O*-tetradecanoylphorbol-13-acetate can stop the increase caused by dioxin). Since many tumors, like breast cancer, are already linked to lifetime levels of estrogens in the blood [4], changes in these levels are likely to affect the overall risk of cancer. Mammals' pineal glands make melatonin found in the blood and different tissues. The liver changes 6-hydroxymelatonin to 6-sulfatoxymelatonin and 6-glucuronylmelatonin, which are then passed out of the body in the urine 6-sulfatoxymelatonin and 6-glucuronylmelatonin. Many things can change the way CYP1A2 works, and some have been shown to change the amount of melatonin in the blood of mammals. These include phenobarbital, 7,12-dimethylbenzanthracene, 17 beta-estradiol, furafylline, and 2,3,7,8-tetrachlorodibenzo-dioxin, among others. As with any change in enzyme activity, these changes could be caused by changes in how the enzyme's genes are expressed or by the substrate binding to the enzyme to block it from breaking down melatonin. Unlike the metabolites of estrogen, which are DNA reactive, the metabolites of melatonin are not likely to increase the risk of cancer because they are not DNA reactive. However, currently, there are no research being done on this topic.

Disruptions in Hormone Response

Most research into the cancer-causing effects of hormones has focused on the tissues that the hormone controls. Since it is thought that receptor-mediated pathways control the carcinogenic response to hormones, hormone mimics, or hormone antagonists, much attention has been paid to how well the hormone or hormone mimic binds to the targeted receptor in the target tissue. In the lab, some tests can be done to see how well different substances bind to important hormone receptors like the estrogen receptors [5] and the androgen receptors [6]. Depending on the type of cancer and tissue type, changes in the way the natural ligand for these receptors binds can either increase [7] or decrease [8] the risk of cancer. How well cofactors attach to the liganded receptor can also change the overall carcinogenic response. A similar effect can be seen when agents upregulate or downregulate the expression of the receptor, cofactors, or other proteins that are important for activating hormonal pathways. This is done through transcriptional regulation or posttranscriptional modification. It is not certain that a decrease or increase in how well melatonin binds to its receptors will directly affect the start, growth, or spread of cancer. However, the melatonin receptor is linked in some cells to important pathways involved in cellular replication [9, 10] and apoptosis [11–13], both of which can play important roles in developing tumors. In some cases, regulation is done by a mix of exposures and receptor cross talk, making it hard to figure out the effect. It is also clear that substances besides melatonin can bind to these receptors with different strengths of attraction and different effects [14–16]. Lastly, in many endocrine systems, the binding of a natural hormone to its receptor or the chain of events that follow this binding acts as a feedback mechanism to control the production and release of more hormones. It is possible that antagonists could trigger this feedback mechanism but not do anything else to the receptor. This kind of feedback would lower the amount of the endogenous hormone in the blood while also making it harder for receptors to bind. In some systems, like the estrogen cycle, this kind of negative feedback loop could increase the chance of cancer.

Gender-Based Sex Hormones and Anticancer Immunity

Cancer risk and survival rates are different for men and women [17]. Generally, men are more prone to get cancer and eventually die of the disease, compare to women of all races and types [18]. Sex chromosomes and sex hormones in both genders affect various biological process of the tumor, including the self-renewal of cancer stem cells, dysregulation of cell metabolism, and immune system [19]. Interestingly, immune system in men and women are different. The hormonal factors that affect innate and adaptive immune responses also differ in both genders [20]. Overall, women's immune systems are stronger. This is shown by the higher rate of autoimmune diseases in women and data on how their bodies react to vaccines and infections [20]. Although estrogen, progesterone, and testosterone are sex hormones, and they primarily function in the regulation of reproductive tissues [19], it is interesting to know that most, if not all, immune cells have receptors for these hormones [21–25]. Among these immune-related genes, many acquire androgen receptor (AR) and estrogen receptor (ER) responsive elements in their promoter region, which could explain why immune responses are different between men and women [26]. These can depend on the type of immune cell, the amount of hormone in the body, and where its receptors are. Depending on the dose and length of time, the same sex hormones can boost the immune system or slow it down [27].

In their adrenal glands and ovaries, women make androgens and their precursors, like dehydroepiandrosterone (DHEA) [28]. Before menopause, women have one-twentieth the amount of testosterone that men do [29, 30]. Testosterone is broken down into DHT in men, which binds to the AR more strongly. In women, the cytochrome P450 aromatase found in fat, skin, bone, and other organs could act upon testosterone and change it into estradiol [31]. Some studies have shown that as men age, their estradiol levels drop along with their testosterone levels [32]. In general, there is a lot of difference between people, which makes it hard to set age-based reference ranges for sex hormones in men and women [32].

Hormone Levels Influence Cancer Immunity

When sex hormone level changes with aging, the risk of getting cancer is higher. This is often overlooked in hormonal therapies. As a prerequisite to fight cancer, the immune system should be equipped. However, with age, with dysregulation of hormone levels, immune system is also affected. However, the hormone level and cancer risk have an ambiguous relationship. For example, menopausal hormone therapies (MHT, estrogen + progesterone, a synthetic analog of progesterone) in women increase risk of breast cancer. This is logical as MHT combined the usage of estrogen and progesterone, and since these two hormones are regulating the female reproductive systems, hormone-sensitive tissues such as breast, ovaries and endometrial cancer are affected [33–35]. Interestingly, (1) this effect varies upon the choice of progesterone, indicating the need for patient stratification [36], (2) this effect is not seen when estrogen usage is combined with natural progesterone, and (3) estrogen treatment only was found to lower breast cancer risk [37]. Its noteworthy that the above result also differs in different patient population (i.e., overweight, genetic factors), could also affect a person's response to MHT. This again, reveals the importance of host inclusion when looking into the optimized treatment of a cancer patient. On the other hand, on effective patients (postmenopausal women), researchers found that MHT could activate the immune system by increasing the number of B-cells and T-cells, while simultaneously lowers the levels of proinflammatory cytokines, TNFα and IL6 [38]. Comprehensive data from 1.8 million women show that different types of hormonal birth control, mostly given as oral combinations of estrogen and progestogen, are linked to a small increase in the risk of breast cancer [39]. This occurs even though the immune system is stimulated, and the number of B and T cells are increased [40], suggesting that the effect of sex hormones to direct and stimulate growth on the reproductive tissues might override their effects on the immune system.

Long-term use of oral hormonal birth control is also linked to a higher risk of cervix adenocarcinoma [41]. Human papillomavirus (HPV) infection and a weakened immune system are known to cause cervix cancer. It is possible that only some oncogenic HPV types, like HPV16, remain after exposure to hormonal contraception [42]. On the other hand, hormonal birth control is linked to a big drop in ovarian cancer risk and this is true even for people with BRCA 1 or 2 gene mutations [43]. Also, people who use hormonal birth control have a lower chance of getting colorectal and endometrial cancer [44]. At the moment, no solid evidence linked to why postmenopausal MHT and hormonal contraception have opposite effects on the risk of ovarian and endometrial cancer, or how interfering with normal sex hormone levels and cycles can selectively change cancer risk in different organs.

In older men, it was not known if testosterone replacement therapy changes how the immune system works. However, because testosterone makes prostate tissue grow faster, there has been a concern that testosterone therapy might be a risk of prostate cancer. A meta-analysis of clinical trials comparing testosterone therapy to a placebo found a slightly higher rate of prostate cancer and prostate-specific antigen (PSA) levels [45], but other reports showed that testosterone therapy is safe [46, 47]. The "saturation model," which says that the prostate is most sensitive to the effects of testosterone at very low concentrations when ARs are open, explains why these results seem to be at odds with each other. Once the AR is full, the presence of more testosterone does not seem to affect prostate tissue anymore [48] (Box 22.1).

Box 22.1 Sex Differences in Immunotherapy Response
Female melanoma patients have been suggested to less likely to response to anti-PD-1 therapy, compared to men [49]. One speculation for this finding could be due to the fact that upon screening, not many female patients presented the partially exhausted PD-1high/CTLA-4–high CD8$^+$ cells, while this phenotype is crucial for responding to combined checkpoint inhibition [50]. However, since there have not been any large clinical trials or analyses based on individual patient data, it is too early to reach firm conclusions. There is not much information about how PD-1/PD-L1 is expressed in male and female cancer patients of different ages or in patients who are getting hormonal treatments. In clinical practice, PD-L1 is a predictor of response to immune checkpoint inhibitors [51], and differences in PD-L1 expression between men

(continued)

> **Box 22.1** (continued)
>
> and women could partly explain why men tend to have a worse prognosis and a better response to immune checkpoint inhibitors. Recently, systematic analysis of some clinical trials' result concluded that men who underwent anti-PD-1 or anti-CTLA-4 therapies have longer lifespan than women who receive the same treatment [52]. Upon reflecting on this finding, one can speculate that the anticancer immunity is indeed different between men and women. This could be due to the generation of different sets of hormones, genes, and the environment. Differences between men and women in innate and adaptive immunity are caused by how sex hormones and genetic and environmental factors talk to each other. Changes in sex hormone levels caused by getting older, being pregnant, or taking medicine can affect how the immune system responds. This can be one reason why women are less likely to get cancer than men. It is still unclear if these differences in how men and women respond to immunotherapy could be because men's and women's tumors use different ways to evade the immune system. Therefore, it is worth looking into whether men and women might respond better to immunotherapy if different approaches can be determined [53].

Hormonal Cancers

Hormone-linked cancers like the ones affecting breasts, endometrium, ovaries, prostate gland, testis, thyroid, and osteosarcoma all have a distinct method of tumorigenesis. Exogenous and endogenous hormones stimulate cellular growth, allowing for the accrual of random genetic abnormalities. The development of malignant attributes is dependent on a range of somatic mutations occurring in the course of cell division, although the exact genes implicated in hormone-linked cancer progression are still unidentified [54]. Herein, we summarized some of the most common hormonal-related carcinogenesis, focusing on breast cancer and endometrial cancer.

Role of Hormones in Endometrial Cancer

Data demonstrates that administering estrogens leads to the likely forecast of endometrial cancer rather than progestin exposure [55]. The likely danger of endometrial cancer can be associated with a mitotic event in the first phase of the menstrual cycle, characterized by uncontested exposure to estrogen as compared to progesterone [56]. The threat of occurrence of endometrial cancer among females increased twofold because of using oral contraceptives (OCs) sequentially, which were withdrawn from the market after 1976. Contrarily, combined oral contraceptives (COCs), administering estrogen, and a high dosage of progesterone for a span of 21 days in a 28-day long cycle reduce the chance of the development of endometrial cancer.

Obesity is a critical risk element for the development of endometrial tumors. The higher risk of cancer in postmenopausal women is thought to be caused by the transformation of adipose tissue-based androstenedione to estrone. Obesity among premenopausal females is hypothesized to be caused by higher anovulatory periods and related deficiency of progesterone [57]. The unchallenged estrogen theory can potentially describe the protective role of parity. Endometrial cancer is more common among nulliparous females, and the risk diminishes with every pregnancy. This is attributed to the justification of the absence of any mitotic process in the course of pregnancy because of high progesterone levels.

Role of Hormones in Breast Cancer

A substantial amount of epidemiological and clinical evidence indicates estrogens in the genesis of breast cancer in humans. Animal experiments have consistently shown the potential of estrogens to cause and exacerbate breast cancers in mice, despite the reverse impact generated due to the removal of the animals' ovaries or providing them with an antiestrogenic medication [58]. The continuous dosage of estrogen administration to breast epithelium commonly acknowledged potential risks causing breast cancer. Even in breast cancer orthotopic models, ER^+ breast cancer could only grow under constant estrogen supplementation for 30–60 days. In human, the frequency of ovulation cycles undergone is maximized with time due to untimely menarche and delayed menopause. Physical exercise, as well as continued nursing, can regulate the frequency of ovulation cycles. Physical exercise tends to postpone the age at which ovulation cycles normally begin, limit the frequency of ovulation cycles, and lower the levels of circulating ovarian hormones [59]. Few studies of lifetime incidences highlighted the preventive impact of physical exercise against breast cancer; however, other investigations of particular time periods found no protective benefits [60]. Using alcohol causes a linear escalation in the likelihood of breast cancer among females having daily consumption of up to 60 g of alcohol [61]. Alcohol is thought to enhance the likelihood of breast cancer through elevated levels of plasma estrogen and IGFs [62]. The transformation of androstenedione to estrone in adipose tissue is the main contributor to estrogen in females after menopause; hence, postmenopausal obesity raises the likelihood of breast cancer by producing estrogen increasingly. Obesity is also linked to lower sex hormone-binding globulin (SHBG) synthesis and higher levels of independent and albumin-linked estrogens. The protective impact of premature birth in first delivery is complicated. The amount of free estradiol grows fast throughout the initial trimester of pregnancy, although the progression of pregnancy is characterized by reduced quantities of prolactin and independent estradiol and increased SHBG levels leading to a net cumulative advantage in terms of endogenous estrogen profiling. Rather more crucially, the first pregnancy may prompt certain premalignant cells to undergo terminal differentiation, allowing them to lose their systemic toxicity.

The most thoroughly conducted international research contrasting estrogen levels of people at varying risks of breast cancer indicates the involvement of estrogens, particularly estradiol, in breast cancer etiology. A set of research was performed on the explorations on teens and young females in Asian countries and North American states in the early 1970s. In an experiment conducted on North American teens, they obtained overnight samples of urine on the morning of the 21st day of the menstrual cycle and observed 36% greater overall urinary estrogen levels in them. Women falling in the age range of 20–39 years showed identical variances [63]. In a research study, estradiol (E2) levels of premenopausal specimens in Los Angeles exceeded by 20% in comparison to Shanghai equivalents [64]. A comparative analysis of post-menopausal women revealed 36% high levels of E2 in females of Los Angeles against Japanese females of identical age group [65]. The causes of these disparities are unknown, although one possibility can be attributed to the genetic abnormalities that alter the production of steroid hormones. A meta-analysis has evaluated the observations of 29 epidemiological investigations based on endogenous hormones and postmenopausal breast cancer. The six prospective experiments reported until now demonstrate that postmenopausal women likely to develop breast cancer had a 15% greater mean blood estradiol content in comparison to healthy women [66].

Although the involvement of high progesterone levels in the genesis of breast cancer is debatable, the latest experimental results highlight the role of progestins as breast mitogens and their likelihood to enhance the risk of breast cancer [67]. A reduction in SHBG levels would mean the existence of higher estrogen levels, which generates an increased risk of breast cancer. Nevertheless, few experiments have shown a favorable link between SHBG and the risk of breast cancer [68], whereas other studies have revealed an opposite link [69, 70]. Likewise, testosterone is found to raise the risk of breast cancer, this result is contradictory. The risk in a few [68, 71] but not all investigation, while studies on the effect of androstenedione are limited [69]. More research is required to reconcile the contradicting results about the involvement of SHBG in breast cancer, as well as to validate the link with testosterone and additional androgens observed in certain studies. The link between blood androgens and the likelihood of breast cancer lies on a scientific foundation since androgens may supply a substantial reservoir of substrates for transforming into estrogens through the activity of aromatase in breast tissues (Box 22.2).

Box 22.2 Heart Hormones as New Anticancer Agent

The heart produces the prohormone atrial natriuretic peptide (ANP), a hormonal peptide. In this family, there are four major members, namely, atrial natriuretic peptide, vessel dilator, kaliuretic peptide, and long-acting natriuretic peptide. These four cardiac hormones can destroy up to 97% of human pancreatic, colon, prostate, breast, ovarian, and kidney adenocarcinoma cells in cell culture [72–77]. They can also inhibit heart angiosarcoma cells, melanomas, medullary thyroid carcinomas, glioblastomas of the brain, [30], small-cell, and squamous cell lung carcinoma cells among many others. Up to 80% of pancreatic adenocarcinomas can be eradicated using heart hormones [78, 79]. When given subcutaneously for 28 days to a breast cancer mouse model, vessel dilator, LANP, KP, and ANP eliminate 67%, 50%, 67%, and 33% of tumor cells, respectively. Mechanistically, these peptides target the ERK1/2, MEK1/2, and RAS signaling pathways in cancer cells. These four cardiac hormones can inhibit up to 95% of the basal activity of RAS, 98% of MEK1/2 kinases phosphorylation, and 96% of the stimulation of the basal activity of ERK1/2 kinases [80]. Through EGF activation, they could successfully block the effects of mitogens, such as ERK and RAS activation. They also effectively block MAPK9 (c-JUN)-terminal kinase 2 and MAPKs. Since these hormones are generated fresh every week at a level of 3 nM per min/kg body weight, these hormones could be the host's inherent army that could strategically help to reduce tumor burden (Fig. 22.2) [81].

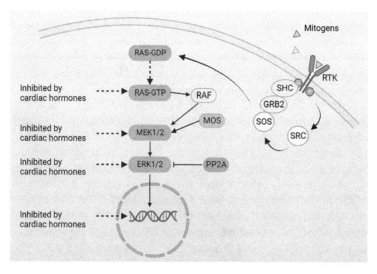

Fig. 22.2 Five metabolic targets of the RAS-MEK1/2-ERK1/2 kinase cascade are blocked by 95–98% by cardiac hormones

Conclusion

It is becoming clear that focusing only on tumor-related characteristics is not be the best way to treat cancer. In this chapter, we looked at the importance of integrating host endocrine factor changes, including hormone dysregulation in cancer. Gender has also been shown to have significant effect on cancer immunotherapy. Therefore, one should consider patient stratification based on multiple factors for creating a more personalized therapeutic regime.

References

1. Portier CJ (2002) Endocrine dismodulation and cancer. Neuro Endocrinol Lett 23(Suppl 2): 43–47
2. Lang-Muritano M, Biason-Lauber A, Gitzelmann C, Belville C, Picard Y, Schoenle EJ (2001) A novel mutation in the anti-müllerian hormone gene as cause of persistent müllerian duct syndrome. Eur J Pediatr 160(11):652–654
3. Goodman MT, McDuffie K, Kolonel LN, Terada K, Donlon TA, Wilkens LR et al (2001) Case-control study of ovarian cancer and polymorphisms in genes involved in catechol estrogen formation and metabolism. Cancer Epidemiol Biomark Prev 10(3):209–216
4. Thomas DB (1983) Factors that promote the development of human breast cancer. Environ Health Perspect 50:209–218
5. Gaido KW, Leonard LS, Lovell S, Gould JC, Babaï D, Portier CJ et al (1997) Evaluation of chemicals with endocrine modulating activity in a yeast-based steroid hormone receptor gene transcription assay. Toxicol Appl Pharmacol 143(1):205–212
6. Wilson VS, Bobseine K, Lambright CR, Gray LE Jr (2002) A novel cell line, MDA-kb2, that stably expresses an androgen- and glucocorticoid-responsive reporter for the detection of hormone receptor agonists and antagonists. Toxicol Sci 66(1):69–81
7. Hodges LC, Hunter DS, Bergerson JS, Fuchs-Young R, Walker CL (2001) An *in vivo/in vitro* model to assess endocrine disrupting activity of xenoestrogens in uterine leiomyoma. Ann N Y Acad Sci 948:100–111
8. Bentrem DJ, Craig Jordan V (2002) Tamoxifen, raloxifene and the prevention of breast cancer. Minerva Endocrinol 27(2):127–139
9. Papazisis KT, Kouretas D, Geromichalos GD, Sivridis E, Tsekreli OK, Dimitriadis KA et al (1998) Effects of melatonin on proliferation of cancer cell lines. J Pineal Res 25(4):211–218
10. Pawlikowski M, Lysoń K, Kunert-Radek J, Stepień H (1988) Effect of benzodiazepines on the proliferation of mouse spleen lymphocytes *in vitro*. J Neural Transm 73(2):161–166
11. Deigner HP, Haberkorn U, Kinscherf R (2000) Apoptosis modulators in the therapy of neurodegenerative diseases. Expert Opin Investig Drugs 9(4):747–764
12. Eck-Enriquez K, Kiefer TL, Spriggs LL, Hill SM (2000) Pathways through which a regimen of melatonin and retinoic acid induces apoptosis in MCF-7 human breast cancer cells. Breast Cancer Res Treat 61(3):229–239
13. Winczyk K, Pawlikowski M, Karasek M (2001) Melatonin and RZR/ROR receptor ligand CGP 52608 induce apoptosis in the murine colonic cancer. J Pineal Res 31(2):179–182
14. Raghavendra V, Kaur G, Kulkarni SK (2000) Anti-depressant action of melatonin in chronic forced swimming-induced behavioral despair in mice, role of peripheral benzodiazepine receptor modulation. Eur Neuropsychopharmacol 10(6):473–481
15. Blumenau C, Berger E, Fauteck JD, Madeja M, Wittkowski W, Speckmann EJ et al (2001) Expression and functional characterization of the mt1 melatonin receptor from rat brain in Xenopus oocytes: evidence for coupling to the phosphoinositol pathway. J Pineal Res 30(3): 139–146

16. Tsotinis A, Panoussopoulou M, Sivananthan S, Sugden D (2001) Synthesis of new tricyclic melatoninergic ligands. Farmaco 56(9):725–729
17. Ozdemir BC, Dotto GP (2019) Sex hormones and anticancer immunity. Clin Cancer Res 25(15):4603–4610
18. Bray F, Ferlay J, Soerjomataram I, Siegel RL, Torre LA, Jemal A (2018) Global cancer statistics 2018: GLOBOCAN estimates of incidence and mortality worldwide for 36 cancers in 185 countries. CA Cancer J Clin 68(6):394–424
19. Clocchiatti A, Cora E, Zhang Y, Dotto GP (2016) Sexual dimorphism in cancer. Nat Rev Cancer 16(5):330–339
20. Klein SL, Flanagan KL (2016) Sex differences in immune responses. Nat Rev Immunol 16(10): 626–638
21. Pierdominici M, Maselli A, Colasanti T, Giammarioli AM, Delunardo F, Vacirca D et al (2010) Estrogen receptor profiles in human peripheral blood lymphocytes. Immunol Lett 132(1–2): 79–85
22. Kovats S (2015) Estrogen receptors regulate innate immune cells and signaling pathways. Cell Immunol 294(2):63–69
23. Mantalaris A, Panoskaltsis N, Sakai Y, Bourne P, Chang C, Messing EM et al (2001) Localization of androgen receptor expression in human bone marrow. J Pathol 193(3):361–366
24. Arruvito L, Giulianelli S, Flores AC, Paladino N, Barboza M, Lanari C et al (2008) NK cells expressing a progesterone receptor are susceptible to progesterone-induced apoptosis. J Immunol 180(8):5746–5753
25. Dosiou C, Hamilton AE, Pang Y, Overgaard MT, Tulac S, Dong J et al (2008) Expression of membrane progesterone receptors on human T lymphocytes and Jurkat cells and activation of G-proteins by progesterone. J Endocrinol 196(1):67–77
26. Hannah MF, Bajic VB, Klein SL (2008) Sex differences in the recognition of and innate antiviral responses to Seoul virus in Norway rats. Brain Behav Immun 22(4):503–516
27. Straub RH (2007) The complex role of estrogens in inflammation. Endocr Rev 28(5):521–574
28. Burger HG (2002) Androgen production in women. Fertil Steril 77(Suppl 4):S3–S5
29. Davison SL, Bell R, Donath S, Montalto JG, Davis SR (2005) Androgen levels in adult females: changes with age, menopause, and oophorectomy. J Clin Endocrinol Metab 90(7):3847–3853
30. Vermeulen AOB (1996) Declining androgens with age: an overview. Parthenon Publishing, New York, NY, pp 3–14
31. Merlotti D, Gennari L, Stolakis K, Nuti R (2011) Aromatase activity and bone loss in men. J Osteoporos 2011:230671
32. Orwoll E, Lambert LC, Marshall LM, Phipps K, Blank J, Barrett-Connor E et al (2006) Testosterone and estradiol among older men. J Clin Endocrinol Metab 91(4):1336–1344
33. Beral V (2003) Breast cancer and hormone-replacement therapy in the Million Women Study. Lancet 362(9382):419–427
34. Grady D, Gebretsadik T, Kerlikowske K, Ernster V, Petitti D (1995) Hormone replacement therapy and endometrial cancer risk: a meta-analysis. Obstet Gynecol 85(2):304–313
35. Lacey JV Jr, Mink PJ, Lubin JH, Sherman ME, Troisi R, Hartge P et al (2002) Menopausal hormone replacement therapy and risk of ovarian cancer. JAMA 288(3):334–341
36. Fournier A, Berrino F, Clavel-Chapelon F (2008) Unequal risks for breast cancer associated with different hormone replacement therapies: results from the E3N cohort study. Breast Cancer Res Treat 107(1):103–111
37. Anderson GL, Limacher M, Assaf AR, Bassford T, Beresford SA, Black H et al (2004) Effects of conjugated equine estrogen in postmenopausal women with hysterectomy: the Women's Health Initiative randomized controlled trial. JAMA 291(14):1701–1712
38. Ghosh M, Rodriguez-Garcia M, Wira CR (2014) The immune system in menopause: pros and cons of hormone therapy. J Steroid Biochem Mol Biol 142:171–175
39. Mørch LS, Skovlund CW, Hannaford PC, Iversen L, Fielding S, Lidegaard Ø (2017) Contemporary hormonal contraception and the risk of breast cancer. N Engl J Med 377(23):2228–2239
40. Auerbach L, Hafner T, Huber JC, Panzer S (2002) Influence of low-dose oral contraception on peripheral blood lymphocyte subsets at particular phases of the hormonal cycle. Fertil Steril 78(1):83–89

41. Madeleine MM, Daling JR, Schwartz SM, Shera K, McKnight B, Carter JJ et al (2001) Human papillomavirus and long-term oral contraceptive use increase the risk of adenocarcinoma in situ of the cervix. Cancer Epidemiol Biomark Prev 10(3):171–177
42. Ghanem KG, Datta SD, Unger ER, Hagensee M, Shlay JC, Kerndt P et al (2011) The association of current hormonal contraceptive use with type-specific HPV detection. Sex Transm Infect 87(5):385–388
43. Iodice S, Barile M, Rotmensz N, Feroce I, Bonanni B, Radice P et al (2010) Oral contraceptive use and breast or ovarian cancer risk in BRCA1/2 carriers: a meta-analysis. Eur J Cancer 46(12): 2275–2284
44. Gierisch JM, Coeytaux RR, Urrutia RP, Havrilesky LJ, Moorman PG, Lowery WJ et al (2013) Oral contraceptive use and risk of breast, cervical, colorectal, and endometrial cancers: a systematic review. Cancer Epidemiol Biomark Prev 22(11):1931–1943
45. Calof OM, Singh AB, Lee ML, Kenny AM, Urban RJ, Tenover JL et al (2005) Adverse events associated with testosterone replacement in middle-aged and older men: a meta-analysis of randomized, placebo-controlled trials. J Gerontol A Biol Sci Med Sci 60(11):1451–1457
46. Feneley MR, Carruthers M (2012) Is testosterone treatment good for the prostate? Study of safety during long-term treatment. J Sex Med 9(8):2138–2149
47. Eisenberg ML, Li S, Betts P, Herder D, Lamb DJ, Lipshultz LI (2015) Testosterone therapy and cancer risk. BJU Int 115(2):317–321
48. Khera M, Crawford D, Morales A, Salonia A, Morgentaler A (2014) A new era of testosterone and prostate cancer: from physiology to clinical implications. Eur Urol 65(1):115–123
49. Nosrati A, Tsai KK, Goldinger SM, Tumeh P, Grimes B, Loo K et al (2017) Evaluation of clinicopathological factors in PD-1 response: derivation and validation of a prediction scale for response to PD-1 monotherapy. Br J Cancer 116(9):1141–1147
50. Loo K, Tsai KK, Mahuron K, Liu J, Pauli ML, Sandoval PM et al (2017) Partially exhausted tumor-infiltrating lymphocytes predict response to combination immunotherapy. JCI Insight 2(14):e93433
51. Maleki Vareki S, Garrigós C, Duran I (2017) Biomarkers of response to PD-1/PD-L1 inhibition. Crit Rev Oncol Hematol 116:116–124
52. Conforti F, Pala L, Bagnardi V, De Pas T, Martinetti M, Viale G et al (2018) Cancer immunotherapy efficacy and patients' sex: a systematic review and meta-analysis. Lancet Oncol 19(6):737–746
53. Barroso-Sousa R, Barry WT, Garrido-Castro AC, Hodi FS, Min L, Krop IE et al (2018) Incidence of endocrine dysfunction following the use of different immune checkpoint inhibitor regimens: a systematic review and meta-analysis. JAMA Oncol 4(2):173–182
54. Henderson BE, Feigelson HS (2000) Hormonal carcinogenesis. Carcinogenesis 21(3):427–433
55. Key TJ, Pike MC (1988) The dose-effect relationship between 'unopposed' oestrogens and endometrial mitotic rate: its central role in explaining and predicting endometrial cancer risk. Br J Cancer 57(2):205–212
56. Hunn J, Rodriguez GC (2012) Ovarian cancer: etiology, risk factors, and epidemiology. Clin Obstet Gynecol 55(1):3–23
57. Potischman N, Hoover RN, Brinton LA, Siiteri P, Dorgan JF, Swanson CA et al (1996) Case-control study of endogenous steroid hormones and endometrial cancer. J Natl Cancer Inst 88(16):1127–1135
58. Rondinelli RH, Haslam SZ, Fluck MM (1995) The role of ovarian hormones, age and mammary gland development in polyomavirus mammary tumorigenesis. Oncogene 11(9):1817–1827
59. Broocks A, Pirke KM, Schweiger U, Tuschl RJ, Laessle RG, Strowitzki T et al (1990) Cyclic ovarian function in recreational athletes. J Appl Physiol 68(5):2083–2086
60. Rockhill B, Willett WC, Hunter DJ, Manson JE, Hankinson SE, Spiegelman D et al (1998) Physical activity and breast cancer risk in a cohort of young women. J Natl Cancer Inst 90(15): 1155–1160
61. Smith-Warner SA, Spiegelman D, Yaun SS, van den Brandt PA, Folsom AR, Goldbohm RA et al (1998) Alcohol and breast cancer in women: a pooled analysis of cohort studies. JAMA 279(7):535–540

62. Coronado GD, Beasley J, Livaudais J (2011) Alcohol consumption and the risk of breast cancer. Salud Publica Mex 53(5):440–447
63. MacMahon B, Cole P, Brown JB, Aoki K, Lin TM, Morgan RW et al (1974) Urine oestrogen profiles of Asian and North American women. Int J Cancer 14(2):161–167
64. Bernstein L, Yuan JM, Ross RK, Pike MC, Hanisch R, Lobo R et al (1990) Serum hormone levels in pre-menopausal Chinese women in Shanghai and white women in Los Angeles: results from two breast cancer case-control studies. Cancer Causes Control 1(1):51–58
65. Shimizu H, Ross RK, Bernstein L, Pike MC, Henderson BE (1990) Serum oestrogen levels in postmenopausal women: comparison of American whites and Japanese in Japan. Br J Cancer 62(3):451–453
66. Thomas HV, Reeves GK, Key TJ (1997) Endogenous estrogen and postmenopausal breast cancer: a quantitative review. Cancer Causes Control 8(6):922–928
67. Cline JM, Soderqvist G, von Schoultz E, Skoog L, von Schoultz B (1996) Effects of hormone replacement therapy on the mammary gland of surgically postmenopausal cynomolgus macaques. Am J Obstet Gynecol 174(1 Pt 1):93–100
68. Dorgan JF, Longcope C, Stephenson HE Jr, Falk RT, Miller R, Franz C et al (1996) Relation of prediagnostic serum estrogen and androgen levels to breast cancer risk. Cancer Epidemiol Biomark Prev 5(7):533–539
69. Lipworth L, Adami HO, Trichopoulos D, Carlstrom K, Mantzoros C (1996) Serum steroid hormone levels, sex hormone-binding globulin, and body mass index in the etiology of postmenopausal breast cancer. Epidemiology 7(1):96–100
70. Berrino F, Muti P, Micheli A, Bolelli G, Krogh V, Sciajno R et al (1996) Serum sex hormone levels after menopause and subsequent breast cancer. J Natl Cancer Inst 88(5):291–296
71. Pike MC, Spicer DV, Dahmoush L, Press MF (1993) Estrogens, progestogens, normal breast cell proliferation, and breast cancer risk. Epidemiol Rev 15(1):17–35
72. Vesely BA, McAfee Q, Gower WR Jr, Vesely DL (2003) Four peptides decrease the number of human pancreatic adenocarcinoma cells. Eur J Clin Investig 33(11):998–1005
73. Vesely BA, Song S, Sanchez-Ramos J, Fitz SR, Solivan SM, Gower WR Jr et al (2005) Four peptide hormones decrease the number of human breast adenocarcinoma cells. Eur J Clin Investig 35(1):60–69
74. Vesely BA, Alli AA, Song SJ, Gower WR Jr, Sanchez-Ramos J, Vesely DL (2005) Four peptide hormones' specific decrease (up to 97%) of human prostate carcinoma cells. Eur J Clin Investig 35(11):700–710
75. Gower WR, Vesely BA, Alli AA, Vesely DL (2005) Four peptides decrease human colon adenocarcinoma cell number and DNA synthesis via cyclic GMP. Int J Gastrointest Cancer 36(2):77–87
76. Vesely BA, Eichelbaum EJ, Alli AA, Sun Y, Gower WR Jr, Vesely DL (2006) Urodilatin and four cardiac hormones decrease human renal carcinoma cell numbers. Eur J Clin Investig 36(11):810–819
77. Vesely BA, Eichelbaum EJ, Alli AA, Sun Y, Gower WR, Vesely DL (2007) Four cardiac hormones cause cell death in 81% of human ovarian adenocarcinoma cells. Cancer Ther 5:97
78. Pitchumoni CS (1998) Pancreatic disease. In: Stein JH (ed) Internal medicine. Mosby, St. Louis, MO, pp 2233–2247
79. Wolff RA, Abbruzzese J, Evans DB (2000) Neoplasms of the exocrine pancreas. In: Holland JF, Frei E III (eds) Cancer medicine. BC Decker Inc., London, pp 1436–1464
80. Vesely DL (2012) New anticancer agents: hormones made within the heart. Anticancer Res 32(7):2515–2521
81. Vesely DL, Vesely BA, Eichelbaum EJ, Sun Y, Alli AA, Gower WR Jr (2007) Four cardiac hormones eliminate up to two-thirds of human breast cancers in athymic mice. In Vivo 21(6): 973–978

Chapter 23
Systemic *Onco-Sphere*: Host Neuronal System in Cancer

Phei Er Saw and Erwei Song

Abstract In human, the nervous system governs vital functional activities of many organs. As tumor is a systemic disease, it does not grow as an independent entity, rather, tumor growth and progression is an integral part of the nervous system. The peripheral nervous system (PNS) is a system of autonomic and sensory nerves outside the central nervous system that helps to integrate and regulate physiological processes at molecular, cellular, and organ level to maintain homeostasis. Indicators of homeostasis, such as blood pressure, pH, and metabolism, are constantly adjusted by the PNS in response to internal and external stimuli. Tumors, likewise, must control these neuronal mechanisms in order to survive. An increasing amount of data implies that tumors adopt and reprogram neuronal interactions to support their development and progression, in a way similar to how healthy tissues recruit and sustain PNS innervation. In this chapter, we highlight the importance of the crosstalk between host PNS system and cancer growth.

P. E. Saw
Guangdong Provincial Key Laboratory of Malignant Tumor Epigenetics and Gene Regulation, Guangdong-Hong Kong Joint Laboratory for RNA Medicine, Medical Research Center, Sun Yat-sen Memorial Hospital, Sun Yat-sen University, Guangzhou, China

Nanhai Translational Innovation Center of Precision Immunology, Sun Yat-sen Memorial Hospital, Sun Yat-sen University, Foshan, China

E. Song (✉)
Guangdong Provincial Key Laboratory of Malignant Tumor Epigenetics and Gene Regulation, Guangdong-Hong Kong Joint Laboratory for RNA Medicine, Medical Research Center, Sun Yat-sen Memorial Hospital, Sun Yat-sen University, Guangzhou, China

Nanhai Translational Innovation Center of Precision Immunology, Sun Yat-sen Memorial Hospital, Sun Yat-sen University, Foshan, China

Breast Tumor Center, Sun Yat-sen Memorial Hospital, Sun Yat-sen University, Guangzhou, China
e-mail: songew@mail.sysu.edu.cn

E. Song (ed.), *Tumor Ecosystem*, https://doi.org/10.1007/978-981-99-1183-7_23

Introduction

The peripheral nervous system (PNS) is a system of autonomic and sensory nerves outside the central nervous system that helps to integrate and regulate physiological processes at molecular, cellular, and organ level to maintain homeostasis. Indicators of homeostasis, such as blood pressure, pH, and metabolism, are constantly adjusted by the PNS in response to internal and external stimuli. Tumors, likewise, must control these neuronal mechanisms in order to survive. An increasing amount of data implies that tumors adopt and reprogram neuronal interactions to support their development and progression, in a way similar to how healthy tissues recruit and sustain PNS innervation [1–4]. The autonomic nervous system (ANS), which is part of the PNS, regulates physiological processes involuntarily and consists of two main regulatory systems: the sympathetic nervous system (SNS) and the parasympathetic nervous system (PSNS) [5]. Despite the differences, both sympathetic and parasympathetic nerves have their cell bodies located outside the CNS and near to the innervation site.

Tumor at the innervation site can substantially influence these postganglionic neurons, prompting them to quickly adapt to changes induced by the cancer cells. Due to the close proximity of the neuronal cell bodies to the tumor in the local *onco-sphere*, the neurons may experience changes in transcription, translation, and even structural alterations in its cytoskeleton. New findings showed that sensory nerves, which are traditionally thought to operate as information relays to the CNS, interact with and regulate the local *onco-sphere* in a similar way [6–10]. The actual effect of the autonomic nervous system on the tumor local environment may be underestimated as tumor profiling studies cannot fully measure the amount of neuronal cell genetic material present. Scientists and physicians have long observed that nerves and blood vessels travel side by side, reaching the conclusion that both components are vital to maintain organ function [11].

In particular, the SNS system governs the operation of practically all organ systems in the human body, via secreting catecholamine neurotransmitters at the synapses of sympathetic nerves, and via circulating catecholamines from the adrenal glands systemically [12–14]. For a long time, physiologists have been interested in understanding the fight-or-flight response, which is represented by surges of SNS activity under a stressful situation, leading to a temporarily improvement in physical strength, agility, perceptual acuity, and body immunity while sacrificing trophic function such as digestion, reproduction, development, and exploration [12–14]. Many studies from the last decade have demonstrated that MMDPs aid cancer growth and metastasis [15–19]. Current pharmacoepidemiology research has connected β-adrenergic antagonists to slower tumor growth, suggesting that SNS activity might have clinically important implications on tumor biology [17, 20]. In this chapter, we discuss the implication of the interaction between host systemic SNS system (systemic neuronal *onco-sphere)* and their close-knit relationship with cancer (Fig. 23.1).

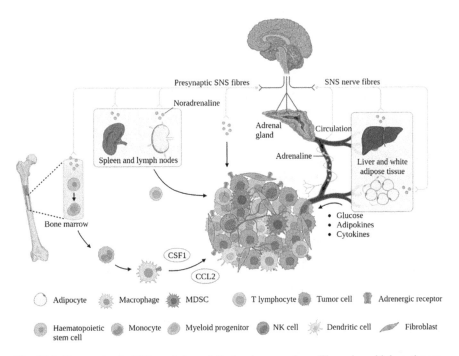

Fig. 23.1 Host systemic SNS regulation of the local *onco-sphere*. Through multiple pathways, activation of SNS can alter gene expression and cellular function in the local *onco-sphere*. SNS exerts its effects directly by releasing catecholamines (i.e., adrenaline and noradrenaline) to target adrenergic receptors that are differentially expressed on cancer cells and the surrounding stromal cells (i.e., TAMs, CAFs, vascular endothelial cells). The effect of catecholamines on the tumor microenvironment is modulated by two major signaling pathways: (1) chemical messengers via noradrenaline released by SNS fibers which directly interact with the cancer cells; and (2) hormonal regulation via adrenaline released by the adrenal gland into the systemic circulation. These catecholamine neuroeffector molecules indirectly regulate tumor biology by influencing the host immune system, by interfering with myelopoiesis, lymphocyte differentiation in secondary lymphoid organs, immunocytes trafficking or modifying tumor growth through altering regulators of metabolism and hormones

Effects of Tumor Innervation at the Local *Onco-Sphere*

Tumors can induce the growth and function of nerves, and in turn, nerves can mediate cancer development via direct or indirect ways. In particular, nerves may promote cancer development through paracrine signaling as the tumor cell membranes consist neurotransmitter-sensitive receptors. As such, neuroactive molecules can be secreted directly into the synaptic space between neurons and tumor cells to communicate an excitatory signal.

Paracrine Mode

Different types of nerve cells, such as neurons and Schwann cells, regulate tumor behavior and affect cancer progression via paracrine signaling. There are three major families of neuroactive molecules involved in the paracrine signaling of tumor–nerve interaction: (1) neurotrophic factors, namely nerve growth factor (NGF), brain-derived neurotrophic factor (BDNF), glial cell line-derived neurotrophic factor, etc.; (2) axon guidance molecules, for example, CCL2, CX3CL1, EphA2, Slit, etc.; (3) neurotransmitters, such as acetylcholine, glutamate, glycine, epinephrine, norepinephrine, dopamine, etc. [21, 22] In turn, tumor cells express different receptors (e.g., tyrosine kinase receptor A (TrkA), TrkB, and NGFR) on its cell membranes to interact with different families of neuroactive molecules and induce the downstream signaling cascade. Numerous studies have showed that neuroactive molecules and tumor-expressed receptors are highly linked with cancer development [23–27]. This tumor–nerve interaction is illustrated in Fig. 23.2. Adrenergic fibers were shown to act through β2- and β3-adrenergic receptors while cholinergic fibers act through cholinergic receptors in experimental models of prostate cancer [28]. Research revealed that cholinergic activation via acetylcholine increases the expression of NGF in the gastric epithelium, which facilitates tumor development [29]. Previous research had demonstrated therapeutic potential of TrkA inhibitors in NTRK fusion-positive cancer [30]. A study demonstrated that acetylcholine promotes tumor cell proliferation in lung cancer through the activation of mitogen-activated protein kinase and AKT pathways, which also strongly facilitates the adhesion, migration, and metastasis of lung cancer cells [31, 32]. Another study found that acetylcholine upregulates MMP9 expression and downregulates E-cadherin expression, which were highly linked to the lung cancer cell type that participates in migration and metastasis [33]. Other evidence revealed that the activation of acetylcholine receptor 7 (α7nAChR) stimulates the JAK2/STAT3 and Ras/Raf/MEK/ERK1/2 pathways and thereby enhances metastasis in pancreatic cancer [34].

Chemical Synapse

Research suggested that the neuron–glioma synapses function in a similar way as the classic synapses between two neurons, by observing the excitatory signals at the postsynaptic cells in glioma. Using gene expression analysis and confocal microscopy, AMPA receptors were detected at the postsynaptic glioma cells, which play a role in mediating glioma cell depolarization and spreading depolarizing across glioma cells via gap junctions. More importantly, this depolarization could enhance cancer growth and promote metastasis. In animal models, the inhibition of this signaling across the chemical synapse could lighten tumor burden and prolong survival time [35–37]. The expression of neuroligin, a molecule that assists in cell

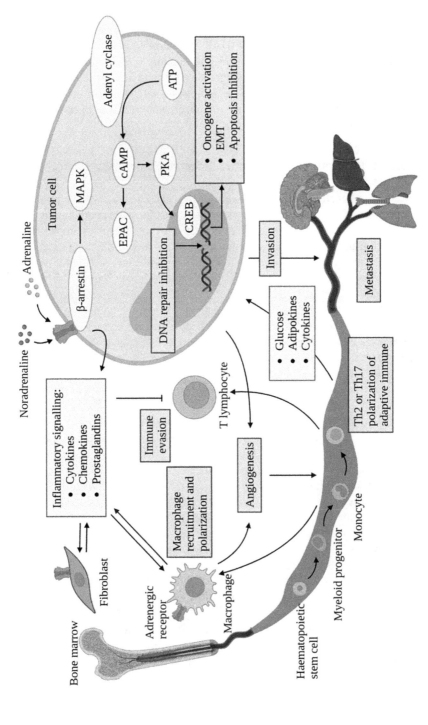

Fig. 23.2 Multi-directional crosstalk of tumor with host systemic neural network. SNS-mediated α-adrenergic and β-adrenergic receptor systems have widespread effects over a range of molecular processes that facilitate tumor progression and metastasis

adhesion, mediates the formation of pseudo-tripartite synapses between neurons in breast-to-brain metastasis [38–40]. Analysis of the transcriptomes revealed that NMDA receptor (NMDAR), especially GLuN2B subunit, was highly expressed. The activity of calcium levels after NMDAR activation was documented. NMDAR synapses have a role in promoting cancer proliferation in brain tumors, as demonstrated in the smaller tumor size and longer survival time after gene knockdown of GLuN2B in mice models. Overall, these findings reveal that tumor–nerve communication can be established through the chemical synapses and, in turn, result in cancer progression [41].

Box 23.1 Perineural Invasion (PNI): Effect of Tumor Cells on Nerves

Opposite from tumor innervation, perineural invasion (PNI) occurs when cancer cells penetrate into or surround nerves and can often occur prior to lymph node or vasculature metastasis [42, 43]. In 2009, a clearer definition for PNI was proposed: "tumor in close proximity to nerve, and involving at least one-third of its circumference or tumor cells within any of the three layers of the nerve sheath." PNI is more often found in aggressive tumors [43, 44]. Also, PNI appears to be a reliable indicator for OS and DFS in cancer patients [45–49]. Cancer-related pain is often caused by PNI, which involves direct nerve injury. Similar to blood vessels and lymphatic system which are regarded as possible routes for cancer metastasis, PNI provides an alternative route for tumor invasion to take place [50]. In the early stage of pancreatic cancer, it was demonstrated that cells originated in the pancreas acinar were detected in the spinal cord, travelling along the sensory neurons into the CNS, indicating that PNI could be a possible pathway of metastasis [10]. Emerging evidence indicates that the neuronal tracking theory is a plausible explanation for PNI process. In the process of nerve damage, cancer cells infiltrate into the perineural space and migrate along or around the nerve structures, thereby inducing neural regeneration. This leads to the establishment of a perineural niche when cancer cells invade and damage the perineurium, thus triggering the generation of inflammatory cytokines in the microenvironment [51–54], and the involvement of other cellular components that regulate neural tracking and further enhance PNI [55, 56]. PNI is a cancer-promoting mechanism in tumor–nerve interaction. However, due to the lack of a suitable model to mimic the complicated tumor–nerve interactions, our knowledge of detailed PNI processes remains restricted.

PNI is especially obvious in PDAC. Results indicated that 80–100% of PDAC patients are positive for PNI, and this has greatly contributed to the poor prognosis of these patients [57]. In a recent study, the connection between PNI and the host immune system has been elucidated in PDACs. Through single cell analysis and transcriptomic expression prolife, researchers observed that in PDAC patients with PNI, immune responses are impaired, as clearly indicated by a decreased in anti-tumoral $CD8^+$ T cells and Th1 cells,

(continued)

> **Box 23.1** (continued)
>
> while an increase in the pro-tumoral Th2 subset. An increment in the level of acetylcholine was also detected in patients with severe PNI, which triggers HDAC-1 to secrete high levels of CCL5, which in turn impedes the ability of PDAC to recruit CD8⁺ T cells. Not only that, in another manner, acetylcholine can directly inhibit the production of IFNγ (from CD8⁺ T cells), while favoring the Th2 phenotype differentiation as compared to Th1 [58]. Taken together, this data suggest that host neuronal system-PNI-host immune-tumor cells axis are complex and should be carefully trodden when implementing PDAC-specific treatments.

SNS Regulation of Cancer Biology in Local *Onco-Sphere*

Clinical data revealed a possible relationship between stress and cancer growth, which prompted researchers to investigate the impact of SNS on cancer biology [16, 18, 59]. Furthermore, recent pharmaco-epidemiological studies demonstrated that cancer patients who were on β-adrenergic antagonists (also known as β-blockers) before the diagnosis had slower disease progression [60–68]. In animal experiments, behavioral stress was proven to speed up various cancer progression, including hematological cancers [69–78]. β-Adrenergic antagonists have demonstrated its effectiveness in inhibiting the biological effects of stress in many experiments while β-agonists could replicate the biological effects of stress [17] (Fig. 23.2).

DNA Repair. Since adrenergic signaling can prevent DNA damage repair and p53-mediated apoptosis, SNS activity could potentially lead to tumor development or chromosomal instability [73]. A few mechanisms associated with β-adrenergic activity were proposed to have implications in inhibiting DNA damage repair, which include (1) activation of the ATR-p21 pathway, (2) activation of AKT pathway, induced by β-arrestin, or (3) degrading p53 protein through E3-ubiquitin ligase MDM2 stimulation [79, 80]. This could result in increased incidence of spontaneous chromosomal abnormalities in organs like the thymus and brain, which could be effectively prevented by β-adrenergic antagonist propranolol [79, 81]. In neuroblastoma cells, propranolol increases p53 levels, induces programmed cell death, and makes cancer cells more susceptible to the actions of the topoisomerase inhibitor SN-38 [73]. However, whether adrenergic suppression of DNA damage repair is enough to enhance spontaneous cancer initiation within the human body is unknown.

Oncogene Activation. Several oncogenic signaling pathways, such as SRC63 and ERBB2-encoded HER2, can be activated by β-adrenergic signaling [82, 83]. β-Adrenergic signaling stimulates STAT3, which then activates the HER-2 (ERBB2) promoter to increase gene transcription of HER2 oncogene. Catecholamine-mediated adrenergic signaling may also stimulate a wide range of oncogenic viruses [16], for example, the Kaposi's sarcoma-associated human herpesvirus 8 (HHV8), which cause B lymphocytes to activate the cellular transcription factor cyclic AMP response element binding protein (CREB) via the PKA-mediated cascade, that lead to the activation of a key viral promoter in HHV8's genome [84]. Consequently, the viral genome of HHV8 increases the gene expression of viral transcription factor that could activate downstream transcription of a number of viral oncogenes, leading to the systemic distribution of the viral genome. Besides contributing to the oncogenesis of Kaposi sarcoma of vascular endothelial cells, HHV8 also causes different kinds of B-cell cancers, suggesting that activation of SNS signaling can cause human cancer through its interaction with oncogenic viruses [85].

Inflammation and Immune Response. In the local *onco-sphere*, the transcription of pro-inflammatory cytokines (e.g., IL-6, IL-8) in cancer cells and myeloid lineage immune cells are upregulated by β-adrenergic signaling [70, 86–89]. Furthermore, adrenergic signaling activates the inflammatory arachidonic acid metabolism, which could result in enhanced cancer growth [90]. SNS activation of the inflammatory signaling has been proven to promote cancer development and metastasis in several in vivo investigations [70, 91]. However, it remains unclear if the role of SNS on inflammatory alone can initiate cancer development. Macrophages have important involvement in facilitating inflammation and regulating the tumor microenvironment, which contributes significantly towards tumor metastasis [70, 91]. β-Adrenergic signaling can stimulate the generation of chemotactic factors (i.e. M-CSF and CCL2), which could considerably boost macrophage recruitment into cancer cells. β-Adrenergic signaling can promote the myelopoiesis of monocytes, which increases the precursor pool of macrophages and results in increased density of tumor-associated macrophages in the local *onco-sphere* [92–94]. After being recruited, β-adrenergic signaling markedly enhances macrophage expression of TGF-β, VEGF, IL-6, MMP9, and PTGS2 to facilitate cancer progression. Adrenergic modulation of macrophage biology plays a key role in SNS-mediated cancer metastasis, suggesting that pharmacologic interventions, such as the use of inhibitors on the CSF-1 or MCP1 signaling pathways, can suppress the progression of metastasis in vivo [70, 91]. On the other hand, SNS signaling may significantly decrease the transcription of type I and type II interferons, which are important in the production of cellular immunity against malignancies and oncogenic viruses [70, 95, 96]. In addition, β-adrenergic signaling can also inhibit the protective effect of cytotoxic T cells and NK cells [78], resulting in greater rates of metastasis—an undesirable outcome that had been observed during surgery [75, 97, 98]. Nevertheless, even without considering the inhibitory effect on NK and cytotoxic T cells, the fact that SNS signaling can drive tumor dissemination has been demonstrated in several studies in SCID and nude mice [4, 69–71].

SNS Regulation of Cancer Biology in EMT and at a Distal *Onco-Sphere*

Several types of mesenchymal cells within the tumor parenchyma, including fibroblasts, pericytes, and mesenchymal stem cells, can be activated by adrenergic signaling [99–103]. Furthermore, adrenergic signaling can also stimulate adipocytes and mesenchymal cells in the bone marrow [104, 105], which can affect cancer biology indirectly by modifying the hematopoiesis of immune cells infiltrating the tumor, thereby regulating the CSCs [15, 106] (Fig. 23.2). According to recent evidence, β-adrenergic stimulation of the SNAIL TF family could increase the tumor-derived expression of mesenchymal gene program, which promotes EMT cancers, and further drive pro-metastatic activities (for example, tumor cell motility and MMP-mediated invasion of basement membrane) [107–113].

Angiogenesis. β-Adrenergic signaling also promotes angiogenesis by activating the transcriptional expression of GFs (i.e. IL-6 and VEGF), which stimulate blood vessel growth that encourages cancer growth and support metastasis [69, 87, 113–117]. Pharmacologic inhibition of angiogenesis has proven to be effective in alleviating the stress effects on cancer growth and metastasis, confirming that SNS-mediated upregulation of angiogenesis has an important role in supporting cancer progression in vivo [69].

Cancer Cell Survival. β-Adrenergic signaling modifies several pathways that influence tumor cells' survival and cell death, namely (1) via focal adhesion kinases (FAK, also called PTK2) to facilitate evasion of anoikis (apoptosis triggered by the detachment of anchorage-dependent cells when it detaches from the ECM, (2) via BCL-2-associated agonist of cell death (BAD), and (3) p53 signaling to aid evasion of apoptosis when subjected to chemotherapy [71–73, 118]. Other factors that maintain cell growth and survival, such as VEGF, IL-6, IL-8, are regulated by β-adrenergic signaling, which confers the ability to resist tyrosine kinase inhibition [117, 119].

Hematopoiesis. β-Adrenergic activity can enhance the development and metastasis of acute lymphoid leukemia in the body [77, 78] through the same molecular mechanisms as to how SNS modulate hematopoiesis [15, 92, 94, 120–122]. Bone marrow is regulated via sympathetic activity to maintain a homeostatically stable stromal cell population and to encourage recovery of the immune system after hematopoietic stem cell transplant [15, 123]. For instance, a research model of AML demonstrated that the administration of β-adrenergic antagonists, or β-blockers, can give rise to the undesirable outcome of advancing disease progression, tipping the balance within the hematopoietic stem cell niche towards a microenvironment that favors uncontrolled stem cell growth [15, 106]. A similar result is observed in the bone marrow when AML degrades sympathetic innervation and provokes leukemic stem cell proliferation, thereby colonizing the bone marrow [15, 106]. However, the scope of understanding the implications of SNS on lymphomas and other hematological cancers remains limited.

Box 23.2 Neoneurogenesis and Cancer

Neoneurogenesis, similar to angiogenesis, is the regeneration of nerves and recruitment of new axons during carcinogenesis. Peripheral nerve cells, unlike those in the CNS, may recover after being injured [124]. Neoneurogenesis is a complicated biological phenomenon that has yet to be fully understood. In different types of tumor tissues, neonerves with different origins have diverse, or even opposing functions. PNS has been associated to neoneurogenesis in cancer. Sympathetic nerve ablation, which may be done chemically or surgically, has been shown to avert prostate cancer progression in mice models. In addition, parasympathetic destruction may slow the spread and metastasis of prostate cancer. When there is more neurogenesis of both sympathetic and parasympathetic tumors, clinical outcomes of cancer patients were found to be poorer. Similar to the findings for prostate cancer, sympathectomy—the resection of superior cervical ganglia on both sides) decreased the progression and aggressiveness of tongue tumors [125]. Surprisingly, activation of sympathetic neurons promoted breast cancer development and progression, but stimulation of parasympathetic nerves inhibited it [7, 126, 127]. Hence, sympathetic and parasympathetic innervation may have varying effects on different types of cancers.

In pancreatic cancer, it was observed that the level of tumor-derived neurotrophic factors increased during the early stages and so did the density of sensory nerves. Cells from the pancreas were then found to migrate to the spinal cord along the sensory ganglia at later stages. The results showed that sensory nerves were involved in the development of pancreatic cancer throughout all stages, including cancer initiation and growth [128]. Similarly, sensory neurons also take part directly in tumorigenesis of basal cell carcinoma [8]. In pancreatic ductal adenocarcinoma and gastric cancer, the vagus nerve has been shown to serve entirely reversed function, which could be due to its duality of containing both parasympathetic and sensory axons [129]. Surgical resection of the vagus nerve or pharmacological denervation of the stomach region can reduce cancer progression and extend survival time in several models of advance gastric cancer [2]. Denervation had notable effect on the regeneration of stem cells in gastric cancers, as well as improving the efficacy of chemotherapy [2]. Also, enteric nerves also have a key role in the onset and development of gastric cancer [29, 130]. Vagus nerve have a protective role against pancreatic cancer, as opposed to its cancer-inducing effect in gastric cancer [131, 132]. Vagotomy, the resection of vagus nerve, attracts TAMs into the TME and induces inflammation and thus promotes carcinogenesis and cancer development in pancreatic cancer [131, 133].

Emerging evidence showed that, in head and neck carcinomas, new adrenergic nerve fibers were derived from sensory neurons rather than from the preexisting adrenergic nerves and were responsible for regulating the signals

(continued)

> **Box 23.2** (continued)
> that promote cancerous growth [134]. Adrenergic differentiation signature was identified in cancer-associated neuron's transcriptome [134]. Furthermore, sensory denervation or pharmacological inhibition of adrenergic receptors was found to suppress cancer development, suggesting that cancer cells are responsible for neuron reprogramming in order to enhance tumor growth. Neurogenesis in tumors could also stem from MSCs that migrated from the bone marrow, which could then differentiate into neurons when reaching the local oncosphere, or when growth conditions are met.

Inter-*Onco-Spherical* Communication: Neurogenesis and Immune System

Nerves acts as the bridge between the tumor in local *onco-sphere* and the host immune system, which the later can play a part in cancer development through promoting inflammatory processes [135]. For example, adrenergic activation in spleen promotes the release of acetylcholine in T cells that express β2-adrenergic receptor (β2-AR) [136]. Reportedly, the function of T-cell-derived ACh is important in the regulation of immune responses and cancer immunity. Acetylcholine released by T cells can bind to the α7 nicotinic Ach receptors on cytokine-producing macrophages, resulting in decrease generation of TNF-α [137]. In lung cancer, acetylcholine also binds to nicotinic and muscarinic receptors in response, which spur cancer proliferation, migration, and metastasis [138]. The enzyme responsible for synthesizing acetylcholine from choline, known as choline acetyltransferase, is potently activated by IL-21 in $CD4^+$ and $CD8^+$ T cells to mediate lymphocytic migration and immunity [139]. To control cancer growth and progression, it is critical for activated immune cells to infiltrate the tumor [140]. The nerve density of SNS and PNS was found to be associated with the expression level of immune checkpoint molecules (e.g., PD1, PD-L1, and FOXP3) and was predictive of the clinical outcomes [126]. However, tumor cells can often resist anti-tumor immune responses by stimulating the immune checkpoint pathways that inhibit these anti-tumor mechanisms, thereby evading immunosurveillance [141, 142].

Both nerve-derived cholinergic and adrenergic activities mediate the recruitment of TAM. For example, adrenergic activity stimulates cancer development and increases the probability of adverse outcomes through TAM recruitment, whereas cholinergic activity does the opposite [132, 143]. Another research demonstrated that vagotomy can influence TNFα secretion via TAMs regulation and promote tumor development in pancreatic cancer, leading to decrease survival time [131]. Furthermore, stress can induce neuroendocrine activation, which can trigger metastasis to secondary sites (such as lungs and lymph nodes). The use of β-agonist activates β-adrenergic signaling and induces similar effect while β-blocker opposes the effect. When adrenergic signaling is activated, the primary tumor site attracts

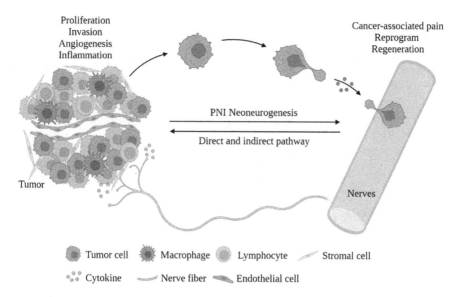

Fig. 23.3 The tumor-nerve crosstalk. Nerves can secrete neuroactive molecules to act on the TME (tumor cells, TAMs, TANs, lymphocytes) to promote every stage of tumorigenesis and progression, invasion, inflammation, and metastasis

CD11b$^+$ F4/80$^+$ macrophages, triggering macrophage differentiation into pro-tumoral M2-like phenotype, which also encourages metastasis. Interestingly, macrophages from endoneurium are also involved in cancer metastasis. Native macrophages that reside in the nervous system, such as microglia, play important role in promoting brain metastasis [144]. A study revealed that endoneural macrophages in the CNS suppress immune responses in brain metastasis by acting through CXCL10. Macrophages could also regulate VISTA—an immune regulatory protein—and PD-L1 [145] to inhibit T-cell activation and thus facilitate brain metastasis. By blocking the functions of microglia, brain metastasis could be controlled with considerable anti-tumor effect. The inhibition of several signaling pathways in macrophages, such as the CCL2, STAT3, CSF-1R, or PI3K, can suppress brain metastasis [146–149]. Similarly, a subset of fibroblast termed endoneural fibroblast-like cells (EFLCs) have been described since a few decades ago; however, their function in cancer is not well defined [150], Fig. 23.3.

Pituitary Neuroendocrine Tumors (PitNETs)

As the name indicates, pituitary neuroendocrine tumors (PitNETs) arise from the pituitary gland, the most important hormone-producing gland found below the hypothalamus in the brain, and can lead to hypersecretion of hormones or local compression of the adjacent intracranial structures and major nerves

[151]. Headaches, vision impairments, and other endocrine disorders are among the comorbidities linked with PitNETs. Cushing disease, which is caused by an excess of adrenocorticotropin (ACTH) produced by pituitary adenomas, is characterized by a series of severe and even fatal symptoms, including diabetes, hypertension, central obesity, osteoporosis, muscle weakness, and psychological disturbances [152]. In addition, PitNETs also trigger aberrant release of growth hormone, thyroid-stimulating hormone, prolactin, follicle-stimulating hormone, and luteinizing hormone; all of which is manifested by its corresponding endocrine disorders, such as acromegaly, thyrotoxicosis, reproductive disorder, and gonadal dysfunction [151].

Paraneoplastic syndromes are often the first indicator of malignancy, where most tumors express a neuroendocrine program that combines both neural and endocrine features, as opposed to PitNETs characteristic internal neuroendocrine disorder. Rather than direct tumor cell invasion, paraneoplastic syndromes are anatomic and functional abnormalities induced by primary tumors at a distant site and the systemic biological effect. These pathological processes are orchestrated by a diverse array of tumor-secreted factors, which separate the syndromes into two major categories: (1) neurological symptoms caused primarily by the production of antineural antibodies, and (2) endocrine symptoms caused by the synthesis of neuroendocrine cell-mediated ectopic hormone [153]. Small-cell-lung cancer (SCLC), for example, is the most common cancer linked to paraneoplastic syndromes [153], with Lambert–Eaten myasthenic syndrome characterized by muscle weakness occurring more frequently than other neurological disorders with an autoimmune cause. This neuromuscular autoimmune disorder is caused by defective antibodies attacking voltage-gated calcium channels (VGCC) found on the presynaptic nerve terminal, as SCLC also express functional VGCC [154]. The common endocrine symptoms of SCLC include ACTH-associated Cushing syndrome and inappropriate antidiuretic hormone secretion (SIADH) [153].

Abnormal neuronal and endocrine signaling in the host macroenvironment plays a part in carcinogenesis and its subsequent progression as well. A solid tumor, like an integrated organ, can receive sympathetic innervation directly where the nerve fibers release neurotransmitter norepinephrine straight into the tumor regions [155]. On the other hand, the SNS regulates tumor biology by the release of epinephrine from the adrenal glands [1, 156]. Stress-responsive signaling pathways can be activated by ligating the neuroeffector molecules to their cognate receptors on cancer cells or the cancer-associated stromal cells, which has far-reaching effect on both the local and systemic *onco-spheres* [157]. Emotional distress and psychiatric syndromes, which are interpreted and integrated by specific regions of the brain, have been shown to cause SNS dysfunction and dysregulation of the hypothalamic–pituitary–adrenal (HPA) axis, resulting in a spike in the release of stress hormones (for example, catecholamines and glucocorticoids) [158, 159]. Chronic stress can be caused by long-term stimulation of the SNS and HPA axis, which in turn accumulates DNA damage and genomic instability, enhances tumor angiogenesis and development, hinders tumor immune surveillance, aggravates inflammatory networks, and eventually speeds up cancer progression [69, 156, 160]. The parasympathetic (cholinergic) division of the peripheral autonomic system, in contrast to the sympathetic (β-adrenergic) nerves' pro-tumor involvement in PCa [1], may ultimately block carcinogenesis and development, as seen in pancreatic cancer [132].

Notably, neuroendocrine disorders caused by tumor may exacerbate emotional disorders, causing vicious loops in both the TME and host macroenvironment, by facilitating malignancy, and by suppressing immunity, promoting metabolic reprogramming, and establishing favorable PMNs in target organs. Within the systemic *onco-sphere*, a deeper knowledge of tumor-neuroendocrine system is critically needed to comprehend how neuroendocrine signals communicate with the tumor through chemical messengers originating from nerve cells, endocrine organs, immune system, and cancer cells. This knowledge would highly benefit the search for newer and better treatment strategies against cancer management.

Box 23.3 Tumor Axonogenesis: An Overlooked Factor in the Local
Onco-Sphere
Previously, axonogenesis—the extension of nerves in the TME, has been disregarded since nerves were not thought to be necessary for cancer development. The fact that nerves are challenging to study in regular histology is another reason why they have been understudied in cancer. Regular histology can reveal large nerve bundles, which are used to determine PNI in pathologic examinations, but most nerves in the TME have microscopic nerve bundles or even single axons, requiring specialized neuronal biomarkers to be identified in immunohistochemistry examinations [43]. PGP9.5, also known as protein gene product 9.5/UCH-L1/PARK5, is a neuronal biomarker that identifies all types of nerve cells in IHC staining. Neurons of the PNS can be identified by other neuronal biomarkers, such as tubulin beta-3 and peripherin (a type III intermediate filament protein biomarker). To identify neurons of the ANS, tyrosine hydroxylase is the biomarker for adrenergic nerves while vesicular acetylcholine transporter (VAChT) is the biomarker of choice for cholinergic nerves. IHC staining for glial fibrillary acidic protein or S100 can also be used to identify peripheral glial cells, also known as Schwann cells, in the TME. Direct microscopic inspection can be used to assess and quantify nerves in tumor by IHC; however, measurement of nerve density may require bioinformatics analysis, as shown in prostate cancer [161]. Employing the neuronal biomarkers and methodology mentioned above, the finding of nerves' regulatory function in tumorigenesis has brought forward more in-depth investigations of the nerve subtype distribution in human cancers. For example, both adrenergic and cholinergic nerves are present in the periphery of the tumors and within the tumor parenchyma, and the nerve density correlates proportionately with malignancy aggressiveness in prostate cancer [4, 162]. Higher histologic grade in prostate cancer demonstrated greater density of nerves when compared to lower grade cancer or benign prostatic hyperplasia. The secretion of neurotrophic growth factors stimulates axonogenesis during

(continued)

Box 23.3 (continued)

embryonic development and tissue regeneration, leading to the migration and formation of more nerve terminals at the site of secretion. A number of neurotrophic growth factors are involved in the mechanisms underlying axonogenesis, including nerve growth factor (NGF), brain-derived neurotrophic factor (BDNF), neutrophin-3 (NT3), and neurotrophin-4/5 (NT4/5), via the activation of tyrosine kinase receptors in nerve terminals [163]. Axon guidance molecules, such as Robo-Slit or semaphorins [164], have also been found in human cancers, suggesting that they may play a role in axonogenesis in cancer [165, 166].

Axonogenesis may be driven by a comparable contribution of both neurotrophic GFs and molecules released by cancer cells. Increased synthesis of proNGF, the precursor of NGF, has been linked to nerve density in the TME of prostate cancer [167]. Furthermore, axonogenesis was successfully replicated in experimental models of prostate cancer, indicating that proNGF/NGF plays mechanistical role in mediating axonogenesis in cancer [167]. G-CSF exerts an off-target effect on the neonerves and seems to enhance carcinogenesis in prostate cancer [168]. The production of NGF from gastric cancer cells caused a similar increase in nerve density in the local *onco-sphere* [29]. Through cholinergic regulation of the WNT signaling pathway, NGF produced from the gastric cancer cells increases parasympathetic innervation of the tumor, which encourages cancer cell proliferation [3]. The tumor-derived leukemia inhibitory factor (LIF) from the IL-6 family also plays a role in tumor innervation in pancreatic cancer [169]. Nerves have been observed in around one-third of invasive ductal carcinomas in breast cancer, and nerve density has been linked to tumor aggressiveness and tumor-derived NGF [127, 170]. Early evidence reveals that sympathetic signaling is involved in the development of breast cancer; however, the mechanism underlying these observations remains unclear [70]. Axonogenesis has also been recognized as an indicator of aggressiveness in colorectal cancer [171, 172].

Axonogenesis is becoming prominent as a new cancer hallmark, and tumor-derived neurotrophic growth factors seem to promote nerve infiltration in the TME. Evidence has demonstrated that neurogenesis in neural ganglia is linked with axonogenesis in prostate cancer, but neurogenesis has not been described in other types of malignancies; hence, the degree of neurogenesis in human cancers remains unknown [28].

Conclusion

The contributions of host nervous system in the systemic *onco-sphere* are indispensable. However, techniques and technologies to manipulate nerves in their location (*i.e.* tumor, metastasized organs) are still preliminary. By comprehensive analysis of the spatial arrangement of tumor innervation, and the effect of host neuronal system to the tumor, we can propose a nerve-targeting therapy that could interfere with tumor–nerve communication, influence their signaling in all stages of tumor progression.

References

1. Zahalka AH, Arnal-Estapé A, Maryanovich M, Nakahara F, Cruz CD, Finley LWS et al (2017) Adrenergic nerves activate an angio-metabolic switch in prostate cancer. Science 358(6361): 321–326
2. Zhao CM, Hayakawa Y, Kodama Y, Muthupalani S, Westphalen CB, Andersen GT et al (2014) Denervation suppresses gastric tumorigenesis. Sci Transl Med 6(250):250ra115
3. Renz BW, Takahashi R, Tanaka T, Macchini M, Hayakawa Y, Dantes Z et al (2018) β2 adrenergic-neurotrophin feedforward loop promotes pancreatic cancer. Cancer Cell 34(5): 863–867
4. Magnon C, Hall SJ, Lin J, Xue X, Gerber L, Freedland SJ et al (2013) Autonomic nerve development contributes to prostate cancer progression. Science 341(6142):1236361
5. Langley J (1921) In: Heffer W (ed) The autonomic nervous system, Part 1. Simpkin, Marshall, Hamilton, Kent & Co, London
6. Erin N, Zhao W, Bylander J, Chase G, Clawson G (2006) Capsaicin-induced inactivation of sensory neurons promotes a more aggressive gene expression phenotype in breast cancer cells. Breast Cancer Res Treat 99(3):351–364
7. Kappos EA, Engels PE, Tremp M, Sieber PK, von Felten S, Madduri S et al (2018) Denervation leads to volume regression in breast cancer. J Plast Reconstr Aesthet Surg 71(6):833–839
8. Peterson SC, Eberl M, Vagnozzi AN, Belkadi A, Veniaminova NA, Verhaegen ME et al (2015) Basal cell carcinoma preferentially arises from stem cells within hair follicle and mechanosensory niches. Cell Stem Cell 16(4):400–412
9. Sinha S, Fu YY, Grimont A, Ketcham M, Lafaro K, Saglimbeni JA et al (2017) PanIN neuroendocrine cells promote tumorigenesis via neuronal cross-talk. Cancer Res 77(8): 1868–1879
10. Saloman JL, Albers KM, Li D, Hartman DJ, Crawford HC, Muha EA et al (2016) Ablation of sensory neurons in a genetic model of pancreatic ductal adenocarcinoma slows initiation and progression of cancer. Proc Natl Acad Sci U S A 113(11):3078–3083
11. Vesalius A (1543) De Humani Corporis Fabrica (The Fabric of the Human Body). Johannes Oporinus, Basel
12. Weiner H (1992) Perturbing the organism: the biology of stressful experience. University of Chicago Press, Chicago
13. Sapolsky RM (1994) Why zebras don't get ulcers: a guide to stress, stress-related diseases, and coping. Freeman, New York
14. Sherwood L (2015) Human physiology: from cells to systems. Cengage Learning, Boston
15. Hanoun M, Maryanovich M, Arnal-Estapé A, Frenette PS (2015) Neural regulation of hematopoiesis, inflammation, and cancer. Neuron 86(2):360–373
16. Antoni MH, Lutgendorf SK, Cole SW, Dhabhar FS, Sephton SE, McDonald PG et al (2006) The influence of bio-behavioural factors on tumour biology: pathways and mechanisms. Nat Rev Cancer 6(3):240–248
17. Cole SW, Sood AK (2012) Molecular pathways: beta-adrenergic signaling in cancer. Clin Cancer Res 18(5):1201–1206
18. Armaiz-Pena GN, Cole SW, Lutgendorf SK, Sood AK (2013) Neuroendocrine influences on cancer progression. Brain Behav Immunity 30(Suppl):S19–S25

19. Cole SW (2013) Nervous system regulation of the cancer genome. Brain Behav Immunity 30 (Suppl):S10–S18
20. Powe DG, Entschladen F (2011) Targeted therapies: using β-blockers to inhibit breast cancer progression. Nat Rev Clin Oncol 8(9):511–512
21. Saloman JL, Albers KM, Rhim AD, Davis BM (2016) Can stopping nerves, stop cancer? Trends Neurosci 39(12):880–889
22. Kuol N, Stojanovska L, Apostolopoulos V, Nurgali K (2018) Role of the nervous system in tumor angiogenesis. Cancer Microenviron 11(1):1–11
23. Arese M, Bussolino F, Pergolizzi M, Bizzozero L, Pascal D (2018) Tumor progression: the neuronal input. Ann Transl Med 6(5):89
24. Deborde S, Wong RJ (2017) How Schwann cells facilitate cancer progression in nerves. Cell Mol Life Sci 74(24):4405–4420
25. Mancino M, Ametller E, Gascón P, Almendro V (2011) The neuronal influence on tumor progression. Biochim Biophys Acta 1816(2):105–118
26. Barquilla A, Pasquale EB (2015) Eph receptors and ephrins: therapeutic opportunities. Annu Rev Pharmacol Toxicol 55:465–487
27. Rehman M, Tamagnone L (2013) Semaphorins in cancer: biological mechanisms and therapeutic approaches. Semin Cell Dev Biol 24(3):179–189
28. Ayala GE, Dai H, Powell M, Li R, Ding Y, Wheeler TM et al (2008) Cancer-related axonogenesis and neurogenesis in prostate cancer. Clin Cancer Res 14(23):7593–7603
29. Hayakawa Y, Sakitani K, Konishi M, Asfaha S, Niikura R, Tomita H et al (2017) Nerve growth factor promotes gastric tumorigenesis through aberrant cholinergic signaling. Cancer Cell 31(1):21–34
30. Cocco E, Scaltriti M, Drilon A (2018) NTRK fusion-positive cancers and TRK inhibitor therapy. Nat Rev Clin Oncol 15(12):731–747
31. Song P, Sekhon HS, Jia Y, Keller JA, Blusztajn JK, Mark GP et al (2003) Acetylcholine is synthesized by and acts as an autocrine growth factor for small cell lung carcinoma. Cancer Res 63(1):214–221
32. Song P, Sekhon HS, Fu XW, Maier M, Jia Y, Duan J et al (2008) Activated cholinergic signaling provides a target in squamous cell lung carcinoma. Cancer Res 68(12):4693–4700
33. Lin G, Sun L, Wang R, Guo Y, Xie C (2014) Overexpression of muscarinic receptor 3 promotes metastasis and predicts poor prognosis in non-small-cell lung cancer. J Thorac Oncol 9(2):170–178
34. Momi N, Ponnusamy MP, Kaur S, Rachagani S, Kunigal SS, Chellappan S et al (2013) Nicotine/cigarette smoke promotes metastasis of pancreatic cancer through α7nAChR-mediated MUC4 upregulation. Oncogene 32(11):1384–1395
35. Rzeski W, Turski L, Ikonomidou C (2001) Glutamate antagonists limit tumor growth. Proc Natl Acad Sci U S A 98(11):6372–6377
36. Savaskan NE, Heckel A, Hahnen E, Engelhorn T, Doerfler A, Ganslandt O et al (2008) Small interfering RNA-mediated xCT silencing in gliomas inhibits neurodegeneration and alleviates brain edema. Nat Med 14(6):629–632
37. Takano T, Lin JH, Arcuino G, Gao Q, Yang J, Nedergaard M (2001) Glutamate release promotes growth of malignant gliomas. Nat Med 7(9):1010–1015
38. Zeng Q, Michael IP, Zhang P, Saghafinia S, Knott G, Jiao W et al (2019) Synaptic proximity enables NMDAR signalling to promote brain metastasis. Nature 573(7775):526–531
39. Gambrill AC, Barria A (2011) NMDA receptor subunit composition controls synaptogenesis and synapse stabilization. Proc Natl Acad Sci U S A 108(14):5855–5860
40. Li L, Hanahan D (2013) Hijacking the neuronal NMDAR signaling circuit to promote tumor growth and invasion. Cell 153(1):86–100
41. Kepper M, Keast J (1995) Immunohistochemical properties and spinal connections of pelvic autonomic neurons that innervate the rat prostate gland. Cell Tissue Res 281(3):533–542
42. Batsakis JG (1985) Nerves and neurotropic carcinomas. Ann Otol Rhinol Laryngol 94(4 Pt 1): 426–427

43. Liebig C, Ayala G, Wilks JA, Berger DH, Albo D (2009) Perineural invasion in cancer: a review of the literature. Cancer 115(15):3379–3391
44. Mavros MN, Economopoulos KP, Alexiou VG, Pawlik TM (2014) Treatment and prognosis for patients with intrahepatic cholangiocarcinoma: systematic review and meta-analysis. JAMA Surg 149(6):565–574
45. Hirai I, Kimura W, Ozawa K, Kudo S, Suto K, Kuzu H et al (2002) Perineural invasion in pancreatic cancer. Pancreas 24(1):15–25
46. Duraker N, Sişman S, Can G (2003) The significance of perineural invasion as a prognostic factor in patients with gastric carcinoma. Surg Today 33(2):95–100
47. He P, Shi JS, Chen WK, Wang ZR, Ren H, Li H (2002) Multivariate statistical analysis of clinicopathologic factors influencing survival of patients with bile duct carcinoma. World J Gastroenterol 8(5):943–946
48. Lee IH, Roberts R, Shah RB, Wojno KJ, Wei JT, Sandler HM (2007) Perineural invasion is a marker for pathologically advanced disease in localized prostate cancer. Int J Radiat Oncol Biol Phys 68(4):1059–1064
49. Schmitd LB, Scanlon CS, D'Silva NJ (2018) Perineural invasion in head and neck cancer. J Dent Res 97(7):742–750
50. Amit M, Na'ara S, Gil Z (2016) Mechanisms of cancer dissemination along nerves. Nat Rev Cancer 16(6):399–408
51. De Oliveira T, Abiatari I, Raulefs S, Sauliunaite D, Erkan M, Kong B et al (2012) Syndecan-2 promotes perineural invasion and cooperates with K-ras to induce an invasive pancreatic cancer cell phenotype. Mol Cancer 11:19
52. Marchesi F, Piemonti L, Fedele G, Destro A, Roncalli M, Albarello L et al (2008) The chemokine receptor CX3CR1 is involved in the neural tropism and malignant behavior of pancreatic ductal adenocarcinoma. Cancer Res 68(21):9060–9069
53. Abiatari I, DeOliveira T, Kerkadze V, Schwager C, Esposito I, Giese NA et al (2009) Consensus transcriptome signature of perineural invasion in pancreatic carcinoma. Mol Cancer Ther 8(6):1494–1504
54. Li X, Wang Z, Ma Q, Xu Q, Liu H, Duan W et al (2014) Sonic hedgehog paracrine signaling activates stromal cells to promote perineural invasion in pancreatic cancer. Clin Cancer Res 20(16):4326–4338
55. Demir IE, Schorn S, Schremmer-Danninger E, Wang K, Kehl T, Giese NA et al (2013) Perineural mast cells are specifically enriched in pancreatic neuritis and neuropathic pain in pancreatic cancer and chronic pancreatitis. PloS One 8(3):e60529
56. Cavel O, Shomron O, Shabtay A, Vital J, Trejo-Leider L, Weizman N et al (2012) Endoneurial macrophages induce perineural invasion of pancreatic cancer cells by secretion of GDNF and activation of RET tyrosine kinase receptor. Cancer Res 72(22):5733–5743
57. Bapat AA, Hostetter G, Von Hoff DD, Han H (2011) Perineural invasion and associated pain in pancreatic cancer. Nat Rev Cancer 11(10):695–707
58. Yang M-W, Tao L-Y, Jiang Y-S, Yang J-Y, Huo Y-M, Liu D-J et al (2020) Perineural invasion reprograms the immune microenvironment through cholinergic signaling in pancreatic ductal adenocarcinoma. Cancer Res 80(10):1991–2003
59. Chida Y, Hamer M, Wardle J, Steptoe A (2008) Do stress-related psychosocial factors contribute to cancer incidence and survival? Nat Clin Pract Oncol 5(8):466–475
60. Barron TI, Connolly RM, Sharp L, Bennett K, Visvanathan K (2011) Beta blockers and breast cancer mortality: a population- based study. J Clin Oncol 29(19):2635–2644
61. Melhem-Bertrandt A, Chavez-Macgregor M, Lei X, Brown EN, Lee RT, Meric-Bernstam F et al (2011) Beta-blocker use is associated with improved relapse-free survival in patients with triple-negative breast cancer. J Clin Oncol 29(19):2645–2652
62. De Giorgi V, Grazzini M, Gandini S, Benemei S, Lotti T, Marchionni N et al (2011) Treatment with β-blockers and reduced disease progression in patients with thick melanoma. Arch Intern Med 171(8):779–781

63. Lemeshow S, Sørensen HT, Phillips G, Yang EV, Antonsen S, Riis AH et al (2011) β-Blockers and survival among Danish patients with malignant melanoma: a population-based cohort study. Cancer Epidemiol Biomarkers Prev 20(10):2273–2279

64. Aydiner A, Ciftci R, Karabulut S, Kilic L (2013) Does beta-blocker therapy improve the survival of patients with metastatic non-small cell lung cancer? Asian Pac J Cancer Prev 14(10):6109–6114

65. Botteri E, Munzone E, Rotmensz N, Cipolla C, De Giorgi V, Santillo B et al (2013) Therapeutic effect of β-blockers in triple-negative breast cancer postmenopausal women. Breast Cancer Res Treat 140(3):567–575

66. De Giorgi V, Gandini S, Grazzini M, Benemei S, Marchionni N, Geppetti P (2013) Effect of β-blockers and other antihypertensive drugs on the risk of melanoma recurrence and death. Mayo Clin Proc 88(11):1196–1203

67. Grytli HH, Fagerland MW, Fosså SD, Taskén KA, Håheim LL (2013) Use of β-blockers is associated with prostate cancer-specific survival in prostate cancer patients on androgen deprivation therapy. Prostate 73(3):250–260

68. Grytli HH, Fagerland MW, Fosså SD, Taskén KA (2014) Association between use of β-blockers and prostate cancer-specific survival: a cohort study of 3561 prostate cancer patients with high-risk or metastatic disease. Eur Urol 65(3):635–641

69. Thaker PH, Han LY, Kamat AA, Arevalo JM, Takahashi R, Lu C et al (2006) Chronic stress promotes tumor growth and angiogenesis in a mouse model of ovarian carcinoma. Nat Med 12(8):939–944

70. Sloan EK, Priceman SJ, Cox BF, Yu S, Pimentel MA, Tangkanangnukul V et al (2010) The sympathetic nervous system induces a metastatic switch in primary breast cancer. Cancer Res 70(18):7042–7052

71. Hassan S, Karpova Y, Baiz D, Yancey D, Pullikuth A, Flores A et al (2013) Behavioral stress accelerates prostate cancer development in mice. J Clin Invest 123(2):874–886

72. Pasquier E, Street J, Pouchy C, Carre M, Gifford AJ, Murray J et al (2013) β-blockers increase response to chemotherapy via direct antitumour and anti-angiogenic mechanisms in neuroblastoma. Br J Cancer 108(12):2485–2494

73. Wolter JK, Wolter NE, Blanch A, Partridge T, Cheng L, Morgenstern DA et al (2014) Anti-tumor activity of the beta-adrenergic receptor antagonist propranolol in neuroblastoma. Oncotarget 5(1):161–172

74. Hasegawa H, Saiki I (2002) Psychosocial stress augments tumor development through beta-adrenergic activation in mice. Jpn J Cancer Res 93(7):729–735

75. Goldfarb Y, Sorski L, Benish M, Levi B, Melamed R, Ben-Eliyahu S (2011) Improving postoperative immune status and resistance to cancer metastasis: a combined perioperative approach of immunostimulation and prevention of excessive surgical stress responses. Ann Surg 253(4):798–810

76. Kim-Fuchs C, Le CP, Pimentel MA, Shackleford D, Ferrari D, Angst E et al (2014) Chronic stress accelerates pancreatic cancer growth and invasion: a critical role for beta-adrenergic signaling in the pancreatic microenvironment. Brain Behav Immun 40:40–47

77. Lamkin DM, Sloan EK, Patel AJ, Chiang BS, Pimentel MA, Ma JC et al (2012) Chronic stress enhances progression of acute lymphoblastic leukemia via β-adrenergic signaling. Brain Behav Immun 26(4):635–641

78. Inbar S, Neeman E, Avraham R, Benish M, Rosenne E, Ben-Eliyahu S (2011) Do stress responses promote leukemia progression? An animal study suggesting a role for epinephrine and prostaglandin-E2 through reduced NK activity. PLoS One 6(4):e19246

79. Hara MR, Kovacs JJ, Whalen EJ, Rajagopal S, Strachan RT, Grant W et al (2011) A stress response pathway regulates DNA damage through β2-adrenoreceptors and β-arrestin-1. Nature 477(7364):349–353

80. Reeder A, Attar M, Nazario L, Bathula C, Zhang A, Hochbaum D et al (2015) Stress hormones reduce the efficacy of paclitaxel in triple negative breast cancer through induction of DNA damage. Br J Cancer 112(9):1461–1470

81. Hara MR, Sachs BD, Caron MG, Lefkowitz RJ (2013) Pharmacological blockade of a β(2) AR-β-arrestin-1 signaling cascade prevents the accumulation of DNA damage in a behavioral stress model. Cell Cycle 12(2):219–224

82. Shi M, Liu D, Duan H, Qian L, Wang L, Niu L et al (2011) The β2-adrenergic receptor and Her2 comprise a positive feedback loop in human breast cancer cells. Breast Cancer Res Treat 125(2):351–362

83. Gu L, Lau SK, Loera S, Somlo G, Kane SE (2009) Protein kinase A activation confers resistance to trastuzumab in human breast cancer cell lines. Clin Cancer Res 15(23): 7196–7206

84. Chang M, Brown HJ, Collado-Hidalgo A, Arevalo JM, Galic Z, Symensma TL et al (2005) beta-Adrenoreceptors reactivate Kaposi's sarcoma-associated herpesvirus lytic replication via PKA-dependent control of viral RTA. J Virol 79(21):13538–13547

85. zur Hausen H (2008) Infections causing human cancer. Wiley, Weinheim

86. Cole SW, Arevalo JM, Takahashi R, Sloan EK, Lutgendorf SK, Sood AK et al (2010) Computational identification of gene-social environment interaction at the human IL6 locus. Proc Natl Acad Sci U S A 107(12):5681–5686

87. Nilsson MB, Armaiz-Pena G, Takahashi R, Lin YG, Trevino J, Li Y et al (2007) Stress hormones regulate interleukin-6 expression by human ovarian carcinoma cells through a Src-dependent mechanism. J Biol Chem 282(41):29919–29926

88. Shahzad MM, Arevalo JM, Armaiz-Pena GN, Lu C, Stone RL, Moreno-Smith M et al (2010) Stress effects on FosB- and interleukin-8 (IL8)-driven ovarian cancer growth and metastasis. J Biol Chem 285(46):35462–35470

89. Yang R, Lin Q, Gao HB, Zhang P (2014) Stress-related hormone norepinephrine induces interleukin-6 expression in GES-1 cells. Braz J Med Biol Res 47(2):101–109

90. Cakir Y, Plummer HK III, Tithof PK, Schuller HM (2002) Beta-adrenergic and arachidonic acid-mediated growth regulation of human breast cancer cell lines. Int J Oncol 21(1):153–157

91. Armaiz-Pena GN, Gonzalez-Villasana V, Nagaraja AS, Rodriguez-Aguayo C, Sadaoui NC, Stone RL et al (2015) Adrenergic regulation of monocyte chemotactic protein 1 leads to enhanced macrophage recruitment and ovarian carcinoma growth. Oncotarget 6(6):4266–4273

92. Powell ND, Sloan EK, Bailey MT, Arevalo JM, Miller GE, Chen E et al (2013) Social stress up-regulates inflammatory gene expression in the leukocyte transcriptome via β-adrenergic induction of myelopoiesis. Proc Natl Acad Sci U S A 110(41):16574–16579

93. Dutta P, Courties G, Wei Y, Leuschner F, Gorbatov R, Robbins CS et al (2012) Myocardial infarction accelerates atherosclerosis. Nature 487(7407):325–329

94. Heidt T, Sager HB, Courties G, Dutta P, Iwamoto Y, Zaltsman A et al (2014) Chronic variable stress activates hematopoietic stem cells. Nat Med 20(7):754–758

95. Collado-Hidalgo A, Sung C, Cole S (2006) Adrenergic inhibition of innate anti-viral response: PKA blockade of Type I interferon gene transcription mediates catecholamine support for HIV-1 replication. Brain Behav Immun 20(6):552–563

96. Cole SW, Korin YD, Fahey JL, Zack JA (1998) Norepinephrine accelerates HIV replication via protein kinase A-dependent effects on cytokine production. J Immunol 161(2):610–616

97. Glasner A, Avraham R, Rosenne E, Benish M, Zmora O, Shemer S et al (2010) Improving survival rates in two models of spontaneous postoperative metastasis in mice by combined administration of a beta-adrenergic antagonist and a cyclooxygenase-2 inhibitor. J Immunol 184(5):2449–2457

98. Lee JW, Shahzad MM, Lin YG, Armaiz-Pena G, Mangala LS, Han HD et al (2009) Surgical stress promotes tumor growth in ovarian carcinoma. Clin Cancer Res 15(8):2695–2702

99. Hori Y, Ishii K, Kanda H, Iwamoto Y, Nishikawa K, Soga N et al (2011) Naftopidil, a selective {alpha}1-adrenoceptor antagonist, suppresses human prostate tumor growth by altering interactions between tumor cells and stroma. Cancer Prev Res 4(1):87–96

100. Calvani M, Pelon F, Comito G, Taddei ML, Moretti S, Innocenti S et al (2015) Norepinephrine promotes tumor microenvironment reactivity through β3-adrenoreceptors during melanoma progression. Oncotarget 6(7):4615–4632

101. Dal Monte M, Casini G, Filippi L, Nicchia GP, Svelto M, Bagnoli P (2013) Functional involvement of β3-adrenergic receptors in melanoma growth and vascularization. J Mol Med 91(12):1407–1419
102. Bruzzone A, Piñero CP, Rojas P, Romanato M, Gass H, Lanari C et al (2011) α(2)-Adrenoceptors enhance cell proliferation and mammary tumor growth acting through both the stroma and the tumor cells. Curr Cancer Drug Targets 11(6):763–774
103. Flint MS, Baum A, Episcopo B, Knickelbein KZ, Liegey Dougall AJ, Chambers WH et al (2013) Chronic exposure to stress hormones promotes transformation and tumorigenicity of 3T3 mouse fibroblasts. Stress 16(1):114–121
104. Cao R, Cao Y (2010) Cancer-associated retinopathy: a new mechanistic insight on vascular remodeling. Cell Cycle 9(10):1882–1885
105. Cao L, During MJ (2012) What is the brain-cancer connection? Annu Rev Neurosci 35:331–345
106. Hanoun M, Zhang D, Mizoguchi T, Pinho S, Pierce H, Kunisaki Y et al (2014) Acute myelogenous leukemia-induced sympathetic neuropathy promotes malignancy in an altered hematopoietic stem cell niche. Cell Stem Cell 15(3):365–375
107. Palm D, Lang K, Niggemann B, Drell TL, Masur K, Zaenker KS et al (2006) The norepinephrine-driven metastasis development of PC-3 human prostate cancer cells in BALB/c nude mice is inhibited by beta-blockers. Int J Cancer 118(11):2744–2749
108. Armaiz-Pena GN, Allen JK, Cruz A, Stone RL, Nick AM, Lin YG et al (2013) Src activation by β-adrenoreceptors is a key switch for tumour metastasis. Nat Commun 4:1403
109. Lang K, Drell TL, Lindecke A, Niggemann B, Kaltschmidt C, Zaenker KS et al (2004) Induction of a metastatogenic tumor cell type by neurotransmitters and its pharmacological inhibition by established drugs. Int J Cancer 112(2):231–238
110. Drell TL, Joseph J, Lang K, Niggemann B, Zaenker KS, Entschladen F (2003) Effects of neurotransmitters on the chemokinesis and chemotaxis of MDA-MB-468 human breast carcinoma cells. Breast Cancer Res Treat 80(1):63–70
111. Landen CN Jr, Lin YG, Armaiz Pena GN, Das PD, Arevalo JM, Kamat AA et al (2007) Neuroendocrine modulation of signal transducer and activator of transcription-3 in ovarian cancer. Cancer Res 67(21):10389–10396
112. Sood AK, Bhatty R, Kamat AA, Landen CN, Han L, Thaker PH et al (2006) Stress hormone-mediated invasion of ovarian cancer cells. Clin Cancer Res 12(2):369–375
113. Yang EV, Sood AK, Chen M, Li Y, Eubank TD, Marsh CB et al (2006) Norepinephrine up-regulates the expression of vascular endothelial growth factor, matrix metalloproteinase (MMP)-2, and MMP-9 in nasopharyngeal carcinoma tumor cells. Cancer Res 66(21):10357–10364
114. Chakroborty D, Sarkar C, Basu B, Dasgupta PS, Basu S (2009) Catecholamines regulate tumor angiogenesis. Cancer Res 69(9):3727–3730
115. Yang EV, Kim SJ, Donovan EL, Chen M, Gross AC, Webster Marketon JI et al (2009) Norepinephrine upregulates VEGF, IL-8, and IL-6 expression in human melanoma tumor cell lines: implications for stress-related enhancement of tumor progression. Brain Behav Immun 23(2):267–275
116. Moretti S, Massi D, Farini V, Baroni G, Parri M, Innocenti S et al (2013) β-adrenoceptors are upregulated in human melanoma and their activation releases pro-tumorigenic cytokines and metalloproteases in melanoma cell lines. Lab Invest 93(3):279–290
117. Liu J, Deng GH, Zhang J, Wang Y, Xia XY, Luo XM et al (2015) The effect of chronic stress on anti-angiogenesis of sunitinib in colorectal cancer models. Psychoneuroendocrinology 52:130–142
118. Sastry KS, Karpova Y, Prokopovich S, Smith AJ, Essau B, Gersappe A et al (2007) Epinephrine protects cancer cells from apoptosis via activation of cAMP-dependent protein kinase and BAD phosphorylation. J Biol Chem 282(19):14094–14100
119. Deng GH, Liu J, Zhang J, Wang Y, Peng XC, Wei YQ et al (2014) Exogenous norepinephrine attenuates the efficacy of sunitinib in a mouse cancer model. J Exp Clin Cancer Res 33(1):21

120. Katayama Y, Battista M, Kao WM, Hidalgo A, Peired AJ, Thomas SA et al (2006) Signals from the sympathetic nervous system regulate hematopoietic stem cell egress from bone marrow. Cell 124(2):407–421
121. Méndez-Ferrer S, Lucas D, Battista M, Frenette PS (2008) Haematopoietic stem cell release is regulated by circadian oscillations. Nature 452(7186):442–447
122. Dar A, Schajnovitz A, Lapid K, Kalinkovich A, Itkin T, Ludin A et al (2011) Rapid mobilization of hematopoietic progenitors by AMD3100 and catecholamines is mediated by CXCR4-dependent SDF-1 release from bone marrow stromal cells. Leukemia 25(8): 1286–1296
123. Lucas D, Scheiermann C, Chow A, Kunisaki Y, Bruns I, Barrick C et al (2013) Chemotherapy-induced bone marrow nerve injury impairs hematopoietic regeneration. Nat Med 19(6): 695–703
124. Makwana M, Raivich G (2005) Molecular mechanisms in successful peripheral regeneration. FEBS J 272(11):2628–2638
125. Raju B, Haug SR, Ibrahim SO, Heyeraas KJ (2007) Sympathectomy decreases size and invasiveness of tongue cancer in rats. Neuroscience 149(3):715–725
126. Kamiya A, Hayama Y, Kato S, Shimomura A, Shimomura T, Irie K et al (2019) Genetic manipulation of autonomic nerve fiber innervation and activity and its effect on breast cancer progression. Nat Neurosci 22(8):1289–1305
127. Huang D, Su S, Cui X, Shen X, Zeng Y, Wu W et al (2014) Nerve fibers in breast cancer tissues indicate aggressive tumor progression. Medicine 93(27):e172
128. Stopczynski RE, Normolle DP, Hartman DJ, Ying H, DeBerry JJ, Bielefeldt K et al (2014) Neuroplastic changes occur early in the development of pancreatic ductal adenocarcinoma. Cancer Res 74(6):1718–1727
129. Berthoud HR, Neuhuber WL (2000) Functional and chemical anatomy of the afferent vagal system. Auton Neurosci 85(1–3):1–17
130. Polli-Lopes AC, Zucoloto S, de Queirós CF, da Silva Figueiredo LA, Garcia SB (2003) Myenteric denervation reduces the incidence of gastric tumors in rats. Cancer Lett 190(1): 45–50
131. Partecke LI, Käding A, Trung DN, Diedrich S, Sendler M, Weiss F et al (2017) Subdiaphragmatic vagotomy promotes tumor growth and reduces survival via TNFα in a murine pancreatic cancer model. Oncotarget 8(14):22501–22512
132. Renz BW, Tanaka T, Sunagawa M, Takahashi R, Jiang Z, Macchini M et al (2018) Cholinergic signaling via muscarinic receptors directly and indirectly suppresses pancreatic tumorigenesis and cancer stemness. Cancer Discov 8(11):1458–1473
133. Zhu Y, Herndon JM, Sojka DK, Kim KW, Knolhoff BL, Zuo C et al (2017) Tissue-resident macrophages in pancreatic ductal adenocarcinoma originate from embryonic hematopoiesis and promote tumor progression. Immunity 47(2):323–38.e6
134. Amit M, Takahashi H, Dragomir MP, Lindemann A, Gleber-Netto FO, Pickering CR et al (2020) Loss of p53 drives neuron reprogramming in head and neck cancer. Nature 578(7795): 449–454
135. Wrona D (2006) Neural-immune interactions: an integrative view of the bidirectional relationship between the brain and immune systems. J Neuroimmunol 172(1-2):38–58
136. Rosas-Ballina M, Olofsson PS, Ochani M, Valdés-Ferrer SI, Levine YA, Reardon C et al (2011) Acetylcholine-synthesizing T cells relay neural signals in a vagus nerve circuit. Science 334(6052):98–101
137. Wang H, Yu M, Ochani M, Amella CA, Tanovic M, Susarla S et al (2003) Nicotinic acetylcholine receptor alpha7 subunit is an essential regulator of inflammation. Nature 421(6921):384–388
138. Friedman JR, Richbart SD, Merritt JC, Brown KC, Nolan NA, Akers AT et al (2019) Acetylcholine signaling system in progression of lung cancers. Pharmacol Ther 194:222–254

139. Cox MA, Duncan GS, Lin GHY, Steinberg BE, Yu LX, Brenner D et al (2019) Choline acetyltransferase-expressing T cells are required to control chronic viral infection. Science 363(6427):639–644
140. Salmon H, Remark R, Gnjatic S, Merad M (2019) Host tissue determinants of tumour immunity. Nat Rev Cancer 19(4):215–227
141. Darvin P, Toor SM, Sasidharan Nair V, Elkord E (2018) Immune checkpoint inhibitors: recent progress and potential biomarkers. Exp Mol Med 50(12):1–11
142. Sharma P, Allison JP (2015) The future of immune checkpoint therapy. Science 348(6230): 56–61
143. Partecke LI, Speerforck S, Käding A, Seubert F, Kühn S, Lorenz E et al (2016) Chronic stress increases experimental pancreatic cancer growth, reduces survival and can be antagonised by beta-adrenergic receptor blockade. Pancreatology 16(3):423–433
144. He BP, Wang JJ, Zhang X, Wu Y, Wang M, Bay BH et al (2006) Differential reactions of microglia to brain metastasis of lung cancer. Mol Med 12(7–8):161–170
145. Guldner IH, Wang Q, Yang L, Golomb SM, Zhao Z, Lopez JA et al (2020) CNS-native myeloid cells drive immune suppression in the brain metastatic niche through Cxcl10. Cell 183(5):1234–48.e25
146. Qian BZ, Li J, Zhang H, Kitamura T, Zhang J, Campion LR et al (2011) CCL2 recruits inflammatory monocytes to facilitate breast-tumour metastasis. Nature 475(7355):222–225
147. Pyonteck SM, Akkari L, Schuhmacher AJ, Bowman RL, Sevenich L, Quail DF et al (2013) CSF-1R inhibition alters macrophage polarization and blocks glioma progression. Nat Med 19(10):1264–1272
148. Blazquez R, Wlochowitz D, Wolff A, Seitz S, Wachter A, Perera-Bel J et al (2018) PI3K: A master regulator of brain metastasis-promoting macrophages/microglia. Glia 66(11): 2438–2455
149. You H, Baluszek S, Kaminska B (2019) Immune microenvironment of brain metastases-are microglia and other brain macrophages little helpers? Front Immunol 10:1941
150. Richard L, Topilko P, Magy L, Decouvelaere AV, Charnay P, Funalot B et al (2012) Endoneurial fibroblast-like cells. J Neuropathol Exp Neurol 71(11):938–947
151. Heaney AP, Melmed S (2004) Molecular targets in pituitary tumours. Nat Rev Cancer 4(4): 285–295
152. Lacroix A, Feelders RA, Stratakis CA, Nieman LK (2015) Cushing's syndrome. Lancet 386(9996):913–927
153. Gazdar AF, Bunn PA, Minna JD (2017) Small-cell lung cancer: what we know, what we need to know and the path forward. Nat Rev Cancer 17(12):725–737
154. Titulaer MJ, Lang B, Verschuuren JJ (2011) Lambert-Eaton myasthenic syndrome: from clinical characteristics to therapeutic strategies. Lancet Neurol 10(12):1098–1107
155. Shi M, Liu D, Yang Z, Guo N (2013) Central and peripheral nervous systems: master controllers in cancer metastasis. Cancer Metastasis Rev 32(3-4):603–621
156. Cole SW, Nagaraja AS, Lutgendorf SK, Green PA, Sood AK (2015) Sympathetic nervous system regulation of the tumour microenvironment. Nat Rev Cancer 15(9):563–572
157. Colon-Echevarria CB, Lamboy-Caraballo R, Aquino-Acevedo AN, Armaiz-Pena GN (2019) Neuroendocrine regulation of tumor-associated immune cells. Front Oncol 9:1077
158. Shin KJ, Lee YJ, Yang YR, Park S, Suh PG, Follo MY et al (2016) Molecular mechanisms underlying psychological stress and cancer. Curr Pharm Des 22(16):2389–2402
159. Holden RJ, Pakula IS, Mooney PA (1998) An immunological model connecting the patho-genesis of stress, depression and carcinoma. Med Hypotheses 51(4):309–314
160. Reiche EM, Nunes SO, Morimoto HK (2004) Stress, depression, the immune system, and cancer. Lancet Oncol 5(10):617–625
161. Bründl J, Schneider S, Weber F, Zeman F, Wieland WF, Ganzer R (2014) Computerized quantification and planimetry of prostatic capsular nerves in relation to adjacent prostate cancer foci. Eur Urol 65(4):802–808

162. Olar A, He D, Florentin D, Ding Y, Ayala G (2014) Biologic correlates and significance of axonogenesis in prostate cancer. Hum Pathol 45(7):1358–1364
163. Park H, Poo MM (2013) Neurotrophin regulation of neural circuit development and function. Nat Rev Neurosci 14(1):7–23
164. Ding Y, He D, Florentin D, Frolov A, Hilsenbeck S, Ittmann M et al (2013) Semaphorin 4F as a critical regulator of neuroepithelial interactions and a biomarker of aggressive prostate cancer. Clin Cancer Res 19(22):6101–6111
165. Biankin AV, Waddell N, Kassahn KS, Gingras MC, Muthuswamy LB, Johns AL et al (2012) Pancreatic cancer genomes reveal aberrations in axon guidance pathway genes. Nature 491(7424):399–405
166. Pinho AV, Van Bulck M, Chantrill L, Arshi M, Sklyarova T, Herrmann D et al (2018) ROBO2 is a stroma suppressor gene in the pancreas and acts via TGF-β signalling. Nat Commun 9(1): 5083
167. Pundavela J, Demont Y, Jobling P, Lincz LF, Roselli S, Thorne RF et al (2014) ProNGF correlates with Gleason score and is a potential driver of nerve infiltration in prostate cancer. Am J Pathol 184(12):3156–3162
168. Dobrenis K, Gauthier LR, Barroca V, Magnon C (2015) Granulocyte colony-stimulating factor off-target effect on nerve outgrowth promotes prostate cancer development. Int J Cancer 136(4):982–988
169. Bressy C, Lac S, Nigri J, Leca J, Roques J, Lavaut MN et al (2018) LIF drives neural remodeling in pancreatic cancer and offers a new candidate biomarker. Cancer Res 78(4): 909–921
170. Pundavela J, Roselli S, Faulkner S, Attia J, Scott RJ, Thorne RF et al (2015) Nerve fibers infiltrate the tumor microenvironment and are associated with nerve growth factor production and lymph node invasion in breast cancer. Mol Oncol 9(8):1626–1635
171. Albo D, Akay CL, Marshall CL, Wilks JA, Verstovsek G, Liu H et al (2011) Neurogenesis in colorectal cancer is a marker of aggressive tumor behavior and poor outcomes. Cancer 117(21):4834–4845
172. Liebl F, Demir IE, Rosenberg R, Boldis A, Yildiz E, Kujundzic K et al (2013) The severity of neural invasion is associated with shortened survival in colon cancer. Clin Cancer Res 19(1): 50–61

Chapter 24
Systemic *Onco-Sphere*: Host Metabolic System and Cancer

Phei Er Saw and Erwei Song

Abstract It is well established that patients with altered metabolism manifesting as obesity, metabolic syndrome and chronic inflammation have an increased incidence of cancer; indicating a crucial relationship between host metabolic system and cancer growth. However, the impact of the systemic metabolic system in the host on the local onco-sphere has not been deeply studied especially on how the host dysregulated metabolism could affect the drug absorption and excertion to have significant effect on tumor has not been studied in detail. Interestingly, more research is now supporting the idea that metabolic states and disorders linked to obesity affect not only the number of people who get cancer but also how well they respond to treatments like radiation and chemotherapy. Therefore, in this chapter, we discuss on the host metabolic diseases and how these changes therapeutic efficacy of cancer-related drugs, and the underlying mechanism which might be responsible to this phenomenon. This chapter details the importance of host metabolic changes in cancer progression.

P. E. Saw
Guangdong Provincial Key Laboratory of Malignant Tumor Epigenetics and Gene Regulation, Guangdong-Hong Kong Joint Laboratory for RNA Medicine, Medical Research Center, Sun Yat-sen Memorial Hospital, Sun Yat-sen University, Guangzhou, China

Nanhai Translational Innovation Center of Precision Immunology, Sun Yat-sen Memorial Hospital, Sun Yat-sen University, Foshan, China

E. Song (✉)
Guangdong Provincial Key Laboratory of Malignant Tumor Epigenetics and Gene Regulation, Guangdong-Hong Kong Joint Laboratory for RNA Medicine, Medical Research Center, Sun Yat-sen Memorial Hospital, Sun Yat-sen University, Guangzhou, China

Nanhai Translational Innovation Center of Precision Immunology, Sun Yat-sen Memorial Hospital, Sun Yat-sen University, Foshan, China

Breast Tumor Center, Sun Yat-sen Memorial Hospital, Sun Yat-sen University, Guangzhou, China
e-mail: songew@mail.sysu.edu.cn

Introduction

Warburg highlighted on the fact that there is a undisputable link between host metabolic system and tumor cells [1]. Since then, most researches are done on how cancer cells manipulate or regulate their environment to sustain their own metabolic changes. In recent years, as economic growth in many developed countries has led to diet changes, major illnesses especially obesity have increased by leaps and bounds. Obesity and obesity-related death (due to high blood pressure, stroke, heart disease, and type II diabetes) are currently at four million, and it is still increasing each year. Cardiovascular disease (due to high blood pressure and metabolic-related diseases) is ranked the number one killer in the world [2]. However, the impact of the systemic metabolic system in the host on the local *onco-sphere* has not been deeply studied especially on how the host dysregulated metabolism could affect the drug ADME to have significant effect on tumor has not been studied in detail [3]. Interestingly, more research is now supporting the idea that metabolic states and disorders linked to obesity affect not only the number of people who get cancer but also how well they respond to treatments like radiation and chemotherapy. Therefore, in this chapter, we discuss on the host metabolic diseases and how this changes therapeutic efficacy of cancer-related drugs, and the underlying mechanism which might be responsible to this phenomenon. This chapter details the importance of host metabolic changes in cancer progression.

In many large-scale epidemiological study, metabolic syndrome affects a large number of population. In the USA alone, 47 million are diagnosed with metabolic syndrome [4]. Recently, many interesting laboratory studies have been published that show a link between the different types of diseases stemming out of metabolic syndrome or metabolic dysfunction and the risk of getting cancer. In some large cohort epidemiological research, studies had been done specifically designed to determine the link between metabolic syndrome and cancer. For example, in gender-specific studies, men with inherent metabolic disease were found to have a higher risk of pancreatic cancer, while in women, metabolic diseases increase the risk of colorectal cancer [5]. Herein, we summarized major metabolic diseases and how these host metabolic dysregulation could affect cancer progression and ultimately cancer therapy (Fig. 24.1).

Metabolic Syndrome and Cancer Occurrence

Obesity and Cancer

Epidemiological research shows that being overweight makes you more likely to be susceptible to almost all cancers [6–11]. In women, these data are true with the addition of breast cancer, ovarian cancer, and endometrial cancer [12, 13]. Being obese means having a large body mass index (BMI), and BMI has been found to be

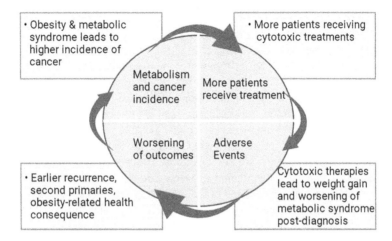

Fig. 24.1 Positive feedback mechanism loop of metabolic diseases and obesity toward cancer incidence. In this positive loop feedback mechanism, patients who receive anti-cancer treatment could present adverse events, which include weight gain and worsening of their inherent metabolic syndrome. This leads to worsening of outcomes, which, again, rises the occurrence of obesity-related health problems, which gives rise to cancer incidence

linked to a higher risk of cancer [14, 15]. In UK, large cohort study in women, it has been proven that a higher BMI leads to higher risk of endometrial cancer, esophageal adenocarcinoma, kidney cancer, leukemia, and multiple myeloma. In the same study, the multivariance analysis of BMI and menopause were also examined. Interestingly, women before menopause had a higher risk of colon cancer and malignant melanoma, while women after menopause had a higher risk of breast cancer and endometrial cancers [16]. Even though we do not fully understand the molecular processes and pathophysiology involved, insulin resistance seems to be the most likely key factor. Chronic insulin rise is linked to having more IGF-I. Oxidative stress is another factor that is linked to obesity, and cancer has been known to have high ROS. ROS has been found to be especially important for kidney cancer in obese population [17].

Insulin Resistance and Cancer

A study found that patients with higher level of blood glucose and insulin have a higher risk of adenoma recurrence [18] Since IGF-1Rs are overexpressed in many human cancers, it is thought that insulin may affect cancer cell growth *in vivo* through IGF-1 stimulation. IGF-1 is a growth hormone produced by the liver. Insulin can communicate with the liver to synthesize more IGF-1 by increasing the amount of IGF-1R. Hyperinsulinemia can also make IGF-1 more bioavailable by lowering the amount of IGF-binding protein (IGFBP)-1 made by the liver. IGF-1 helps cells grow and divide and prevent cell death. IGF-1 also increases the production of VEGF to include and promote angiogenesis in breast and colon cancer cell lines.

Mechanistically, when IGF-R is activated, both the PI3K/AKT and p21ras/MAPK pathways are also activated. Both pathways are crucial for cell growth and cell survival [19, 20]. In a crosstalk mechanism, IGF-1 could also halt the production of sex hormone-binding globulin (SHBG), which the latter is responsible to bind to sex hormone. When the SHBG is decreased, the concentration of free sex hormones would also increase, leading to the increment of hormone-based cancers (*i.e.,* breast cancers, endometrial cancers, prostate cancers) [21]. In a recent study, castration therapies used for prostate cancer could be the reason for increasing hyperinsulinemia, which raises concerns about the risk of cancer recurrence [22]. Many population-based studies on humans link insulin resistance or high insulin levels and different epithelial cancers. Initial studies on prostate cancer showed a link between IGF-1 levels in the blood and the disease [23]. Since then, many studies have confirmed that high levels of IGF-1 and insulin are linked to an increased risk of getting prostate cancer [24–26].

Hyperglycemia and Cancer

Malignancies have been linked to hyperglycemia in recent years. In a study in the USA, after considering age, BMI, serum cholesterol, systolic blood pressure, and treatment for high blood pressure, hyperglycemia was linked to death from cancer in men but not in women [27]. Since then, several studies have shown that the same results are true for both men and women [28, 29]. The fact that hyperglycemia is the main feature of diabetes, there could be an association between hyperglycemia and diabetic cancer patients. Mechanistically, hyperglycemia can activate multiple pathways due to lack of nutrient or starvation of cancer cells, leading to a malignant phenotype of cancers [30]. Two studies have found a version (allele) of a mutation in the HNF1B gene which is responsible for type II diabetes susceptibility. Moreover, the risk of colorectal cancer is increased with people with type II diabetes, regardless of gender [31, 32]. The hyperinsulinemia hypothesis says that high levels of insulin and free IGF-1 in the blood stimulate the growth of colon cells and help colon cancer cells survive after they have changed [33, 34].

Dyslipidemia and Cancer

Dysregulation of lipid metabolism or dyslipidemia has been linked to many cancer risks. In the USA, a prospective study looked at the link between baseline plasma high-density lipoprotein cholesterol (HDL-C) levels and the rate of lung cancer. Low level of HDL was calculated to be an independent risk ratio for lung cancer [35]. Low HDL levels (≤ 20 mg/dL) are linked to a higher risk of cancer [36], while low levels of serum low-density lipoprotein cholesterol (LDL-C) (≤ 70 mg/dL) are linked to a 15-fold higher risk of hematological malignancy [37]. Multiple studies have linked high TG levels to increased postmenopausal breast and prostate cancer risk [38, 39].

Molecular Changes in Host during Metabolic Dysregulation

Transcription Factors

One of the most important transcription factors involved in metabolism is the peroxisome proliferator-activated receptors (PPARs) family. PPAR TFs are turned on by ligands and are part of the superfamily of nuclear hormone receptors. There are three subtypes of PPARs: PPARα, PPARδ (also called PPARβ), and PPARγ. The sequences of each subtype are very similar across different species. Metabolic disorders are linked to PPARs, which make them interesting drug targets [40–42]. PPARα is mostly found in the liver, functions to break down fatty acids, and lowers the TG concentration in blood; therefore, it is an effective drug for dyslipidemia. PPARδ is found everywhere and is involved in the oxidation of fatty acids and the differentiation of keratinocytes. PPARδ agonists could be used to make drugs that treat obesity, heart disease, and diabetes. PPARγ is involved in glucose metabolism by making insulin more sensitive and therefore could be a therapeutic target for people with type II diabetes. One of the subset, PPARγ2, is only found in adipose tissue, and it is an important part of how adipocytes develop. Therefore, PPARs are molecular targets that can be used to make drugs that treat metabolic syndrome. PPARs also help control the growth of cancer cells. Many studies have shown that PPARγ activation is an antitumorigenic and prodifferentiation factor [41]. There are clues pointing toward the collaboration between the nuclear receptor PPAR works with transcriptional factors to change how cytokines are made and how they work in immune systems, inflammation, autoimmune diseases, and tumors. PPARs are responsible to orchestrate multiple changes in the gene expression in cancer cells and immune cells, induces different cytokines and their receptors, to create an active network of cytokine-mediated signaling pathways, and enhances tumor growth.

Cyclooxygenase-2 (COX-2) and Prostaglandins

Cyclooxygenase-2 (COX-2), a subtype of the cyclooxygenase family, has long been considered a target for pain relief and treatment of inflammation [43, 44]. COX-2 has been shown to be overexpressed in a variety of cancers and plays a crucial role in promoting cancer cell proliferation, angiogenesis, invasion, and metastasis [45]. Multiple signals contribute to the regulation of cancer cell function via COX-2. Meanwhile, COX2-centered-related pathways play a key role in tumor cell metabolism. COX-2 catalyzes metabolic pathway involving the transformation of arachidonic acid to PGE2 (an important active product and bioactive lipid of COX-2), which promotes the growth and survival of tumor cells [46, 47]. COX2/ PGE2 axis is one of the important pathways in cancer metabolism and development. A recent study had shown that COX-2/PGE2 pathway might promote tumor escape in colorectal adenomas [48]. In addition, studies have shown that COX1/2-PGE2 facilitates tumorigenesis by disrupting the malate-aspartate shuttle system through activation of the cAMP-PKA pathway, leading to a reduction in multiple enzymes and intermediate metabolites as well as growth arrest of CD8+ T cells [49].

Adiponectin

Adiponectin, a 244-amino acid, an adipokine protein, and a hormone, is known to affect several metabolic processes. Adiponectin is secreted by adipocytes [50], and it is mostly known for its anti-inflammatory effect. Adiponectin is also an insulin sensitizer, which entails glucose-level regulation, apart from being able to moderate lipid metabolism. All these metabolic processes are mediated by AdipoR1 and AdipoR2 [51]. In a recent study, host physiological changes, such as weight loss, lead to an increment in adiponectin, which in turn leads to an increased insulin sensitivity [51]. Since adiponectin is favoring host health, it is not surprising that adiponectin levels are lower in obese people or those with type II diabetes. In a clinical study involving women, a strong negative link was found between obesity and adiponectin levels, in all range of age, regardless of menopause or estradiol level [52]. It was found that adiponectin acts on preneoplastic colon ECs to control cell growth through two different pathways, which was undocumented. The first one is through leptin-induced NF-κB-dependent autocrine IL-6 production; or two, through trans-IL-6 signaling [53]. Adiponectin levels can induce the increment of 17β-estradiol, causing breast cancer cell growth, and therefore have been linked to breast cancer in several epidemiological studies [54]. Epidemiological studies show that the amount of adiponectin in the blood is inversely related to the number of cases of endometrial carcinoma. A recent study examined the direct effects of adiponectin on endometrial cancer cell lines. Both types of cells stopped growing when they were treated with adiponectin. This was thought to be mostly because the number of cells in the G1/G0 phase grew and because apoptosis was triggered [55]. Plasma levels of adiponectin were much lower in 30 men with prostate cancer than in 41 men with benign prostatic hyperplasia and 36 healthy people who served as controls. Also, the levels of adiponectin were inversely related to the size of the tumor and the stage of the disease [56]. All the above studies indicated on the importance of adiponectin as a metabolic regulator, to regulate host metabolic system to influence cancer growth.

Proinflammatory Cytokines

Adipocytes release cytokines that cause inflammation, such as TNF-α, IL-6, IL-8, IL-10, macrophage inflammatory protein 1 (MIP-1), and monocyte chemoattractant protein-1 (MCP-1). It is known that these cytokines, which are released by adipocytes, make insulin resistance worse and increase circulating TG. Both of these are signs of metabolic syndrome. Cancers of the stomach, pancreas, esophagus, liver, bladder, and colon have also been linked to inflammation [3]. This is because inflammation affects how tumor and stromal cells grow, die, and multiply. Increased cytokines in the blood from adipocytes help cancer spread by causing inflammation and ROS to form. Multiple myeloma (MM) cells require IL-6 to grow and to avoid cell death. It is also involved in the growth of both healthy and cancerous plasma cells and MM cell resistance [4]. In hepatocellular carcinoma, for example, tumor-derived cytokines (*i.e.,* interleukins, including IL-6, 1L-15, and TNF-α) are crucial for cancer development. In lung adenocarcinoma, there is a signature of eleven cytokines that could be used to predict lymph node metastasis and cancer prognosis. IL-8 and TNF-α especially were the key cytokines for predicting cancer prognosis. IL-8 can act as a positive autocrine GF that could stimulate angiogenesis and encouraging the formation of new blood vessels in the tumor, resulting in enhanced tumor growth. In skin cancer and lymphoma, when stimulated with a chemical carcinogen, IL-6 and TNF-α expression was elevated, leading to a proinflammatory environment, also favoring tumor growth. In hormonal-dependent cancer, such as breast cancer and endometrial cancers, there could be a positive feedback looks between inflammatory factors (secreted by tumor, stromal, or infiltrated immune cells) and estrogen, which could trigger ER+-mediated pathways that could help breast cancer growth and metastasis [57]. In turn, tumor-derived cytokines can also increase the the aromatase expression and the hormone activity (especially 17-β-hydroxysteroid dehydrogenase activity) in breast tissue, leading to an increment of E2 synthesis by the host [57]. Proinflammatory cytokines like TNF-α or IL-1β also turn up the level of prostaglandin E synthase (PTGES), which is also a crucial factor for cancer growth (mentioned in the previous paragraph) (Fig. 24.2).

Inter-*Onco-Spherical* Crosstalk: Metabolic Alterations and Host Inflammation

Chronic inflammation is linked to both the growth of cancer and the development of diseases linked to obesity. More epidemiological research has shown that tumor cells often use chronic inflammatory mediators to support malignant traits like cell growth and spreading to other parts of the body [58]. For a long time, it has been known that adipose tissue has a lot of autocrine, paracrine, and endocrine proteins called adipokines. These proteins work with proinflammatory cytokines to cause chronic inflammation throughout the body. Inflammation caused by obesity seems to have a wide range of effects on tumor growth, immune responses against tumors, and may be even the effectiveness of immunotherapy [59–61]. Detailed summary of host inflammatory system and cancer has been described in Chapter 21.

The adipose tissues in immune environment vary significantly in comparing non-obese and obese people, also in terms of how cytokines are expressed and their behavior. The most obvious examples of this are the expression of monocytes

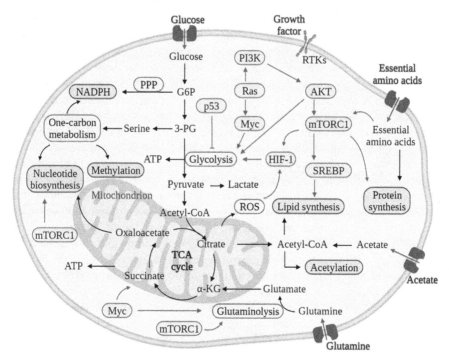

Fig. 24.2 Overview of normal metabolic pathways in a cell. A dysfunction in one or many of these pathways would lead to metabolic syndrome which ultimately leads to cancer

and macrophages in adipose tissue. In non-obese people, these cells are mostly consisting of the regulatory M2 phenotype. In obese people, they are more likely to be of the M1 phenotype, which is marked by the production of proinflammatory cytokines like TNFα, IL-6, and IL-1β, and MCP-1 and macrophage inhibitory factor. Interestingly, the overexpression of PAMPS/DAMPS can also activate Toll-like receptors (TLRs) may then push these macrophages toward the M1 phenotype [62]. TLR activation turns on NF-κB signaling, which speeds up the production and release of proinflammatory cytokines [63–66]. The inflammatory adipose tissues of obese people affect the whole body and can affect immune homeostasis in distant places, such as in malignant tumors. People who are overweight, for example, have more cytokines in their blood, such as IL-6 and TNFα [67]. In immune cells and tumor cells, IL-6 encourages STAT3 signaling, pushing myeloid cell differentiation toward immunosuppressive phenotypes [68, 69]. People who eat fewer calories and work out regularly have lower levels of IL-6 and TNF-α in their blood and lower activity of tumor-promoting transcription factors like activator protein (AP)-1, STAT3, and NF-κB [70–73]. As mentioned in previous chapters, extracellular vesicles (EVs) are being studied as a way for cell–cell communication that affects host inflammation, insulin sensitivity, and lipid metabolism. These EVs carry proteins, lipids, and nucleic acids like mRNAs, tRNAs, and miRNAs to many parts of the body as a way of communication [74, 75]. Obesity has been linked to more extracellular vesicles circulating in the blood [76, 77]. This mimics the development of monocytes into active macrophages and causes the release of proinflammatory cytokines like IL-1 and TNF-α [78].

Obesity changes immunological homeostasis in many ways, including the spatiotemporal arrangement of immune cell populations in both tumor tissues and circulation system. Researchers have found that obese people have more MDSCs in their peripheral blood [79]. MDSCs have been linked to suppressing antitumor immune responses in cancer patients in several ways, such as by stopping the growth and function of tumor-infiltrating T cells, bringing in Tregs, and stopping NK cells from doing their job [80]. It has been shown that pathologically high levels of obesity-induced leptin and IL-6 are able to regulate NK cells and reducing their toxicity, making them lesser a threat to cancer cells [81]. When mice were obese and had tumors, there were more circulating DCs [82] and intratumoral MDSCs [83]. This has been linked to less effective immunotherapy responses [84]. Other types of regulatory immune cells, like Th1, Th17, and Treg lymphocytes, are also increased in the adipose tissue of obese people [85–87]. Not only that these key molecules also secrete soluble factors that could be having autocrine or paracrine effect on surrounding tumor tissues, leading to procancerous environment (Fig. 24.3). These results support the idea that having too much adipose tissue has systemic effects on both the innate and adaptive immune systems, making it harder for the immune system to fight cancer.

Altered Metabolism and Cancer Outcomes

Only in the USA, 85,000 cases of cancer are caused by being overweight every year, and this number is expected to rise to 500,000 cases by 2030 [88]. The number of people who get cancer because they are overweight has also gone up a lot in the UK. This rise in cancers linked to obesity is happening simultaneously with an estimated 20% increase in total cancer deaths [89], and this is true for many cancers [90, 91]. More information shows that people who get metabolic disorders during and after cancer treatment are also more likely to be overweight [92, 93]. Many people gain weight after being told they have cancer, especially in the first year of diagnosis. An increase of 10–20 pounds is common, and these weight gains are linked to disease progression. In a study with 5204 women who had invasive breast cancer that had not spread, the effect of gaining weight after a diagnosis was looked at. A higher BMI during treatment was linked to more deaths from breast cancer, recurrences far away, and deaths from all causes [94]. A randomized, multi-institutional, phase III clinical trial of breast cancer patients found that reducing lipid intake was linked to a big improvement in relapse-free survival [95, 96]. It is not clear what makes people gain weight after being told they have cancer, but it seems to be a combination of things. People may do less physical activity and eat more food to help them deal with their diagnosis [97–99]. Also, cancer treatment has

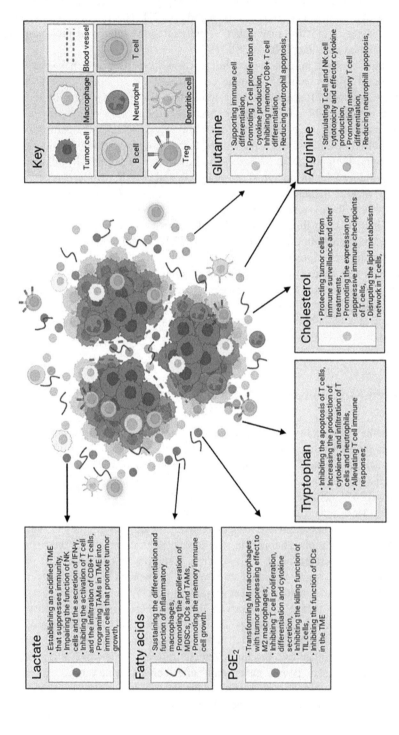

Fig. 24.3 Detailed understanding of each molecular mechanism and their importance in the offset of metabolic syndrome, which ultimately leads to cancer. All important molecules important in metabolic regulation of a tumor is presented in each box

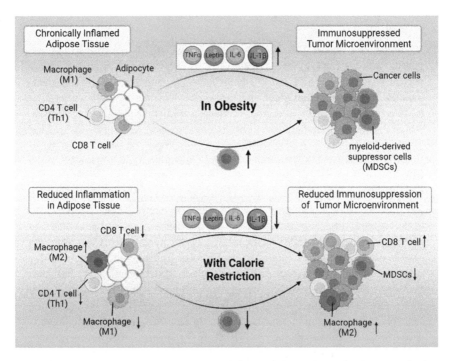

Fig. 24.4 Schematic analysis of how calorie restriction could be used as a stimulatory mechanism against cancer growth and progression. Calorie restriction leads to the reduction of inflammation in adipose tissue, which leads to a decrease in TNF-α, leptin, IL-6, and IL-1β. This will in turn activate anti-tumoral CD8 T cells, reducing MDSCs, and increase the M2 phenotype of macrophages

a bad effect on the patient's metabolism, making them gain weight. For example, people often take a dose of steroids before chemotherapy. Even in small amounts, there seems to be a link between using steroids as part of a treatment plan and gaining weight [100, 101]. As mentioned briefly above, anti-estrogen drugs used to treat breast cancer and androgen deprivation therapy used to treat prostate cancer have been shown to change a patient's metabolism, causing weight gain, that could lead to the development of metabolic syndrome [102–104]. This is a negative feedback mechanism loop where metabolic problems help cancer cells stay alive and grow, making it harder for treatment to work. Together, these discoveries show how important it is to find breakthroughs to solve host's inherent metabolic problems before and during cancer treatment (Fig. 24.4).

Box 24.1 Altered Metabolism Influences Radiotherapy Outcome
People who are overweight or obese have worse treatment outcomes than non-obese people. This could be partly since obese patients could have difficulties in navigating therapeutic equipment that are generally designed

(continued)

Box 24.1 (continued)

for non-obese people [105]. However, this link still holds true for people getting normal care. In obese patients, it is worth noting that due to the patient's size, it could be hard to control, set up, and repeat radiation treatments to the prostate and other high-risk areas. However, people with a high BMI who had prostate cancer were treated with brachytherapy, a technic which allows accurate radiation to be sent to the organ without being affected by body size [106]. Across different cancers, both obesity and diabetes increase the risk of side effects during and after radiotherapy. If a breast cancer patient with a ≥ 30 kg/m^2 BMI receives radiation therapy, they would have a higher chance of developing adverse effects, most notably lymphedema [107]. Also, obese male patients are more likely to have adverse effects related to pelvic symptoms after radiation for prostate cancer, such as rectal bleeding and frequent urination [108]. In the same way, the average BMI was linked to higher-grade gynecologic and skin side effects from radiation treatment for endometrial cancer in women [109]. Not only that, stereotactic body radiation therapy (SBRT), a specialized therapy for pulmonary tumors (especially for tumor that resides only about 2.5 cm from chest wall), BMI seems to be the best predictor of pain a post-treatment. In another similar study, results revealed that overweight patients (BMI > 29) have double probability of having the risk chronic chest wall pain [110]. In another interesting study, changes in the white matter after whole brain irradiation for brain metastases show that people with poor blood sugar control had more cognitive and functional decline [111]. All the results above indicated that specialized patients (such as patients with metabolic diseases, overweight, or obese patients) should be treated with care and practitioners should be able to come out with a modification on therapeutic regime that these patients could benefit from.

Conclusion

Since obesity is a global problem, we need to pay more attention to how the metabolic state of the host affects cancer risk, treatment outcomes, and the way tumors grow. Combining the pleiotropic effects of metabolically targeted interventions with modern cancer treatments may be possible to control the growth of tumors better locally, reduce damage to healthy tissue, and improve patient outcomes. Due to the fast growth of immunotherapy, these efforts are likely to focus a lot on the effects of metabolic dysregulation on antitumor immune responses. It is hoped that these studies will show how useful current dietary approaches are before and during cancer treatment and show if pharmacological modifiers of metabolism can help even more. Using unique factors for both the host and the tumor is an exciting way to improve cancer treatments.

References

1. Warburg O, Wind F, Negelein E (1927) The metabolism of tumors in the body. J Gen Physiol 8(6):519–530
2. Afshin A, Forouzanfar MH, Reitsma MB, Sur P, Estep K, Lee A et al (2017) Health effects of overweight and obesity in 195 countries over 25 years. N Engl J Med 377(1):13–27
3. Wright CM, Shastri AA, Bongiorno E, Palagani A, Rodeck U, Simone NL (2020) Is host metabolism the missing link to improving cancer outcomes? Cancer 12(9):2338
4. Pothiwala P, Jain SK, Yaturu S (2009) Metabolic syndrome and cancer. Metab Syndr Relat Disord 7(4):279–288
5. Russo A, Autelitano M, Bisanti L (2008) Metabolic syndrome and cancer risk. Eur J Cancer 44(2):293–297
6. Larsson SC, Wolk A (2007) Obesity and colon and rectal cancer risk: a meta-analysis of prospective studies. Am J Clin Nutr 86(3):556–565
7. Larsson SC, Wolk A (2007) Overweight, obesity and risk of liver cancer: a meta-analysis of cohort studies. Br J Cancer 97(7):1005–1008
8. Larsson SC, Wolk A (2007) Body mass index and risk of multiple myeloma: a meta-analysis. Int J Cancer 121(11):2512–2516
9. Larsson SC, Wolk A (2007) Obesity and the risk of gallbladder cancer: a meta-analysis. Br J Cancer 96(9):1457–1461
10. Larsson SC, Orsini N, Wolk A (2007) Body mass index and pancreatic cancer risk: a meta-analysis of prospective studies. Int J Cancer 120(9):1993–1998
11. Larsson SC, Wolk A (2008) Overweight and obesity and incidence of leukemia: a meta-analysis of cohort studies. Int J Cancer 122(6):1418–1421
12. Olsen CM, Nagle CM, Whiteman DC, Purdie DM, Green AC, Webb PM (2008) Body size and risk of epithelial ovarian and related cancers: a population-based case-control study. Int J Cancer 123(2):450–456
13. Jensen A, Sharif H, Olsen JH, Kjaer SK (2008) Risk of breast cancer and gynecologic cancers in a large population of nearly 50,000 infertile Danish women. Am J Epidemiol 168(1):49–57
14. McCourt CK, Mutch DG, Gibb RK, Rader JS, Goodfellow PJ, Trinkaus K et al (2007) Body mass index: relationship to clinical, pathologic and features of microsatellite instability in endometrial cancer. Gynecol Oncol 104(3):535–539
15. Patel AV, Feigelson HS, Talbot JT, McCullough ML, Rodriguez C, Patel RC et al (2008) The role of body weight in the relationship between physical activity and endometrial cancer: results from a large cohort of US women. Int J Cancer 123(8):1877–1882
16. Reeves GK, Pirie K, Beral V, Green J, Spencer E, Bull D (2007) Cancer incidence and mortality in relation to body mass index in the Million Women Study: cohort study. BMJ 335(7630):1134
17. Gago-Dominguez M, Castelao JE, Yuan JM, Ross RK, Yu MC (2002) Lipid peroxidation: a novel and unifying concept of the etiology of renal cell carcinoma (United States). Cancer Causes Control 13(3):287–293
18. Flood A, Mai V, Pfeiffer R, Kahle L, Remaley AT, Lanza E et al (2007) Elevated serum concentrations of insulin and glucose increase risk of recurrent colorectal adenomas. Gastroenterology 133(5):1423–1429
19. Hoeben A, Landuyt B, Highley MS, Wildiers H, Van Oosterom AT, De Bruijn EA (2004) Vascular endothelial growth factor and angiogenesis. Pharmacol Rev 56(4):549–580
20. Ibrahim YH, Yee D (2004) Insulin-like growth factor-I and cancer risk. Growth Horm IGF Res 14(4):261–269
21. Calle EE, Kaaks R (2004) Overweight, obesity and cancer: epidemiological evidence and proposed mechanisms. Nat Rev Cancer 4(8):579–591
22. Smith MR, Lee H, Nathan DM (2006) Insulin sensitivity during combined androgen blockade for prostate cancer. J Clin Endocrinol Metab 91(4):1305–1308

23. Chan JM, Stampfer MJ, Giovannucci E, Gann PH, Ma J, Wilkinson P et al (1998) Plasma insulin-like growth factor-I and prostate cancer risk: a prospective study. Science 279(5350): 563–566
24. Giovannucci E, Rimm EB, Liu Y, Willett WC (2004) Height, predictors of C-peptide and cancer risk in men. Int J Epidemiol 33(1):217–225
25. Harman SM, Metter EJ, Blackman MR, Landis PK, Carter HB (2000) Serum levels of insulin-like growth factor I (IGF-I), IGF-II, IGF-binding protein-3, and prostate-specific antigen as predictors of clinical prostate cancer. J Clin Endocrinol Metab 85(11):4258–4265
26. Kaaks R, Lukanova A, Rinaldi S, Biessy C, Söderberg S, Olsson T et al (2003) Interrelationships between plasma testosterone, SHBG, IGF-I, insulin and leptin in prostate cancer cases and controls. Eur J Cancer Prev 12(4):309–315
27. Levine W, Dyer AR, Shekelle RB, Schoenberger JA, Stamler J (1990) Post-load plasma glucose and cancer mortality in middle-aged men and women. 12-year follow-up findings of the Chicago Heart Association Detection Project in Industry. Am J Epidemiol 131(2):254–262
28. Jee SH, Ohrr H, Sull JW, Yun JE, Ji M, Samet JM (2005) Fasting serum glucose level and cancer risk in Korean men and women. JAMA 293(2):194–202
29. Rapp K, Schroeder J, Klenk J, Ulmer H, Concin H, Diem G et al (2006) Fasting blood glucose and cancer risk in a cohort of more than 140,000 adults in Austria. Diabetologia 49(5): 945–952
30. Duan W, Shen X, Lei J, Xu Q, Yu Y, Li R et al (2014) Hyperglycemia, a neglected factor during cancer progression. Biomed Res Int 2014:461917
31. Berster JM, Göke B (2008) Type 2 diabetes mellitus as risk factor for colorectal cancer. Arch Physiol Biochem 114(1):84–98
32. Yang YX, Hennessy S, Lewis JD (2005) Type 2 diabetes mellitus and the risk of colorectal cancer. Clin Gastroenterol Hepatol 3(6):587–594
33. Chung YW, Han DS, Park KH, Eun CS, Yoo KS, Park CK (2008) Insulin therapy and colorectal adenoma risk among patients with Type 2 diabetes mellitus: a case-control study in Korea. Dis Colon Rectum 51(5):593–597
34. Yang YX, Hennessy S, Lewis JD (2004) Insulin therapy and colorectal cancer risk among type 2 diabetes mellitus patients. Gastroenterology 127(4):1044–1050
35. Kucharska-Newton AM, Rosamond WD, Schroeder JC, McNeill AM, Coresh J, Folsom AR (2008) HDL-cholesterol and the incidence of lung cancer in the Atherosclerosis Risk in Communities (ARIC) study. Lung Cancer 61(3):292–300
36. Shor R, Wainstein J, Oz D, Boaz M, Matas Z, Fux A et al (2008) Low HDL levels and the risk of death, sepsis and malignancy. Clin Res Cardiol 97(4):227–233
37. Shor R, Wainstein J, Oz D, Boaz M, Matas Z, Fux A et al (2007) Low serum LDL cholesterol levels and the risk of fever, sepsis, and malignancy. Ann Clin Lab Sci 37(4):343–348
38. Gaard M, Tretli S, Urdal P (1994) Risk of breast cancer in relation to blood lipids: a prospective study of 31,209 Norwegian women. Cancer Causes Control 5(6):501–509
39. Wuermli L, Joerger M, Henz S, Schmid HP, Riesen WF, Thomas G et al (2005) Hypertriglyceridemia as a possible risk factor for prostate cancer. Prostate Cancer Prostatic Dis 8(4):316–320
40. Glazer RI, Yuan H, Xie Z, Yin Y (2008) PPARgamma and PPARdelta as modulators of neoplasia and cell fate. PPAR Res 2008:247379
41. Sertznig P, Seifert M, Tilgen W, Reichrath J (2007) Present concepts and future outlook: function of peroxisome proliferator-activated receptors (PPARs) for pathogenesis, progression, and therapy of cancer. J Cell Physiol 212(1):1–12
42. Tachibana K, Yamasaki D, Ishimoto K, Doi T (2008) The Role of PPARs in cancer. PPAR Res 2008:102737
43. Wong JH, Ho KH, Nam S, Hsu WL, Lin CH, Chang CM et al (2017) Store-operated Ca(2+) entry facilitates the lipopolysaccharide-induced cyclooxygenase-2 expression in gastric cancer cells. Sci Rep 7(1):12813

44. Ferrer MD, Busquets-Cortés C, Capó X, Tejada S, Tur JA, Pons A et al (2019) Cyclooxygenase-2 inhibitors as a therapeutic target in inflammatory diseases. Curr Med Chem 26(18):3225–3241
45. Hashemi Goradel N, Najafi M, Salehi E, Farhood B, Mortezaee K (2019) Cyclooxygenase-2 in cancer: a review. J Cell Physiol 234(5):5683–5699
46. Trikha P, Carson WE III (2014) Signaling pathways involved in MDSC regulation. Biochim Biophys Acta 1846(1):55–65
47. Van Dross RT (2009) Metabolism of anandamide by COX-2 is necessary for endocannabinoid-induced cell death in tumorigenic keratinocytes. Mol Carcinog 48(8): 724–732
48. Wei J, Zhang J, Wang D, Cen B, Lang JD, DuBois RN (2022) The COX-2-PGE2 pathway promotes tumor evasion in colorectal adenomas. Cancer Prev Res (Phila) 15(5):285–296
49. Böttcher JP, Bonavita E, Chakravarty P, Blees H, Cabeza-Cabrerizo M, Sammicheli S et al (2018) NK cells stimulate recruitment of cDC1 into the tumor microenvironment promoting cancer immune control. Cell 172(5):1022–37.e14
50. Scherer PE, Williams S, Fogliano M, Baldini G, Lodish HF (1995) A novel serum protein similar to C1q, produced exclusively in adipocytes. J Biol Chem 270(45):26746–26749
51. Nguyen TMD (2020) Adiponectin: role in physiology and pathophysiology. Int J Prev Med 11:136
52. Gavrila A, Chan JL, Yiannakouris N, Kontogianni M, Miller LC, Orlova C et al (2003) Serum adiponectin levels are inversely associated with overall and central fat distribution but are not directly regulated by acute fasting or leptin administration in humans: cross-sectional and interventional studies. J Clin Endocrinol Metab 88(10):4823–4831
53. Fenton JI, Birmingham JM, Hursting SD, Hord NG (2008) Adiponectin blocks multiple signaling cascades associated with leptin-induced cell proliferation in Apc Min/+ colon epithelial cells. Int J Cancer 122(11):2437–2445
54. Pfeiler GH, Buechler C, Neumeier M, Schäffler A, Schmitz G, Ortmann O et al (2008) Adiponectin effects on human breast cancer cells are dependent on 17-beta estradiol. Oncol Rep 19(3):787–793
55. Cong L, Gasser J, Zhao J, Yang B, Li F, Zhao AZ (2007) Human adiponectin inhibits cell growth and induces apoptosis in human endometrial carcinoma cells, HEC-1-A and RL95 2. Endocr Relat Cancer 14(3):713–720
56. Baillargeon J, Platz EA, Rose DP, Pollock BH, Ankerst DP, Haffner S et al (2006) Obesity, adipokines, and prostate cancer in a prospective population-based study. Cancer Epidemiol 15(7):1331–1335
57. Frasor J, Weaver AE, Pradhan M, Mehta K (2008) Synergistic up-regulation of prostaglandin E synthase expression in breast cancer cells by 17beta-estradiol and proinflammatory cytokines. Endocrinology 149(12):6272–6279
58. Coussens LM, Werb Z (2002) Inflammation and cancer. Nature 420(6917):860–867
59. Brocco D, Florio R, De Lellis L, Veschi S, Grassadonia A, Tinari N et al (2020) The role of dysfunctional adipose tissue in pancreatic cancer: a molecular perspective. Cancer 12(7):1849
60. Singh M, Benencia F (2019) Inflammatory processes in obesity: focus on endothelial dysfunction and the role of adipokines as inflammatory mediators. Int Rev Immunol 38(4): 157–171
61. Himbert C, Delphan M, Scherer D, Bowers LW, Hursting S, Ulrich CM (2017) Signals from the adipose microenvironment and the obesity-cancer link-a systematic review. Cancer Prev Res (Phila) 10(9):494–506
62. Pal D, Dasgupta S, Kundu R, Maitra S, Das G, Mukhopadhyay S et al (2012) Fetuin-A acts as an endogenous ligand of TLR4 to promote lipid-induced insulin resistance. Nat Med 18(8): 1279–1285
63. Baker RG, Hayden MS, Ghosh S (2011) NF-κB, inflammation, and metabolic disease. Cell Metab 13(1):11–22

64. Vandanmagsar B, Youm YH, Ravussin A, Galgani JE, Stadler K, Mynatt RL et al (2011) The NLRP3 inflammasome instigates obesity-induced inflammation and insulin resistance. Nat Med 17(2):179–188
65. Fantuzzi G (2005) Adipose tissue, adipokines, and inflammation. J Allergy Clin Immunol 115(5):911–919. quiz 20
66. Axelsson J, Heimbürger O, Lindholm B, Stenvinkel P (2005) Adipose tissue and its relation to inflammation: the role of adipokines. J Ren Nutr 15(1):131–136
67. Solinas G, Vilcu C, Neels JG, Bandyopadhyay GK, Luo JL, Naugler W et al (2007) JNK1 in hematopoietically derived cells contributes to diet-induced inflammation and insulin resistance without affecting obesity. Cell Metab 6(5):386–397
68. Cheng P, Corzo CA, Luetteke N, Yu B, Nagaraj S, Bui MM et al (2008) Inhibition of dendritic cell differentiation and accumulation of myeloid-derived suppressor cells in cancer is regulated by S100A9 protein. J Exp Med 205(10):2235–2249
69. Vasquez-Dunddel D, Pan F, Zeng Q, Gorbounov M, Albesiano E, Fu J et al (2013) STAT3 regulates arginase-I in myeloid-derived suppressor cells from cancer patients. J Clin Invest 123(4):1580–1589
70. Font-Burgada J, Sun B, Karin M (2016) Obesity and cancer: the oil that feeds the flame. Cell Metab 23(1):48–62
71. Park EJ, Lee JH, Yu GY, He G, Ali SR, Holzer RG et al (2010) Dietary and genetic obesity promote liver inflammation and tumorigenesis by enhancing IL-6 and TNF expression. Cell 140(2):197–208
72. Pendyala S, Neff LM, Suárez-Fariñas M, Holt PR (2011) Diet-induced weight loss reduces colorectal inflammation: implications for colorectal carcinogenesis. Am J Clin Nutr 93(2): 234–242
73. Bai Y, Sun Q (2015) Macrophage recruitment in obese adipose tissue. Obes Rev 16(2): 127–136
74. Valadi H, Ekström K, Bossios A, Sjöstrand M, Lee JJ, Lötvall JO (2007) Exosome-mediated transfer of mRNAs and microRNAs is a novel mechanism of genetic exchange between cells. Nat Cell Biol 9(6):654–659
75. Kim A, Shah AS, Nakamura T (2018) Extracellular vesicles: a potential novel regulator of obesity and its associated complications. Children 5(11):152
76. Stepanian A, Bourguignat L, Hennou S, Coupaye M, Hajage D, Salomon L et al (2013) Microparticle increase in severe obesity: not related to metabolic syndrome and unchanged after massive weight loss. Obesity 21(11):2236–2243
77. Ferrante SC, Nadler EP, Pillai DK, Hubal MJ, Wang Z, Wang JM et al (2015) Adipocyte-derived exosomal miRNAs: a novel mechanism for obesity-related disease. Pediatr Res 77(3): 447–454
78. Deng ZB, Poliakov A, Hardy RW, Clements R, Liu C, Liu Y et al (2009) Adipose tissue exosome-like vesicles mediate activation of macrophage-induced insulin resistance. Diabetes 58(11):2498–2505
79. Bao Y, Mo J, Ruan L, Li G (2015) Increased monocytic CD14+HLADR low/- myeloid-derived suppressor cells in obesity. Mol Med Rep 11(3):2322–2328
80. Gabrilovich DI, Nagaraj S (2009) Myeloid-derived suppressor cells as regulators of the immune system. Nat Rev Immunol 9(3):162–174
81. Bähr I, Spielmann J, Quandt D, Kielstein H (2020) Obesity-associated alterations of natural killer cells and immunosurveillance of cancer. Front Immunol 11:245
82. James BR, Tomanek-Chalkley A, Askeland EJ, Kucaba T, Griffith TS, Norian LA (2012) Diet-induced obesity alters dendritic cell function in the presence and absence of tumor growth. J Immunol 189(3):1311–1321
83. Hale M, Itani F, Buchta CM, Wald G, Bing M, Norian LA (2015) Obesity triggers enhanced MDSC accumulation in murine renal tumors via elevated local production of CCL2. PLoS One 10(3):e0118784

84. James BR, Anderson KG, Brincks EL, Kucaba TA, Norian LA, Masopust D et al (2014) CpG-mediated modulation of MDSC contributes to the efficacy of Ad5-TRAIL therapy against renal cell carcinoma. Cancer Immunol Immunother 63(11):1213–1227

85. Pacifico L, Di Renzo L, Anania C, Osborn JF, Ippoliti F, Schiavo E et al (2006) Increased T-helper interferon-gamma-secreting cells in obese children. Eur J Endocrinol 154(5): 691–697

86. Zúñiga LA, Shen WJ, Joyce-Shaikh B, Pyatnova EA, Richards AG, Thom C et al (2010) IL-17 regulates adipogenesis, glucose homeostasis, and obesity. J Immunol 185(11):6947–6959

87. Deiuliis J, Shah Z, Shah N, Needleman B, Mikami D, Narula V et al (2011) Visceral adipose inflammation in obesity is associated with critical alterations in regulatory cell numbers. PLoS One 6(1):e16376

88. Basen-Engquist K, Chang M (2011) Obesity and cancer risk: recent review and evidence. Curr Oncol Rep 13(1):71–76

89. Calle EE, Rodriguez C, Walker-Thurmond K, Thun MJ (2003) Overweight, obesity, and mortality from cancer in a prospectively studied cohort of U.S. adults. N Engl J Med 348(17): 1625–1638

90. Dahlberg SE, Schiller JH, Bonomi PB, Sandler AB, Brahmer JR, Ramalingam SS et al (2013) Body mass index and its association with clinical outcomes for advanced non-small-cell lung cancer patients enrolled on Eastern Cooperative Oncology Group clinical trials. J Thorac Oncol 8(9):1121–1127

91. Yuan C, Bao Y, Wu C, Kraft P, Ogino S, Ng K et al (2013) Prediagnostic body mass index and pancreatic cancer survival. J Clin Oncol 31(33):4229–4234

92. Fredslund SO, Gravholt CH, Laursen BE, Jensen AB (2019) Key metabolic parameters change significantly in early breast cancer survivors: an explorative PILOT study. J Transl Med 17(1): 105

93. Westerink NL, Nuver J, Lefrandt JD, Vrieling AH, Gietema JA, Walenkamp AM (2016) Cancer treatment induced metabolic syndrome: Improving outcome with lifestyle. Crit Rev Oncol Hematol 108:128–136

94. Kroenke CH, Chen WY, Rosner B, Holmes MD (2005) Weight, weight gain, and survival after breast cancer diagnosis. J Clin Oncol 23(7):1370–1378

95. Chlebowski RT, Blackburn GL, Thomson CA, Nixon DW, Shapiro A, Hoy MK et al (2006) Dietary fat reduction and breast cancer outcome: interim efficacy results from the Women's Intervention Nutrition Study. J Natl Cancer Inst 98(24):1767–1776

96. Blackburn GL, Wang KA (2007) Dietary fat reduction and breast cancer outcome: results from the Women's Intervention Nutrition Study (WINS). Am J Clin Nutr 86(3):s878–s881

97. Camoriano JK, Loprinzi CL, Ingle JN, Therneau TM, Krook JE, Veeder MH (1990) Weight change in women treated with adjuvant therapy or observed following mastectomy for node-positive breast cancer. J Clin Oncol 8(8):1327–1334

98. Gadéa E, Thivat E, Planchat E, Morio B, Durando X (2012) Importance of metabolic changes induced by chemotherapy on prognosis of early-stage breast cancer patients: a review of potential mechanisms. Obes Rev 13(4):368–380

99. Gadéa É, Thivat É, Wang-Lopez Q, Viala M, Paulon R, Planchat É et al (2013) [Poor prognostic value of weight change during chemotherapy in non-metastatic breast cancer patients: causes, mechanisms involved and preventive strategies]. Bull Cancer 100(9): 865–870

100. Vardy J, Chiew KS, Galica J, Pond GR, Tannock IF (2006) Side effects associated with the use of dexamethasone for prophylaxis of delayed emesis after moderately emetogenic chemotherapy. Br J Cancer 94(7):1011–1015

101. Kulkarni SK, Kaur G (2001) Pharmacodynamics of drug-induced weight gain. Drugs Today 37(8):559–571

102. Cleary MP, Grossmann ME (2009) Minireview: obesity and breast cancer: the estrogen connection. Endocrinology 150(6):2537–2542

103. Timilshina N, Breunis H, Alibhai SM (2012) Impact of androgen deprivation therapy on weight gain differs by age in men with nonmetastatic prostate cancer. J Urol 188(6): 2183–2188

104. Braunstein LZ, Chen MH, Loffredo M, Kantoff PW, D'Amico AV (2014) Obesity and the odds of weight gain following androgen deprivation therapy for prostate cancer. Prostate Cancer 2014:230812

105. Moszyńska-Zielińska M, Chałubińska-Fendler J, Gottwald L, Żytko L, Bigos E, Fijuth J (2014) Does obesity hinder radiotherapy in endometrial cancer patients? The implementation of new techniques in adjuvant radiotherapy - focus on obese patients. Prz Menopauzalny 13(2):96–100

106. Cao Y, Ma J (2011) Body mass index, prostate cancer-specific mortality, and biochemical recurrence: a systematic review and meta-analysis. Cancer Prev Res (Phila) 4(4):486–501

107. Togawa K, Ma H, Sullivan-Halley J, Neuhouser ML, Imayama I, Baumgartner KB et al (2014) Risk factors for self-reported arm lymphedema among female breast cancer survivors: a prospective cohort study. Breast Cancer Res 16(4):414

108. Thomas RJ, Holm M, Williams M, Bowman E, Bellamy P, Andreyev J et al (2013) Lifestyle factors correlate with the risk of late pelvic symptoms after prostatic radiotherapy. Clin Oncol 25(4):246–251

109. Dandapani SV, Zhang Y, Jennelle R, Lin YG (2015) Radiation-associated toxicities in obese women with endometrial cancer: more than just BMI? Scientific World Journal 2015:483208

110. Welsh J, Thomas J, Shah D, Allen PK, Wei X, Mitchell K et al (2011) Obesity increases the risk of chest wall pain from thoracic stereotactic body radiation therapy. Int J Radiat Oncol Biol Phys 81(1):91–96

111. Szerlip N, Rutter C, Ram N, Yovino S, Kwok Y, Maggio W et al (2011) Factors impacting volumetric white matter changes following whole brain radiation therapy. J Neurooncol 103(1):111–119

Chapter 25
Systemic *Onco-Sphere*: Host Microbiome and Cancer

Phei Er Saw and Erwei Song

Abstract In recent years, it has been found that gut microbiota is involved in the metabolism of the host and cancer cells. Interestingly, gut microbiome and their metabolites have been demonstrated great influence on the tumor formation, prognosis and treatment, leading researchers to elucidate the underlying mechanisms of the host microbiome axis in cancer. This chapter looks at various oncogenic microbes and how they affect the host systemic onco-sphere and their link with cancer progression.

Introduction

Cancer has been linked to a vast body of bacterial pathogens. By 1772, it was believed that *Mycobacterium tuberculosis* caused malignancy [1]. Bronchogenic carcinomas were reported to develop across regions of pulmonary scarring, supposedly tuberculosis. Lung cancer patients also suffered from active tuberculosis more frequently than the general population. Unlike numerous instances that associated cancer with specific

P. E. Saw
Guangdong Provincial Key Laboratory of Malignant Tumor Epigenetics and Gene Regulation, Guangdong-Hong Kong Joint Laboratory for RNA Medicine, Medical Research Center, Sun Yat-sen Memorial Hospital, Sun Yat-sen University, Guangzhou, China

Nanhai Translational Innovation Center of Precision Immunology, Sun Yat-sen Memorial Hospital, Sun Yat-sen University, Foshan, China

E. Song (✉)
Guangdong Provincial Key Laboratory of Malignant Tumor Epigenetics and Gene Regulation, Guangdong-Hong Kong Joint Laboratory for RNA Medicine, Medical Research Center, Sun Yat-sen Memorial Hospital, Sun Yat-sen University, Guangzhou, China

Nanhai Translational Innovation Center of Precision Immunology, Sun Yat-sen Memorial Hospital, Sun Yat-sen University, Foshan, China

Breast Tumor Center, Sun Yat-sen Memorial Hospital, Sun Yat-sen University, Guangzhou, China
e-mail: songew@mail.sysu.edu.cn

infectious agents, the hypothesis on tuberculosis did not stand the scrutiny of time. Most cases of bronchogenic carcinomas in tuberculosis patients emerge in other areas of the lung. Moreover, scars seen at sites of tumors are currently ascribed to malignancy, as opposed to the origin. Whatever connection between malignancy and tuberculosis is attributed to infection reactivation within cancer patients with immunocompromise, rather than a cause-and-effect association between neoplasm and infection [2–4]. This chapter looks at various oncogenic microbes and how they affect the host systemic *onco-sphere* and their link with cancer progression.

Microbial Oncogenesis: An Overview

Tumors and microbial agents tend to be diverse and many principles can be used to inform considerations in the future. Oncogenic microbes are found to remain for years within their hosts. There may be resolution of acute infections, but scars that facilitate neoplasia might be left behind. However, this process appears to be remarkable. More commonly, persisting microbes that have failed to be eliminated by the host involves the host in a constant battle that inflicts damage on tissue [5]. Instead of a singular pathogen, a cluster of colonizing organisms has been known to instigate such instances of inflammations. Next, there are differences as far as oncogenic potential is concerned in microbial species for HPV, some variations which lead to most cancers, *H. pylori* as well as hepatitis viruses, where certain genotypes have high virulence [6–9]. Third, the microbial load is usually important, as demonstrated by schistosomes and the hepatitis viruses [6, 7]. Also, the interplay of microbial genotypes and load could be synergistic, leading to considerably heightened risks of diseases [10, 11]. Fifth, the microbial genotype–load interaction and controls risk include host phenotypes and genotype [8, 12–14]. Sixth, as microbes are communicable agents, their prevalence in subsequent generations will be affected by the prevalence in a prior generation. Hence, tendencies of amplification (inter-generational) can evolve within a population in the absence of any recognized rise in exposure, as opposed to chemical carcinogenesis, as a case in point (Fig. 25.1).

Bacterial Cell–Surface Components

Bacteria's outer surface directly establishes contact with host cells and is made up of intricate structures which include numerous antigenic moieties triggering adaptive/innate responses. Consequently, pathogenic bacteria accommodate a significant number of outer surface changes conferring immune evasion tendencies, leading to key opportunities for survival. To obliterate immune clearance/recognition, the intricate macromolecules (outer surface) are safeguarded by polysaccharide-rich capsule in Gram-negative bacteria. This, in turn, safeguards structures located on pathogenic variations' membranes as far as *E. coli, Neisseria meningitidis,*

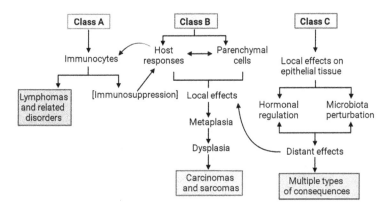

Fig. 25.1 General classification of microbes is divided into three major classes (A, B, and C). Class A microbes are related to lymphomas. Class B microbes are usually linked to carcinomas and sarcomas while class C is linked to a diverse type of consequences, including being able to have a distant effect on class B microbes. This has been reviewed in detail in [15]. In this chapter, we will not discuss deeper into each class, rather, focusing on the mechanism in which the bacteria could influence host to encourage cancer growth

Streptococcus pneumoniae, and *Haemophilus influenzae* type, among others are concerned. Thereafter, professional phagocytes help curtail engulfment [16–19]. Mutations of these bacteria which are unencapsulated seldom lead to invasive infections and are greatly attenuated in numerous models of infection as a result of improved opsonophagocytic clearance [17, 20, 21].

Many bacterial pathogens such as flagella and lipopolysaccharides (LPS) have showcased how their molecule (surface-exposed) have been modified to curb recognition of immune. To illustrate, *H. pylori* possesses surface molecules of LPS, accommodating lipid A molecules which subsequently elude sensing of innate immunity [22, 23]. *H. pylori* also generates altered flagellin molecules that can evade TLR5 recognition, hence preventing the secretion of TLR5-mediated IL-8 signaling pathway [24]. *Salmonella typhimurium* demonstrates expression of lipid A palmitoyl-transferase PagP and lipid A deacetylase PagL to alter lipid A, causing a 100-fold reduction in TLR4 activation mediated by lipid A and activation of NF-κB [25]. These illustrations show how bacterial pathogens are able to alter their other surfaces to evade the recognition of immune. Pathogenic bacteria lending support to intracellular lifestyles witness proteins facilitating attachment and internalization to host cells. As a case in point, the Neisseria family's pathogenic species expresses an assortment of adhesins (surface) that affect interplay with specific types of cells, hence enabling specific host cell niches' exploitation [26]. Analogously, the fibronectin-binding proteins expressed by *Borrelia burgdorferi* and *Staphylococcus aureus* exhibit mediation of the interplay between host cells' fibronectin and bacterium by generating tandem β-zippers [27, 28].

Generally, these surface-mediated assault tactics are targeted toward the promotion of bacterial survival in the host via both host invasion and immune evasion. Nevertheless, to better modulate the machinery of host cells, bacteria's surface molecules exploit signaling cascades of host cells before affecting their integrity, potentially provoking cellular malignancies by coincidence. Not only ascertains *H. pylori* attachment to gastric epithelial cells but also deals with a signaling cascade stimulating secretion upregulation of gastric acid. The resulting hypergastrinemia is a significant risk for gastric adenocarcinoma's progression. The outer inflammatory protein A that *H. pylori* possesses initiates EGFR besides encouraging β-catenin as well as Akt signaling, a commonly observed phenotype in various cancers [29, 30]. The *Fusobacterium nucleatum's* (*F. nucleatum*) fusobacterium adhesion A (FadA) showcases binding of E-cadherin extracellular domain, thus leading to E-cadherin internalization/phosphorylation, eventually inducing the release of β-catenin to modulate gene transcription related to cell proliferation, apoptosis, and transformation [31]. Sufferers of colon adenomas/ adenocarcinomas often suffer from high expression levels of *F. nucleatum* fadA. This, in turn, has been associated with inflammatory/oncogenic genes' upregulated expression concerning the pathway of Wnt signaling [32, 33].

LPS, which is an important surface-exposed constituent of Gram-negative bacteria, also triggers signaling cascades which facilitate the development of cancer. It manifests in commensal as well as pathogenic bacteria, playing a vital role in activating TLR4. Signaling mediated by TLR4 is imperative for several signaling pathways' downstream activation, besides being able to facilitate the development of inflammation-associated colorectal cancers as well as adenomatous polyposis coli (Apc)-dependent colorectal cancers within mice. Tumor tissue from mice which lacked MyD88 demonstrated reduced COX2 gene expression; this gene is implicated during inflammation, signifying its function in reducing tumor development [34]. Moreover, COX2 inhibitors including aspirin lowers the hazard of colorectal cancer among individuals with 15-PGDH gene overexpression that encodes an enzyme impeding COX2 activities [35]. According to investigations of wild-type and germ-free mice, LPS' ability to activate TLR4 activation from the pool of intestinal microbiota facilitates inflammation and the activation of antiapoptotic and proliferative signals in HCC [36].

Crosstalk in the Local *Onco-Sphere*: Bacterial Toxin-Mediated Host Cell Transformation

The interaction between the host and protein toxins usually takes place in an organized set of events as evidenced by diphtheria toxins suppressing the synthesis of host cell protein by deactivating elongation factor 2 (EF-2) protein. This diphtheria toxin comprising three subunits gets released as a single polypeptide chain by *Corynebacterium diphtheriae*. Subsequently, diphtheria toxin binds to the host's EGFR that then gets internalized within the endosomal system. At this point, the transmembrane domain of the toxin unfolds, leading to the toxin's translocation. Subsequently, the C-domain releases inside the cytoplasm and gets refolded into a conformation which facilitates ADP-ribosylation. Protein synthesis is then inhibited,

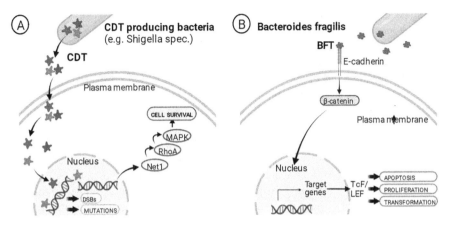

Fig. 25.2 (**a**) CDT toxin's CdtB subunit conveyed to the nucleus, leading to DSBs and impaired feature of DNA DDR sensor. Simultaneously, RhoA and NET1 are triggered, which results in MAPK upregulation as well as cellular survival. (**b**) Bacteroides fragilis BFT is implicated in cellular signaling, proliferation, and transformation by triggering the NF-κB and β-catenin/Wnt signaling pathways

which eventually leads to the targeted cells; death [37]. While pathogenic bacteria mainly use toxin-mediated assault to develop a favorable environment of host cells, their toxins are capable of providing support to carcinogenesis. It is possible for carcinogenesis mediated by toxins to arise via several ways, including by genomic instability, proliferative signaling inducting, and the signaling of cell death resistance [38]. Genomic instability can be easily created by protein toxins capable of disturbing double-stranded DNA, including cytolethal distending toxin (CDT), colibactin, the Shiga toxin, as well as endonucleases. Host cell binding as well as internalization is particularly responsive to such toxins. Consequently, immune cells can be locally eliminated by this toxin, supplying a clear benefit for the bacteria. Nevertheless, continued exposure to CDT's sublethal doses can harm the DDR sensor's functionality, leading to compromised DNA damage detection and mutation aggregation. Simultaneously, the stimulation of GTPase RhoA and the neuroepithelial cell-transforming gene 1 protein (NET1) upregulates mitogen-activated protein kinase (MAPK) activity, allowing the toxin-exposed cells to survive. As a result, these cells are capable of proliferating with DNA mutations/deletions that have emerged through repair, thus leading to genomic errors which forms the base for developing cancer (Fig. 25.2).

As an adverse event, bacteria that produce colibactin get chromosomal instability triggered, repair DNA incorrectly, and form colonies that is anchorage-dependent, which are phenotypes capable of facilitating formation of cancer [39, 40]. This is additionally corroborated by epidemiological research which demonstrated that *E. coli* which produced colibactin appeared with increased prevalence in biopsies of human colorectal tumor patients [41, 42]. Furthermore, IL-10-deficient mice which were susceptible to colitis exhibited heightened invasive carcinoma formation upon *E. coli's* colonization which secreted colibactin [43]. In addition to toxins that facilitate carcinogenesis by presenting genomic instability and DSBs, there have been reports of toxins that facilitate carcinogenesis by triggering resistance by encouraging proliferative signaling. Usually, these toxins are formed by pathogenic bacteria that prefer intracellular host cell life as some aspects of their infectious lifecycle, thus reaping direct benefits of host cell survival. An example of such a toxin is *Bacteroides fragilis* (abbreviated as *B. fragilis*) toxin (BFT) demonstrating the ability to bind cell receptors (intestinal epithelial) and stimulate the proliferation of cells by joining E-cadherin [44, 45], which, in turn, generates intercellular adhesion junctions and gets implicated in differentiation, signaling, and proliferation of cells by getting NF-κB as well as β-catenin/Wnt signaling pathways triggered [46–48]. BFT induced both acute and chronic colitis in six mice, apart from colon tumors in multiple intestinal neoplasia (mouse model) for colon carcinoma in humans. It is this mouse model wherein *H. pylori* led to a multi-step, pro-carcinogenic cascade of inflammation necessitating signaling of NF-κB, IL-17R, and STAT3 in epithelial cells of colon [49, 50]. Epidemiology corroborates these experiments, which implies that infections in *B. fragilis'* enterotoxigenic variants feature a higher prevalence in colorectal cancer patients. More specifically, the variant (enterotoxigenic) exists in a maximum of 20% of the healthy population, while enterotoxigenic *B. fragilis* is demonstrated in the feces of 40% of patients with CRC [51]. Besides BFT, various biologically reasonable mechanisms have been published regarding the explanation of how *H. pylori's* vacuolating cytotoxin A heightens the risk of gastric cancer. In comparison with OipA of *H. pylori*, VacA gets the EGFR receptor stimulated that then activates PI3K–Akt signaling, while deactivating glycogen synthase kinase 3β [30, 52]. Consequently, degradation of β-catenin is halted, facilitating transcription controlled by Tcf/LEF that then augments cell growth [30, 52, 53]. Both unphosphorylated and phosphorylated CagA are also capable of interacting with several ERK, MEK, β-catenin, and NF-κB-implicate host proteins that play a key role in cancer's genesis [54, 55], detailed in Fig. 25.3.

Bacterial Effector Mediating Transformation of Host Cells

Numerous pathogens (intracellular bacterial) form molecular means for guaranteeing relentless infection within the environment that host cells provide. This necessitates management of host cells at many phases, such as internalization of host cell through phagocytosis mediated by receptors or endocytosis, cellular survival, and growth, apart from release from the problematic host cell. After internalization of host cell, bacterial cargo gets directed via the endosomal system, generally ending in the phagolysosome, an extremely degradative organelle. To evade degradation by phagolysosomes, a multitude of mechanisms has evolved from intracellular bacterial pathogens, which can be generally categorized into pathways that allow pathogenic bacteria to avert the phagosome or enter the cytosol. Cytosolic pathogens like *Listeria, Francisella,* and *Shigella flexneri* (*S. flexneri*) get recognized so that they can quickly avert the introduction of phagosomes inside the host cytosol

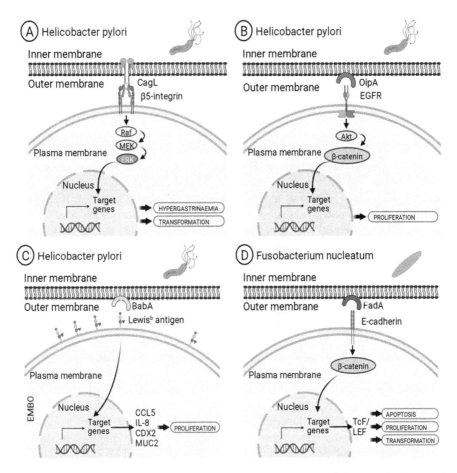

Fig. 25.3 Detailed mechanism of the effect of microbes on the host cell by *H. Pylori* (**a–c**) and *fusobacterium nucleatum* (**d**)

[56]. Typically, this requires the formation of bacterial effector proteins stimulating pore formation on the vacuole and resulting in a rupture. As a case in point, *S. flexneri* releases plasmid antigen B, generating ion channels while also controlling potassium influx along with the resultant endolysosomal leakage [57]. Additionally, listeriolysin-O protein can be secreted by Listeria, which stimulates small membrane perforations, resulting in leakage of Ca^{2+} from vacuoles and the corresponding increase in vacuolar pH. Thereafter, maturation of vacuoles is hindered [58, 59]. In addition, *Francisella tularensis (F. tularensis)* evades in host cells' cytoplasm as well.

Following phagocytic ingestion on the part of macrophages, it is shown that *F. tularensis* stays inside the phagosome containing Francisella that develops from a premature endosomal character, namely phagosome. Considering that the FCP acidification inhibition curtails the *F. tularensis'* evasion in the cytosol, further acidification ostensibly impels *F. tularensis* to form undefined and exceptional factors so that the phagosomal membrane can be impeded [60–62]. Contrary to bacteria that evade phagosomes, some pathogenic bacteria get the phagosome hijacked to ensure a beneficial replication niche. One such model is *Legionella pneumophila*, shunting the aforementioned phagosome by forming proteins (bacterial) through the Dot-Icm secretion system, thus curtailing degradation of lysosome and safeguarding Legionella's replication [63, 64]. Phagosomal maturation manipulation on the past of bacteria has been shown for a pathogen called *Salmonella*. After the internalization of host cells, Salmonella makes its presence felt via a vacuolar compartment that appears like phagosome and is called the Salmonella-containing vacuole (SCV). SCV maturation occurs, resulting in acquisition of the features of late endocytic compartments such as acidification. However, it does not turn bactericidal. Under modulation of the Salmonella effectors, SifA, SseF, SseG, SseJ, SopD2, and PipB2, cellular host processes are controlled to alter SCV into a container that promotes replication of *Salmonella* [65]. Being a crucial process, SifA interacts with SifA and kinesin-interacting protein SKIP, the host cell effector of the GTPase Arl8b [66]. This interplay leads to the generation of Salmonella-induced filaments that assume great significance for supplying nutrients to the SCV and curtailing endosomal antimicrobial operations as a result of continuous mixing with late lysosomes and endosomes [67, 68].

Pathogenic bacteria (intracellular) entailing effector proteins during their life cycle significantly showcase host cell integrity manipulation. In this context, some infections are linked to specific cancer types. For example, infections caused by *Salmonella serovars*, *S. Enteritidis,* and *S. Typhi*, are associated with colon cancer and gallbladder carcinoma [69, 70]. They feature a gamut of effectors proteins inside the host cell to get host cell biology manipulate and accelerate cancer formation. To illustrate, a Salmonella effector protein is acetyltransferase AvrA, thus modifying several pathways of host signaling and controlling apoptosis [71, 72]. AvrA transforms β-catenin, thereby enhancing signaling and catalyzing epithelial cells' proliferation [73–75]. Additionally, AvrA subdues the host's immune system and the apoptotic defenses [76]. Besides AvrA, three other AvrA orthologues have also been found, which demonstrates similar interaction with crucial host cell signaling pathways. Nevertheless, unlike AvrA, they mainly inhibit the immune system of the host. *Yersinia pestis* expresses YopJ, which demonstrated attenuation of the p38, ERK, JNK, and IκB kinase (IKK) pathways which concern the generation of cytokines in addition to anti-apoptotic factors [77]. Similarly, *Vibrio parahaemolyticus* expresses VopA, which inhibits host p38, ERK, and JNK signaling, with exception of the IKK pathway [78, 79], whereas AopP expressed by *Aeromonas salmonicida* demonstrates interaction with the IKK pathway [80].

Within *S. typhimurium*-infected epithelial cells, SopB, SopE, and SopE2 are capable of controlling host Rho-family GTPases, ABL tyrosine kinase, and p21-activated kinase (PAK) to trigger the activation of STAT3 and modify transcription regulation, which can moderate cell transformation [81]. Additionally, cellular transformation can take place via Salmonella effectors SopB, SopE, and SopE2, in addition to SptP-mediated triggering of the AKT and MAPK pathways

[82]. Triggering of these signaling pathways leads to the alteration of gallbladder organoids and fibroblasts that contain a pre-transformed phenotype where the MYC oncogene is overexpressed and the tumor suppressor gene p53 is deactivated. These results are endorsed by pathological findings from gallbladder carcinoma samples derived from Indian patients that include the DNA of *S. Typhi* as well as the alterations recorded within lab experiments and also by an ApcMin/$^+$ model (of mouse) wherein *S. typhimurium*-induced oral infection forms colorectal adenocarcinomas [70].

Inter-*Onco Spherical* Communication: Cancer and the Gut Microbiota

The human intestine consists of 100 trillion organisms—mostly bacteria—collectively called the gut microbiota [83]. Microbiota in the gut flourishes in the host, reflecting a remarkable degree of coevolution (eubiosis) [84]. On its part, the intestine provides resident microbes with a warm and protective environment. The immune system maintains immunosurveillance against invasive infections while tolerating the typical gut flora. Additionally, mounting data suggests that the gut microbiota is vital for an immune system's overall development [85]. The gut microbiota and anticancer medications interact in both directions during cancer treatment. On the one hand, various treatments for neoplastic disorders currently have cytotoxic benefits on gut microorganisms, encouraging dysbiosis [86]. Options such as allogeneic stem cell transplantation and radiation therapy can alter the composition of gut microbiota, including by getting an immune response induced [87–89]. Meanwhile, growing data suggest that it affects pharmacodynamic [90, 91] and immunological processes that control the negative effects and therapeutic effectiveness of anticancer drugs [92–94].

Previous studies have discovered molecular and genomic biomarkers associated with the host that are linked to ICB [95–100] response. In fact, certain gut microbial signatures separate healthy people from cancer patients and responders from non-responders in several ICB-treated cancer cohorts [101–103], suggesting that the gut microbiome's makeup could entail both prognostic and predictive applications for ICB. These discoveries have ignited the formation as well as use of brand-new microbiome-based therapeutic approaches that attempt to alter gut microbes of patients and the related activities in relation to ICB [104–106] and mitigate therapy toxicity [107–109]. Many interventional tactics have demonstrated promise as gut microbiome modulators, including dietary interventions/antibiotic therapies/prebiotic/probiotic options (Fig. 25.4). As evidenced so far, the interaction between facets of systemic immunity as well as indicators related to inflammation, immunology related to tissues and tumors, and microbiomes concerning the gut can affect overall health and disease pattern, including specific cancer types, at a systematic level [110–112]. Poignantly, the most current version of the "Hallmarks of Cancer" now recognizes the microbiome as an important hallmark in cancer growth and progression [113].

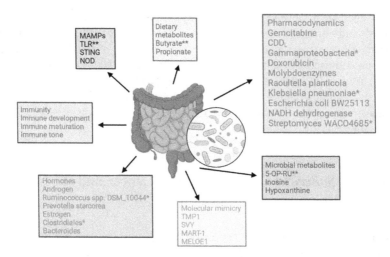

Fig. 25.4 How the gut microbiomes are affecting the host via activation of immune system, regulation of hormones, and genes. The gut microbiota's potential to positively influence systemic immunity and the general health of the host, as well as its functional state, are what determine its final therapeutic role. As a result, it will be essential to characterize the systemic biological processes linked to the gut microbiota and the underlying molecular pathways to identify new, practicable targets for future intervention and clinical assessment

Mechanisms of Action on Systemic Immunity and Cancer Treatment Response

An abundance of research shows the relationship between ICB response and the gut microbiome [102, 103, 106, 114–116]. Through numerous distinctive methods, gut microbes affect host immunity and cancer treatment response. They consist of the following: (a) ecological changes brought on by impacts on other gut microbes [117]; impacts over enterocytes (autophagy and death) as well as the lymphoid tissue connected with the gut [110, 111]; pattern-recognition receptors that trace locally or systemically adjuvant signals [112, 118]; impact on the neuroendocrine system by gut hormone release [119]; metabolic impacts using the production of polyamine and vitamin B [120]; and the activation of immunological defenses against microbes that exhibit cross-reactivity with antigens associated with tumors [121–146]. The significance of considering tumor/patient-specific factors when assessing the role of the microbiome in cancer treatment is underscored as follows: hallmarks depend on the context although they do affect resistance as well as response to cancer therapies.

Preclinical evidence. Preclinical research demonstrates how gut microbes affect systemic immunity. For instance, gnotobiotic mice (grown in an environment devoid of germs) have an undeveloped immune system, thus compromising their resistance to infections [147]. There is a variety of antibiotics that reduce the diversity of bacteria in the GI tract, which has a negative effect on the effectiveness of chemotherapy drugs like cyclophosphamide [92] and oxaliplatin [93]. This also remains valid for mice residing in specific conditions devoid of pathogens. In preclinical models, administering broad-spectrum antibiotics curtails the impact of therapy with ICB targeting CTLA-4 [50] or PD1/PD-L1 [102, 103, 116]. Notably, FMT transforms mice who have had antibiotic treatment into "avatars" that may be able to predict whether or not a patient will respond to PD-1 blocking [102, 116], despite the fact that this method is uncommon and needs further research and confirmation.

Clinical evidence. Several studies demonstrate that cancer patients on generic antibiotics just prior to or amid ICB therapy had lower OS and PFS [102, 103, 148, 149]. This supports the idea that a microbiota out of balance has detrimental effects on the cycle of cancer and immunity [117]. Although there are no casual linkages between carcinogenesis and these gut microorganisms, it is necessary to conduct further research. In fact, prior research showed a heightened abundance of specific microbial taxa within cancer patients' guts when compared with their cancer-free counterparts across various cancer types [101]. Additionally, distinct microbial taxa have been linked to ICB response [23, 25–27, 150–159], and there are some bacterial taxa that resemble these cohorts. Although there is some overlap in the gut microbes linked to ICB response spanning many kinds of cancer in extant literature, it remains minimal and cannot be justified by changes in sequencing methods [160]. This emphasizes the potential to characterize the gut microbiome's immune-activating and response-related traits from a functional viewpoint and via more incisive human cohorts' characterization in preclinical models.

Treatment-related toxicity. Specific gut microbial taxa and dysbiosis are associated with toxicity related to treatment, apart from uncovering response-linked microbial signatures [107, 108, 161–166]. With FMT treatment or targeted microbial-modulating therapy, these results have opened up options to target certain bacteria or re-establish healthy microbiota to lessen medication-related toxicity. FMT, for instance, lessens the side effects of chemotherapy based on 5-fluorouracil in preclinical models of CRC [167]. In preclinical models, both FMT as well as indole 3-propionic acid combat toxicity related to radiation [168, 169], and the administration of Bifidobacterium has been linked to a reduction in CTLA-4-related intestinal toxicity [170].

Tissue-Resident and Intratumoral Microorganisms: Friend or Foe?

Microorganisms in different habitats may have a significant impact on host physiology in addition to those in the gut [94, 171–174]. This comprises microbes on mucosal and surface areas and tissue-resident microbes [175]. Although some knowledge has been gathered about how microorganisms affect carcinogenesis and therapeutic response, much more has to be discovered. Although there are challenges in mining NGS data for other reasons [176–178], recent developments have significantly enhanced microbes' identification in tissues and how they impact illness, including cancer. For instance, poly(A) mRNA capture curbs the value of classical RNA-seq datasets to collect more information on microbiome as they lack useful prokaryotic transcripts [179]. Because the relative biomass in these peripheral areas is much smaller than that in the gut, additional difficulties still remain even when NGS methods are explicitly utilized to detect bacteria in tissues and tumors [180]. Another significant obstacle to accurately evaluating microbial presence is ambient sources-induced contamination during tissue collecting as well as sequencing [177], even though sophisticated *in silico* "decontamination" techniques are being developed to surmount this impediment [181].

Tissue-Based and Tumor-Based Microorganisms and Carcinogenesis

In a local *onco-sphere* of a solid tumor, characterization across tumor types has led to the identification of unique intratumoral microbiomes for various malignancy forms [94]. Typically, intracellular intratumoral bacteria of the TME invade cancer, stromal, and immune cells [182]. It is interesting to note that historical data have shown many processes by which intratumoral bacteria promote carcinogenesis. To begin with, tissue-resident bacteria could stimulate cancer by modifying various parts of the DNA of the host. To illustrate, bacteria that produce genotoxins may directly cause DNA damage. Notably, strains *F. nucleatum* [183] cause DNA oxidative stress via the production of reactive oxygen species, while *C. jejuni* [184] is known to cause double-stranded DNA breaks. Furthermore, microorganisms residing in tissues could impede processes of DNA mismatch, including EspF-expressing *E. coli* [185] as well as *H. pylori* [186, 187], which worsens genomic instability and promotes carcinogenesis. Separately, the HPV-driven and EBV-driven cancers show that tissue-resident viruses may potentially directly disturb the cell cycle to induce carcinogenesis [188].

Tissue-based bacteria could spur tumor growth by triggering an inflammatory milieu that is tumorigenic in the tissue. A number of species, such as enterotoxigenic Bacteroides fragilis (ETBF) [189], *F. nucleatum* [190], *E. coli* [191], and *Stenotrophomonas/Selenomonas,* can trigger reactions pertaining to inflammation and promulgate tissue hyperproliferation. *B. fragilis* toxin causes a pro-inflammatory signaling cascade in colonocytes that relies on the secretion of cytokines that leads to the activation of STAT3/NF-κB signaling pathway [189]. Furthermore, *H. pylori* has been shown to cause gastric tissue-related hyperproliferative inflammation by expressing CagA [54]. On the other hand, *F. nucleatum* induces this phenotype within colorectal tissue by expressing FadA [31]. It has also been shown that certain MAMPs (microorganism-associated molecular patterns) encourage cancer. For instance, in a chemically induced skin cancer model, flagellin-dependent TLR5 activation in bone marrow-derived leukocytes increased carcinogenesis [192]. Beyond bacteria, other microorganisms may potentially affect the development of tumors. PDACs have been linked to the mycobiome, which consists of the fungi in a particular microenvironment [193]. Finally, metabolites of microbial metabolism may play a role in cancer development. Acetate and butyrate are examples of catabolites that enhance cell proliferation or epithelial–mesenchymal transition across several models of cancer [144, 194]. Secondary metabolites and bile acids have also been shown to demonstrate a carcinogenic role [195]. In high-fat diets, deoxycholic acid level is elevated [196], further establishing a rationale for the connection between specific high-risk diets and the emergence of gastrointestinal cancer.

Microorganisms Found in Tissues and Tumors and Their Significance in the Antitumor Immune Response

Tissue-based bacteria may affect the immunological environment inside a cancer lesion and play a role in the carcinogenesis of particular tissue types by changing the local cytokine and immune cell profiles. Various microorganisms have been found to polarize contrastingly distinct forms of local immune responses that may either support or prevent tumor development makes it important to recognize that these effects are very context-dependent. Intratumoral bacteria often encourage tolerogenic immunity, which promotes tumor development. The main mechanism is usually by conditionally activating pattern-recognition receptors. For instance, bacterial LPS, which has been identified in both immune and cancer cells in the local *onco-sphere* [182], can bind to TLR4 on infiltrating monocytes to skew their differentiation to an immunosuppressive M2-like phenotype [197, 198] as well as on tumor cells to encourage recruitment of CD11b$^+$Gr1$^+$ MDSCs and CD1d$^+$CD5$^+$ Breg cells, which collectively are immunosuppressive [199]. Additionally, in CRC, microbial peptidoglycan activation of NOD1 has been demonstrated to cause immunosuppression that is mediated by myeloid-derived suppressor cells in an arginase 1-dependent manner [200].

Another method to increase immunosuppression is to increase the expression of immunoregulatory ligands on tumor cells. By increasing immunoregulatory cytokines like IL-10, proteobacteria in PDAC encourage immune evasion by reducing the polarization of IFNγ+ Th1 cells and shifting the growth of monocytes that infiltrate within the tumor toward an M2 phenotype [201]. Separate studies have shown improved and effective immunosurveillance of the malignant lesion when intratumoral activation of TLR2 [202], TLR6 [203], STING [204], and NOD1 [205] by MAMPs. A growing body of research also points to the possibility that microbes might operate centrally for activating local lymphocyte, leading to the formation of very beneficial tertiary lymphoid structures (TLSs). Notably, experimental colonization using *Helicobacter hepaticus* (Hhep) lowered a rat model's tumor burden by creating TLSs with a classical, germinal center [206]. Notably, these typical TLSs comprised Hhep as well as Hhep-specific T follicular helper (Tfh) cells, indicating

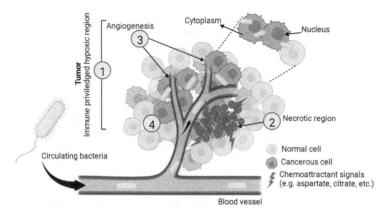

Fig. 25.5 Model of bacterial colonization in tumor tissue. Due to tumor tissue's intrinsic properties, the tumor foci provide a permissive environment to facilitate bacteria invasion, survival, and growth. (1) A hypoxic environment is common in tumor masses with low levels of oxygen which provides an advantage to the growth of certain bacterial species; (2) both the rapid cell proliferation and survival of bacteria are greatly benefited by necrotic tissue which are rich in nutrients (*i.e.,* purines). Similarly, the bacteria's extravasation is facilitated by many chemoattractant signals emerging from tumor necrotic areas; (3) new blood vessels surround the growing tissues as the tumor develops. Leaky vasculature around the tumor cells is a result of this angiogenic process which circulating bacteria take advantage of entering the tissues. Bacteria can proliferate both in intracellular and in extracellular compartments; (4) tumors evade the host immune surveillance by surrounding itself with immune cells which prevent tumor necrotic regions from expanding. This immune-privileged status is taken advantage by the colonizing bacteria to proliferate at ease while undisturbed by the host immune system

that intratumoral Hhep served as the main target of TLS-derived antitumor immunity. Compared to HPV-negative HNSCC, microbe-associated cancers like HPV-positive HNSCC feature a longer survival, heightened frequencies of TLS, and increased B-cell activities. Additionally, it has been shown that microbial peptides displayed on melanoma tumor cells' surface are identified by T cells [207]. According to these findings, the TME contains intratumoral microbial antigens which, in turn, could trigger strong immune responses locally, particularly in the TLS, where highly therapeutic and cross-functional immunity might be primed (Fig. 25.5).

Conclusion

To conquer the pathophysiological challenges in battling cancers, scientists should take every weapon within the arsenal of cancer therapy into account. Although conventional cancer treatments possess several benefits, based on the intricacy behind cancer pathophysiology, traditional treatments are still unsuccessful, leading to less than stellar cancer therapy; however, conventional treatments still possess precedence for the treatment of cancer. In light of the ecological view of cancer ecosystem, we should discover the purpose of microbiome in host, and how changes in the flora of host microbiome are directed toward cancer growth and metastasis. Although current improvements in single cell sequencing have increased our knowledge in this field, there are still many questions remaining, such as how did the microbiome changes in cancer progression? Are they directly involved in metastasis? What was the major communication pathway between microbiomes and cancer? Is microbiome-cancer a causal–effect relationship or vice versa? All these questions should be solved in order for us to fully understand the impact of host microbiome in cancer, and how to specifically target these microbiomes in cancer therapy.

References

1. Onuigbo WI (1975) Some nineteenth century ideas on links between tuberculous and cancerous diseases of the lung. Br J Dis Chest 69:207–210
2. Kung IT, Lui IO, Loke SL, Khin MA, Mok CK, Lam WK et al (1985) Pulmonary scar cancer. A pathologic reappraisal. Am J Surg Pathol 9(6):391–400
3. Browne M, Healy TM (1982) Coexisting carcinoma and active tuberculosis of the lung: 24 patients. Ir J Med Sci 151(3):75–78
4. Flance IJ (1991) Scar cancer of the lung. JAMA 266(14):2003–2004
5. Blaser MJ, Kirschner D (2007) The equilibria that allow bacterial persistence in human hosts. Nature 449(7164):843–849
6. Sun CA, Wu DM, Lin CC, Lu SN, You SL, Wang LY et al (2003) Incidence and cofactors of hepatitis C virus-related hepatocellular carcinoma: a prospective study of 12,008 men in Taiwan. Am J Epidemiol 157(8):674–682
7. Yu MW, Yeh SH, Chen PJ, Liaw YF, Lin CL, Liu CJ et al (2005) Hepatitis B virus genotype and DNA level and hepatocellular carcinoma: a prospective study in men. J Natl Cancer Inst 97(4):265–272
8. Bruno S, Crosignani A, Maisonneuve P, Rossi S, Silini E, Mondelli MU (2007) Hepatitis C virus genotype 1b as a major risk factor associated with hepatocellular carcinoma in patients with cirrhosis: a seventeen-year prospective cohort study. Hepatology 46(5):1350–1356
9. Figueiredo C, Machado JC, Pharoah P, Seruca R, Sousa S, Carvalho R et al (2002) Helicobacter pylori and interleukin 1 genotyping: an opportunity to identify high-risk individuals for gastric carcinoma. J Natl Cancer Inst 94(22):1680–1687
10. Castle PE, Jeronimo J, Schiffman M, Herrero R, Rodríguez AC, Bratti MC et al (2006) Age-related changes of the cervix influence human papillomavirus type distribution. Cancer Res 66(2):1218–1224
11. Wu HC, Wang Q, Wang LW, Yang HI, Ahsan H, Tsai WY et al (2007) Urinary 8-oxodeoxyguanosine, aflatoxin B1 exposure and hepatitis B virus infection and hepatocellular carcinoma in Taiwan. Carcinogenesis 28(5):995–999
12. Hsieh CC, Tzonou A, Zavitsanos X, Kaklamani E, Lan SJ, Trichopoulos D (1992) Age at first establishment of chronic hepatitis B virus infection and hepatocellular carcinoma risk. A birth order study. Am J Epidemiol 136(9):1115–1121
13. Blaser MJ, Nomura A, Lee J, Stemmerman GN, Perez-Perez GI (2007) Early-life family structure and microbially induced cancer risk. PLoS Med 4(1):e7
14. Chang YJ, Wu MS, Lin JT, Pestell RG, Blaser MJ, Chen CC (2006) Mechanisms for Helicobacter pylori CagA-induced cyclin D1 expression that affect cell cycle. Cell Microbiol 8(11):1740–1752
15. Blaser MJ (2008) Understanding microbe-induced cancers. Cancer Prev Res (Phila) 1(1): 15–20

16. Winkelstein JA, Tomasz A (1978) Activation of the alternative complement pathway by pneumococcal cell wall teichoic acid. J Immunol 120(1):174–178
17. Brown EJ, Hosea SW, Frank MM (1983) The role of antibody and complement in the reticuloendothelial clearance of pneumococci from the bloodstream. Rev Infect Dis 5(suppl 4):S797–S805
18. Abeyta M, Hardy GG, Yother J (2003) Genetic alteration of capsule type but not PspA type affects accessibility of surface-bound complement and surface antigens of Streptococcus pneumoniae. Infect Immun 71(1):218–225
19. Pluschke G, Mayden J, Achtman M, Levine RP (1983) Role of the capsule and the O antigen in resistance of O18:K1 Escherichia coli to complement-mediated killing. Infect Immun 42(3): 907–913
20. Geno KA, Gilbert GL, Song JY, Skovsted IC, Klugman KP, Jones C et al (2015) Pneumococcal capsules and their types: past, present, and future. Clin Microbiol Rev 28(3):871–899
21. Watson DA, Musher DM (1990) Interruption of capsule production in Streptococcus pneumonia serotype 3 by insertion of transposon Tn916. Infect Immun 58(9):3135–3138
22. Tran AX, Stead CM, Trent MS (2005) Remodeling of Helicobacter pylori lipopolysaccharide. J Endotoxin Res 11(3):161–166
23. Mattsby-Baltzer I, Mielniczuk Z, Larsson L, Lindgren K, Goodwin S (1992) Lipid A in Helicobacter pylori. Infect Immun 60(10):4383–4387
24. Gewirtz AT, Yu Y, Krishna US, Israel DA, Lyons SL, Peek RM Jr (2004) Helicobacter pylori flagellin evades toll-like receptor 5-mediated innate immunity. J Infect Dis 189(10): 1914–1920
25. Kawasaki K, Ernst RK, Miller SI (2004) 3-O-deacylation of lipid A by PagL, a PhoP/PhoQ-regulated deacylase of Salmonella typhimurium, modulates signaling through Toll-like receptor 4. J Biol Chem 279(19):20044–20048
26. Popp A, Billker O, Rudel T (2001) Signal transduction pathways induced by virulence factors of Neisseria gonorrhoeae. Int J Med Microbiol 291(4):307–314
27. Raibaud S, Schwarz-Linek U, Kim JH, Jenkins HT, Baines ER, Gurusiddappa S et al (2005) Borrelia burgdorferi binds fibronectin through a tandem beta-zipper, a common mechanism of fibronectin binding in staphylococci, streptococci, and spirochetes. J Biol Chem 280(19): 18803–18809
28. Meenan NA, Visai L, Valtulina V, Schwarz-Linek U, Norris NC, Gurusiddappa S et al (2007) The tandem beta-zipper model defines high affinity fibronectin-binding repeats within Staphylococcus aureus FnBPA. J Biol Chem 282(35):25893–25902
29. Polk DB, Peek RM Jr (2010) Helicobacter pylori: gastric cancer and beyond. Nat Rev Cancer 10(6):403–414
30. Tabassam FH, Graham DY, Yamaoka Y (2009) Helicobacter pylori activate epidermal growth factor receptor- and phosphatidylinositol 3-OH kinase-dependent Akt and glycogen synthase kinase 3beta phosphorylation. Cell Microbiol 11(1):70–82
31. Rubinstein MR, Wang X, Liu W, Hao Y, Cai G, Han YW (2013) Fusobacterium nucleatum promotes colorectal carcinogenesis by modulating E-cadherin/β-catenin signaling via its FadA adhesin. Cell Host Microbe 14(2):195–206
32. Castellarin M, Warren RL, Freeman JD, Dreolini L, Krzywinski M, Strauss J et al (2012) Fusobacterium nucleatum infection is prevalent in human colorectal carcinoma. Genome Res 22(2):299–306
33. Kostic AD, Gevers D, Pedamallu CS, Michaud M, Duke F, Earl AM et al (2012) Genomic analysis identifies association of Fusobacterium with colorectal carcinoma. Genome Res 22(2):292–298
34. Abreu MT (2010) Toll-like receptor signalling in the intestinal epithelium: how bacterial recognition shapes intestinal function. Nat Rev Immunol 10(2):131–144
35. Fink SP, Yamauchi M, Nishihara R, Jung S, Kuchiba A, Wu K et al (2014) Aspirin and the risk of colorectal cancer in relation to the expression of 15-hydroxyprostaglandin dehydrogenase (HPGD). Sci Transl Med 6(233):233re2

36. Adlercreutz H, Martin F, Pulkkinen M, Dencker H, Rimér U, Sjöberg NO et al (1976) Intestinal metabolism of estrogens. J Clin Endocrinol Metab 43(3):497–505
37. Murphy JR (2011) Mechanism of diphtheria toxin catalytic domain delivery to the eukaryotic cell cytosol and the cellular factors that directly participate in the process. Toxins 3(3): 294–308
38. Rosadi F, Fiorentini C, Fabbri A (2016) Bacterial protein toxins in human cancers. Pathog Dis 74(1):ftv105
39. Cuevas-Ramos G, Petit CR, Marcq I, Boury M, Oswald E, Nougayrède JP (2010) Escherichia coli induces DNA damage *in vivo* and triggers genomic instability in mammalian cells. Proc Natl Acad Sci U S A 107(25):11537–11542
40. Nougayrède JP, Homburg S, Taieb F, Boury M, Brzuszkiewicz E, Gottschalk G et al (2006) Escherichia coli induces DNA double-strand breaks in eukaryotic cells. Science 313(5788): 848–851
41. Dejea CM, Fathi P, Craig JM, Boleij A, Taddese R, Geis AL et al (2018) Patients with familial adenomatous polyposis harbor colonic biofilms containing tumorigenic bacteria. Science 359(6375):592–597
42. Buc E, Dubois D, Sauvanet P, Raisch J, Delmas J, Darfeuille-Michaud A et al (2013) High prevalence of mucosa-associated E. coli producing cyclomodulin and genotoxin in colon cancer. PloS One 8(2):e56964
43. Arthur JC, Perez-Chanona E, Mühlbauer M, Tomkovich S, Uronis JM, Fan TJ et al (2012) Intestinal inflammation targets cancer-inducing activity of the microbiota. Science 338(6103): 120–123
44. Sears CL (2009) Enterotoxigenic Bacteroides fragilis: a rogue among symbiotes. Clin Microbiol Rev 22(2):349–369, Table of Contents
45. Wu S, Rhee KJ, Zhang M, Franco A, Sears CL (2007) Bacteroides fragilis toxin stimulates intestinal epithelial cell shedding and gamma-secretase-dependent E-cadherin cleavage. J Cell Sci 120(pt 11):1944–1952
46. Nelson WJ, Nusse R (2004) Convergence of Wnt, beta-catenin, and cadherin pathways. Science 303(5663):1483–1487
47. Wu S, Powell J, Mathioudakis N, Kane S, Fernandez E, Sears CL (2004) Bacteroides fragilis enterotoxin induces intestinal epithelial cell secretion of interleukin-8 through mitogen-activated protein kinases and a tyrosine kinase-regulated nuclear factor-kappaB pathway. Infect Immun 72(10):5832–5839
48. Wu S, Lim KC, Huang J, Saidi RF, Sears CL (1998) Bacteroides fragilis enterotoxin cleaves the zonula adherens protein, E-cadherin. Proc Natl Acad Sci U S A 95(25):14979–14984
49. Rhee KJ, Wu S, Wu X, Huso DL, Karim B, Franco AA et al (2009) Induction of persistent colitis by a human commensal, enterotoxigenic Bacteroides fragilis, in wild-type C57BL/6 mice. Infect Immun 77(4):1708–1718
50. Wu S, Rhee KJ, Albesiano E, Rabizadeh S, Wu X, Yen HR et al (2009) A human colonic commensal promotes colon tumorigenesis via activation of T helper type 17 T cell responses. Nat Med 15(9):1016–1022
51. Toprak NU, Yagci A, Gulluoglu BM, Akin ML, Demirkalem P, Celenk T et al (2006) A possible role of Bacteroides fragilis enterotoxin in the aetiology of colorectal cancer. Clin Microbiol Infect 12(8):782–786
52. Nakayama M, Hisatsune J, Yamasaki E, Isomoto H, Kurazono H, Hatakeyama M et al (2009) Helicobacter pylori VacA-induced inhibition of GSK3 through the PI3K/Akt signaling pathway. J Biol Chem 284(3):1612–1619
53. Sokolova O, Bozko PM, Naumann M (2008) Helicobacter pylori suppresses glycogen synthase kinase 3beta to promote beta-catenin activity. J Biol Chem 283(43):29367–29374
54. Wang F, Meng W, Wang B, Qiao L (2014) Helicobacter pylori-induced gastric inflammation and gastric cancer. Cancer Lett 345(2):196–202

55. Xu X, Liu Z, Fang M, Yu H, Liang X, Li X et al (2012) Helicobacter pylori CagA induces ornithine decarboxylase upregulation via Src/MEK/ERK/c-Myc pathway: implication for progression of gastric diseases. Exp Biol Med (Maywood) 237(4):435–441
56. Fredlund J, Enninga J (2014) Cytoplasmic access by intracellular bacterial pathogens. Trends Microbiol 22(3):128–137
57. Senerovic L, Tsunoda SP, Goosmann C, Brinkmann V, Zychlinsky A, Meissner F et al (2012) Spontaneous formation of IpaB ion channels in host cell membranes reveals how Shigella induces pyroptosis in macrophages. Cell Death Dis 3(9):e384
58. Shaughnessy LM, Lipp P, Lee KD, Swanson JA (2007) Localization of protein kinase C epsilon to macrophage vacuoles perforated by Listeria monocytogenes cytolysin. Cell Microbiol 9(7):1695–1704
59. Henry R, Shaughnessy L, Loessner MJ, Alberti-Segui C, Higgins DE, Swanson JA (2006) Cytolysin-dependent delay of vacuole maturation in macrophages infected with Listeria monocytogenes. Cell Microbiol 8(1):107–119
60. Chong A, Wehrly TD, Nair V, Fischer ER, Barker JR, Klose KE et al (2008) The early phagosomal stage of Francisella tularensis determines optimal phagosomal escape and Francisella pathogenicity island protein expression. Infect Immun 76(12):5488–5499
61. Ozanic M, Marecic V, Abu Kwaik Y, Santic M (2015) The divergent intracellular lifestyle of Francisella tularensis in evolutionarily distinct host cells. PLoS Pathog 11(12):e1005208
62. Santic M, Asare R, Skrobonja I, Jones S, Abu KY (2008) Acquisition of the vacuolar ATPase proton pump and phagosome acidification are essential for escape of Francisella tularensis into the macrophage cytosol. Infect Immun 76(6):2671–2677
63. Tilney LG, Harb OS, Connelly PS, Robinson CG, Roy CR (2001) How the parasitic bacterium Legionella pneumophila modifies its phagosome and transforms it into rough ER: implications for conversion of plasma membrane to the ER membrane. J Cell Sci 114(pt 24):4637–4650
64. Nagai H, Kagan JC, Zhu X, Kahn RA, Roy CR (2002) A bacterial guanine nucleotide exchange factor activates ARF on Legionella phagosomes. Science 295(5555):679–682
65. Rajashekar R, Liebl D, Chikkaballi D, Liss V, Hensel M (2014) Live cell imaging reveals novel functions of Salmonella enterica SPI2-T3SS effector proteins in remodeling of the host cell endosomal system. PLoS One 9(12):e115423
66. Beuzón CR, Méresse S, Unsworth KE, Ruíz-Albert J, Garvis S, Waterman SR et al (2000) Salmonella maintains the integrity of its intracellular vacuole through the action of SifA. EMBO J 19(13):3235–3249
67. Stein MA, Leung KY, Zwick M, Garcia-del Portillo F, Finlay BB (1996) Identification of a Salmonella virulence gene required for formation of filamentous structures containing lysosomal membrane glycoproteins within epithelial cells. Mol Microbiol 20(1):151–164
68. Sindhwani A, Arya SB, Kaur H, Jagga D, Tuli A, Sharma M (2017) Salmonella exploits the host endolysosomal tethering factor HOPS complex to promote its intravacuolar replication. PLoS Pathog 13(10):e1006700
69. Mughini-Gras L, Schaapveld M, Kramers J, Mooij S, Neefjes-Borst EA, Pelt WV et al (2018) Increased colon cancer risk after severe Salmonella infection. PloS One 13(1):e0189721
70. Scanu T, Spaapen RM, Bakker JM, Pratap CB, Wu LE, Hofland I et al (2015) Salmonella manipulation of host signaling pathways provokes cellular transformation associated with gallbladder carcinoma. Cell Host Microbe 17(6):763–774
71. Lu R, Bosland M, Xia Y, Zhang YG, Kato I, Sun J (2017) Presence of Salmonella AvrA in colorectal tumor and its precursor lesions in mouse intestine and human specimens. Oncotarget 8(33):55104–55115
72. Lu R, Wu S, Zhang YG, Xia Y, Zhou Z, Kato I et al (2016) Salmonella protein AvrA activates the STAT3 signaling pathway in colon cancer. Neoplasia 18(5):307–316
73. Sun J, Hobert ME, Rao AS, Neish AS, Madara JL (2004) Bacterial activation of beta-catenin signaling in human epithelia. Am J Physiol Gastrointest Liver Physiol 287(1):G220–G227
74. Ye Z, Petrof EO, Boone D, Claud EC, Sun J (2007) Salmonella effector AvrA regulation of colonic epithelial cell inflammation by deubiquitination. Am J Pathol 171(3):882–892

75. Lu R, Wu S, Zhang YG, Xia Y, Liu X, Zheng Y et al (2014) Enteric bacterial protein AvrA promotes colonic tumorigenesis and activates colonic beta-catenin signaling pathway. Oncogenesis 3(6):e105

76. Jones RM, Wu H, Wentworth C, Luo L, Collier-Hyams L, Neish AS (2008) Salmonella AvrA coordinates suppression of host immune and apoptotic defenses via JNK pathway blockade. Cell Host Microbe 3(4):233–244

77. Orth K, Palmer LE, Bao ZQ, Stewart S, Rudolph AE, Bliska JB et al (1999) Inhibition of the mitogen-activated protein kinase kinase superfamily by a Yersinia effector. Science 285(5435):1920–1923

78. Trosky JE, Li Y, Mukherjee S, Keitany G, Ball H, Orth K (2007) VopA inhibits ATP binding by acetylating the catalytic loop of MAPK kinases. J Biol Chem 282(47):34299–34305

79. Trosky JE, Mukherjee S, Burdette DL, Roberts M, McCarter L, Siegel RM et al (2004) Inhibition of MAPK signaling pathways by VopA from Vibrio parahaemolyticus. J Biol Chem 279(50):51953–51957

80. Fehr D, Casanova C, Liverman A, Blazkova H, Orth K, Dobbelaere D et al (2006) AopP, a type III effector protein of Aeromonas salmonicida, inhibits the NF-kappaB signalling pathway. Microbiology 152(pt 9):2809–2818

81. Hannemann S, Gao B, Galán JE (2013) Salmonella modulation of host cell gene expression promotes its intracellular growth. PLoS Pathog 9(10):e1003668

82. Kuijl C, Savage ND, Marsman M, Tuin AW, Janssen L, Egan DA et al (2007) Intracellular bacterial growth is controlled by a kinase network around PKB/AKT1. Nature 450(7170): 725 730

83. Zitvogel L, Galluzzi L, Viaud S, Vetizou M, Daillere R, Merad M et al (2015) Cancer and the gut microbiota: an unexpected link. Sci Transl Med 7(271):271ps1

84. Schwabe RF, Jobin C (2013) The microbiome and cancer. Nat Rev Cancer 13(11):800–812

85. Maynard CL, Elson CO, Hatton RD, Weaver CT (2012) Reciprocal interactions of the intestinal microbiota and immune system. Nature 489(7415):231–241

86. Touchefeu Y, Montassier E, Nieman K, Gastinne T, Potel G, Bruley des Varannes S et al (2014) Systematic review: the role of the gut microbiota in chemotherapy- or radiation-induced gastrointestinal mucositis - current evidence and potential clinical applications. Aliment Pharmacol Ther 40(5):409–421

87. Von Bültzingslöwen I, Adlerberth I, Wold AE, Dahlén G, Jontell M (2003) Oral and intestinal microflora in 5-fluorouracil treated rats, translocation to cervical and mesenteric lymph nodes and effects of probiotic bacteria. Oral Microbiol Immunol 18(5):278–284

88. Jenq RR, Ubeda C, Taur Y, Menezes CC, Khanin R, Dudakov JA et al (2012) Regulation of intestinal inflammation by microbiota following allogeneic bone marrow transplantation. J Exp Med 209(5):903–911

89. Nam YD, Kim HJ, Seo JG, Kang SW, Bae JW (2013) Impact of pelvic radiotherapy on gut microbiota of gynecological cancer patients revealed by massive pyrosequencing. PloS One 8(12):e82659

90. Lam W, Bussom S, Guan F, Jiang Z, Zhang W, Gullen EA et al (2010) The four-herb Chinese medicine PHY906 reduces chemotherapy-induced gastrointestinal toxicity. Sci Transl Med 2(45):45ra59

91. Wallace BD, Wang H, Lane KT, Scott JE, Orans J, Koo JS et al (2010) Alleviating cancer drug toxicity by inhibiting a bacterial enzyme. Science 330(6005):831–835

92. Viaud S, Saccheri F, Mignot G, Yamazaki T, Daillère R, Hannani D et al (2013) The intestinal microbiota modulates the anticancer immune effects of cyclophosphamide. Science 342(6161):971–976

93. Iida N, Dzutsev A, Stewart CA, Smith L, Bouladoux N, Weingarten RA et al (2013) Commensal bacteria control cancer response to therapy by modulating the tumor microenvironment. Science 342(6161):967–970

94. Park EM, Chelvanambi M, Bhutiani N, Kroemer G, Zitvogel L, Wargo JA (2022) Targeting the gut and tumor microbiota in cancer. Nat Med 28(4):690–703

95. Dong ZY, Zhong WZ, Zhang XC, Su J, Xie Z, Liu SY et al (2017) Potential predictive value of TP53 and KRAS mutation status for response to PD-1 blockade immunotherapy in lung adenocarcinoma. Clin Cancer Res 23(12):3012–3024
96. Bodor JN, Boumber Y, Borghaei H (2020) Biomarkers for immune checkpoint inhibition in non-small cell lung cancer (NSCLC). Cancer 126(2):260–270
97. Liu D, Schilling B, Liu D, Sucker A, Livingstone E, Jerby-Arnon L et al (2019) Integrative molecular and clinical modeling of clinical outcomes to PD1 blockade in patients with metastatic melanoma. Nat Med 25(12):1916–1927
98. Ayers M, Lunceford J, Nebozhyn M, Murphy E, Loboda A, Kaufman DR et al (2017) IFN-γ-related mRNA profile predicts clinical response to PD-1 blockade. J Clin Invest 127(8):2930–2940
99. Le DT, Uram JN, Wang H, Bartlett BR, Kemberling H, Eyring AD et al (2015) PD-1 blockade in tumors with mismatch-repair deficiency. N Engl J Med 372(26):2509–2520
100. Morad G, Helmink BA, Sharma P, Wargo JA (2021) Hallmarks of response, resistance, and toxicity to immune checkpoint blockade. Cell 184(21):5309–5337
101. Yonekura S, Terrisse S, Alves Costa Silva C, Lafarge A, Iebba V, Ferrere G et al (2022) Cancer induces a stress ileopathy depending on β-adrenergic receptors and promoting dysbiosis that contributes to carcinogenesis. Cancer Discov 12(4):1128–1151
102. Routy B, Le Chatelier E, Derosa L, Duong CPM, Alou MT, Daillere R et al (2018) Gut microbiome influences efficacy of PD-1-based immunotherapy against epithelial tumors. Science 359(6371):91–97
103. Gopalakrishnan V, Spencer CN, Nezi L, Reuben A, Andrews MC, Karpinets TV et al (2018) Gut microbiome modulates response to anti-PD-1 immunotherapy in melanoma patients. Science 359(6371):97–103
104. Baruch EN, Youngster I, Ben-Betzalel G, Ortenberg R, Lahat A, Katz L et al (2021) Fecal microbiota transplant promotes response in immunotherapy-refractory melanoma patients. Science 371(6529):602–609
105. Davar D, Dzutsev AK, McCulloch JA, Rodrigues RR, Chauvin JM, Morrison RM et al (2021) Fecal microbiota transplant overcomes resistance to anti-PD-1 therapy in melanoma patients. Science 371(6529):595–602
106. Spencer CN, McQuade JL, Gopalakrishnan V, McCulloch JA, Vetizou M, Cogdill AP et al (2021) Dietary fiber and probiotics influence the gut microbiome and melanoma immunotherapy response. Science 374(6575):1632–1640
107. Blake SJ, James J, Ryan FJ, Caparros-Martin J, Eden GL, Tee YC et al (2021) The immunotoxicity, but not anti-tumor efficacy, of anti-CD40 and anti-CD137 immunotherapies is dependent on the gut microbiota. Cell Rep Med 2(12):100464
108. Andrews MC, Duong CPM, Gopalakrishnan V, Iebba V, Chen WS, Derosa L et al (2021) Gut microbiota signatures are associated with toxicity to combined CTLA-4 and PD-1 blockade. Nat Med 27(8):1432–1441
109. Wang DD, Nguyen LH, Li Y, Yan Y, Ma W, Rinott E et al (2021) The gut microbiome modulates the protective association between a Mediterranean diet and cardiometabolic disease risk. Nat Med 27(2):333–343
110. Goubet AG, Wheeler R, Fluckiger A, Qu B, Lemaître F, Iribarren K et al (2021) Multifaceted modes of action of the anticancer probiotic Enterococcus hirae. Cell Death Differ 28(7): 2276–2295
111. Roberti MP, Yonekura S, Duong CPM, Picard M, Ferrere G, Tidjani Alou M et al (2020) Chemotherapy-induced ileal crypt apoptosis and the ileal microbiome shape immunosurveillance and prognosis of proximal colon cancer. Nat Med 26(6):919–931
112. Griffin ME, Espinosa J, Becker JL, Luo JD, Carroll TS, Jha JK et al (2021) Enterococcus peptidoglycan remodeling promotes checkpoint inhibitor cancer immunotherapy. Science 373(6558):1040–1046
113. Hanahan D (2022) Hallmarks of Cancer: new dimensions. Cancer Discov 12(1):31–46

114. Vétizou M, Pitt JM, Daillère R, Lepage P, Waldschmitt N, Flament C et al (2015) Anticancer immunotherapy by CTLA-4 blockade relies on the gut microbiota. Science 350(6264): 1079–1084

115. Sivan A, Corrales L, Hubert N, Williams JB, Aquino-Michaels K, Earley ZM et al (2015) Commensal Bifidobacterium promotes antitumor immunity and facilitates anti-PD-L1 efficacy. Science 350(6264):1084–1089

116. Matson V, Fessler J, Bao R, Chongsuwat T, Zha Y, Alegre ML et al (2018) The commensal microbiome is associated with anti-PD-1 efficacy in metastatic melanoma patients. Science 359(6371):104–108

117. Derosa L, Routy B, Desilets A, Daillère R, Terrisse S, Kroemer G et al (2021) Microbiota-centered interventions: the next breakthrough in immuno-oncology? Cancer Discov 11(10): 2396–2412

118. Plovier H, Everard A, Druart C, Depommier C, Van Hul M, Geurts L et al (2017) A purified membrane protein from Akkermansia muciniphila or the pasteurized bacterium improves metabolism in obese and diabetic mice. Nat Med 23(1):107–113

119. Yoon HS, Cho CH, Yun MS, Jang SJ, You HJ, Kim JH et al (2021) Akkermansia muciniphila secretes a glucagon-like peptide-1-inducing protein that improves glucose homeostasis and ameliorates metabolic disease in mice. Nat Microbiol 6(5):563–573

120. Grajeda-Iglesias C, Durand S, Daillère R, Iribarren K, Lemaitre F, Derosa L et al (2021) Oral administration of Akkermansia muciniphila elevates systemic antiaging and anticancer metabolites. Aging 13(5):6375–6405

121. Fluckiger A, Daillère R, Sassi M, Sixt BS, Liu P, Loos F et al (2020) Cross-reactivity between tumor MHC class I-restricted antigens and an enterococcal bacteriophage. Science 369(6506): 936–942

122. Bessell CA, Isser A, Havel JJ, Lee S, Bell DR, Hickey JW et al (2020) Commensal bacteria stimulate antitumor responses via T cell cross-reactivity. JCI Insight 5(8):e135597

123. Bouskra D, Brézillon C, Bérard M, Werts C, Varona R, Boneca IG et al (2008) Lymphoid tissue genesis induced by commensals through NOD1 regulates intestinal homeostasis. Nature 456(7221):507–510

124. Chen GY, Shaw MH, Redondo G, Núñez G (2008) The innate immune receptor Nod1 protects the intestine from inflammation-induced tumorigenesis. Cancer Res 68(24):10060–10067

125. Lam KC, Araya RE, Huang A, Chen Q, Di Modica M, Rodrigues RR et al (2021) Microbiota triggers STING-type I IFN-dependent monocyte reprogramming of the tumor microenvironment. Cell 184(21):5338–56 e21

126. Ge Y, Wang X, Guo Y, Yan J, Abuduwaili A, Aximujiang K et al (2021) Gut microbiota influence tumor development and alter interactions with the human immune system. J Exp Clin Cancer Res 40(1):42

127. Huhta H, Helminen O, Lehenkari PP, Saarnio J, Karttunen TJ, Kauppila JH (2016) Toll-like receptors 1, 2, 4 and 6 in esophageal epithelium, Barrett's esophagus, dysplasia and adenocarcinoma. Oncotarget 7(17):23658–23667

128. Abt MC, Osborne LC, Monticelli LA, Doering TA, Alenghat T, Sonnenberg GF et al (2012) Commensal bacteria calibrate the activation threshold of innate antiviral immunity. Immunity 37(1):158–170

129. Kamada N, Seo SU, Chen GY, Núñez G (2013) Role of the gut microbiota in immunity and inflammatory disease. Nat Rev Immunol 13(5):321–335

130. Lathrop SK, Bloom SM, Rao SM, Nutsch K, Lio CW, Santacruz N et al (2011) Peripheral education of the immune system by colonic commensal microbiota. Nature 478(7368): 250–254

131. Pabst O, Herbrand H, Friedrichsen M, Velaga S, Dorsch M, Berhardt G et al (2006) Adaptation of solitary intestinal lymphoid tissue in response to microbiota and chemokine receptor CCR7 signaling. J Immunol 177(10):6824–6832

132. Bauer H, Horowitz RE, Levenson SM, Popper H (1963) The response of the lymphatic tissue to the microbial flora. Studies on germfree mice. Am J Pathol 42(4):471–483

133. Flores R, Shi J, Fuhrman B, Xu X, Veenstra TD, Gail MH et al (2012) Fecal microbial determinants of fecal and systemic estrogens and estrogen metabolites: a cross-sectional study. J Transl Med 10:253
134. Fuhrman BJ, Feigelson HS, Flores R, Gail MH, Xu X, Ravel J et al (2014) Associations of the fecal microbiome with urinary estrogens and estrogen metabolites in postmenopausal women. J Clin Endocrinol Metab 99(12):4632–4640
135. Pernigoni N, Zagato E, Calcinotto A, Troiani M, Mestre RP, Calì B et al (2021) Commensal bacteria promote endocrine resistance in prostate cancer through androgen biosynthesis. Science 374(6564):216–224
136. Mager LF, Burkhard R, Pett N, Cooke NCA, Brown K, Ramay H et al (2020) Microbiome-derived inosine modulates response to checkpoint inhibitor immunotherapy. Science 369(6510):1481–1489
137. Legoux F, Bellet D, Daviaud C, El Morr Y, Darbois A, Niort K et al (2019) Microbial metabolites control the thymic development of mucosal-associated invariant T cells. Science 366(6464):494–499
138. Ruf B, Catania VV, Wabitsch S, Ma C, Diggs LP, Zhang Q et al (2021) Activating mucosal-associated invariant T cells induces a broad antitumor response. Cancer Immunol Res 9(9): 1024–1034
139. Westman EL, Canova MJ, Radhi IJ, Koteva K, Kireeva I, Waglechner N et al (2012) Bacterial inactivation of the anticancer drug doxorubicin. Chem Biol 19(10):1255–1264
140. Yan A, Culp E, Perry J, Lau JT, MacNeil LT, Surette MG et al (2018) Transformation of the anticancer drug doxorubicin in the human gut microbiome. ACS Infect Dis 4(1):68–76
141. Geller LT, Barzily-Rokni M, Danino T, Jonas OH, Shental N, Nejman D et al (2017) Potential role of intratumor bacteria in mediating tumor resistance to the chemotherapeutic drug gemcitabine. Science 357(6356):1156–1160
142. Bindels LB, Porporato P, Dewulf EM, Verrax J, Neyrinck AM, Martin JC et al (2012) Gut microbiota-derived propionate reduces cancer cell proliferation in the liver. Br J Cancer 107(8):1337–1344
143. Kim K, Kwon O, Ryu TY, Jung CR, Kim J, Min JK et al (2019) Propionate of a microbiota metabolite induces cell apoptosis and cell cycle arrest in lung cancer. Mol Med Rep 20(2): 1569–1574
144. Belcheva A, Irrazabal T, Robertson SJ, Streutker C, Maughan H, Rubino S et al (2014) Gut microbial metabolism drives transformation of MSH2-deficient colon epithelial cells. Cell 158(2):288–299
145. Bultman SJ (2014) Molecular pathways: gene-environment interactions regulating dietary fiber induction of proliferation and apoptosis via butyrate for cancer prevention. Clin Cancer Res 20(4):799–803
146. He Y, Fu L, Li Y, Wang W, Gong M, Zhang J et al (2021) Gut microbial metabolites facilitate anticancer therapy efficacy by modulating cytotoxic CD8(+) T cell immunity. Cell Metab 33(5):988–1000.e7
147. Mazmanian SK, Liu CH, Tzianabos AO, Kasper DL (2005) An immunomodulatory molecule of symbiotic bacteria directs maturation of the host immune system. Cell 122(1):107–118
148. Khan U, Ho K, Hwang EK, Peña C, Brouwer J, Hoffman K et al (2021) Impact of use of antibiotics on response to immune checkpoint inhibitors and tumor microenvironment. Am J Clin Oncol 44(6):247–253
149. Huemer F, Rinnerthaler G, Lang D, Hackl H, Lamprecht B, Greil R (2019) Association between antibiotics use and outcome in patients with NSCLC treated with immunotherapeutics. Ann Oncol 30(4):652–653
150. Zheng Y, Wang T, Tu X, Huang Y, Zhang H, Tan D et al (2019) Gut microbiome affects the response to anti-PD-1 immunotherapy in patients with hepatocellular carcinoma. J Immunother Cancer 7(1):193

151. Peng Z, Cheng S, Kou Y, Wang Z, Jin R, Hu H et al (2020) The gut microbiome is associated with clinical response to anti-PD-1/PD-L1 immunotherapy in gastrointestinal cancer. Cancer Immunol Res 8(10):1251–1261
152. Mao J, Wang D, Long J, Yang X, Lin J, Song Y et al (2021) Gut microbiome is associated with the clinical response to anti-PD-1 based immunotherapy in hepatobiliary cancers. J Immunother Cancer 9(12):e003334
153. Salgia NJ, Bergerot PG, Maia MC, Dizman N, Hsu J, Gillece JD et al (2020) Stool microbiome profiling of patients with metastatic renal cell carcinoma receiving anti-PD-1 immune checkpoint inhibitors. Eur Urol 78(4):498–502
154. Derosa L, Routy B, Fidelle M, Iebba V, Alla L, Pasolli E et al (2020) Gut bacteria composition drives primary resistance to cancer immunotherapy in renal cell carcinoma patients. Eur Urol 78(2):195–206
155. Jin Y, Dong H, Xia L, Yang Y, Zhu Y, Shen Y et al (2019) The diversity of gut microbiome is associated with favorable responses to anti-programmed death 1 immunotherapy in Chinese patients with NSCLC. J Thorac Oncol 14(8):1378–1389
156. Cascone T, William WN Jr, Weissferdt A, Leung CH, Lin HY, Pataer A et al (2021) Neoadjuvant nivolumab or nivolumab plus ipilimumab in operable non-small cell lung cancer: the phase 2 randomized NEOSTAR trial. Nat Med 27(3):504–514
157. Hakozaki T, Richard C, Elkrief A, Hosomi Y, Benlaïfaoui M, Mimpen I et al (2020) The gut microbiome associates with immune checkpoint inhibition outcomes in patients with advanced non-small cell lung cancer. Cancer Immunol Res 8(10):1243–1250
158. Derosa L, Routy B, Thomas AM, Iebba V, Zalcman G, Friard S et al (2022) Intestinal Akkermansia muciniphila predicts clinical response to PD-1 blockade in patients with advanced non-small-cell lung cancer. Nat Med 28(2):315–324
159. Lee KA, Thomas AM, Bolte LA, Björk JR, de Ruijter LK, Armanini F et al (2022) Cross-cohort gut microbiome associations with immune checkpoint inhibitor response in advanced melanoma. Nat Med 28(3):535–544
160. Gharaibeh RZ, Jobin C (2019) Microbiota and cancer immunotherapy: in search of microbial signals. Gut 68(3):385–388
161. Holler E, Butzhammer P, Schmid K, Hundsrucker C, Koestler J, Peter K et al (2014) Metagenomic analysis of the stool microbiome in patients receiving allogeneic stem cell transplantation: loss of diversity is associated with use of systemic antibiotics and more pronounced in gastrointestinal graft-versus-host disease. Biol Blood Marrow Transplant 20(5):640–645
162. Jenq RR, Taur Y, Devlin SM, Ponce DM, Goldberg JD, Ahr KF et al (2015) Intestinal Blautia is associated with reduced death from graft-versus-host disease. Biol Blood Marrow Transplant 21(8):1373–1383
163. Biagi E, Zama D, Nastasi C, Consolandi C, Fiori J, Rampelli S et al (2015) Gut microbiota trajectory in pediatric patients undergoing hematopoietic SCT. Bone Marrow Transplant 50(7):992–998
164. Biagi E, Zama D, Rampelli S, Turroni S, Brigidi P, Consolandi C et al (2019) Early gut microbiota signature of aGvHD in children given allogeneic hematopoietic cell transplantation for hematological disorders. BMC Med Genomics 12(1):49
165. Wang A, Ling Z, Yang Z, Kiela PR, Wang T, Wang C et al (2015) Gut microbial dysbiosis may predict diarrhea and fatigue in patients undergoing pelvic cancer radiotherapy: a pilot study. PloS One 10(5):e0126312
166. Mitra A, Grossman Biegert GW, Delgado AY, Karpinets TV, Solley TN, Mezzari MP et al (2020) Microbial diversity and composition is associated with patient-reported toxicity during chemoradiation therapy for cervical cancer. Int J Radiat Oncol Biol Phys 107(1):163–171
167. Chang CW, Lee HC, Li LH, Chiang Chiau JS, Wang TE, Chuang WH et al (2020) Fecal microbiota transplantation prevents intestinal injury, upregulation of toll-like receptors, and 5-fluorouracil/oxaliplatin-induced toxicity in colorectal cancer. Int J Mol Sci 21(2):386

168. Xiao HW, Cui M, Li Y, Dong JL, Zhang SQ, Zhu CC et al (2020) Gut microbiota-derived indole 3-propionic acid protects against radiation toxicity via retaining acyl-CoA-binding protein. Microbiome 8(1):69

169. Cui M, Xiao H, Li Y, Zhou L, Zhao S, Luo D et al (2017) Faecal microbiota transplantation protects against radiation-induced toxicity. EMBO Mol Med 9(4):448–461

170. Wang F, Yin Q, Chen L, Davis MM (2018) Bifidobacterium can mitigate intestinal immuno-pathology in the context of CTLA-4 blockade. Proc Natl Acad Sci U S A 115(1):157–161

171. Ma B, Forney LJ, Ravel J (2012) Vaginal microbiome: rethinking health and disease. Annu Rev Microbiol 66:371–389

172. Schommer NN, Gallo RL (2013) Structure and function of the human skin microbiome. Trends Microbiol 21(12):660–668

173. Dickson RP, Huffnagle GB (2015) The lung microbiome: new principles for respiratory bacteriology in health and disease. PLoS Pathog 11(7):e1004923

174. O'Dwyer DN, Dickson RP, Moore BB (2016) The lung microbiome, immunity, and the pathogenesis of chronic lung disease. J Immunol 196(12):4839–4847

175. Pflughoeft KJ, Versalovic J (2012) Human microbiome in health and disease. Annu Rev Pathol 7:99–122

176. Glassing A, Dowd SE, Galandiuk S, Davis B, Chiodini RJ (2016) Inherent bacterial DNA contamination of extraction and sequencing reagents may affect interpretation of microbiota in low bacterial biomass samples. Gut Pathog 8:24

177. Eisenhofer R, Minich JJ, Marotz C, Cooper A, Knight R, Weyrich LS (2019) Contamination in low microbial biomass microbiome studies: issues and recommendations. Trends Microbiol 27(2):105–117

178. Laurence M, Hatzis C, Brash DE (2014) Common contaminants in next-generation sequencing that hinder discovery of low-abundance microbes. PloS One 9(5):e97876

179. Colgan DF, Manley JL (1997) Mechanism and regulation of mRNA polyadenylation. Genes Dev 11(21):2755–2766

180. Sender R, Fuchs S, Milo R (2016) Revised estimates for the number of human and bacteria cells in the body. PLoS Biol 14(8):e1002533

181. Davis NM, Proctor DM, Holmes SP, Relman DA, Callahan BJ (2018) Simple statistical identification and removal of contaminant sequences in marker-gene and metagenomics data. Microbiome 6(1):226

182. Nejman D, Livyatan I, Fuks G, Gavert N, Zwang Y, Geller LT et al (2020) The human tumor microbiome is composed of tumor type-specific intracellular bacteria. Science 368(6494): 973–980

183. Barrett M, Hand CK, Shanahan F, Murphy T, O'Toole PW (2020) Mutagenesis by microbe: the role of the microbiota in shaping the cancer genome. Trends Cancer 6(4):277–287

184. He Z, Gharaibeh RZ, Newsome RC, Pope JL, Dougherty MW, Tomkovich S et al (2019) Campylobacter jejuni promotes colorectal tumorigenesis through the action of cytolethal distending toxin. Gut 68(2):289–300

185. Maddocks OD, Scanlon KM, Donnenberg MS (2013) An Escherichia coli effector protein promotes host mutation via depletion of DNA mismatch repair proteins. MBio 4(3):e00152–e00113

186. Kim JJ, Tao H, Carloni E, Leung WK, Graham DY, Sepulveda AR (2002) Helicobacter pylori impairs DNA mismatch repair in gastric epithelial cells. Gastroenterology 123(2):542–553

187. Santos JC, Brianti MT, Almeida VR, Ortega MM, Fischer W, Haas R et al (2017) Helicobacter pylori infection modulates the expression of miRNAs associated with DNA mismatch repair pathway. Mol Carcinog 56(4):1372–1379

188. Yin H, Qu J, Peng Q, Gan R (2019) Molecular mechanisms of EBV-driven cell cycle progression and oncogenesis. Med Microbiol Immunol 208(5):573–583

189. Chung L, Thiele Orberg E, Geis AL, Chan JL, Fu K, DeStefano Shields CE et al (2018) Bacteroides fragilis toxin coordinates a pro-carcinogenic inflammatory cascade via targeting of colonic epithelial cells. Cell Host Microbe 23(2):203–14.e5

190. Lee JA, Yoo SY, Oh HJ, Jeong S, Cho NY, Kang GH et al (2021) Differential immune microenvironmental features of microsatellite-unstable colorectal cancers according to Fusobacterium nucleatum status. Cancer Immunol Immunother 70(1):47–59
191. Lopès A, Billard E, Casse AH, Villéger R, Veziant J, Roche G et al (2020) Colibactin-positive Escherichia coli induce a procarcinogenic immune environment leading to immunotherapy resistance in colorectal cancer. Int J Cancer 146(11):3147–3159
192. Hoste E, Arwert EN, Lal R, South AP, Salas-Alanis JC, Murrell DF et al (2015) Innate sensing of microbial products promotes wound-induced skin cancer. Nat Commun 6:5932
193. Aykut B, Pushalkar S, Chen R, Li Q, Abengozar R, Kim JI et al (2019) The fungal mycobiome promotes pancreatic oncogenesis via activation of MBL. Nature 574(7777):264–267
194. Yao L, Jiang L, Zhang F, Li M, Yang B, Zhang F et al (2020) Acetate promotes SNAI1 expression by ACSS2-mediated histone acetylation under glucose limitation in renal cell carcinoma cell. Biosci Rep 40(6):BSR20200382
195. Rossi T, Vergara D, Fanini F, Maffia M, Bravaccini S, Pirini F (2020) Microbiota-derived metabolites in tumor progression and metastasis. Int J Mol Sci 21(16):5786
196. Yoshimoto S, Loo TM, Atarashi K, Kanda H, Sato S, Oyadomari S et al (2013) Obesity-induced gut microbial metabolite promotes liver cancer through senescence secretome. Nature 499(7456):97–101
197. Vitiello GA, Cohen DJ, Miller G (2019) Harnessing the microbiome for pancreatic cancer immunotherapy. Trends Cancer 5(11):670–676
198. Seifert L, Werba G, Tiwari S, Giao Ly NN, Alothman S, Alqunaibit D et al (2016) The necrosome promotes pancreatic oncogenesis via CXCL1 and Mincle induced immune suppression. Nature 532(7598):245–249
199. Das S, Shapiro B, Vucic EA, Vogt S, Bar-Sagi D (2020) Tumor cell-derived IL1β promotes desmoplasia and immune suppression in pancreatic cancer. Cancer Res 80(5):1088–1101
200. Maisonneuve C, Tsang DKL, Foerster EG, Robert LM, Mukherjee T, Prescott D et al (2021) Nod1 promotes colorectal carcinogenesis by regulating the immunosuppressive functions of tumor-infiltrating myeloid cells. Cell Rep 34(4):108677
201. Pushalkar S, Hundeyin M, Daley D, Zambirinis CP, Kurz E, Mishra A et al (2018) The pancreatic cancer microbiome promotes oncogenesis by induction of innate and adaptive immune suppression. Cancer Discov 8(4):403–416
202. Deng Y, Yang J, Qian J, Liu R, Huang E, Wang Y et al (2019) TLR1/TLR2 signaling blocks the suppression of monocytic myeloid-derived suppressor cell by promoting its differentiation into M1-type macrophage. Mol Immunol 112:266–273
203. Kim JH, Kordahi MC, Chac D, DePaolo RW (2020) Toll-like receptor-6 signaling prevents inflammation and impacts composition of the microbiota during inflammation-induced colorectal cancer. Cancer Prev Res (Phila) 13(1):25–40
204. Shi Y, Zheng W, Yang K, Harris KG, Ni K, Xue L et al (2020) Intratumoral accumulation of gut microbiota facilitates CD47-based immunotherapy via STING signaling. J Exp Med 217(5):e20192282
205. da Silva CJ, Miranda Y, Austin-Brown N, Hsu J, Mathison J, Xiang R et al (2006) Nod1-dependent control of tumor growth. Proc Natl Acad Sci U S A 103(6):1840–1845
206. Overacre-Delgoffe AE, Bumgarner HJ, Cillo AR, Burr AHP, Tometich JT, Bhattacharjee A et al (2021) Microbiota-specific T follicular helper cells drive tertiary lymphoid structures and anti-tumor immunity against colorectal cancer. Immunity 54(12):2812–24.e4
207. Kalaora S, Nagler A, Nejman D, Alon M, Barbolin C, Barnea E et al (2021) Identification of bacteria-derived HLA-bound peptides in melanoma. Nature 592(7852):138–143

Chapter 26
Systemic *Onco-Spheres*: Viruses in Cancer

Phei Er Saw and Erwei Song

Abstract It was recently estimated that a virus infection is the central cause of more than 1,400,000 cancer cases annually, representing approximated 10% of the worldwide cancer burden. DNA viruses that have been confirmed to cause cancer are Epstein–Barr virus (EBV), hepatitis B virus (HBV), human papillomavirus (HPV), and human herpesvirus 8 (HSV-8). Some examples of cancer-causing RNA viruses are the human T lymphotropic virus type 1 (HTLV-1) and hepatitis C virus (HCV). The study of viruses and human cancer has sparked hope for developing novel ways to prevent cancer-causing viral infection. In this chapter, we decipher the general mechanism of cancer-causing virus and their general principles. We also summarize the common mechanism of direct and indirect carcinogenesis caused by virus infection.

P. E. Saw
Guangdong Provincial Key Laboratory of Malignant Tumor Epigenetics and Gene Regulation, Guangdong-Hong Kong Joint Laboratory for RNA Medicine, Medical Research Center, Sun Yat-sen Memorial Hospital, Sun Yat-sen University, Guangzhou, China

Nanhai Translational Innovation Center of Precision Immunology, Sun Yat-sen Memorial Hospital, Sun Yat-sen University, Foshan, China

E. Song (✉)
Guangdong Provincial Key Laboratory of Malignant Tumor Epigenetics and Gene Regulation, Guangdong-Hong Kong Joint Laboratory for RNA Medicine, Medical Research Center, Sun Yat-sen Memorial Hospital, Sun Yat-sen University, Guangzhou, China

Nanhai Translational Innovation Center of Precision Immunology, Sun Yat-sen Memorial Hospital, Sun Yat-sen University, Foshan, China

Breast Tumor Center, Sun Yat-sen Memorial Hospital, Sun Yat-sen University, Guangzhou, China
e-mail: songew@mail.sysu.edu.cn

Introduction

Viruses are thought to be responsible for around 15% of all human malignancies globally, accounting for a substantial quantity of the global cancer burden. It has been demonstrated that human cancers may be caused by DNA and RNA viruses. DNA viruses that have been confirmed to cause cancer are Epstein–Barr virus (EBV), hepatitis B virus (HBV), human papillomavirus (HPV), and human herpesvirus 8 (HSV-8). Some examples of cancer-causing RNA viruses are the human T lymphotropic virus type 1 (HTLV-1) and hepatitis C virus (HCV). The study of viruses and human cancer has sparked hope for developing novel ways to prevent cancer-causing viral infection in the first place. The accumulation of viral gene copies in the cancer cells—which are crucial in allowing uncontrolled cancer proliferation—can serve as the key targets in targeted treatments and as gene markers to differentiate cancer cells from healthy cells. Standard cancer therapies including chemotherapy and radiation treatment are limited by its failure to discriminate healthy cells from cancer cells, which pose as a major side effect for patients. On the other hand, targeted treatments or immune therapy only destroys cancer cells infected with viral genes while preserving the healthy cells, therefore presenting greater potential for more effective and tolerable treatments [1].

Viruses: A History in Epidemiology

At the start of the twentieth century, scientists began to notice a possible etiological relationship between cancer and viral infection [2]. Ellermann and Bang in 1908, and Peyton Rous in 1911, both succeeded in transmitting cancer (avian leukemia and sarcomas, respectively) via tumor agents; this indicated that cancer could have a viral etiology [3–5]. The first human cancer-causing virus was found half a century later. The Epstein–Barr virus (EBV) was named after its discoverers, Sir Anthony Epstein, Bert Achong, and Yvonne Barr, who isolated the virus particles in cultured lymphoblasts from equatorial African pediatric patients with Burkitt's lymphoma [6]. Further experiments proved that endemic Burkitt's lymphoma and other tumors were caused by EBV in the subsequent years. Scientists today have a clear understanding that several types of viruses are carcinogenic to humans by the virtue of decades of research work put into the study of cancer virology.

Harald zur Hausen was awarded the Medicine Nobel Prize in 2008 for discovering HPV as the cause of cervical cancer, marking the end of the first century of cancer virology researcher [7, 8]. The International Agency for Research on Cancer (IARC) has categorized EBV, Kaposi's sarcoma-associated herpesvirus (KSHV), high-risk HPV, Merkel cell polyomavirus (MCPV), HBV, HCV, and HTLV1 as Group 1 human carcinogens, which are most likely to cause cancers [9]. Viral infections are thought to account for around 15% of cancer incidences globally and one-fifth of the cases in developing regions [10]. It is highly plausible that incidence of cancer will continue to rise as new technologies to identify genetic information become more commonly available. Oncogenic viruses coordinate multiple premalignant events that are associated with its life cycle and thereby mediate the development of cancer.

The biological framework gained from the study of cancer virology can be applied in understanding cancer pathogenesis of both infectious and non-infectious etiology. However, changing the conventional scientific thinking to embrace the role of oncogenic viruses in carcinogenesis proved challenging, owing to the biological mechanisms involved not conforming to Koch's postulates [11]. Due to cancer's complicated origin and the fact that oncogenic viruses are prevalent but dormant in the general population, Koch's initial discoveries concerning the spread of acute infectious agents are hardly applicable to cancer. The relationship between oncogenic virus and cancer can be better explained using the Bradford–Hill criteria, which were first suggested to prove a causal association between smoking and lung cancer [12].

Scientists also acknowledged that none of the Bradford–Hill criteria can conclusively prove causality on their own and that compliance with all of them is not required to accept the relationship between oncogenic virus and cancer. In fact, if we look at the global geographical distribution of Burkitt's lymphoma and EBV, they do not match that of each other. But we do know that malaria—endemic to equatorial Africa just like Burkitt's lymphoma—is a major trigger to the development of Burkitt's lymphoma [13]. If the oncogenic virus is detectable in the cancer cells and not in the adjacent cells, and if there is valid evidence linking the viral infection to cancer, then according to Bradford–Hill criteria, the causality between the oncogenic virus and cancer is deemed established. EBV is found in B lymphocytes of the upper gastrointestinal tract, which has been linked to B-cell lymphomas and tumors in gastric cavity, tongue, and nasopharynx. Furthermore, transgenic animals with EBV latent proteins also develop tumors [14]. Such findings fulfilled the logical reasoning required in the Bradford–Hill criteria.

Viruses Associated with Human Cancers

Human tumor viruses are conveniently grouped and studied together despite belonging to different viral families that have highly distinct life cycles and genomes. The progression from infection to cancer is slow and only occurs in a small proportion of the infected population, taking up to years or decades to manifest after the initial infection. Merely infected with oncogenic viruses are largely insufficient for cancer to develop. Additional oncogenic hits are required for oncogenesis, such as host genetics, contact with carcinogens, mutations, and immunosuppression.

Hepatitis B and C Viruses

Hepatitis B virus (HBV) is a member of the Hepadnaviridae family, a DNA virus that also infects liver cells. HBV also is transmitted via blood route, leading to both acute and chronic hepatitis in infected individuals. HBV or HCV infection that is longer than 3 months is considered as chronic hepatitis and can lead to cirrhosis, liver failure, and development of hepatocellular carcinoma [15]. Each year, about 2 billion individuals are infected with HBV and roughly 1.2 million died from consequences of the infection, including hepatitis, cirrhosis, and hepatocellular carcinoma, marking HBV infection as a major health concern worldwide [16]. Hepatitis C virus (HCV) is a human flavivirus, an enveloped RNA virus that infects liver cells and causes acute and chronic hepatitis in human, and roughly 3% of the global population are carriers [14]. Long-term HCV infection is a major cause of cirrhosis, which can result in the development of hepatocellular carcinoma. About 1% to 2% of HCV patients with compensated cirrhosis develop hepatocellular carcinoma every year [17]. HCV is transmitted primarily via exposure to blood, sharing of intravenous drug-use needles, sexual activities, and during birth from mother to child.

Hepatocellular carcinoma is an invasive primary tumor of the liver that can develop in the presence of chronic liver illness caused by HBV or HCV infection, albeit the specific mechanism is unknown. Generally, patients with HCC are diagnosed only until the later stages of the disease and their median survival are about 6–20 months after diagnosis [18]. The conventional treatment for HCC is surgery, such as resection of tumor or liver transplantation. Depending on the severity of the disease and the patient's remaining liver function, other treatment options for HCC include percutaneous injection of ethanol, transarterial chemoembolization (TACE), local ablation with radiofrequency, and radiation therapy [19, 20]. Targeted therapy and virus-based immunotherapy are novel treatment approaches that focus on avoiding oncogenic infection. However, in the case of HCV, vaccines against HCV yield poor result due to its highly mutagenic viral genome, particularly in the envelope proteins which could be unrecognizable by vaccine-induced immune response. Currently, eleven distinct genotypes of HCV have been identified. In contrast, vaccines against HBV have yielded great success, setting a milestone in history as the "first cancer prevention vaccine" in the 1980s with effective prevention against hepatitis.

According to the World Health Organization (WHO), over 110 countries have started immunization programs against HBV for all infants, and a sharp drop in carrier rate and infection rate was observed in the fully immunized population [21]. Unfortunately, HBV immunization coverage remains low in many developing nations because of limited healthcare resources to administer vaccines, financial challenges, and logistic challenges to deliver all three doses over a period of 6 months. Universal immunization program has not been introduced, even in developed countries, due to the notion that it is a minor public health issue for which the cost is not justified [22, 23]. Between 2005 and 2010, the World Health Organization predicts that $8 to $12 billion would be required to immunize children in the poorest nations, spurring governmental and private efforts to campaign for funding. Interferon is used to treat hepatitis B by inhibiting viral replication, and those who respond to treatment will have lower risk of developing severe complications of hepatitis [24]. IFN-α treatment can effectively induce shedding of HBV antigen in 20% to 30% of HBV patients. But the effect of IFN-α therapy on HCC development is unclear [25, 26]. The limitations of interferon therapy include its side effects and cost, which have been partially mitigated with the introduction of targeted antiviral agents. Lamivudine, anti-HBV agents, has been demonstrated to be associated with lower rate of hepatic decompensation and lower risk of developing HCC in large multi-center randomized controlled trial [27]. Adefovir, entecavir, and telbivudine are among other effective anti-HBV agents used clinically to treat hepatitis B. Nucleotide analogs represent a class of antiviral agents that targets the DNA replication machinery of HBV, specifically the reverse transcriptase, and is better tolerated as oral medications are available. Despite that genotypic resistance could be caused by long-term use of lamivudine [28], the benefits of lamivudine therapy in lowering HCC risk outweigh its side effects.

Patients with HBV-induced severe cirrhosis can now be treated and transplanted without developing HBV in the transplanted liver owning to the efficacy of these antiviral agents. In contrast, pharmacological therapeutics for HCV advances at a slower rate. Studies have shown that pegylated interferon with ribavirin, an anti-HCV agent, may operate as a nucleoside analog and also block the RNA-dependent RNA polymerase of HCV, has effectively eliminated HCV infection in 50% of the cases [29]. The drawbacks of this therapy include its high cost and substantial adverse effects. Oral antivirals like protease inhibitors and polymerase inhibitors are now undergoing Phase II studies [30]. In contrast to HBV, HCC caused by HCV infection nearly always led to recurrence of HCV infection in the transplanted liver [31]. For many years, the absence of an efficient experimental infection model for HCV, such as in vitro cell culture or animal models, has hindered progress in developing targeted drugs against HCV viral replication. Recently, the discovery of viral replicons—viral RNAs at sub-genomic level that are capable of self-replication—has allowed researchers to investigate HCV replication in human hepatoma cells [32] and to develop mouse models for HCV [33, 34]. These breakthroughs should pave the way for faster development of virally targeted medicines, including drugs that can specifically inhibit HCV proteases and polymerases.

Epstein–Barr Virus (EBV) and Human Herpesvirus 8 (HHV-8)

EBV (or HHV-4) and HHV-8 (or Kaposi's sarcoma-associated herpesvirus, KSHV) belongs to the herpesvirus family. Similar to all members of the herpesvirus family, both EBV and HHV-8 have a large double-stranded DNA genome, encode enzymes for replicating viral DNA and synthesizing proteins, and can persist latently in B cells for later reactivation into the lytic cycle. These two herpesviruses are also known to cause cancers in human. EBV is highly prevalent in the human population and is popularly known for causing infectious mononucleosis. Although about 95% of the adult population is EBV+, most infection are asymptomatic. EBV has been linked to several types of human cancer, including lymphomas (B-cell, T-cell, or Hodgkin's lymphoma), post-transplant lymphoproliferative disease, leiomyosarcomas, and nasopharyngeal carcinomas. Immunosurveillance has been suggested to strongly influence malignant transformation as immunocompromised patients exhibit higher risk of developing Burkitt's lymphoma, post-transplant lymphoproliferative disease or leiomyosarcomas. EBV infection primarily targets the oropharyngeal cavity, in which both B cells and epithelial cells could be infected [35]. Gp350/220 is the major surface glycoprotein on EBV envelope and it specifically binds to cellular receptor CD21 of B cells. EBV can efficiently transform B cells, utilizing a significant proportion of its genome during the process. EBV genome circularizes during latency and replication. With the lytic cycle suppressed, EBV will enter the latent gene expression stage, producing latent gene products which immortalized B cells.

To circumvent the traditional therapy of using multi-agent chemotherapy, radiation, and surgery, researchers have been focusing on developing immunotherapy for EBV-associated tumors. This new strategy involves the adoptive transfer of EBV-specific cytotoxic T cells into the patient [36, 37] and has demonstrated success albeit several issues remain to be solved, including the risk of developing graft versus host disease, and therapeutic resistance caused by EBV epitope mutation [38]. Currently, vaccines that can prevent EBV infection or increase immune responses against EBV-related malignancies are still in development. Most of the vaccines in development target the gp350/220 subunits [39] because the subunits are present in great quantity on the EBV viral envelope and they are also the target site of the neutralizing antibody of the host immune system [40]. Another approach is to produce an EBV membrane antigen using a recombinant vaccinia virus vector [41]. An effective vaccination would be most impactful in areas of the world where certain cancers are more common.

For instance, Burkitt's lymphoma has the highest incidence among childhood cancers found in Africa, in which its cancer development is highly associated with EBV and malaria infection. Data showed that up to 95% of children in Africa are infected by 3 years old, whereas in the United States, infection generally occurs later in adolescents [42]. Another example is nasopharyngeal carcinoma, which has a strikingly high incidence in southern China as compared to the rest of the world, with an incidence rate of almost 20 times that of the other population [43]. Kaposi sarcoma was relatively rare before AIDS became prevalent, but in 1994, the gene products of HHV-8 were isolated from tumor samples obtained from a Kaposi sarcoma patient [44]. This suggested that HHV-8 infection is likely to contribute to the development of Kaposi sarcoma. Furthermore, other studies suggested that HHV-8 is involved in the pathogenesis of Castleman's disease and primary effusion lymphoma [45]. These tumors express viral genes which encode for transforming proteins and anti-apoptotic factors and promote the growth of microvascular endothelial cells [46]. EBV mostly infects B cells, and in this case, the lytic cycle is induced. This suggests that we can potentially alter the disease development of Kaposi sarcoma through influencing the production of viral and host cytokines that drive cell growth, angiogenesis, and viral propagation.

Antiviral drugs that target viral DNA replication, such as ganciclovir, have drastically reduced the incidence of Kaposi sarcoma in AIDS patients, both as treatment and as prevention [47]. Ganciclovir is phosphorylated to produce a GTP analog, which competitively inhibits the viral DNA polymerase, causing viral DNA elongation to stop. In addition, in HHV-8-infected cells, a G protein-coupled receptor (vGPCR) has been discovered as a viral oncogene that can use cell signaling pathways to drive carcinogenesis and angiogenesis [48]. Because of its critical role in cancer development, vGPCR has also been recommended as a target for innovative molecular therapeutics [49]. However, given it was the introduction of HIV that led to the growing prevalence of Kaposi sarcoma, the effectiveness of highly active antiretroviral treatment (HAART) regimens targeting HIV may possibly be the therapeutic regimen most liable for the lowering incidence of Kaposi sarcoma [50].

Human Papillomavirus (HPV)

Benign papilloma and warts in human are commonly caused by human papillomavirus (HPV), a small DNA virus without viral envelope, and chronic HPV infection with high-risk subtypes is often related to cervical cancer development [51]. HPV infection begins when the virus enters epithelial cells and integrates its DNA into the host genome, and produces oncoproteins, primarily E6 and E7, which impair the normal tumor suppressor mechanism and allow cervical cancer cells to proliferate [52]. Furthermore, HPV is postulated to have a role in the development of other cancers in human, including cancers of the head and neck region, skin of immunocompromised patients, and the anogenital area.

Cervical cancer is the second leading cause of cancer death in women globally, claiming the lives of 240,000 women each year [53]. More than 80% of the 490,000 cases reported each year occur in underdeveloped countries due to the lack of Pap smear screening test which are highly effective but expensive. Pap smears can reveal early precancerous changes and malignancies, which can be efficiently managed and healed with surgical intervention or ablation. Without an effective screening program, cervical diseases and malignancies are diagnosed late, and the available treatment options for cervical cancers that have progressed beyond definitive surgical treatment are chemotherapy and radiation, but these options come with a slew of side effects and do not provide a long-term cure. The latency of chronic HPV infection and its advancement of precancerous lesions are largely dependent on the response of our immune system. HPV per se is a poor immunogen. Since HPV is a double-stranded DNA virus, it does not need to produce RNA intermediate or trigger cytolysis during infection, and this allows for innate immune response to occur [54]. The majority of viral proteins produced by HPV are non-secretory nucleoproteins, which exhibit poor uptake and cross-presentation by antigen-presenting cells. HPV expresses relatively low levels of non-structural proteins. Insufficient immune cell responses may also result in the inability to remove diseased cells infected with HPV. A higher rate of HPV persistency, anogenital lesions, and cervical cancer is often observed in patients with acquired immunodeficiency syndrome (AIDS), transplant patients on immunosuppressants, and those with T-cell deficiency [55–58].

In 2006, FDA approved the use of prophylactic HPV vaccines against subtype-16 and subtype-18, which was engineered based on virus-like particles (VLP) of the major capsid protein recombinant L1 to induce production of high levels of neutralizing antibodies [59, 60] and had displayed almost 100% effectiveness in preventing persistent infection in clinical trials. As these two subtypes of HPV are responsible for around 70% of cervical malignancies, developing an effective vaccination offers a lot of potential for cervical cancer prevention. Surgical excision or ablation is the standard treatment for early cervical cancer and precancerous lesions. The goal of therapeutic vaccination is to create a population of cytotoxic T lymphocytes that can detect and kill cancer cells. As patients with T-cell deficiency are more vulnerable to HPV infection and malignant transformation, increasing T-cell responses to HPV might be critical in a therapeutic immunological approach. In cervical cancer, E6 and E7 oncoproteins are exclusively expressed in all cancer cells but not in uninfected healthy cells. As a result, E6 and E7 are good candidates for a therapeutic immune response and different ways to elicit immune responses to these antigens are being researched. In addition to E6 and E7 oncoproteins, viral and bacterial vectors have also been used in mouse models to elicit immune responses. HPV16/18-E6/E7 proteins delivered via vaccinia virus had indicated safety and targeted immune responses in early clinical studies [61]. Treatment approaches using DNA vaccine are also being researched, with a number of them in different stages of clinical trials. When administered in individuals with high-grade cervical dysplasia, vaccines based on plasmid DNA enveloped in biodegradable microparticles showed histological and immunological responses [62–64].

Human T Lymphotropic Virus Type I (HTLV-1)

HTLV-1 is a single-stranded RNA retrovirus that is linked to adult T-cell leukemia (ATL), involving a slow transformation process [65]. Like other retroviruses, HTLV-1 has a diploid genome which consists of two long terminal repeats surrounding the gag, pol, and env genes, regulatory genes, and other accessory genes. HTLV-1 is found all over the world with approximately 12 to 25 million cases of infection globally, but it is only symptomatic in less than 5% of the infected cases. The mode of transmission of HTLV-1 is through blood transfusion, sexual contact, and during birth from the mother. HTLV-1 has a distinct affinity for CD4 cells, which clonally expand in adult T-cell leukemia, despite the mechanism is still unclear. The latency period for HTLV-1 infection is 20 to 30 years; however, once tumor growth begins, it progresses quickly. An initial response with a partial or complete remission can be achieved with standard chemotherapy, but ATL patients are likely to relapse and the median survival is around 8 months. Tax gene of the HTLV-1 virus has been hypothesized to have a key role in carcinogenesis [66] by promoting the transcription of viral genes and hijacking of host cell machinery to regulate cellular growth and cell division, although the exact pathway that leads to adult T-cell leukemia remains unclear. Some suggested that the carcinogenesis process to transform into adult T-cell leukemia requires more than mere HTLV-1 infection, and new findings have pointed toward HTLV-1-specific CD8 T cells that exhibit reduced diversity, frequency, and function [67]. To elicit neutralizing antibodies against HTLV-1 and to induce a multivalent cytotoxic T-cell response to Tax proteins, various targeted therapeutics are being investigated, including those using peptide, recombinant protein, DNA, and viral vectors [1, 68].

Merkel Cell Polyomavirus (MCV)

In 2008, Merkel cell polyomavirus (MCV) from Merkel cell carcinoma (MCC), a rare type of aggressive skin tumor was identified. Epidemiological data record around 1600 new cases of MCC every year in the United States, which translates to an annual incidence rate of 0.06% (0.6 case in a population of 100,000 individuals), and a 5-year mortality rate of around 46%. The median age of MCC diagnosis is above 70 years old, and it is exceedingly rare in children and is seldom identified below 50 years old (approximately 4% of cases). MCV's oncogenic mechanism is unknown, although the rise in MCC cases in response to UV irradiation suggests that faulty DNA repair mechanisms may be involved in the transformation process. Furthermore, the higher prevalence of MCC seen in AIDS patients or solid organ transplant recipients, as well as reports of tumor regression following improved immune function, has suggested that decreased immunity may play a role in the development of MCC. MCV requires additional co-factors and induction of immunosuppression to cause MCC, and further research is necessary to assess its oncogenic potential [69].

General Principles of Viral Oncogenic Mechanisms

Oncogenic viruses usually cause chronic infection and remain latent in the lifetime of the host, maintaining its insidious presence by synthesizing minimal or no viral products. This characteristic viral latency parallels the key mechanism of cancer development, where infected cells evade apoptosis during the lytic phase and escape from host immune surveillance for a long time, by integrating its viral genetic information into the host cell genome or by synthesizing viral proteins that distribute the viral genome evenly among daughter cells during cell partitioning. Oncogenic viruses sustain infection in a regulated number of cells by expressing proteins that govern cellular growth and death; in this way, oncogenic viruses establish a balanced virus-host relationship and persist chronically in host tissue. Cell transformation is an uncommon occurrence in the relationship between virus and host cells, rather than an approach developed from generations of evolution. Host death due to cancer also signifies the death of the virus. The occurrence of viral oncogenes is discussed in the context of the mechanism of viral latency, whereby cancer development is only initiated when certain conditions are met. Cancer caused by oncogenic viruses is the consequence of a complex chain of events that includes more than just chronic infection and viral transformation, that is, further oncogenic hits are required to achieve full-fledged malignant transformation. Mutations that convert (viral or host) protooncogenes into oncogenes are essential during the development of cancer, consistent with this view, infected cells have a higher mutation rate than healthy cells [70, 71]. Cells infected by oncogenic virus may be more vulnerable to further oncogenic hits such as carcinogen exposure, smoking, and poor diet. The stress load of viral infection on the host cells and the host cells' response by spiking up inflammation, together, culminate in malignant transformation and propel host tissue toward cancer growth.

Direct and Indirect Viral Carcinogenesis

Cancer-causing infectious pathogens can be divided into two groups based on their mechanism of carcinogenesis: direct or indirect (Figs. 26.1 and 26.2, respectively). Under the direct mechanism, oncogenic viruses within the cancer cells are usually present in monoclonal form and serve to preserve the cancer phenotype through

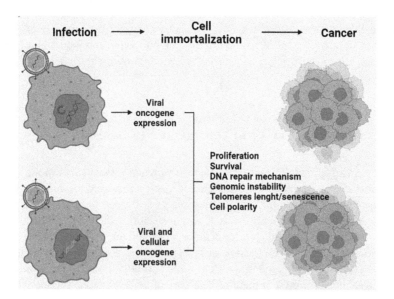

Fig. 26.1 Direct mechanisms of viral carcinogenesis. First, oncogenic viruses infect target host cells and preserve itself as viral genome in either two forms, as an episome like herpesviruses (as shown in the upper panel) or as part of the host genome via integration (as shown in the lower panel) for retroviruses and HBV. Under the indirect mechanism, the oncogenic virus does not generate or effect cancer directly from the host cell it resides; instead, it exerts its carcinogenic influence via two pathways: (1) inducing chronic inflammation and oxidative stress, which harm local tissues over time, and (2) causing immunosuppression, which lower or remove the host's immune surveillance. Notable examples of inflammation-inducing oncogenic virus are HBV and HCV, which produce chronic hepatitis infection in human and contribute to high risk factor for hepatocellular cancer. Concomitant infection of HIV with EBV or KSV suppresses the host's immunity and significantly diminishes the CD4 count, leading to the development of lymphomas

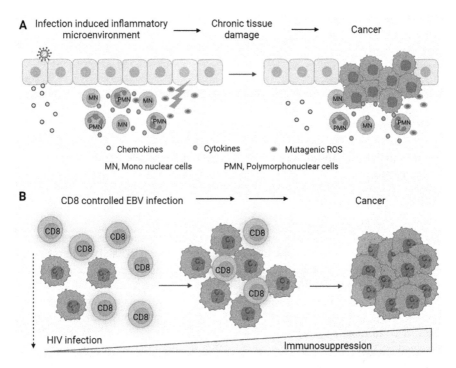

Fig. 26.2 Indirect mechanisms of viral carcinogenesis. (**a**) Chronic inflammation. Chemokines produced by virus-infected host cells trigger an inflammatory response and recruit immune cells to the site of infection. This established a chronically inflamed microenvironment where local tissues are constantly being injured and repairing itself, allowing cancer to arise from the tissue damaged-repaired cycles. (**b**) Immunosuppression. HIV is the classic virus for causing immunosuppression. Generally, EBV infection can be well managed by cytotoxic CD8 T cells in immunocompetent individuals. But in immunocompromised individuals like those infected with HIV, their immunity deteriorates significantly; if such individuals acquire EBV infection, they are at a higher risk of developing lymphomas

expressing the viral or cellular oncogenes [9]. One example is retroviruses, which integrate its viral genome into the host genome during replication, and frequently undergo transformation as insertional mutagenesis takes place when the retrovirus inserts into the sequence of oncogenes or tumor suppressor genes. Another example is EBV, which on the contrary, transforms via expressing its own viral oncogenes without integrating and hijacking the host's oncogenes.

Previously, oncogenic viruses were thought to act through either direct or indirect mechanism, but some viruses like HBV and HCV can employ both direct and indirect mechanisms in its carcinogenesis [72, 73]. *H. pylori*, a classic oncogenic pathogen that causes cancer via indirect mechanism (by inducing chronic inflammation) [74], also directly encodes its own oncoproteins—CagA oncoprotein, which translocates to the epithelial cells through a protein complex across the bacterium cell envelope call type IV secretion systems [75]. As a result, direct and indirect mechanisms may be complementary strategies of the oncogenic pathogens to induce malignant transformation in organs like liver and stomach.

Common Mechanisms of Direct Carcinogenesis

Viral Oncogenes and Oncoproteins

p53 and pRb Inactivation and Other Targets of Increased Proliferation and Survival

Viral oncogenes frequently boost cell growth and resistance to cell death. This results in changes to DNA repair and jeopardize genomic stability, in which accelerated rate of mutation shifts cell polarity, leading to uncontrolled cell proliferation and accumulation of genotypes that enables cell migration, and encourages the acquisition of malignant traits required for mature cancer to develop. Similar mechanisms may be employed by different viruses to cause these biological alterations, and they frequently share overlapping signaling pathways or transcription factors. The mechanism of inactivating p53 and pRb tumor suppressor genes, for example, takes place in most human and animal viral oncogenesis [76–78]. When DNA is damaged, p53 induces cell cycle arrest for DNA repair; if the repair is not initiated or incomplete, p53 will trigger cell death or senescence [79, 80]. On the other hand, pRb blocks the cell cycle by inhibiting transcription factors from the E2F family; specifically, pRb stops the cell cycle from transitioning from G1 phase to S phase when DNA is damaged [78]. The inactivation of p53 and pRb tumor suppressor genes, therefore, allows genetic mutations and chromosomal abnormalities to accumulate easily. Oncogenic viruses rely on accelerated cell proliferation to enlarge their existing pool of infected cells because they are not generally linked to huge generation of viral infectious molecules that usually define viruses that cause acute infection. If p53 and pRb proteins are not inactivated, they may detect the terminal ends of the viral genome (nick DNA) and trigger cell death shortly after viral infection. The viral E6 and E7 oncoproteins of HPV cause p53 and pRb tumor suppressor proteins to be degraded, respectively. E6 oncoprotein binds to the E6-associated protein (E6AP) to form the E6/E6AP complex, which can then bind to p53, resulting in ubiquitination-mediated degradation of p53 [81, 82]; E6 also accelerates cell growth by suppressing p16INK4, an inhibitor of cell cycle [83]. On the other hand, E7 interacts with the pRb/E2F1–3 complex and frees E2F1–3, in which E2F1–3 transcription factors promote the transcription of cell cycle-related genes including cyclin E and A [84, 85]. pRb is hyperphosphorylated by HTVL-1 Tax, which promotes its breakdown in the proteosome [86]. Although less well known, Tax alters p53 activity in a variety of ways, including hyperphosphorylation, indirect competitive binding with cellular co-activators, and NFκB-mediated direct binding [87]. The expression level of cyclins and cyclin-dependent kinases is altered by the viral Tax protein [88–90]. HBZ, another HTLV-1-encoded protein, stimulates T-cell proliferation by causing overexpression of E2F1 target genes [91]. Through its interaction with CDK6, LANA-1 protein of KSHV inactivates p53 and pRb tumor suppressor proteins via triggering phosphorylation of pRb [92–94]. The majority of the latency III proteins produced by EBV-infected cells inactivate p53 and pRb and interact with a set of cell proliferation-mediating proteins, namely HA95, HAX1, cyclin A and D, p27kip1, p16INK4A, and c-Myc [95]. The processes that control cell cycle progression and cell survival are intertwined. In addition to targeting p53 and pRb inactivation, oncogenic viruses usually activate numerous pathways to ensure their survival. In EBV-infected cells, the NFκB and PI3K/Akt signaling pathways were activated by LMP-1 and LMP-2A viral proteins to increase expression of antiapoptotic proteins Bcl-2, Bcl-X, Mcl-1, and A20 [96–98]. BHRF1, a viral Bcl-2 homologue encoded by EBV, appears to block the proapoptotic activity of c-Myc in a subset of Burkitt's lymphoma [99]. In individuals infected with HTLV-1, the viral proteins p12 and p13 control the activity of Bcl-2 and caspase 3 and 9, while Tax proteins activate the NFκB and PI3K/Akt signaling pathways [100]. In HPV-infected individuals, E6 and E7 proteins increase the expression of antiapoptotic proteins (c-IAP2 and surviving) while decreasing the number of proapoptotic proteins (pro-caspase 8, FADD and BAK) [101–105]. E6 proteins degrade proapoptotic proteins through associating with E6AP ubiquitin ligase, which attracts proapoptotic proteins to the proteasome. HBx protein encoded by HBV binds to cellular damaged DNA binding protein 1 (DDB1) to evade apoptosis through blocking the function of proteasome [106]. Protein cores and NS5A protein of HCV have been reported to play key roles in the antiapoptotic mechanism [107]. Developing multiple antiapoptotic mechanisms is the first step to escape purging by the host's defense, which is crucial to the viral latency and cancer formation.

Genomic Instability

Genomic instability, which results in gene amplification and deletion, alterations in chromosome numbers (such as polyploidy and aneuploidy), and abnormal fusion of non-homologous chromosomes (translocation), is another typical carcinogenic mechanism favored by oncogenic viruses. HPV-16 E6 and E7 proteins, for example, cause aneuploidy and polyploidy by promoting gene amplification, structural changes in chromosomes, and defects in centrosome replication. As a result, HPV-infected cells show addition or deletion of entire chromosomes [108–111] and aneuploidy can be detected in HPV-related lesions before metastasis [112]. HBV HBx protein influences genomic instability by forming HBx/HBXIP complexes which modifies the formation of mitotic spindles, leading to abnormality in centrosome function. In EBV-infected cells, viral protein EBNA-1 triggers genomic instability by activating recombinase-activating genes RAG-1 and RAG-2 [9], which are thought to induce translocation of the Myc chromosome in Burkitt's lymphoma [113]. EBV-mediated expression of activation-induced cytidine deaminase (AID) enzyme is highly associated with genomic instability, evident by the increase in mutation rate at variable areas of heavy and light chains following EBV infection [114]. It is likely that AID enzyme also promotes EBV-induced transformation, although it is still unclear whether AID enzyme targets other areas of the host genome. In HTLV-1-infected cells, Tax protein has been linked to a mutator phenotype, with both minor and major alterations in DNA and chromosomes frequently observed [115, 116]. Tax proteins affect genomic instability in two mechanisms: by impairing DNA repair during the transition phase from G2 to M phase via multiple targets, which allow cells to accumulate mutations [117]; and by inducing chromosomal instability via inhibition of transcriptional factors involved in DNA repair during cell cycle, such as the DNA polymerase β enzyme which is responsible for base-excision repair. Tax proteins also inhibit the nucleotide excision repair pathway, which is typically activated by ultraviolet ray exposure [118]. Tax proteins are hypothesized to cause aneuploidy in adult T-cell lymphoma (ATL) cells, by the inactivation of the spindle assembly checkpoint (SAC) kinetochore protein (MAD-1) that mediates chromosomal segregation during mitosis [119]. In cells infected with HTLV-1, Tax proteins prematurely activate the CDC20-associated anaphase promoting complex in the cell cycle [120]. All these mechanisms would contribute to the failure of proper chromosomal segregation during mitosis, leading to an abnormal number of chromosomes in HTLV-1-infected cells.

Interfering with Telomere Shortening

Normal cells undergo telomere shortening with every cycle of DNA replication and eventual cell senescence, but oncogenic viruses are capable of maintaining the telomere length of the host chromosome, potentially permitting unlimited cell turnover. The length of the telomere is maintained in equilibrium by regulatory proteins and the telomerase enzyme [121]. Under normal circumstances, telomerase do not function in differentiated cells and only lengthens the telomere of stem cells. A group of viral-induced oncoproteins have demonstrated the ability to trigger telomerase expression, including HPV E6, EBV LMP-1, KSHV LANA, HTLV-1 Tax protein, and HBV HBx protein, although the exact mechanism remains unclear [122–125]. Oncogenic viruses grant its infected cells with the ability to escape cell cycle regulatory checkpoints, interfere with telomere length, and disrupt cell senescence processes regulated by p53 and pRb, which ultimately result in genomic instability and a defective DNA repair mechanism [126]. Therefore, oncogenic viruses have developed with these capabilities to attain limitless cell replication and consequently to induce long latent infection in its host.

Interfering with Cell Polarity

Human virus oncoproteins may interfere with cell polarity by inhibiting regulatory proteins and this helps to facilitate carcinogenesis. In cells infected with adenovirus-9, the viral oncoprotein E4-ORF1 was first reported to have a class I PDZ-binding motif (PBM) that can target and bind PDZ domains. PDZ domain-containing proteins structurally support membranous and cytosolic supramolecular complexes, control cell-to-cell interaction, and regulate cell signaling through interaction with PBM. PBM was later reported in HPV E6 and HTLV-1 Tax protein [127–130]. The HPV E6 PBM is required for E6-mediated transformation in experimental models in vivo and in vitro [131, 132]. The HTVL-1 Tax protein PBM, however, could lower Tax-mediated transformation if the binding domain becomes mutated, and diminish HTVL-1's ability to cause chronic infection [133, 134]. Oncogenic viruses inactivate and inhibit the underlying proteins responsible for maintaining cell polarity, resulting in abnormal cell growth, cell division, cell migration, and cell differentiation, which ultimately create an environment conducive to the development of cancer.

Viral miRNAs

The normal expression of miRNAs has been tampered with in practically all types of cancer [135, 136]. Currently, virus-encoded oncogenic miRNAs are a topic of concern in the field of viral oncology and were first identified in the EBV B95 cell line. More than 40 miRNAs derived from EBV BARTs and BHFR1 transcripts have been discovered thus far [137, 138]. Some of these miRNAs were shown to target tumor suppressor genes (such as WIF1, PUMA, Bin, and TOMM22 genes) and facilitate the infected cells in escaping programmed cell death [139–142]. In EBV-infected gastric carcinoma cells, the lesion could achieve anchorage independence—a malignant feature—without viral proteins. This suggests that viral miRNAs from EBV play a critical role in its carcinogenesis [143].

Insertional Mutagenesis

The life cycle of retroviruses involves the integration of its genetic sequence into the host cell genome (known as a provirus following this process) and the replication of viral gene as part of the host genome. Long terminal repeats (LTRs), which are potent transcriptional activators that frequently influence the activation of cellular genes in the insertion region, control the expression of the provirus. LTRs increase the expression of a host protooncogene when the provirus inserts itself nearby, resulting in oncogenic consequences. Although protooncogene overexpression is the most well-known cause of cell transformation, retroviruses have the capacity to disrupt tumor suppressor genes with comparable results [144]. When the provirus is replicated along with the host genome, its progeny often contains host oncogenes near the insertion area, which are transduced to new host cells under LTR's regulation. Retroviruses typically transduce the genes of cell receptors (i.e., ErbB and Fms), kinases (i.e., Src and Abl), and transcriptional factors (i.e., Jun, Fos, and Myc). These oncogene-carrying retroviruses (also termed chimeric viruses) lose their ability to cause lytic infection and become ineffective after a few days. In compensation, such viruses have an enhanced transformation capability, marking retroviruses as acute transformers. Hotspots are sequence of genes favored by oncogenic viruses during insertion. In murine models of breast cancer induced by the murine mammary tumor virus (MMTV), it was found the gene sequence near Wnt and Notch protooncogenes are the hotspots of MMTV [145]. However, there is inadequate evidence of insertional mutation or protooncogenes transduction in human retroviruses so far. For instance, human retrovirus HTLV-1 induces cell transformation by expressing Tax protein [146]. On the other hand, next-generation sequencing analysis revealed that HBV preferentially integrates into cancerous cells rather than healthy cells in the HBV-infected liver. The liver cancer cells integrated with HBV provirus also demonstrate dysregulated oncogene expression in TERT, MLL4, and CCNE [147]. The mechanism of insertional mutagenesis in HBV has been compared with animal retroviruses due to its similarities. Although integration is necessary for HPV and MCPV to become carcinogenic, the biological outcomes are more akin to acute transforming retroviruses in these circumstances, where proviruses become dysfunctional and could not yield infectious progeny when the viral regulatory regions are lost. As a result, viral integration often results in viral latency, upregulation of oncogenes expression, and host cell transformation.

Crosstalk of Viruses with Host Inflammation and Immune System

Increasing evidence of virally driven modulation in cancer has been found. For example, HCMV infection is highly prevalent with a global incidence of at least 50% and up to 100% in adults. In most people, HCMV infection is asymptomatic, but could cause morbidity and mortality in immunosuppressed individuals. To date, there is insufficient proof that HCMV itself can induce malignant transformation. But the viral proteins produced from HCMV infection could modulate and augment malignancy through influencing signaling pathways critical for regulating cell proliferation, migration, apoptosis, vascular changes, and immunosurveillance [148–152]. High-grade gliomas, a brain cancer with poor prognosis, have reported HCMV's involvement; more evidence of HCMV proteins and genetic materials was discovered in high-grade gliomas than in brain tissues of other diseases, such as epilepsy [153–155]. Although HCMV can be detected in the tumor, the infection only involves a minor proportion of the cancer cells without causing overt viral monoclonality. Thus, the relationship between HCMV and high-grade gliomas does

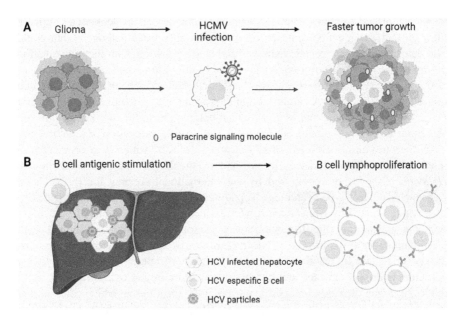

Fig. 26.3 Crosstalk of virus-mediated carcinogenesis. (**a**) and chronic antigen-driven lymphoproliferation (**b**). (**a**) It is proposed that HCMV only participates after the formation of a glioma, where the virus only transforms a minor percentage of the cancer cells to activate signaling networks that upregulate cell proliferation. (**b**) HCV antigens produced by HCV-infected hepatocytes chronically stimulate HCV-specific B cells, resulting in higher risk of uncontrolled lymphoproliferation and lymphoma development

not meet Bradford–Hill criteria of temporality, implying that HCMV infection only occurred after malignant transformation (Fig. 26.3).

Chronic Inflammation

Despite the mechanisms in place to escape immune surveillance, long-term viral infection often leads to chronic inflammation at the local tissue. Chronic inflammation generates consistent and increasing local tissue injury, places the tissue under a repair-injury cycle, and upregulates the expression of genes involved in the inflammatory response (including those of proinflammatory cytokines, chemokines, adhesion factors, growth factors, and antiapoptotic proteins). This results in leukocytes recruitment and proliferation of fibroblasts and endotheliocytes, leading to tissue remodeling and neovascularization at the local injury site [156]. Under physiological conditions, an inflammatory response resolves on its own by halting the chemoattraction of immune cells, inducing programmed cell death and phagocytosis of proinflammatory cells, and restoring normal hemodynamic at the site of inflammation. However, the inflammatory response is protracted in the presence of persistent infection, keeping immune cells at the site of inflammation and resisting apoptosis of the immune cells. The immune cells, such as leukocytes, release nitrogen and oxygen free radicals to remove the infectious pathogens, but could also damage the host's genetic materials and cause mutation. Chronic inflammation promotes the formation of a malignant clone in this setting, and here, tissue repair also contributes to carcinogenesis by facilitating cell growth, tissue invading and tumor metastasis [157]. A classic example of an indirect carcinogen is the bacteria Helicobacter pylori that causes persistent inflammation in the stomach. Untreated Helicobacter infection often leads to gastric cancer via a succession of inflammatory lesions, from non-atrophic gastritis to atrophic gastritis, which then progresses to intestinal metaplasia, tissue dysplasia, and eventually in situ gastric carcinoma. Helicobacter pylori is recognized by the International Agency for Research on Cancer (IARC) as a type I carcinogenic pathogen [158]. The gastric mucosa releases IL-8 when infected by Helicobacter pylori, which recruits neutrophils to the infection site, facilitating the formation of a leukocyte-rich milieu saturated with proinflammatory cytokines (i.e., TNF-α, IL-6, IL-1β, and IL-12) [159]. Neutrophils also generate harmful reactive oxygen species (such as superoxide anions, hydrogen peroxide, hydroxyl radicals, and hydroperoxyl) and nitrogen oxides (namely nitric oxides, nitrogen dioxides, and peroxynitrite) at the local tissue, which could potentially cause the gastric cells to mutate [160]. Those who have IL-8, IL-1, or TNF-α polymorphisms have a higher chance of developing stomach cancer [161–164]. Notably, pharmaceutical eradication of Helicobacter pylori in individuals with premalignant lesions restores tissue injury and delays the onset of cancer, adding to the evidence for microorganism's role in the development of stomach cancer. The function of inflammatory response in cancer development is not fully understood, despite the fact that all oncogenic viruses sustain chronic infection. Inflammation caused by HCV and HBV is associated with necrosis and tissue repair, which leads to liver pathologies including steatosis, fibrosis, and cirrhosis, culminating in the development of liver cancer. The liver is extensively invaded by inflammatory cells during steatosis and fibrosis, forming a milieu saturated with cytokines and chemokines, especially TGF-β and IL-1β [165]. In addition, increased EBV reactivation has been linked to significant inflammation in gastric tissue and subsequent tissue destruction, from which premalignant lesions develop. This suggests that inflammation plays a key role in the EBV-induced transformation of mucosa lining in the stomach [166, 167].

Immunosuppression

Since AIDS become prevalent worldwide, the immune system's function in onco-surveillance has been well-established. Despite the fact that HIV cannot cause malignancy in its host cells, two out of five AIDS patients acquire cancer as a result of HIV-induced severe immunosuppression, which indirectly facilitates carcinogenesis [168, 169]. Immunocompromised AIDS patients with very low CD8 T-cell count are more susceptible to cancers of infectious etiology [168], for example, lymphomas induced by EBV and KSHV infection, KSHV-associated sarcomas,

HPV-associated cervical cancers, MCPV Merkel cell carcinomas. As such, HIV is categorized as an indirect carcinogen, and in the presence of EBV, KSHV, HPV, or MCPV infection, the direct carcinogenic mechanisms of these oncogenic viruses continue to operate. Immunosuppression could also be observed in patients after bone marrow or organ transplantation due to pharmacological interventions to suppress rejection reaction. These immunosuppressed patients may develop post-transplant lymphoproliferative disorder (PTLD), where EBV-infected B cells undergo uncontrolled polyclonal proliferation which could likely develop into advanced monoclonal lymphomas [170, 171]. The majority of PTLD originates in the host cells, and on rarer occasions, in the donor cells. T-cell-depleting agents, a class of immunosuppressant, increases the risk to acquiring EBV-associated PTLD, emphasizing the role of T cells in the anticancer immunosurveillance landscape [172]. Autologous T-cell immunotherapy targeting the EBV nuclear antigen 3 (EBNA-3) family proteins, i.e., EBNA-3A/-3B/-3C, has shown to be a highly effective treatment [173, 174].

Chronic Antigen-Driven Lymphoproliferation

Immune cells, especially B cells, multiply and proliferate in response to an infection. B cells proliferate substantially by two mechanisms during germinal center (GC) reaction: antigen receptor class switching and somatic hypermutation (for affinity maturation), regulated by the enzyme activation-induced cytidine deaminase (AID) modification of B-cell antigen receptor. Due to augmented B-cell proliferation and abnormally encoded AID enzymes, B-cell lymphoma usually arise from GC reaction. EBV proteins LMP1 and LMP2A send decoy signals to EBV-infected B cells, causing them to undergo GC reaction and become memory cells, which allow lifelong latency of EBV in the host cell. This type of EBV-induced GC reaction may lead to development of lymphomas [114]. Latent infections caused by other pathogens can also trigger chronic antigen-driven lymphoproliferation, such as *H. pylori, B. burgdorferi, C. jejuni, C. psittaci,* and HCV, which could lead to an increased risk of developing lymphomas. In HCV-infected patients, it was found that clonal B-cell expansions are closely associated with a longer period of latency and with HCV viral protein-specific receptors [175–177]. The pharmacological eradication of HCV, which is commonly linked with lymphoma remission, is still the most convincing proof for a causative relationship between the two [178]. In a similar fashion, the pharmacological eradication of *H. pylori* is associated with remission of gastric mucosa-associated lymphoid tissue (MALT) lymphomas [179].

Conclusion

Host has been accommodating bacteria and viruses for a long time. It is obvious that virus residing in the host is an important factor that triggers carcinogenesis. Despite this, not much studies were done on the prevention of these viruses to invade host.

Since virus and bacteria (highlighted in previous chapter) could co-exist in the host, we should identify and stratify patients that could benefit from virus-directed onco-therapeutics, such as HPV or HCV vaccine. More in-depth studies should be done on the therapeutic effects of these vaccines in cancer patients.

References

1. Liao JB (2006) Viruses and human cancer. Yale J Biol Med 79(3–4):115–122
2. Morales-Sanchez A, Fuentes-Panana EM (2014) Human viruses and cancer. Viruses 6(10): 4047–4079
3. Rous P (1979) A transmissible avian neoplasm. (Sarcoma of the common fowl) by Peyton Rous, M.D., Experimental Medicine for Sept. 1, 1910, vol. 12, pp.696-705. J Exp Med 150(4): 738–753
4. Rous P (1911) A sarcoma of the fowl transmissible by an agent separable from the tumor cells. J Exp Med 13(4):397–411
5. Ellerman V, Bang O (1908) Experimentelle leukämie bei hühnern. II. Zent Bakteriol ParasitenkdInfectionskr Hyg Abt Orig 63:595–609
6. Epstein MA, Achong BG, Barr YM (1964) Virus particles in cultured lymphoblasts from Burkitt's lymphoma. Lancet 1(7335):702–703
7. Dürst M, Gissmann L, Ikenberg H, zur Hausen H (1983) A papillomavirus DNA from a cervical carcinoma and its prevalence in cancer biopsy samples from different geographic regions. Proc Natl Acad Sci U S A 80(12):3812–3815
8. Boshart M, Gissmann L, Ikenberg H, Kleinheinz A, Scheurlen W, zur Hausen H. (1984) A new type of papillomavirus DNA, its presence in genital cancer biopsies and in cell lines derived from cervical cancer. EMBO J 3(5):1151–1157
9. Moore PS, Chang Y (2010) Why do viruses cause cancer? Highlights of the first century of human tumour virology. Nat Rev Cancer 10(12):878–889
10. Parkin DM (2006) The global health burden of infection-associated cancers in the year 2002. Int J Cancer 118(12):3030–3044
11. Koch R (1876) Untersuchungen über bakterien: V. Die ätiologie der milzbrand-krankheit, begründet auf die entwicklungsgeschichte des bacillus anthracis [investigations into bacteria: V. The etiology of anthrax, based on the ontogenesis of bacillus anthracis]. Beitr Biol Pflanz 2(2):277–310
12. Hill AB (1965) The environment and disease: association or causation? Proc R Soc Med 58(5): 295–300
13. Thompson MP, Kurzrock R (2004) Epstein-Barr virus and cancer. Clin Cancer Res 10(3): 803–821
14. Kulwichit W, Edwards RH, Davenport EM, Baskar JF, Godfrey V, Raab-Traub N (1998) Expression of the Epstein-Barr virus latent membrane protein 1 induces B cell lymphoma in transgenic mice. Proc Natl Acad Sci U S A 95(20):11963–11968
15. Beasley RP (1988) Hepatitis B virus. The major etiology of hepatocellular carcinoma. Cancer 61(10):1942–1956
16. Lavanchy D (2004) Hepatitis B virus epidemiology, disease burden, treatment, and current and emerging prevention and control measures. J Viral Hepat 11(2):97–107
17. Fattovich G, Giustina G, Degos F, Tremolada F, Diodati G, Almasio P et al (1997) Morbidity and mortality in compensated cirrhosis type C: a retrospective follow-up study of 384 patients. Gastroenterology 112(2):463–472
18. The Cancer of the Liver Italian Program (CLIP) Investigators (1998) A new prognostic system for hepatocellular carcinoma: a retrospective study of 435 patients: the Cancer of the Liver Italian Program (CLIP) investigators. Hepatology 28(3):751–755

19. Okuda K, Ohtsuki T, Obata H, Tomimatsu M, Okazaki N, Hasegawa H et al (1985) Natural history of hepatocellular carcinoma and prognosis in relation to treatment. Study of 850 patients. Cancer 56(4):918–928

20. Llovet JM, Burroughs A, Bruix J (2003) Hepatocellular carcinoma. Lancet 362(9399): 1907–1917

21. Ni YH, Chang MH, Huang LM, Chen HL, Hsu HY, Chiu TY et al (2001) Hepatitis B virus infection in children and adolescents in a hyperendemic area: 15 years after mass hepatitis B vaccination. Ann Intern Med 135(9):796–800

22. Ramsay M, Gay N, Balogun K, Collins M (1998) Control of hepatitis B in the United Kingdom. Vaccine 16(Suppl):S52–S55

23. Iwarson S (1998) Report from working group 3 (The Czech Republic, Denmark, Finland, Norway, The Netherlands, Slovakia, Sweden and the UK). Vaccine 16(Suppl):S63–S64

24. Niederau C, Heintges T, Lange S, Goldmann G, Niederau CM, Mohr L et al (1996) Long-term follow-up of HBeAg-positive patients treated with interferon alfa for chronic hepatitis B. N Engl J Med 334(22):1422–1427

25. Lampertico P, Del Ninno E, Viganò M, Romeo R, Donato MF, Sablon E et al (2003) Long-term suppression of hepatitis B e antigen-negative chronic hepatitis B by 24-month interferon therapy. Hepatology 37(4):756–763

26. Yuen MF, Hui CK, Cheng CC, Wu CH, Lai YP, Lai CL (2001) Long-term follow-up of interferon alfa treatment in Chinese patients with chronic hepatitis B infection: The effect on hepatitis B e antigen seroconversion and the development of cirrhosis-related complications. Hepatology 34(1):139–145

27. Liaw YF, Sung JJ, Chow WC, Farrell G, Lee CZ, Yuen H et al (2004) Lamivudine for patients with chronic hepatitis B and advanced liver disease. N Engl J Med 351(15):1521–1531

28. Lai CL, Dienstag J, Schiff E, Leung NW, Atkins M, Hunt C et al (2003) Prevalence and clinical correlates of YMDD variants during lamivudine therapy for patients with chronic hepatitis B. Clin Infect Dis 36(6):687–696

29. Manns MP, Wedemeyer H, Cornberg M (2006) Treating viral hepatitis C: efficacy, side effects, and complications. Gut 55(9):1350–1359

30. Schiff ER (2006) Prevention of mortality from hepatitis B and hepatitis C. Lancet 368(9539): 896–897

31. Terrault NA, Berenguer M (2006) Treating hepatitis C infection in liver transplant recipients. Liver Transpl 12(8):1192–1204

32. Bartenschlager R (2002) Hepatitis C virus replicons: potential role for drug development. Nat Rev Drug Discov 1(11):911–916

33. Mercer DF, Schiller DE, Elliott JF, Douglas DN, Hao C, Rinfret A et al (2001) Hepatitis C virus replication in mice with chimeric human livers. Nat Med 7(8):927–933

34. Meuleman P, Libbrecht L, De Vos R, de Hemptinne B, Gevaert K, Vandekerckhove J et al (2005) Morphological and biochemical characterization of a human liver in a uPA-SCID mouse chimera. Hepatology 41(4):847–856

35. Borza CM, Hutt-Fletcher LM (2002) Alternate replication in B cells and epithelial cells switches tropism of Epstein-Barr virus. Nat Med 8(6):594–599

36. Papadopoulos EB, Ladanyi M, Emanuel D, Mackinnon S, Boulad F, Carabasi MH et al (1994) Infusions of donor leukocytes to treat Epstein-Barr virus-associated lymphoproliferative disorders after allogeneic bone marrow transplantation. N Engl J Med 330(17):1185–1191

37. Haque T, Wilkie GM, Taylor C, Amlot PL, Murad P, Iley A et al (2002) Treatment of Epstein-Barr-virus-positive post-transplantation lymphoproliferative disease with partly HLA-matched allogeneic cytotoxic T cells. Lancet 360(9331):436–442

38. Gottschalk S, Ng CY, Perez M, Smith CA, Sample C, Brenner MK et al (2001) An Epstein-Barr virus deletion mutant associated with fatal lymphoproliferative disease unresponsive to therapy with virus-specific CTLs. Blood 97(4):835–843

39. Jackman WT, Mann KA, Hoffmann HJ, Spaete RR (1999) Expression of Epstein-Barr virus gp350 as a single chain glycoprotein for an EBV subunit vaccine. Vaccine 17(7–8):660–668

40. Thorley-Lawson DA, Poodry CA (1982) Identification and isolation of the main component (gp350-gp220) of Epstein-Barr virus responsible for generating neutralizing antibodies *in vivo*. J Virol 43(2):730–736
41. Gu SY, Huang TM, Ruan L, Miao YH, Lu H, Chu CM et al (1995) First EBV vaccine trial in humans using recombinant vaccinia virus expressing the major membrane antigen. Dev Biol Stand 84:171–177
42. Donati D, Espmark E, Kironde F, Mbidde EK, Kamya M, Lundkvist A et al (2006) Clearance of circulating Epstein-Barr virus DNA in children with acute malaria after antimalaria treatment. J Infect Dis 193(7):971–977
43. Ho JH (1978) An epidemiologic and clinical study of nasopharyngeal carcinoma. Int J Radiat Oncol Biol Phys 4(3–4):182–198
44. Chang Y, Cesarman E, Pessin MS, Lee F, Culpepper J, Knowles DM et al (1994) Identification of herpesvirus-like DNA sequences in AIDS-associated Kaposi's sarcoma. Science 266(5192):1865–1869
45. Sarid R, Olsen SJ, Moore PS (1999) Kaposi's sarcoma-associated herpesvirus: epidemiology, virology, and molecular biology. Adv Virus Res 52:139–232
46. Flore O, Rafii S, Ely S, O'Leary JJ, Hyjek EM, Cesarman E (1998) Transformation of primary human endothelial cells by Kaposi's sarcoma-associated herpesvirus. Nature 394(6693): 588–592
47. Martin DF, Kuppermann BD, Wolitz RA, Palestine AG, Li H, Robinson CA (1999) Oral ganciclovir for patients with cytomegalovirus retinitis treated with a ganciclovir implant. Roche ganciclovir study group. N Engl J Med 340(14):1063–1070
48. Bais C, Santomasso B, Coso O, Arvanitakis L, Raaka EG, Gutkind JS et al (1998) G-protein-coupled receptor of Kaposi's sarcoma-associated herpesvirus is a viral oncogene and angiogenesis activator. Nature 391(6662):86–89
49. Montaner S, Sodhi A, Ramsdell AK, Martin D, Hu J, Sawai ET et al (2006) The Kaposi's sarcoma-associated herpesvirus G protein-coupled receptor as a therapeutic target for the treatment of Kaposi's sarcoma. Cancer Res 66(1):168–174
50. Gingues S, Gill MJ (2006) The impact of highly active antiretroviral therapy on the incidence and outcomes of AIDS-defining cancers in Southern Alberta. HIV Med 7(6):369–377
51. Wallin KL, Wiklund F, Angström T, Bergman F, Stendahl U, Wadell G et al (1999) Type-specific persistence of human papillomavirus DNA before the development of invasive cervical cancer. N Engl J Med 341(22):1633–1638
52. von Knebel DM, Oltersdorf T, Schwarz E, Gissmann L (1988) Correlation of modified human papilloma virus early gene expression with altered growth properties in C4-1 cervical carcinoma cells. Cancer Res 48(13):3780–3786
53. Generation of heart muscle cells from blood or skin cells of breast cancer patients. https:// ClinicalTrials.gov/show/NCT02772367
54. Frazer IH (2004) Prevention of cervical cancer through papillomavirus vaccination. Nat Rev Immunol 4(1):46–54
55. Palefsky JM, Holly EA (2003) Immunosuppression and co-infection with HIV. J Natl Cancer Inst Monogr 31:41–46
56. Halpert R, Fruchter RG, Sedlis A, Butt K, Boyce JG, Sillman FH (1986) Human papillomavirus and lower genital neoplasia in renal transplant patients. Obstet Gynecol 68(2):251–258
57. Petry KU, Scheffel D, Bode U, Gabrysiak T, Köchel H, Kupsch E et al (1994) Cellular immunodeficiency enhances the progression of human papillomavirus-associated cervical lesions. Int J Cancer 57(6):836–840
58. Frisch M, Biggar RJ, Goedert JJ (2000) Human papillomavirus-associated cancers in patients with human immunodeficiency virus infection and acquired immunodeficiency syndrome. J Natl Cancer Inst 92(18):1500–1510
59. Koutsky LA, Ault KA, Wheeler CM, Brown DR, Barr E, Alvarez FB et al (2002) A controlled trial of a human papillomavirus type 16 vaccine. N Engl J Med 347(21):1645–1651
60. Harper DM, Franco EL, Wheeler C, Ferris DG, Jenkins D, Schuind A et al (2004) Efficacy of a bivalent L1 virus-like particle vaccine in prevention of infection with human papillomavirus types 16 and 18 in young women: a randomised controlled trial. Lancet 364(9447):1757–1765

61. Kaufmann AM, Stern PL, Rankin EM, Sommer H, Nuessler V, Schneider A et al (2002) Safety and immunogenicity of TA-HPV, a recombinant vaccinia virus expressing modified human papillomavirus (HPV)-16 and HPV-18 E6 and E7 genes, in women with progressive cervical cancer. Clin Cancer Res 8(12):3676–3685

62. Garcia F, Petry KU, Muderspach L, Gold MA, Braly P, Crum CP et al (2004) ZYC101a for treatment of high-grade cervical intraepithelial neoplasia: a randomized controlled trial. Obstet Gynecol 103(2):317–326

63. Sheets EE, Urban RG, Crum CP, Hedley ML, Politch JA, Gold MA et al (2003) Immuno-therapy of human cervical high-grade cervical intraepithelial neoplasia with microparticle-delivered human papillomavirus 16 E7 plasmid DNA. Am J Obstet Gynecol 188(4):916–926

64. Klencke B, Matijevic M, Urban RG, Lathey JL, Hedley ML, Berry M et al (2002) Encapsu-lated plasmid DNA treatment for human papillomavirus 16-associated anal dysplasia: a phase I study of ZYC101. Clin Cancer Res 8(5):1028–1037

65. Gallo RC, Kalyanaraman VS, Sarngadharan MG, Sliski A, Vonderheid EC, Maeda M et al (1983) Association of the human type C retrovirus with a subset of adult T-cell cancers. Cancer Res 43(8):3892–3899

66. Duggan DB, Ehrlich GD, Davey FP, Kwok S, Sninsky J, Goldberg J et al (1988) HTLV-I-induced lymphoma mimicking Hodgkin's disease. Diagnosis by polymerase chain reaction amplification of specific HTLV-I sequences in tumor DNA. Blood 71(4):1027–1032

67. Kozako T, Arima N, Toji S, Masamoto I, Akimoto M, Hamada H et al (2006) Reduced frequency, diversity, and function of human T cell leukemia virus type 1-specific CD8+ T cell in adult T cell leukemia patients. J Immunol 177(8):5718 5726

68. Lynch MP, Kaumaya PT (2006) Advances in HTLV-1 peptide vaccines and therapeutics. Curr Protein Pept Sci 7(2):137–145

69. Zella D, Gallo RC (2021) Viruses and bacteria associated with cancer: an overview. Viruses 13(6):1039

70. Loeb LA, Springgate CF, Battula N (1974) Errors in DNA replication as a basis of malignant changes. Cancer Res 34(9):2311–2321

71. Prindle MJ, Fox EJ, Loeb LA (2010) The mutator phenotype in cancer: molecular mechanisms and targeting strategies. Curr Drug Targets 11(10):1296–1303

72. Coleman WB (2003) Mechanisms of human hepatocarcinogenesis. Curr Mol Med 3(6): 573–588

73. Zucman-Rossi J, Laurent-Puig P (2007) Genetic diversity of hepatocellular carcinomas and its potential impact on targeted therapies. Pharmacogenomics 8(8):997–1003

74. Correa P, Piazuelo MB (2012) The gastric precancerous cascade. J Dig Dis 13(1):2–9

75. Hatakeyama M, Higashi H (2005) Helicobacter pylori CagA: a new paradigm for bacterial carcinogenesis. Cancer Sci 96(12):835–843

76. Hollstein M, Sidransky D, Vogelstein B, Harris CC (1991) p53 mutations in human cancers. Science 253(5015):49–53

77. Levine AJ, Momand J, Finlay CA (1991) The p53 tumour suppressor gene. Nature 351(6326): 453–456

78. Khidr L, Chen PL (2006) RB, the conductor that orchestrates life, death and differentiation. Oncogene 25(38):5210–5219

79. Lee JM, Bernstein A (1995) Apoptosis, cancer and the p53 tumour suppressor gene. Cancer Metastasis Rev 14(2):149–161

80. Amundson SA, Myers TG, Fornace AJ Jr (1998) Roles for p53 in growth arrest and apoptosis: putting on the brakes after genotoxic stress. Oncogene 17(25):3287–3299

81. Scheffner M, Werness BA, Huibregtse JM, Levine AJ, Howley PM (1990) The E6 oncoprotein encoded by human papillomavirus types 16 and 18 promotes the degradation of p53. Cell 63(6):1129–1136

82. Scheffner M, Huibregtse JM, Vierstra RD, Howley PM (1993) The HPV-16 E6 and E6-AP complex functions as a ubiquitin-protein ligase in the ubiquitination of p53. Cell 75(3): 495–505

83. Reznikoff CA, Yeager TR, Belair CD, Savelieva E, Puthenveettil JA, Stadler WM (1996) Elevated p16 at senescence and loss of p16 at immortalization in human papillomavirus 16 E6, but not E7, transformed human uroepithelial cells. Cancer Res 56(13):2886–2890

84. Ghittoni R, Accardi R, Hasan U, Gheit T, Sylla B, Tommasino M (2010) The biological properties of E6 and E7 oncoproteins from human papillomaviruses. Virus Genes 40(1):1–13

85. Dyson N, Howley PM, Münger K, Harlow E (1989) The human papilloma virus-16 E7 oncoprotein is able to bind to the retinoblastoma gene product. Science 243(4893):934–937

86. Giam CZ, Jeang KT (2007) HTLV-1 tax and adult T-cell leukemia. Front Biosci 12:1496–1507

87. Pise-Masison CA, Brady JN (2005) Setting the stage for transformation: HTLV-1 Tax inhibition of p53 function. Front Biosci 10:919–930

88. Haller K, Wu Y, Derow E, Schmitt I, Jeang KT, Grassmann R (2002) Physical interaction of human T-cell leukemia virus type 1 Tax with cyclin-dependent kinase 4 stimulates the phosphorylation of retinoblastoma protein. Mol Cell Biol 22(10):3327–3338

89. Suzuki T, Narita T, Uchida-Toita M, Yoshida M (1999) Down-regulation of the INK4 family of cyclin-dependent kinase inhibitors by tax protein of HTLV-1 through two distinct mechanisms. Virology 259(2):384–391

90. Suzuki T, Kitao S, Matsushime H, Yoshida M (1996) HTLV-1 tax protein interacts with cyclin-dependent kinase inhibitor p16INK4A and counteracts its inhibitory activity towards CDK4. EMBO J 15(7):1607–1614

91. Satou Y, Yasunaga J, Yoshida M, Matsuoka M (2006) HTLV-I basic leucine zipper factor gene mRNA supports proliferation of adult T cell leukemia cells. Proc Natl Acad Sci U S A 103(3):720–725

92. Cai QL, Knight JS, Verma SC, Zald P, Robertson ES (2006) EC5S ubiquitin complex is recruited by KSHV latent antigen LANA for degradation of the VHL and p53 tumor suppressors. PLoS Pathog 2(10):e116

93. Friborg J Jr, Kong W, Hottiger MO, Nabel GJ (1999) p53 inhibition by the LANA protein of KSHV protects against cell death. Nature 402(6764):889–894

94. Si H, Robertson ES (2006) Kaposi's sarcoma-associated herpesvirus-encoded latency-associated nuclear antigen induces chromosomal instability through inhibition of p53 function. J Virol 80(2):697–709

95. Klein G, Klein E, Kashuba E (2010) Interaction of Epstein-Barr virus (EBV) with human B-lymphocytes. Biochem Biophys Res Commun 396(1):67–73

96. Spender LC, Cannell EJ, Hollyoake M, Wensing B, Gawn JM, Brimmell M et al (1999) Control of cell cycle entry and apoptosis in B lymphocytes infected by Epstein-Barr virus. J Virol 73(6):4678–4688

97. Mei YP, Zhou JM, Wang Y, Huang H, Deng R, Feng GK et al (2007) Silencing of LMP1 induces cell cycle arrest and enhances chemosensitivity through inhibition of AKT signaling pathway in EBV-positive nasopharyngeal carcinoma cells. Cell Cycle 6(11):1379–1385

98. Portis T, Longnecker R (2004) Epstein-Barr virus (EBV) LMP2A mediates B-lymphocyte survival through constitutive activation of the Ras/PI3K/Akt pathway. Oncogene 23(53):8619–8628

99. Desbien AL, Kappler JW, Marrack P (2009) The Epstein-Barr virus Bcl-2 homolog, BHRF1, blocks apoptosis by binding to a limited amount of bim. Proc Natl Acad Sci U S A 106(14):5663–5668

100. Saggioro D, Silic-Benussi M, Biasiotto R, D'Agostino DM, Ciminale V (2009) Control of cell death pathways by HTLV-1 proteins. Front Biosci 14(9):3338–3351

101. Underbrink MP, Howie HL, Bedard KM, Koop JI, Galloway DA (2008) E6 proteins from multiple human betapapillomavirus types degrade Bak and protect keratinocytes from apoptosis after UVB irradiation. J Virol 82(21):10408–10417

102. Garnett TO, Filippova M, Duerksen-Hughes PJ (2006) Accelerated degradation of FADD and procaspase 8 in cells expressing human papilloma virus 16 E6 impairs TRAIL-mediated apoptosis. Cell Death Differ 13(11):1915–1926

103. Yuan H, Fu F, Zhuo J, Wang W, Nishitani J, An DS et al (2005) Human papillomavirus type 16 E6 and E7 oncoproteins upregulate c-IAP2 gene expression and confer resistance to apoptosis. Oncogene 24(32):5069–5078
104. Filippova M, Parkhurst L, Duerksen-Hughes PJ (2004) The human papillomavirus 16 E6 protein binds to Fas-associated death domain and protects cells from Fas-triggered apoptosis. J Biol Chem 279(24):25729–25744
105. Du J, Chen GG, Vlantis AC, Chan PK, Tsang RK, van Hasselt CA (2004) Resistance to apoptosis of HPV 16-infected laryngeal cancer cells is associated with decreased Bak and increased Bcl-2 expression. Cancer Lett 205(1):81–88
106. Becker SA, Lee TH, Butel JS, Slagle BL (1998) Hepatitis B virus X protein interferes with cellular DNA repair. J Virol 72(1):266–272
107. Aweya JJ, Tan YJ (2011) Modulation of programmed cell death pathways by the hepatitis C virus. Front Biosci 16(2):608–618
108. Plug-DeMaggio AW, Sundsvold T, Wurscher MA, Koop JI, Klingelhutz AJ, McDougall JK (2004) Telomere erosion and chromosomal instability in cells expressing the HPV oncogene 16E6. Oncogene 23(20):3561–3571
109. Duensing S, Münger K (2002) The human papillomavirus type 16 E6 and E7 oncoproteins independently induce numerical and structural chromosome instability. Cancer Res 62(23): 7075–7082
110. Duensing S, Duensing A, Crum CP, Münger K (2001) Human papillomavirus type 16 E7 oncoprotein-induced abnormal centrosome synthesis is an early event in the evolving malignant phenotype. Cancer Res 61(6):2356–2360
111. Duensing S, Lee LY, Duensing A, Basile J, Piboonniyom S, Gonzalez S et al (2000) The human papillomavirus type 16 E6 and E7 oncoproteins cooperate to induce mitotic defects and genomic instability by uncoupling centrosome duplication from the cell division cycle. Proc Natl Acad Sci U S A 97(18):10002–10007
112. Chen JJ (2010) Genomic instability induced by human papillomavirus oncogenes. N Am J Med Sci (Boston) 3(2):43–47
113. Bornkamm GW (2009) Epstein-Barr virus and its role in the pathogenesis of Burkitt's lymphoma: an unresolved issue. Semin Cancer Biol 19(6):351–365
114. Heath E, Begue-Pastor N, Chaganti S, Croom-Carter D, Shannon-Lowe C, Kube D et al (2012) Epstein-Barr virus infection of naïve B cells *in vitro* frequently selects clones with mutated immunoglobulin genotypes: implications for virus biology. PLoS Pathog 8(5): e1002697
115. Marriott SJ, Lemoine FJ, Jeang KT (2002) Damaged DNA and miscounted chromosomes: human T cell leukemia virus type I tax oncoprotein and genetic lesions in transformed cells. J Biomed Sci 9(4):292–298
116. Lemoine FJ, Marriott SJ (2002) Genomic instability driven by the human T-cell leukemia virus type I (HTLV-I) oncoprotein, Tax. Oncogene 21(47):7230–7234
117. Chandhasin C, Ducu RI, Berkovich E, Kastan MB, Marriott SJ (2008) Human T-cell leukemia virus type 1 tax attenuates the ATM-mediated cellular DNA damage response. J Virol 82(14): 6952–6961
118. Kao SY, Lemoine FJ, Marriott SJ (2001) p53-independent induction of apoptosis by the HTLV-I tax protein following UV irradiation. Virology 291(2):292–298
119. Jin DY, Spencer F, Jeang KT (1998) Human T cell leukemia virus type 1 oncoprotein tax targets the human mitotic checkpoint protein MAD1. Cell 93(1):81–91
120. Liu B, Hong S, Tang Z, Yu H, Giam CZ (2005) HTLV-I tax directly binds the Cdc20-associated anaphase-promoting complex and activates it ahead of schedule. Proc Natl Acad Sci U S A 102(1):63–68
121. Cohen SB, Graham ME, Lovrecz GO, Bache N, Robinson PJ, Reddel RR (2007) Protein composition of catalytically active human telomerase from immortal cells. Science 315(5820): 1850–1853
122. Terrin L, Dal Col J, Rampazzo E, Zancai P, Pedrotti M, Ammirabile G et al (2008) Latent membrane protein 1 of Epstein-Barr virus activates the hTERT promoter and enhances telomerase activity in B lymphocytes. J Virol 82(20):10175–10187

123. Zhang X, Dong N, Zhang H, You J, Wang H, Ye L (2005) Effects of hepatitis B virus X protein on human telomerase reverse transcriptase expression and activity in hepatoma cells. J Lab Clin Med 145(2):98–104
124. Verma SC, Borah S, Robertson ES (2004) Latency-associated nuclear antigen of Kaposi's sarcoma-associated herpesvirus up-regulates transcription of human telomerase reverse transcriptase promoter through interaction with transcription factor Sp1. J Virol 78(19): 10348–10359
125. Gewin L, Myers H, Kiyono T, Galloway DA (2004) Identification of a novel telomerase repressor that interacts with the human papillomavirus type-16 E6/E6-AP complex. Genes Dev 18(18):2269–2282
126. Chen X, Kamranvar SA, Masucci MG (2014) Tumor viruses and replicative immortality--avoiding the telomere hurdle. Semin Cancer Biol 26:43–51
127. Ohashi M, Sakurai M, Higuchi M, Mori N, Fukushi M, Oie M et al (2004) Human T-cell leukemia virus type 1 tax oncoprotein induces and interacts with a multi-PDZ domain protein, MAGI-3. Virology 320(1):52–62
128. Glaunsinger BA, Lee SS, Thomas M, Banks L, Javier R (2000) Interactions of the PDZ-protein MAGI-1 with adenovirus E4-ORF1 and high-risk papillomavirus E6 oncoproteins. Oncogene 19(46):5270–5280
129. Rousset R, Fabre S, Desbois C, Bantignies F, Jalinot P (1998) The C-terminus of the HTLV-1 tax oncoprotein mediates interaction with the PDZ domain of cellular proteins. Oncogene 16(5):643–654
130. Lee SS, Weiss RS, Javier RT (1997) Binding of human virus oncoproteins to hDlg/SAP97, a mammalian homolog of the Drosophila discs large tumor suppressor protein. Proc Natl Acad Sci U S A 94(13):6670–6675
131. Spanos WC, Hoover A, Harris GF, Wu S, Strand GL, Anderson ME et al (2008) The PDZ binding motif of human papillomavirus type 16 E6 induces PTPN13 loss, which allows anchorage-independent growth and synergizes with ras for invasive growth. J Virol 82(5): 2493–2500
132. Spanos WC, Geiger J, Anderson ME, Harris GF, Bossler AD, Smith RB et al (2008) Deletion of the PDZ motif of HPV16 E6 preventing immortalization and anchorage-independent growth in human tonsil epithelial cells. Head Neck 30(2):139–147
133. Xie L, Yamamoto B, Haoudi A, Semmes OJ, Green PL (2006) PDZ binding motif of HTLV-1 tax promotes virus-mediated T-cell proliferation *in vitro* and persistence *in vivo*. Blood 107(5): 1980–1988
134. Hirata A, Higuchi M, Niinuma A, Ohashi M, Fukushi M, Oie M et al (2004) PDZ domain-binding motif of human T-cell leukemia virus type 1 tax oncoprotein augments the transforming activity in a rat fibroblast cell line. Virology 318(1):327–336
135. Calin GA, Croce CM (2006) MicroRNA signatures in human cancers. Nat Rev Cancer 6(11): 857–866
136. Lu J, Getz G, Miska EA, Alvarez-Saavedra E, Lamb J, Peck D et al (2005) MicroRNA expression profiles classify human cancers. Nature 435(7043):834–838
137. Cai X, Schäfer A, Lu S, Bilello JP, Desrosiers RC, Edwards R et al (2006) Epstein-Barr virus microRNAs are evolutionarily conserved and differentially expressed. PLoS Pathog 2(3):e23
138. Pfeffer S, Zavolan M, Grässer FA, Chien M, Russo JJ, Ju J et al (2004) Identification of virus-encoded microRNAs. Science 304(5671):734–736
139. Choy EY, Siu KL, Kok KH, Lung RW, Tsang CM, To KF et al (2008) An Epstein-Barr virus-encoded microRNA targets PUMA to promote host cell survival. J Exp Med 205(11): 2551–2560
140. Dölken L, Malterer G, Erhard F, Kothe S, Friedel CC, Suffert G et al (2010) Systematic analysis of viral and cellular microRNA targets in cells latently infected with human gamma-herpesviruses by RISC immunoprecipitation assay. Cell Host Microbe 7(4):324–334
141. Marquitz AR, Mathur A, Nam CS, Raab-Traub N (2011) The Epstein-Barr virus BART microRNAs target the pro-apoptotic protein Bim. Virology 412(2):392–400

142. Marquitz AR, Raab-Traub N (2012) The role of miRNAs and EBV BARTs in NPC. Semin Cancer Biol 22(2):166–172
143. Marquitz AR, Mathur A, Shair KH, Raab-Traub N (2012) Infection of Epstein-Barr virus in a gastric carcinoma cell line induces anchorage independence and global changes in gene expression. Proc Natl Acad Sci U S A 109(24):9593–9598
144. Blattner WA (1999) Human retroviruses: their role in cancer. Proc Assoc Am Physicians 111(6):563–572
145. Kim HH, van den Heuvel AP, Schmidt JW, Ross SR (2011) Novel common integration sites targeted by mouse mammary tumor virus insertion in mammary tumors have oncogenic activity. PLoS One 6(11):e27425
146. Sourvinos G, Tsatsanis C, Spandidos DA (2000) Mechanisms of retrovirus-induced oncogenesis. Folia Biol 46(6):226–232
147. Sung WK, Zheng H, Li S, Chen R, Liu X, Li Y et al (2012) Genome-wide survey of recurrent HBV integration in hepatocellular carcinoma. Nat Genet 44(7):765–769
148. Boldogh I, Huang ES, Rady P, Arany I, Tyring S, Albrecht T (1994) Alteration in the coding potential and expression of H-ras in human cytomegalovirus-transformed cells. Intervirology 37(6):321–329
149. Geder KM, Lausch R, O'Neill F, Rapp F (1976) Oncogenic transformation of human embryo lung cells by human cytomegalovirus. Science 192(4244):1134–1137
150. Geder L, Kreider J, Rapp F (1977) Human cells transformed *in vitro* by human cytomegalovirus: tumorigenicity in athymic nude mice. J Natl Cancer Inst 58(4):1003–1009
151. Geder L, Laychock AM, Gorodecki J, Rapp F (1978) Alterations in biological properties of different lines of cytomegalovirus-transformed human embryo lung cells following *in vitro* cultivation. IARC Sci Publ 24 Pt 2:591–601
152. Cinatl J, Scholz M, Kotchetkov R, Vogel JU, Doerr HW (2004) Molecular mechanisms of the modulatory effects of HCMV infection in tumor cell biology. Trends Mol Med 10(1):19–23
153. Scheurer ME, Bondy ML, Aldape KD, Albrecht T, El-Zein R (2008) Detection of human cytomegalovirus in different histological types of gliomas. Acta Neuropathol 116(1):79–86
154. Cobbs CS, Soroceanu L, Denham S, Zhang W, Kraus MH (2008) Modulation of oncogenic phenotype in human glioma cells by cytomegalovirus IE1-mediated mitogenicity. Cancer Res 68(3):724–730
155. Maussang D, Verzijl D, van Walsum M, Leurs R, Holl J, Pleskoff O et al (2006) Human cytomegalovirus-encoded chemokine receptor US28 promotes tumorigenesis. Proc Natl Acad Sci U S A 103(35):13068–13073
156. Chimal-Ramírez GK, Espinoza-Sánchez NA, Fuentes-Pananá EM (2013) Protumor activities of the immune response: insights in the mechanisms of immunological shift, oncotraining, and oncopromotion. J Oncol 2013:835956
157. Elinav E, Nowarski R, Thaiss CA, Hu B, Jin C, Flavell RA (2013) Inflammation-induced cancer: crosstalk between tumours, immune cells and microorganisms. Nat Rev Cancer 13(11):759–771
158. IARC Working Group (1994) Schistosomes, liver flukes and helicobacter pylori. IARC Monogr Eval Carcinog Risks Hum 61:1–241. IARC working group on the evaluation of carcinogenic risks to humans. Lyon, 7–14 June 1994
159. Fuentes-Pananá E, Camorlinga-Ponce M, Maldonado-Bernal C (2009) Infection, inflammation and gastric cancer. Salud Publica Mex 51(5):427–433
160. Kusters JG, van Vliet AH, Kuipers EJ (2006) Pathogenesis of helicobacter pylori infection. Clin Microbiol Rev 19(3):449–490
161. Xu J, Yin Z, Cao S, Gao W, Liu L, Yin Y et al (2013) Systematic review and meta-analysis on the association between IL-1B polymorphisms and cancer risk. PLoS One 8(5):e63654
162. Xue H, Lin B, Ni P, Xu H, Huang G (2010) Interleukin-1B and interleukin-1 RN polymorphisms and gastric carcinoma risk: a meta-analysis. J Gastroenterol Hepatol 25(10):1604–1617

163. Crusius JB, Canzian F, Capellá G, Peña AS, Pera G, Sala N et al (2008) Cytokine gene polymorphisms and the risk of adenocarcinoma of the stomach in the European prospective investigation into cancer and nutrition (EPIC-EURGAST). Ann Oncol 19(11):1894–1902

164. Cheng D, Hao Y, Zhou W, Ma Y (2013) Positive association between Interleukin-8 -251A > T polymorphism and susceptibility to gastric carcinogenesis: a meta-analysis. Cancer Cell Int 13(1):100

165. Poli G (2000) Pathogenesis of liver fibrosis: role of oxidative stress. Mol Asp Med 21(3): 49–98

166. Cárdenas-Mondragón MG, Carreón-Talavera R, Camorlinga-Ponce M, Gomez-Delgado A, Torres J, Fuentes-Pananá EM (2013) Epstein Barr virus and Helicobacter pylori co-infection are positively associated with severe gastritis in pediatric patients. PLoS One 8(4):e62850

167. Cárdenas-Mondragón MG, Flores-Luna L, Camorlinga-Ponce M, Gómez-Delgado A, Torres J, Fuentes-Pananá E (2014) Epstein barr virus reactivation is an important trigger of gastric inflammation and progression to intestinal type gastric cancer. In: Proceedings of the Epstein Barr virus 50th anniversary conference. Keble College, Oxford

168. Chadburn A, Abdul-Nabi AM, Teruya BS, Lo AA (2013) Lymphoid proliferations associated with human immunodeficiency virus infection. Arch Pathol Lab Med 137(3):360–370

169. Bernstein WB, Little RF, Wilson WH, Yarchoan R (2006) Acquired immunodeficiency syndrome-related malignancies in the era of highly active antiretroviral therapy. Int J Hematol 84(1):3–11

170. Young LS, Murray PG (2003) Epstein-Barr virus and oncogenesis: from latent genes to tumours. Oncogene 22(33):5108–5121

171. Young L, Alfieri C, Hennessy K, Evans H, O'Hara C, Anderson KC et al (1989) Expression of Epstein-Barr virus transformation-associated genes in tissues of patients with EBV lymphoproliferative disease. N Engl J Med 321(16):1080–1085

172. Nourse JP, Jones K, Gandhi MK (2011) Epstein-Barr virus-related post-transplant lymphoproliferative disorders: pathogenetic insights for targeted therapy. Am J Transplant 11(5):888–895

173. Gandhi MK, Wilkie GM, Dua U, Mollee PN, Grimmett K, Williams T et al (2007) Immunity, homing and efficacy of allogeneic adoptive immunotherapy for posttransplant lymphoproliferative disorders. Am J Transplant 7(5):1293–1299

174. Haque T, Wilkie GM, Jones MM, Higgins CD, Urquhart G, Wingate P et al (2007) Allogeneic cytotoxic T-cell therapy for EBV-positive posttransplantation lymphoproliferative disease: results of a phase 2 multicenter clinical trial. Blood 110(4):1123–1131

175. Vallat L, Benhamou Y, Gutierrez M, Ghillani P, Hercher C, Thibault V et al (2004) Clonal B cell populations in the blood and liver of patients with chronic hepatitis C virus infection. Arthritis Rheum 50(11):3668–3678

176. Quinn ER, Chan CH, Hadlock KG, Foung SK, Flint M, Levy S (2001) The B-cell receptor of a hepatitis C virus (HCV)-associated non-Hodgkin lymphoma binds the viral E2 envelope protein, implicating HCV in lymphomagenesis. Blood 98(13):3745–3749

177. Chan CH, Hadlock KG, Foung SK, Levy S (2001) V (H)1-69 gene is preferentially used by hepatitis C virus-associated B cell lymphomas and by normal B cells responding to the E2 viral antigen. Blood 97(4):1023–1026

178. Hermine O, Lefrère F, Bronowicki JP, Mariette X, Jondeau K, Eclache-Saudreau V et al (2002) Regression of splenic lymphoma with villous lymphocytes after treatment of hepatitis C virus infection. N Engl J Med 347(2):89–94

179. Zullo A, Hassan C, Cristofari F, Andriani A, De Francesco V, Ierardi E et al (2010) Effects of Helicobacter pylori eradication on early stage gastric mucosa-associated lymphoid tissue lymphoma. Clin Gastroenterol Hepatol 8(2):105–110

Part IV
Holistic Approach in Cancer Ecosystem Diagnosis and Prognosis

Chapter 27
Visualizing and Subtyping Tumor Ecosystem

Phei Er Saw and Erwei Song

Abstract A revolutionary way of classifying malignancies based on molecular markers and classification models is referred to as "molecular subtyping of cancer." This method allows us to classify cancer in a molecular level, where researchers rely heavily on specific biomarkers and classifiers, that are either over-expressed or under-expressed in cancer. Unlike traditional histology cancer classifications, biomarkers include informative coding genetic changes, non-coding RNA profile (such as miRNAs, circRNAs, lncRNAs), post-genetic modification (such as DNA methylation, sumoylation, phosphorylation) among others. Biomarkers and classifiers can be constructed using machine-learning techniques like hypothesis testing for microarrays (PAM), support vector machines (SVMs), and various others. The latest recent imaging techniques regarding the visualization and subtyping of cancer are summarized in this chapter.

P. E. Saw
Guangdong Provincial Key Laboratory of Malignant Tumor Epigenetics and Gene Regulation, Guangdong-Hong Kong Joint Laboratory for RNA Medicine, Medical Research Center, Sun Yat-sen Memorial Hospital, Sun Yat-sen University, Guangzhou, China

Nanhai Translational Innovation Center of Precision Immunology, Sun Yat-sen Memorial Hospital, Sun Yat-sen University, Foshan, China

E. Song (✉)
Guangdong Provincial Key Laboratory of Malignant Tumor Epigenetics and Gene Regulation, Guangdong-Hong Kong Joint Laboratory for RNA Medicine, Medical Research Center, Sun Yat-sen Memorial Hospital, Sun Yat-sen University, Guangzhou, China

Nanhai Translational Innovation Center of Precision Immunology, Sun Yat-sen Memorial Hospital, Sun Yat-sen University, Foshan, China

Breast Tumor Center, Sun Yat-sen Memorial Hospital, Sun Yat-sen University, Guangzhou, China
e-mail: songew@mail.sysu.edu.cn

Introduction

The identification of distinct subpopulations of tumor cells and/or stromal cells inside distinct oncospheres is necessary for defining tumor heterogeneity and ecosystemic complexity. However, traditional immunohistochemistry and cytometry analyses are inefficient, owing to the restricted number of antibodies that may be utilized concurrently. Multiplex staining by sequential immunostaining may gain more characteristics, with the drawbacks of time-consuming operation, substantial tissue manipulation, and antigen perturbation over numerous staining cycles. Via a single tissue slice, emerging mass cytometry imaging technologies allow the analysis of 40 parameters at the subcellular resolution, yielding a pathology image to directly visualize the *onco-sphere* networks' topography. Large-scale genomic data have been developed following recent advancements in genome-wide profiling techniques, and novel calculation systems, especially improvement in artificial intelligence (AI), have been integrated into machine learning to improve biochemical and clinical software analyses. With this advancement, we can now propose a large-scale utilization of these methods to process, quantify, classify, and understand these data [1–6]. As we mentioned in the previous chapters, various imaging systems have been improved for us to visualize the specific interactions of cancer cells with their surrounding tissue, infiltrated immune cells, and how they are arranged in a spatio-temporal manner, which gave researchers important clue of how these cells behave in their local *onco-sphere*.

A revolutionary way of classifying malignancies based on molecular markers and classification models is referred to as "molecular subtyping of cancer." This method allows us to classify cancer in a molecular level, where researchers rely heavily on specific biomarkers and classifiers, that are either over-expressed or under-expressed in cancer. Unlike traditional histology cancer classifications, biomarkers include informative coding genetic changes, non-coding RNA profile (such as miRNAs, circRNAs, lncRNAs), post-genetic modification (such as DNA methylation, sumoylation, phosphorylation) among others [7, 8]. Biomarkers and classifiers can be constructed using machine-learning techniques like hypothesis testing for microarrays (PAM), support vector machines (SVMs), and various others [9, 10]. The latest recent imaging techniques regarding the visualization and subtyping of cancer are summarized in this chapter.

Focused Ion Beam Scanning Electron Microscopy (FIB-SEM)

The focused ion beam scanning electron microscopy (FIB/SEM) is used in relation to biological tissues. FIB/SEM is bolstered with a gallium ion beam that mills the sample surface sequentially along with a backscattered electron (BSE) detector, for getting the milled services imaged, yielding myriad images capable of being combined to form a three-dimensional image of embedded/stained biological tissues. It is feasible to derive structural information related to thousands of cubed micrometers, exhibiting complex microanatomy with precision (subcellular). The process for processing tissues, BSE imaging, enhancing contrast with potassium ferricyanide/osmium tetroxide, and platinum preparation and deposition across a chosen site within an embedded tissue block coupled with data gathering (sequential) takes ~90 h. Also detailed are the imaging settings, methods for alternating milling as well as data collection, processing methods, 3D dataset dividing, which consumes ~30 h. This technique is applied to the developing chick cornea wherein cells get collagen fibril bundles arrange into multilamellar structures to ensure transparency in the matrix of mature connective tissue. In addition to pathology, developmental biology, regenerative medicine, microstructural anatomy as well as other outlined approaches could be used in many other domains [11].

High-Throughput Imaging

High-throughput imaging is making transformational changes in cellular imaging by employing high-precision/capacity and automatic microscopes allowing for fast-paced imagining for myriad samples. It also allows for quantitative evaluation of morphological phenotypes by means of intricate datasets, and methods of computational image analysis, thus facilitating the emergence of novel experimental approaches for treating cancer. With HTI uncommon occurrences can be identified, such as cells' stochastic behavior, sparse stem cells, or certain attributes associated with the heterogeneity of tumor. Contrastingly, it is possible to simultaneously examine copious amounts of cellular targets in a sample that uses thousands of DNA probes/antibodies. Furthermore, HTI allows RNAi as well as CRISPRi screens capable of utilizing any distinction (phenotypic) between cancer cells and normal ones within an assay. Having revolutionized cellular imaging within the field of cancer research, HTI is yet to reach its full potential; its combination with super-resolution imaging, coupled with the development of novel kinds of imaging probes, its adaption to imaging of tissues, as well as the utilization of artificial intelligence (AI) would allow new patterns of tissue/cellular organization to become quantifiable and visible [12].

HTI methods are classified into these categories: profiling, deep imaging, and screening, which is the most frequently form of using HTI. Among the earliest perturbing reagents employed in conjunction with HTI for screening purposes were chemical compounds [13]. Ever since, HTI screening of chemically heterogeneous compounds has emerged as a popular drug discovery technique [14]. Chemical genetics screening is an operationally similar but conceptually distinct method that uses HTI to find pathways/genes utilized to control the phenotype of cells. This method's examples include screens for examining ways to ascertain the susceptibility of bacterial infection [15] as well as the creation of cellular stress granules [16]. The second most frequently used group of reagents within HTI screens is

RNAi [17, 18]. Previous studies have extensively applied arrayed RNAi screens to examine several cellular pathways. In the recent past, genome editing reagents based on CRISPR/Cas9 were employed with siRNA oligos in the capacity of perturbing treatments for discovering variables that control nuclear areas within the cell lines of colon cancer [19]. Although with CRISPR/Cas9 reagents, this study obtained screening results that were found to be more consistent in comparison with siRNA oligo, there remains a paucity of research on using CRISPR/Cas9 concerning the arrayed screen, thus underscoring the need for more studies so that the findings can be extrapolated to other types of cells as well as HTI assays. Another possible option is to use pooled screens of CRISPR/Cas9 to HTI screens [20, 21]. In pooled screenings, a large single-cell population is infected with libraries of lentiviral vectors expressing. Unlike arrayed HTI screens, CRISPR/Cas9 screens make it possible to use genome-wide libraries. These include a series of per gene targeting reagents without the need for automated liquid handling equipment or expensive microplates [22].

HTI for Visualizing Cancer

Through phenotypic screening, HTI is a powerful method for discovering new genetic and chemical vulnerabilities of malignancies. RNAi search for neuroblastoma (NB) cell proliferation found the KMT5A (SETD8) lysine-methyltransferase enzyme as a vital element of NB maintenance [23]. As a surrogate, HTI examined the number of nuclei regarding the ability of NB cells to proliferate along with the overall neurite length. To ascertain this screening hit, KMT5A expression's RNAi knockdown lowered the proliferation of NB cells, improved the production of neurite production, and caused death through a p53-dependent mechanism using RNAi knockdown, leading to a drop in tumor growth within a mice model of neuroblastoma [23]. This provided independent validation of the hit.

Live-cell HTI uncovered and analyzed drugs that suppress cell development of glioblastoma multiforme (GBM) [24] as part of a similar strategy to determine the vulnerabilities of certain brain cancers. Patients with GBM exhibit genetic as well as phenotypic intra/inter-tumor heterogeneity. GBM cell lines neither totally capture the underlying variability, nor mirror the characteristics of illness in cell culture, which is why they denote a less-than-satisfactory surrogate cancer [25]. To circumvent this problem, glioblastoma neuronal stem cell lines sourced from 3 patients having distinct subtypes of molecular GBM and an embryonal neural stem cell line were tested against a panel of 160 kinase inhibitors in a live-cell HTI experiment [24]. Multiple glioblastoma neuronal stem cell (GNS) cell lines comprising distinct cell subtypes were used to identify potential compounds with broad-spectrum action against GBM. J101, an initially annotated PDGFR kinase IV inhibitor, emerged for all GNS cell lines albeit that was not the case for NS cell line, thus reflecting a vulnerability specific to cancer within GBM. Based on its cellular phenotype, J101 was shown to result in cytostasis by curbing PLK1, whereas more particular PLK1 helped curtail the growth of GNS within cell cultures [24].

These observations are supported by an apoptosis enhancer in a model of chronic lymphocytic leukemia (CLL) [26]. As far as cell culture is concerned, unstimulated CLL cells derived from patients respond to venetoclax-induced death, but stimulation via IL2 and TLR7 or TLR8, a therapy replicating the patients' leukemic milieu, reduces their resistance to this medication without altering the experimental settings. Notably, an HTI assay that used the combination of cellular attributes pertaining to mitochondrial potential underwent refinement for evaluating venetoclax death sensitization in IL2 as well as TLR7/8-stimulated cells (2S cells). This approached was used to identify positive synergistic drug–drug interactions by screening 320 kinase inhibitors in relation to 2S cells from 13 patients. By inhibiting the axis of Bcl-xl/Mcl-1 anti-apoptotic, FDA-approved medication sunitinib was identified to potentiate venetoclax action in 8 2S cell lines. To develop successful cancer treatments, HTI cellular assays must be designed that can capture the patient-to-patient heterogeneity in responding to cancer treatments.

Optical Metabolic Imaging (OMI)

To assess cell redox status as well as the activity of binding enzymes, OMI uses photon fluorescence lifetime microscopy of Nicotinamide *adenine dinucleotide* phosphate (abbreviated NADPH) and flavin adenine dinucleotide (abbreviated FAD) within three-dimensional samples to pre-existing fluorophores. In this manner, metabolism can be monitored using the resolution of a single cell. OMI was created using image analysis methods to evaluate cellular heterogeneity before linking it with tumor progression and the accompanying treatment. In recent years, these methods have measured the metabolic diversity of diverse cell groups, such as fibroblasts/immune cells/tumor cells. OMI can better illuminate the underlying metabolic differences between resistant and responsive cells in a single tumor. OMI approaches play a key role in enhancing and assessing medications aimed at minority cell subpopulations resistant to treatment that could result in the reoccurrence of tumors [27].

Positron Emission Tomography (PET)

As a result of extraordinary technological advancements and a rising awareness of accurate, sensitive indicators of human function in health and illness, PET plays a key role in research as well as clinical applications. A significant portion of the physics and technical work in PET during the last three decades has been inspired by cancer, the major clinical use during that time period. This has resulted in significant advances, including the development of techniques such as whole-body PET,

PET/CT, time-of-flight PET, as well as 3D PET, among others. Despite the impressive improvements in image quality made possible by these advancements, it is necessary to understand that the capacity of PET to quantify tracer kinetics-based parameters that are biologically relevant is yet to be utilized. Recent innovations have made it possible to tackle a vast range of novel research topics, which is likely to lead to further development of radiotracers as well as applications. At least initially, many new applications will require quantitative studies that use PET's exquisite sensitivity along with the tracer principle in a significant manner. Additionally, they are expected to need more advanced quantitative analytic techniques than are now accessible.

Quantitative PET

The utilization of PET imaging in relation to radionuclide therapy, oftentimes called theranostics [28], is the second requirement for quantitative PET in cancer. In recent years, many novel theranostic compounds have been licensed in a number of nations throughout the globe, and more are on the way. SPECT has been used for conventional calculating diagnostic imaging/dosimetry; however, PET has become increasingly popular in this regard owing to its enhanced quantitative accuracy, sensitivity, and availability of positron-emitting isotopes for PET imaging (e.g., ^{124}I and positron-emitting radiometals) feasible for longer-lived therapeutic nuclei. With the understanding that tailored therapy may have a significant effect on end outcomes, it is necessary to discover new agents of PET molecular imaging which assess clinically significant targets acting as predictors or surrogates of the disease. A fast-expanding corpus of research identifies the epithelial-specific cell surface receptor integrin $\alpha v \beta 6$ as one such target, which remains very high within a large spectrum of malignancies. Meanwhile for a number of difficult cancers, $\alpha v \beta 6$ is identified in the capacity of a prognostic biomarker and corresponds with the metastatic phenotype, rendering it feasible for both cancer diagnosis and therapy. Combined with other approaches, radio-labeled peptides were created for PET imaging (non-invasive) of integrin $\alpha v \beta 6$ expression in vivo. This agent has been administered to individuals with different types of cancers, such as pancreas, breast, and lung. PET/CT scans demonstrated minimal background uptake across normal metastatic disease places but their uptake was shown to be high in not only primary lesions but also metastases, inclusive of sub-centimeter metastases. In addition to the immediate clinical effect on pre-treatment molecular imaging, the ligand could possibly function as a platform for delivering therapeutic option for some very serious tumors [29].

Multi-Plex Imaging

Intravital Microscopy

Intravital microscopy has transformed how we understand a tumor's microenvironment. Due to easy access to the calvarium with minimum surgery, bone marrow could get scanned at high resolution across time. This method has been used by our group to see the presence of fluorescent hematopoietic cells in dark bone cavities. Subsequently, a sophisticated/dynamic multicellular unit that lent support to both normal and malignant hematopoiesis was found. Intravital microscopy is mostly used to examine cancer cells' dynamic activity in their original environment. Simultaneously, researchers have developed pipelines and procedures to examine intricate attributes, such as vascular functioning/metabolite flow/intercellular exchange. The challenging multipara metric tissue map could throw up myriad challenges. The next challenge of this research is to reduce the complex network's dimensionality using image pattern recognition techniques and processing algorithms to broaden our horizons about cancer biology.

In the past, intravital microscopy (abbreviated as IVM) of small-sized animals has been undertaken for examining many aspects of tumor metastasis to determine pre-existing phenotypes of tumors in vivo and the manner in which they engage with one another. These include invasion, extravasation, and intravasation. Due to the emergence of new biosensors as well as fluorescent proteins, researchers are able to examine how different cell types interact with each other, thus widening the study's scope to include diverse cellular compartments. Combining mouse models with implanted windows of anatomical imaging has facilitated an examination of the location of tumor on metastatic organs across many days for long time periods. The next step would entail further enhancing model-based preclinical imaging methods and convert them into a clinical context in order to obtain real-time data on tumor characteristics in patients. Based on direct monitoring of tumors in patients, this strategy might possibly inform future therapeutic choices to improve the treatment of primary and metastatic cancer [30, 31].

Intravital Multiphoton Microscopy (IV-MPM)

During the last decade, IV-MPM investigations have led to key breakthroughs in cancer cell biology. However, maintaining this rate of discovery is becoming more difficult due to these reigns: (1) the need to image large and multiple arrears; (2) the variation of time ranging from milliseconds to weeks without affecting high spatial resolution needed for resolving subcellular structures; (3) IV-MPM leads to the formation of big 5D datasets that unsupported by current tools of image processing; and (4) optical/informatics advancements are swiftly implemented to cancer biology to better understand the underlying intricacy of cancer and broaden our insights into this illness, which, is opening up new dimensions of IV-MPM in the context of cancer treatment.

First, current developments in microscopy equipment and image processing techniques simultaneously detect various interactions between tumor microenvironment components and tumor cells. Next, molecular biosensors as well as protein chimeras are formed to observe activities of protein along with subcellular structures in cells and get them linked to metastatic behavior. Thirdly, IV-MPM may be integrated with other imaging modalities for correlating cell activity with its genotype or metabolic condition. Lastly, the expanding preclinical/clinical usages of IV-MPM imply that IV-MPM will play an increasing role in customized medicine. Each part also provides a few assumptions about the future evolution of IV-MPM [30].

Intravital CLEM

Recently, in partnership with metastasis imaging specialists, correlative techniques were formed and applied to link the dynamic recordings of (in vivo) tumorigenic processes to the most precise ultrastructure. The technique is called intravital correlative light and electron microscopy (intravital CLEM) and combines the innate ability of intravital imaging together with electron microscopy. It is employed in man models, such as those relating to zebrafish and mice [31]. It is also possible to use this method to examine the formation and invasion of tumors, metastatic niches' priming by means of extracellular vesicles, as well as means of metastatic extravasation. It is adaptable, supplants high-end techniques, and is capable of uncovering vital metastatic programs which may pave the way for therapeutic targeting.

Combining image of live multicellular model systems and electron microscopy (EM), intravital CLEM provides total ultrastructural information on transitory processes in vivo. Intravital microscopy is one of the many functional methods that may be used to comprehend certain phenomena in vivo (IVM), which enables the display of particular events within yearly model systems at optimum temporal resolution across extended time periods, if necessary [32–35]. In contrast, EM remains the only technique showing the high-resolution image of the subcellular world. Given that EM could also be able to address ultrastructural background, it is possible to examine cellular interactions with surroundings within tissues. CLEM combines the two imaging modalities' advantages, facilitating the focusing on a given event in time and space with light microscopy before getting the same region imaged with high-resolution EM. CLEM yields substantial findings (in vitro) using organotypic tissue slices or cultivated cells [36–40], resulting in the emergence of many correlation mechanisms between EM and dynamic fluorescence microscopy (FM) [41–47]. Within an organism that is intact, linking IVM with EM via intravital CLEM permits high-resolution assessments (temporal and geographical) of vital biological processes in their natural surroundings. IVM permits monitoring of behavior or the evaluation of function, owing to the availability of functional probes such as in vivo sensors.

Intravital CLEM in Cancer Biology

At the subatomic level, intravital CLEM has considerable promise for treating animal models of human illnesses. IVM has often investigated cancer biology [48], yielding significant insights on critical elements of tumor cell metastasis or invasion [49–53]. Recent advancements in intravital CLEM gathered invasive tumor cells in mice skin [54]. Here, a subcutaneous tumor xenograft was implanted inside the animal's ear, followed by EM/IVM. The method exhibited, in great detail, tumor invasion's subcellular characteristics, such as protrusions of tumor cell, interaction among tumor cells as well as the adjoining extracellular matrix. MicroCT-driven CLEM drastically shortened the time needed to recover tumor cells that were microscopic invasive at high resolution, probably resulting in new findings that would be imperative to explicate the molecular mechanisms behind the invasion of tumor cells [55]. Such an approach may yield ultrastructural information on invasive tumor cells' adaptability as well as their microenvironment at a tumor xenograft's stromal border [55]. This work demonstrates that an uncommon occurrence such as tumor cell extravasation may be evaluated in vivo with high resolution in its metastatic habitat.

In live tissue, IVM can only detect ephemeral metastatic events, including invasion, extravasation, as well as intravasation. IVM could be used to determine an event's location and time as well as trace tumor cells' behavior over a period of time. Nevertheless, IVM's resolution is incapable of revealing the precise architecture of tumor cells, or how they interact with the milieu, something that only EM is capable of doing. For example, it is only the ability of EM to discern the cytoskeletal structure's intricacy or intracellular organelles' diversity necessary for cell signaling. Intravital CLEM is known to provide rare inputs about metastatic processes. In the future, it could also be able to divulge further attributes of invading tumor cells, including extracellular vesicle uptake/shedding [35], tumor crosstalk, and nuclear squeezing resulting in nuclear envelope rupture [56].

zipSeq

The spatial heterogeneity of the tumor microenvironment is substantial, since a particular cell being's placement is essential in predicting the growth of tumors and related therapeutic response. In this context, ZipSeq, which is a mechanism to carry out live cells' spatial barcoding (on-demand) to map scRNA-seq data, was introduced recently [57]. Blends of barcodes bound on surface identify many interest areas for the purpose of transcriptome analysis following myriad illuminations (spatially modulated) liberating DNA. This, in turn, enables scientists to superimpose scRNA-seq data over imaging data and display genes, the expression of which alters spatially inside a specific cell population. In the present study, authors identified gene expression inside a lymph node, whereas a tumor model denotes a linkage between the depth of tumor infiltration and the differentiation between myeloid and lymphoid cells. Broadening the scope of this strategy to patient samples would yield key information on pathways which cause immunotherapy resistance. As mentioned in the previous chapters, simply categorizing tumors as cold or hot immunologically cannot capture the whole picture, given that tumors could have diverse immune-active or immune-excluded areas. ZipSeq will enable researchers to clearly and precisely examine the cell compartments' constituents within hot and cold areas, thus exposing the cell–cell interactions underpinning this heterogeneity [57].

Put succinctly, the authors successfully mapped gene expression in three conditions using ZipSeq (1) in vitro wound healing, (2) live lymph node sections, as well as (3) a live tumor microenvironment (TME). In all the aforementioned instance, the authors were able to identify new gene expression patterns concerning distinct histological features. This indicated an inward progression of both myeloid as well as T-cell development in the TME. A variant of ZipSeq effectively scales various designated areas, enabling comprehensive mapping of living tissues in the aftermath of real-time imaging or perturbation. In another study, the authors show the capacity of assigning single-cell transcriptomes to areas that were established at the same time with fluorescent imaging within in vitro wound healing model, in ex vivo tissue sections (lymph node and tumor), as well as by using ZipSeq. Using a wound healing model, this method found unique transcriptional programs active in fibroblasts, with immunofluorescence validation of many targets [57], revealing an inadequacy in current live imaging system in quantifying the spatial arrangement of the cells in TME.

Against the backdrop of lymph nodes, this approach illuminates spatially dependent gene expression verified by previous research, including Klf2, Ccr7, as well as S100a6 expression [58–60]. As the number of regions increases, this strategy facilitates the discovery of genes mapping similarly or dissimilarly to a known gene throughout space, of which some are not known. At the same time, this technique enables the advancement of T cell/myeloid differentiation mapped to the depth of physical infiltration within a tumor model's setting. As demonstrated earlier in numerous tumor models, myeloid differentiation is congruent with recruited monocytes receiving local signals which go on to skew their differentiation trajectories at the edge of tumors [61, 62].

In addition to macrophage differentiation, we detected upregulation of genes related to T-cell fatigue in tumor-specific CD8 T cells when comparing tumor core to tumor margins. Tcf1, a vital component in mainlining an exhausted stem-like phenotype, was abundantly found in marginal T cells rather than core T cells [63, 64]. The scattered T cells were farther down the exhaustion route than the T cells at the margins, based on imaging data collected prior to barcoding. The mechanical connection between depth and dedication to exhaustion merits more exploration. Interestingly, expression of chemokines/receptors, such as CCL4/5 and receptor CCR5, is increased in CD8 T cells from the tumor's center relative to those from the tumor's periphery [65–67]. To connect with a variety of hitherto unrecognized spatially varied gene expression patterns in the TME, further high-resolution transcriptional profiling techniques, such as FISH or CODEX, are necessary.

Numerous spatial transcriptomics techniques employ barcoded poly-dT grids or poly-dT-bearing barcoded beads to collect all transcripts inside the grid position [68–70]. Despite the high spatial resolution of these methods, it will not be easy to implement them straight away to tissue following either live imaging or disturbances. The comparatively low read depth of many of these methods ($\sim1^{e4}$ reads per 150 μm grid square for spatial transcriptomics and 2^{e2} per 10 μm bead for SLIDE-seq) would make it difficult to analyze expression patterns in either rarer cell types or the ones with RNA levels. This is because during the capture step, their transcripts would be diluted. ZipSeq integrates into scRNA-Seq procedures based on droplets, which is why it can potentially exploit a higher number of read depth per cell and allow the formation of transcriptomes without requiring deconvolution of transcripts derived from manly cells. ZipSeq is capable of being readily combined with contemporaneous surface epitope labeling by means of immune repertoire sequencing single-cell [57, 71, 72].

Next-Generation Monitoring Systems for the Immune System

Mass Cytometry (CyTOF)

Imaging mass cytometry (IMC) makes it possible to in situ investigation of cell phenotyping in a single tissue segment's architecture. As of now, it is possible to simultaneously examine 50 protein markers simultaneously. IMC's application in cancer research could aid in defining biomarkers of prognostic as well as theragnostic importance for both existing and future treatments against new and established therapeutic targets while improving how we understand the progression of cancer along with its resistance to immune systems, as well as ways of surmounting them [73]. Diagnostic techniques like cytometer as well as immuno-histochemistry/immunofluorescence (IHC/IF) are routinely used for profiling cells in tissue samples. Both techniques use antibodies that target these protein markers' epitopes to get protein markers highlighted within tissues as well as cells. The conjugation of Abs enables the measurement and tracing of Abs-fixed within the tissues and cells, to denote the localization/amount of these protein markers. Nevertheless, the markers that simultaneously utilize these diagnostic approaches remain modest due to the limited number of revelation channels that can be used concurrently, hence curtailing the number of Abs labeled differently that can be simultaneously utilized. Standard cytometry as well as IF methods based on fluorescence is curtailed in their multiplexing capabilities owing to certain fluorochromes' overlapping spectra, due to which signals cannot be distinguished from each another [73].

In order to enhance the number of concurrently evaluable markers, new revelation methods of the various Abs without overlapping spectra and detecting signals were used. Using mass spectrometry and time-of-flight (TOF) measurements, each metal isotope may be detected individually based on its correct mass. Consequently, it is possible to detect several metal isotopes with TOF-based identification techniques. By creating cytometry using TOF (CyTOF) technology of mass spectrometry, the concept of employing metal-tagged Abs and mass spectrometry to identify them has been used for the first time in cytometry [74]. Using mass spectrometry to detect numerous metal isotopes coupled to diverse antibodies targeting multiple proteins enables significant multiplexing capabilities for detecting concomitantly distinct indicators. The overall metal isotopes that are accessible (around so far) determine the number of markers that may be co-analyzed using this technique [75]. Accordingly, CyTOF's multiplexing capability surpasses fluorochrome-based cytometry's capabilities.

The combination of CyTOF technology with cell–/tissue-material's laser ablation deposited over glass slides led to IMC technique, leading to the addition of tissue architectural information to data based on CyTOF. Thus, IMC has exemplified a key advancement in multiple markers' multiplexed immunodetection in tissue samples [74] and is capable of simultaneously assessing around 50 protein markers along with 50 antibodies on all cells [75] located inside the tissue. In doing so, it is able to comfortably surpass IHC/IF's multiplexing capabilities. Apart from examining cells in their respective tissues, the IMC facilitates the localization of proteins inside the nuclear, membrane cell, as well as cytoplasmic compartments. Fluidigm Corporation (South San Francisco, CA, USA) had commercialized the IMC technology in 2011 under Hyperion Imaging System. This approach, in turn, enabled IMC's application to each sample type placed over glass slides, which was also inclusive of cells [76] and snap-frozen tissues [77]. For this reason, IMC is well suited to examining tiny, valuable archival pathology samples including biopsies [78]. Like IHC/IF, it involves the same mechanism whereby specimen undergoes pre-treatment before antibody incubation as well as washing prior to detecting Abs signals.

Multiplexed Ion Beam Imaging (MIBI)

Fluorophore-labeled probes are used by laser scanning cytometry as well as fluorescent microscopy [79, 80] for visualizing tissue stained using 6–8 markers. Utilizing cyclical rounds of staining, imaging, and stripping a single formalin-fixed paraffin-embedded (FFPE) tissue piece, multiplex immunohistochemistry (mIHC) is accomplished to cover a higher number of targets. Generally, all cycles are known to utilize antigen retrieval induced by heat and alcohol dehydration, potentially harming the tissue along with the accompanying antigens found in the FFPE sample. This leads to long processing times and challenges related to picture co-registration. Recent advancements in CO-Detection by indEXing make it possible for the tissue to get tagged with a large panel of antibodies with unique DNA barcodes and before proceeding with cycling processing.

Recent studies have typified the immunological infiltrates in both normal as well as lupus (MRL/lpr) mouse spleens [81]. Multiplexing has also been allowed by utilizing metal-labeled antibodies simultaneously traced by an image mass cytometer. This device employs an atmospheric laser ablation chamber along with a mass cytometer [82, 83]. However, the widespread implementation of these systems is impeded by sample preparation, sensitivity, image quality, and throughput issues. A recent advancement includes multiplexed ion beam imaging (MIBI) that simultaneously traces more than 40 markers at subcellular resolution. In turn, this allows for cell type classification based on markers, single-cell segmentation, as well as spatial analysis of the cells present in the TME [84–86]. Tissue is stained with a panel of metal-labeled antibodies, followed by the use of secondary ion mass spectrometry (time-of-flight; MS-TOF) for imaging the stained tissue. Then, the masses of identified species are allocated to target biomolecules based on each antibody's unique metal isotope label, resulting in the creation of multiplex pictures.

Subtyping Cancer Ecosystem

High-Throughput Screening Method to Obtain Precise Molecular Data

Profiling Gene Expression

The two most used profiling techniques for producing significant gene expression data include microarray and RNA-Seq. Microarrays can characterize and categorize not only the expression level, but also the expression patterns of up to 10^6 of selected genes in a single experiment. A sequencing-based method for figuring out how various genes are present throughout the entire genome is called RNA-Seq. RNA-Seq has several advantages over microarray [87]. To begin with, RNA-Seq measures gene expression more precisely than microarrays that use hybridization. In contrast to microarray, RNA-Seq has the potential to detect both coding and non-coding novel transcripts, single-nucleotide variants, changes in non-coding RNA profile, and other modifications. The minimal background signal and broad dynamic range of RNA-Seq are its final advantages. Microarray is the most extensively used technology for producing massive amounts of molecular data for various years [88]. The only bottleneck with this technic is high cost. However, with the quick advancement of sequencing and analytical techniques, sequencing costs will drop significantly. As more RNA-Seq statistical tools will be developed, RNA-Seq is likely to replace microarray technology [89].

Profiling Low- and Medium-Throughput Molecular Data

The therapeutic application of biomarkers identified through subtyping research is possible. To reduce testing time and costs, only a few hundred of these well-established biomarkers are often examined in clinical settings [90]. Only a few newly processed or snap-frozen cancer specimens are present, the majority being formalin-fixed paraffin-embedded (FFPE) [91]. Contrary to the high-throughput approaches described above, several low- and medium-throughput techniques, including qPCR, NanoString, and TMA, are ideally suited for clinical biomarker as they allow for a significant study of clinical material. These methods are often used when time is of essence, and sample size and cost are maintained to a minimum [92, 93].

CNV analysis and measuring biomarker expression levels are two frequent applications of qPCR. It consumes few resources since the PCR amplification stage might greatly improve the nucleic acid intake. The speed, sensitivity, specificity, and accuracy of qPCR are further advantages that have helped to establish it as the go-to method for verifying the results of high-throughput systems like microarray and RNA-Seq [94]. QPCR-based tests can only assay a small proportion of biomarkers in a single experiment, in contrast to the approach that can assay large quantities of biomarkers in a specific experiment. Fresh-frozen tissue is frequently necessary because qPCR-based diagnostics demand the finest nucleic acids while sampling the material. Up to 800 genes can have their expression measured by the NanoString nCounter analytical tool [95]. The nCounter technology is comparable to qPCR and much more precise than microarrays [96]. This method uses electronic molecular barcoding and microscopic imaging to measure the amounts of gene expression in a single experiment without the use of enzymatic procedures [96, 97]. Another advantage of this strategy is its exceptional specificity and precision [98]. One of the drawbacks is the expensive, but necessary chemicals and equipment [95].

One paraffin block can hold up to 1000 tumor specimens that can be examined concurrently using the histology-based test tissue microarray (TMA) [99, 100]. The DNA, mRNA, and protein levels can all be examined to examine molecular targets. If the depth of each core is sufficient, a TMA block may get sectioned repeatedly, with the ability to analyze biomarkers in each segment. The array samples are all processed uniformly, which is the main advantage of TMA [101]. TMA also has the advantage of being reasonably priced. Only a tiny amount of reagent is required to analyze all of the specimens on a single slide [101]. FFPE tissues are required for TMA, whereas fresh-frozen tissues are needed for qPCR, which is the primary source of resources in a clinic. TMA has its own limitations. For instance, a TMA test has subpar sensitivity, specificity, and precision [102]. Other downsides include the fact that only a few analytes may be examined, that the analyzed specimen fraction is too tiny to accurately reflect the entire tumor, and that it normally takes several days to acquire the analysis results [101]. Additionally, fewer tissues will be present during the TMA staining process [103].

Subtype Identification and Characterization

The technique of arranging data items so that those in a similar cluster are more comparable to those in other clusters is known as molecular subtyping (or molecular classification). Current classification technic is divided into supervised (with predetermined labels, i.e., tumors or healthy tissues) and unsupervised (no prior classification). Subtyping, which can be either supervised or unsupervised, is a more general term for categorization. In biological research, unsupervised classification has been more and more prevalent [104] and has been applied in various cancer studies [105–110]. Based on these studies, we summarized an approach for molecular subtyping of cancer as detailed below.

Subtype Identifications

A common way to arrange high-throughput molecular data is as a matrix, with the x-axis rows denoting traits (indicators specific to this study including genes, non-coding RNAs, or DNA methylation indicators) and the y-axis columns denoting samples, a common 2D way used in current research, and these two features mentioned above are standardized and are usually used in clustering analysis [111]. A more advanced setting called "biclustering," also known as subspace clustering, is important in identifying certain feature subsets that are only active or suppressed in specific conditions [112]. It is now possible to have multiple samples of different qualities across various times or experimental settings because of the quick development of data profiling technologies. Therefore, the addition of the z-axis is vital, as such information (time or experimental condition) could be added on top of the 2D matrices above (samples, attributes) [113]. In this tri-cluster data mining, feature groups that are specific in time or specific condition must be input into the system, so that the mathematical analysis could accurately calculate the data for quantitative analysis [114, 115] has been developed as an alternative for analyzing such longitudinal and geographic data.

To determine the ideal number of clusters that should be included in an analysis, measurements such as gap statistics [116], cophenetic coefficients [117], and the cumulative distribution function (CDF) are utilized [118]. The computed results of cluster sizes and assignments vary because different algorithms are used in different cluster analysis methodologies [118]. The findings from repeated testing of clustering algorithms are combined into a single consensus outcome in the cluster ensemble technique, which was developed to increase the durability of clustering [118]. When simultaneously used with resampling technic, agreement clustering provides a consensus after numerous iterations of the clustering procedure [119]. Ensemble clustering further integrates various cluster analysis from results, but consensus clustering allows resampling and replicates one specific type of clustering strategy. Biclustering and triclustering can benefit from ensembles and consensus clustering methodologies, which are extensively used in cancer subtyping investigations [120–123].

Subtype Characterizations

Studying the links between newly identified subtypes and their molecular/clinical significance is one goal. Subtype characterizations generally depend on genomic and clinical data [124]. Characterizations of subtypes may be useful in locating consensus subtypes both within and within cancers. Subtyping of a tumor allows researcher to study specific changes that are seen in different signaling pathways, mutations that occur during cancer progression, methylation patterns across malignancies. This information is crucial as clinicians would then know how these data fit into the subtype classification that can be accurately used for patient stratification. A subtyping "visualizing" tool is therefore developed, named StratomeX. This system was created as a comprehensive visualization tool that enables researchers to examine the relationships between subtypes and other genomic data sources such as CNV, different epigenetic changes, post-translational modification, and copy number information [125]. These data could be incorporated using StratomeX, to generate useful comprehensive data to identify unique cancer subtypes as well as to have a better understanding on how to interpret these molecular changes in a cancer subtype. Furthermore, the biology behind the identified subtypes is frequently defined using gene set enrichment analysis (GSEA). Gene sets, which are collections of genes with the same bioactivity, chromosomal location, or regulatory mechanism, are groups in which expression data are analyzed by GSEA [126]. Databases like KEGG and Gene Ontology (GO) [56] provide access to most recent data that have annotated gene sets [127].

In order to characterize the detected subtypes clinically, clinicians must be able to extract all clinical data must contain patient including inclusion of clinical information, such as background data (name, gender, race), current tumor condition (tumor grade, tumor size, time of discovery), epidemiology data (smoking history), and clinical treatment plans (relapse data, follow-up time), and so forth. These data closely relate to a common method for analyzing differences in survival times among subtypes is survival analysis. The Kaplan–Meier plot can be used to create the survival curve that enables a statistical comparison between two subtypes (also possible using Log-rank test) [128, 129]. Subtype characterization is essential. They provide a subtype validation mechanism and help us better understand the subtype features. As mentioned above, recognized subtypes should ideally have distinct biological molecular features which lead to an obvious change in clinical characteristics. It is important to note that sometimes, subtypes frequently differ statistically but not phenotypically, and therefore could be easily passed off as patient-to-patient variation. In these cases, re-clustering and categorization (or using multi-variate analysis) should be carried out until more comprehensible results are generated.

Immunogenomics in Tumor Subtyping

Over the past 20 years, next-genome sequencing (NGS), which includes whole-genome sequencing (WGS), whole-exome sequencing (WES), and RNA sequencing (RNA-seq, mentioned above), has been successfully developed and applied to gather whole-genome data in individuals. NGS, in contrast to Sanger sequencing, provides significant genomic and transcriptome datasets, laying the foundation for the investigation of the multi-step immune response. Through the use of bioinformatic techniques, immunogenomics research findings in the NGS era provide a global perspective of the immune cell compositions of tumor-immune environment in the local *onco-sphere*. NGS also helps identify immunogenic proteins through the prediction of aberrant peptides, HLA types, and MHC-peptide binding affinities [130].

Quantification of Immune Cells

Tumor-immune environment is made up of innate and adaptive immune cells, as mentioned in previous chapters. Due to many reasons, including high cost, time-consuming, and scarce tissue supply, profiling immune cells through flow cytometry, FACs and immunohistochemistry (IHC) is not practical. NGS allows in silico analysis as a viable alternative approach for solving this issue. Gene expression patterns differed widely among different types of immune cells due to the high cellular heterogeneity, and they may in some ways represent immune cell types. Since NGS data have been verified to be reliable, we can use it to predict the prevalence of hundreds of different immune cell types. These studies mostly rely on DNA and RNA profile analysis, but mainly RNAs [131]. Exemplary GSEA-based algorithms include ESTIMATE, xCell, and MCP counter are summarized in Table 27.1 below.

Immunogenomics and Artificial Intelligence (AI)

In order to diagnose illnesses, anticipate prognoses, and predict treatment outcomes, scientists and medical professionals are concentrating on computer science or, at a higher level, deep learning [139]. A newly developed program called CN-learn has been created to find CNVs in addition to the numerous established methods for detecting SNVs, and preliminary results are encouraging [140–142]. The entire mass spectrometry deep learning approach EDGE [143], which was verified in NSCLC patients, may be trained using a sizable integrated dataset of HLA variants and peptides from various cancer tissues that were developed and made available. Recently, two prominent computational deep learning methods, MARIA and

Table 27.1 GSEA-based algorithm and their merits

Exemplary GSEA-based algorithms	Advantages	Disadvantages	Ref
ESTIMATE	Determine the number and distribution of immune cells and stromal cells. The ESTIMATE algorithm produces an immunity score and a stromal score dependent on the gene signature and single sample GSEA (ssGSEA)	However, specific immune cell types cannot be distinguished using the ESTIMATE score	[132]
xCELL	ssGSEA-based method that gathers gene sets to characterize diverse cell types from a variety of RNA-seq and microarray-based datasets, enhancing robustness to reduce noise disruptions	The requirement for a unique gene set for each target immunocyte subpopulation	[133]
MCP counter	Determines an abundance score for each TIME cell group (such as immune cells, endothelial cells, and fibroblasts) in each sample based on the geometric mean of marker gene expression levels	The requirement for a unique gene set for each target immunocyte subpopulation	[134]
Deconvolution method (functions)			
CIBERSORT	Employs a gene expression signature matrix and linear support vector regression		[135]
QuanTIseq	Consists of finite least-squares regression-based deconvolution, raw RNA-seq data preparation, and gene expression analysis. Integrated imaging information obtained from H&E, IHC, and IF-stained plates is employed to support gene expression deconvolution, enabling immune profiling of the relative cell fraction and unique immune cell densities		[136]
FARDEEP	Concentrates on a significant issue that earlier algorithms have not addressed, including how outlier contamination of gene expression affects deconvolution accuracy. For datasets with significant tail noise, Builds a robust model using the least trimmed square (LTS) approach		[137]
MuSiC	Makes use of cross-subject scRNA-seq, which considers cross-subject and cross-cell consistency, to create cell type-specific gene sequences for bulk RNA-seq deconvolution analysis		[138]

MixMHC2pred, were introduced, greatly enhancing MHC-II prediction accuracy. MARIA then uses a recurrent neural network to generate a presentation score (RNN). The deep learning MHC-II peptide classifier MixMHC2pred was trained using the MoDec motif deconvolution technique. The neoantigens anticipated by both systems have been demonstrated to activate responsive $CD4^+$ T cells, and these two deep learning algorithms beat the previously employed NetMHCII pan program [144].

Radiomics in Cancer Immunity

With the evolution of AI in medical imageology, scanning is now a vast amount of digital data rather than just a picture. Areas of interest (ROIs), which frequently include tumor sites, can be used to obtain quantitative and qualitative data that can be used to describe tumor biological activity and possibly link it to clinical outcomes. Radiomics is a method for analyzing visual data with the aid of artificial intelligence [145]. Additionally, a new clinical model for identifying NSCLC patients either having a high or low tumor mutation burden (TMB), with different clinical outcomes, was developed. This new model called the tumor mutational burden radiomics biomarker (TMBRB) outperformed previous clinical models [146]. To differentiate between responders and non-responders, researchers looked at variations in radiomic texture (DelRADx) between baseline and post-treatment CT imaging [147]. The radiomics signature was identified as an immunotherapy response indicator in validation cohorts. Instead of employing T-cell infiltration to demonstrate correlations between radiomic properties and clinical responses, a radiomics biomarker was created and validated using images and clinical data [148]. To predict the effectiveness of immunotherapy and overall survival, this biomarker has shown to have an advantage over calculating lesion volume [149]. With ICB therapy, certain peculiar effects have been noted. One illustration is hyperprogression (HP), which is an abnormally quick development following the beginning of immunotherapy [150, 151]. The poor prognosis of the disease necessitates the urgent need for predictive biomarkers. To distinguish HPs from respondents and nonrespondents, textural and distinctive quantitative vascular tortuosity features were applied [152]. Overall, radiomics technology enables the non-invasive prediction of therapeutic results, stratification of patient immunotherapy sensitivity, and early identification of changes in malignancies. These results must be confirmed in larger cohorts and prospective studies, though, as the majority of existing research is retrospective.

Computational Pathology in Tumor Immunity

The goal of pathologists, as opposed to radiologists, is to identify microscopic histological alterations. To differentiate between the different cell types, pathologists employ H&E staining, IHC, and IF. Artificial intelligence in pathology, also referred to as digital pathology, uses computer analysis to provide new information on the relationship between crucial aspects of cancer biology and the interplay of immune cells and tumor cells. To explore the quantity and geographic distribution of immune cells that infiltrate tumors on H&E or IHC staining slides, deep learning algorithms based on CNN have been created [153–156]. A deep learning algorithm was developed to evaluate the TIME's spatial architecture, and it discovered that the prognosis depends on the proportion of "immune-cold" patches and that immune infiltration varies between samples from patients with comparable clinical characteristics. The spatial complexity of TIL and TIME is related to evolutionary dynamics, clonal neoantigens, and antigen presentation [157]. Similar to radiomics, which enables us to perceive TIME at the cellular or molecular level, digital pathology draws out hidden information from images [74, 85, 158]. In computational pathology, deep learning is a paradigm for vast detection, which indicates that AI can look at multiple suspicious slides at once. Significant improvements in radiomics have been made in clinical practice over the past 10 years. Radiomics can forecast immune infiltration and the effectiveness of immunotherapy. On the other hand, deep learning is used in digital pathology to examine spatial architecture. Although they need intrusive examination, pathological slides may provide more accurate immunological data than imaging; as a result, radiomics and computational pathology work best together when examining the immune environment.

Conclusion

In terms of visualizing cancer ecosystem, imaging has had a profound impact on our ability to understand and treat cancer. State-of-the-art technology has increased our knowledge in visualizing cancer using various imaging approaches. It has also broadened our horizon on the inherent complexity of the tumor and their relationship with their local, distal, and systemic *onco-sphere*. These imaging technics are now used in various aspects of cancer research, from investigating the complexity and diversity of cancer cells and their environments to guiding clinical decision-making. In terms of subtyping cancer ecosystem, a crucial stage is the characterization of subgroups. The unique subgroups must have both statistical and physiological significance. This suggests that to adequately explain the identified subgroups, clinical and molecular data must be gathered. Additionally, the performance of classifiers may be evaluated using publicly available data sets. By enhancing statistical techniques and data interpretation, the distance between findings (identified subgroups) and clinical applications can be bridged. When cancers are correctly identified by visualization techniques and divided into subtypes, the crucial next step is to correctly interpret these subgroups from a biological perspective, after which the focus shifts to therapeutic applications.

References

1. Eisen MB, Spellman PT, Brown PO, Botstein D (1998) Cluster analysis and display of genome-wide expression patterns. Proc Natl Acad Sci U S A 95(25):14863–14868
2. Tibshirani R, Hastie T, Narasimhan B, Chu G (2002) Diagnosis of multiple cancer types by shrunken centroids of gene expression. Proc Natl Acad Sci U S A 99(10):6567–6572
3. Lee DD, Seung HS (1999) Learning the parts of objects by non-negative matrix factorization. Nature 401(6755):788–791

4. Breiman L (2001) Random forests. Mach Learn 45(1):5–32
5. Pena JM, Lozano JA, Larranaga P (1999) An empirical comparison of four initialization methods for the K-means algorithm. Pattern Recogn Lett 20(10):1027–1040
6. Hearst MA, Dumais ST, Osman E, Platt J, Scholkopf B (1998) Support vector machines. IEEE Intell Syst 13(4):18–28
7. Zhao L, Lee VHF, Ng MK, Yan H, Bijlsma MF (2019) Molecular subtyping of cancer: current status and moving toward clinical applications. Brief Bioinform 20(2):572–584
8. Hoadley KA, Yau C, Wolf DM, Cherniack AD, Tamborero D, Ng S et al (2014) Multiplatform analysis of 12 cancer types reveals molecular classification within and across tissues of origin. Cell 158(4):929–944
9. Tan CS, Ting WS, Shahreen K, Saberi MM, Chan WH, Safaai D et al (2015) A review of cancer classification software for gene expression data. Int J Biol Biotechnol 7(4):89–108
10. Tan CS, Soon TIW, Kasim S, Mohamad MS, Ibrahim Z (2015) A review of cancer classification software for gene expression data. Int J Biol Biotechnol 7(4):89–108
11. Baena V, Conrad R, Friday P, Fitzgerald E, Kim T, Bernbaum J et al (2021) FIB-SEM as a volume electron microscopy approach to study cellular architectures in sars-cov-2 and other viral infections: a practical primer for a virologist. Viruses 13(4):611
12. Pegoraro G, Misteli T (2017) High-throughput imaging for the discovery of cellular mechanisms of disease. Trends Genet 33(9):604–615
13. Haggarty SJ, Mayer TU, Miyamoto DT, Fathi R, King RW, Mitchison TJ et al (2000) Dissecting cellular processes using small molecules: identification of colchicine-like, taxol-like and other small molecules that perturb mitosis. Chem Biol 7(4):275–286
14. Bickle M (2010) The beautiful cell: high-content screening in drug discovery. Anal Bioanal Chem 398(1):219–226
15. Kuijl C, Savage ND, Marsman M, Tuin AW, Janssen L, Egan DA et al (2007) Intracellular bacterial growth is controlled by a kinase network around PKB/AKT1. Nature 450(7170): 725–730
16. Wippich F, Bodenmiller B, Trajkovska MG, Wanka S, Aebersold R, Pelkmans L (2013) Dual specificity kinase DYRK3 couples stress granule condensation/dissolution to mTORC1 signaling. Cell 152(4):791–805
17. Boutros M, Heigwer F, Laufer C (2015) Microscopy-based high-content screening. Cell 163(6):1314–1325
18. Conrad C, Gerlich D, W. (2010) Automated microscopy for high-content RNAi screening. J Cell Biol 188(4):453–461
19. Tan J, Martin SE (2016) Validation of synthetic CRISPR reagents as a tool for arrayed functional genomic screening. PLoS One 11(12):e0168968
20. Wang T, Wei JJ, Sabatini DM, Lander ES (2014) Genetic screens in human cells using the CRISPR-Cas9 system. Science 343(6166):80–84
21. Shalem O, Sanjana NE, Hartenian E, Shi X, Scott DA, Mikkelson T et al (2014) Genome-scale CRISPR-Cas9 knockout screening in human cells. Science 343(6166):84–87
22. Wade M (2015) High-throughput silencing using the CRISPR-Cas9 system: a review of the benefits and challenges. J Biomol Screen 20(8):1027–1039
23. Veschi V, Liu Z, Voss TC, Ozbun L, Gryder B, Yan C et al (2017) Epigenetic siRNA and chemical screens identify SETD8 inhibition as a therapeutic strategy for p53 activation in high-risk Neuroblastoma. Cancer Cell 31(1):50–63
24. Danovi D, Folarin A, Gogolok S, Ender C, Elbatsh AM, Engström PG et al (2013) A high-content small molecule screen identifies sensitivity of glioblastoma stem cells to inhibition of polo-like kinase 1. PLoS One 8(10):e77053
25. Pollard SM, Yoshikawa K, Clarke ID, Danovi D, Stricker S, Russell R et al (2009) Glioma stem cell lines expanded in adherent culture have tumor-specific phenotypes and are suitable for chemical and genetic screens. Cell Stem Cell 4(6):568–580

26. Oppermann S, Ylanko J, Shi Y, Hariharan S, Oakes CC, Brauer PM et al (2016) High-content screening identifies kinase inhibitors that overcome venetoclax resistance in activated CLL cells. Blood 128(7):934–947
27. Walsh AJ, Skala MC (2015) Optical metabolic imaging quantifies heterogeneous cell populations. Biomed Opt Express 6(2):559–573
28. Loke KS, Padhy AK, Ng DC, Goh AS, Divgi C (2011) Dosimetric considerations in radioimmunotherapy and systemic radionuclide therapies: a review. World J Nucl Med 10(2):122–138
29. Meikle SR, Sossi V, Roncali E, Cherry SR, Banati R, Mankoff D et al (2021) Quantitative PET in the 2020s: a roadmap. Phys Med Biol 66(6):06RM1
30. Perrin L, Bayarmagnai B, Gligorijevic B (2020) Frontiers in intravital multiphoton microscopy of cancer. Cancer Rep (Hoboken) 3(1):e1192
31. Karreman MA, Hyenne V, Schwab Y, Goetz JG (2016) Intravital correlative microscopy: imaging life at the nanoscale. Trends Cell Biol 26(11):848–863
32. Lämmermann T, Afonso PV, Angermann BR, Wang JM, Kastenmüller W, Parent CA et al (2013) Neutrophil swarms require LTB4 and integrins at sites of cell death *in vivo*. Nature 498(7454):371–375
33. Chèvre R, González-Granado JM, Megens RT, Sreeramkumar V, Silvestre-Roig C, Molina-Sánchez P et al (2014) High-resolution imaging of intravascular atherogenic inflammation in live mice. Circ Res 114(5):770–779
34. Erami Z, Herrmann D, Warren SC, Nobis M, McGhee EJ, Lucas MC et al (2016) Intravital FRAP imaging using an E-cadherin-GFP mouse reveals disease- and drug-dependent dynamic regulation of cell-cell junctions in live tissue. Cell Rep 14(1):152–167
35. Zomer A, Maynard C, Verweij FJ, Kamermans A, Schäfer R, Beerling E et al (2015) *In vivo* imaging reveals extracellular vesicle-mediated phenocopying of metastatic behavior. Cell 161(5):1046–1057
36. Van Engelenburg SB, Shtengel G, Sengupta P, Waki K, Jarnik M, Ablan SD et al (2014) Distribution of ESCRT machinery at HIV assembly sites reveals virus scaffolding of ESCRT subunits. Science 343(6171):653–656
37. Kukulski W, Schorb M, Kaksonen M, Briggs JA (2012) Plasma membrane reshaping during endocytosis is revealed by time-resolved electron tomography. Cell 150(3):508–520
38. Briggman KL, Helmstaedter M, Denk W (2011) Wiring specificity in the direction-selectivity circuit of the retina. Nature 471(7337):183–188
39. Avinoam O, Schorb M, Beese CJ, Briggs JA, Kaksonen M (2015) ENDOCYTOSIS. Endocytic sites mature by continuous bending and remodeling of the clathrin coat. Science 348(6241):1369–1372
40. Al Jord A, Lemaître AI, Delgehyr N, Faucourt M, Spassky N, Meunier A (2014) Centriole amplification by mother and daughter centrioles differs in multiciliated cells. Nature 516(7529):104–107
41. Müller-Reichert T, Verkade P (2014) Correlative light and electron microscopy. Methods Cell Biol 124:xvii–xviii
42. Muller-Reichert T (2012) Correlative light and electron microscopy: correlative light and electron microscopy. Methods Cell Biol 111:xvii–xix
43. Loussert Fonta C, Humbel BM (2015) Correlative microscopy. Arch Biochem Biophys 581: 98–110
44. de Boer P, Hoogenboom JP, Giepmans BN (2015) Correlated light and electron microscopy: ultrastructure lights up! Nat Methods 12(6):503–513
45. Mironov AA, Beznoussenko GV (2009) Correlative microscopy: a potent tool for the study of rare or unique cellular and tissue events. J Microsc 235(3):308–321
46. Caplan J, Niethammer M, Taylor RM 2nd, Czymmek KJ (2011) The power of correlative microscopy: multi-modal, multi-scale, multi-dimensional. Curr Opin Struct Biol 21(5): 686–693

47. Meisslitzer-Ruppitsch C, Röhrl C, Neumüller J, Pavelka M, Ellinger A (2009) Photooxidation technology for correlated light and electron microscopy. J Microsc 235(3):322–335
48. Ellenbroek SI, van Rheenen J (2014) Imaging hallmarks of cancer in living mice. Nat Rev Cancer 14(6):406–418
49. Lohela M, Casbon AJ, Olow A, Bonham L, Branstetter D, Weng N et al (2014) Intravital imaging reveals distinct responses of depleting dynamic tumor-associated macrophage and dendritic cell subpopulations. Proc Natl Acad Sci U S A 111(47):E5086–E5095
50. Provenzano PP, Cuevas C, Chang AE, Goel VK, Von Hoff DD, Hingorani SR (2012) Enzymatic targeting of the stroma ablates physical barriers to treatment of pancreatic ductal adenocarcinoma. Cancer Cell 21(3):418–429
51. Kienast Y, von Baumgarten L, Fuhrmann M, Klinkert WE, Goldbrunner R, Herms J et al (2010) Real-time imaging reveals the single steps of brain metastasis formation. Nat Med 16(1):116–122
52. Alexander S, Weigelin B, Winkler F, Friedl P (2013) Preclinical intravital microscopy of the tumor-stroma interface: invasion, metastasis, and therapy response. Curr Opin Cell Biol 25(5): 659–671
53. Hirata E, Girotti MR, Viros A, Hooper S, Spencer-Dene B, Matsuda M et al (2015) Intravital imaging reveals how BRAF inhibition generates drug-tolerant microenvironments with high integrin β1/FAK signaling. Cancer Cell 27(4):574–588
54. Karreman MA, Mercier L, Schieber NL, Shibue T, Schwab Y, Goetz JG (2014) Correlating intravital multi-photon microscopy to 3D electron microscopy of invading tumor cells using anatomical reference points. PLoS One 9(12):e114448
55. Karreman MA, Mercier L, Schieber NL, Solecki G, Allio G, Winkler F et al (2016) Fast and precise targeting of single tumor cells in vivo by multimodal correlative microscopy. J Cell Sci 129(2):444–456
56. Denais CM, Gilbert RM, Isermann P, McGregor AL, te Lindert M, Weigelin B et al (2016) Nuclear envelope rupture and repair during cancer cell migration. Science 352(6283):353–358
57. Hu KH, Eichorst JP, McGinnis CS, Patterson DM, Chow ED, Kersten K et al (2020) ZipSeq: barcoding for real-time mapping of single cell transcriptomes. Nat Methods 17(8):833–843
58. Zemmour D, Zilionis R, Kiner E, Klein AM, Mathis D, Benoist C (2018) Single-cell gene expression reveals a landscape of regulatory T cell phenotypes shaped by the TCR. Nat Immunol 19(3):291–301
59. Weber JP, Fuhrmann F, Feist RK, Lahmann A, Al Baz MS, Gentz LJ et al (2015) ICOS maintains the T follicular helper cell phenotype by down-regulating Krüppel-like factor 2. J Exp Med 212(2):217–233
60. Lee JY, Skon CN, Lee YJ, Oh S, Taylor JJ, Malhotra D et al (2015) The transcription factor KLF2 restrains CD4+ T follicular helper cell differentiation. Immunity 42(2):252–264
61. Franklin RA, Liao W, Sarkar A, Kim MV, Bivona MR, Liu K et al (2014) The cellular and molecular origin of tumor-associated macrophages. Science 344(6186):921–925
62. Movahedi K, Laoui D, Gysemans C, Baeten M, Stangé G, Van den Bossche J et al (2010) Different tumor microenvironments contain functionally distinct subsets of macrophages derived from Ly6C (high) monocytes. Cancer Res 70(14):5728–5739
63. Lin YD, Arora J, Diehl K, Bora SA, Cantorna MT (2019) Vitamin D is required for ILC3 derived IL-22 and protection from Citrobacter rodentium infection. Front Immunol 10:1
64. Im SJ, Hashimoto M, Gerner MY, Lee J, Kissick HT, Burger MC et al (2016) Defining CD8+ T cells that provide the proliferative burst after PD-1 therapy. Nature 537(7620):417–421
65. de Oliveira CE, Gasparoto TH, Pinheiro CR, Amôr NG, Nogueira MRS, Kaneno R et al (2017) CCR5-dependent homing of T regulatory cells to the tumor microenvironment contributes to skin squamous cell carcinoma development. Mol Cancer Ther 16(12):2871–2880
66. González-Martín A, Mira E, Mañes S (2012) CCR5 in cancer immunotherapy: more than an "attractive" receptor for T cells. Onco Targets Ther 1(1):106–108

67. Parsonage G, Machado LR, Hui JW, McLarnon A, Schmaler T, Balasothy M et al (2012) CXCR6 and CCR5 localize T lymphocyte subsets in nasopharyngeal carcinoma. Am J Pathol 180(3):1215–1222

68. Rodriques SG, Stickels RR, Goeva A, Martin CA, Murray E, Vanderburg CR et al (2019) Slide-seq: a scalable technology for measuring genome-wide expression at high spatial resolution. Science 363(6434):1463–1467

69. Vickovic S, Eraslan G, Salmén F, Klughammer J, Stenbeck L, Schapiro D et al (2019) High-definition spatial transcriptomics for in situ tissue profiling. Nat Methods 16(10):987–990

70. Ståhl PL, Salmén F, Vickovic S, Lundmark A, Navarro JF, Magnusson J et al (2016) Visualization and analysis of gene expression in tissue sections by spatial transcriptomics. Science 353(6294):78–82

71. Hartmann FJ, Bendall SC (2020) Immune monitoring using mass cytometry and related high-dimensional imaging approaches. Nat Rev Rheumatol 16(2):87–99

72. Stoeckius M, Hafemeister C, Stephenson W, Houck-Loomis B, Chattopadhyay PK, Swerdlow H et al (2017) Simultaneous epitope and transcriptome measurement in single cells. Nat Methods 14(9):865–868

73. Le Rochais M, Hemon P, Pers JO, Uguen A (2022) Application of high-throughput imaging mass cytometry hyperion in cancer research. Front Immunol 13:859414

74. Giesen C, Wang HA, Schapiro D, Zivanovic N, Jacobs A, Hattendorf B et al (2014) Highly multiplexed imaging of tumor tissues with subcellular resolution by mass cytometry. Nat Methods 11(4):417–422

75. Baharlou H, Canete NP, Cunningham AL, Harman AN, Patrick E (2019) Mass cytometry imaging for the study of human diseases-applications and data analysis strategies. Front Immunol 10:2657

76. Bouzekri A, Esch A, Ornatsky O (2019) Multidimensional profiling of drug-treated cells by imaging mass cytometry. FEBS Open Bio 9(9):1652–1669

77. Elaldi R, Hemon P, Petti L, Cosson E, Desrues B, Sudaka A et al (2021) High dimensional imaging mass cytometry panel to visualize the tumor immune microenvironment contexture. Front Immunol 12:666233

78. Mavropoulos ALD, Lam B, Bisgrove D, Ornatsky O (2012) Equivalence of imaging mass cytometry and immunofluorescence on FFPE tissue sections, vol 12. Fluidigm Company, South San Francisco, CA, pp 1–12

79. Gorris MAJ, Halilovic A, Rabold K, van Duffelen A, Wickramasinghe IN, Verweij D et al (2018) Eight-color multiplex immunohistochemistry for simultaneous detection of multiple immune checkpoint molecules within the tumor microenvironment. J Immunol 200(1): 347–354

80. Harnett MM (2007) Laser scanning cytometry: understanding the immune system in situ. Nat Rev Immunol 7(11):897–904

81. Goltsev Y, Samusik N, Kennedy-Darling J, Bhate S, Hale M, Vazquez G et al (2018) Deep profiling of mouse splenic architecture with CODEX multiplexed imaging. Cell 174(4): 968–81.e15

82. Chang Q, Ornatsky OI, Siddiqui I, Loboda A, Baranov VI, Hedley DW (2017) Imaging mass cytometry. Cytometry A 91(2):160–169

83. Nuñez J, Renslow R, Cliff JB 3rd, Anderton CR (2017) NanoSIMS for biological applications: current practices and analyses. Biointerphases 13(3):03b301

84. Rost S, Giltnane J, Bordeaux JM, Hitzman C, Koeppen H, Liu SD (2017) Multiplexed ion beam imaging analysis for quantitation of protein expression in cancer tissue sections. Lab Investig 97(8):992–1003

85. Angelo M, Bendall SC, Finck R, Hale MB, Hitzman C, Borowsky AD et al (2014) Multiplexed ion beam imaging of human breast tumors. Nat Med 20(4):436–442

86. Keren L, Bosse M, Marquez D, Angoshtari R, Jain S, Varma S et al (2018) A structured tumor-immune microenvironment in triple negative breast cancer revealed by multiplexed ion beam imaging. Cell 174(6):1373–87.e19

87. Newman AM, Steen CB, Liu CL, Gentles AJ, Chaudhuri AA, Scherer F et al (2019) Determining cell type abundance and expression from bulk tissues with digital cytometry. Nat Biotechnol 37(7):773–782
88. Clark DJ, Dhanasekaran SM, Petralia F, Pan J, Song X, Hu Y et al (2019) Integrated proteogenomic characterization of clear cell renal cell carcinoma. Cell 179(4):964–83.e31
89. Gillette MA, Satpathy S, Cao S, Dhanasekaran SM, Vasaikar SV, Krug K et al (2020) Proteogenomic characterization reveals therapeutic vulnerabilities in lung adenocarcinoma. Cell 182(1):200–25.e35
90. Wang Y (2015) Development of cancer diagnostics—from biomarkers to clinical tests. Transl Cancer Res 4(3):270–279
91. Corless CL, Spellman PT (2012) Tackling formalin-fixed, paraffin-embedded tumor tissue with next-generation sequencing. Cancer Discov 2(1):23–24
92. Ghaaliq LA, Anthony MC (2008) Clinical tests: sensitivity and specificity. Cont Educ Anaesth Crit Care Pain 6:221–223
93. Linnet K, Bossuyt PM, Moons KG, Reitsma JB (2012) Quantifying the accuracy of a diagnostic test or marker. Clin Chem 58(9):1292–1301
94. Prokopec SD, Watson JD, Waggott DM, Smith AB, Wu AH, Okey AB et al (2013) Systematic evaluation of medium-throughput mRNA abundance platforms. RNA 19(1):51–62
95. Kulkarni MM (2011) Digital multiplexed gene expression analysis using the NanoString nCounter system. Curr Protoc Mol Biol Chapter 25:Unit25B.10
96. Geiss GK, Bumgarner RE, Birditt B, Dahl T, Dowidar N, Dunaway DL et al (2008) Direct multiplexed measurement of gene expression with color-coded probe pairs. Nat Biotechnol 26(3):317–325
97. Payton JE, Grieselhuber NR, Chang LW, Murakami M, Geiss GK, Link DC et al (2009) High throughput digital quantification of mRNA abundance in primary human acute myeloid leukemia samples. J Clin Invest 119(6):1714–1726
98. Veldman-Jones MH, Brant R, Rooney C, Geh C, Emery H, Harbron CG et al (2015) Evaluating robustness and sensitivity of the NanoString technologies nCounter platform to enable multiplexed gene expression analysis of clinical samples. Cancer Res 75(13): 2587–2593
99. Kononen J, Bubendorf L, Kallioniemi A, Bärlund M, Schraml P, Leighton S et al (1998) Tissue microarrays for high-throughput molecular profiling of tumor specimens. Nat Med 4(7):844–847
100. Shergill IS, Shergill NK, Arya M, Patel HR (2004) Tissue microarrays: a current medical research tool. Curr Med Res Opin 20(5):707–712
101. Rimm DL, Camp RL, Charette LA, Olsen DA, Provost E (2001) Amplification of tissue by construction of tissue microarrays. Exp Mol Pathol 70(3):255–264
102. Schmidt LH, Biesterfeld S, Kümmel A, Faldum A, Sebastian M, Taube C et al (2009) Tissue microarrays are reliable tools for the clinicopathological characterization of lung cancer tissue. Anticancer Res 29(1):201–209
103. Hoos A, Cordon-Cardo C (2001) Tissue microarray profiling of cancer specimens and cell lines: opportunities and limitations. Lab Investig 81(10):1331–1338
104. Xu R, Wunsch DC 2nd (2010) Clustering algorithms in biomedical research: a review. IEEE Rev Biomed Eng 3:120–154
105. Moffitt RA, Marayati R, Flate EL, Volmar KE, Loeza SG, Hoadley KA et al (2015) Virtual microdissection identifies distinct tumor- and stroma-specific subtypes of pancreatic ductal adenocarcinoma. Nat Genet 47(10):1168–1178
106. Verhaak RG, Hoadley KA, Purdom E, Wang V, Qi Y, Wilkerson MD et al (2010) Integrated genomic analysis identifies clinically relevant subtypes of glioblastoma characterized by abnormalities in PDGFRA, IDH1, EGFR, and NF1. Cancer Cell 17(1):98–110
107. Garber ME, Troyanskaya OG, Schluens K, Petersen S, Thaesler Z, Pacyna-Gengelbach M et al (2001) Diversity of gene expression in adenocarcinoma of the lung. Proc Natl Acad Sci U S A 98(24):13784–13789

108. Zhao L, Fong AHW, Liu N, Cho WCS (2018) Molecular subtyping of nasopharyngeal carcinoma (NPC) and a microRNA-based prognostic model for distant metastasis. J Biomed Sci 25(1):16
109. Golub TR, Slonim DK, Tamayo P, Huard C, Gaasenbeek M, Mesirov JP et al (1999) Molecular classification of cancer: class discovery and class prediction by gene expression monitoring. Science 286(5439):531–537
110. Guinney J, Dienstmann R, Wang X, de Reyniès A, Schlicker A, Soneson C et al (2015) The consensus molecular subtypes of colorectal cancer. Nat Med 21(11):1350–1356
111. Madeira SC, Oliveira AL (2004) Biclustering algorithms for biological data analysis: a survey. IEEE/ACM Trans Comput Biol Bioinform 1(1):24–45
112. Cheng Y, Church GM (2000) Biclustering of expression data. Proc Int Conf Intell Syst Mol Biol 8:93–103
113. Michailidis G, Mankad S (2014) Biclustering three-dimensional data arrays with plaid models. J Comput Graph Stat 23(4):943–965
114. Luo Y, Wang F, Szolovits P (2017) Tensor factorization toward precision medicine. Brief Bioinform 18(3):511–514
115. Li Y, Ngom A (2011) Classification of clinical gene-sample-time microarray expression data via tensor decomposition methods. In: CIBB 2010; International meeting on computational intelligence methods for bioinformatics and biostatistics
116. Tibshirani R, Hastie WT (2001) Estimating the number of clusters in a data set via the gap statistic. J R Stat Soc 63(2):411–423
117. Brunet JP, Tamayo P, Golub TR, Mesirov JP (2004) Metagenes and molecular pattern discovery using matrix factorization. Proc Natl Acad Sci U S A 101(12):4164–4169
118. Vega-Pons S, Ruiz-Shulcloper J (2011) A survey of clustering ensemble algorithms. Int J Pattern Recognit Artif Intell 25(3):337–372
119. Monti S, Tamayo P, Mesirov JP, Golub TR (2003) Consensus clustering: a resampling-based method for class discovery and visualization of gene expression microarray data. Mach Learn 52(1–2):91–118
120. Mukhopadhyay A, Bandyopadhyay S, Maulik U (2010) Multi-class clustering of cancer subtypes through SVM based ensemble of pareto-optimal solutions for gene marker identification. PLoS One 5(11):e13803
121. Marisa L, de Reyniès A, Duval A, Selves J, Gaub MP, Vescovo L et al (2013) Gene expression classification of colon cancer into molecular subtypes: characterization, validation, and prognostic value. PLoS Med 10(5):e1001453
122. De Sousa EMF, Wang X, Jansen M, Fessler E, Trinh A, de Rooij LP et al (2013) Poor-prognosis colon cancer is defined by a molecularly distinct subtype and develops from serrated precursor lesions. Nat Med 19(5):614–618
123. Collisson EA, Sadanandam A, Olson P, Gibb WJ, Truitt M, Gu S et al (2011) Subtypes of pancreatic ductal adenocarcinoma and their differing responses to therapy. Nat Med 17(4): 500–503
124. Wang X, Markowetz F, De Sousa EMF, Medema JP, Vermeulen L (2013) Dissecting cancer heterogeneity--an unsupervised classification approach. Int J Biochem Cell Biol 45(11): 2574–2579
125. Lex A, Streit M, Schulz HJ, Partl C, Schmalstieg D, Park PJ et al (2012) StratomeX: visual analysis of large-scale heterogeneous genomics data for cancer subtype characterization. Comput Graph Forum 31(33):1175–1184
126. Subramanian A, Tamayo P, Mootha VK, Mukherjee S, Ebert BL, Gillette MA et al (2005) Gene set enrichment analysis: a knowledge-based approach for interpreting genome-wide expression profiles. Proc Natl Acad Sci U S A 102(43):15545–15550
127. Kanehisa M, Goto S, Hattori M, Aoki-Kinoshita KF, Itoh M, Kawashima S et al (2006) From genomics to chemical genomics: new developments in KEGG. Nucleic Acids Res 34(Database issue):D354–D357

128. Mantel N (1966) Evaluation of survival data and two new rank order statistics arising in its consideration. Cancer Chemother Rep 50(3):163–170

129. Kaplan EL, Meier P (1958) Nonparametric estimation from incomplete observations. J Am Stat Assoc 53:457–481

130. Xu Y, Su GH, Ma D, Xiao Y, Shao ZM, Jiang YZ (2021) Technological advances in cancer immunity: from immunogenomics to single-cell analysis and artificial intelligence. Signal Transduct Target Ther 6(1):312

131. Finotello F, Trajanoski Z (2018) Quantifying tumor-infiltrating immune cells from transcriptomics data. Cancer Immunol Immunother 67(7):1031–1040

132. Yoshihara K, Shahmoradgoli M, Martínez E, Vegesna R, Kim H, Torres-Garcia W et al (2013) Inferring tumor purity and stromal and immune cell admixture from expression data. Nat Commun 4:2612

133. Aran D, Hu Z, Butte AJ (2017) xCell: digitally portraying the tissue cellular heterogeneity landscape. Genome Biol 18(1):220

134. Becht E, Giraldo NA, Lacroix L, Buttard B, Elarouci N, Petitprez F et al (2016) Estimating the population abundance of tissue-infiltrating immune and stromal cell populations using gene expression. Genome Biol 17(1):218

135. Newman AM, Liu CL, Green MR, Gentles AJ, Feng W, Xu Y et al (2015) Robust enumeration of cell subsets from tissue expression profiles. Nat Methods 12(5):453–457

136. Plattner C, Finotello F, Rieder D (2020) Deconvoluting tumor-infiltrating immune cells from RNA-seq data using quanTIseq. Methods Enzymol 636:261–285

137. Hao Y, Yan M, Heath BR, Lei YL, Xie Y (2019) Fast and robust deconvolution of tumor infiltrating lymphocyte from expression profiles using least trimmed squares. PLoS Comput Biol 15(5):e1006976

138. Wang X, Park J, Susztak K, Zhang NR, Li M (2019) Bulk tissue cell type deconvolution with multi-subject single-cell expression reference. Nat Commun 10(1):380

139. Rajkomar A, Dean J, Kohane I (2019) Machine learning in medicine. N Engl J Med 380(14): 1347–1358

140. Poplin R, Chang PC, Alexander D, Schwartz S, Colthurst T, Ku A et al (2018) A universal SNP and small-indel variant caller using deep neural networks. Nat Biotechnol 36(10): 983–987

141. Gerstung M, Beisel C, Rechsteiner M, Wild P, Schraml P, Moch H et al (2012) Reliable detection of subclonal single-nucleotide variants in tumor cell populations. Nat Commun 3: 811

142. Pounraja VK, Jayakar G, Jensen M, Kelkar N, Girirajan S (2019) A machine-learning approach for accurate detection of copy number variants from exome sequencing. Genome Res 29(7):1134–1143

143. Bulik-Sullivan B, Busby J, Palmer CD, Davis MJ, Murphy T, Clark A et al (2018) Deep learning using tumor HLA peptide mass spectrometry datasets improves neoantigen identification. Nat Biotechnol 37:55. https://doi.org/10.1038/nbt.4313

144. Racle J, Michaux J, Rockinger GA, Arnaud M, Bobisse S, Chong C et al (2019) Robust prediction of HLA class II epitopes by deep motif deconvolution of immunopeptidomes. Nat Biotechnol 37(11):1283–1286

145. Gillies RJ, Kinahan PE, Hricak H (2016) Radiomics: images are more than pictures, they are data. Radiology 278(2):563–577

146. He B, Dong D, She Y, Zhou C, Fang M, Zhu Y et al (2020) Predicting response to immunotherapy in advanced non-small-cell lung cancer using tumor mutational burden radiomic biomarker. J Immunother Cancer 8(2):e000550

147. Khorrami M, Prasanna P, Gupta A, Patil P, Velu PD, Thawani R et al (2020) Changes in CT radiomic features associated with lymphocyte distribution predict overall survival and response to immunotherapy in non-small cell lung cancer. Cancer Immunol Res 8(1):108–119

148. Sun R, Limkin EJ, Vakalopoulou M, Dercle L, Champiat S, Han SR et al (2018) A radiomics approach to assess tumor-infiltrating CD8 cells and response to anti-PD-1 or anti-PD-L1

immunotherapy: an imaging biomarker, retrospective multicohort study. Lancet Oncol 19(9): 1180–1191

149. Trebeschi S, Drago SG, Birkbak NJ, Kurilova I, Călin AM, Delli Pizzi A et al (2019) Predicting response to cancer immunotherapy using noninvasive radiomic biomarkers. Ann Oncol 30(6):998–1004

150. García-Figueiras R, Baleato-González S, Luna A, Muñoz-Iglesias J, Oleaga L, Vallejo Casas JA et al (2020) Assessing immunotherapy with functional and molecular imaging and radiomics. Radiographics 40(7):1987–2010

151. Nishino M, Hatabu H, Hodi FS (2019) Imaging of cancer immunotherapy: current approaches and future directions. Radiology 290(1):9–22

152. Vaidya P, Bera K, Patil PD, Gupta A, Jain P, Alilou M et al (2020) Novel, non-invasive imaging approach to identify patients with advanced non-small cell lung cancer at risk of hyperprogressive disease with immune checkpoint blockade. J Immunother Cancer 8(2): e001343

153. Klauschen F, Müller KR, Binder A, Bockmayr M, Hägele M, Seegerer P et al (2018) Scoring of tumor-infiltrating lymphocytes: from visual estimation to machine learning. Semin Cancer Biol 52(Pt 2):151–157

154. Krijgsman D, van Leeuwen MB, van der Ven J, Almeida V, Vlutters R, Halter D et al (2021) Quantitative whole slide assessment of tumor-infiltrating CD8-positive lymphocytes in ER-positive breast cancer in relation to clinical outcome. IEEE J Biomed Health Inform 25(2):381–392

155. Lu Z, Xu S, Shao W, Wu Y, Zhang J, Han Z et al (2020) Deep-learning-based characterization of tumor-infiltrating lymphocytes in breast cancers from histopathology images and multiomics data. JCO Clin Cancer Inform 4:480–490

156. Saltz J, Gupta R, Hou L, Kurc T, Singh P, Nguyen V et al (2018) Spatial organization and molecular correlation of tumor-infiltrating lymphocytes using deep learning on pathology images. Cell Rep 23(1):181–93.e7

157. AbdulJabbar K, Raza SEA, Rosenthal R, Jamal-Hanjani M, Veeriah S, Akarca A et al (2020) Geospatial immune variability illuminates differential evolution of lung adenocarcinoma. Nat Med 26(7):1054–1062

158. Keren L, Bosse M, Thompson S, Risom T, Vijayaragavan K, McCaffrey E et al (2019) MIBI-TOF: a multiplexed imaging platform relates cellular phenotypes and tissue structure. Sci Adv 5(10):eaax5851

Chapter 28
Tumor Ecosystem-Mimicking Bioengineering Methods

Phei Er Saw and Erwei Song

Abstract Biomedical research has improved by leaps and bounds due to the creation of first cell line models, followed by animal models, to various bioengineering methods such as organoids and organ-on-a-chip. A successful translation of a drug candidate always starts from chemical drug screening in a 2D in vitro cell culture, followed by verification in animal models prior to clinical trials. Although feasible, 2D monolayer cell culture does not represent the fullness of an in vivo cancer environment, leading to a constant deviation of drug efficacy when tested in non-primate and primate models. Even in animal models, the exact tumor environment in a human host cannot be represented in animal models. Therefore, attempts have been made to model the human organs in vitro, giving rise to the technics known as bioprinting, organoids, and "organ-on-a-chip." In this chapter, we will look into current developments in humanized 3D platforms in realizing personalized medicine in terms of drug screening, diagnosis, and prognosis of cancer.

P. E. Saw
Guangdong Provincial Key Laboratory of Malignant Tumor Epigenetics and Gene Regulation, Guangdong-Hong Kong Joint Laboratory for RNA Medicine, Medical Research Center, Sun Yat-sen Memorial Hospital, Sun Yat-sen University, Guangzhou, China

Nanhai Translational Innovation Center of Precision Immunology, Sun Yat-sen Memorial Hospital, Sun Yat-sen University, Foshan, China

E. Song (✉)
Guangdong Provincial Key Laboratory of Malignant Tumor Epigenetics and Gene Regulation, Guangdong-Hong Kong Joint Laboratory for RNA Medicine, Medical Research Center, Sun Yat-sen Memorial Hospital, Sun Yat-sen University, Guangzhou, China

Nanhai Translational Innovation Center of Precision Immunology, Sun Yat-sen Memorial Hospital, Sun Yat-sen University, Foshan, China

Breast Tumor Center, Sun Yat-sen Memorial Hospital, Sun Yat-sen University, Guangzhou, China
e-mail: songew@mail.sysu.edu.cn

Introduction

Biomedical research has improved by leaps and bounds due to the creation of first cell line models, followed by animal models, to various bioengineering methods such as organoids and organ-on-a-chip. These techniques have helped us tremendously in identifying potential drug targets, especially to guide the design of candidate drugs for major diseases, including cancer. A successful translation of a drug candidate always starts from chemical drug screening in a 2D in vitro cell culture, followed by verification in animal models prior to clinical trials [1]. Although feasible, 2D monolayer cell culture does not represent the fullness of an in vivo cancer environment, leading to a constant deviation of drug efficacy when tested in non-primate and primate models. Apparently, even in animal models, the exact tumor environment in a human host cannot be represented in animal models. Therefore, attempts have been made to model the human organs in vitro, giving rise to the technics known as bioprinting, organoids, and "organ-on-a-chip." In this chapter, we will look into current developments in humanized 3D platforms in realizing personalized medicine in terms of drug screening, diagnosis, and prognosis of cancer (Fig. 28.1).

2D Cell Culture

Over the past decades, our understanding of cancer biology is largely based on our observation on 2D cell culture model [2]. Though simple, high-throughput screening (HTS) of many drug candidates was successfully done on this system and therefore contributed much to pharmacological testing. However, there are substantial differences between 2D and 3D cancer models, and these include (1) the lack of molecular signaling, (2) communication between different cell types, (3) inherent expressions of gene, protein, cytokines, chemokines, enzymes, etc. and (4) cell proliferation and migration; just to name a few [3–5]. Certainly, in a 3D system, a platform serves as a scaffold, providing mechanical strength to the cells, which in turn encourages the cells to secrete cytokines, GFs, chemokines, and others for a sustained period of time [6, 7].

3D Cell Culture

Comparing to 2D method, 3D cell culture system is an improvement toward a better representation of tissue environment, in terms of spatiotemporal distribution of cancer cells [8]. There are multiple advantages of 3D culture model, including the utilization of cells from biopsies to develop tumor-mimicking models for chemo-drug testing. Researchers have proven that the simplest model of tumor spheroid is

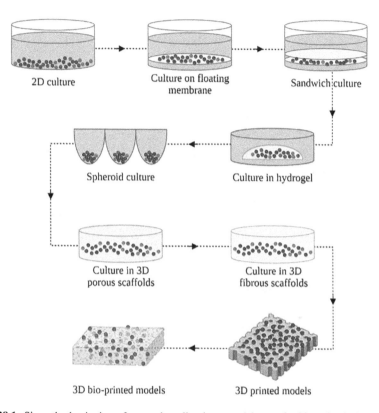

Fig. 28.1 Since the beginning of research, cell culture model started with a simple 2D in vitro monolayer culture. This then evolves into a culture in 3D matrix, such as hydrogel, spheroid culture. Finally, 3D culture are introduced as the most complex, tumor environment mimicking cell culture models available

better than a 2D culture system. For example, by using a 3D model of a prostate cancer cell line, the 3D spheroids could mimic the prostate tumor environment, stimulating tumor cells, and their microenvironment for the toxicity evaluation of ruthenium complexes [9].

Advancement of 3D Spheroid Culture System

3D Spheroid System

Since 3D spheroid models are formed by spontaneous aggregation of cells, the cell–cell contact and cell–matrix contact must be enhanced through the secretion of ECM-stimulating factors. In the spheroid culture, upon cell–cell contact, these tumor cells then upregulate E-cadherin to accumulate on cell surface, to produce a compact and robust spheroid. Of course, this spheroid-forming process differs in each cancer model, the availability of nutrients, and other factors (such as the additional cytokines, chemokines, GFs, and amino acids) that could lead to different spheroids formed [10–12].

Multicellular Tumor Spheroids

In an upgrade version of spheroid, multicellular tumor spheroids were introduced. Since these spheroids are composed of different cell lines, they possess the advantages such as simple expansion into large quantity, making it a suitable model for high-throughput screening (HTS) system [13]. Histologically, MCTs show very minimal resemblance to tumor; however, they do possess basic proliferation and metabolic changes that are close to the tumor setting.

Tumor-Derived Spheroids

In an attempt to have closer mimicry to tumor, spheroids were derived from primary tumor from the patients. This was done to preserve the tumor environment as much as possible, even though cells were grown in a synthetic method. Tumor-derived spheroids are prepared from mechanical or enzymatic dissociation of tumor tissue into a single cell suspension, followed by in vitro culture. This method has been deemed successful, as many tumor-derived spheroids have been prepared from various tumors [14–20].

Organotypic Multicellular Tumor Spheroids

Similar to ex vivo explant cultures, tumor was also used. The tumor is first sliced into cube-like 0.3 mm or as mentioned above, partially dissociated using enzymatic assay or mechanical force. The tumor slice/cube is then cultured on agar-coated plates and in the presence of serum-containing media [21] (Fig. 28.2).

Organoids

Different from a simple aggregation of cells in a 3D spheroid culture system, an organoid is defined as a structure that contains most (if not all) the cells represented in the original organ, while preserving the capability of self-organization in their specific compartments [22]. Most organoids are created to closely mimic a histologically and functionally similar in situ organs [23–29]. All organoids (to date) are

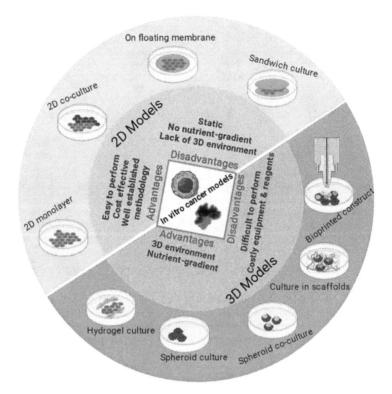

Fig. 28.2 Evolution of cancer cell culture models. From a conventional 2D monolayer mono-cell culture to a co-culture to sandwich culture, these 2D culture models represented an important source of screening method in early pharmacological testing of chemotherapeutics. The emergence of 3D culture widens the horizon of cancer-mimicking culture, where advancement can be continuously observed from a mono-spheroid culture, to co-culture, scaffold-based culture. Both systems have their advantages and disadvantages and should be used after deep consideration on the purpose and the final aim of their usage

made from either (1) pluripotent stem cells (PSCs) or (2) adult stem cells (AdSCs, also known as tissue stem cells) [30]. One undisputable advantage of organoid culture is that data generated from organoid could provide details regarding the mechanism behind the close-knit interactions between cellular compartments, soluble factors, secreted EVs, and inter-cellular communications. These data are priceless to both the advancement of molecular medicine and drug testing for pharmaceutical companies. Therefore, organoids are now becoming the top choice as a model system for medical research, as it is becoming more widely accepted by the researchers worldwide [1]. We summarized the difference between 2D cultures, 3D cultures, 2D culture from primary cells, and organoid culture from primary cells in Fig. 28.3.

As mentioned above, there are two major sources of organoid culture: (1) embryonic pluripotent stem cells (PSCs) or (2) adult stem cells (AdSCs). Both sources

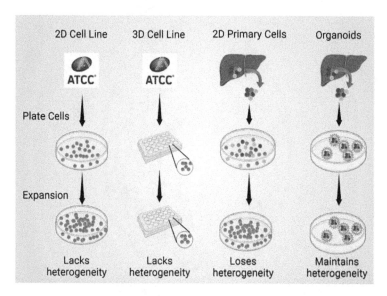

Fig 28.3 Comparison of four major cell culture system. The most obvious difference between a cell line and primary cell culture us the lack of heterogeneity, regardless of a 2D or 3D culture system. In 2D culture of primary cells, the cells could lose heterogeneity after expansion, or a few rounds of culture. Only primary cells cultured in an organoid form are able to maintain heterogeneity

have their own advantages and disadvantages, which are summarized in Table 28.1 below.

Molecular Cues in Organoids

Recently, an AdSC-based organoid was developed to mimic intestines. This group found that Lgr5 is a biomarker for adult stem cells in the gut, which is activated by Wnt signaling. Location wise, these Lgr5+ cells were found to be embedded in the basal membrane, and they are capable to grow and self-organize into an intestine-mimicking callus-like crypt structure, given the appropriate cocktails of GFs [23]. However, it is worth noting that the GFs required for the stem cell niche varies, depending on the tissue. For epithelial cell-based organoid, their outgrowth requires the following cocktails: Wnt activators (such as Wnt3a, R-spondin), tyrosine kinase ligand receptor, BMP inhibitor (noggin), and TGF-β inhibitor [40]. This protocol has been proven successful in many epithelial-based organoid models [26, 33, 41–52]. Recently, development has been seen in the usage of patient tumor as the primary cells for organoids, known as patient-derived tumor organoid. Break-throughs are seen in the creating of organoids in major cancer types, such as breast, pancreatic, colon, prostate, hepatobiliary cancers, among others [29, 50–

Table 28.1 Major differences between pluripotent stem cells and adult stem cells in organoids

	Pluripotent stem cells [27, 31–38]	Adult stem cells (AdSCs) [23, 39]
Similarity		
	Form structures through developmental processes	
	Requires ECM as basal lamina	
Differences		
Culture process	Step 1: Expansion	Similar culture process to PSC, only the time frame is shortened
	Step 2: Multi-step differentiation	
	Requires a longer process (2–3 months), depending on the complexity of structure, and the GFs used in the culture	
Organoid characteristics		
Advantages	Inherent complex structure	Fully resembles parental cells in terms of histopathological and genetical characteristics
	Able to mimic organ development	
	Contains all types of cells (endothelial, epithelial, and mesenchymal)	
Disadvantages		
	Less efficient organoid differentiation	Lower complexity compared to PSC organoids
	Retain fetal resemblance	Can only be made from tissue or compartments that possess regenerative capacity
	Do not possess adult gene expression	
Recommended applications		
	The study of organogenesis genetic pathology	Can only be made from tissue or compartments that possess regenerative capacity
	Infectious diseases	
	Organ-specific diseases (i.e., brain model, as it has little or zero regenerative capacity)	

63]. Interestingly, several groups have also initiated studies to employ these patient-derived organoids in drug development and precision medicine-related studies, including research on patients' responses to chemotherapies and chemoradiation [64–70]. However, this field is still in its infancy, and with lack of consistent and standardized protocols, these studies have yet to show a pan-cancer generalizability [71] (Box 28.1).

Box 28.1 Artificial Lymph Node Organoid

Immunocompetency is the key factor of a patient's response to immunotherapy. Since lymph node is the location that prime adaptive immune cells in the host, creating an immunocompetent lymph node would be providing an alternative to boost immunotherapeutic outcomes. Cancer patients, however, often possess less vigorous immune system, as the tumor has re-educated the host's adaptive immune cells into regulatory or exhausted phenotypes. To

(continued)

Box 28.1 (continued)

overcome the severe immunocompetency problems in tumor immunotherapy, we seek for approaches to rebuild benign environment for anti-tumor immunity by implantation of artificial lymph node. Instead of a soldier, we send an army. Lymphoid tissue inducer cells (LTiCs), gathering in specific sites during embryonic development, interact with stromal cells to produce positive feedback to form lymph node primordial. Lymphohocyte recruitment and organization are specific to their site and structure, such as T zone and B zone. LTiCs are the initiators of lymph node embryogenesis. However, the number of primary LTiCs is small and the isolation is largely inaccessible (Fig. 28.4).

Tissue regeneration techniques are introduced to generate induced LTiCs from induce pluripotent stem cells (iPSCs). Therefore, the expression profiles of iPSCs and primary LTiCs were compared by Smart-seq and ATAC-seq, we found that three core transcription factors are exclusively expressed in LTiC. By enforced over-expression of these 3 transcription factors in iPSCs, we induce iPS cells to exhibit the phenotype of primary lymphoid tissue initiators. The obtained LTiCs are co-cultured with stromal cells in vitro and showed the ability to upregulate the expression of the adhesion molecules ICAM1, VCAM1, MadCAM1, and chemokine CXCL13 of stromal cells, a process resembled the molecular events of lymph node primordial formation in embryonic stages. The induced LTiCs and mesenchymal cells were inoculated in biomaterial and implanted subcutaneously into the lymph node-deficient Rorcgfp/gfp transgenic mice, which lacked lymph nodes due to lack of Rorγt transcription factors leading to defects in LTiC cell development. After a period of time, flow cytometry analysis of the implant showed cellular contents including T, B, DC, macrophage, NK, etc., as well as a small number of stromal cells expressing CD31 or PDPN. Immunofluorescence staining showed there were T-cell-rich regions, B-cell aggregations, and vascular-like structures expressing PNAd. After inoculation of OVA-expressing tumor cells to implanted mice, DC cells within this structure can response molecular events similar to bulk lymph nodes, including antigen presentation by DC cells to SIINFEKL polypeptides, T cells produced specific killing against OVA antigens, B cells differentiated to CD138$^+$ plasma cells, and memory B cells (Fig. 28.5).

Organ-on-a-Chip (OOAC)

The first OOAC can be traced back to more than 30 years ago, when microfluidics start to penetrate the biological analysis and cell culture method [72–75]. One of the most distinct properties of OOAC is the fact that it is designed with reductionism in mind, meaning that OOCA is not going to be more complex, requiring more cells, tissues, or organs; in contrast, this technic aims to mimic the most important cell

Fig. 28.4 Induction of
iPSC-derived LTiCs using
fibroblast-derived iPSC and
lymph node LTiCs

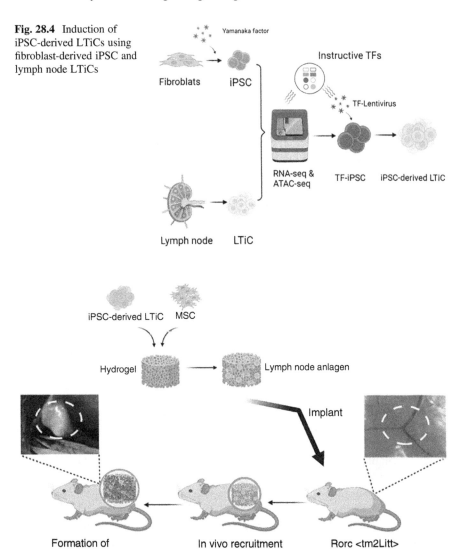

Fig. 28.5 Formation of artificial functional lymph node in a mouse model. iPSC-derived LTiC and MSC are both encapsulated in a hydrogel to form a lymph node anlagen. After a few days, the formation of functional immune niche can be seen in the implant

functionality and architecture [75, 76]. Since OOAC is derived from a microfluidic device, one fully functional OOAC could be done in a micro-sized chip. These chips were designed with multiple micro-channels that could be adjusted according to physiological condition, including pH, flow rate, oxygen, pressure, etc. [72–75]. The focus of "Organ-on-Chip (OOAC)" models aim to create a near wholesome ex situ organ environment, with similar functions of native tissues [77]. Since the organ is now translated into a chip, all required communications among various cells in the organs, including similar physiological biophysical forces, could be accurately captured by an OOAC model [78–81]. The most recent advancement of OOAC includes the attachment of the microfluidic compartment, also termed microphysiological system. This system can accurately mimic both the functionality of human organs, with full retainment of their physiological properties. Since this is a fully artificial system, microfluidic OOAC has been nominated as the next paradigm shift in personalized medicine, replacing animal testing that not only costly, but also removed ethical problems that surrounds animal-based research [82]. Nevertheless, although OOAC could revolutionize the way we do pharmacological testing, the overall impact of this system has yet to be verified, and there is still a huge gap between pre-clinical to clinical study [83]. One prominent study was the remarkable Lung-on-a-Chip model built by researchers in Harvard Medical School [77, 84]. This group uses two sides of a porous membrane to represent the lung alveolar and capillary cells, respectively. In this way, they could now closely learn about the breathing mechanisms that occur at the interface of human lungs (the alveoli-capillary interface). This model also provided a proof of concept as a biomimetic model to decode many pathological mechanisms in the lung, especially in respiratory diseases [58]. Since then, many others have proven that the OOAC could be reproduced in major organs [25, 85–98] (BBB) chips [99, 100] and even bone marrow chips [101–103].

Although single-organ chip is sufficient to analyze biological mechanism or to test drug efficacy/toxicity, a more comprehensive multi-organ chips would provide a more wholesome detail. Single-organ chips can only mimic one individual organs, while a multi-organ chip could integrate two or more organ-mimicking chips to closely resemble the compartmentalized functions of human organs. For example, liver-chip could be used to test drug metabolism, the gut-chip could be used for analyzing drug absorbance, while kidney-chip could be used to analyze drug elimination. Providing an integrated chips could prove to be more cost-efficient, while resulting in a more accurate representation of the drug ADME, similar to physiological condition [104, 105]. In a revolutionized study, a 13-organ chip system was recently developed. These chips have various cells lining different chips, representing the main organs and physiological barriers in human [106]. In an attempt to design a fully functional multi-chips, a more advanced version of "Body-on-a-Chip" or "Human-on-a-Chip" is being developed. If successful, this Humanized chips could mimic the entire physiological condition of a human body. In short, future pharmacological testing could be realized through one system [107–109].

3D Bioprinting

As the name implies, 3D bioprinting is a printing technic that could realize a three-dimensional model by using a computer-aided design to construct a highly sophisticated tissue structure [110, 111]. To date, bioprinting can create massive architectures that are similar to the ECM and also the tumor microenvironment. Since the CAD is controlled by artificial intelligence (AI) and detailed programming system, it is plausible to create a fully automated model with functional vascular networks that could be used in biological research [112]. On a more sophisticated model, bioprinting is able to construct a complex internal tissue structure with varying dimensions, at different spatiotemporal arrangements [113, 114]. It is important to note that in bioprinting, theoretically, any cells could be printed at any specific location, at any given time point. Therefore, this model could be the closest to human physiological condition.

3D Bioprinting for Modeling Cancer

To model a cancer environment that is truly personalized, the bioprinting construct should take into account the diversity of cells in the solid tumor. Generally, a solid tumor comprises cancer cells, stromal cells (fibroblast, adipocytes, ECMs), CSCs, CTCs, and infiltrating immune cells. Recently, a bioprinted tumor was constructed using a Matrigel-alginate-gelatin bioink embedded with intrahepatic cholangiocarcinoma cells derived from the patient [115]. Interestingly, after this tumor model is successfully constructed, the tumor showed elevated expression of cancer-associated biomarkers, CSC markers, and more importantly, a hint of EMT progression. As the first proof-of-principle construct, this cancer-bioprinting model could be an example of personalized cancer therapeutic diagnostic and drug testing platform, where a patient can derive a whole tumor model using their own cells to predict their possible reaction to chemotherapeutic drugs [116]. Nevertheless, it is important to note that a bioprinted tumor model should always adhere to these rules: (1) contain suitable stromal cells and ECM that could mimic the real tumor environment, (2) the selection of bioink (the raw materials for cell embedding) should be considered carefully, as various cells have different biological and chemical characteristics, and (3) the environment should include a fraction of normal (non-tumoral) cells to better represent a wholesome tumor environment. The different choice of cells should always adhere to the tumor's original location. For example, a bioprinting construct of a breast cancer should include mammary cells, ECs, adipocytes, and fibroblasts while a construct of a brain tumor must include neurons, astrocytes, glial cells, and microvascular ECs [117–120].

Conclusion

Currently, many technics are being explored to mimic the real human physiological condition. Not only this diminishes the current limitation of current in vitro and in vivo cancer models, using organoids, OOAC and bioprinting, could, to some extent, re-create the in vivo condition that makeup the genetic, biology, chemistry, and physiology of cancer cells. Not only these bioengineering methods could enhance the precision of drug screening, they could also redefine personalized drug screening methods. Impedes their applicability in the screening of chemotherapeutic drugs and precision medicine. Nevertheless, none of these technics are perfect and could fully represent a human physiological condition. Therefore, one should consider integrating various bioengineering method to create a holistic methodology that could be translated into clinical use in the near future.

References

1. Kim J, Koo BK, Knoblich JA (2020) Human organoids: model systems for human biology and medicine. Nat Rev Mol Cell Biol 21(10):571–584
2. Augustine R, Kalva SN, Ahmad R, Zahid AA, Hasan S, Nayeem A et al (2021) 3D bioprinted cancer models: revolutionizing personalized cancer therapy. Transl Oncol 14(4):101015
3. Knowlton S, Onal S, Yu CH, Zhao JJ, Tasoglu S (2015) Bioprinting for cancer research. Trends Biotechnol 33(9):504–513
4. Wang C, Tang Z, Zhao Y, Yao R, Li L, Sun W (2014) Three-dimensional *in vitro* cancer models: a short review. Biofabrication 6(2):022001
5. Zhao Y, Yao R, Ouyang L, Ding H, Zhang T, Zhang K et al (2014) Three-dimensional printing of Hela cells for cervical tumor model *in vitro*. Biofabrication 6(3):035001
6. Ricci-Vitiani L, Pallini R, Biffoni M, Todaro M, Invernici G, Cenci T et al (2010) Tumour vascularization via endothelial differentiation of glioblastoma stem-like cells. Nature 468(7325):824–828
7. Amini A, Masoumi Moghaddam S, Morris DL, Pourgholami MH (2012) The critical role of vascular endothelial growth factor in tumor angiogenesis. Curr Cancer Drug Targets 12(1): 23–43
8. Rodrigues J, Heinrich MA, Teixeira LM, Prakash J (2021) 3D *in vitro* model (R)evolution: unveiling tumor-stroma interactions. Trends Cancer 7(3):249–264
9. De Grandis RA, Santos P, Oliveira KM, Machado ART, Aissa AF, Batista AA et al (2019) Novel lawsone-containing ruthenium(II) complexes: synthesis, characterization and anticancer activity on 2D and 3D spheroid models of prostate cancer cells. Bioorg Chem 85:455–468
10. Steinberg MS (2007) Differential adhesion in morphogenesis: a modern view. Curr Opin Genet Dev 17(4):281–286
11. Lin RZ, Chou LF, Chien CC, Chang HY (2006) Dynamic analysis of hepatoma spheroid formation: roles of E-cadherin and beta1-integrin. Cell Tissue Res 324(3):411–422
12. Bates RC, Edwards NS, Yates JD (2000) Spheroids and cell survival. Crit Rev Oncol Hematol 36(2–3):61–74
13. Kunz-Schughart LA, Freyer JP, Hofstaedter F, Ebner R (2004) The use of 3-D cultures for high-throughput screening: the multicellular spheroid model. J Biomol Screen 9(4):273–285
14. Quereda V, Hou S, Madoux F, Scampavia L, Spicer TP, Duckett D (2018) A cytotoxic three-dimensional-spheroid, high-throughput assay using patient-derived glioma stem cells. SLAS Discov 23(8):842–849

15. Halfter K, Hoffmann O, Ditsch N, Ahne M, Arnold F, Paepke S et al (2016) Testing chemotherapy efficacy in HER2 negative breast cancer using patient-derived spheroids. J Transl Med 14(1):112

16. Della Corte CM, Barra G, Ciaramella V, Di Liello R, Vicidomini G, Zappavigna S et al (2019) Antitumor activity of dual blockade of PD-L1 and MEK in NSCLC patients derived three-dimensional spheroid cultures. J Exp Clin Cancer Res 38(1):253

17. Jeppesen M, Hagel G, Glenthoj A, Vainer B, Ibsen P, Harling H et al (2017) Short-term spheroid culture of primary colorectal cancer cells as an *in vitro* model for personalizing cancer medicine. PLoS One 12(9):e0183074

18. Linxweiler J, Hammer M, Muhs S, Kohn M, Pryalukhin A, Veith C et al (2019) Patient-derived, three-dimensional spheroid cultures provide a versatile translational model for the study of organ-confined prostate cancer. J Cancer Res Clin Oncol 145(3):551–559

19. Tomás-Bort E, Kieler M, Sharma S, Candido JB, Loessner D (2020) 3D approaches to model the tumor microenvironment of pancreatic cancer. Theranostics 10(11):5074–5089

20. Raghavan S, Mehta P, Ward MR, Bregenzer ME, Fleck EMA, Tan L et al (2017) Personalized medicine-based approach to model patterns of chemoresistance and tumor recurrence using ovarian cancer stem cell spheroids. Clin Cancer Res 23(22):6934–6945

21. Ryu NE, Lee SH, Park H (2019) Spheroid culture system methods and applications for mesenchymal stem cells. Cell 8(12):1620

22. Corro C, Novellasdemunt L, Li VSW (2020) A brief history of organoids. Am J Physiol Cell Physiol 319(1):C151–CC65

23. Sato T, Vries RG, Snippert HJ, van de Wetering M, Barker N, Stange DE et al (2009) Single Lgr5 stem cells build crypt-villus structures *in vitro* without a mesenchymal niche. Nature 459(7244):262–265

24. Sato T, Stange DE, Ferrante M, Vries RG, Van Es JH, Van den Brink S et al (2011) Long-term expansion of epithelial organoids from human colon, adenoma, adenocarcinoma, and Barrett's epithelium. Gastroenterology 141(5):1762–1772

25. Fujii M, Matano M, Toshimitsu K, Takano A, Mikami Y, Nishikori S et al (2018) Human intestinal organoids maintain self-renewal capacity and cellular diversity in niche-inspired culture condition. Cell Stem Cell 23(6):787–93.e6

26. Lancaster MA, Renner M, Martin CA, Wenzel D, Bicknell LS, Hurles ME et al (2013) Cerebral organoids model human brain development and microcephaly. Nature 501(7467): 373–379

27. Takasato M, Er PX, Chiu HS, Maier B, Baillie GJ, Ferguson C et al (2015) Kidney organoids from human iPS cells contain multiple lineages and model human nephrogenesis. Nature 526(7574):564–568

28. Hu H, Gehart H, Artegiani B, Löpez-Iglesias C, Dekkers F, Basak O et al (2018) Long-term expansion of functional mouse and human hepatocytes as 3D organoids. Cell 175(6): 1591–606.e19

29. Turco MY, Gardner L, Hughes J, Cindrova-Davies T, Gomez MJ, Farrell L et al (2017) Long-term, hormone-responsive organoid cultures of human endometrium in a chemically defined medium. Nat Cell Biol 19(5):568–577

30. Huch M, Koo BK (2015) Modeling mouse and human development using organoid cultures. Development 142(18):3113–3125

31. McCauley HA, Wells JM (2017) Pluripotent stem cell-derived organoids: using principles of developmental biology to grow human tissues in a dish. Development 144(6):958–962

32. Spence JR, Mayhew CN, Rankin SA, Kuhar MF, Vallance JE, Tolle K et al (2011) Directed differentiation of human pluripotent stem cells into intestinal tissue *in vitro*. Nature 470(7332): 105–109

33. Bartfeld S, Bayram T, van de Wetering M, Huch M, Begthel H, Kujala P et al (2015) *In vitro* expansion of human gastric epithelial stem cells and their responses to bacterial infection. Gastroenterology 148(1):126–36.e6

34. Garcez PP, Loiola EC, Madeiro da Costa R, Higa LM, Trindade P, Delvecchio R et al (2016) Zika virus impairs growth in human neurospheres and brain organoids. Science 352(6287): 816–818
35. Takebe T, Sekine K, Enomura M, Koike H, Kimura M, Ogaeri T et al (2013) Vascularized and functional human liver from an iPSC-derived organ bud transplant. Nature 499(7459): 481–484
36. Dutta D, Heo I, Clevers H (2017) Disease Modeling in stem cell-derived 3D organoid systems. Trends Mol Med 23(5):393–410
37. Clevers H (2016) Modeling development and disease with organoids. Cell 165(7):1586–1597
38. Wu H, Uchimura K, Donnelly EL, Kirita Y, Morris SA, Humphreys BD (2018) Comparative analysis and refinement of human PSC-derived kidney organoid differentiation with single-cell transcriptomics. Cell Stem Cell 23(6):869–81.e8
39. Schutgens F, Clevers H (2020) Human organoids: tools for understanding biology and treating diseases. Annu Rev Pathol 15:211–234
40. Kaushik G, Ponnusamy MP, Batra SK (2018) Concise review: current status of three-dimensional organoids as preclinical models. Stem Cells 36(9):1329–1340
41. Jacob F, Salinas RD, Zhang DY, Nguyen PTT, Schnoll JG, Wong SZH et al (2020) A patient-derived glioblastoma organoid model and biobank recapitulates inter- and intra-tumoral heterogeneity. Cell 180(1):188–204.e22
42. Kasagi Y, Chandramouleeswaran PM, Whelan KA, Tanaka K, Giroux V, Sharma M et al (2018) The esophageal organoid system reveals functional interplay between notch and cytokines in reactive epithelial changes. Cell Mol Gastroenterol Hepatol 5(3):333–352
43. Barkauskas CE, Chung MI, Fioret B, Gao X, Katsura H, Hogan BL (2017) Lung organoids: current uses and future promise. Development 144(6):986–997
44. Huch M, Gehart H, van Boxtel R, Hamer K, Blokzijl F, Verstegen MM et al (2015) Long-term culture of genome-stable bipotent stem cells from adult human liver. Cell 160(1–2):299–312
45. Li X, Nadauld L, Ootani A, Corney DC, Pai RK, Gevaert O et al (2014) Oncogenic transformation of diverse gastrointestinal tissues in primary organoid culture. Nat Med 20(7):769–777
46. Cruz NM, Song X, Czerniecki SM, Gulieva RE, Churchill AJ, Kim YK et al (2017) Organoid cystogenesis reveals a critical role of microenvironment in human polycystic kidney disease. Nat Mater 16(11):1112–1119
47. Pringle S, Maimets M, van der Zwaag M, Stokman MA, van Gosliga D, Zwart E et al (2016) Human salivary gland stem cells functionally restore radiation damaged salivary glands. Stem Cells 34(3):640–652
48. Maenhoudt N, Defraye C, Boretto M, Jan Z, Heremans R, Boeckx B et al (2020) Developing organoids from ovarian cancer as experimental and preclinical models. Stem Cell Rep 14(4): 717–729
49. Kessler M, Hoffmann K, Brinkmann V, Thieck O, Jackisch S, Toelle B et al (2015) The notch and Wnt pathways regulate stemness and differentiation in human fallopian tube organoids. Nat Commun 6:8989
50. Sachs N, de Ligt J, Kopper O, Gogola E, Bounova G, Weeber F et al (2018) A living biobank of breast cancer organoids captures disease heterogeneity. Cell 172(1–2):373–86.e10
51. van de Wetering M, Francies HE, Francis JM, Bounova G, Iorio F, Pronk A et al (2015) Prospective derivation of a living organoid biobank of colorectal cancer patients. Cell 161(4): 933–945
52. Gao D, Vela I, Sboner A, Iaquinta PJ, Karthaus WR, Gopalan A et al (2014) Organoid cultures derived from patients with advanced prostate cancer. Cell 159(1):176–187
53. Fujii M, Shimokawa M, Date S, Takano A, Matano M, Nanki K et al (2016) A colorectal tumor organoid library demonstrates progressive loss of niche factor requirements during tumorigenesis. Cell Stem Cell 18(6):827–838
54. Boj SF, Hwang CI, Baker LA, Chio II, Engle DD, Corbo V et al (2015) Organoid models of human and mouse ductal pancreatic cancer. Cell 160(1–2):324–338

55. Romero-Calvo I, Weber CR, Ray M, Brown M, Kirby K, Nandi RK et al (2019) Human organoids share structural and genetic features with primary pancreatic adenocarcinoma tumors. Mol Cancer Res 17(1):70–83

56. Tiriac H, Belleau P, Engle DD, Plenker D, Deschênes A, Somerville TDD et al (2018) Organoid profiling identifies common responders to chemotherapy in pancreatic cancer. Cancer Discov 8(9):1112–1129

57. Huang L, Holtzinger A, Jagan I, BeGora M, Lohse I, Ngai N et al (2015) Ductal pancreatic cancer modeling and drug screening using human pluripotent stem cell- and patient-derived tumor organoids. Nat Med 21(11):1364–1371

58. Broutier L, Mastrogiovanni G, Verstegen MM, Francies HE, Gavarró LM, Bradshaw CR et al (2017) Human primary liver cancer-derived organoid cultures for disease modeling and drug screening. Nat Med 23(12):1424–1435

59. Sachs N, Papaspyropoulos A, Zomer-van Ommen DD, Heo I, Böttinger L, Klay D et al (2019) Long-term expanding human airway organoids for disease modeling. EMBO J 38(4):e100300

60. Boretto M, Maenhoudt N, Luo X, Hennes A, Boeckx B, Bui B et al (2019) Patient-derived organoids from endometrial disease capture clinical heterogeneity and are amenable to drug screening. Nat Cell Biol 21(8):1041–1051

61. Kijima T, Nakagawa H, Shimonosono M, Chandramouleeswaran PM, Hara T, Sahu V et al (2019) Three-dimensional organoids reveal therapy resistance of Esophageal and oropharyngeal squamous cell carcinoma cells. Cell Mol Gastroenterol Hepatol 7(1):73–91

62. Li X, Francies HE, Secrier M, Perner J, Miremadi A, Galeano-Dalmau N et al (2018) Organoid cultures recapitulate esophageal adenocarcinoma heterogeneity providing a model for clonality studies and precision therapeutics. Nat Commun 9(1):2983

63. Nanki K, Toshimitsu K, Takano A, Fujii M, Shimokawa M, Ohta Y et al (2018) Divergent routes toward Wnt and R-spondin niche independency during human gastric carcinogenesis. Cell 174(4):856–69.e17

64. de Witte CJ, Espejo Valle-Inclan J, Hami N, Lõhmussaar K, Kopper O, Vreuls CPH et al (2020) Patient-derived ovarian cancer organoids mimic clinical response and exhibit heterogeneous inter- and Intrapatient drug responses. Cell Rep 31(11):107762

65. Driehuis E, Kolders S, Spelier S, Lõhmussaar K, Willems SM, Devriese LA et al (2019) Oral mucosal organoids as a potential platform for personalized cancer therapy. Cancer Discov 9(7):852–871

66. Ferguson FM, Nabet B, Raghavan S, Liu Y, Leggett AL, Kuljanin M et al (2020) Discovery of a selective inhibitor of doublecortin like kinase 1. Nat Chem Biol 16(6):635–643

67. Narasimhan V, Wright JA, Churchill M, Wang T, Rosati R, Lannagan TRM et al (2020) Medium-throughput drug screening of patient-derived organoids from colorectal peritoneal metastases to direct personalized therapy. Clin Cancer Res 26(14):3662–3670

68. Ooft SN, Weeber F, Dijkstra KK, McLean CM, Kaing S, van Werkhoven E et al (2019) Patient-derived organoids can predict response to chemotherapy in metastatic colorectal cancer patients. Sci Transl Med 11(513):eaay2574

69. Ganesh K, Wu C, O'Rourke KP, Szeglin BC, Zheng Y, Sauvé CG et al (2019) A rectal cancer organoid platform to study individual responses to chemoradiation. Nat Med 25(10):1607–1614

70. Yao Y, Xu X, Yang L, Zhu J, Wan J, Shen L et al (2020) Patient-derived organoids predict chemoradiation responses of locally advanced rectal cancer. Cell Stem Cell 26(1):17–26.e6

71. Wensink GE, Elias SG, Mullenders J, Koopman M, Boj SF, Kranenburg OW et al (2021) Patient-derived organoids as a predictive biomarker for treatment response in cancer patients. NPJ Precis Oncol 5(1):30

72. Xia Y, Whitesides GM (1998) Soft lithography. Angew Chem Int Ed Engl 37(5):550–575

73. Duffy DC, McDonald JC, Schueller OJ, Whitesides GM (1998) Rapid prototyping of microfluidic systems in Poly (dimethylsiloxane). Anal Chem 70(23):4974–4984

74. Whitesides GM (2006) The origins and the future of microfluidics. Nature 442(7101):368–373

75. Bhatia SN, Ingber DE (2014) Microfluidic organs-on-chips. Nat Biotechnol 32(8):760–772

76. Langer R, Vacanti JP (1993) Tissue engineering. Science 260(5110):920–926

77. Huh D, Matthews BD, Mammoto A, Montoya-Zavala M, Hsin HY, Ingber DE (2010) Reconstituting organ-level lung functions on a chip. Science 328(5986):1662–1668
78. Kasendra M, Luc R, Yin J, Manatakis DV, Kulkarni G, Lucchesi C et al (2020) Duodenum intestine-chip for preclinical drug assessment in a human relevant model. Elife 9:e50135
79. Kasendra M, Tovaglieri A, Sontheimer-Phelps A, Jalili-Firoozinezhad S, Bein A, Chalkiadaki A et al (2018) Development of a primary human small intestine-on-a-chip using biopsy-derived organoids. Sci Rep 8(1):2871
80. Gayer CP, Basson MD (2009) The effects of mechanical forces on intestinal physiology and pathology. Cell Signal 21(8):1237–1244
81. Kerns SJ, Belgur C, Petropolis D, Kanellias M, Barrile R, Sam J et al (2021) Human immunocompetent organ-on-chip platforms allow safety profiling of tumor-targeted T-cell bispecific antibodies. Elife 10:e67106
82. Zhang B, Korolj A, Lai BFL, Radisic M (2018) Advances in organ-on-a-chip engineering. Nat Rev Mater 3(8):257–278
83. Ma C, Peng Y, Li H, Chen W (2021) Organ-on-a-chip: A new paradigm for drug development. Trends Pharmacol Sci 42(2):119–133
84. Huh D, Fujioka H, Tung YC, Futai N, Paine R 3rd, Grotberg JB et al (2007) Acoustically detectable cellular-level lung injury induced by fluid mechanical stresses in microfluidic airway systems. Proc Natl Acad Sci U S A 104(48):18886–18891
85. Ma C, Zhao L, Zhou EM, Xu J, Shen S, Wang J (2016) On-chip construction of liver lobule-like microtissue and its application for adverse drug reaction assay. Anal Chem 88(3): 1719–1727
86. Ma C, Tian C, Zhao L, Wang J (2016) Pneumatic-aided micro-molding for flexible fabrication of homogeneous and heterogeneous cell-laden microgels. Lab Chip 16(14):2609–2617
87. Mu X, Zheng W, Xiao L, Zhang W, Jiang X (2013) Engineering a 3D vascular network in hydrogel for mimicking a nephron. Lab Chip 13(8):1612–1618
88. Musah S, Mammoto A, Ferrante TC, Jeanty SSF, Hirano-Kobayashi M, Mammoto T et al (2017) Mature induced-pluripotent-stem-cell-derived human podocytes reconstitute kidney glomerular-capillary-wall function on a chip. Nat Biomed Eng 1:0069
89. Shik Mun K, Arora K, Huang Y, Yang F, Yarlagadda S, Ramananda Y et al (2019) Patient-derived pancreas-on-a-chip to model cystic fibrosis-related disorders. Nat Commun 10(1): 3124
90. Glieberman AL, Pope BD, Zimmerman JF, Liu Q, Ferrier JP, Kenty JHR et al (2019) Synchronized stimulation and continuous insulin sensing in a microfluidic human islet on a Chip designed for scalable manufacturing. Lab Chip 19(18):2993–3010
91. Ahn S, Ardoña HAM, Lind JU, Eweje F, Kim SL, Gonzalez GM et al (2018) Mussel-inspired 3D fiber scaffolds for heart-on-a-chip toxicity studies of engineered nanomaterials. Anal Bioanal Chem 410(24):6141–6154
92. Marsano A, Conficconi C, Lemme M, Occhetta P, Gaudiello E, Votta E et al (2016) Beating heart on a chip: a novel microfluidic platform to generate functional 3D cardiac microtissues. Lab Chip 16(3):599–610
93. Ugolini GS, Visone R, Cruz-Moreira D, Mainardi A, Rasponi M (2018) Generation of functional cardiac microtissues in a beating heart-on-a-chip. Methods Cell Biol 146:69–84
94. Zhang X, Wang T, Wang P, Hu N (2016) High-throughput assessment of drug cardiac safety using a high-speed impedance detection technology-based heart-on-a-chip. Micromachines 7(7):122
95. Sheehy SP, Grosberg A, Qin P, Behm DJ, Ferrier JP, Eagleson MA et al (2017) Toward improved myocardial maturity in an organ-on-chip platform with immature cardiac myocytes. Exp Biol Med (Maywood) 242(17):1643–1656
96. Shim KY, Lee D, Han J, Nguyen NT, Park S, Sung JH (2017) Microfluidic gut-on-a-chip with three-dimensional villi structure. Biomed Microdevices 19(2):37
97. Poceviciute R, Ismagilov RF (2019) Human-gut-microbiome on a chip. Nat Biomed Eng 3(7): 500–501

98. Guo Y, Li Z, Su W, Wang L, Zhu Y, Qin J (2018) A biomimetic human gut-on-a-chip for modeling drug metabolism in intestine. Artif Organs 42(12):1196–1205
99. Wevers NR, Kasi DG, Gray T, Wilschut KJ, Smith B, van Vught R et al (2018) A perfused human blood-brain barrier on-a-chip for high-throughput assessment of barrier function and antibody transport. Fluids Barriers CNS 15(1):23
100. Koo Y, Hawkins BT, Yun Y (2018) Three-dimensional (3D) tetra-culture brain on chip platform for organophosphate toxicity screening. Sci Rep 8(1):2841
101. Marturano-Kruik A, Nava MM, Yeager K, Chramiec A, Hao L, Robinson S et al (2018) Human bone perivascular niche-on-a-chip for studying metastatic colonization. Proc Natl Acad Sci U S A 115(6):1256–1261
102. Hao S, Ha L, Cheng G, Wan Y, Xia Y, Sosnoski DM et al (2018) A spontaneous 3D bone-on-a-chip for bone metastasis study of breast cancer cells. Small 14(12):e1702787
103. Torisawa YS, Mammoto T, Jiang E, Jiang A, Mammoto A, Watters AL et al (2016) Modeling Hematopoiesis and responses to radiation countermeasures in a bone marrow-on-a-chip. Tissue Eng Part C Methods 22(5):509–515
104. Pires de Mello CP, Carmona-Moran C, McAleer CW, Perez J, Coln EA, Long CJ et al (2020) Microphysiological heart-liver body-on-a-chip system with a skin mimic for evaluating topical drug delivery. Lab Chip 20(4):749–759
105. Maschmeyer I, Lorenz AK, Schimek K, Hasenberg T, Ramme AP, Hübner J et al (2015) A four-organ-chip for interconnected long-term co-culture of human intestine, liver, skin and kidney equivalents. Lab Chip 15(12):2688–2699
106. Miller PG, Shuler ML (2016) Design and demonstration of a pumpless 14 compartment microphysiological system. Biotechnol Bioeng 113(10):2213–2227
107. Abaci HE, Shuler ML (2015) Human-on-a-chip design strategies and principles for physiologically based pharmacokinetics/pharmacodynamics modeling. Integr Biol 7(4):383–391
108. Zhang C, Zhao Z, Abdul Rahim NA, van Noort D, Yu H (2009) Towards a human-on-chip: culturing multiple cell types on a chip with compartmentalized microenvironments. Lab Chip 9(22):3185–3192
109. Sung JH, Wang YI, Narasimhan Sriram N, Jackson M, Long C, Hickman JJ et al (2019) Recent advances in body-on-a-chip systems. Anal Chem 91(1):330–351
110. Ashammakhi N, Hasan A, Kaarela O, Byambaa B, Sheikhi A, Gaharwar AK et al (2019) Advancing frontiers in bone bioprinting. Adv Healthc Mater 8(7):e1801048
111. Murphy SV, Atala A (2014) 3D bioprinting of tissues and organs. Nat Biotechnol 32(8): 773–785
112. Datta P, Dey M, Ataie Z, Unutmaz D, Ozbolat IT (2020) 3D bioprinting for reconstituting the cancer microenvironment. NPJ Precis Oncol 4:18
113. Stanton MM, Samitier J, Sánchez S (2015) Bioprinting of 3D hydrogels. Lab Chip 15(15): 3111–3115
114. Mandrycky C, Wang Z, Kim K, Kim DH (2016) 3D bioprinting for engineering complex tissues. Biotechnol Adv 34(4):422–434
115. Mao S, He J, Zhao Y, Liu T, Xie F, Yang H et al (2020) Bioprinting of patient-derived in vitro intrahepatic cholangiocarcinoma tumor model: establishment, evaluation and anti-cancer drug testing. Biofabrication 12(4):045014
116. Ringeisen BR, Kim H, Barron JA, Krizman DB, Chrisey DB, Jackman S et al (2004) Laser printing of pluripotent embryonal carcinoma cells. Tissue Eng 10(3–4):483–491
117. O'Brien ER, Howarth C, Sibson NR (2013) The role of astrocytes in CNS tumors: pre-clinical models and novel imaging approaches. Front Cell Neurosci 7:40
118. Paolillo M, Schinelli S (2016) Brain infiltration by cancer cells: different roads to the same target? J Cancer Metastasis Treat 2:90–100
119. Mao Y, Keller ET, Garfield DH, Shen K, Wang J (2013) Stromal cells in tumor microenvironment and breast cancer. Cancer Metastasis Rev 32(1–2):303–315
120. Wu SZ, Roden DL, Wang C, Holliday H, Harvey K, Cazet AS et al (2020) Stromal cell diversity associated with immune evasion in human triple-negative breast cancer. EMBO J 39(19):e104063

Chapter 29
Classification and Evolution of Tumor Ecosystem

Phei Er Saw and Erwei Song

Abstract The development of neoplasms has been documented since decades ago, and this documentation illustrates the mechanisms of acquired treatment resistance and carcinogenesis. The natural selection forces put on neoplasms by their micro-environmental ecology shape the tumors' ongoing metamorphosis. Tumors may, however, show variances in the dynamics of cancer ecology and evolution, including the rates of emergence and extinction of new clones, the degree of divergence among the clones, and whether they develop at a more periodic pace or in bursts, both within and across forms of cancer. Many ecological and evolutionary traits of a neoplasm have clinical significance, and in most instances, their clinical significance has not been explored. There is a need for conceptual frameworks and a shared lingo for creating clinical distinctions that reflect the relevant environmental, genetic, and kinetic factors that influence tumor adaption, progression, and therapeutic response. In this chapter, we introduce the quantification of neoplasm using Evo and Eco-index in measuring cancer diversity and how these cancer changes over time.

P. E. Saw
Guangdong Provincial Key Laboratory of Malignant Tumor Epigenetics and Gene Regulation, Guangdong-Hong Kong Joint Laboratory for RNA Medicine, Medical Research Center, Sun Yat-sen Memorial Hospital, Sun Yat-sen University, Guangzhou, China

Nanhai Translational Innovation Center of Precision Immunology, Sun Yat-sen Memorial Hospital, Sun Yat-sen University, Foshan, China

E. Song (✉)
Guangdong Provincial Key Laboratory of Malignant Tumor Epigenetics and Gene Regulation, Guangdong-Hong Kong Joint Laboratory for RNA Medicine, Medical Research Center, Sun Yat-sen Memorial Hospital, Sun Yat-sen University, Guangzhou, China

Nanhai Translational Innovation Center of Precision Immunology, Sun Yat-sen Memorial Hospital, Sun Yat-sen University, Foshan, China

Breast Tumor Center, Sun Yat-sen Memorial Hospital, Sun Yat-sen University, Guangzhou, China
e-mail: songew@mail.sysu.edu.cn

Introduction

Since early 70s, the development of neoplasms has been documented, and this documentation illustrates the mechanisms of acquired treatment resistance and carcinogenesis [1, 2]. The selection forces put on neoplasms by their microenvironmental ecology shape the tumors' ongoing metamorphosis. Tumors may, however, show variances in the dynamics of cancer ecology and evolution, including the rates of emergence and extinction of new clones, the degree of divergence among the clones, and whether they develop at a more periodic pace or in bursts, both within and across forms of cancer. Many ecological and evolutionary traits of a neoplasm have clinical significance [3–14], although this is not always the case [4, 14, 15], and in most instances, their clinical significance has not been explored. There is a need for conceptual frameworks and a shared lingo for creating clinical distinctions that reflect the relevant environmental, genetic, and kinetic factors that influence tumor adaption, progression, and therapeutic response.

Quantifying Changes in Neoplasm: A Classification System

Researchers and clinicians would have a better foundation for establishing superior predictive and prognostic assessments of tumor behavior, such as how well the tumor will respond to a particular treatment, with the help of a classification system that considers the ecology and evolution of neoplasms. Delivering an expressive tool that may improve clinical care regarding patient quality of life and overall survival is the clear goal of a categorization system for the ecology and development of neoplasms. Additionally, it would advance knowledge and research in oncology and cancer biology. The ecological index (**Eco-index**) shows potential selection forces brought about by the surrounding microenvironment. In contrast, the evolutionary index (**Evo-index**) illustrates the innate adaptability held by the population of neoplastic cells. These two indexes are reviewed in detail here [1].

The Evo-Index

The Evo-index and the Eco-index (mentioned later in this chapter) are built upon a consensus in 2017 [1]. The Evo-index ($D\#\Delta\#$) is an amalgamation of two elementary components: the diversity (D) or intratumoral heterogeneity of the neoplasm and the nature of its alteration over time (Δ). To put it another way, the Evo-index measures spatial and temporal heterogeneity (Fig. 29.1). Pre-clinical research or clinical trials may be used to assess the variety of malignancies and changes in the clonal organization over time.

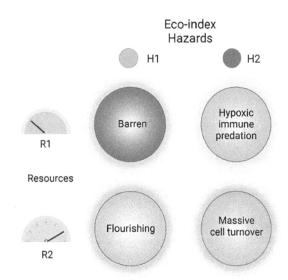

Fig. 29.1 Categorizing tumors using Eco-index. Eco-index is composed of two factors: hazards (H) and resources (R), which are available to the tumor cells. For example, tumor with low hazards (H1) and low resources (R1) might be barren (i.e., few TILs, poor perfusion, few supporting cells). High levels of hazards (H2) would lead to rapid proliferation, evasion of predation, migration away from the hazards. High levels of resources allow cancer cells to proliferate rapidly

Diversity in Cancer Population and Heterogeneity

Diversity refers to a population's heterogeneity, affecting how well it adapts to population-level selection forces. The gasoline that drives the engine of natural selection is this variety. There are many variables, including phenotypic, functional, genetic, and epigenetic diversity. Cancer survival and recurrence rates, as well as the emergence of invasive tumors, may all be predicted by genetic diversity [3–7, 10, 11, 14]. The relationship between variety and clinical outcomes may be complicated and not universally consistent across all cancer types [4, 14]. Diversity could serve as a stand-in for the likelihood that a resistant clone is present inside a tumor. At this time, we are not fully aware of all the epigenetic changes and mutations that give cancer cells their resistance to certain treatments. Those that we are aware of are difficult to spot if they are present in just a small portion of the tumor. Diverse neoplasms have a larger likelihood of hiding resistant clones than homogeneous neoplasms do and thus may be more likely to acquire resistance in the long run. Different sorts of variety that a neoplasm exhibits may be clinically meaningful, as the drive behind natural selection and clinically actionable indicators of dynamics. For instance, the means of suppression within the cell that act as a buffer against the above-mentioned deleterious effects, such as chaperone proteins, should preferably target neoplastic cells if elevated levels of genetic diversity represent elevated levels of reasonably deleterious passenger mutations [16, 17]. Alternatively, via processes like cross-feeding, variety could be indicative of cooperation between clones [18–22]. By themselves, these cooperative systems represent potential therapeutic targets. According to theory, cytotoxic medicines should provide a better selection for resistance than those that target the cooperation of cancer cells [23]. It is possible that not all diversity constructs are created equal; thus, future studies should look at which have therapeutic use.

Measuring Diversity in Cancer

The assessment of diversity (intratumoral heterogeneity), one of the four components of the categorization framework, has yielded the highest number of methods [11, 20, 24]. There is a ton of literature in ecology that discusses how to measure diversity [25]. The differences between local *onco-sphere* (alpha diversity) and between regions, distal *onco-sphere* (beta diversity), may be further subdivided from the overall variety of a large area or landscape, systemic *onco-sphere* (gamma diversity) [26]. The idea that assessing variety necessitates defining the geographical scale under consideration is crucial to this definition. While between-region diversity accounts for differences across biopsy specimens in multi-region sampling studies, within-region diversity may be defined as the diversity measured inside a biopsy sample [3, 4, 27]. It is still not quite clear how ecological statistics may be used to quantify between-region diversity within tumors. The assessment of discrepancies between biopsy samples may use conventional metrics of differences between microbial populations [28]. Diversity may be measured in a variety of ways, and evaluating diversity within neoplasms has presented a number of obstacles.

Cancer Population Changes Over Time

There is no doubt that different mutation rates are brought about by diverse epigenetic and genetic alteration mechanisms, including non-homologous recombination, telomerase degradation, CpG methylation, histone alterations, and other types of chromosomal instability [29]. The relevant processes would vary across various tumor clones and would rely on the specific tumor. It is assumed that mutations happen at a constant pace when discussing mutation rates and their quantification. These are what evolutionary scientists refer to as "molecular clocks" [30]. However, catastrophic mitosis is possible to produce chromosomal changes over the whole genome in a single event [31, 32]. From slow, consistent, clocklike minute variations to jarring, irregular, large shifts, there is a continuum. For instance, different mutation rates may emerge throughout the course of a lineage's history, much as the evolution shown by the mutator phenotype [33, 34]. Additionally, single nucleotide variations have shown that higher mutation rates may result in detrimental mutations, which deteriorate the fitness of neoplastic cell lineages via Muller's ratchet [16, 35]. This may sometimes even lead to tumor regression [16, 17]. A key element of the future therapeutic care of tumors may develop to be the finding and monitoring of natural selection. We should renew our perspective on how cancer develops, and their progress over time. The categorization should at least include the pace of change, whether its epigenetic or genetic mutations, or phenotypical changes, which include the rate at which clones spread via natural selection (gradual to punctuated). The rate of change over time would determine the appropriate sample intervals [36]. It should be highlighted that since selection pressures fluctuate over

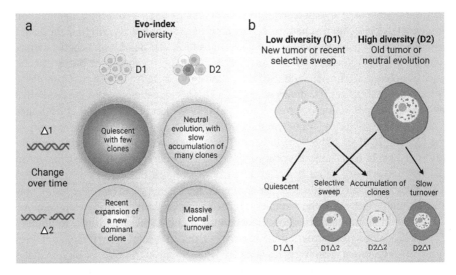

Fig. 29.2 The Evo-index and how it evolves. (**a**) Two parameters that represent heterogeneity over time (change over time, Δ) and heterogeneity over space (diversity, D) make up the evolutionary index (Evo-index). "Change" was used to refer to both changes in the population's epigenetic, genetic, and phenotypic modifications as well as changes in the frequencies of those changes within the population of neoplastic cells. It is unclear which values of D and Δ are the best. Furthermore, it is still unclear how these elements should be divided into two, three, or more groups. Here, for the sake of clarity, we provide examples of the many dynamics that may be categorized in a straight-forward 2 × 2 manner. (**b**) TA tumor's genetic makeup may change in a variety of ways, either slowly (Δ1) or quickly (Δ2). Due to its recent homogenizing clonal proliferation or the fact that it is a fresh tumor, the tumor on the left may have low diversity (D1) at time 0. The tumor may exhibit quiescence and hence manifest considerably at time 1 (D1Δ1), or it may accumulate clones, some of which spread and expand, to generate a varied tumor by time 1 (D2Δ2). On the other hand, because of its age or the presence of a higher mutation rate owing to neutral evolution, a tumor may exhibit diversity (D2) at time 0. That tumor may have undergone homogeneity at time 1 by a selective sweep (D1Δ2) or may have continued on its present course with a gradual turnover of its clones (D2Δ1)

time, particularly after the start of treatment, neutral or "passenger" mutations cannot be ignored in these estimates. Therefore, resistance mutations that might be benefi-cial or harmful in the absence of treatment can provide neoplastic cells a selective advantage in the presence of therapy [37].

Measuring Change Over Time in Cancer Population

No matter whether the change is phenotypic or genetic, measuring change through time is difficult. A simple representation of how the Evo-index might show evolu-tionary changes within tumor cell populations is shown in Fig. 29.2. It is possible for change to occur throughout time, yet diversity is still stable thanks to the emergence and extinction of a dynamic equilibrium of clones [12]. According to mutation frequencies, past genetic changes across time may be indirectly inferred for single samples [15, 38]. In molecular population genetics, the degree of genetic variety among samples—referred to as "nucleotide diversity"—provides a proxy for the pace of evolution. The percentage of the genome that differs between two samples is often referred to as genetic divergence [10–12]. This statistic provides the predictive ability for the prediction of progression that is not bound by the number of clones [10, 11], which helps the framework embrace both change over time and diversity in the Evo-index. It should be noted that different clonal structures may exhibit wildly different levels of genetic diversity (Fig. 29.2). Researchers calculated the mean pairwise divergence score between all pairs of samples taken from a tumor [10–12]. The mean pairwise divergence combines the degree of divergence with measures of clone size since the likelihood of two samples deriving from a single clone (resulting in minimum divergence) depends on the clone size (thus combining D with Δ). When reconstructing the history of a tumor, one of the primary strategies used in evolutionary biology to quantify change through time is phylogenetic inference [39, 40]. Phylogenetic methods may be used to measure diversity patterns, as well as rates of evolution through time and place, and to characterize them. Recently, a variety of phylogenetic techniques have been developed to examine the development of tumors within patients, for both single-cell and bulk data, and from a variety of data formats [41, 42]. From a single timepoint, all of the previously stated methods may be calculated. Undoubtedly, superior measures of the kind and extent of change across time may be obtained immediately by longitudinal sampling. Sequencing cfDNA from longitudinal blood samples is one less invasive technology that may reveal if a patient has undergone natural or artificial selection. The inclusion of the Evo-index in clinical trials may enhance the way that the evolutionary causes of intervention failure are described. Most human cancers include many big clones at the time of clinical manifestation, in addition, to probably many smaller clones [4, 14], and relapse in the absence of variety may reflect inherent resistance or enhanced mutagenesis as a result of an intervention. Relapse with lesser diversity (D1), on the other hand, points to a bottleneck effect where just a limited number of tumor cells were able to withstand the intervention, potentially pointing to selection for one or more resistant clones.

Factoring in the Cancer Ecosystem: The Eco-Index

Hazards (H) and resources (R) may be used to describe an ecosystem from the perspective of a cancer cell or an organism [43–46] (Fig. 29.2) The elements that may cause a cell to die are referred to here as dangers. The relevant resources required for cell development and maintenance are many and varied, and they include anything that could be able to stop the formation of the neoplastic cell population [43]. Ecology teaches us that we may better comprehend population responses and evolution when we take one organism inside the population into account [47]. From an ecological perspective, a species' risk and resource profiles are chosen according to the unique life-history strategies that apply to that species. Similar theories apply to neoplastic cells [48]. The life-history strategies of species that are exposed to higher levels of risk tend to develop quickly, reproduce quickly, and spend less on maintenance and survival. Hazard-exposed organisms often leave behind larger amounts of untapped resources. Ecosystems with increasing or fluctuating resource availability are advantageous to species that can reproduce quickly to take advantage of those changes. There is a tendency to prioritize speed above efficiency, which may result in variable levels of underutilized resources as well as very high population densities [49].

Hazards

Neoplastic cells may be at risk from various things, including toxins, immune cells, microbes, waste materials, and anticancer treatments. Reliable data have shown that immune predation is associated with a better outcome for cancer [50–59]. Furthermore, individuals who underwent immune checkpoint blockade therapy had higher survival rates and elevated mutation burdens that resulted in the production of neo-antigens [60–62]. Additionally, in patients with lung cancer treated with checkpoint inhibitors, a higher load of subclonal neo-antigens was linked to worse outcomes [63]. These findings suggest that subclonal neo-antigens may inhibit cytotoxic immune responses directed toward the neo-antigens present in every tumor cell. Neoplastic cells also face risks from accumulating waste products in their microenvironments [44, 46, 64, 65]. This might entail the buildup of reactive oxygen species brought on by excessive cellular growth and lactate and lactic acid from glycolysis [64, 66, 67]. Advanced glycation end products [68, 69], nitric oxide [70, 71], and methylglyoxal [72, 73] have all been linked to cancer microenvironments as hazardous waste products. The microbiome's role in cancer is complicated and mostly unstudied. Although certain bacteria may contribute to the development of tumors [74, 75], others have anticancer properties [98], which increase the effectiveness of chemotherapy [76]. Therefore, microbes may act as threats to and suppliers of material for cancerous cells.

Measuring Hazards

The most effective safeguards against cancerous cells now in use depend on measures to prevent immunological predation. Numerous studies have examined the relationship between infiltrating lymphocytes and a good prognosis for cancer [50–59]. Furthermore, a pan-cancer investigation revealed that T-cell signatures were very reliable prognostic indicators for 25 different cancer types [77]. It was found that a profile of activated T cells from bulk tumor samples was highly indicative of increased survival [52–54, 59]. Breast cancer patients who show that lymphocytes and cancerous cells are co-localized within tumors have a better prognosis than patients whose tumors show that lymphocytes and cancerous cells are not connected [51]. This was consistent with the usual ecological statistic known as the Morisita–Horn index [78], which measures statistically significant colocalization for the identification of ecological interactions (in this instance, predation). These findings suggested that immunological predation poses a considerable threat to neoplastic cells and that the ecological index should include indicators of the aforementioned predation. While numerous research has looked at the possible toxicity of low pH [79, 80], fewer have looked at the effects of various metabolites on the fitness of cancer cells. The effects of various quantities of hypothesized hazardous metabolites on the survival and growth of cancer cells in both cell culture experiments and mice models should be studied further [81].

Resources

The future behavior of tumors depends on resources including glucose, oxygen, micronutrients, growth signals, survival signals, and space. The linkages between the availability of critical nutrients and cell metabolism, which ecologists refer to as the organism's "foraging ecology," are surprisingly little understood. Because almost all malignancies rely on glycolytic metabolism rather than aerobic metabolism, resources may be able to choose certain tumor characteristics [82, 83]. Natural selection favors feeding strategies that balance efficiency, speed, and safety, as we have learned from the environment [84]. Therefore, a strong selection for cancer cells to behave similarly is necessary (for example, by overexpression of transporters like glucose transporter type 1, GLUT1) is vital for their survival [85]. Resources are often depleted at levels far lower than what is typically available in normal tissue as a result of all cells' cumulative use [86]. In fact, glucose is depleted at levels below what most studies can detect [87]. However, under certain circumstances, variations in the availability of resources and immune predation might obstruct the complete consumption of resources [88, 89], leaving behind patches of unused resources that are still available for use in the future [90].

The material in plasma, as well as the produced and released metabolites from normal tumor cells and the microenvironment, is potential source for malignancies. The list thus includes glucose, proteins (albumins, fibrinogens, and globulins), fatty acids, amino acids, electrolytes, hormones, oxygen, and trace elements. Nutritional interactions impact the value of resources to consumers and the practical response [91]. Lack of a resource may result in stagnation in certain conditions, but it may also trigger cell death or dispersion in other situations [92]. There are currently a number of unanswered problems surrounding the intratumoral cycle of important nutrients other than carbon and nitrogen (such as iron, phosphate, and copper) [93]. These nutritional cycles may include valuable therapeutic targets [94, 95]. Nutrients may also come from the stroma. Fibroblast activation may transport lactate and pyruvate to cancer cells, whereas stimulation of adipocytes may supply fatty acids [96, 97]. CAFs, which are known to play a critical role in the formation and control of tumors, particularly solid tumors, interact directly with cancer cells during this stage [95, 98] and support both treatment resistance and cancer development and growth [99–101].

The vasculature is the crucial connection between tumor invasion and metastasis with angiogenesis, realizing that preventing the creation of new blood vessels would provide a straightforward way to stop tumor growth [102, 103]. Hypoxia and necrosis, which are important angiogenesis drivers and are present in many cancers, confirm that resource constraint in tumors is of the highest relevance. Additionally, research has shown that necrosis is a prognostic factor in a number of malignancies [104]. Resources' effects on tumor evolution are not only limited by their supply, availability, and depletion. Diverse resource availability might be crucial. There is a variation depending on whether resources are homogeneous (exhibiting gradients or "patchy") across space or not [105]. Patchy resources (and risks) lead to a variety of habitats (such as sparse and rich areas), which may exert selection for certain clones that can live there and may exhibit particular reactions to (along with particular exposure to) treatments. Furthermore, researches have shown that if the aforementioned patchy resources are altered over time, cells will experience selection pressure to move away from areas with low resources and use transitory places with abundant nutrients [88, 89, 106–108]. Therefore, according to ecological theory, diverse resources should favor invasion and metastasis [106, 107], and there is evidence in favor of that idea in the case of cancer [109–115]. Additionally, resource gradients often drive fast evolution because species that can adapt to increasingly challenging conditions may survive the competition and prosper [116].

Measuring Resources

Examining temporal and geographical scales is necessary for the measuring of resources (and dangers). How to combine measurements of resource degree, stability through time, and geographical variation into a single statistic is still unclear. There are several tools and resources to measure them, and doing so might have predictive value, such as PET-CT, or measurement of blood vessel density may be utilized to determine the proportion of a tumor that is poorly perfused or necrotic [117–119]. Additionally, molecular biomarkers such as antibodies against HIF1α [90], or CA9; measuring their binding within tumor tissue can be used to assess the amount and patchiness of hypoxia in FFPE specimens [120]. The ability to bind EF5 and related techniques has been shown to be useful in the clinical context for the identification of hypoxic areas, assessment of therapeutic response, and prognosis determination [121]. Evaluation of ATP may potentially provide a useful indirect indicator of the amount of resources accessible to cancer cells [122]. Pyruvate, glutamine, fatty acids, lactate, calcium, phosphate, potassium, and many trace metals might potentially be limiting elements and are crucial to evaluate, although this area is still not well-studied [123–125].

In natural habitats, there is often a close relationship between the habitat and the traits and species. Similar to this, just identifying the many habitat types inside a tumor may be predictive of the cancer cell population and the results of treatment. For instance, regardless of tumor size, the evaluation of fluid-attenuated inversion recovery (FLAIR), T1 and T2 from MRI exams after administration of gadolinium was able to differentiate several habitats that were connected to treatment results [124]. Texture analysis of MRI images has been used to identify regional differences and spatial heterogeneity due to microenvironmental factors such as tissue stiffness, cell density, nutrition dispersion, and blood flow [123, 125]. These variables might potentially be used to calculate the functional diversity (D) of tumors. Although there is a wealth of literature on ecology and geographic information systems (GIS) [126–128], and these are the sources of tools for the analysis of spatial resource information, these fields are not typically employed in cancer research [50, 129]. In addition to T-cell infiltration, conventional histopathology may provide measurements of lymphatic and vascular density [53]. In histological samples of breast cancer, digital pathology to examine the spatial distributions of estrogen receptor (ER) expression was used in relation to tissue necrosis and vascular density. Significant regional variations in the cancer proliferation phenotypes, which were accompanied by immune response and vascularity, were indicated [90, 130]. The spatial interactions between fibroblasts and cancerous cells were also depicted using digital pathology [131] (Box 29.1).

Box 29.1 Important Concerns in the Measurement of Diversity in Cancer
The measuring of variety in cancer raises a number of significant issues and unanswered topics, including the following: What is the best way to gauge diversity? How are clones determined to be clones? How are the measurements scaled up for genomic assays? Exist non-linear relationships between diversity and therapeutic results? Functional diversity or genetic diversity is more predictive, right? Does measuring the variety of the main tumor enough, or are measurements of the diversity of the metastases also necessary? Is it enough to estimate diversity using bulk biopsy tests, or are studies of diversity at the single-cell level also necessary? One must first identify the unit being assessed if one wants to quantify diversity. Clones are often formed when cells group together; however, there is currently no accepted definition of a clone. For simplicity's sake, clones are often described as a group of cells that have descended from a single ancestor cell and have a common modification of interest. According to some tests, a collection of cells with a similar genotype is considered to be a clone [10, 11]. Despite this, since each neoplastic cell probably has a distinct genome, this definition does not scale well to whole-

(continued)

Box 29.1 (continued)

genome experiments. On the other hand, estimates of sample divergence only get more accurate when tests are scaled up to the genome level [10–12, 34]. Although this is not simple, another method would be to rebuild the cell lineage (phylogeny) of a neoplasm and then define clones in accordance with the cell lineage topology. Bacterial and viral phylogenetics have addressed a similar problem, and methods from these domains may be used here [132, 133]. Which modifications should be used to gauge diversity is still up for debate. Compared to other kinds of variety, some may be more clinically significant than others, such as changes in copy number and exon mutations. Despite this, it was found that defining a clone based on selectively beneficial mutations and defining a clone based on evolutionarily neutral mutations both predicted the development of cancer [11]. The assessment of variety might be carried out in accordance with RNA expression or other behavioral traits rather than genetics [134, 135]. This may be a better indicator of a tumor's ability to evolve than genetic measurements of variety because of how selection operates on phenotypes [136, 137]. However, just a few research have tested this concept, and it is still debatable [138, 139].

Dynamics of Tumor Ecosystem in Equilibria

A favorable habitat provides a safe harbor for considerable population expansion in a stable-state ecology, also known as equilibrium (or alternatively, carrying capacity), when the growth rate is equal to the species' mortality rate. However, according to the Allee effects in ecology, a species' population size must at least reach a certain threshold (the Allee threshold) in order to start moving in an upward direction. A new species has a high chance of collapsing and becoming extinct if its population size or density is too small (not meeting the Allee threshold). It is interesting to note that cancer biology also exhibits similar phenomena. For instance, establishing a cancer cell line's metastatic model successfully requires a particular number of cells. It was also mentioned that CTCs in breast cancer patients might have a significantly higher potential for metastasis if circulation as a cluster took place [1].

Allee Effects

Evolutionary modeling has provided crucial insights into how cancer develops, although many of the models' presumptions still need to be verified. In particular, our understanding of the ecological dynamics inside the tumor is still restricted, especially in the case of tiny tumors that have not yet been detected or that have undergone therapy. Most models assume that tumors (or pre-cancerous lesions) develop exponentially or maintain a constant size in the absence of experimental evidence. A logistic growth curve may be used to represent these dynamics, in which a population first exhibits exponential growth before stabilizing at the carrying capacity. But logistic growth is only one of the plausible population dynamics that may be seen in both lab-based and wild populations. The inverse density dependency, sometimes referred to as the Allee effect, is a typical deviation from logistic growth [140–142].

Strong Allee effects show populations that can expand at a medium population density but suffer when there are either too few or too many organisms. Due to the tremendous difficulty of intervening in and conserving a population that has shrunk below the threshold population size, these Allee effects highlight a fundamental problem in conservation biology. The Allee effect, however, implies that there may be a growth threshold in the context of cancer that may be examined in therapies. Allee effects are the consequence of several processes, including coordinated feeding and defense [140–142], which may be important to cancer. Cooperation is often ineffective when there are few organisms, leading to a growth threshold in population dynamics because an appropriate growth rate is required to outpace inevitable mortality brought on by external forces. Many different types of creatures use cooperative feeding tactics, from African wild canines that hunt and feed their young in large packs to baker's yeast that digests sugar in a communal pool outside of the cell [143, 144]. In the case of cancer, cooperation between cells may be necessary to produce the adequate density of diffusible growth factors needed for tumor growth or pro-angiogenic growth factors, such as VEGFA, which promotes the recruitment of blood vessels to perfuse the tumor [145].

Cell culture experiments often yield the Allee effect. In most cases, growing a single cancer cell in isolation is difficult unless the medium has been prepared by the secretions of other cells [18]. Micrometastases also have growth thresholds, and a large number of them are protracted-dormant [18]. Additionally, many species work together to protect one another from harmful environmental factors or predators. Examples include the general warming of Emperor penguin colonies, schools of fish avoiding predators, and the formation of protective biofilms, which are surface-attached bacterial populations that are closely packed [140, 146, 147]. Similar to biofilm bacteria, which are much harder to treat than free-living bacteria, bigger tumors are more challenging to treat with radiation or medications, which might have an Allee effect [147, 148].

The Allee effect's presence and scope have received very little attention, much like several elements of population dynamics in cancer. Despite this, growth thresholds within the population dynamics of malignancies remain consistent in many of the current investigations. For instance, when more cancer cells are given to a mouse with a fully functioning immune system, xenograft transplantation of cancer cells has a higher success rate. This may imply that in these models, cell cooperation is essential for effective initiation [149]. The lower rates of cancer start, invasion, and metastasis may also be explained by the Allee effects. Numerous microscopic tumors may form, but they almost always disappear before becoming clinically relevant or even before identification is possible [150]. Successful cancers develop when the Allee effects are present because of exceptionally large population size variations that push tumors over the Allee threshold. Allee effects appear after the formation of the tumor because unique cancer subclones are created, which are more fit at greater densities but are subject to the Allee effect at lower densities. Despite the persistence of a very small number of cancerous cells, certain tumors show recurrence following therapy. This phenomenon, also known as minimum residual disease (MRD), shows that the Allee effects for such tumors are either negligible or may be removed by further cancer cell development while the patient is in remission [151]. Similarly, in certain transgenic mice models designed for strong cancer initiation, cancer may be able to emerge from a single progenitor cell, making them unique from human malignancies that often take years to establish.

Conclusion

The understanding of evolutionary biology of cancer is vital. In this chapter, we have dwelve into the core of how a tumor may evolve, and how this could be calculated or predicted using multiple algorithm. The Eco- and Evo-index should be taken into account when diagnosing and classifying tumor, not only based on their tissue of origin and staging, one should also take into account the spatiotemporal changes in the environment (for example, a breast primary tumor would be different compared to breast metastatic tumor) as their hazards and resources could be varying significantly. However, currently, there is no standard for classifying the comprehensive ecological markers of a tumor. Evolutionary oncology should be taken into consideration when considering patients' therapeutic intervention.

References

1. Maley CC, Aktipis A, Graham TA, Sottoriva A, Boddy AM, Janiszewska M et al (2017) Classifying the evolutionary and ecological features of neoplasms. Nat Rev Cancer 17(10): 605–619
2. Greaves M, Maley CC (2012) Clonal evolution in cancer. Nature 481(7381):306–313
3. Mroz EA, Tward AD, Pickering CR, Myers JN, Ferris RL, Rocco JW (2013) High intratumor genetic heterogeneity is related to worse outcome in patients with head and neck squamous cell carcinoma. Cancer 119(16):3034–3042
4. Andor N, Graham TA, Jansen M, Xia LC, Aktipis CA, Petritsch C et al (2016) Pan-cancer analysis of the extent and consequences of intratumor heterogeneity. Nat Med 22(1):105–113
5. Wangsa D, Chowdhury SA, Ryott M, Gertz EM, Elmberger G, Auer G et al (2016) Phylogenetic analysis of multiple FISH markers in oral tongue squamous cell carcinoma suggests that a diverse distribution of copy number changes is associated with poor prognosis. Int J Cancer 138(1):98–109
6. Schwarz RF, Ng CK, Cooke SL, Newman S, Temple J, Piskorz AM et al (2015) Spatial and temporal heterogeneity in high-grade serous ovarian cancer: a phylogenetic analysis. PLoS Med 12(2):e1001789

7. Urbschat S, Rahnenführer J, Henn W, Feiden W, Wemmert S, Linsler S et al (2011) Clonal cytogenetic progression within intratumorally heterogeneous meningiomas predicts tumor recurrence. Int J Oncol 39(6):1601–1608

8. Birkbak NJ, Eklund AC, Li Q, McClelland SE, Endesfelder D, Tan P et al (2011) Paradoxical relationship between chromosomal instability and survival outcome in cancer. Cancer Res 71(10):3447–3452

9. Roylance R, Endesfelder D, Gorman P, Burrell RA, Sander J, Tomlinson I et al (2011) Relationship of extreme chromosomal instability with long-term survival in a retrospective analysis of primary breast cancer. Cancer Epidemiol Biomarkers Prev 20(10):2183–2194

10. Maley CC, Galipeau PC, Finley JC, Wongsurawat VJ, Li X, Sanchez CA et al (2006) Genetic clonal diversity predicts progression to esophageal adenocarcinoma. Nat Genet 38(4):468–473

11. Merlo LM, Shah NA, Li X, Blount PL, Vaughan TL, Reid BJ et al (2010) A comprehensive survey of clonal diversity measures in Barrett's esophagus as biomarkers of progression to esophageal adenocarcinoma. Cancer Prev Res (Phila) 3(11):1388–1397

12. Martinez P, Timmer MR, Lau CT, Calpe S, Sancho-Serra Mdel C, Straub D et al (2016) Dynamic clonal equilibrium and predetermined cancer risk in Barrett's oesophagus. Nat Commun 7:12158

13. Lipinski KA, Barber LJ, Davies MN, Ashenden M, Sottoriva A, Gerlinger M (2016) Cancer evolution and the limits of predictability in precision cancer medicine. Trends Cancer 2(1):49–63

14. Morris LG, Riaz N, Desrichard A, Şenbabaoğlu Y, Hakimi AA, Makarov V et al (2016) Pan-cancer analysis of intratumor heterogeneity as a prognostic determinant of survival. Oncotarget 7(9):10051–10063

15. Williams MJ, Werner B, Barnes CP, Graham TA, Sottoriva A (2016) Identification of neutral tumor evolution across cancer types. Nat Genet 48(3):238–244

16. McFarland CD, Korolev KS, Kryukov GV, Sunyaev SR, Mirny LA (2013) Impact of deleterious passenger mutations on cancer progression. Proc Natl Acad Sci U S A 110(8):2910–2915

17. McFarland CD, Mirny LA, Korolev KS (2014) Tug-of-war between driver and passenger mutations in cancer and other adaptive processes. Proc Natl Acad Sci U S A 111(42):15138–15143

18. Axelrod R, Axelrod DE, Pienta KJ (2006) Evolution of cooperation among tumor cells. Proc Natl Acad Sci U S A 103(36):13474–13479

19. Marusyk A, Tabassum DP, Altrock PM, Almendro V, Michor F, Polyak K (2014) Non-cell-autonomous driving of tumor growth supports sub-clonal heterogeneity. Nature 514(7520):54–58

20. Marusyk A, Almendro V, Polyak K (2012) Intra-tumor heterogeneity: a looking glass for cancer? Nat Rev Cancer 12(5):323–334

21. Chapman A, Fernandez del Ama L, Ferguson J, Kamarashev J, Wellbrock C, Hurlstone A (2014) Heterogeneous tumor subpopulations cooperate to drive invasion. Cell Rep 8(3):688–695

22. Cleary AS, Leonard TL, Gestl SA, Gunther EJ (2014) Tumor cell heterogeneity maintained by cooperating subclones in Wnt-driven mammary cancers. Nature 508(7494):113–117

23. Driscoll WW, Pepper JW (2010) Theory for the evolution of diffusible external goods. Evolution 64(9):2682–2687

24. Alizadeh AA, Aranda V, Bardelli A, Blanpain C, Bock C, Borowski C et al (2015) Toward understanding and exploiting tumor heterogeneity. Nat Med 21(8):846–853

25. Magurran AE (2004) Measuring biological diversity. Blackwell, Durham

26. Whittaker RH (1972) Evolution and measurement of species diversity. Taxon 21:213–251

27. Mroz EA, Tward AD, Hammon RJ, Ren Y, Rocco JW (2015) Intra-tumor genetic heterogeneity and mortality in head and neck cancer: analysis of data from the cancer genome atlas. PLoS Med 12(2):e1001786

28. Lozupone C, Lladser ME, Knights D, Stombaugh J, Knight R (2011) UniFrac: an effective distance metric for microbial community comparison. ISME J 5(2):169–172
29. Krüger S, Piro RM (2019) decompTumor2Sig: identification of mutational signatures active in individual tumors. BMC Bioinformatics 20(Suppl 4):152
30. dos Reis M, Donoghue PC, Yang Z (2016) Bayesian molecular clock dating of species divergences in the genomics era. Nat Rev Genet 17(2):71–80
31. Stephens PJ, Greenman CD, Fu B, Yang F, Bignell GR, Mudie LJ et al (2011) Massive genomic rearrangement acquired in a single catastrophic event during cancer development. Cell 144(1):27–40
32. Stevens JB, Abdallah BY, Liu G, Ye CJ, Horne SD, Wang G et al (2011) Diverse system stresses: common mechanisms of chromosome fragmentation. Cell Death Dis 2(6):e178
33. Dewhurst SM, McGranahan N, Burrell RA, Rowan AJ, Grönroos E, Endesfelder D et al (2014) Tolerance of whole-genome doubling propagates chromosomal instability and accelerates cancer genome evolution. Cancer Discov 4(2):175–185
34. Li X, Galipeau PC, Paulson TG, Sanchez CA, Arnaudo J, Liu K et al (2014) Temporal and spatial evolution of somatic chromosomal alterations: a case-cohort study of Barrett's esophagus. Cancer Prev Res (Phila) 7(1):114–127
35. Haigh J (1978) The accumulation of deleterious genes in a population—Muller's Ratchet. Theor Popul Biol 14(2):251–267
36. Drummond AJ, Pybus OG, Rambaut A, Forsberg R, Rodrigo AG (2003) Measurably evolving populations. Trends Ecol 18:481–488
37. Chmielecki J, Foo J, Oxnard GR, Hutchinson K, Ohashi K, Somwar R et al (2011) Optimization of dosing for EGFR-mutant non-small cell lung cancer with evolutionary cancer modeling. Sci Transl Med 3(90):90ra59
38. Maley CC, Galipeau PC, Li X, Sanchez CA, Paulson TG, Reid BJ (2004) Selectively advantageous mutations and hitchhikers in neoplasms: p16 lesions are selected in Barrett's esophagus. Cancer Res 64(10):3414–3427
39. Gerlinger M, Horswell S, Larkin J, Rowan AJ, Salm MP, Varela I et al (2014) Genomic architecture and evolution of clear cell renal cell carcinomas defined by multiregion sequencing. Nat Genet 46(3):225–233
40. Gerlinger M, Rowan AJ, Horswell S, Math M, Larkin J, Endesfelder D et al (2012) Intratumor heterogeneity and branched evolution revealed by multiregion sequencing. N Engl J Med 366(10):883–892
41. Beerenwinkel N, Schwarz RF, Gerstung M, Markowetz F (2015) Cancer evolution: mathematical models and computational inference. Syst Biol 64(1):e1–e25
42. Schwartz R, Schäffer AA (2017) The evolution of tumor phylogenetics: principles and practice. Nat Rev Genet 18(4):213–229
43. Amend SR, Pienta KJ (2015) Ecology meets cancer biology: the cancer swamp promotes the lethal cancer phenotype. Oncotarget 6(12):9669–9678
44. Amend SR, Roy S, Brown JS, Pienta KJ (2016) Ecological paradigms to understand the dynamics of metastasis. Cancer Lett 380(1):237–242
45. Pienta KJ, Robertson BA, Coffey DS, Taichman RS (2013) The cancer diaspora: metastasis beyond the seed and soil hypothesis. Clin Cancer Res 19(21):5849–5855
46. Yang KR, Mooney SM, Zarif JC, Coffey DS, Taichman RS, Pienta KJ (2014) Niche inheritance: a cooperative pathway to enhance cancer cell fitness through ecosystem engineering. J Cell Biochem 115(9):1478–1485
47. Brown JSK, B. P. (2004) Hazardous duty pay and the foraging cost of predation. Ecol Lett 7: 999–1014
48. Aktipis CA, Boddy AM, Gatenby RA, Brown JS, Maley CC (2013) Life history trade-offs in cancer evolution. Nat Rev Cancer 13(12):883–892
49. de Groot AE, Roy S, Brown JS, Pienta KJ, Amend SR (2017) Revisiting seed and soil: examining the primary tumor and cancer cell foraging in metastasis. Mol Cancer Res 15(4): 361–370

50. Lloyd MC, Rejniak KA, Brown JS, Gatenby RA, Minor ES, Bui MM (2015) Pathology to enhance precision medicine in oncology: lessons from landscape ecology. Adv Anat Pathol 22(4):267–272
51. Maley CC, Koelble K, Natrajan R, Aktipis A, Yuan Y (2015) An ecological measure of immune-cancer colocalization as a prognostic factor for breast cancer. Breast Cancer Res 17(1):131
52. Kirilovsky A, Marliot F, El Sissy C, Haicheur N, Galon J, Pagès F (2016) Rational bases for the use of the Immunoscore in routine clinical settings as a prognostic and predictive biomarker in cancer patients. Int Immunol 28(8):373–382
53. Mlecnik B, Bindea G, Kirilovsky A, Angell HK, Obenauf AC, Tosolini M et al (2016) The tumor microenvironment and Immunoscore are critical determinants of dissemination to distant metastasis. Sci Transl Med 8(327):327ra26
54. Galon J, Costes A, Sanchez-Cabo F, Kirilovsky A, Mlecnik B, Lagorce-Pages C et al (2006) Type, density, and location of immune cells within human colorectal tumors predict clinical outcome. Science 313(5795):1960–1964
55. Sato E, Olson SH, Ahn J, Bundy B, Nishikawa H, Qian F et al (2005) Intraepithelial CD8+ tumor-infiltrating lymphocytes and a high CD8+/regulatory T cell ratio are associated with favorable prognosis in ovarian cancer. Proc Natl Acad Sci U S A 102(51):18538–18543
56. Loi S, Sirtaine N, Piette F, Salgado R, Viale G, Van Eenoo F et al (2013) Prognostic and predictive value of tumor-infiltrating lymphocytes in a phase III randomized adjuvant breast cancer trial in node-positive breast cancer comparing the addition of docetaxel to doxorubicin with doxorubicin-based chemotherapy: BIG 02-98. J Clin Oncol 31(7):860–867
57. Adams S, Gray RJ, Demaria S, Goldstein L, Perez EA, Shulman LN et al (2014) Prognostic value of tumor-infiltrating lymphocytes in triple-negative breast cancers from two phase III randomized adjuvant breast cancer trials: ECOG 2197 and ECOG 1199. J Clin Oncol 32(27): 2959–2966
58. Motz GT, Coukos G (2013) Deciphering and reversing tumor immune suppression. Immunity 39(1):61–73
59. Galon J, Angell HK, Bedognetti D, Marincola FM (2013) The continuum of cancer immunosurveillance: prognostic, predictive, and mechanistic signatures. Immunity 39(1): 11–26
60. Rizvi NA, Hellmann MD, Snyder A, Kvistborg P, Makarov V, Havel JJ et al (2015) Cancer immunology. Mutational landscape determines sensitivity to PD-1 blockade in non-small cell lung cancer. Science 348(6230):124–128
61. Van Allen EM, Miao D, Schilling B, Shukla SA, Blank C, Zimmer L et al (2015) Genomic correlates of response to CTLA-4 blockade in metastatic melanoma. Science 350(6257): 207–211
62. Snyder A, Makarov V, Merghoub T, Yuan J, Zaretsky JM, Desrichard A et al (2014) Genetic basis for clinical response to CTLA-4 blockade in melanoma. N Engl J Med 371(23): 2189–2199
63. McGranahan N, Furness AJ, Rosenthal R, Ramskov S, Lyngaa R, Saini SK et al (2016) Clonal neoantigens elicit T cell immunoreactivity and sensitivity to immune checkpoint blockade. Science 351(6280):1463–1469
64. Carmona-Fontaine C, Bucci V, Akkari L, Deforet M, Joyce JA, Xavier JB (2013) Emergence of spatial structure in the tumor microenvironment due to the Warburg effect. Proc Natl Acad Sci U S A 110(48):19402–19407
65. Fang JS, Gillies RD, Gatenby RA (2008) Adaptation to hypoxia and acidosis in carcinogenesis and tumor progression. Semin Cancer Biol 18(5):330–337
66. Gatenby RA, Gawlinski ET (2003) The glycolytic phenotype in carcinogenesis and tumor invasion: insights through mathematical models. Cancer Res 63(14):3847–3854
67. Vander Heiden MG, Cantley LC, Thompson CB (2009) Understanding the Warburg effect: the metabolic requirements of cell proliferation. Science 324(5930):1029–1033

68. Riehl A, Németh J, Angel P, Hess J (2009) The receptor RAGE: bridging inflammation and cancer. Cell Commun Signal 7:12
69. Lv L, Shao X, Chen H, Ho CT, Sang S (2011) Genistein inhibits advanced glycation end product formation by trapping methylglyoxal. Chem Res Toxicol 24(4):579–586
70. Grimm EA, Sikora AG, Ekmekcioglu S (2013) Molecular pathways: inflammation-associated nitric-oxide production as a cancer-supporting redox mechanism and a potential therapeutic target. Clin Cancer Res 19(20):5557–5563
71. Fukumura D, Kashiwagi S, Jain RK (2006) The role of nitric oxide in tumor progression. Nat Rev Cancer 6(7):521–534
72. Antognelli C, Mezzasoma L, Fettucciari K, Talesa VN (2013) A novel mechanism of methylglyoxal cytotoxicity in prostate cancer cells. Int J Biochem Cell Biol 45(4):836–844
73. Ghosh M, Talukdar D, Ghosh S, Bhattacharyya N, Ray M, Ray S (2006) In vivo assessment of toxicity and pharmacokinetics of methylglyoxal. Augmentation of the curative effect of methylglyoxal on cancer-bearing mice by ascorbic acid and creatine. Toxicol Appl Pharmacol 212(1):45–58
74. Schwabe RF, Jobin C (2013) The microbiome and cancer. Nat Rev Cancer 13(11):800–812
75. Swidsinski A, Khilkin M, Kerjaschki D, Schreiber S, Ortner M, Weber J et al (1998) Association between intraepithelial Escherichia coli and colorectal cancer. Gastroenterology 115(2):281–286
76. Perez-Chanona E, Trinchieri G (2016) The role of microbiota in cancer therapy. Curr Opin Immunol 39:75–81
77. Gentles AJ, Newman AM, Liu CL, Bratman SV, Feng W, Kim D et al (2015) The prognostic landscape of genes and infiltrating immune cells across human cancers. Nat Med 21(8): 938–945
78. Horn HS (1966) Measurement of "Overlap" in comparative ecological studies. Am Nat 100(914):419–424
79. Swietach P, Vaughan-Jones RD, Harris AL, Hulikova A (2014) The chemistry, physiology and pathology of pH in cancer. Philos Trans R Soc Lond Ser B Biol Sci 369(1638):20130099
80. Damaghi M, Tafreshi NK, Lloyd MC, Sprung R, Estrella V, Wojtkowiak JW et al (2015) Chronic acidosis in the tumor microenvironment selects for overexpression of LAMP2 in the plasma membrane. Nat Commun 6:8752
81. Burns MB, Lynch J, Starr TK, Knights D, Blekhman R (2015) Virulence genes are a signature of the microbiome in the colorectal tumor microenvironment. Genome Med 7(1):55
82. Gatenby RA, Gillies RJ (2004) Why do cancers have high aerobic glycolysis? Nat Rev Cancer 4(11):891–899
83. Shiraishi T, Verdone JE, Huang J, Kahlert UD, Hernandez JR, Torga G et al (2015) Glycolysis is the primary bioenergetic pathway for cell motility and cytoskeletal remodeling in human prostate and breast cancer cells. Oncotarget 6(1):130–143
84. Stephens DW, Brown JS, Ydenberg RC (2007) Foraging: behavior and ecology. University of Chicago Press, Chicago
85. Schmidt M, Voelker HU, Kapp M, Krockenberger M, Dietl J, Kammerer U (2010) Glycolytic phenotype in breast cancer: activation of Akt, up-regulation of GLUT1, TKTL1 and down-regulation of M2PK. J Cancer Res Clin Oncol 136(2):219–225
86. Perera RM, Bardeesy N (2015) Pancreatic cancer metabolism: breaking it down to build it back up. Cancer Discov 5(12):1247–1261
87. Jung B, Lee S, Yang IH, Good T, Coté GL (2002) Automated on-line noninvasive optical glucose monitoring in a cell culture system. Appl Spectrosc 56:51–57
88. Chen J, Sprouffske K, Huang Q, Maley CC (2011) Solving the puzzle of metastasis: the evolution of cell migration in neoplasms. PLoS One 6(4):e17933
89. Aktipis CA, Maley CC, Pepper JW (2012) Dispersal evolution in neoplasms: the role of dysregulated metabolism in the evolution of cell motility. Cancer Prev Res (Phila) 5(2): 266–275

90. Lloyd MC, Cunningham JJ, Bui MM, Gillies RJ, Brown JS, Gatenby RA (2016) Darwinian dynamics of Intratumoral heterogeneity: not solely random mutations but also variable environmental selection forces. Cancer Res 76(11):3136–3144

91. Vincent TLS, Scheel. (1996) Trade-offs and coexistence in consumer-resource models: it all depends on what and where you eat. Am Nat 148(6):1038–1058

92. Ferreira SC Jr, Martins ML, Vilela MJ (2002) Reaction-diffusion model for the growth of avascular tumor. Phys Rev E Stat Nonlinear Soft Matter Phys 65(2 Pt 1):021907

93. DeNicola GM, Cantley LC (2015) Cancer's fuel choice: new flavors for a picky eater. Mol Cell 60(4):514–523

94. Ornitz DM, Itoh N (2015) The fibroblast growth factor signaling pathway. Wiley Interdiscip Rev Dev Biol 4(3):215–266

95. Hanahan D, Coussens LM (2012) Accessories to the crime: functions of cells recruited to the tumor microenvironment. Cancer Cell 21(3):309–322

96. Martinez-Outschoorn UE, Sotgia F, Lisanti MP (2012) Power surge: supporting cells "fuel" cancer cell mitochondria. Cell Metab 15(1):4–5

97. Nieman KM, Kenny HA, Penicka CV, Ladanyi A, Buell-Gutbrod R, Zillhardt MR et al (2011) Adipocytes promote ovarian cancer metastasis and provide energy for rapid tumor growth. Nat Med 17(11):1498–1503

98. Kalluri R (2016) The biology and function of fibroblasts in cancer. Nat Rev Cancer 16(9): 582–598

99. Ostman A, Augsten M (2009) Cancer-associated fibroblasts and tumor growth—bystanders turning into key players. Curr Opin Genet Dev 19(1):67–73

100. Franco OE, Shaw AK, Strand DW, Hayward SW (2010) Cancer associated fibroblasts in cancer pathogenesis. Semin Cell Dev Biol 21(1):33–39

101. Hirata E, Girotti MR, Viros A, Hooper S, Spencer-Dene B, Matsuda M et al (2015) Intravital imaging reveals how BRAF inhibition generates drug-tolerant microenvironments with high integrin β1/FAK signaling. Cancer Cell 27(4):574–588

102. Folkman J (1971) Tumor angiogenesis: therapeutic implications. N Engl J Med 285(21): 1182–1186

103. Folkman J, Watson K, Ingber D, Hanahan D (1989) Induction of angiogenesis during the transition from hyperplasia to neoplasia. Nature 339(6219):58–61

104. Richards CH, Mohammed Z, Qayyum T, Horgan PG, McMillan DC (2011) The prognostic value of histological tumor necrosis in solid organ malignant disease: a systematic review. Future Oncol 7(10):1223–1235

105. Anderson AR, Weaver AM, Cummings PT, Quaranta V (2006) Tumor morphology and phenotypic evolution driven by selective pressure from the microenvironment. Cell 127(5): 905–915

106. Ferriere II, Belthoff JR, Olivieri II, Krackow II (2000) Evolving dispersal: where to go next? Trends Ecol Evol 15(1):5–7

107. Johnson ML, Gaines MS (1990) Evolution of dispersal: theoretical models and empirical tests using birds and mammals. Annu Rev Ecol Syst 21(1):449–480

108. Bowler DE, Benton TG (2005) Causes and consequences of animal dispersal strategies: relating individual behaviour to spatial dynamics. Biol Rev Camb Philos Soc 80(2):205–225

109. Brizel DM, Scully SP, Harrelson JM, Layfield LJ, Bean JM, Prosnitz LR et al (1996) Tumor oxygenation predicts for the likelihood of distant metastases in human soft tissue sarcoma. Cancer Res 56(5):941–943

110. Cairns RA, Hill RP (2004) Acute hypoxia enhances spontaneous lymph node metastasis in an orthotopic murine model of human cervical carcinoma. Cancer Res 64(6):2054–2061

111. Hockel M, Schlenger K, Aral B, Mitze M, Schaffer U, Vaupel P (1996) Association between tumor hypoxia and malignant progression in advanced cancer of the uterine cervix. Cancer Res 56(19):4509–4515

112. Nordsmark M, Bentzen SM, Rudat V, Brizel D, Lartigau E, Stadler P et al (2005) Prognostic value of tumor oxygenation in 397 head and neck tumors after primary radiation therapy. An international multi-center study. Radiol Oncol 77(1):18–24
113. Rofstad EK, Galappathi K, Mathiesen B, Ruud EB (2007) Fluctuating and diffusion-limited hypoxia in hypoxia-induced metastasis. Clin Cancer Res 13(7):1971–1978
114. Mazzone M, Dettori D, de Oliveira RL, Loges S, Schmidt T, Jonckx B et al (2009) Heterozygous deficiency of PHD2 restores tumor oxygenation and inhibits metastasis via endothelial normalization. Cell 136(5):839–851
115. Goel S, Duda DG, Xu L, Munn LL, Boucher Y, Fukumura D et al (2011) Normalization of the vasculature for treatment of cancer and other diseases. Physiol Rev 91(3):1071–1121
116. Zhang Q, Lambert G, Liao D, Kim H, Robin K, Tung CK et al (2011) Acceleration of emergence of bacterial antibiotic resistance in connected microenvironments. Science 333(6050):1764–1767
117. Tatum JL, Kelloff GJ, Gillies RJ, Arbeit JM, Brown JM, Chao KS et al (2006) Hypoxia: importance in tumor biology, noninvasive measurement by imaging, and value of its measurement in the management of cancer therapy. Int J Radiat Biol 82(10):699–757
118. Inai T, Mancuso M, Hashizume H, Baffert F, Haskell A, Baluk P et al (2004) Inhibition of vascular endothelial growth factor (VEGF) signaling in cancer causes loss of endothelial fenestrations, regression of tumor vessels, and appearance of basement membrane ghosts. Am J Pathol 165(1):35–52
119. Wikström P, Lissbrant IF, Stattin P, Egevad L, Bergh A (2002) Endoglin (CD105) is expressed on immature blood vessels and is a marker for survival in prostate cancer. Prostate 51(4):268–275
120. Evans SM, Judy KD, Dunphy I, Jenkins WT, Nelson PT, Collins R et al (2004) Comparative measurements of hypoxia in human brain tumors using needle electrodes and EF5 binding. Cancer Res 64(5):1886–1892
121. Ljungkvist AS, Bussink J, Kaanders JH, van der Kogel AJ (2007) Dynamics of tumor hypoxia measured with bioreductive hypoxic cell markers. Radiat Res 167(2):127–145
122. Chida J, Yamane K, Takei T, Kido H (2012) An efficient extraction method for quantitation of adenosine triphosphate in mammalian tissues and cells. Anal Chim Acta 727:8–12
123. Chaudhury B, Zhou M, Goldgof DB, Hall LO, Gatenby RA, Gillies RJ et al (2015) Heterogeneity in intratumoral regions with rapid gadolinium washout correlates with estrogen receptor status and nodal metastasis. J Magn Reson Imaging 42(5):1421–1430
124. Zhou M, Hall L, Goldgof D, Russo R, Balagurunathan Y, Gillies R et al (2014) Radiologically defined ecological dynamics and clinical outcomes in glioblastoma multiforme: preliminary results. Transl Oncol 7(1):5–13
125. Gatenby RA, Grove O, Gillies RJ (2013) Quantitative imaging in cancer evolution and ecology. Radiology 269(1):8–15
126. Kozak KH, Graham CH, Wiens JJ (2008) Integrating GIS-based environmental data into evolutionary biology. Trends Ecol Evol 23(3):141–148
127. Chan LM, Brown JL, Yoder AD (2011) Integrating statistical genetic and geospatial methods brings new power to phylogeography. Mol Phylogenet Evol 59(2):523–537
128. Millington AC, Walsh SJ, Osborne PE (2013) GIS and remote sensing applications in biogeography and ecology. Springer, Cham
129. Nawaz S, Heindl A, Koelble K, Yuan Y (2015) Beyond immune density: critical role of spatial heterogeneity in estrogen receptor-negative breast cancer. Mod Pathol 28(6):766–777
130. Lloyd MC, Alfarouk KO, Verduzco D, Bui MM, Gillies RJ, Ibrahim ME et al (2014) Vascular measurements correlate with estrogen receptor status. BMC Cancer 14:279
131. Yuan Y, Failmezger H, Rueda OM, Ali HR, Gräf S, Chin SF et al (2012) Quantitative image analysis of cellular heterogeneity in breast tumors complements genomic profiling. Sci Transl Med 4(157):157ra43

132. Fujisawa T, Barraclough TG (2013) Delimiting species using single-locus data and the generalized mixed yule coalescent approach: a revised method and evaluation on simulated data sets. Syst Biol 62(5):707–724
133. Prosperi MC, Prosperi L, Bruselles A, Abbate I, Rozera G, Vincenti D et al (2011) Combinatorial analysis and algorithms for quasispecies reconstruction using next-generation sequencing. BMC Bioinformatics 12:5
134. Amir el AD, Davis KL, Tadmor MD, Simonds EF, Levine JH, Bendall SC et al (2013) viSNE enables visualization of high dimensional single-cell data and reveals phenotypic heterogeneity of leukemia. Nat Biotechnol 31(6):545–552
135. Macosko EZ, Basu A, Satija R, Nemesh J, Shekhar K, Goldman M et al (2015) Highly parallel genome-wide expression profiling of individual cells using nanoliter droplets. Cell 161(5): 1202–1214
136. Gatenby RA, Gillies RJ, Brown JS (2011) Of cancer and cave fish. Nat Rev Cancer 11(4): 237–238
137. Gatenby RA, Cunningham JJ, Brown JS (2014) Evolutionary triage governs fitness in driver and passenger mutations and suggests targeting never mutations. Nat Commun 5:5499
138. Win T, Miles KA, Janes SM, Ganeshan B, Shastry M, Endozo R et al (2013) Tumor heterogeneity and permeability as measured on the CT component of PET/CT predict survival in patients with non-small cell lung cancer. Clin Cancer Res 19(13):3591–3599
139. Chicklore S, Goh V, Siddique M, Roy A, Marsden PK, Cook GJ (2013) Quantifying tumor heterogeneity in 18F-FDG PET/CT imaging by texture analysis. Eur J Nucl Med Mol Imaging 40(1):133–140
140. Courchamp F, Clutton-Brock T, Grenfell B (1999) Inverse density dependence and the allee effect. Trends Ecol Evol 14(10):405–410
141. Allee WC (1978) Animal aggregations: a study in general sociology. AMS Press, Brooklyn
142. Kramer AM, Dennis B, Liebhold AM, Drake JM (2009) The evidence for allee effects. Popul Ecol 51:341–354
143. Weinberg R (2013) The biology of cancer. Garland Science, New York
144. Greig D, Travisano M (2004) The Prisoner's dilemma and polymorphism in yeast SUC genes. Proc Biol Sci 271(Suppl 3(Suppl 3)):S25–S26
145. Gore J, Youk H, van Oudenaarden A (2009) Snowdrift game dynamics and facultative cheating in yeast. Nature 459(7244):253–256
146. West SA (2007) The social lives of microbes. Annu Rev Ecol Evol Syst 38:53–77
147. Elias S, Banin E (2012) Multi-species biofilms: living with friendly neighbors. FEMS Microbiol Rev 36(5):990–1004
148. Thomlinson RH, Gray LH (1955) The histological structure of some human lung cancers and the possible implications for radiotherapy. Br J Cancer 9(4):539–549
149. Li C, Heidt DG, Dalerba P, Burant CF, Zhang L, Adsay V et al (2007) Identification of pancreatic cancer stem cells. Cancer Res 67(3):1030–1037
150. Frank SA (2007) Dynamics of cancer: incidence, inheritance, and evolution. Princeton University Press, Princeton
151. Szczepański T, Orfão A, van der Velden VH, San Miguel JF, van Dongen JJ (2001) Minimal residual disease in leukaemia patients. Lancet Oncol 2(7):409–417

Chapter 30
Tumor Ecosystem-Directed Therapeutic Strategies

Phei Er Saw and Erwei Song

Abstract We have finally reached the end of this book. Having a comprehensive summary of how to understand cancer as an ecosystem, how to view cancer as an ecological entity, and understanding how each component in the local onco-sphere, inter-communications among onco-spheres, including how the host environment could affect the tumor behavior; has led us to grow in deeper understanding of the core biology and mechanisms of cancer occurrence, growth, and metastasis. Therefore, it is high time to treat tumors as an ecological network, finding solutions to modify the systemic or the distal onco-sphere that can have detrimental effect toward the local onco-sphere. In this chapter, we emphasize on targeting specific niches in the local, distal and systemic onco-sphere.

Introduction

We have finally reached the end of this book. Having a comprehensive summary of how to understand cancer as an ecosystem, how to view cancer as an ecological entity, and understanding how each component in the local *onco-sphere*, inter-

P. E. Saw
Guangdong Provincial Key Laboratory of Malignant Tumor Epigenetics and Gene Regulation, Guangdong-Hong Kong Joint Laboratory for RNA Medicine, Medical Research Center, Sun Yat-sen Memorial Hospital, Sun Yat-sen University, Guangzhou, China

Nanhai Translational Innovation Center of Precision Immunology, Sun Yat-sen Memorial Hospital, Sun Yat-sen University, Foshan, China

E. Song (✉)
Guangdong Provincial Key Laboratory of Malignant Tumor Epigenetics and Gene Regulation, Guangdong-Hong Kong Joint Laboratory for RNA Medicine, Medical Research Center, Sun Yat-sen Memorial Hospital, Sun Yat-sen University, Guangzhou, China

Nanhai Translational Innovation Center of Precision Immunology, Sun Yat-sen Memorial Hospital, Sun Yat-sen University, Foshan, China

Breast Tumor Center, Sun Yat-sen Memorial Hospital, Sun Yat-sen University, Guangzhou, China
e-mail: songew@mail.sysu.edu.cn

communications among *onco-spheres*, including how the host environment could affect the tumor behavior; has led us to grow in deeper understanding of the core biology and mechanisms of cancer occurrence, growth, and metastasis. One bottle-neck in the cancer therapy system is that there is no perfect drug that can possibly kill all the cancer cells. The cells that did not die during the chemo/radiotherapy can lead to resistance of these cells, leading to a new generation of resistant cancer [1, 2]. Therefore, it is high time to treat tumors as an ecological network, finding solutions to modify the systemic or the distal *onco-sphere* that can have detrimental effect toward the local *onco-sphere*.

Targeting Specific Niches in the Local *Onco-Sphere*

Targeting Tumor–Immune Cells Interactions

As we mentioned earlier in this book, solid tumor ecosystem is complex, with the support system branching from infiltration of various immune cells, CAFs, ECs, adipocytes, MDSCs, TAMs, and effector T and NK cells [3]. Although immune system and the recognition of TSA by the TILs are crucial, unfortunately, cancers have developed ways to avoid the immune system. There are two main strategies for this: (1) to target tumor's avoidance of immune surveillance and (2) reactivating the immune system, re-educating these cells to recognize the tumor cells as for and not friends (initiating attack). Antibodies inhibiting immunological checkpoint pro-teins on the cell surface make up many of the traditional immunotherapeutic drugs, including anti-CTLA-4 treatment and anti-PD-1 therapy. Normally, these check-point proteins work to reduce the immune system's reaction. Consequently, antibody-based checkpoint inhibition promotes more T-cell activation and a potent anticancer immune response [3]. Despite the potential of immunotherapy, only a small percentage of patients have persistent responses [4, 5], and treatment failure may be caused by changes in ITH, tumor evolution, or the microenvironment around the tumor [6]. Another reason for the observed variation in responsiveness to checkpoint blockade immunotherapy is the heterogeneity of neoantigens [3]. Under-standing whether individuals have immunologically "cold" malignancies that will never react or acquire resistance, as opposed to those with tumors that can be rendered immunologically "hot," is clearly necessary.

Adaptive Containment Strategies

In cancers with several competing heterogenous phenotypes, including drug resis-tance clones, adaptive containment therapy aims to control clonal evolution. The idea that treatment resistance has a fitness cost is a fundamental tenet of adaptive therapy. In a resistant clone, these cells must overexpress membrane efflux pump (i.e., MDR gene, ABC transporters) to remove chemotherapeutics actively from inside the cells [7]. Adaptive therapy is specifically cornering these resistance cells, where treatments were given as pulses, with specific on-and-off periods of therapy. Their main hypothesis is that if both populations (normal and resistance subclone) are kept stable, their development is competitively restricted by one another(s), one classic example of competitive behavior in cancer ecosystem. Adaptive treatment has received support from preclinical research. In in vitro breast cancer models, pulsated vemurafenib treatment has effectively slow down the cancer progression [8]. Despite the fact that adaptive treatment is still not widely used in patient care, some first achievements have been made. A clinical study has reported steady balance of tumor loads in patients ($n = 10$) when given a pulsated adaptive therapy, a significant 50% drop of usual abiraterone usage in metastatic CRPC [9]. This clinical trial's adaptive therapy treatment plan was developed using a precise calculation using a mathematical model that takes into account the importance of "eco-evolutionary interactions" between subclones, in the context of evolution, and their constant changes during the therapy; underscoring the value of modeling to inform initial hypotheses that will be tested in vivo. These case studies emphasize the significance of comprehending how sensitive and resistant subclones evolve both on and off treatment.

Targeting Biochemical Changes in Local *Onco-Sphere*

As we mentioned in Chap. 8, there are certain biochemical changes in the local *onco-sphere* that is unique to the tumor. Within these modifications, we can utilize these changes as a targeting modality to suppress tumor growth [10–12]. Herein, we summarize various targeting modality that could be used to change or normalize the tumor local environment in order to inhibit cancer growth (Table 30.1).

Targeting Specific Niches in Distal *Onco-Sphere*

Targeting Exosomes

Owing to the attractive medicinal delivery capabilities of exosomes and their engagement in metastatic cycles, we will thoroughly discuss the existing exosome-based treatment techniques having strongly prospective clinical relevance in a further section. Reduced synthesis, secretion, and absorption of exosomes is indeed a promising and feasible strategy for preventing metastasis. For example, it was discovered the significant metastasis inhibiting potential of heparin by lowering the absorption of tumor-produced exosomes in OSCC [36]. Additionally, an antibody that reduces the generation of tumor-produced exosomes was created, and treatment of these antibodies resulting in a reduction in remote metastasis of breast cancer in a murine model

Table 30.1 Targeting various biochemical pathways in the local *onco-sphere*

Acidosis related pathways	Family members	Functions	Ref
Proton-pump inhibitors (PPIs) prodrugs that are activated by a proton-catalyzed process to generate a sulfenamide	Omeprazole and esomeprazole	Interacts with the sulfhydryl groups of cysteine residues in the extracellular domain of the H^+/K^+-ATPase, thereby inhibiting its activity	[11–16]
	Bafilomycin A1	Highly specific inhibitor of V-ATPase Disrupt autophagic flux through inhibition of lysosome acidification and associated autophagosome–lysosome fusion	[17, 18]
Carbonic anhydrase (CAs)	CAIX and CAXII	CAIX- and CAXII-specific chemical inhibitors (i.e., sulfonamide- and coumarin-derived compounds) have shown positive preclinical evaluations on the formation of primary tumors and metastases in several cancer mouse models CAIX-specific antibodies (BAY-79-4620 and girentuximab) are currently under clinical evaluation	[19–23]

Lactate-metabolism related pathways	Family members	Functions	Ref
Monocarboxylate transporters (MCTs)	MCT1 and MCT4	AZD3965, a dual inhibitor of MCT1 and MCT2, showed potent antitumor effects in mouse models, currently under clinical evaluation	[24–26]

Imbalance of cellular pH	Family members	Functions	Ref
Sodium/hydro-gen exchanger	NHE-1	Genetic disruption of NHE1 reduces tumor growth in multiple mouse cancer models Anticancer effects were observed with selective pharmacological inhibitors of NHE1 (i.e., amiloride and cariporide)	[27–32]
Bi-carbonate inhibitors	NBC	Compounds S0859 and S3705, developed as NBC inhibitors, were reported to reduce tumor growth multiple breast cancer cell lines	[33–35]

[37]. Furthermore, a unique gadget has been developed to prevent or redirect the propagation of tumor cells. The development of an imitation pre-metastatic niche via implantation of tumor exosomes in a 3D matrix followed by its transplantation in the peritoneal cavity of a mouse assisted the researchers in collecting ovarian tumor cells from the peritoneum and diverting them away from their source-target areas. This method effectively reduced tumor metastasis remotely [38]. This treatment technique, however, requires further investigations under in vivo trials [39].

The impact of extracellular acidity on the cancer cells' productivity of exosomes has been reflected in multiple research data. Originally, it was shown that melanoma cells cultivated under acidic circumstances (pH 6.7) secreted a greater quantity of exosomes as compared to the cells cultivated in physiological settings (pH 7.4). This pattern was eventually proven in various forms of human tumors, including prostate cancer, melanoma, osteosarcoma, colon cancer, and breast cancer [40]. Although the processes underlying enhanced exosomal release in acidic settings remain unknown, some studies have suggested that releasing more exosomes under low-pH circumstances may be a method of reducing intracellular hazardous substance buildup [40]. Similar proton-pump blockers have been created on the basis of this notion to reduce levels of exosome in the plasma of xenograft mice [41]. As a result, patients suffering from tumor metastases may look up to the alkalinizing technique as a viable antitumor treatment [42].

Exosomal miRNAs

Exosomes comprise a number of miRNAs that can be directed for exosome-facilitated metastasis prevention [43]. CRC-generated exosomal miRNAs are found to increase tumor cell growth in colorectal cancer (CRC) [44, 45], allowing gene therapy to be used to reduce tumor metastasis by altering exosomal miRNA. For example, miR-375 could inhibit BCL-2 and reducing the metastasis capability of tumor to metastasize in a colon cancer model [46]. In another example, exosomal miR193a has been closely linked to liver metastasis in colon cancer. Some had further been proposed that the potential of major vault protein (MVP) to reduce the circulatory level of exosomal miR-193a has further been anticipated, which in turn sets a base for a novel medicinal approach to treat colon cancer metastasis [47].

Vaccination

Exosomes weaken the immune system, according to accumulating evidence. The exosomes could block NK cell cytotoxicity and DC maturation, as well as stimulate cytotoxic T-cell death and macrophage M2-like polarization, all of which accelerate tumor metastasis [48, 49]. The first-in-kind Phase I clinical trials of exosome reveal that exosome therapy did not induce large-scale serious adverse events in the 15 metastatic melanoma patients, indicating the feasibility of producing exosomes at a large scale for medicinal reasons due to their superior safety attributes [50]. Interestingly, in a phase I study at Duke University in advanced lung cancer of non-small cells, the effectiveness of corresponding DC-produced exosomes and MHC class I peptides extended the survivability of the patient [51].

Targeting Cancer Stem Cells: Strategies to Target Resistance and Niche Interactions

Ultimately, adaptability and heterogeneity—both heavily influenced by the microenvironment—are the key factors contributing to treatment resistance in solid tumors that are still incurable. Targeting a single niche or marker is often inadequate, and developing new and successful therapies will require combinatorial techniques [52]. Hypoxic environments trigger immunosuppressive signaling, probably partly because CSCs take up nutrients preferentially and autophagy is elevated. Therefore, cytotoxic T-cell therapy or anti-PD-L1 therapy alone may not be enough to treat solid tumors that include a hypoxic niche effectively. Immunotherapeutic targeting in hypoxic areas may be enhanced by altering CAR T cells to boost glucose absorption or by using autophagic inhibitors in combination with other therapies. It is well known that CSCs in the hypoxic niche are highly resistant to conventional radiation and chemotherapy. Pleiotropic HIF factors route numerous signaling alterations brought on by hypoxic stress. Several HIF-1 inhibitors have advanced to phase III studies; however, they have not successfully extended life [53].

The development of methods to improve immune-mediated tumor suppression includes a widening range of adoptive immunotherapeutic approaches involving both autologous and allogeneic cells and an increasing number of immune checkpoint inhibitors. These strategies, which predominantly rely on CAR T cells or dendritic cells, are intended to target CSC markers like CD133 and ROR1 [54, 55]. Other approaches can concentrate on boosting class I MHC expression to account for CSCs increased immune evasion. In resectable solid tumors, infiltrative CSCs are perhaps the most important group to target therapeutically. Integrin signaling molecules may regularly act in these cells as both CSC markers and initiators of migration and infiltration. Antiangiogenic medicines, such as anti-VEGF medications, have been used in efforts to address the perivascular microenvironment [56]. Although certain malignancies responded well to these treatments, therapeutic effectiveness is typically undermined by alternative vascularization signals and CSCs' increased ability to co-opt the regular vasculature and survive in hypoxic environments. Antiangiogenic approaches must consider the mechanisms via which CSCs might promote vascularization, such as HIF-mediated signaling, as shown by anti-VEGF treatments.

Interventions in Systemic *Onco-Sphere*

Targeting Host Immune System

Immune Checkpoint Blockades

In immunotherapy, ICBs are the main players of the class of cancer immunotherapy. ICBs are designed to enhance antitumor efficacy by blocking immune checkpoints, particularly by activated T cells [57], though recent studies are now revealing that these checkpoints could also be found in tumor-infiltrated immune cells, such as NK cells, B cells, TAMs, TANs, DCs, and MDSCs [58, 59]. T-cell effector activity is crucial for effective cancer therapy. However, evidences have shown that tumor-infiltrated T cells presented increased levels of these receptors (such as CTLA-4, PD-1, TIM-3, BTLA, and LAG-3) [60]. Binding of these receptors with their respective ligands on tumor leads to T-cell exhaustion, diminishing T-cell activity to kill the tumor cells. By using the intervention of ICB, these receptor–ligand interaction could be blocked, therefore restoring T-cell effector function and boosting anticancer efficacy [61]. The first FDA-approved ICB therapy is in 2011, by the name of Yervoy (or ipilimumab), developed by Bristol-Myers Squibb, for the treatment of metastatic melanoma. Since then, more than 100 ICB-related drugs are currently being tested in clinical trials [62].

Adoptive Cell Therapy

In general, adoptive cell therapy (ACT) is an act of isolating various immune cells from donors or patients, genetically modifying these cells to include ligands specific to TSA, then transferring these cells back to cancer patients [63, 64]. The first ever evidence of ACT is done in 1988, where a patient's TILs are isolated, expanded, and re-infused into the patient to treat metastatic melanoma [65, 66]. Through several decades, ACT has been improving, with more specific changes are required on immune cells. There is also an expansion in the types of immune cells used in the study. Some of the famously known cells are as follows: (1) non-specific lympho-kine-activated killer (LAK) cells, (2) adoptive T cells, (3) CAR-T, (4) TCR-engineered T cells, and (5) CAR-NK cells [67, 68].

Among these cells, there are still non-specific antitumor effects seen in the therapy, especially with LAK cells and TILs. Furthermore, one of the bottlenecks of ACT is to obtain sufficient cells after expansions to be able to exert their effect. Therefore, the development of TCR-engineered T cells, CAR-T, and CAR-NK cells was designed to overcome this bottleneck, as they possess target-specific antigens on cancer cells and could be expanded easily [69], as summarized in Table 30.2 below.

Cancer Vaccines

To pre-induce the host to cancer-specific antigens, cancer vaccines have been proposed. The administration of cancer vaccine is similar to standardized vaccines, the only difference is that antigen presented in the vaccine is tumor-specific, thereby called tumor-specific antigens (TSAs) [78]. However, there are also therapeutic cancer vaccines, where patient-specific TSAs could be injected into the host after cancer occurrence. The advantages of therapeutic vaccine are that the vaccine could be designed specifically to the tumor in the patients, leading to higher specificity and efficacy [79]. There are various kinds of cancer vaccines based on different

Table 30.2 Different methods in engineering effector cells for personalized immunotherapy

Engineered cells	Methods	Functions	Refs
TCR-T	Transfecting cloned antigen-specific TCR genes into the T cells isolated from cancer patients, using either lentivirus or retrovirus	To eradicate specific tumor cells TCR-T cells showed optimistic results in sarcoma, metastatic melanoma, lymphoma, and leukemia patients	[70–75]
CAR-T	Compose of an antigen-binding single-chain variable fragment (scFv) domain, a signal transduction domain, and a transmembrane domain Allow CAR-T cells to recognize tumor cells in MHC-unrestricted manner	Overcoming the limitations raised by MHC restriction in the TCR-T	[76, 77]
CAR-NK	Similar CAR-T, but genetically modified NK cells	Cytotoxicity against tumor cells, Infusion of CAR-NK cells will not induce graft-versus-host disease in cancer patients	[68]

biomolecules delivered, namely peptide, DNA, RNA, or DC vaccines [80–82]. To date, several cancer vaccines have been approved by FDA, including HBV-vaccine Provenge and HPV vaccines [80, 83, 84]. The application of cancer vaccine is numerous, and many clinical trials are ongoing to investigate liposomal delivery of DNA/RNA vaccines, which could lead to a paradigm shift in cancer therapeutic in the near future [85–87].

Oncolytic Virus

Naturally occurring or genetically engineered virus could also be used as a class of immunotherapy. These oncolytic viruses may work (at least partially) by triggering a host immune response against the cancer by this underlying mechanism: (1) virus infects tumor cells after introduction to host, (2) after infection, virus makes many copies of itself in the cells leading to cell burst and death, (3) cancer cell bursting (death) leads to release cytoplasmic materials (i.e., tumor-specific antigens, cell death proteins, "eat-me" signals), and (4) immune system recognizes these as non-self and destroys the tumors surrounding this dead tumor cells. In clinical trials, it has been shown that oncolytic virus can selectively lyse cancer cells, while eliciting potent adaptive immune system as they could active DCs with DAMPs (produced by dead tumor cells), while having very minimal side effects to surrounding normal cells [88]. One most recent example is T-VEC, the first oncolytic virus approved by the US FDA in 2015 [89]. To date, a number of clinical trials are ongoing, with some pending FDA approval, indicating the feasibility and safety of this treatment modality [90–97].

Cytokine Therapy

As the name implies, cytokine therapy is the administration of various antitumoral-related cytokines that could activate various pathways to destroy cancer cells. Cytokines could act directly at the tumor cells by inhibiting their cellular growth by activating apoptosis, reducing angiogenesis, or modifying the cell's differentiation profile (i.e., reducing EMT phenotype change, or inhibit CSC formation) [98, 99]. Some studies have shown favorable results using cytokine therapy alone; however, cytokine therapy should be used in caution, as some cytokines do possess dual-behavioral properties, where it could be a pro-tumoral agent at certain point of tumor growth. It is speculated that cytokine therapy could be used in combination with ICBs, vaccines, or adoptive cell therapy to significantly boost the efficacy of these immunotherapeutic [100, 101].

Targeting Host Inflammation

Much data show that utilization of NSAIDs lessens colon cancer risk by around 40–50% and could have preventive functions for lung, esophagus, and stomach cancers [102, 103]. The ability of NSAIDs to hinder cyclo-oxygenase (COX-1 and -2) underlies their processes of chemoprevention. COX-2 changes arachidonic acid to prostaglandins, which in turn secretes inflammatory reactions in inflicted tissues [104]. Aspirin is a classic example of COX-2 inhibitor, which causes non-selective suppression of platelet function by acetylating and irreversibly inactivating both COX-1 and COX-2 [105]. Not only that, NSAIDs can also trigger antitumor activity including cytochrome C release from mitochondria after NSAID treatment, which are important for the activation of caspase 3 and caspase 9, both are vital in inducing apoptosis [106]. Furthermore, as we mention in the earlier chapters, inflammation has a close connection with immunosurveillance. Therefore, blocking the increment of inflammatory-related cytokines, chemokines, proteases, and other soluble factors could be important in reducing inflammation, therefore inhibiting tumor growth [107, 108]. For example, targeting a selectin-specific receptor sialyl-Lewis X epitope may reduce metastasis [109]. The MMPs are secreted by inflammatory cells and by stromal cells reacting to chemokines and cytokines produced by inflammatory cells within the tumor microenvironments [110]. Similarly, an increment in MMP secretion can increase the inflammatory cell infiltration, simultaneously producing GFs and other cytokines. It is important to note, however, that although MMPs have pro-angiogenic activity, they are crucial in generating basement-membrane collagens as well as plasminogen, which are angiogenesis inhibitors. These dual and contradicting phenotypes should be taken into consideration when using MMP inhibitors as a target [111, 112].

Targeting Nervous System: Tumor Axonogenesis

Tumor axonogenesis may have therapeutic implications in cancer in terms of its diagnosis, prognosis, and therapy. At present time, large clinical trials are needed to determine the degree of nerve infiltration in human cancers, as well as to explore how it is related to cancer diagnosis and prognosis. Current approaches involve more in-depth studies of the nerve, but to apply the knowledge of nerves in cancer to a clinical setting will need a thorough understanding of the neural landscape across a wide range of human cancers.

Targeting Nerves and Neurotrophic Factors

Multiple large retrospective and prospective studies of cancer patients have been done to investigate how the measurement of nerve infiltration by pathology of clinical samples can be used to predict prognosis and treatment response. When cancer diagnosis and prognosis are closely related, measurement of nerve density may also assist in distinguishing between benign tumors or indolent cancer and aggressive cancer. One clear example is the link of highly innervated prostate cancer, where comparing to benign prostatic hyperplasia, had higher aggressiveness than indolent ones, quantifying autonomic nerve density in prostate cancer might enhance histologic grading and cancer prognosis [113, 114]. In addition, detecting and quantifying neurotrophic growth factors that drive tumor axonogenesis may also contribute to cancer diagnosis and predicting prognosis. For example, the proNGF expression in prostate cancer cells drives axonogenesis in the TME, which also corresponds to histologic grade. Also, the proNGF level in thyroid cancer cells is higher than adjacent normal cells [115, 116]. The significance of NGF as a predictive biomarker should be studied in pancreatic [117] and gastric cancers [118], where NGF synthesis by cancer cells also stimulates axonogenesis. NGF expression corresponds to lymph node invasion in breast cancer while BDNF synthesis induces adrenergic nerve infiltration in ovarian cancer [119, 120]. Neurotrophic factors may thus be utilized as biomarkers in the diagnosis and prognosis of cancer due to their functions in tumor innervation. Furthermore, as neurotrophic factors can be circulated in the bloodstream, there is a need to study whether the cancer-induced increased expression of neurotrophic factors can be reflected and measured from the result of blood test of cancer patients. Most neuroproteins are becoming more widely recognized as possible cancer biomarkers [121].

Tumor Denervation-Based Cancer Therapies

As a modality in cancer treatments, surgical denervation has been successfully tested in various animal models, but is likely to be difficult to replicate similar results in humans. This is because, in human, the innervation of a single organ comes from multiple levels of the neuronal network (including the spinal cord and neural plexus outside of CNS), and neuronal inputs control the metabolic and physiologic changes of most organs; thus, surgical denervation might have unintended negative consequences. Administration of injectable neurotoxic drugs into the tumors, on the other hand, may be more viable since it can target specific neuron subtypes while keeping adverse effects to a minimal level. For example, botulinum toxin (Botox) is a type of neurotoxin that inhibits cholinergic activity (which could be applied in cosmetics to reduce wrinkles, and also control muscle spasms) might be used to simulate autonomic denervation without impairing sensory or motor afferences. In animal experiments, neurotoxin denervation of gastric tumors has been tested using botulinum toxin, and further clinical trials to evaluate this strategy in human gastric cancer are currently underway [122]. The results of phase I clinical study of botulinum toxin in the denervation of prostate cancer are now published, and it showed that botulinum toxin injection reduced nerve density in prostate tumors, resulting in higher cancer cell apoptosis [123].

Targeting Neurotrophic Factors

To prevent tumor innervation, targeting neurotrophic factors involved in tumor axonogenesis may be a better treatment method than surgical or chemical denervation since preexisting innervation of the organ would be preserved. Neurotrophic growth factors like NGF are required for neuron growth and proliferation throughout the peripheral nervous system, but they are not engaged in neuronal maintenance once the tissue is fully innervated. This is best shown by NGF, where it has limited neurotrophic effect in adults and instead functions as a pain mediator by stimulating the tyrosine kinase receptor TrkA in sensory neurons [124]. Anti-NGF antibodies injected systemically have little effect on neuronal and cognitive processes based on results of animal models and clinical trials. An approach to curb nerve outgrowth in the TME is to target NGF, which has neurotrophic impact and plays a part in tumor axonogenesis [117–119, 125]. Anti-NGF blocking antibodies and TrkA inhibitors, as well as NGF-targeting siRNA enclosed in nanoparticles, have previously been shown to reduce cancer development and metastasis in animal experiments, and further clinical studies are needed [9, 126]. Currently, anti-NGF blocking antibodies are being tested in clinical trials to treat chronic and arthritis pain, but they might be repurposed to prevent tumor axonogenesis, which ultimately helps to control cancer development [124]. Furthermore, anti-NGF antibodies may reduce cancer pain, and animal studies have previously demonstrated the efficacy of targeting NGF for the relief of cancer-induced pain [127]. Although the studies of targeting neurotrophic factors are still at an early stage in humans, but the current findings indicated that neurotrophic factors as a target in cancer treatment offer a possibility to tackle both cancer progression and cancer-induced pain at the same time [128, 129].

Targeting Vasculo-Lymphatic System: Vascular Normalization and VEGF Inhibitors

VEGF Signaling Inhibitors

The FDA has approved the anti-VEGF-A monoclonal antibody, bevacizumab, whose varying synergistic properties in conventional radiotherapies or chemotherapies have been assessed across various therapies and tumor models [130]. The overall response and survival without progression were found to have significantly improved in patients with gastric cancer who were undergoing a combinatorial treatment that utilized both chemotherapies as well as bevacizumab [131]. Bevacizumab, combined with gemcitabine or cisplatin, demonstrated outcomes that resembled the same in a non-small cell lung cancer [132]; many similar results were noted as an effect of paclitaxel and bevacizumab in women with metastatic breast cancer [133]. The FDA has also approved the use of sorafenib and sunitinib, among other inhibitors that target VEGFRs, to treat metastatic renal cell carcinoma [134]. The type of tumor has been determined as a significant determinant for the successes and failures of the VEGF blockade [135]. While tumors such as renal carcinoma demonstrate increased sensitivity to VEGH inhibitors (wherein the prevention of metastatic spread typically requires antiangiogenic drugs), pancreatic and prostate cancers are characterized by refractory responses to angiogenesis modulators [135]. According to empirical research, the increase in metastatic potential in vivo, tumor cell migration, and invasion, as well as the heightened expression of PlGF, VEGFR-1, and VEGFR-1 phosphorylation, VEGF-C, VEGF-B, and VEGF-A occurs as a result of chronic exposure of tumor cells to VEGF inhibitors [136]. Certain significant toxicities have been found to exist in the context of anti-VEGF therapies, exemplified by hypertension and other venous thromboembolic issues [137].

Vascular Normalization

The maturation effect on blood vessels has been outlined by vascular normalization as the probable underlying cause of improvements in chemotherapy treatments, when combined with VEGF signaling inhibitors [138]. Insufficient pericyte coverage is represented by immature vessels that are formed due to the increase in VEGF secretion from tumor cells [139]. The active recruitment of pericytes and the reduced permeability by tightening junctions between cells are caused by the restoration of angiogenic signals in tumors, due to the careful dosage administration of VEGF inhibitors, resulting in the increased perfusion among tumors [140]. The activation of Ang-1/Tie2 signaling is partially responsible for the recruitment of pericytes to the blood vessels, which is a consequence of VEGFR2 blockade [141]. Similarly, the facilitation of pericyte maturation and recruitment, in addition to an increase in PDGFRβ signaling, occurs due to VEGF inhibition [139]. The dosage and point in time associated with the administration of VEGF inhibitors to normalize the blood vessels of tumor tend to be narrow and are dependent on the schedule, type of inhibitor, and tumor targeted, thereby posing a challenge to its use [142]. Further, based on the type of the tumor and the kind of drug used, the effect may last up to four months, although it is generally not prolonged [143]. Marked vascular regression replaces vascular normalization when VEGF activity is highly neutralized, as demonstrated by long durations of exposition or increased doses; this, in turn, increases the risk of metastatic spread due to higher potential for tumor hypoxia and since the invasive tumor cells are favored in terms of selection [144, 145]. As the therapeutic index of various approaches necessitates the persistence of vascular normalization over longer periods, strategies that effectuate long-term and effective stabilization of the blood vessels of the tumor are in urgent demand [146]. The benefits of treatments against cancer can be enhanced and hypoxia can be alleviated through the vital role of appropriate vascular normalization, as supported by gene expression and imaging studies [147]. The ideal regimen that can be adopted for the achievement of normalization is determined using the functionality of tumor blood vessels following antiangiogenic treatments, which can be determined using DCE-MRI (dynamic contrast-enhanced magnetic resonance imaging) or radiotracer ^{18}F-MISO, developed for positron emission tomography (PET), both of which are techniques characterized by their non-invasiveness [148, 149].

Targeting Metabolism

When it comes to therapy, the focus should be on lowering the risk factors. People, in general, are less likely to get cancer if they lose weight and live a healthy lifestyle, which has been linked to several different therapies. A recent study on mortality after bariatric surgery found that deaths from cancer were much less common in the group that had bariatric surgery [150]. For example, metformin is the insulin sensitizer most often used to treat type 2 diabetes. Compared to other insulin secretagogues like sulfonylurea or insulin, it seems to protect diabetics from getting cancer. This is thought to be because it lowers insulin resistance [151], as proven by data from a population-based large cohort study. The data showed that people with type 2 diabetes who were given sulfonylureas and exogenous insulin had a much higher risk of dying from cancer than those given metformin [152]. Similarly, pancreatic cancer could be prevented or treated with anti-cytokine vaccines, proinflammatory NF-κB and COX-2 pathways inhibitors, thiazolidinediones, and antioxidants. Epidemiological studies have shown that people who take nonsteroidal anti-inflammatory drugs have a 40–50% lower chance of getting colorectal cancer (NSAIDs) (Fig. 30.1).

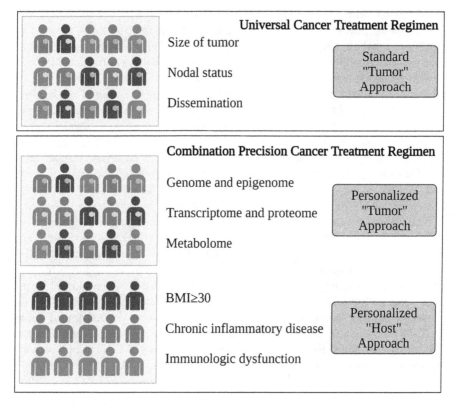

Fig. 30.1 Example of a treatment plan for the future that combines personalized therapies taking host (systemic *onco-sphere*) and tumor (local *onco-sphere*) into consideration. Traditional cancer treatment plans use alphanumeric codes to describe the size of the primary tumor, the involvement of nearby (regional) lymph nodes, and the spread of cancer to other parts of the body (metastases). In the future, treatments should try to combine "local-tumor" medicine with "systemic-host" medicine to obtain the best clinical results, based on the molecular profile of the tumor, precision medicine tries to personalize treatment. This should be combined with an approach that considers each patient's unique characteristics, such as body mass, disease states that cause chronic inflammation, and immune system, as we clearly discussed in previous chapters of this book

Targeting the Endocrine System

Endocrine treatments that target endogenous estrogen have mostly but not entirely been used to treat breast cancer in oncology [153]. Three primary categories exist: luteinizing hormone-releasing hormone agonists and, more recently, antagonists [154] for premenopausal women and aromatase inhibitors (AIs) for postmenopausal women are examples of interventions that could effectively lower the estrogen levels, without severe side effects. ER modifiers, like tamoxifen, bind competitively to ER to modulate the estrogen signaling [155, 156]. Additionally, the pure anti-estrogen treatment, fulvestrant, binds competitively to ER. Similar to women, males may be castrated surgically or chemically to target androgens on a systemic level, and they can be treated locally by using antiandrogens like flutamide and bicalutamide [157]. Additionally, castrate individuals who use the lyase inhibitor abiraterone acetate [158, 159] may reduce their adrenal androgen production [160, 161].

New Targeting Strategies for Disrupting Tumor Ecosystem

Core Principle: Allee Effects

Allee effect is an ecologic concept that manifests the association between population size and individual fitness in species, with cooperative feeding and defense as underlying biological mechanisms [162]. A population needs to get beyond the Allee threshold, namely the critical population size, to avoid getting declined, and even extinction. Otherwise, a small population might lead to loss of genetic variability and reduced fitness to survival, which further cause lower production, higher mortality rate, and smaller population, forming a vicious cycle called extinction vortex [163].

The existence of Allee effects has been comprehensively reviewed in the field of cancer researches [164], as exemplified by the cooperative behaviors among breast cancer cells at low cell density [165]. As the standard treatment for early-stage breast cancer patients, breast-conserving surgery (BCS) aims at achieving negative surgical margins. However, a negative surgical margin never indicates zero residual cancer cell, but just an implication that the residual cancer burden could be controlled by adjuvant therapies [166]. In early development of breast cancer, BCS has similar clinical outcomes compared to mastectomy [167–169], while a real-world study in 2016 demonstrated improved 10-year survival after BCS plus radiotherapy relative to mastectomy [170]. From the ecological perspective, surgery for early breast cancer might be able to minimize the tumor burden, leaving the residual ones vulnerable to adjuvant therapies such as radiotherapy and chemotherapy. Crucially, BCS followed by radiotherapy might rebuild a primary *onco-sphere* favorable for adjuvant therapies. For middle-stage cancer, neoadjuvant therapy could also render the remnant of tumor burden more suited to surgical eradication. Moreover, series of studies from our group have illustrated that neoadjuvant trastuzumab therapy could induce PD-L1/IDO-orchestrated immunosuppression, while neoadjuvant chemotherapy would elicit a lncRNA-driven pro-tumoral inflammation, implying that neoadjuvant therapy holds potential to reprogram the systemic *onco-sphere* to favor immunotherapy or other targeted therapy [171, 172]. Decreasing the tumor burden to a level below the Allee threshold is the core of any successful cancer treatments. Herein, three strategies are proposed to achieve this goal.

Strategy 1: One Strike to Success

An ancient Chinese saying from the Zuo's Commentary on Spring and Autumn Annals goes in battles, "The most important in battle depends on (soldiers') courage. The first drumming cheers them up, then second weakens, while third exhausted." Similarly in cancer treatment, a "one strike to success" strategy could be decisive to reduce cancer burden below the Allee threshold so as to prevent tumor recurrence and/or distant metastasis. To a degree, higher dose of chemotherapy tends to correlate with better clinical outcomes. The nanoparticle albumin-bound paclitaxel has significantly less toxicity and therefore can be delivered in a higher dosing level (260 mg/m^2), when compared with standard paclitaxel (175 mg/m^2), obtaining an improved efficacy [173]. The CONFIRM trial also revealed that fulvestrant 500 mg was superior to 250 mg in prolonging PFS of postmenopausal patients with estrogen receptor-positive advanced breast cancer [174]. However, a higher dose might evoke severe or even fatal adverse events, including myelosuppression and cardiotoxicity, that could be far beyond patients' tolerance. Even if well tolerated, a harder strike is not necessarily associated with a favorable outcome, as demonstrated by the discovery that the extent of surgery has no impact on the OS of early breast cancer patients [169, 175]. Thus, the first-strike strategy seems more feasible in low-risk patients with low tumor burden. For example, for phyllodes tumor and ductal carcinoma in situ, surgical treatment only is adequate to achieve tumor control, whereas for more aggressive tumor like invasive ductal carcinoma, a "second strike" is warranted for further tumor management.

Strategy 2: Second-Strike Strategy

Post-operative adjuvant systemic therapies could be clinically beneficial, as even in early breast cancer, CTCs can be detected pre-operatively, which were significantly associated with long-term survival [176]. During the past 40 years, the extent of surgery remains largely unchanged, while the drastic development of modern chemotherapy, endocrine therapy, and trastuzumab greatly contributes to the improving outcome of breast cancer [177]. Administrating chemotherapy after/before surgical first strike in patients with localized Ewing's sarcoma also increases the OS from 10% to 70% [178].

However, successful second strike is not casual as cancer cells may mutate, evolve resistance, and relapse. Paralleling to the Predator Facilitation in ecology [179], a phenomenon called collateral sensitivity occurs in tumors, that is, drug-resistant ones may be specifically hypersensitive to other drugs [180]. In a dynamic eco-evolutionary context, a novel concept termed "temporal collateral sensitivity" was further developed, suggesting that during tumor clonal selection of resistant subpopulations under the initial induction treatments (e.g., BCR-ABL1-targeted inhibitors), an intermediate stage exists, in which tumor will be sensitized to small molecules that might be initially not effective (e.g., non-classical BCR-ABL1 drugs) [181]. More implications of eco-evolutionary dynamics of background extinctions in designing second-strike strategy have been reviewed extensively in metastatic cancer, in which sequential therapies or drug combinations that are individually effective but noncurative should be considered for tumor eradication. In tumor ecosystem, a strategic second strike empirically involves demographic perturbations of the population (hormone and chemotherapeutic agents), disruption of the metabolic balance (metabolism modulators), intervention of its habitat (antiangiogenic therapy), and introduction of a predator (immunotherapy) [182].

Strategy 3: Adaptive Therapy

The "first strike–second strike" strategy tends to be curative in patients with lower tumor burden, or with tumor that is more homogenous. However, for those with high cancer burden (e.g., primary stage IV cancers), or with relapsed and resistant tumors after a period of disease-free survival, curable treatment seems unlikely. A novel ecologically inspired strategy termed "adaptive therapy" thus emerges for treating tumors with higher heterogeneity as well as capability of evolution and adaptation. Learning from pest management, competitive release [183] could apply to the interaction between drug-sensitive and drug-resistant subclones in cancer treatment [184]. Based on that, the adaptive cancer therapy was proposed [185] and suggested a "treatment-for-control" strategy, which is to allow a substantial treatment-sensitive population to survive and thus confer growth inhibition to the less-fit resistant clones via resource competition. In an orthotopic mouse model of breast cancer, researchers compared the effectiveness of tumor control of conventional maximum dose density with two adaptive treatments: one is to maintain the dosing frequency while diminishing the doses according to the tumor response (variable-dosing algorithms), and the other is to maintain the dose but to skip the dosing as tumor responds (dose-skipping algorithms) [186]. They observed that relative to conventional treatment, the variable-dosing algorithms markedly restrained the tumor growth and prolonged the survival, which might be associated with vascular normalization and less necrosis. The adaptive therapy was also tested in a clinical trial of metastatic PCa [187, 188], in which abiraterone as antiandrogen treatment was administrated only until the *serum prostate*-specific *antigen* (PSA) declined to 50% of the pre-treatment value and was resumed when PSA restored to the original level. This proof-of-concept trial showed a significantly longer median PFS (30 months) than that in the AA-302 trial (16.5 months) [189]. More studies have been initiated to explore the feasibility of adaptive therapy across a series of solid tumors [190].

Conclusion

As tumors evolve, it remains challenging to steer tumor evolution toward a desired direction. The deficiency in monitoring methods as well as optional drugs becomes the bottleneck of current adaptive therapy clinical trials. Several critical issues, in detail, should be addressed for designing a therapy. What is the reliable biomarker to monitor the dynamic changing tumor burden? What is the triggering threshold to stop/re-start the treatment? What is the optimal therapeutic dose? Are there any biomarkers to monitor whether the treatment-resistant clone is not proliferating or become more invasive during the treatment? In-depth collaboration between oncologist, biologist, bio-statistician, and mathematician is necessary for developing long-term, multi-adaptive therapies toward extended tumor control. As we come to the end of the book, these are the questions that still lingers, which we hope to solve in the near future to come up with a comprehensive, personalized, patient-directed cancer therapeutic approach.

References

1. Holohan C, Van Schaeybroeck S, Longley DB, Johnston PG (2013) Cancer drug resistance: an evolving paradigm. Nat Rev Cancer 13(10):714–726
2. Borst P (2012) Cancer drug pan-resistance: pumps, cancer stem cells, quiescence, epithelial to mesenchymal transition, blocked cell death pathways, persisters or what? Open Biol 2(5): 120066
3. Schumacher TN, Schreiber RD (2015) Neoantigens in cancer immunotherapy. Science 348(6230):69–74
4. Robert C, Schachter J, Long GV, Arance A, Grob JJ, Mortier L et al (2015) Pembrolizumab versus Ipilimumab in advanced melanoma. N Engl J Med 372(26):2521–2532
5. Reck M, Rodríguez-Abreu D, Robinson AG, Hui R, Csőszi T, Fülöp A et al (2016) Pembrolizumab versus chemotherapy for PD-L1-positive non-small-cell lung cancer. N Engl J Med 375(19):1823–1833
6. Riaz N, Havel JJ, Makarov V, Desrichard A, Urba WJ, Sims JS et al (2017) Tumor and microenvironment evolution during immunotherapy with nivolumab. Cell 171(4):934–49.e16
7. Szakács G, Hall MD, Gottesman MM, Boumendjel A, Kachadourian R, Day BJ et al (2014) Targeting the Achilles heel of multidrug-resistant cancer by exploiting the fitness cost of resistance. Chem Rev 114(11):5753–5774
8. Silva AS, Kam Y, Khin ZP, Minton SE, Gillies RJ, Gatenby RA (2012) Evolutionary approaches to prolong progression-free survival in breast cancer. Cancer Res 72(24): 6362–6370
9. Lei Y, Tang L, Xie Y, Xianyu Y, Zhang L, Wang P et al (2017) Gold nanoclusters-assisted delivery of NGF siRNA for effective treatment of pancreatic cancer. Nat Commun 8:15130
10. Parks SK, Chiche J, Pouysségur J (2013) Disrupting proton dynamics and energy metabolism for cancer therapy. Nat Rev Cancer 13(9):611–623
11. Spugnini E, Fais S (2017) Proton pump inhibition and cancer therapeutics: a specific tumor targeting or it is a phenomenon secondary to a systemic buffering? Semin Cancer Biol 43:111–118
12. Neri D, Supuran CT (2011) Interfering with pH regulation in tumors as a therapeutic strategy. Nat Rev Drug Discov 10(10):767–777
13. Fais S, Venturi G, Gatenby B (2014) Microenvironmental acidosis in carcinogenesis and metastases: new strategies in prevention and therapy. Cancer Metastasis Rev 33(4):1095–1108
14. De Milito A, Iessi E, Logozzi M, Lozupone F, Spada M, Marino ML et al (2007) Proton pump inhibitors induce apoptosis of human B-cell tumors through a caspase-independent mechanism involving reactive oxygen species. Cancer Res 67(11):5408–5417

15. Luciani F, Spada M, De Milito A, Molinari A, Rivoltini L, Montinaro A et al (2004) Effect of proton pump inhibitor pretreatment on resistance of solid tumors to cytotoxic drugs. J Natl Cancer Inst 96(22):1702–1713
16. Taylor S, Spugnini EP, Assaraf YG, Azzarito T, Rauch C, Fais S (2015) Microenvironment acidity as a major determinant of tumor chemoresistance: proton pump inhibitors (PPIs) as a novel therapeutic approach. Drug Resist Updat 23:69–78
17. Yuan N, Song L, Zhang S, Lin W, Cao Y, Xu F et al (2015) Bafilomycin A1 targets both autophagy and apoptosis pathways in pediatric B-cell acute lymphoblastic leukemia. Haematologica 100(3):345–356
18. Yan Y, Jiang K, Liu P, Zhang X, Dong X, Gao J et al (2016) Bafilomycin A1 induces caspase-independent cell death in hepatocellular carcinoma cells via targeting of autophagy and MAPK pathways. Sci Rep 6:37052
19. Lou Y, McDonald PC, Oloumi A, Chia S, Ostlund C, Ahmadi A et al (2011) Targeting tumor hypoxia: suppression of breast tumor growth and metastasis by novel carbonic anhydrase IX inhibitors. Cancer Res 71(9):3364–3376
20. Doyen J, Parks SK, Marcié S, Pouysségur J, Chiche J (2012) Knock-down of hypoxia-induced carbonic anhydrases IX and XII radiosensitizes tumor cells by increasing intracellular acidosis. Front Oncol 2:199
21. McIntyre A, Patiar S, Wigfield S, Li JL, Ledaki I, Turley H et al (2012) Carbonic anhydrase IX promotes tumor growth and necrosis in vivo and inhibition enhances anti-VEGF therapy. Clin Cancer Res 18(11):3100–3111
22. Petrul HM, Schatz CA, Kopitz CC, Adnane L, McCabe TJ, Trail P et al (2012) Therapeutic mechanism and efficacy of the antibody-drug conjugate BAY 79-4620 targeting human carbonic anhydrase 9. Mol Cancer Ther 11(2):340–349
23. Siebels M, Rohrmann K, Oberneder R, Stahler M, Haseke N, Beck J et al (2011) A clinical phase I/II trial with the monoclonal antibody cG250 (RENCAREX®) and interferon-alpha-2a in metastatic renal cell carcinoma patients. World J Urol 29(1):121–126
24. Bola BM, Chadwick AL, Michopoulos F, Blount KG, Telfer BA, Williams KJ et al (2014) Inhibition of monocarboxylate transporter-1 (MCT1) by AZD3965 enhances radiosensitivity by reducing lactate transport. Mol Cancer Ther 13(12):2805–2816
25. Hong CS, Graham NA, Gu W, Espindola Camacho C, Mah V, Maresh EL et al (2016) MCT1 modulates cancer cell pyruvate export and growth of tumors that co-express MCT1 and MCT4. Cell Rep 14(7):1590–1601
26. Polański R, Hodgkinson CL, Fusi A, Nonaka D, Priest L, Kelly P et al (2014) Activity of the monocarboxylate transporter 1 inhibitor AZD3965 in small cell lung cancer. Clin Cancer Res 20(4):926–937
27. Lagarde AE, Franchi AJ, Paris S, Pouysségur JM (1988) Effect of mutations affecting Na+: H + antiport activity on tumorigenic potential of hamster lung fibroblasts. J Cell Biochem 36(3):249–260
28. Parks SK, Cormerais Y, Durivault J, Pouyssegur J (2017) Genetic disruption of the pHi-regulating proteins Na+/H+ exchanger 1 (SLC9A1) and carbonic anhydrase 9 severely reduces growth of colon cancer cells. Oncotarget 8(6):10225–10237
29. Pouysségur J, Sardet C, Franchi A, L'Allemain G, Paris S (1984) A specific mutation abolishing Na+/H+ antiport activity in hamster fibroblasts precludes growth at neutral and acidic pH. Proc Natl Acad Sci U S A 81(15):4833–4837
30. Rich IN, Worthington-White D, Garden OA, Musk P (2000) Apoptosis of leukemic cells accompanies reduction in intracellular pH after targeted inhibition of the Na(+)/H(+) exchanger. Blood 95(4):1427–1434
31. Harley W, Floyd C, Dunn T, Zhang XD, Chen TY, Hegde M et al (2010) Dual inhibition of sodium-mediated proton and calcium efflux triggers non-apoptotic cell death in malignant gliomas. Brain Res 1363:159–169
32. Masereel B, Pochet L, Laeckmann D (2003) An overview of inhibitors of Na(+)/H(+) exchanger. Eur J Med Chem 38(6):547–554

33. McIntyre A, Hulikova A, Ledaki I, Snell C, Singleton D, Steers G et al (2016) Disrupting hypoxia-induced bicarbonate transport acidifies tumor cells and suppresses tumor growth. Cancer Res 76(13):3744–3755
34. Wong P, Kleemann HW, Tannock IF (2002) Cytostatic potential of novel agents that inhibit the regulation of intracellular pH. Br J Cancer 87(2):238–245
35. Corbet C, Feron O (2017) Tumor acidosis: from the passenger to the driver's seat. Nat Rev Cancer 17(10):577–593
36. Sento S, Sasabe E, Yamamoto T (2016) Application of a persistent heparin treatment inhibits the malignant potential of oral squamous carcinoma cells induced by tumor cell-derived exosomes. PLoS One 11(2):e0148454
37. Nishida-Aoki N, Tominaga N, Takeshita F, Sonoda H, Yoshioka Y, Ochiya T (2017) Disruption of circulating extracellular vesicles as a novel therapeutic strategy against cancer metastasis. Mol Ther 25(1):181–191
38. de la Fuente A, Alonso-Alconada L, Costa C, Cueva J, Garcia-Caballero T, Lopez-Lopez R et al (2015) M-trap: exosome-based capture of tumor cells as a new technology in peritoneal metastasis. J Nat Cancer Inst 107(9):djv184
39. Tkach M, Théry C (2016) Communication by extracellular vesicles: where we are and where we need to go. Cell 164(6):1226–1232
40. Logozzi M, Mizzoni D, Angelini DF, Di Raimo R, Falchi M, Battistini L et al (2018) Microenvironmental pH and exosome levels interplay in human cancer cell lines of different histotypes. Cancers 10(10):370
41. Federici C, Petrucci F, Caimi S, Cesolini A, Logozzi M, Borghi M et al (2014) Exosome release and low pH belong to a framework of resistance of human melanoma cells to cisplatin. PLoS One 9(2):e88193
42. Zhao H, Achreja A, Iessi E, Logozzi M, Mizzoni D, Di Raimo R et al (2018) The key role of extracellular vesicles in the metastatic process. Biochim Biophys Acta Rev Cancer 1869(1): 64–77
43. Zhang Y, Yang P, Wang XF (2014) Microenvironmental regulation of cancer metastasis by miRNAs. Trends Cell Biol 24(3):153–160
44. Cheshomi H, Matin MM (2018) Exosomes and their importance in metastasis, diagnosis, and therapy of colorectal cancer. J Cell Biochem 120(2):2671–2686
45. Hong BS, Cho JH, Kim H, Choi EJ, Rho S, Kim J et al (2009) Colorectal cancer cell-derived microvesicles are enriched in cell cycle-related mRNAs that promote proliferation of endothelial cells. BMC Genomics 10:556
46. Zaharie F, Muresan MS, Petrushev B, Berce C, Gafencu GA, Selicean S et al (2015) Exosome-carried microRNA-375 inhibits cell progression and dissemination via Bcl-2 blocking in colon cancer. J Gastrointestin Liver Dis 24(4):435–443
47. Teng Y, Ren Y, Hu X, Mu J, Samykutty A, Zhuang X et al (2017) MVP-mediated exosomal sorting of miR-193a promotes colon cancer progression. Nat Commun 8:14448
48. Lobb RJ, Lima LG, Möller A (2017) Exosomes: key mediators of metastasis and pre-metastatic niche formation. Semin Cell Dev Biol 67:3–10
49. Weidle UH, Birzele F, Kollmorgen G, Rüger R (2017) The multiple roles of exosomes in metastasis. Cancer Genomics Proteomics 14(1):1–15
50. Escudier B, Dorval T, Chaput N, André F, Caby MP, Novault S et al (2005) Vaccination of metastatic melanoma patients with autologous dendritic cell (DC) derived-exosomes: results of the first phase I clinical trial. J Transl Med 3(1):10
51. Morse MA, Garst J, Osada T, Khan S, Hobeika A, Clay TM et al (2005) A phase I study of dexosome immunotherapy in patients with advanced non-small cell lung cancer. J Transl Med 3(1):9
52. Pei S, Minhajuddin M, D'Alessandro A, Nemkov T, Stevens BM, Adane B et al (2016) Rational design of a parthenolide-based drug regimen that selectively eradicates acute myelogenous leukemia stem cells. J Biol Chem 291(42):21984–22000

53. Schito L, Semenza GL (2016) Hypoxia-inducible factors: master regulators of cancer progression. Trends Cancer 2(12):758–770
54. Berger C, Sommermeyer D, Hudecek M, Berger M, Balakrishnan A, Paszkiewicz PJ et al (2015) Safety of targeting ROR1 in primates with chimeric antigen receptor-modified T cells. Cancer Immunol Res 3(2):206–216
55. Zhu TS, Costello MA, Talsma CE, Flack CG, Crowley JG, Hamm LL et al (2011) Endothelial cells create a stem cell niche in glioblastoma by providing NOTCH ligands that nurture self-renewal of cancer stem-like cells. Cancer Res 71(18):6061–6072
56. Jain RK, Duda DG, Clark JW, Loeffler JS (2006) Lessons from phase III clinical trials on anti-VEGF therapy for cancer. Nat Clin Pract Oncol 3(1):24–40
57. Chen Q, Wang J, Liu WN, Zhao Y (2019) Cancer immunotherapies and humanized mouse drug testing platforms. Transl Oncol 12(7):987–995
58. Dyck L, Mills KHG (2017) Immune checkpoints and their inhibition in cancer and infectious diseases. Eur J Immunol 47(5):765–779
59. Pardoll DM (2012) The blockade of immune checkpoints in cancer immunotherapy. Nat Rev Cancer 12(4):252–264
60. Marin-Acevedo JA, Dholaria B, Soyano AE, Knutson KL, Chumsri S, Lou Y (2018) Next generation of immune checkpoint therapy in cancer: new developments and challenges. J Hematol Oncol 11(1):39
61. Wei SC, Duffy CR, Allison JP (2018) Fundamental mechanisms of immune checkpoint blockade therapy. Cancer Discov 8(9):1069–1086
62. Ribas A, Wolchok JD (2018) Cancer immunotherapy using checkpoint blockade. Science 359(6382):1350–1355
63. Rohaan MW, Wilgenhof S, Haanen J (2019) Adoptive cellular therapies: the current landscape. Virchows Archiv 474(4):449–461
64. Perica K, Varela JC, Oelke M, Schneck J (2015) Adoptive T cell immunotherapy for cancer. Rambam Maimonides Med J 6(1):e0004
65. Schmitt TM, Stromnes IM, Chapuis AG, Greenberg PD (2015) New strategies in engineering T-cell receptor gene-modified T cells to more effectively target malignancies. Clin Cancer Res 21(23):5191–5197
66. Sukari A, Nagasaka M, Al-Hadidi A, Lum LG (2016) Cancer immunology and immunotherapy. Anticancer Res 36(11):5593–5606
67. Rezvani K, Rouce RH (2015) The application of natural killer cell immunotherapy for the treatment of cancer. Front Immunol 6:578
68. Mehta RS, Rezvani K (2018) Chimeric antigen receptor expressing natural killer cells for the immunotherapy of cancer. Front Immunol 9:283
69. Iyer RK, Bowles PA, Kim H, Dulgar-Tulloch A (2018) Industrializing autologous adoptive immunotherapies: manufacturing advances and challenges. Front Med 5:150
70. D'Angelo SP, Melchiori L, Merchant MS, Bernstein D, Glod J, Kaplan R et al (2018) Antitumor activity associated with prolonged persistence of adoptively transferred NY-ESO-1 (c259)T cells in synovial sarcoma. Cancer Discov 8(8):944–957
71. Robbins PF, Morgan RA, Feldman SA, Yang JC, Sherry RM, Dudley ME et al (2011) Tumor regression in patients with metastatic synovial cell sarcoma and melanoma using genetically engineered lymphocytes reactive with NY-ESO-1. J Clin Oncol 29(7):917–924
72. Ochi T, Fujiwara H, Okamoto S, An J, Nagai K, Shirakata T et al (2011) Novel adoptive T-cell immunotherapy using a WT1-specific TCR vector encoding silencers for endogenous TCRs shows marked antileukemia reactivity and safety. Blood 118(6):1495–1503
73. Mastaglio S, Genovese P, Magnani Z, Ruggiero E, Landoni E, Camisa B et al (2017) NY-ESO-1 TCR single edited stem and central memory T cells to treat multiple myeloma without graft-versus-host disease. Blood 130(5):606–618
74. Legut M, Dolton G, Mian AA, Ottmann OG, Sewell AK (2018) CRISPR-mediated TCR replacement generates superior anticancer transgenic T cells. Blood 131(3):311–322

75. Miyazaki Y, Fujiwara H, Asai H, Ochi F, Ochi T, Azuma T et al (2013) Development of a novel redirected T-cell-based adoptive immunotherapy targeting human telomerase reverse transcriptase for adult T-cell leukemia. Blood 121(24):4894–4901
76. Levine BL, Miskin J, Wonnacott K, Keir C (2017) Global manufacturing of CAR T cell therapy. Mol Ther Methods Clin Dev 4:92–101
77. Harris DT, Kranz DM (2016) Adoptive T cell therapies: A comparison of T cell receptors and chimeric antigen receptors. Trends Pharmacol Sci 37(3):220–230
78. Guo C, Manjili MH, Subjeck JR, Sarkar D, Fisher PB, Wang XY (2013) Therapeutic cancer vaccines: past, present, and future. Adv Cancer Res 119:421–475
79. Roden R, Wu TC (2003) Preventative and therapeutic vaccines for cervical cancer. Expert Rev Vaccines 2(4):495–516
80. Palucka K, Banchereau J (2013) Dendritic-cell-based therapeutic cancer vaccines. Immunity 39(1):38–48
81. Li J, Valentin A, Beach RK, Alicea C, Felber BK, Pavlakis GN (2015) DNA is an efficient booster of dendritic cell-based vaccine. Hum Vaccin Immunother 11(8):1927–1935
82. Hirayama M, Nishimura Y (2016) The present status and future prospects of peptide-based cancer vaccines. Int Immunol 28(7):319–328
83. Cheever MA, Higano CS (2011) PROVENGE (Sipuleucel-T) in prostate cancer: the first FDA-approved therapeutic cancer vaccine. Clin Cancer Res 17(11):3520–3526
84. Chang MH, Shau WY, Chen CJ, Wu TC, Kong MS, Liang DC et al (2000) Hepatitis B vaccination and hepatocellular carcinoma rates in boys and girls. JAMA 284(23):3040–3042
85. Schwartzentruber DJ, Lawson DH, Richards JM, Conry RM, Miller DM, Treisman J et al (2011) gp100 peptide vaccine and interleukin-2 in patients with advanced melanoma. N Engl J Med 364(22):2119–2127
86. U'Ren L, Kedl R, Dow S (2006) Vaccination with liposome—DNA complexes elicits enhanced antitumor immunity. Cancer Gene Ther 13(11):1033–1044
87. Yang R, Xu J, Xu L, Sun X, Chen Q, Zhao Y et al (2018) Cancer cell membrane-coated adjuvant nanoparticles with mannose modification for effective anticancer vaccination. ACS Nano 12(6):5121–5129
88. Prestwich RJ, Harrington KJ, Pandha HS, Vile RG, Melcher AA, Errington F (2008) Oncolytic viruses: a novel form of immunotherapy. Expert Rev Anticancer Ther 8(10):1581–1588
89. Rehman H, Silk AW, Kane MP, Kaufman HL (2016) Into the clinic: Talimogene laherparepvec (T-VEC), a first-in-class intratumoral oncolytic viral therapy. J Immunother Cancer 4:53
90. Russell L, Peng KW (2018) The emerging role of oncolytic virus therapy against cancer. Chin Clin Oncol 7(2):16
91. Goshima F, Esaki S, Luo C, Kamakura M, Kimura H, Nishiyama Y (2014) Oncolytic viral therapy with a combination of HF10, a herpes simplex virus type 1 variant and granulocyte-macrophage colony-stimulating factor for murine ovarian cancer. Int J Cancer 134(12):2865–2877
92. Ramesh N, Ge Y, Ennist DL, Zhu M, Mina M, Ganesh S et al (2006) CG0070, a conditionally replicating granulocyte macrophage colony-stimulating factor—armed oncolytic adenovirus for the treatment of bladder cancer. Clin Cancer Res 12(1):305–313
93. Fan J, Jiang H, Cheng L, Liu R (2016) The oncolytic herpes simplex virus vector, G47Δ, effectively targets tamoxifen-resistant breast cancer cells. Oncol Rep 35(3):1741–1749
94. Noonan AM, Farren MR, Geyer SM, Huang Y, Tahiri S, Ahn D et al (2016) Randomized phase 2 trial of the oncolytic virus pelareorep (Reolysin) in upfront treatment of metastatic pancreatic adenocarcinoma. Mol Ther 24(6):1150–1158
95. Taguchi S, Fukuhara H, Todo T (2019) Oncolytic virus therapy in Japan: progress in clinical trials and future perspectives. Jpn J Clin Oncol 49(3):201–209

96. Tanoue K, Wang Y, Ikeda M, Mitsui K, Irie R, Setoguchi T et al (2014) Survivin-responsive conditionally replicating adenovirus kills rhabdomyosarcoma stem cells more efficiently than their progeny. J Transl Med 12:27
97. Saga K, Kaneda Y (2015) Oncolytic Sendai virus-based virotherapy for cancer: recent advances. Oncolytic Virother 4:141–147
98. Schooltink H, Rose-John S (2002) Cytokines as therapeutic drugs. J Interferon Cytokine Res 22(5):505–516
99. Feldmann M (2008) Many cytokines are very useful therapeutic targets in disease. J Clin Invest 118(11):3533–3536
100. Ma Z, Li W, Yoshiya S, Xu Y, Hata M, El-Darawish Y et al (2016) Augmentation of immune checkpoint cancer immunotherapy with IL18. Clin Cancer Res 22(12):2969–2980
101. Dammeijer F, Lau SP, van Eijck CHJ, van der Burg SH, Aerts J (2017) Rationally combining immunotherapies to improve efficacy of immune checkpoint blockade in solid tumors. Cytokine Growth Factor Rev 36:5–15
102. Baron JA, Sandler RS (2000) Nonsteroidal anti-inflammatory drugs and cancer prevention. Annu Rev Med 51:511–523
103. García-Rodríguez LA, Huerta-Alvarez C (2001) Reduced risk of colorectal cancer among long-term users of aspirin and nonaspirin nonsteroidal antiinflammatory drugs. Epidemiology 12(1):88–93
104. Williams CS, Mann M, DuBois RN (1999) The role of cyclooxygenases in inflammation, cancer, and development. Oncogene 18(55):7908–7916
105. Mamytbeková A, Rezábek K, Kacerovská H, Grimová J, Svobodová J (1986) Antimetastatic effect of flurbiprofen and other platelet aggregation inhibitors. Neoplasma 33(4):417–421
106. Moore MA (2001) The role of chemoattraction in cancer metastases. Bioessays 23(8):674–676
107. Balkwill F, Mantovani A (2001) Inflammation and cancer: back to virchow? Lancet 357(9255):539–545
108. Balkwill F (2002) Tumor necrosis factor or tumor promoting factor? Cytokine Growth Factor Rev 13(2):135–141
109. Borsig L, Wong R, Hynes RO, Varki NM, Varki A (2002) Synergistic effects of L- and P-selectin in facilitating tumor metastasis can involve non-mucin ligands and implicate leukocytes as enhancers of metastasis. Proc Natl Acad Sci U S A 99(4):2193–2198
110. Coussens LM, Tinkle CL, Hanahan D, Werb Z (2000) MMP-9 supplied by bone marrow-derived cells contributes to skin carcinogenesis. Cell 103(3):481–490
111. Egeblad M, Werb Z (2002) New functions for the matrix metalloproteinases in cancer progression. Nat Rev Cancer 2(3):161–174
112. Overall CM, López-Otín C (2002) Strategies for MMP inhibition in cancer: innovations for the post-trial era. Nat Rev Cancer 2(9):657–672
113. Magnon C, Hall SJ, Lin J, Xue X, Gerber L, Freedland SJ et al (2013) Autonomic nerve development contributes to prostate cancer progression. Science 341(6142):1236361
114. Olar A, He D, Florentin D, Ding Y, Ayala G (2014) Biologic correlates and significance of axonogenesis in prostate cancer. Hum Pathol 45(7):1358–1364
115. Pundavela J, Demont Y, Jobling P, Lincz LF, Roselli S, Thorne RF et al (2014) ProNGF correlates with Gleason score and is a potential driver of nerve infiltration in prostate cancer. Am J Pathol 184(12):3156–3162
116. Faulkner S, Roselli S, Demont Y, Pundavela J, Choquet G, Leissner P et al (2016) ProNGF is a potential diagnostic biomarker for thyroid cancer. Oncotarget 7(19):28488–28497
117. Renz BW, Takahashi R, Tanaka T, Macchini M, Hayakawa Y, Dantes Z et al (2018) β2 Adrenergic-Neurotrophin Feedforward Loop Promotes Pancreatic Cancer. Cancer Cell 33(1):75–90.e7
118. Hayakawa Y, Sakitani K, Konishi M, Asfaha S, Niikura R, Tomita H et al (2017) Nerve growth factor promotes gastric tumorigenesis through aberrant cholinergic signaling. Cancer Cell 31(1):21–34

119. Pundavela J, Roselli S, Faulkner S, Attia J, Scott RJ, Thorne RF et al (2015) Nerve fibers infiltrate the tumor microenvironment and are associated with nerve growth factor production and lymph node invasion in breast cancer. Mol Oncol 9(8):1626–1635

120. Allen JK, Armaiz-Pena GN, Nagaraja AS, Sadaoui NC, Ortiz T, Dood R et al (2018) Sustained adrenergic signaling promotes intratumoral innervation through BDNF induction. Cancer Res 78(12):3233–3242

121. Li X, Dun MD, Faulkner S, Hondermarck H (2018) Neuroproteins in cancer: assumed bystanders become culprits. Proteomics 18(14):e1800049

122. Zhao CM, Hayakawa Y, Kodama Y, Muthupalani S, Westphalen CB, Andersen GT et al (2014) Denervation suppresses gastric tumorigenesis. Sci Transl Med 6(250):250ra115

123. Coarfa C, Florentin D, Putluri N, Ding Y, Au J, He D et al (2018) Influence of the neural microenvironment on prostate cancer. Prostate 78(2):128–139

124. Denk F, Bennett DL, McMahon SB (2017) Nerve growth factor and pain mechanisms. Annu Rev Neurosci 40:307–325

125. Griffin N, Faulkner S, Jobling P, Hondermarck H (2018) Targeting neurotrophin signaling in cancer: the renaissance. Pharmacol Res 135:12–17

126. Bapat AA, Munoz RM, Von Hoff DD, Han H (2016) Blocking nerve growth factor signaling reduces the neural invasion potential of pancreatic cancer cells. PLoS One 11(10):e0165586

127. Buehlmann D, Ielacqua GD, Xandry J, Rudin M (2019) Prospective administration of anti-nerve growth factor treatment effectively suppresses functional connectivity alterations after cancer-induced bone pain in mice. Pain 160(1):151–159

128. Faulkner S, Jobling P, March B, Jiang CC, Hondermarck H (2019) Tumor neurobiology and the war of nerves in cancer. Cancer Discov 9(6):702–710

129. Viallard C, Larrivee B (2017) Tumor angiogenesis and vascular normalization: alternative therapeutic targets. Angiogenesis 20(4):409–426

130. Crawford Y, Ferrara N (2009) VEGF inhibition: insights from preclinical and clinical studies. Cell Tissue Res 335(1):261–269

131. Ohtsu A, Shah MA, Van Cutsem E, Rha SY, Sawaki A, Park SR et al (2011) Bevacizumab in combination with chemotherapy as first-line therapy in advanced gastric cancer: a randomized, double-blind, placebo-controlled phase III study. J Clin Oncol 29(30):3968–3976

132. Reck M, von Pawel J, Zatloukal P, Ramlau R, Gorbounova V, Hirsh V et al (2009) Phase III trial of cisplatin plus gemcitabine with either placebo or bevacizumab as first-line therapy for nonsquamous non-small-cell lung cancer: AVAiL. J Clin Oncol 27(8):1227–1234

133. Miller K, Wang M, Gralow J, Dickler M, Cobleigh M, Perez EA et al (2007) Paclitaxel plus bevacizumab versus paclitaxel alone for metastatic breast cancer. N Engl J Med 357(26): 2666–2676

134. Escudier B, Eisen T, Stadler WM, Szczylik C, Oudard S, Siebels M et al (2007) Sorafenib in advanced clear-cell renal-cell carcinoma. N Engl J Med 356(2):125–134

135. Jayson GC, Kerbel R, Ellis LM, Harris AL (2016) Antiangiogenic therapy in oncology: current status and future directions. Lancet 388(10043):518–529

136. Fan F, Samuel S, Gaur P, Lu J, Dallas NA, Xia L et al (2011) Chronic exposure of colorectal cancer cells to bevacizumab promotes compensatory pathways that mediate tumor cell migration. Br J Cancer 104(8):1270–1277

137. Widakowich C, de Castro G Jr, de Azambuja E, Dinh P, Awada A (2007) Review: side effects of approved molecular targeted therapies in solid cancers. Oncologist 12(12):1443–1455

138. Jain RK (2001) Normalizing tumor vasculature with anti-angiogenic therapy: a new paradigm for combination therapy. Nat Med 7(9):987–989

139. Greenberg JI, Shields DJ, Barillas SG, Acevedo LM, Murphy E, Huang J et al (2008) A role for VEGF as a negative regulator of pericyte function and vessel maturation. Nature 456(7223):809–813

140. Tolaney SM, Boucher Y, Duda DG, Martin JD, Seano G, Ancukiewicz M et al (2015) Role of vascular density and normalization in response to neoadjuvant bevacizumab and chemotherapy in breast cancer patients. Proc Natl Acad Sci U S A 112(46):14325–14330

141. Winkler F, Kozin SV, Tong RT, Chae SS, Booth MF, Garkavtsev I et al (2004) Kinetics of vascular normalization by VEGFR2 blockade governs brain tumor response to radiation: role of oxygenation, angiopoietin-1, and matrix metalloproteinases. Cancer Cell 6(6):553–563

142. Jain RK (2014) Antiangiogenesis strategies revisited: from starving tumors to alleviating hypoxia. Cancer Cell 26(5):605–622

143. Batchelor TT, Sorensen AG, di Tomaso E, Zhang WT, Duda DG, Cohen KS et al (2007) AZD2171, a pan-VEGF receptor tyrosine kinase inhibitor, normalizes tumor vasculature and alleviates edema in glioblastoma patients. Cancer Cell 11(1):83–95

144. Graeber TG, Osmanian C, Jacks T, Housman DE, Koch CJ, Lowe SW et al (1996) Hypoxia-mediated selection of cells with diminished apoptotic potential in solid tumors. Nature 379(6560):88–91

145. Ebos JM, Kerbel RS (2011) Antiangiogenic therapy: impact on invasion, disease progression, and metastasis. Nat Rev Clin Oncol 8(4):210–221

146. Huang Y, Yuan J, Righi E, Kamoun WS, Ancukiewicz M, Nezivar J et al (2012) Vascular normalizing doses of antiangiogenic treatment reprogram the immunosuppressive tumor microenvironment and enhance immunotherapy. Proc Natl Acad Sci U S A 109(43): 17561–17566

147. Martin JD, Fukumura D, Duda DG, Boucher Y, Jain RK (2016) Reengineering the tumor microenvironment to alleviate hypoxia and overcome cancer heterogeneity. Cold Spring Harb Perspect Med 6(12):a027094

148. Chen BB, Lu YS, Lin CH, Chen WW, Wu PF, Hsu CY et al (2016) A pilot study to determine the timing and effect of bevacizumab on vascular normalization of metastatic brain tumors in breast cancer. BMC Cancer 16:466

149. Lin A, Hahn SM (2012) Hypoxia imaging markers and applications for radiation treatment planning. Semin Nucl Med 42(5):343–352

150. Adams TD, Gress RE, Smith SC, Halverson RC, Simper SC, Rosamond WD et al (2007) Long-term mortality after gastric bypass surgery. N Engl J Med 357(8):753–761

151. Bowker SL, Majumdar SR, Veugelers P, Johnson JA (2006) Increased cancer-related mortality for patients with type 2 diabetes who use sulfonylureas or insulin. Diabetes Care 29(2): 254–258

152. Evans JM, Donnelly LA, Emslie-Smith AM, Alessi DR, Morris AD (2005) Metformin and reduced risk of cancer in diabetic patients. BMJ 330(7503):1304–1305

153. Folkerd EJ, Dowsett M (2010) Influence of sex hormones on cancer progression. J Clin Oncol 28(26):4038–4044

154. Crawford ED, Hou AH (2009) The role of LHRH antagonists in the treatment of prostate cancer. Oncology 23(7):626–630

155. Smith CL, Nawaz Z, O'Malley BW (1997) Coactivator and corepressor regulation of the agonist/antagonist activity of the mixed antiestrogen, 4-hydroxytamoxifen. Mol Endocrinol 11(6):657–666

156. Dutertre M, Smith CL (2000) Molecular mechanisms of selective estrogen receptor modulator (SERM) action. J Pharmacol Exp Ther 295(2):431–437

157. Schellhammer PF, Sharifi R, Block NL, Soloway MS, Venner PM, Patterson AL et al (1997) Clinical benefits of bicalutamide compared with flutamide in combined androgen blockade for patients with advanced prostatic carcinoma: final report of a double-blind, randomized, center trial. Casodex Combination Study Group. Urology 50(3):330–336

Stanczyk FZ, Longcope C, Stephenson HE Jr, Chang L, Miller R et al (1997) serum dehydroepiandrosterone (DHEA), DHEA sulfate, and 5-androstene-3 to risk of breast cancer in postmenopausal women. Cancer Epidemiol 177–181

B, O'Malley BW (1999) Nuclear receptor coregulators: cellular and ocr Rev 20(3):321–344

159. McKenna NJ, Lanz R molecular biology. End 7 beta-dio up o Biomarkers Prev 6(3)

160. Attard G, Reid AH, Yap TA, Raynaud F, Dowsett M, Settatree S et al (2008) Phase I clinical trial of a selective inhibitor of CYP17, abiraterone acetate, confirms that castration-resistant prostate cancer commonly remains hormone driven. J Clin Oncol 26(28):4563–4571

161. Attard G, Reid AH, A'Hern R, Parker C, Oommen NB, Folkerd E et al (2009) Selective inhibition of CYP17 with abiraterone acetate is highly active in the treatment of castration-resistant prostate cancer. J Clin Oncol 27(23):3742–3748

162. Courchamp F, Clutton-Brock T, Grenfell B (1999) Inverse density dependence and the allee effect. Trends Ecol Evol 14(10):405–410

163. Palomares F, Godoy JA, Lopez-Bao JV, Rodriguez A, Roques S, Casas-Marce M et al (2012) Possible extinction vortex for a population of Iberian lynx on the verge of extirpation. Conserv Biol 26(4):689–697

164. Korolev KS, Xavier JB, Gore J (2014) Turning ecology and evolution against cancer. Nat Rev Cancer 14(5):371–380

165. Johnson KE, Howard G, Mo W, Strasser MK, Lima E, Huang S et al (2019) Cancer cell population growth kinetics at low densities deviate from the exponential growth model and suggest an allee effect. PLoS Biol 17(8):e3000399

166. Morrow M, Harris JR, Schnitt SJ (2012) Surgical margins in lumpectomy for breast cancer—bigger is not better. N Engl J Med 367(1):79–82

167. Lichter AS, Lippman ME, Danforth DN Jr, d'Angelo T, Steinberg SM, deMoss E et al (1992) Mastectomy versus breast-conserving therapy in the treatment of stage I and II carcinoma of the breast: a randomized trial at the National Cancer Institute. J Clin Oncol 10(6):976–983

168. van Dongen JA, Bartelink H, Fentiman IS, Lerut T, Mignolet F, Olthuis G et al (1992) Factors influencing local relapse and survival and results of salvage treatment after breast-conserving therapy in operable breast cancer: EORTC trial 10801, breast conservation compared with mastectomy in TNM stage I and II breast cancer. Eur J Cancer 28a(4–5):801–805

169. Fisher B, Anderson S, Bryant J, Margolese RG, Deutsch M, Fisher ER et al (2002) Twenty-year follow-up of a randomized trial comparing total mastectomy, lumpectomy, and lumpectomy plus irradiation for the treatment of invasive breast cancer. N Engl J Med 347(16):1233–1241

170. van Maaren MC, de Munck L, de Bock GH, Jobsen JJ, van Dalen T, Linn SC et al (2016) 10 year survival after breast-conserving surgery plus radiotherapy compared with mastectomy in early breast cancer in The Netherlands: a population-based study. Lancet Oncol 17(8):1158–1170

171. Liu J, Lao L, Chen J, Li J, Zeng W, Zhu X et al (2021) The IRENA lncRNA converts chemotherapy-polarized tumor-suppressing macrophages to tumor-promoting phenotypes in breast cancer. Nat Cancer 2(4):457–473

172. Su S, Zhao J, Xing Y, Zhang X, Liu J, Ouyang Q et al (2018) Immune checkpoint inhibition overcomes ADCP-induced immunosuppression by macrophages. Cell 175(2):442–57.e23

173. Gradishar WJ, Tjulandin S, Davidson N, Shaw H, Desai N, Bhar P et al (2005) Phase III trial of nanoparticle albumin-bound paclitaxel compared with polyethylated castor oil-based paclitaxel in women with breast cancer. J Clin Oncol 23(31):7794–7803

174. Di Leo A, Jerusalem G, Petruzelka L, Torres R, Bondarenko IN, Khasanov R et al (2010) Results of the CONFIRM phase III trial comparing fulvestrant 250 mg with fulvestrant 500 mg in postmenopausal women with estrogen receptor-positive advanced breast cancer. J Clin Oncol 28(30):4594–4600

175. Fisher B, Jeong JH, Anderson S, Bryant J, Fisher ER, Wolmark N (2002) Twenty-five-year follow-up of a randomized trial comparing radical mastectomy, total mastectomy, and total mastectomy followed by irradiation. N Engl J Med 347(8):567–575

176. Magbanua MJM, Yau C, Wolf DM, Lee JS, Chattopadhyay Synchronous detection of circulating tumor cells in blood and bone marrow predicts adverse outcome in early breast cancer 5388–5397

177. Perez EA, Romond EH, Suman VJ, Jeong JH, Sledge G, Geyer CE Jr et al (2014) Trastuzumab plus adjuvant chemotherapy for human epidermal growth factor receptor 2-positive breast cancer: planned joint analysis of overall survival from NSABP B-31 and NCCTG N9831. J Clin Oncol 32(33):3744–3752
178. Balamuth NJ, Womer RB (2010) Ewing's sarcoma. Lancet Oncol 11(2):184–192
179. Kotler BP, Blaustein L, Brown JS (1992) Predator facilitation: the combined effect of snakes and owls on the foraging behavior of gerbils. Ann Zool Fenn 29(4):199–206
180. Efferth T, Saeed MEM, Kadioglu O, Seo EJ, Shirooie S, Mbaveng AT et al (2020) Collateral sensitivity of natural products in drug-resistant cancer cells. Biotechnol Adv 38:107342
181. Zhao B, Sedlak JC, Srinivas R, Creixell P, Pritchard JR, Tidor B et al (2016) Exploiting temporal collateral sensitivity in tumor clonal evolution. Cell 165(1):234–246
182. Gatenby RA, Zhang J, Brown JS (2019) First strike-second strike strategies in metastatic cancer: lessons from the evolutionary dynamics of extinction. Cancer Res 79(13):3174–3177
183. Zeilinger AR, Olson DM, Andow DA (2016) Competitive release and outbreaks of non-target pests associated with transgenic Bt cotton. Ecol Appl 26(4):1047–1054
184. Gatenby RA (2009) A change of strategy in the war on cancer. Nature 459(7246):508–509
185. Gatenby RA, Silva AS, Gillies RJ, Frieden BR (2009) Adaptive therapy. Cancer Res 69(11): 4894–4903
186. Enriquez-Navas PM, Kam Y, Das T, Hassan S, Silva A, Foroutan P et al (2016) Exploiting evolutionary principles to prolong tumor control in preclinical models of breast cancer. Science Transl Med 8(327):327ra24
187. Zhang J, Cunningham JJ, Brown JS, Gatenby RA (2017) Integrating evolutionary dynamics into treatment of metastatic castrate-resistant prostate cancer. Nat Commun 8(1):1816
188. Zhang J, Fishman MN, Brown J, Gatenby RA (2019) Integrating evolutionary dynamics into treatment of metastatic castrate-resistant prostate cancer (mCRPC): updated analysis of the adaptive abiraterone (abi) study (NCT02415621). J Clin Oncol 37:5041
189. Ryan CJ, Smith MR, de Bono JS, Molina A, Logothetis CJ, de Souza P et al (2013) Abiraterone in metastatic prostate cancer without previous chemotherapy. N Engl J Med 368(2):138–148
190. West J, You L, Zhang J, Gatenby RA, Brown JS, Newton PK et al (2020) Towards multidrug adaptive therapy. Cancer Res 80(7):1578–1589

CPSIA information can be obtained
at www.ICGtesting.com
Printed in the USA
LVHW052300230723
753220LV00006B/335

9 789819 911820